CHANDLER

$\longleftarrow$ and $\longrightarrow$

GRANT'S

GLAUCOMA

FIFTH EDITION

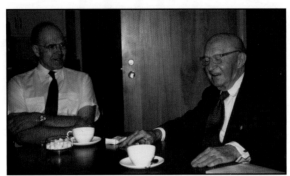

W. Morton Grant, MD and Paul A. Chandler, MD in their weekly meeting in the laboratory. (Reprinted with permission from Marshall N. Cyrlin, MD.)

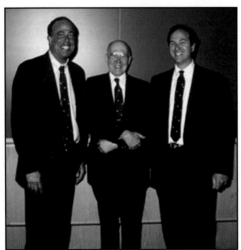

David L. Epstein, MD, MMM (left), W. Morton Grant, MD (center), and Joel S. Schuman, MD, FACS (right).

CHANDLER and GRANT'S

GLAUCOMA
FIFTH EDITION

Edited by
Malik Y. Kahook, MD
Professor of Ophthalmology
Director of Clinical and Translational Research
Chief, Glaucoma Service at the University of Colorado Eye Center
University of Colorado School of Medicine
Aurora, Colorado

Joel S. Schuman, MD, FACS
Eye and Ear Foundation Professor and Chairman of Ophthalmology
University of Pittsburgh School of Medicine
Professor of Bioengineering, Swanson School of Engineering, University of Pittsburgh
Director, UPMC Eye Center
Pittsburgh, Pennsylvania

Consulting Editor
David L. Epstein, MD, MMM
Joseph A.C. Wadsworth Clinical Professor and Chairman
Department of Ophthalmology
Duke University School of Medicine
Durham, North Carolina

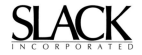

www.Healio.com/books

ISBN: 978-1-55642-954-5

Published by: SLACK Incorporated
                  6900 Grove Road
                  Thorofare, NJ 08086 USA
                  Telephone: 856-848-1000
                  Fax: 856-848-6091
                  www.Healio.com/books

Contact SLACK Incorporated for more information about other books in this field or about the availability of our books from distributors outside the United States.

Library of Congress Cataloging-in-Publication Data

Chandler and Grant's glaucoma. -- 5th ed. / Malik Y. Kahook, Joel S. Schuman, editors ; David L. Epstein, contributing editor.
     p. ; cm.
  Glaucoma
  Rev. ed. of: Chandler and Grant's glaucoma / David L. Epstein ; with R. Rand Allingham, Joel S. Schuman. 4th ed. 1997.
  Includes bibliographical references and index.
  ISBN 978-1-55642-954-5 (alk. paper)
  I. Kahook, Malik Y. II. Schuman, Joel S. III. Epstein, David L. IV. Chandler, Paul A. (Paul Austin), 1896- V. Title: Glaucoma.
  [DNLM: 1. Glaucoma. WW 290]

  617.7'41--dc23
                          2012045362

For permission to reprint material in another publication, contact SLACK Incorporated. Authorization to photocopy items for internal, personal, or academic use is granted by SLACK Incorporated provided that the appropriate fee is paid directly to Copyright Clearance Center. Prior to photocopying items, please contact the Copyright Clearance Center at 222 Rosewood Drive, Danvers, MA 01923 USA; phone: 978-750-8400; website: www.copyright.com; email: info@copyright.com

Printed in the United States of America.

Last digit is print number: 10   9   8   7   6   5   4   3   2   1

DEDICATION

We dedicate this textbook to our families for their constant support,
our residents and fellows for allowing us the privilege of passing on the teachings of Drs. Chandler and Grant,
and our patients for the honor of being entrusted with their care.

CONTENTS

Acknowledgments

We would like to acknowledge David L. Epstein, MD, MMM for his mentorship and wisdom during the process of completing the work on this Fifth Edition of *Chandler and Grant's Glaucoma*.

We would also like to acknowledge Dr. Paul Lee for his advice, as well as contributions to previous editions of *Chandler and Grant's Glaucoma*.

ABOUT THE EDITORS

Malik Y. Kahook, MD is Professor of Ophthalmology and Director of Clinical and Translational Research in the Department of Ophthalmology at the University of Colorado. He also directs the glaucoma service and glaucoma fellowship. Dr. Kahook specializes in the medical and surgical treatment of glaucoma and cataracts. He is active within the ophthalmology community, including memberships in the American Academy of Ophthalmology, American Glaucoma Society, American Society of Refractive and Cataract Surgeons, and the Association for Research in Vision and Ophthalmology. Dr. Kahook has authored more than 200 peer-reviewed manuscripts, abstracts, and book chapters, and is editor of 4 textbooks, including *Essentials of Glaucoma Surgery* (SLACK Incorporated). He is on the editorial board of the *American Journal of Ophthalmology* and *International Glaucoma Review,* among others. He was awarded an American Glaucoma Society Clinician-Scientist Fellowship Award for 2007, as well as the American Glaucoma Society Compliance Grant for 2006, and was named New Inventor of the Year for the University of Colorado in 2009 and Inventor of the Year for 2010. Dr. Kahook received the American Academy of Ophthalmology Achievement Award in 2011. He has filed for more than 12 patents, several of which have been licensed by companies for development and commercialization. He currently serves as a consultant to the US Food and Drug Administration's Ophthalmic Device Division.

Dr. Kahook completed his residency training at the University of Colorado, Rocky Mountain Lions Eye Institute in Denver, Colorado, where he was named Chief Resident. He then went on to complete his fellowship in glaucoma from the University of Pittsburgh Medical Center in Pittsburgh, Pennsylvania.

Joel S. Schuman, MD, FACS is the Eye and Ear Foundation Professor and Chairman of Ophthalmology, the Eye and Ear Institute, University of Pittsburgh School of Medicine and Director of the University of Pittsburgh Medical Center (UPMC) Eye Center. He is also Professor of Bioengineering at the Swanson School of Engineering, University of Pittsburgh, and a Founder of the Louis J. Fox Center for Vision Restoration of UPMC and the University of Pittsburgh. He is a member of the McGowan Institute for Regenerative Medicine and the Center for the Neural Basis of Cognition, Carnegie Mellon University and University of Pittsburgh. Dr. Schuman is a native of Roslyn, New York; he graduated from Columbia University (BA, 1980) and Mt. Sinai School of Medicine (MD, 1984). Following his internship at New York's Beth Israel Medical Center (1985), he completed residency training at Medical College of Virginia (1988) and glaucoma fellowship at Massachusetts Eye & Ear Infirmary (clinical 1989; research 1990), where he was a Heed Fellow. After just over a year on the Harvard faculty, he moved to the New England Medical Center, Tufts University, to co-found the New England Eye Center in 1991, where he was Residency Director and Glaucoma and Cataract Service Chief. In 1998, he became Professor of Ophthalmology, and Vice Chair in 2001.

Dr. Schuman and his colleagues were the first to identify a molecular marker for human glaucoma, as published in *Nature Medicine* in 2001. He has been continuously funded by the National Eye Institute as a principal investigator since 1995, is principal investigator of a National Institutes of Health (NIH) grant to study novel glaucoma diagnostics, and is co-investigator of NIH grants for research into novel optical diagnostics and short pulse laser surgery and for advanced imaging in glaucoma. He is an inventor of optical coherence tomography (OCT), used world-wide for ocular diagnostics. Dr. Schuman has published more than 250 peer-reviewed scientific journal articles, has authored or edited 8 books, and has contributed more than 50 book chapters.

In 2002, Dr. Schuman received the Alcon Research Institute Award, as well as the New York Academy of Medicine's Lewis Rudin Glaucoma Prize. In 2003, he received the Senior Achievement Award from the American Academy of Ophthalmology. In 2004, he was elected into the American Society for Clinical Investigation. In 2006, he received the Association for Research in Vision and Ophthalmology (ARVO) Translational Research Award. He was elected to the American Ophthalmological Society in 2008. He received a 2006-2009 American Medical Association Physician's Recognition Award with Commendation. In 2010, he became a silver Fellow of ARVO. In 2011, Dr. Schuman was the Clinician-Scientist Lecturer of the American Glaucoma Society. In 2012, he received the Carnegie Science Center's Award in Life Sciences and was a co-recipient of the Champalimaud Award.

Contributing Authors

Ron A. Adelman, MD, MPH, MBA, FACS (Chapter 33)
Professor of Ophthalmology and Visual Science
Director of Retina Center
Yale University School of Medicine
New Haven, Connecticut

Iqbal "Ike" K. Ahmed, MD, FRCSC (Chapter 66)
Assistant Professor
University of Toronto
Toronto, Canada

Lama A. Al-Aswad, MD (Chapter 71)
Harkness Eye Institute
Columbia University Medical Center
New York, New York

R. Rand Allingham, MD (Chapters 11, 17, 27, 39, 42, 60)
Duke Eye Center
Durham, North Carolina

Michael A. Alunni, MD (Chapter 67)
Allegheny Ophthalmic & Orbital Associates, PC
Department of Ophthalmology
Allegheny General Hospital
Pittsburgh, Pennsylvania

Cristan M. Arena, MD (Chapter 57)
Glaucoma and Comprehensive Ophthalmology
Chester County Eye Care
West Chester, Pennsylvania

Sanjay Asrani, MD (Chapter 72)
Duke Eye Center
Durham, North Carolina

Ramesh S. Ayyala, MD, FRSC(E), FRCOphth(Lon)
(Chapter 66)
Professor of Ophthalmology
Director of Glaucoma Services
Tulane School of Medicine
New Orleans, Louisiana

Priti Batta, MD (Chapter 49)
New York Eye and Ear Infirmary
New York, New York

Carla I. Bourne, MD (Chapters 43, 61)
Assistant Professor
University of South Florida
Tampa, Florida

Zvia Burgansky-Eliash, MD (Chapters 30, 42)
Ophthalmology Department
The Edith Wolfson Medical Center
Holon, Israel
Sackler School of Medicine
Tel-Aviv University
Tel-Aviv, Israel

Pratap Challa, MD, MS (Chapters 12-15, 17, 20)
Director, Residency Training Program
Associate Professor of Ophthalmology
Duke University Eye Center
Durham, North Carolina

Vicki M. Chen, MD (Chapter 69)
Assistant Professor
Pediatric Ophthalmology and Strabismus
New England Eye Center
Tufts Medical Center
Boston, Massachusetts

Garry P. Condon, MD (Chapter 67)
Chairman, Department of Ophthalmology
Allegheny General Hospital
Associate Professor of Ophthalmology
Drexel University College of Medicine
Clinical Assistant Professor of Ophthalmology
University of Pittsburgh
Pittsburgh, Pennsylvania

Ian P. Conner, MD, PhD (Chapters 5, 8, 19, 21, 23, 29, 34, 39, 46, 47)
UPMC Eye Center
Pittsburgh, Pennsylvania

Daniel Cotlear, MD (Chapter 53)
Consultant
The Sam Rothberg Glaucoma Center
Goldschleger Eye Institute
Sheba Medical Center
Tel Hashomer, Israel

Marshall N. Cyrlin, MD (Chapter 54)
Professor of Ophthalmology
Oakland University William Beaumont School of Medicine
Clinical Professor of Biomedical Sciences
Eye Research Institute
Oakland University
Rochester, Michigan
Emeritus Director, Glaucoma Service
Beaumont Eye Institute
Royal Oak, Michigan

David K. Dueker, MD (Chapter 31)
Senior Consultant
Surgery-Ophthalmology
Hamad Medical Corp
Doha, Qatar

Jay S. Duker, MD (Chapter 41)
Chairman, Department of Ophthalmology
Tufts University School of Medicine
Director, Tufts New England Eye Center
Boston, Massachusetts

David L. Epstein, MD, MMM (Chapters 1, 3-5, 8, 12-14, 18-29, 34-40, 45-48, 63, 64)
Joseph A.C. Wadsworth Clinical Professor
Chairman, Department of Ophthalmology
Duke University School of Medicine
Durham, North Carolina

Lindsey S. Folio, MS, MBA (Chapter 9)
UPMC Eye Center, Eye & Ear Institute
Ophthalmology and Visual Science Research Center
Department of Ophthalmology
University of Pittsburgh School of Medicine
Pittsburgh, Pennsylvania

Gretta Fridman, MD (Chapter 74)
New Tampa Eye Institute
Tampa, Florida

Lisa S. Gamell, MD (Chapters 7, 55, 57, 74)
Glaucoma Fellowship Director
USF Eye Institute
Associate Professor of Ophthalmology
USF Health Morsani College of Medicine
Tampa, Florida

Morton F. Goldberg, MD (Chapter 43)
Director Emeritus and Joseph Green Professor of Ophthalmology
Wilmer Eye Institute
Johns Hopkins Hospital
Baltimore, Maryland

Modi Goldenfeld, MD (Chapter 53)
Consultant
The Sam Rothberg Glaucoma Center
Goldschleger Eye Institute
Sheba Medical Center
Tel Hashomer, Israel

Leon W. Herndon Jr, MD (Chapter 70)
Associate Professor of Ophthalmology
Medical Director, Duke Eye Center
Durham, North Carolina

Richard W. Hertle, MD, FAAO, FACS, FAAP (Chapter 68)
Chief of Pediatric Ophthalmology
Director, Children's Vision Center
Akron Children's Hospital
Akron, Ohio
Professor, Department of Surgery
College of Medicine
Northeast Ohio Medical College
Rootstown, Ohio

Michael B. Horsley, MD (Chapter 75)
Private Practice
Phoenix, Arizona

Farhan A. Irshad, MD (Chapter 66)
Clinical Assistant Professor of Ophthalmology
Tulane School of Medicine
New Orleans, Louisiana

Annisa L. Jamil, MD (Chapter 59)
Glaucoma Consultants Northwest
Seattle, Washington

Murray A. Johnstone, MD (Chapter 59)
Clinical Professor
Department of Ophthalmology
University of Washington
Seattle, Washington

Deval Joshi, MD (Chapter 7)
Retina Fellow
Department of Ophthalmology
University of Florida
Gainesville, Florida

Mahmoud A. Khaimi, MD (Chapters 58-60)
Clinical Associate Professor of Ophthalmology
Dean McGee Eye Institute
The University of Oklahoma College of Medicine
Oklahoma City, Oklahoma

David A. Lee, MD, MS, MBA, FACS, FARVO (Chapter 59)
Clinical Professor
Ruiz Department of Ophthalmology
University of Texas Medical School at Houston
Robert Cizik Eye Clinic
Houston, Texas

Cynthia Mattox, MD (Chapter 49)
New England Eye Center
Tufts University School of Medicine
Boston, Massachusetts

Stuart J. McKinnon, MD, PhD (Chapter 73)
Duke Eye Center
Durham, North Carolina

Shlomo Melamed, MD (Chapter 53)
Professor of Ophthalmology
Director, The Sam Rothberg Glaucoma Center
Goldschleger Eye Institute
Sheba Medical Center
Tel Hashomer, Israel

Kimberly V. Miller, MD (Chapters 18, 19, 21)
Department of Ophthalmology
UPMC Eye Center, Eye & Ear Institute
University of Pittsburgh
Pittsburgh, Pennsylvania

Peter A. Netland, MD, PhD (Chapter 19)
Vernah Scott Moyston Professor and Chair
Department of Ophthalmology
University of Virginia School of Medicine
Charlottesville, Virginia

Yvonne Ou, MD (Chapters 72, 73)
University of California San Francisco
San Francisco, California

Mina B. Pantcheva, MD (Chapters 10, 25, 37, 44, 56)
Ophthalmology Department
University of Colorado School of Medicine
Aurora, Colorado

Marcos Reyes, MD (Chapters 59, 60, 65)
Assistant Professor of Clinical Ophthalmology
Mason Eye Institute
The University of Missouri School of Medicine
Columbia, Missouri

Douglas J. Rhee, MD (Chapter 16)
Harvard Medical School
Massachusetts Eye and Ear Infirmary
Boston, Massachusetts

Claudia U. Richter, MD (Chapter 53)
Clinical Instructor in Ophthalmology
Harvard Medical School
Boston, Massachusetts

Sarwat Salim, MD, FACS (Chapters 32, 62)
Associate Professor of Ophthalmology
Director, Glaucoma Service
Hamilton Eye Institute
Memphis, Tennessee

Steven R. Sarkisian Jr, MD (Chapter 65)
Glaucoma, Cataract, and Anterior Segment Eye Surgeon
Glaucoma Fellowship Director
Dean McGee Eye Institute
Clinical Associate Professor
University of Oklahoma College of Medicine
Oklahoma City, Oklahoma

Timothy Saunders, MD (Chapter 55)
Retina Fellow
USF Eye Institute
Tampa, Florida

Sumit P. Shah, MD (Chapter 41)
Vitreoretinal Specialist
New England Retina Associates
Hamden, Connecticut
Clinical Instructor
Yale University School of Medicine
New Haven, Connecticut

M. Bruce Shields, MD (Chapter 32)
Professor and Chairman Emeritus
Department of Ophthalmology
Yale University School of Medicine
New Haven, Connecticut

Bradford J. Shingleton, MD (Chapters 43, 61)
Ophthalmic Consultants of Boston, Inc
Tufts New England Medical Center
Massachusetts Eye and Ear Infirmary
Harvard Medical School
Boston, Massachusetts

Richard J. Simmons, MD (Chapter 30)
Simmons Eye Associates of Boston
Associate Clinical Professor of Ophthalmology
Harvard Medical School
Surgeon in Ophthalmology
Massachusetts Eye and Ear Infirmary
Boston, Massachusetts

Brian J. Song, MD (Chapter 71)
UCLA Jules Stein Eye Institute
Los Angeles, California

Jeffrey R. SooHoo, MD (Chapter 31)
Department of Ophthalmology
University of Colorado Denver School of Medicine
Aurora, Colorado

Joshua D. Stein, MD, MS (Chapters 11, 17)
University of Michigan
W.K. Kellogg Eye Center
Ann Arbor, Michigan

David P. Tingey, BA, MD, FRCSC (Chapter 59)
Associate Professor of Ophthalmology
Western University
London, Ontario, Canada

Angela V. Turalba, MD (Chapter 16)
Harvard Medical School
Massachusetts Eye and Ear Infirmary
Boston VA Healthcare System
Boston, Massachusetts

George Ulrich, MD, FACS (Chapters 22, 23, 24)
Private Practice
Colorado Springs, Colorado

E. Michael Van Buskirk, MD (Chapter 2)
Clinical Professor of Ophthalmology, Retired
Oregon Health and Sciences University
Portland, Oregon

David S. Walton, MD (Chapter 69)
Massachusetts Eye and Ear Infirmary
Boston, Massachusetts

Martin Wand, MD (Chapter 33)
Clinical Professor of Ophthalmology
University of Connecticut School of Medicine
Farmington, Connecticut

Guy Aharon Weiss, MD (Chapter 42)
Department of Medicine
State University of New York at Buffalo
Buffalo, New York

Janey L. Wiggs, MD, PhD (Chapter 50)
Paul Austin Chandler Associate Professor of Ophthalmology
Harvard Medical School
Massachusetts Eye and Ear Infirmary
Boston, Massachusetts

M. Roy Wilson, MD, MS (Chapter 75)
Chancellor Emeritus
University of Colorado Denver
Denver, Colorado

Jeremy B. Wingard, MD (Chapters 6, 51, 52)
Glaucoma and Cataract Consultant
Wheaton Eye Clinic
Wheaton, Illinois
Adjunct Assistant Professor
Department of Ophthalmology
University of Pittsburgh School of Medicine
Pittsburgh, Pennsylvania

Gadi Wollstein, MD (Chapter 9)
UPMC Eye Center, Eye & Ear Institute
Ophthalmology and Visual Science Research Center
Department of Ophthalmology
University of Pittsburgh School of Medicine
Pittsburgh, Pennsylvania

PREFACE

There is no greater obligation, but also joy, than to help perpetuate the wisdom of one's teachers for ensuing generations. Therefore, when Drs. Chandler and Grant asked me to author the Third Edition of this book in 1986 (the "green book") I was thrilled, but also very concerned. As I wrote in the Preface:

> On re-reading the Second Edition I was almost awestruck by the wisdom and veracity of what was written. Even where there had been incomplete understanding of the mechanism for a particular occurrence, the practical concepts of management were still true and fully applicable. The integrity of what was written was extraordinary. It was thus with great trepidation that this student of PAC and WMG attempted to update their wisdom and understanding in this Third Edition.

So I was subsequently pleased when both Drs. Chandler and Grant approved of my efforts!

When it came time for a further update in the Fourth Edition (the "blue book"), I became very focused on a specific goal for this book. As I wrote in the Preface to the "blue book" in 1997:

> I wanted to try to write a book on glaucoma that would give practical clinical information to the clinician dealing with an individual patient, and yet at the same time, stimulate us all to ask "why," ie, what is the mechanism for the clinical observation, and how might we be better able to treat the condition in the future. Drs. Chandler and Grant had taught me to strive to think this way. Glaucoma is a discipline commonly of subtleties and nuances with the detailed clinical observation of an individual patient quite important.

Again it was a source of great satisfaction to me when Dr. Grant (Dr. Chandler unfortunately had passed away) told me that he enjoyed this emphasis and that it was a fitting continuation of the "Chandler-Grant tradition."

It is now 16 years since the last [Fourth] Edition of the book and although I am struck by how the wisdom of the clinical observations (mostly of Drs. Chandler and Grant, themselves) have endured in their accuracy and practical wisdom, it is clearly time for this important core of glaucoma knowledge to be updated, amplified, and further modernized. I am so grateful to Malik Y. Kahook, MD and Joel S. Schuman, MD, FACS for undertaking this needed "modernization," and I am very impressed with the exceptionally high quality of their achievement. They have greatly improved the textbook with expertise well beyond my capabilities. I believe Drs. Chandler and Grant would be so proud of them and pleased that their heritage and legacy of glaucoma thought have been so well perpetuated for the next generation.

The fundamental truths of *Chandler and Grant's Glaucoma* have been preserved in this Fifth Edition by Kahook and Schuman, and I am also very pleased that my goals of practical clinical information for the clinician dealing with the individual patient with glaucoma have not only been achieved, but actually improved upon. My thanks and congratulations to Drs. Kahook and Schuman for their extraordinary achievement in maintaining the Chandler-Grant tradition of practical wisdom about glaucoma, while also simultaneously stimulating inquisitiveness and innovation.

David L. Epstein, MD, MMM

INTRODUCTION

The teachings of Drs. Chandler and Grant have shaped the course of glaucoma diagnosis and treatment for decades. The lessons they forged through careful clinical observation and laboratory research have lived on through several editions of this comprehensive textbook and have managed to remain relevant despite a massive amount of new knowledge and rapid pace of research and development since their passing. We believe that *Chandler and Grant's Glaucoma* is more relevant today than ever because it provides the framework and guidance to apply newly learned knowledge to any clinical or surgical scenario while still holding to the values of inquisitiveness and sound judgment that direct superior patient care.

In this book, we endeavor to maintain the historical teachings that were present since the first lectures on glaucoma given by Drs. Chandler and Grant at the New England Ophthalmological Society more than 50 years ago. In some circumstances passages are included to provide reference to older techniques and therapies that help us understand how modern methods evolved. Chapters on current and potential future classes of medications are included to guide therapeutic choices for the practicing physician. Minimally invasive surgical techniques are covered with the hope that future editions of this text will elucidate how they best fit in our surgical decision making. New imaging chapters contain a wealth of information on basic interpretation skills as well as explanations on how new devices are influencing clinical practice. Explanations of common clinical and surgical pitfalls are covered to help the clinician avoid suboptimal outcomes. Decision trees, tables, and figures can be found throughout each chapter and help augment the information provided in the text in a clear and concise manner. Basic clinical decision making and sound surgical principles are carefully detailed and remain the focus of this comprehensive reference.

It is only by looking to the past that we can learn how best to move forward. The teachings of Drs. Chandler and Grant are ever present in each page of this book. We hope the reader will take time to read each lesson and internalize the essence of the philosophy shared by these two giants of ophthalmology.

Malik Y. Kahook, MD
Joel S. Schuman, MD, FACS

THE BASICS

1

Introduction

Joel S. Schuman, MD, FACS and David L. Epstein, MD, MMM

THE PROBLEM

The study of glaucoma can be both clinically satisfying and intellectually stimulating. Yet, it is also the most humbling of disciplines, both because of our clinical failures but even more because of our lack of real understanding. In truth, if one looks at ophthalmic knowledge in the last century, despite new medications, surgeries, and sophisticated measurement techniques, the field of glaucoma has shown the least progress.

Why is this? Chronic glaucomas are, in general, slowly progressive diseases that develop over time. This time factor creates substantial difficulties in achieving meaningful clinical deductions and insight. One of the major reasons for this book is the fact that long-term clinical observations can provide a basis for meaningful knowledge. This is the true Chandler-Grant tradition.

Those caring for glaucoma patients bear the curse of long-term follow-up. However, such perspective is important both for practical patient care and as a template for new knowledge, but this experience requires long periods of clinical observation. Experienced clinicians have a great deal to contribute to our knowledge of glaucoma. The fields of glaucoma are littered with relics of short-term enthusiasms for certain procedures and techniques.

OUR METHODS

In addition to the time factor, our methods in glaucoma have been very crude and provide inadequate information. The measurement of intraocular pressure (IOP) is inaccurate, and it indicates the IOP at only one instant of time. We know there is both a diurnal and seasonal variation in IOP.[1] Patients often only take their antiglaucoma medication just before coming to the ophthalmologist's office. Each of us measures the IOP, and because it is the only data we have, we generalize that this must be the representative IOP for that patient during the entire time interval since we have last seen the patient. This is often not true. Our office IOP measurement is a single snapshot.

This often contributes to fuzzy thinking about primary open-angle glaucoma (POAG). There are many population survey studies in which patients who demonstrate POAG-related field loss do not have elevated IOP at the time of sampling.[2-4] This has led to avenues of thought, especially abroad, that IOP is not involved in glaucomatous optic neuropathy, even though most studies have shown that the risk for field loss in POAG increases linearly with the level of IOP.[5] Much effort has been spent pursuing these non-IOP-related glaucoma hypotheses, even though, at the same time, early filtration surgery for patients with glaucoma has been simultaneously proposed by many of the same investigators (presumably the only known efficacy of filtration surgery for glaucoma is to consistently lower the IOP). Some insight into possible pathogenic mechanisms in glaucoma has come from population studies in which a second IOP has been measured[6]: the prevalence of at least one increased IOP measurement is substantially higher; that is, discovered glaucoma patients with normal IOP at the time of initial evaluation may demonstrate an elevated IOP at a subsequent visit. What this means to us is that, although IOP can be accurately measured, we have vast expanses of missing data points for evaluation of glaucoma patients. A Holter monitor or glycosylated hemoglobin approach, if possible, might revolutionize understanding.

All this does not detract from the clinical fact from long-term clinical observations that there is varying susceptibility of the optic nerve to given levels of IOP. But what is the quality of data about this end organ, the optic nerve, concerning damage in glaucoma? Again, methods of clinical analysis are crude. Descriptions of optic discs, cup/disc ratios, and disc drawings are notoriously inaccurate. The best advice one could give the beginning ophthalmic resident is to make drawings of optic nerves on all

Kahook MY, Schuman JS, eds.
Chandler and Grant's Glaucoma, Fifth Edition (pp 3-6).
© 2013 SLACK Incorporated.

glaucoma patients and then later compare these to actual disc photographs and imaging. Stereo disc photographs should be obtained on all glaucoma patients, especially as a baseline, if at all feasible. Although there are artifacts if a true stereo image is not photographed, the newer cameras can perform this adequately.[7] Regardless, a photograph, even if Nonstereo, is the most objective way to obtain this snapshot of the optic nerve at one point in time; however, the assessment of this objective snapshot is still subjective. For that reason, it is also important that we include ocular imaging of the retina and optic nerve in our assessment of the glaucoma patient, because this can provide objective, quantitative analysis of the patient's ocular structure. The degree of optic nerve damage at that given point in time can be accurately and reproducibly measured.[8-19]

It is still another matter to detect a change in appearance of the optic nerve. Direct meticulous comparison by the clinician of 2 photographs performed with the same camera at different points in time, or comparison by clinical examination techniques of the current appearance with the previous baseline photograph, is no longer the best that we can do. It is difficult with our subjective evaluation of such objective data to be sure of progression. Computerized technologies now allow us to measure progression, and several devices now provide this ability. Confocal scanning laser ophthalmoscopy, scanning laser polarimetry, and optical coherence tomography have all been validated as methods to measure progressive structural change in glaucoma.[18-23]

What of visual fields? Although great strides have been made in the reproducibility of data with modern automated perimeter machines, these still remain subjective tests that depend on a patient pressing a button in response to a stimulus. These are subjective data. The system cries out for objective measurements. An objective visual field, perhaps made by recording an optic nerve response to a light stimulus placed on the retina, would yield more accurate and more sensitive data.

OUR BASIS OF
UNDERSTANDING GLAUCOMA

What of glaucoma science? When one looks at all the wonderful progress in the understanding of diseases on a cellular and molecular level, it is humbling to see how little true-progress has been made in glaucoma. Investigators do not even agree on what should be studied. There are many problems and it is a small scientific field that is fragmented both as to the areas of study (trabecular meshwork [TM], ciliary body, or optic nerve) and what to study. The tissues involved are difficult to study experimentally either because of their size or complexity. Animal models of the disease do not reproduce clinical human glaucoma. The clinical debate in glaucoma between an IOP disease or an optic neuropathy (rather than involvement of both) has added to the confusion.

A Concept

In the glaucoma field, the questions remain the same, but the answers keep on changing. One cannot be dogmatic, especially with so few real data. But, at our current level of understanding, we would frame the chronic glaucomas the following way:

- In almost all cases, an abnormality in drainage of aqueous humor through the outflow pathway tissue, potentially at many sites in the TM, leads to elevation of IOP and causes damage to the optic nerve end organ, which demonstrates varying susceptibility to different levels of IOP (including statistically normal IOP).

- The 2 main scientific questions are as follows:

  1. In the open-angle glaucomas, what is the cause of obstruction to trabecular outflow and how can this trabecular glaucoma be best treated?

  2. What is the cause of the optic nerve damage and especially its varying susceptibility (a feature that can appropriately be termed an *optic neuropathy*), and are there any specific remedies for the optic nerve beyond consistently lowering the IOP?

Both of these questions are very important. These 2 schools of scientific inquiry should be complementary rather than competitive.

Clinical Implications of These Basic Concepts

For the student of glaucoma, framing these concepts this way is not an academic exercise but it does have clinical relevance. Students should strive to understand why the IOP is elevated (why there is the obstruction to outflow), especially on comparative examinations, and why the optic nerve cupping is occurring at a specific IOP.

Elevated IOP is due to impaired drainage through the TM and is probably never due to above-normal aqueous humor formation. When doing gonioscopy, the diseased tissue involved in the hydrodynamic component of glaucoma is visible. If there were an understanding of what was going on in the visible tissue, much advancement might be possible. And although for POAG, nothing unusual may be detected in the open angle, a sleuth-like style in glaucoma sometimes does provide insight. Are there occult inflammatory precipitates? Exfoliation material? Abnormal vessels? Partial angle closure? When a patient with open-angle glaucoma returns for follow-up and an even higher IOP is measured, one should approach the problem from the point-of-view of the TM and always through repeat gonioscopy, strive to answer why the IOP is now further elevated.

This tissue-oriented approach may also help conceptually in understanding certain clinical phenomena. For example, the term *steroid responder* refers to a steroid-induced decrease in facility of aqueous humor drainage by the TM. It may indicate latent POAG. In acute uveitides, when steroids are used and there is prompt and subsequent elevation of IOP, this most often is not due to a steroid-induced further decrease in TM function (which is impaired due to inflammation in the TM), but rather to the steroid restoring aqueous humor formation toward normal by suppressing inflammation in the ciliary body. TM function may not, in fact, have worsened from the steroid; therefore, from a clinical point-of-view, the patient should not be labeled as a steroid responder. In fact, steroids may not need to be discontinued, and continued steroid therapy might actually improve the impairment in TM function caused by the inflammation. Similarly, by trying to explain a late-onset IOP elevation after penetrating keratoplasty from the point-of-view of the TM, a diagnosis of steroid-induced secondary open-angle glaucoma may be identified that was not at first appreciated. (It is surprising how often this diagnosis is not correctly made because of the usual very-low dosage of topical steroids, which have a cumulative effect).

There is also clearly more to optic nerve cupping than IOP alone. What are the factors that contribute to this varying susceptibility? Are they local or systemic? Could certain systemic medications prescribed for nonophthalmologic purposes increase the susceptibility of the optic nerve to glaucomatous cupping? When looking at the optic nerve of a patient who is progressing despite reasonable IOP, step back and take a look at the whole patient, and consider whether there are any systemic or other local influences. At the present time, we really do not have such understanding, but we predict that when we eventually do, it will have originated with a clinical observation by an ophthalmologist, who was attempting to answer these questions. (For example, if there truly is increased susceptibility to optic nerve cupping in exfoliation syndrome and in systemic amyloidosis, then such a clinical observation might represent this type of important clinical insight.)

The latter possibility is what makes clinical glaucoma so exciting and often so satisfying. It is a real clinical disease, where clinicians can make meaningful observations that even in this new high-tech era can be original and unique. There is room for tremendous advancement in understanding starting with clinical observation, especially as methods of examination will hopefully improve in the future. These new clinical observations and unique insights can lead to specific new hypotheses that can be tested by both clinical and laboratory investigation. Medical doctors can be both clinicians and scientists in the discipline of glaucoma and in the end, make a difference to patients with this treacherous, chronic-progressive disease.

Glaucoma is a wonderful field for the young ophthalmologist to enter. It is both an intellectual- and a practical-clinical challenge. We have gained much new knowledge and expect a great deal more in coming years. The new talent and evolving science will finally bring new methods of cellular and molecular inquiry to the discipline.

In some ways then, the glaucoma field today is both the worst and best of times.

GOAL OF THIS BOOK

The goal of this book is to provide practical clinical information about the management of all patients with glaucoma. We have tried to frame the current understanding in such a way as to stimulate the reader and the editors to ask the question, Why is this glaucoma occurrence happening in this patient, and how might I be able to treat this better?

REFERENCES

1. Epstein DL, Krug Jr JH, Hertzmark E, et al. A long-term clinical trial of timolol therapy versus no treatment in the management of glaucoma suspects. *Ophthalmology.* 1989;96:1460-1467.
2. Hollows FC, Graham PA. Intra-ocular pressure glaucoma and glaucoma suspects in a defined population. *Br J Ophthalmol.* 1966;50:570-586.
3. Bengtsson B. The prevalence of glaucoma. *Br J Ophthalmol.* 1981;65:46-49.
4. Dielemans I, Vingerling JR, Wolfs RCW, et al. The prevalence of primary open angle glaucoma in a population-based study in the Netherlands. *Ophthalmology.* 1994;101:1851-1855.
5. American Academy of Ophthalmology Quality of Care Committee Glaucoma Panel. *Preferred Practice Patterns: Primary Open Angle Glaucoma.* San Francisco, CA: The Academy; 1992.
6. Sommer A, Tielsch JM, Katz J, et al. Relationship between intraocular pressure and primary open angle glaucoma among white and black Americans: the Baltimore Eye Survey. *Arch Ophthalmol.* 1991;109:1090-1095
7. Greenfield DS, Zacharia PT, Schuman JS. Comparison of Nidek 3DX vs. Donaldson simultaneous stereoscopic disc photography. *Am J Ophthalmol.* 1993;116:741-747.
8. Schuman JS, Hee MR, Puliafito CA, et al. Quantification of nerve fiber layer thickness in normal and glaucomatous eyes using optical coherence tomography. *Arch Ophthalmol.* 1995;113(5):586-596.
9. Schuman JS, Pedut-Kloizman T, Hertzmark E, et al. Reproducibility of nerve fiber layer thickness measurements using optical coherence tomography. *Ophthalmology.* 1996;103:1889-1898.
10. Paunescu LA, Schuman JS, Price LL, et al. Reproducibility of nerve fiber thickness, macular thickness, and optic nerve head measurements using Stratus OCT. *Invest Ophthalmol Vis Sci.* 2004;45:1716-1724.
11. Budenz DL, Michael A, Chang RT, McSoley J, Katz J. Sensitivity and specificity of the Stratus OCT for perimetric glaucoma. *Ophthalmology.* 2005;112:3-9.
12. Medeiros FA, Alencar LM, Zangwill LM, Bowd C, Sample PA, Weinreb RN. Prediction of functional loss in glaucoma from progressive optic disc damage. *Arch Ophthalmol.* 2009;127(10):1382-1383.
13. Kim JS, Sung KR, Xu J, et al. Retinal nerve fiber layer thickness measurement reproducibility improved with spectral domain optical coherence tomography. *Br J Ophthalmol.* 2009;93:1057-1063.
14. Weinreb RN. Evaluating the retinal nerve fiber layer in glaucoma with scanning laser polarimetry. *Arch Ophthalmol.* 1999;117(10):1403-1406.

15. Ohkubo S, Takeda H, Higashide T, Sasaki T, Sugiyama K. A pilot study to detect glaucoma with confocal scanning laser ophthalmoscopy compared with nonmydriatic stereoscopic photography in a community health screening. *J Glaucoma.* 2007;16(6): 531-538.

16. Girkin CA, DeLeon-Ortega JE, Xie A, McGwin G, Arthur SN, Monheit BE. Comparison of the Moorfields classification using confocal scanning laser ophthalmoscopy and subjective optic disc classification in detecting glaucoma in blacks and whites. *Ophthalmology.* 2006;113(12):2144-2149.

17. Zangwill LM, Weinreb RN, Beiser JA, et al. Baseline topographic optic disc measurements are associated with the development of primary open-angle glaucoma: the Confocal Scanning Laser Ophthalmoscopy Ancillary Study to the Ocular Hypertension Treatment Study. *Arch Ophthalmol.* 2005;123(9):1188-1197.

18. Townsend KA, Wollstein G, Schuman JS. Imaging of the retinal nerve fibre layer for glaucoma. *Br J Ophthalmol.* 2009;93(2):139-143.

19. Sharma P, Sample PA, Zangwill LM, Schuman JS. Diagnostic tools for glaucoma detection and management. *Surv Ophthalmol.* 2008;53(suppl 1):S17-S32.

20. Wollstein G, Schuman JS, Price LL, et al. Optical coherence tomography longitudinal evaluation of retinal nerve fiber layer thickness in glaucoma. *Arch Ophthalmol.* 2005;123(4):464-470.

21. Bowd C, Balasubramanian M, Weinreb RN, et al. Performance of confocal scanning laser tomograph Topographic Change Analysis (TCA) for assessing glaucomatous progression. *Invest Ophthalmol Vis Sci.* 2009;50(2):691-701.

22. Medeiros FA, Alencar LM, Zangwill LM, et al. Detection of progressive retinal nerve fiber layer loss in glaucoma using scanning laser polarimetry with variable corneal compensation. *Invest Ophthalmol Vis Sci.* 2009;50(4):1675-1681.

23. Giangiacomo A, Garway-Heath D, Caprioli J. Diagnosing glaucoma progression: current practice and promising technologies. *Curr Opin Ophthalmol.* 2006;17(2):153-162.

2

Anatomy

Malik Y. Kahook, MD and E. Michael Van Buskirk, MD

The human eye is bound by 3 concentric, virtually spherical layers or coats: the outer fibrous layer, the cornea and sclera; the middle vascular layer, the uveal tract; and the inner neurosensory layer, the retina. The interior of the globe is divided into 3 compartments: the anterior chamber between iris and cornea, the posterior chamber between lens and posterior iris, and the vitreous cavity, posterior to the lens, comprising most of the ocular volume. The aqueous humor is contained by the posterior chamber and the anterior chamber and has a volume of about 200 microliters.[1] Aqueous humor flows from the ciliary processes at about 2 to 2.5 microliters per minute.[1]

The uveal tract attaches to the sclera at 3 sites: the optic nerve, the vortex veins, and the chamber angle. The latter consists of an inward roll of collagenous tissue, the scleral spur, that serves as the partial insertion of the ciliary muscle fibers that are important for maintenance of aqueous humor outflow and accommodation. These attachments can become clinically relevant especially after blunt trauma when shear forces between the ocular layers tear the ciliary muscle and uvea away from the scleral spur, leading to cyclodialysis, iridodialysis, or angle recession and secondary glaucoma.

AQUEOUS HUMOR OUTFLOW PATHWAYS

Aqueous humor leaves the eye primarily through the so-called conventional outflow pathways: the trabecular meshwork (TM), Schlemm's canal, the aqueous humor collector channels, and the aqueous veins, to the episcleral veins, orbital veins, and the intracranial cavernous venous sinus. A substantial portion leaves by means of the uveoscleral outflow pathways, through the anterior chamber angle, the anterior extreme of the ciliary muscle,

the posterior uvea, the suprachoroidal space, the sclera (perhaps along perforations for veins and nerves), and into the orbital tissues.[2,3] In contrast to conventional outflow, which is dependent upon the intraocular pressure, uveoscleral outflow is relatively pressure independent. It is enhanced by certain prostaglandins and can become significant in the inflamed eye, possibly contributing to the low intraocular pressure sometimes seen in uveitis. In addition, pharmacologic prostaglandin analog compounds, administered topically, appear to stimulate uveoscleral outflow and reduce intraocular pressure in glaucomatous eyes, even in those typically resistant to outflow-stimulating drugs, such as cholinergic agents. In addition, some absorption takes place through the iris, but this may not be physiologically or clinically significant.

CONVENTIONAL AQUEOUS HUMOR OUTFLOW PATHWAYS

A thorough understanding of the anatomy of the anterior chamber angle is essential for any clinician treating glaucoma as well as for scientists investigating this tiny but complex region. The precise proportions and relations of the various structures of the chamber angle are dependent on anatomic characteristics, such as size of the globe, the refractive error, the size and position of the lens, and physiologic factors associated with aqueous secretion, accommodative tone, venous pressure, and postural position. The peripheral iris, or iris root, blends with the anterior and medial fibers of the ciliary muscle to form the apex of the anterior chamber angle, posterior to the true TM and scleral spur (Figure 2-1). The ciliary muscle fibers then pass anteriorly to insert into scleral spur and TM to complete the angle. Thus, the anterior chamber angle typically subtends about 30 degrees with the iris making one arm and the scleral spur, TM, and cornea

Kahook MY, Schuman JS, eds.
Chandler and Grant's Glaucoma, Fifth Edition (pp 7-15).
© 2013 SLACK Incorporated.

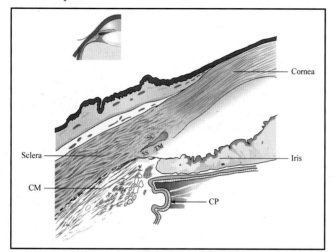

Figure 2-1. Drawing of the anterior chamber angle, bound superiorly by the cornea, inferiorly by the iris with the trabecular meshwork (TM), scleral spur (SS), and ciliary muscle (CM) at the apex. Schlemm's canal (SC) lies within the apex of the angle, just external to the TM, its inner wall contiguous with the outer wall of the meshwork.

comprising the other. The iris plane may vary from flat to slightly concave or convex, but is typically convex, with a smooth transition from the mid-iris to the angle apex.

THE TRABECULAR MESHWORK

The TM lies in the corneoscleral arm of the chamber angle, just anterior to the angle apex. It extends between the scleral spur posteriorly and the peripheral cornea or Schwalbe's line anteriorly. Functionally, the scleral spur, ciliary muscle, TM, and Schlemm's canal work as a single unit to comprise the conventional aqueous outflow pathways. The TM in cross-section is triangular in shape, its apex at the corneal periphery, in effect suspended from the peripheral extreme of Decemet's membrane, Schwalbe's line. The base of the triangular mesh is then formed by the scleral spur and the inner fibers of the ciliary muscle.

The inner wall of the meshwork faces the anterior chamber, and the outer comprises the inner wall of Schlemm's canal. The TM may be divided into 3 histologically identifiable components: the most inner aspect, the uveal meshwork; the central component, the corneoscleral meshwork; and the outer aspect, the juxtacanalicular (JXT) tissue-inner wall of Schlemm's canal (see Figure 2-1). Outgoing aqueous humor passes through each element sequentially, from the uveal meshwork, through the corneoscleral meshwork, and then the JXT tissue to enter Schlemm's canal.

The uveal meshwork is perhaps most variable from eye to eye and hence, most difficult to define. During fetal development, an intact tissue layer extends from cornea over the angle to the iris surface. During the final trimester, this layer undergoes a dissolution process as the remainder of the TM matures to accommodate aqueous outflow.[4] The uveal

meshwork contains large spaces between tissue lamellae and thus, typically contributes little if any significant resistance to aqueous humor outflow. When the iridocorneal fetal tissue layer fails to undergo normal developmental dissolution in the final gestational trimester, this tissue (anomalous uveal meshwork) can block aqueous humor outflow, leading to so-called primary congenital glaucoma. Such membranes can be incised surgically to restore physiologic aqueous outflow. In other unusual circumstances, such persistent tissue layers apparently are sufficiently permeable to permit adequate intraocular pressure in early childhood but become clinically significant in adolescence with a visible uveal tissue layer covering the normal TM. The remaining uveal tissue remnants become the uveal meshwork and typically consist of strands of uveal tissue from peripheral iris to the mid or anterior corneoscleral meshwork. These are sometimes called iris processes, may contain melanin, and can be variably pigmented. In some cases, uveal meshwork strands extend all the way to Schwalbe's line. Prominent uveal meshwork with iris processes are not particularly associated with glaucoma but are sometimes seen with various forms of congenital glaucoma. In other subjects, the uveal meshwork has a diaphanous membranous quality. Usually, the uveal meshwork does not form a significant component to aqueous humor outflow resistance, but when substantial, probably can contribute, for example, in some congenital or juvenile-onset glaucomas.

The bulk of the TM consists of the corneoscleral portion, of about 10 to 15 perforated collagenous sheets, or layers, suspended between Schwalbe's line or the peripheral cornea anteriorly and ciliary muscle or scleral spur posteriorly. The outer layers arise directly from scleral spur, but the inner layers directly arise from insertions of the inner fibers of the ciliary muscle. Each lamella consists of a central collagen core, overlain by basement membrane and endothelial type trabecular cells and a complex extracellular macromolecular interstitium. Trabecular cells form a variably intact monolayer to line the interstices of the meshwork. They are multipotential cells with great phagocytic and migratory capabilities in response to physiologic, pathologic, and injurious stimuli.[5] The trabecular cells gradually diminish in density throughout life.[6] This trabecular depopulation is accelerated in primary open-angle glaucoma.[6] Stimulation of the trabeculum with some forms of mild injury, such as laser trabeculoplasty, appear to enhance trabecular cell division and migration, temporarily repopulating the tissue with newly formed cells.[7,8] The relative mechanical tension of the ciliary muscle fibers on the corneoscleral lamella plays a major role in modulating resistance to aqueous humor outflow, but the exact mechanism of this modulation is not well understood. The insertion of the longitudinal ciliary muscle fibers into the scleral spur and corneoscleral sheets is vital for maintenance and modulation of aqueous humor outflow. Shearing forces associated with the global distortion during blunt ocular trauma can disrupt the ciliary muscle insertion, leading to collapse of the TM against the scleral wall, increased trabecular outflow resistance, and severe glaucoma, known as *angle recession*. Because of the disinsertion of the ciliary muscle, conventional cyclotonic therapy with cholinergic-stimulating agents like pilocarpine become ineffective with angle recession.

The JXT tissue (or cribriform meshwork) comprises the most-outer portion of the trabeculum and lies between the most-outer corneoscleral lamella and Schlemm's canal. This tissue is a more loosely organized, reticulated connective tissue composed of variable amounts of collagen, proteoglycans, glycoproteins, and hyaluronic acid.[9] It is hypocellular compared to the corneoscleral meshwork. The outer aspect of the JXT tissue consists of the endothelial cells lining the inner wall of Schlemm's canal. These are joined by tight junctions, but appear to be highly distendable, forming giant vacuoles in response to a pressure gradient across the TM.[10-13] The exact route by which aqueous humor passes from the interstices of the corneoscleral meshwork to the lumen of Schlemm's canal is a topic of great research efforts. Arguments[11,12] have been advanced that pores develop between or through endothelial cells. Some[10,13] believe the formation and collapse of the giant vacuoles to be important to maintenance of aqueous humor outflow. In the JXT tissue, the outflowing aqueous humor directly encounters an extracellular tissue barrier through which it must percolate without access to open spaces. Thus, anatomically, this tissue, with the inner wall endothelial lining of Schlemm's canal, appears to account for the principal component of aqueous humor outflow resistance, and experimental studies in monkeys and eyebank eyes confirm its primary importance.[14] Moreover, accumulation in this JXT tissue of extracellular material, appearing as plaques in electron microscopic sections, is associated with open-angle glaucoma.[15] Thus, the precise site of resistance to outflow in the normal and glaucomatous eye is not completely understood, but the peripheral JXT connective tissue and Schlemm's canal inner wall appear to be the most likely location. Many of the pathophysiologic mechanisms cited, for example, cellular depopulation and plaque accumulation, also are associated with aging, but are accelerated and exaggerated in the glaucomatous eye.

Schlemm's canal is an endothelial-lined aqueous conducting channel lying circumferentially parallel to, and contiguous with, the outer aspect of the TM; its inner wall endothelium comprises the outer lining of the JXT tissue (see Figure 2-1). The canal is oval shaped cross-sectionally, its posterior aspect determined by the scleral sulcus, lying within the scleral spur internally and posteriorly, and with the scleral wall externally. Most of the inner aspect lies adjacent to the TM and anteriorly is bordered by the junction of the anterior meshwork and the cornea. Although the canal usually forms an intact circumferential channel, it is crossed by numerous septae from inner to outer wall and branches to multiple lumens in some locations. The outer wall is perforated by about 30 to 35 collector channels whose endothelium is contiguous with that of intrascleral veins. Although one can commonly observe retrograde flow of blood from these veins into the lumen of Schlemm's canal, in the adult

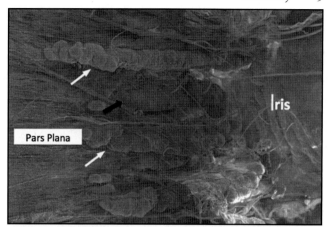

Figure 2-2. Scanning electron micrograph of the ciliary body showing the ciliary processes with alternate major process (white arrows) with the smaller minor processes (black arrow) between them. The posterior surface of the iris lies to the right side of the photograph, the pars plana of the ciliary body to the left.

eye, most aqueous humor appears to travel radially across the lumen of the canal with little circumferential flow in the canal lumen.[16]

CILIARY BODY ANATOMY

The ciliary body lies posterior to the iris and comprises the ciliary muscle and ciliary processes (see Figure 2-1). Both structures possess unique morphologic features that are essential to their specialized functions for accommodation, outflow facility regulation, and aqueous humor formation.

The ciliary muscle subtends a triangular, cross-sectional profile with its apex pointing posteriorly, ending at the ora serrata. The outermost longitudinal fibers insert as tendinous bands into the corneoscleral TM and scleral spur, whereas the middle-radial and inner-circular fibers are only loosely adherent to the adjacent sclera via sparse collagen fibers. Ciliary muscle contraction decreases the resistance to outflow of aqueous humor, apparently through mechanical tension on the TM.

Lying internal to the ciliary muscle, the ciliary processes form the pars plicata, that along with the more posterior pars plana, constitute the lateral wall of the posterior chamber (see Figure 2-1). Approximately 70 to 80 radially arrayed major ciliary processes project into the posterior chamber (Figure 2-2). Their anterior borders arise from the iris root, sweeping behind the iris to form the ciliary sulcus (see Figure 2-1). These major processes measure approximately 2-mm long, 0.5-mm wide, and 1-mm high and possess an irregular surface. Smaller, minor ciliary processes lie between the major processes and do not project as far into the posterior chamber.

In cross-section, the major ciliary processes manifest 3 components (Figure 2-3): an inner capillary core, a surrounding loose stroma, and a double-layered epithelium

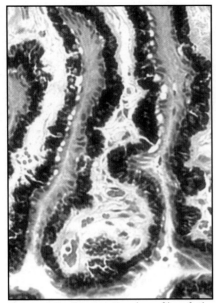

Figure 2-3. Cross-sectional profile of the · human ciliary process showing the capillary core, stromal connective tissue, and the bilayer ciliary epithelium.

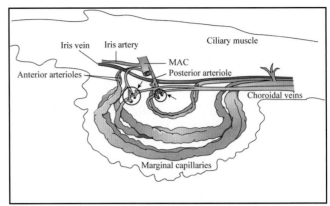

Figure 2-4. Schematic drawing of the vasculature of the major ciliary processes in profile showing the anterior and posterior arterioles arising from the discontinuous major arterial circle (MAC).

continuous with that of the pars plana. These components each possess unique morphologic features that underpin their contribution to aqueous humor formation, a 2-stage process that begins with passive ultrafiltration of plasma from the capillaries into the stroma followed by movement through the ciliary epithelium into the posterior chamber. Because the aqueous humor derives from the ciliary processes, reduction of intraocular pressure can be accomplished by disturbing the ciliary body pharmacologically or surgically. Many drugs block aqueous humor inflow by interfering with the normal secretory process in the epithelium or by reducing arteriolar perfusion of regional ciliary processes. Most of the pharmacologic agents, such as carbonic anhydrase inhibitors (CAIs), beta-adrenergic antagonists, or alpha-2 adrenergic agonists, appear to act in this manner directly on the ciliary epithelium. Some of the vasoactive adrenergic agents also can induce localized arteriolar constriction in the anterior ciliary processes.[17]

Aqueous humor inflow can also be inhibited by destruction of some or all of the ciliary processes with cryotherapy or laser photocoagulation. The treating clinician must be aware of the anatomic location of the processes at the anterior portion of the ciliary body, about 1.5- to 2-mm posterior to the corneoscleral limbus, to achieve the most effective result with the least tissue destruction when using a transscleral approach.

Ciliary Body Microvasculature

The ciliary body receives blood from 2 sources: the anterior ciliary arteries and the long posterior ciliary arteries.

Branches from all of these arteries anastomose freely with each other to produce a complex, redundant system characterized by numerous collateral channels that ensure consistent anterior segment perfusion even after partial interruption of its arterial supply, such as following strabismus and retinal detachment surgery.[18] Derived from the ophthalmic artery, 2 anterior ciliary arteries approach the limbus from the border of each rectus muscle with the exception of the lateral rectus, which contributes only one. Within the episclera, these arteries commonly branch and then interconnect, often forming a nearly complete anastomotic vascular ring that can occasionally be observed clinically.

At the limbus, several branches from each anterior ciliary artery turn inward, perforating the limbal sclera to enter the capillary bed of the ciliary muscle. These branches arborize within the ciliary muscle and interconnect with each other and with branches from the nasal and temporal long posterior ciliary arteries.[18] These interconnections form a second anastomotic vascular ring, the intramuscular circle, representing the major source of collateral blood flow to the ciliary body between the anterior and long posterior ciliary arterial systems.

Branches from the intramuscular arterial circle supply capillaries to the ciliary muscle, which are densely packed and oriented parallel to the muscle fibers. Venous blood from the ciliary muscle drains primarily to the choroidal veins.

Other branches from the intramuscular circle pass anteriorly to the root of the iris, where they bend and branch at right angles to form the major arterial circle that lies tangential to the limbus. The major arterial circle is often discontinuous and may constitute the only minor contributor to anterior segment collateral blood flow (Figure 2-4).

The ciliary processes receive their arterial supply from 2 types of arterioles—anterior and posterior—that emanate from the major arterial circle.[19] Anterior arterioles arise in tufts and often show focal constrictions as they span the ciliary sulcus. As they enter the processes, they rapidly dilate into irregular, large, vein-like capillaries that are initially directed anteriorly toward the ciliary process tip. These capillaries then turn and pass posteriorly within the internal margin of the process to empty into the choroidal veins. The posterior arterioles, generally less numerous and less constricted than the anterior, enter the basal regions of the ciliary processes, apparently to serve the basal and posterior regions of the ciliary processes. These capillaries also travel in a posterior direction, concentric to those from the anterior arterioles. Thus, capillaries derived from anterior arterioles serve the margins of the ciliary process, and those arising more posteriorly are situated within the base of the process. Interprocess connections also arise from the posterior arterioles and serve the minor ciliary processes on either side and the basal regions of neighboring major processes.

THE CILIARY EPITHELIUM

The ciliary epithelium actively secretes some components of aqueous humor and provides the barrier that prevents macromolecules from reaching the posterior chamber. The ciliary epithelium consists of 2 layers of cells, the outer pigmented and the inner nonpigmented, facing the posterior chamber. Despite its bilayered structure, the ciliary epithelium is not compound but consists of 2 simple epithelia joined apex to apex with the basal lamina of the pigmented layer resting on the stroma of the ciliary body and that of the nonpigmented layer lining the posterior chamber. This unusual arrangement results from invagination of the optic vesicle to form the optic cup during embryonic development.

The inner nonpigmented ciliary epithelium is continuous anteriorly with the pigment epithelium of the iris and posteriorly with the neurosensory retina at the ora serrata. The pigmented epithelium continues anteriorly as the anterior myoepithelium of the iris and posteriorly as the retinal pigment epithelium. The nonpigmented ciliary epithelial cells lack melanin and, compared with the cells of the pigmented epithelium, have more and larger mitochondria and rough endoplasmic reticulum, indicating a greater metabolic capacity. These features are amplified in the cells of the nonpigmented layer that lie in the anterior pars plicata whence derives the greater contribution overall to the production of aqueous humor.[20]

Both the pigmented and nonpigmented epithelial cells are interconnected by specialized intercellular junctions that control the passage of water, ions, and macromolecules into the aqueous humor.[21,22] Desmosomes and gap junctions lie within and between both layers of the ciliary epithelium, and the desmosomes appear to maintain adjacent cells, approximately 17-nm apart. The resulting intercellular cleft is spanned by branching filaments connecting the cytoplasmic surfaces of the adjoining cells. Near their apical surfaces, nonpigmented ciliary epithelial cells are joined by zonula occludens, or tight junctions, that constitute the blood-aqueous barrier of the ciliary body.[15,20] Zonula occludens appear as one or more areas of direct contact between intramembranous proteins of the adjacent plasma membranes, to block the intercellular spaces between adjacent plasma membranes, thus occluding the intercellular cleft.

The tight junctions located between the nonpigmented epithelial cells represent a selective barrier that allows diffusion of water and small molecules into the posterior chamber, while maintaining the osmotic and electrical gradients across the ciliary epithelium that are required for the final, active step in aqueous humor production. These junctions permit and modulate electrical and metabolic coupling of ciliary epithelial cells, permitting the 2 layers to operate as a functional unit for aqueous humor production.

THE OPTIC NERVE

The optic nerve transmits visual and other photopic stimuli between the neurosensory retina and the lateral geniculate body and the cerebral visual pathways. The nerve is primarily composed of neural fibers (the retinal ganglion cell axons), glial cells, extracellular matrix supportive tissue, and vascular elements.[23-27] The optic nerve head refers to the anterior surface of the optic nerve, which is seen en face during clinical funduscopic examination. When viewed stereoscopically in clinical examination, the nerve head assumes a bagel-like configuration, convex in the periphery, as the nerve fibers bend from the axis of the nerve to comprise the nerve fiber layer of the retina. This neural component manifests an orange-pink tint on funduscopy. Because the fibers so abruptly change direction, bending centrifugally, a central concavity, or optic nerve cup, is created, the base of which appears more yellow because of the collagenous fibers of the lamina cribrosa underlying the supporting tissue. The central cupped zone typically occupies about 30% of the diameter of the nerve head, but the proportions are highly dependent on the size of the eye and the diameter of the scleral canal. Glaucomatous eyes that lose nerve fiber tissue gradually develop progressively larger cup sizes until virtually no neural tissue persists in the final stages of the disease.

The neural component of the optic nerve is composed of approximately 1.2 to 1.5 million axons. The intraorbital optic nerve is divided into the anterior and the posterior components. The anterior optic nerve extends from the retinal surface to the retrolaminar region, just as the nerve exits the posterior aspect of the globe. The posterior optic nerve transits the orbit from the globe to the optic canal. The diameter of the optic nerve head and anterior portion of the optic nerve is approximately 1.5 mm.[28] The optic nerve expands to approximately 3 to 4 mm in diameter upon exiting the globe, with the glial tissue, the leptomeninges (optic nerve sheath), and the beginning of the axonal myelination.

Retinal ganglion cell axons, composed of retinal nerve fiber layers, converge radially to form the optic nerve as they abruptly turn posteriorly to exit the eye through the lamina cribrosa. The nerve fibers enter the optic nerve from the retina in a characteristic anatomic pattern. Fibers entering

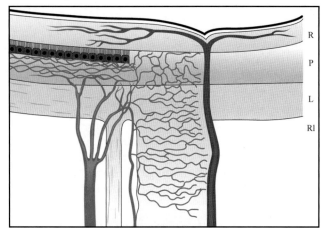

Figure 2-5. Schematic drawing of the anterior optic nerve head showing the arterial blood supply and the 4 anatomic layers: the retinal (R), prelaminar (P), laminar (L; lamina cribrosa), and the retrolaminar (Rl) zones.

the superior and inferior temporal aspects of the optic nerve arise from the peripheral temporal retina.[29,30] These arcuate nerve fibers originate either superior to or inferior to the medial raphe of the temporal neurofiber layer and assume an arcuate course around, above, or below the fovea. These are the fibers most susceptible to damage in early glaucomatous optic neuropathy. Careful, well-focused funduscopic examination of the posterior pole of the human eye will permit visualization of the striations of the retinal nerve fiber layer in the clinical situation, especially when the striations are enhanced by red-free illumination. Loss of neural fibers as in glaucoma can also be seen clinically by the loss of striations in the affected location. When sufficient fibers are lost from a specific location, the clinician expects to correlate the location of visual field defects with the anatomic findings in the fundus. Hence, loss of superior arcuate neural fibers leads to an inferior defect in the visual field, also subscribing an arcuate pattern corresponding to the zone of reduced retinal function. Because the arcuate neural fibers terminate along an anatomically defined raphe in the temporal retina, such arcuate visual field defects also respect the anatomy and produce a nasal stepped defect ending along the horizontal axis. Fibers originating from the macular region, or the papillomacular fibers, occupy approximately one-third of the temporal optic nerve head. Papillomacular fibers take a more direct course from the macular and perimacular region to the optic nerve. Other nerve fibers from the superior, inferior, and nasal retina radially converge at the nerve.

The anterior optic nerve conveniently divides into 4 anatomic regions (Figure 2-5).[26,31,32] The most anterior zone is the superficial region of the nerve fiber layer that is continuous with the nerve fiber layer of the retina. This region is primarily composed of the axons of the retinal ganglion cells in transition from the superficial retina to the neuronal component of the optic nerve. Immediately posterior to the nerve fiber layer is the prelaminar region, which lies contiguous with the peripapillary choroid. Next posteriorly, the laminar

region is adjacent to the sclera, where the axons pass out of the eye through the lamina cribrosa. This complex, collagenous, and relatively elastic structure consists of fenestrated, connective tissue lamellae that allow the transit of neural fibers through the scleral coat.[23,26,31,32] The lamina cribrosa is composed of a series of fenestrated sheets of connective tissue and provides the main support for the optic nerve as it exits the eye and penetrates the scleral coat. Between the optic nerve and the adjacent peripapillary tissue lies a rim of connective tissue, the border tissue of Elschnig.[33] The connective tissue beams of the lamina cribrosa extend from this surrounding connective tissue border and are arranged in a series of parallel stacked plates. The beams of connective tissue are composed primarily of collagen and other extracellular matrix components, including elastin, laminin, and fibronectin. These connective tissue layers are perforated by various-sized fenestrations through which the neural elements of the optic nerve pass. Central, larger fenestrae allow transit of the central retinal artery and central retinal vein. The neural fenestrations within the lamina are, histologically, larger superiorly and inferiorly as compared to the temporal and nasal aspects of the optic nerve. These differences have been suggested to play a role in the development of glaucomatous optic neuropathy. Alteration of the shape of the optic nerve head, enlargement of the physiologic cup both peripherally and posteriorly, most characterizes the neuropathy of glaucoma. Thus, not only is neural tissue lost, but also the connective tissue becomes distorted with posterior bowing of the lamina. Whether this shape change causes or derives from the glaucomatous damage is uncertain, but clearly, alterations in the connective tissue in this region seem a likely contributor to the pathophysiology of this unique neuropathy.[31] The fenestrations of the lamina cribrosa can be seen clinically in the base of the optic nerve head cup on ophthalmoscopic examination. The retrolaminar region lies posterior to the lamina cribrosa, is marked by the beginning of axonal myelination, and is surrounded by the leptomeninges of the central nervous system.

VASCULATURE OF THE OPTIC NERVE

The arterial supply of the anterior optic nerve derives entirely from branches of the ophthalmic artery. One to 5 posterior ciliary arteries divide in the posterior orbit from the ophthalmic artery, itself a branch of the internal carotid artery.[26,27,34,35] Typically, between 2 and 4 posterior ciliary arteries course anteriorly before dividing into approximately 10 to 20 short posterior ciliary arteries, just prior to entering the globe posteriorly. Often, the posterior ciliary arteries separate into a medial and a lateral group before branching into the short posterior ciliary arteries. In addition, the long posterior ciliary arteries, which are also branches of the posterior ciliary arteries, course anteriorly along the outside of the globe before penetrating the sclera to supply the iris, ciliary body, and anterior region of the choroid.

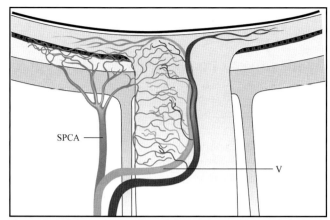

Figure 2-6. Schematic drawing of the microvasculature of the optic nerve head showing the arterial supply primarily derived from branches of the short posterior ciliary arteries (SPCA) and the venous drainage by way of the central retinal vein (V).

The short posterior ciliary arteries penetrate the sclera surrounding the optic nerve to supply the peripapillary choroid and the majority of the anterior optic nerve. Some short posterior ciliary arteries course, without branching, through the sclera directly into the choroid; others divide within the sclera to provide branches to both the choroid and the optic nerve. Often, a noncontinuous, arterial circle exists within the perineural sclera, known as the circle of Zinn-Haller.[36] This structure is formed by the confluence of branches of the short posterior ciliary arteries. This arterial circle may completely encircle the optic nerve and often is, or may be, interrupted along its course. Multiple branches from this arterial circle penetrate the various regions of the anterior optic nerve, to the peripapillary choroid, and to the pial arterial system. The central retinal artery, also a posterior orbital branch of the ophthalmic artery, penetrates the optic nerve approximately 10 to 15 mm behind the globe, but has few if any intraneural branches—the exception being an occasional small branch within the retrolaminar region.

MICROVASCULATURE OF SPECIFIC OPTIC NEURAL REGIONS

The superficial nerve fiber layer is supplied principally by recurrent retinal arterioles branching from the central retinal artery. As the central retinal artery emerges from within the optic nerve, it branches into a superior and an inferior trunk. From these major trunks, as well as from more distal branches, small arterioles emerge to supply the superficial nerve fiber layer of the optic nerve and peripapillary retina (Figure 2-6). The capillary branches from these vessels are continuous with the retinal capillaries at the disc margin, but they also have posterior anastomoses with the prelaminar capillaries of the optic nerve.

The prelaminar region is principally supplied by direct branches of the short posterior ciliary arteries and by branches of the circle of Zinn-Haller, when it is present.

PERIPAPILLARY ATROPHY
Joel S. Schuman, MD, FACS and Malik Y. Kahook, MD

A significant controversy exists with regard to peripapillary atrophy and its relationship to glaucomatous optic neuropathy. These atrophic areas, which often take the form of crescents, sometimes correlate with areas of nerve fiber layer atrophy and cupping, as well as with visual field loss.[1-4] Peripapillary atrophy may progress and may precede the development of cupping and visual field loss in a given region.[5]

Peripapillary atrophy may be related to impaired optic nerve or choroidal circulation, and this has spurred speculation with regard to the relationship between this phenomenon and damage to the optic nerve.[2,3,6] Should vascular factors play a significant role in glaucomatous optic neuropathy, as well as in the development of peripapillary atrophy, regions of peripapillary atrophy could be used as predictors of future optic nerve damage.

Recent evidence has shown that changes in neuroretinal rim area and peripapillary atrophy are not coupled temporally,[7] and different forms of glaucoma might be more or less likely to be associated with changes in peripapillary atrophy.[8,9]

REFERENCES
1. Wilensky JT, Kolker AE. Peripapillary changes in glaucoma. *Am J Ophthalmol.* 1976;81:341.
2. Anderson DR. Correlation of the peripapillary anatomy with the disc damage and field abnormalities in glaucoma. In: Greve EL, Heijl A, eds. *Fifth International Visual Field Symposium.* The Netherlands: Dr. W Junk Publishers; 1983.
3. Anderson DR. Relationship of peripapillary haloes and crescents to glaucomatous cupping. In: Krieglstein GK, ed. *Glaucoma Update III.* Berlin: Springer-Verlag; 1987.
4. Heijl A, Samander C. Peripapillary atrophy and glaucomatous visual field defects. In: Greve EL, Heijl A, eds. *Sixth International Visual Field Symposium.* The Netherlands: Dr. W Junk Publishers; 1985.
5. Airaksinen PJ, Juvala PA, Tuulonen A, et al. Change of peripapillary atrophy in glaucoma. In: Krieglstein GK, ed. *Glaucoma Update III.* Berlin: Springer-Verlag; 1987.
6. Airaksinen PJ, Tuulonen A, Werner EB. Clinical evaluation of the optic disc and retinal nerve fiber layer. In: Ritch R, Shields MB, Krupin T, eds. *The Glaucomas.* St Louis, MO: CV Mosby Co; 1989:467-494.
7. See JL, Nicolela MT, Chauhan BC. Rates of neuroretinal rim and peripapillary atrophy area change: a comparative study of glaucoma patients and normal controls. *Ophthalmology.* 2009;116(5):840-847.
8. Lee KY, Rensch F, Aung T, et al. Peripapillary atrophy after acute primary angle closure. *Br J Ophthalmol.* 2007;91(8):1059-1061.
9. Jonas JB. Clinical implications of peripapillary atrophy in glaucoma. *Curr Opin Ophthalmol.* 2005;16(2):84-88.

In eyes with a well-developed circle of Zinn-Haller, fine arterial branches supply both the prelaminar and laminar regions. Most of these vessels do not arise from the choroid but merely pass through it from this short posterior ciliary arterial origin. Branches from the circle of Zinn-Haller and from the short posterior ciliary arteries course through the choroid and ultimately supply the optic nerve in this region. Occasional small centripetal arteries or arterioles do branch from the larger vessels of the peripapillary choroid, but direct arterial supply to the prelaminar region arising from the choroidal vasculature is minimal. No direct connection exists between the peripapillary choriocapillaris and the prelaminar region.

The lamina cribrosa region also receives its blood supply from branches of the short posterior ciliary arteries or from branches of the circle of Zinn-Haller and is similar to the prelaminar region (see Figure 2-6). These precapillary branches perforate the outer aspects of the lamina cribrosa before branching into an intraseptal capillary network. As in the prelaminar region, the larger vessels of the peripapillary choroid may contribute occasional small arterioles to this region, although there is no connection between the peripapillary choriocapillaris and the capillaries of the optic nerve.

The retrolaminar region is also supplied by branches from the short posterior ciliary arteries, but also by pial arterial branches (see Figure 2-6). The pial arteries originate from both the central retinal artery, before it pierces the retrobulbar optic nerve, and branches of the short posterior ciliary arteries more anteriorly.

Thus, with the exceptions of the superficial nerve fiber layer branches of the central retinal artery, the occasional retrolaminar branches of the central retinal artery, and the small contribution of the choroidal vasculature to the prelaminar and laminar regions, the principal arterial supply to the anterior optic nerve is derived from the short posterior ciliary arteries.

The rich capillary beds of each of the 4 anatomic regions within the anterior optic nerve are anatomically confluent. These capillary interconnections anatomically unite the microvasculature along the length of the anterior optic nerve, but appear to be such fine, resistent capillaries that there is probably little physiologic confluence among them. Capillaries in the nerve fiber layer region are continuous with the retinal capillaries at the disc margin. More posteriorly, the capillaries of the nerve fiber layer region form a complicated plexus that interconnects with the capillaries of the prelaminar regions. The capillaries of the laminar region conform to the pattern of the connective tissue septae, which compose the laminar supportive architecture. Capillaries in the laminar region are organized in the polygonal pattern of the laminar septae.

The arterioles along the periphery of the optic nerve have a limited smooth muscle layer surrounding the endothelial layer. The capillary network of the anterior optic nerve is composed of nonfenestrated vessels, similar to the capillaries of the retina. These capillaries are composed of a single layer of tight-junctioned endothelial cells surrounded by supportive glial tissue and intermittent pericytes.

The venous drainage of the anterior optic nerve is almost exclusively via the central retinal vein (see Figure 2-6). In the nerve fiber layer, blood is drained directly into the retinal veins, which then join to form the central retinal vein. In the prelaminar, laminar, and retrolaminar regions, venous drainage also occurs via the central retinal vein or axial tributaries to the central retinal vein. Occasionally, small venules connecting the optic nerve and the peripapillary choroid can be identified, mainly within the prelaminar region.

VARIABILITY OF VASCULAR PATTERNS

There is marked inter-individual variation in the precise vascular patterns of the anterior optic nerve and peripapillary region. Among individuals, the predominant variability is observed in the arterial supply. The posterior ciliary arteries vary in number, distribution, and caliber. These arteries may be distributed only medially and laterally, or a third superior grouping may be present.[35-39] The grouping of these vessels into lateral and medial groups could play a role in the clinical presentations subsequent to an ischemic event. The distribution of the posterior ciliary arteries may explain the altitudinal visual field defects seen following anterior ischemic optic neuropathy, the nasal visual field loss seen in glaucoma, and the arcuate field loss seen in acute optic nerve infarction.[40,41] These hypotheses rely heavily on physiologic inference from anatomic findings and thus remain unproven, if attractive, speculations.

REFERENCES

1. Brubaker RF. The flow of aqueous humor in the human eye. *Trans Am Ophthalmol Soc.* 1982;80:391-474.
2. Bill A, Phillips S. Uveoscleral drainage of aqueous humor in human eyes. *Exp Eye Res.* 1971;12:275.
3. Pederson JE, Gaasterland DE, MacLellan HM. Uveoscleral aqueous outflow in the rhesus monkey: importance of uveal reabsorption. *Invest Ophthalmol Vis Sci.* 1977;16:1008-1017.
4. Van Buskirk EM. Clinical implications of iridocorneal angle development. *Ophthalmology.* 1981;88:361-367.
5. Rohen JW, van der Zypen E. The phagocytic activity of the trabecular meshwork endothelium: an electron microscopic study of the verve (Cercopithesus aethiops). *Albrecht Von Graefes Arch Klin Exp Ophthalmol.* 1968;175:143-160.
6. Alvarado J, Murphy C, Polansky J, Juster R. Trabecular meshwork cellularity in primary open-angle glaucoma and nonglaucomatous normals. *Ophthalmology.* 1984;91:564-579.
7. Stein JD, Challa P. Mechanisms of action and efficacy of argon laser trabeculoplasty and selective laser trabeculoplasty. *Curr Opin Ophthalmol.* 2007;18(2):140-145.
8. Acott TS, Samples JR, Bradley BS, Bacon DR, Bylsma SS, Van Buskirk EM. Trabecular repopulation by anterior trabecular meshwork cells after laser trabeculoplasty. *Am J Ophthalmol.* 1989;107:1-6.
9. Acott TS. Biochemistry of aqueous humor outflow. In: Podos SM Yanoff M, eds. *Textbook of Ophthalmology. Vol 7. Glaucoma.* Philadelphia, PA: Mosby, 1991.
10. Tripathi RC. The functional morphology of the outflow systems of the ocular and cerebrospinal fluids. *Exp Eye Res.* 1977;25(suppl):65-116.
11. Bill A, Svedbergh B. Scanning electron microscopic studies of the trabecular meshwork and the canal of Schlemm. An attempt to localize the main resistance to outflow of aqueous humor in man. *Acta Ophthalmol.* 1972;50:295-320.
12. Epstein DL, Rohen JW. Morphology of the trabecular meshwork and inner wall endothelium after cationized ferritin perfusion in the monkey eye. *Invest Ophthalmol Vis Sci.* 1991;32:160-171.
13. Fink AL, Feliz MD, Fletcher RC. Schlemm's canal and adjacent structures in glaucomatous patients. *Am J Ophthalmol.* 1972;74:893-906.

14. Maepea O, Bill A. The pressure in the episcleral veins, Schlemm's canal and the trabecular meshwork in monkeys: Effects of changes in intraocular pressure. *Exp Eye Res.* 1989;49:645-663.

15. Rohen JW, Witmer R. Electron microscope studies on the trabecular meshwork in glaucoma simplex. *Graefes Arch Clin Exp Ophthalmol.* 1972;83:251-266.

16. Van Buskirk EM. Trabeculotomy in the immature, enucleated human eye. *Invest Ophthalmol Vis Sci.* 1977;16:63-66.

17. Van Buskirk EM, Bacon DR, Fahrenbach WH. Replication of ciliary vasomotor effects with controlled intravascular corrosion casting. *Trans Am Ophthalmol Soc.* 1990;87:124-142.

18. Morrison JC, Van Buskirk EM. Anterior collateral circulation in the primate eye. *Ophthalmology.* 1983;90:707-715.

19. Morrison JC, Van Buskirk EM. Ciliary process microvasculature of the primate eye. *Am J Ophthalmol.* 1984;97:372-383.

20. Hara K, Lütjen-Drecoll E, Prestle H, Rohen JW. Structural differences between regions of the ciliary body in primates. *Invest Ophthalmol Vis Sci.* 1977;16:912-924.

21. Raviola G. The structural basis of the blood-ocular barriers. *Exp Eye Res.* 1977;25(suppl):27-63.

22. Raviola G, Raviola E. Intercellular junctions in the ciliary epithelium. *Invest Ophthalmol Vis Sci.* 1978;17:958-981.

23. Hernandez MR, Lua XX, Igoe F, Neufeld AH. Extracellular matrix of the human lamina cribrosa. *Am J Ophthalmol.* 1987;104:567-576.

24. Kronfeld PC. Normal variations of the optic disc as observed by conventional ophthalmoscopy and their anatomic correlations. *Trans Sect Ophthalmol Am Acad Phthalmol Otolaryngol.* 1976:81(2):214-216

25. Hayreh SS. Anatomy and physiology of the optic nerve head. *Trans Am Acad Ophthalmol Otolaryngol* 1974;78:240-254.

26. Anderson DR. Ultrastructure of human and monkey lamina cribrosa and optic nerve head. *Arch Ophthalmol.* 1969;82:800-814.

27. Liebermann MF, Maumenee AE, Green WR. Histologic studies of the vasculature of the anterior optic nerve. *Am J Ophthalmol.* 1976;82:405-423.

28. Jonas JB, Gusek GC, Guggenmoos-Holtzmann I, Naumann GOH. Size of the optic nerve scleral canal and comparison with intravital determination of optic disc dimensions. *Graefes Arch Clin Exp Ophthalmol.* 1988;226:213-215.

29. Radius RL, Anderson DR. The histology of retinal nerve fiber layer bundles and bundle defects. *Arch Ophthalmol.* 1979;97:948-950.

30. Radius RL, Anderson DR. The course of axons through the retina and optic nerve head. *Arch Ophthalmol.* 1979;97:1154-1158.

31. Quigley HA, Addicks EM. Regional differences in the structure of the lamina cribrosa and their relation to glaucomatous optic nerve damage. *Arch Ophthalmol.* 1981;99:137-143.

32. Radius RL, Gonzales M. Anatomy at the lamina cribrosa in human eyes. *Arch Ophthalmol.* 1981;99:2159-2162.

33. Elschnig A. *Der normal Sehnerveneintritt des menschlichen Auges, Denkschriften der Mathematisch-Naturwissenschaftliche Classe der Kaiserlichen Akademie der Wissenschaften in Wien.* 1901;70:219-303.

34. Hayreh SS. Blood supply of the optic nerve head and its role in optic atrophy, glaucoma and oedema of the optic disc. *Br J Ophthalmol.* 1969;53:721-748.

35. Cioffi GA, Van Buskirk EM. Vasculature anatomy of the optic nerve. In: Ritch R, Shields MR, Krupin T, eds. *The Glaucomas.* St. Louis, MO: CV Mosby;1994:8.

36. Zinn IGL. *Descriptio Anatomica Ocuoli Humani.* 1st ed. Gottingen: Abrami Vandenhoeck; 1755:216-217.

37. Hayreh SS. Inter-individual variation in blood supply of the optic nerve head. Its importance in various ischemic disorders of the nerve head, and glaucoma, low-tension glaucoma and allied disorders. *Doc Ophthalmol.* 1985;59:217-246.

38. Hayreh SS. Anterior ischemic optic neuropathy. *Arch Neurol.* 1981;38:675-678.

39. Geijssen HC. *Studies on Normal Pressure Glaucoma.* New York, NY: Kugler;1991:8-31.

40. Lichter PR, Henderson JW. Optic nerve infarction. *Am J Ophthalmol.* 1978;85:302-310.

41. Olver JM, Spalton DJ, McCartney ACE. Microvascular study of the retrolaminar optic nerve in man; the possible significance in anterior ischemic optic neuropathy. *Eye.* 1990;4:7-24.

Practical Aqueous Humor Dynamics

Joel S. Schuman, MD, FACS; Malik Y. Kahook, MD; and David L. Epstein, MD, MMM

CLINICAL RELEVANCE

Aqueous Humor Formation

Aqueous humor is produced by the ciliary body and flows into the posterior chamber at a rate of approximately 2 to 3 microliters per minute.[1] It is believed that at least a majority of this aqueous humor production derives from active secretion of the ciliary epithelium bilayer, which is in continuity posteriorly with the adjacent retinal and, anteriorly, the iris epithelia. The outer (sclerad) pigmented ciliary epithelial cell layer lies apex-to-apex to the inner (vitread) nonpigmented ciliary epithelial cell layer. The base of the latter cells faces the posterior chamber. (Exfoliation material may occur on the base of this cell layer.)

The stroma of the ciliary body (sclerad to the pigmented ciliary epithelium) contains numerous capillaries. Potentially, both this blood supply area as well as the secreting ciliary epithelial cells themselves may be sites of drug or laser obliterative actions. Although the nonpigmented ciliary epithelium has frequently been identified as containing the enzymatic machinery involved in active aqueous humor secretion,[2-4] the actual process may require the coupling of both the nonpigmented and pigmented cell layers.[5]

It is believed that bicarbonate is actively secreted into the posterior chamber by the ciliary epithelium, carrying water with it and thus representing part of the active secretion of aqueous humor.[6] This is under the control of the enzyme, carbonic anhydrase, in the ciliary epithelium (presumably nonpigmented). Thus, carbonic anhydrase inhibitors (CAIs) can reduce aqueous humor formation (up to 40% to 50%).

Beta-adrenergic agonist activity has been believed to be involved in active secretion of aqueous humor,[1] such that beta blockade will result in a decrease in this secretion. Many investigators have thought that the site of beta-blocker activity is at the level of the ciliary epithelium, but a vascular site has not been totally ruled out. The effects of beta blockade and carbonic anhydrase inhibition are not fully additive, suggesting that there are some linkage and interrelated effects.[7]

Apraclonidine, an alpha-2 agonist, reduces aqueous humor formation[8] and is also partially additive to both CAIs and beta-blockers, but it is not certain whether the site of action is ciliary epithelial or vascular. (The vasoconstriction that the drug produces might suggest the latter.) Brimonidine is a relatively selective alpha-2 adrenergic receptor agonist. Fluorophotometric studies suggest that brimonidine tartrate has a dual mechanism of action by reducing aqueous humor production and increasing uveoscleral outflow.

The part of aqueous humor formation that is not active transport has in previous times been called *ultrafiltration*. However, whether this is a passive pressure-driven process (presumably under vascular control) or some other ciliary epithelial cell process (eg, uncatalyzed hydration of CO_2) is unclear.

Aqueous humor moves from the ciliary epithelium into the posterior chamber, and then through the pupil into the anterior chamber (AC) (Figure 3-1). Because there is usually some pupillary resistance to forward fluid flow (which is termed *relative pupillary block*), the pressure is slightly higher in the posterior chamber than the AC, resulting in forward iris convexity. In the extreme, this can cause the peripheral iris to move over the front of the trabecular meshwork (TM) and thus cause angle-closure glaucoma (usually due to pupillary block) (see Chapter 22). Iris convexity or concavity is thus a useful indicator of relative pressures in the posterior and ACs. (See later discussions of iris concavity in pigmentary glaucoma [Chapter 21] and also various iris retraction syndromes where, for example, there is posterior movement of fluid out of the eye through a retinal hole.)

Kahook MY, Schuman JS, eds.
Chandler and Grant's Glaucoma, Fifth Edition (pp 17-23).
© 2013 SLACK Incorporated.

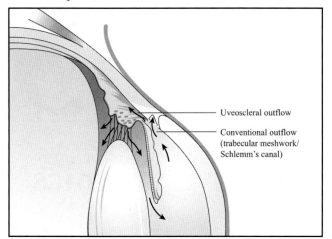

Figure 3-1. Aqueous humor is actively secreted by the ciliary epithelium into the posterior chamber, flows through the pupil into the anterior chamber, and drains through the conventional and unconventional pathways.

The amount of aqueous humor in the posterior chamber acts as a force (vector) to move the iris forward in a convex configuration. Agents that decrease aqueous humor formation can, by themselves, act to decrease this iris convexity (see Chapter 22). Thus, these agents are effective in treating the process of angle-closure glaucoma due to pupillary block (independent of the obvious intraocular pressure [IOP] effect itself), but, just as importantly, can lead to confusion in evaluating (usually asymptomatic) narrow-angled eyes by lessening this posterior chamber vector and thereby deepening the angle.

The aqueous humor in the posterior chamber is likely in equilibrium with fluid in the vitreous cavity (see Chapter 29). With retinal tears and detachments, the resulting hypotony most likely occurs because there is net fluid movement out of the eye through the retinal hole. The hyaloid is involved in this fluid exchange between vitreous and posterior chamber. In malignant glaucoma, fluid is retained in an expanded vitreous chamber, and it is commonly required to disrupt the hyaloid barrier (with a yttrium-aluminum-garnet [YAG] laser or surgically), in order to restore the normal anatomy, and allow fluid exchange between the posterior and anterior segments (see Chapter 29).

Diurnal Variation of Intraocular Pressure

We know that there is a diurnal variation in IOP that is believed to be mostly or entirely due to changes in the rate of aqueous humor formation.[1] Although the studies of Kronfeld[9,10] suggested that there might be a small fluctuation in tonographic outflow facility as well, we believe that such possible changes are small and may be explained, at least in part, by the noise in the tonographic technique. There is also a small seasonal variation in IOP,[11] but the

mechanism behind this has not been determined. IOP tends to be higher in winter and lower in summer.

What causes the varying rate of aqueous humor production during the day has not been fully determined. It is most common for the highest IOP to occur in the early morning, and, in fact, an IOP spike upon awakening is believed to occur commonly in primary open-angle glaucoma (POAG). On the other hand, the literature describes many patients with other diurnal patterns, and there is much individual variation. The systemic catecholamine burst upon awakening might be implicated in the morning IOP elevation because beta-adrenergic agonists are believed to slightly stimulate aqueous humor formation[1] (see Chapter 12; thus beta-blockers interfere with this and, therefore, act to diminish aqueous humor production), but this has not been unequivocally resolved. Although systemic cortisol levels have been proposed to relate to the diurnal variation of aqueous humor production, recent evidence does not support this.[12]

The lowest IOP was previously believed to occur during sleep, again due to decreased aqueous humor formation.[1,13] One might over-simplify this and conceptualize that the pumps in the ciliary body have similarly gone to sleep. However, recent data from sleep labs have contradicted this concept by showing a rise in IOP that happens during the nocturnal period prior to a slow dip in IOP in the early morning hours. See Chapter 71 for further details on 24-hour IOP curves.[14]

Some investigators have proposed that patients with glaucoma can show elevated spikes of IOP at odd hours, including while asleep. One of the problems with these data is that it is possible that the act of performing these measurements, by waking people up to take their IOP, may not accurately reflect their true IOP steady-state while asleep. There is a need for new, noninvasive measurements of IOP during the course of a day or during several days in order to provide this important information. As discussed in Chapter 1, our IOP measurements, although extremely accurate, are only one snapshot in time, and the field of glaucoma would benefit from a Holter monitor equivalent for IOP measurements.

Another problem with such diurnal IOP data is that the common technique used to obtain it is to do a diurnal curve; that is, to have the patient come to the office (or worse, inpatient setting) for these measurements. It really has not been established that these measurements reflect the patient's true diurnal curve during the patient's normal, active day's schedule.

Conventional Outflow Pathway (Trabecular Meshwork–Schlemm's Canal)

In adult humans, more than 90% of the aqueous humor fluid in the AC exits the eye via the trabecular–Schlemm's canal system (the conventional outflow pathway) with the remaining 10% existing through the uveoscleral outflow system (see Figure 3-1).[15,16] It is important to note that recent work suggests that the percentage of outflow through the uveoscleral route may be higher than 10%, but that this remains uncertain and appears to be age related.[17,18] Schlemm's canal communicates via a series of collector channels with the aqueous veins, part of the venous system, which are apparent on the outside of the eye (aqueous veins are much less frequently observed in eyes with glaucoma than in normal eyes).[19] There is a resistance and a pressure decrease across the inner wall of Schlemm's canal (either at or just proximal to the inner wall in the juxtacanalicular [JXT] tissue),[20-24] such that the pressure in the TM just proximal to the canal (toward the AC) is higher than that in the canal. Thus, at elevated IOP, the TM distends, and the inner wall moves toward the outer wall of Schlemm's canal.[25,26] The locus of abnormal resistance in POAG is believed to be at the same general location (JXT-inner wall Schlemm's canal)[20] as a normal eye, but, theoretically, abnormal resistance in the various glaucomas can be added at any place along the aqueous humor outflow pathway.

Relation of Episcleral Venous Pressure to Intraocular Pressure

In conditions with elevated episcleral venous pressure (eg, dural shunt or some cases of Sturge-Weber syndrome), this elevated venous pressure is transmitted back to Schlemm's canal and then into the AC (and therefore the whole eye; see Chapter 46). Although IOP is elevated, the resistance across the inner wall of Schlemm's canal may be unchanged, and tonographic outflow facility may thus be normal (in fact, normal outflow facility is observed in fresh cases of dural shunt quite commonly). Put another way, if the afterload is elevated, the pressure at all proximal points in the system are elevated without need for any change in coefficient of outflow across the normal resistance site. (Outflow facility [C value] is the inverse of resistance.)

Segmental Nature of Outflow: Implications for Angle-Closure Glaucoma

Although Schlemm's canal extends for 360 degrees inside the limbus, there is considerable resistance to circumferential flow in Schlemm's canal, at least in adult eyes. It has been calculated that aqueous humor exiting through 1 hour of the Schlemm's canal circumference effectively has access to only approximately 1 additional hour of circumference of Schlemm's canal on either side.[27] The TM-Schlemm's canal aqueous drainage system behaves as several separate segmental outflow pathways rather than a freely communicating single-circumferential entity. Thus, in progressive chronic angle-closure glaucoma (due to relative pupillary block), the amount of IOP elevation is roughly proportional (in a

---

---

progressive way) to the amount of angle closure. Aqueous humor moving through the open portions of the angle cannot move freely into the entire circumference of Schlemm's canal. Irreversible changes in the TM and Schlemm's canal can occur as a consequence of peripheral anterior synechiae (PAS) formation in this condition or possibly after chronic iris touch to the TM without synechia formation, most commonly after pupillary block is alleviated. In this case, areas of prior appositional closure now become open and once again segmentally drain a portion of aqueous humor, and IOP can thereby be normalized. In fact, with fresh PAS formation, using an argon laser to break the synechiae (gonioplasty) can restore normal outflow function.

Thus, by evaluating the amount of open functional angle (full width TM) in narrow-angled eyes with partial appositional or synechial closure, one can relate the number of presumably functionally closed hours of angle to the magnitude of the IOP elevation (Table 3-1).

For example, if 6 of 12 hours of the angle are functionally closed, one would expect the outflow (and thus outflow facility) to be halved (the resistance to be doubled). From the Goldmann equation, one can estimate the expected IOP elevation:

$$P = (F/C) + P_e$$

where P is intraocular pressure; F is flow; C is outflow facility; and P_e is episcleral venous pressure.

For example, assume F=2 μl/minute; C=0.2 μl/min/mm Hg; and P_e=8 mm Hg; then:

$$P = (2/0.2) + 8 = 18$$

$$P = 18 \text{ mm Hg}$$

	(mm Hg)		(µl/min)		(µl/min/mm Hg)		(mm Hg)
	P	=	(F	÷	C)	+	P_e
Normal	15		1.5		0.25		9
	13 to 17		1 to 2		0.25		9
	14		1.5		0.30		9
Glaucoma	39		1.5		0.05		9
	29 to 49		1 to 2		0.05		9
	24		1.5		0.10		9
Good normal	14		1.5		0.30		9
½ angle closed	19		1.5		0.15		9
¾ angle closed	29		1.5		0.075		9
Poor normal	19		1.5		0.15		9
½ angle closed	29		1.5		0.075		9
¾ angle closed	49		1.5		0.0375		9

TABLE 3-1. EXAMPLES OF DIFFERENCE IN THE DEGREE TO WHICH THE INTRAOCULAR PRESSURE (P) IS CALCULATED TO BE AFFECTED BY CHANGES IN FLOW (F) AND FACILITY OF OUTFLOW (C) IN DIFFERENT TYPES OF EYES, ASSUMING CONSTANT EPISCLERAL VENOUS PRESSURE (P_e)

If half of the angle becomes closed, outflow facility is halved, then:

$$P = (2/0.1) + 8 = 28 \text{ mm Hg}$$

That is, in this example, closure of 6 hours of the angle results in a 10-mm Hg IOP elevation.

Obviously, the initial inherent outflow facility of the 12 hours of open TM-Schlemm's canal may vary among different individuals and will influence this calculation, as will the rate of aqueous humor formation and the true value of P_e (which may possibly be lower than 8 mm Hg). Nevertheless, in patients without any open-angle glaucoma disease, one would, for example, most likely not expect IOP levels into the 30s with only 3 hours of the angle functionally closed. On the other hand, patients with exfoliation open-angle glaucoma not uncommonly can develop an additional angle-closure component to their glaucoma (as, in fact, Paul Chandler, MD, did). If the open portions of the angle have impaired outflow (reduced C value), then lesser amounts of superimposed functional angle closure can result in more substantial IOP elevation.

For example, let C = 0.08 µl/min/mm Hg for 12 hours of open-angle due to exfoliation. Then

$$P = (2/0.08) + 8 = 33 \text{ mm Hg}$$

If 3 of 12 hours subsequently become functionally closed, C = 0.06. Then

$$P = (2/0.06) + 8 = 41.3 \text{ mm Hg}$$

In contrast, if 12 hours of open angle had normal outflow facility (C = 0.20), then 3 hours of closure would result only in an IOP elevation from 18 to 21.3 mm Hg.

Another clinical implication from this type of analysis is that for greater amounts of angle closure beyond 6 hours, the amount of IOP elevation expected for each additional hour of closure dramatically increases. For example, for C = 0.20 µl/min/mm Hg and the above parameters:

$$P = (2/0.2) + 18 = 18 \text{ mm Hg}$$

For 6 hours of closure: P = 2/0.10 + 8 = 28 mm Hg. That is, there is an increase of 10 mm Hg for the 6 hours that are closed. But assume now that an additional 3 hours become closed:

$$P = (2/0.05) + 8 = 48 \text{ mm Hg}$$

That is, there is an additional increase in IOP of 20 mm Hg for the 3 additional hours of closure (now totaling 9 hours of closure), whereas the initial 6 hours of closure only resulted in a 10-mm Hg IOP elevation.

Thus, knowledge of Goldmann's equation and the segmental nature of aqueous outflow through the TM-Schlemm's canal pathway allows one to make reasonable predictions from gonioscopic observations (as well as allows reasonable information for the patient and physician about the chances for residual OAG after iridectomy [see Chapter 38]). This important subject is further discussed in Chapter 7.

Ciliary Muscle Tension

The longitudinal part of the ciliary muscle inserts not only on the scleral spur (see Figure 2-1) but also sends extensions of the tendons into the TM and JXT tissue.[28] Thus, the outflow pathway tissue is under mechanical tension normally. Under the influence of a cycloplegic drug, this tension is diminished, and, in fact, approximately one-third of POAG patients (not on pilocarpine therapy) will show an increase in IOP[29] (and a decrease in tonographic outflow facility) after cycloplegic drug administration. This cycloplegic IOP rise by an open-angle mechanism is rare in the normal population[30] (approximately 1%). It raises the question as to whether ciliary muscle tone might be involved in the mechanism of POAG. Is POAG really a disease of the ciliary muscle instead of the TM-Schlemm's canal?

The onset of increased prevalence of POAG is similar to that of presbyopia. Yet, in the majority of patients with POAG (not on pilocarpine therapy), there is no worsening of outflow facility after instillation of a cycloplegic, and although pilocarpine, a cholinergic agonist that causes ciliary muscle contraction, is a useful drug for glaucoma and improves outflow facility, the disease process of POAG nevertheless continues.

One might hypothesize instead that, with a primary abnormality in the TM-Schlemm's canal system in POAG, ciliary muscle tension becomes even more important as a factor to increase outflow (eg, by widening the spaces in the outflow pathway that are somehow partially compromised by the POAG process). Still, we should not dismiss the importance of ciliary muscle tension normally for the proper function of the outflow pathway,[31] and there may be more of a role for ciliary muscle dysfunction in POAG than we perhaps now realize. For example, contraction of cells in the outflow pathway may be important in outflow regulation,[32] and the tethering of cells by their mechanical suspension to extensions of ciliary muscle tendons thus may be a critical phenomenon. Perhaps, if plasma-derived proteins are constantly seeping into the TM from the root of the iris,[33,34] ciliary muscle tension, perhaps intermittent, might be important in stirring functions to prevent protein aggregation and deposition.

As mentioned, the cholinergic drug pilocarpine works to decrease the IOP by an outflow effect that is mediated by the ciliary muscle. No direct effects of cholinergic drugs on the TM-Schlemm's canal cells have been demonstrated. Disinserting the ciliary muscle from the scleral spur in experimental animals prevents pilocarpine's effects on outflow.[35] Morphologically, pilocarpine leads to widening of the spaces in the JXT tissue and TM,[36] and this is believed to occur by the increase in mechanical tension that is transmitted through the extensions of the ciliary muscle tendons into the TM.[28]

TESTING OF NEW GLAUCOMA DRUGS
David L. Epstein, MD, MMM

An important implication of this usual diurnal variation in IOP relates to the testing of potentially new antiglaucoma agents for efficacy. The best studies are those where a baseline diurnal curve is obtained without active drug first. Then, on another day, over the same time interval, the experimental medication is applied to one eye only, and IOP effects are determined in relation to the baseline visit, comparing similar hours of the 2 days.

A common, potentially fallacious technique instead is to put the drop in one (or sometimes both) eye and measure the IOP several hours later, and then compare the measurements to the baseline time zero measurement on the single testing day, thus ignoring the endogenous diurnal rhythm of IOP in the patient. The fellow eye in a unilateral administration trial does have some utility as a control (the diurnal change in aqueous humor formation under systemic influence is likely very similar for the 2 eyes). However, the outflow status in patients with POAG may not be symmetrical in both eyes, and thus the magnitude of the observed IOP change may be different, although in the same direction, in the two eyes during the course of a single day. Regardless, many medications have contralateral effects through undefined mechanisms that can obscure these drug effects. Thus, a single drop, then look and see protocol is really justified only in the very first such human applications, especially when evaluating safety.

Unfortunately, so far it has not proven possible to separate pharmacologically the contraction of only selected portions of the ciliary muscle. Therefore, pilocarpine and other direct cholinergic antiglaucomatous agents, such as carbachol, necessarily can cause an increase in accommodation as well as pupillary sphincter contraction and thus miosis (see Chapter 13). It would be advantageous if a cholinergic drug could be developed that could cause selective contraction of the longitudinal portion of the ciliary muscle and, thus, have an isolated outflow effect by this mechanism. The main limitations in the use of pilocarpine clinically are the presence of these additional cholinergic side effects (as well as a need for relatively frequent instillation as with most eye drop formulations).

There is much merit conceptually in treating POAG with an outflow drug,[37] even perhaps a mechanical one such as pilocarpine, but there is no evidence that pilocarpine alters the natural history of progressive impairment in outflow facility with time that characterizes the disease of POAG. The latter is presumably due to the slowly progressive changes that occur as a primary event within the outflow pathway.

OUTFLOW DRUGS

These are discussed in more detail in Chapter 16, but are included here because of their relationship to aqueous humor dynamics.

Uveoscleral Outflow (Nonconventional Outflow)

There is reportedly a steady, low-level seepage of aqueous humor out from the AC through the face of the ciliary body, through the ciliary muscle, and ultimately leaving the eye either through the sclera or uveal blood vessels (see Chapter 2). This has been termed either *uveoscleral outflow* or *uveovascular-scleral outflow*, the latter to indicate the ultimate fluid movement, which is believed by some to be into the uveal vasculature.[38] Although this unconventional outflow pathway may represent up to 40% of outflow in certain species such as nonhuman primates,[39] in adult humans, it is believed to represent no more than 10% of total outflow.[15,16,38] Studies[40,41] of mouse aqueous production and outflow as well as the effects of prostaglandin analogs on aqueous flow are allowing for an increased understanding of uveoscleral drainage that continues to evolve. Contraction of the ciliary muscle by cholinergic agents is believed to decrease outflow by this pathway,[39,42] whereas cycloplegics can act, by relaxing the ciliary muscle, to increase such outflow.[43,44] Although there are isolated anecdotal case reports where this pathway through such pharmacological manipulation may have had important effects on IOP (where trabecular-Schlemm's canal outflow was impaired), it is still difficult to be certain that the normal seepage of aqueous humor through this pathway has clinically important effects on IOP.

In contrast, when the barriers to this nonconventional outflow pathway are diminished either in ocular disease, such as uveitis, or under the influence of certain drugs, such as prostaglandins,[45-47] IOP can be lowered substantially, sometimes to near hypotonous levels. It previously has been taught that IOP is low in uveitis because of inflammation in the ciliary body that diminishes active aqueous humor secretion. Although this is still believed to be true, an additional mechanism likely is enhanced uveovascular-scleral outflow. Chapter 16 on prostaglandin analogs will add to the understanding of these issues.

Classically, it has been described that this pathway is pressure independent (and, more recently, minimally pressure dependent[38]). That is, at elevated IOP, such seepage in terms of volume of fluid movement minimally increases. Conceptually, it is as if it were a constant seepage. Thus, tonography, in which the IOP is experimentally elevated and the decay curve measured, does not appreciably measure such pressure-independent (or minimally pressure-dependent) outflow.

In cyclodialysis, a communication is created either surgically or as a result of trauma from the AC posterior to the scleral spur into the suprachoroidal space. Classically, it was believed that this detachment of the ciliary body resulted in impaired aqueous humor production. However, an additional mechanism for the decreased IOP might be enhanced uveovascular-scleral outflow as a result of this new pathway into the suprachoroidal space.

Trabecular Outflow Drugs

Because the locus of abnormal resistance to aqueous humor outflow in POAG resides in the TM, drug therapy specifically targeted at this tissue makes a great deal of sense. It is rational medicine to try to intervene within the diseased tissue and attempt to reverse the abnormality in aqueous humor outflow.[37] This is an area of exciting active investigation, with the potential for many novel trabecular drugs that could be developed to treat glaucoma.[48,49]

REFERENCES

1. Brubaker RF. Flow of aqueous humor in humans: the Friedenwald lecture. *Invest Ophthalmol Vis Sci.* 1991;32:3145-3166.
2. Lüttjen-Drecoll E, Lonnerholm G, Eichhorn M. Carbonic anhydrase distribution in the human and monkey eye by light and electron microscopy. *Graefes Arch Clin Exp Ophthalmol.* 1983;220:285-291.
3. Lüttjen-Drecoll E, Eichhorn M. Morphologische Grundlagen des Kammerwassersekretionssystems und seine Veranderungen durch antiglau-komatose Pharmaka. *Fortschr Ophthalmol.* 1988;85:25-32.
4. Polansky JR, Lui GM, Alvarado JA, et al. Receptor characterization of cultured human nonpigmented and pigmented ciliary epithelial cells using cyclic nucleotide responses. In: Lutjen-Drecoll E, ed. *Basic Aspects of Glaucoma Research III.* New York, NY: Schattauer; 1993:243-256.
5. Chen J, Lui G, Wood I, et al. Localization of the "blood-aqueous barrier" in cultured human ciliary epithelial cells. *Invest Ophthalmol Vis Sci.* 1994;35(suppl):1849.
6. Maren TH. The rates of movement of Na, Cl, and HCO₃ from plasma to posterior chamber: effect of acetazolamide and relation to the treatment of glaucoma. *Invest Ophthalmol.* 1976;15:356-364.
7. Berson FG, Epstein DL. Separate and combined effects of timolol maleate and acetazolamide in open angle glaucoma. *Am J Ophthalmol.* 1981;92:788-791.
8. Gharagozloo NZ, Relf SJ, Brubaker RF. Aqueous flow is reduced by the alpha-adrenergic agonist, apraclonidine hydrochloride (ALO 2145). *Ophthalmology.* 1988;95:1217-1220.
9. Kronfeld PC. Tonography. *Arch Ophthalmol.* 1952;48:393-404.
10. Kronfeld PC. Some basic statistics of clinical tonography. *Invest Ophthalmol.* 1968;7:319-327.
11. Epstein DL, Krug JH Jr, Hertzmark E, et al. A long-term clinical trial of timolol therapy versus no treatment in the management of glaucoma suspects. *Ophthalmology.* 1989;96:1460-1767.
12. Sheridan PT, Brubaker RF, Larsson L-I, et al. The effect of oral dexamethasone on the circadian rhythm of aqueous humor flow in humans. *Invest Ophthalmol Vis Sci.* 1994;35:1150-1156.
13. Larsson L-I, Rettig ES, Brubaker RF. Aqueous flow in open angle glaucoma. *Arch Ophthalmol.* 1995;113:283-286.
14. Liu JH, Sit AJ, Weinreb RN. Variation of 24-hour IOP in healthy individuals: right eye versus left eye. *Ophthalmology.* 2005;112(10):1670-1675.
15. Bill A, Phillips CI. Uveoscleral drainage of aqueous humour in human eyes. *Exp Eye Res.* 1971;12:275-281.
16. Bill A. The drainage of aqueous humor via Schlemm's canal and uveoscleral routes. *Ophthal Res.* 1980;12:130.
17. Fautsch MP, Johnson DH, Second ARVO/Pfizer Research Institute Working Group. Aqueous humor outflow. What do we know? Where will it lead us? *Invest Ophthalmol Vis Sci.* 2006;47(10):4181-4187.

18. Nilsson SF. The uveoscleral outflow routes. *Eye.* 1997;11:149-154.

19. Ascher KW. *The Aqueous Veins.* Springfield, IL: Thomas; 1961:269.

20. Grant WM. Experimental aqueous perfusion in enucleated human eyes. *Arch Ophthalmol.* 1963;69:783-801.

21. Ellingsen BA, Grant WM. Trabeculotomy and sinusotomy in enucleated human eyes. *Invest Ophthalmol.* 1972;11:21-28.

22. Ellingsen BA, Grant WM. Influences in intraocular pressure and trabeculotomy on aqueous outflow in enucleated monkey eyes. *Invest Ophthalmol.* 1971;10:705-709.

23. Peterson WS, Jocson VL, Sears ML. Resistance to aqueous outflow in the rhesus monkey eye. *Am J Ophthalmol.* 1971;72:445-451.

24. Maepa O, Bill A. Pressures in the juxtacanalicular tissue and Schlemm's canal in monkeys. *Exp Eye Res.* 1992;54:879-883.

25. Johnstone MA, Grant WM. Pressure dependent changes in structures of the outflow system of human and monkey eyes. *Am J Ophthalmol.* 1973;75:365-383.

26. Grierson I, Lee WR. Pressure-induced changes in the ultrastructure of the endothelium lining Schlemm's canal. *Am J Ophthalmol.* 1975;80:863-884.

27. Van Buskirk EM, Grant WM. Lens depression and aqueous outflow in enucleated primate eyes. *Am J Ophthalmol.* 1973;76:632-640.

28. Rohen JW. Why is intraocular pressure elevated in chronic simple glaucoma? Anatomical considerations. *Ophthalmology.* 1983;90:758-765.

29. Harris LS, Galin MA. Cycloplegic provocative testing. *Arch Ophthalmol.* 1969;81:544-547.

30. Harris LS, Galin MA, Mittag TW. Cycloplegic provocative testing and topical administration of steroids. *Arch Ophthalmol.* 1971;86:12-14.

31. Kaufman PL, Gabelt BT. Aging, accommodation and outflow facility. In: Lutjen-Drecoll E, ed. *Basic Aspects of Glaucoma Research III.* New York, NY: Schattauer; 1993:257-274.

32. Epstein DL, de Kater AW, Erickson-Lamy K, et al. The search for a sulfhydryl drug for glaucoma: From chemistry to the cytoskeleton. In: Lutjen-Drecoll E, ed. *Basic Aspects of Glaucoma Research III.* New York, NY: Schattauer; 1993:345-354.

33. Barsotti M, Bartels SP, Freddo TF, et al. The source of proteins in the aqueous humor of the normal monkey eye. *Invest Ophthalmol Vis Sci.* 1992;33:581-595.

34. Johnson M, Gong H, Freddo TF, et al. Serum proteins and aqueous outflow resistance in bovine eyes. *Invest Ophthalmol Vis Sci.* 1993;34:3549-3557.

35. Kaufman PL, Bárány EH. Loss of acute pilocarpine effect on outflow facility following surgical disinsertion and retrodisplacement of the ciliary muscle from the scleral spur in the cynomolgus monkey. *Invest Ophthalmol.* 1977;15:793-807.

36. Grierson I, Lee WR, Abraham S. The effects of pilocarpine on the morphology of the human outflow apparatus. *Br J Ophthalmol.* 1978;62:302-313.

37. Epstein DL. Will there be a remedy to reverse the changes in the trabecular meshwork and the optic nerve? A personal point-of-view on glaucoma therapy. *J Glaucoma.* 1993;2:138-140.

38. Pederson JE, Gaasterland DE, MacLellan HM. Uveoscleral aqueous outflow in the rhesus monkey: Importance of uveal reabsorption. *Invest Ophthalmol Vis Sci.* 1977;16:1008-1017.

39. Bill A. Aqueous humor dynamics in monkeys. *Exp Eye Res.* 1971;11:195-206.

40. Aihara M, Lindsey JD, Weinreb RN. Aqueous humor dynamics in mice. *Invest Ophthalmol Vis Sci.* 2003;44(12):5168-5173.

41. Weinreb RN, Toris CB, Gabelt BT, Lindsey JD, Kaufman PL. Effects of prostaglandins on the aqueous humor outflow pathways. *Surv Ophthalmol.* 2002;47(suppl 1):S53-S64.

42. Bill A. Effect of atropine and pilocarpine on aqueous humor dynamics in cynomolgus monkeys (Macaca irus). *Exp Eye Res.* 1967;6:120-125.

43. Bill A, Wålinder P-E. The effects of pilocarpine on the dynamics of aqueous humor in a primate (Macaca irus). *Invest Ophthalmol.* 1966;5:170-175.

44. Bill A. Effects of atropine on aqueous humor dynamics in the vervet monkey (Cercopithecus ethiops). *Exp Eye Res.* 1969;8:284-291.

45. Toris CB, Camras CB, Yablonski ME. Effects of PhXA41, a new prostaglandin F_{2a} analog, on aqueous humor dynamics in human eyes. *Ophthalmology.* 1993;100:1297-1304.

46. Racz P, Ruzsonyi MR, Nagy ZT, et al. Maintained intraocular pressure reduction with once-a-day application of a new prostaglandin F_{2a} analogue (PhXA4l). An in hospital, placebo-controlled study. *Arch Ophthalmol.* 1993;111:657-661.

47. Ziai N, Dolan JW, Kacere RD, et al. The effects on aqueous dynamics of PhXA41, a new prostaglandin F_{2a} analogue, after topical application in normal and ocular hypertensive human eyes. *Arch Ophthalmol.* 1993;111:1351-1358.

48. Kumar J, Epstein DL. Rho GTPase-mediated cytoskeletal organization in Schlemm's canal cells play a critical role in the regulation of aqueous humor outflow facility. *J Cell Biochem.* 2011;112(2):600-606.

49. Okka M, Tian B, Kaufman PL. Effects of latrunculin B on outflow facility, intraocular pressure, corneal thickness, and miotic and accommodative responses to pilocarpine in monkeys. *Trans Am Ophthalmol Soc.* 2004;102:251-257; discussion 257-259.

4

The Patient's History
Symptoms of Glaucoma

Joel S. Schuman, MD, FACS and David L. Epstein, MD, MMM

SYMPTOMS

Blurred Vision With Haloes

When IOP is suddenly elevated from any cause, fluid moves into the cornea, exceeding the capacity of the corneal endothelial pumps to remove it. Resulting corneal epithelial edema can produce symptoms of blurred vision and the perception of colored haloes around lights. (The presence of colored haloes is important, for noncolored haloes around lights are a common symptom simply of myopia, astigmatism, and other refractive problems with no intraocular pressure [IOP] implication.) Colored haloes are also common symptoms of patients with nuclear sclerotic lens changes, especially early, without any elevation of IOP. Although such symptoms are more common in various forms of angle-closure glaucoma (especially subacute forms) in which there is rapid elevation of IOP when the iris moves into apposition with the surface of the trabecular meshwork (TM), colored haloes can also be seen in open-angle forms of glaucoma with similarly rapid elevation of IOP, such as with glaucomato-cyclitic crisis, postcataract surgery, pigmentary glaucoma, and juvenile open-angle glaucoma. However, in primary open-angle glaucoma (POAG), except for cases with very high IOP, there are usually no such symptoms. This is what makes the disease so treacherous. Most patients with POAG are unaware of any symptoms until there is substantial visual field loss, at which time visual function is compromised.

Colored haloes with blurred vision upon arising in the morning is a common symptom in patients with Chandler's syndrome, an iridocorneal endothelial (ICE) syndrome variant. It can also be seen in patients with nonglaucomatous primary corneal disease where edema accumulates in the corneal epithelium overnight because of the lack of helpful evaporation when the eyelids are closed.

Pain

Rapid elevation of IOP can also be accompanied by pain. Although some of this pain may be due to corneal edema or irregularity of the epithelial surface, it characteristically behaves as if it were more global in origin, as perhaps from stretching of the ocular coats. Topical anesthetics typically do not totally alleviate this symptom. With long-standing elevation of IOP, the corneal endothelium may be able to prevent corneal epithelial edema presumably due to the compensatory pumping action of the endothelium. Nevertheless, patients with sustained elevation of IOP to levels of 50 mm Hg or greater often complain of pain even in the absence of corneal edema. Ocular pain may be accompanied by nausea and vomiting.

Blurred Vision (Without Haloes)

In some forms of secondary angle-closure glaucoma, such as malignant glaucoma or uveal effusion syndromes in which there is a forward shift of the crystalline lens, symptoms of myopia can occur. A fascinating entity in this category is myopia due to sensitivity to systemic sulfonamides and other medications, where either forward-shift of the crystalline lens and/or lens swelling (or at least increased anterior-posterior lens thickness) can result in temporary myopia.

Rarely, if the retina and choroid are elevated due to suprachoroidal fluid, such as may occur following filtration surgery or in certain uveal effusion syndromes (usually when there is minimal change in position of the crystalline lens), a hyperopic shift can be observed.

Kahook MY, Schuman JS, eds.
Chandler and Grant's Glaucoma, Fifth Edition (pp 25-31).
© 2013 SLACK Incorporated.

Subjective Visual Field Defects

Because the chronic POAGs usually produce peripheral visual field loss (without regular symmetry between the 2 eyes), most patients are unaware of their visual field defects and do not demonstrate symptoms until the disease is far advanced. However, in certain forms of glaucoma, such as low-tension glaucoma or open-angle glaucoma associated with myopia, early field defects of considerable density can occur close to fixation and may be symptomatic to the patient. Because loss of visual acuity in glaucoma is especially debilitating, patients with field loss close to fixation need to be monitored closely with central field programs that measure actual sensitivity levels around fixation. When patients have little or no margin to follow in remaining central points of their visual field, one is justified to move to filtration surgery without documented further field progression (unless medical or laser therapy results in target IOPs close to or at what one might expect with filtration surgery).

Sometimes, patients with open-angle glaucoma (eg, POAG, low-tension, and exfoliation) give a very reliable history of a sudden onset of a subjective paracentral scotoma. It makes the clinician contemplate whether some acute mini-event has occurred in the chronic progressive natural history of the open-angle glaucoma. One wonders about some final small vascular event at the level of the optic nerve.[1]

Subjective Loss of Vision (Acuity)

With high sustained IOP in angle-closure glaucoma but also in certain forms of open-angle glaucoma, optic atrophy can develop with accompanying loss of visual acuity and pallor of the optic nerve without the contour changes in the disc rim that characterize the cupping that is more commonly seen in chronic glaucoma.

However, when a patient complains about a subjective loss of acuity and has advanced glaucomatous field loss or dense field loss above and below close to fixation, as commonly is seen in low-tension glaucoma or OAG associated simply with myopia, this is a dangerous warning sign that, at a minimum, indicates the need to advance therapy in order to further reduce IOP. As mentioned earlier, this is often an indication for urgent filtration surgery. In patients with such visual field changes, it is often useful to have the patient test his or her subjective acuity at home between visits by viewing objects on the wall or by using an Amsler grid.

Loss of Color Vision

Subjective loss of color vision is not uncommon in patients with long-standing POAG, and objective measures of color vision often demonstrate abnormalities in such patients. Clinically, though, it is difficult to relate progression of the disease with measured progressive changes in color vision.

Patient's Own Sense of (Painless) Pressure in the Eye

Many patients insist that they can sense what the pressure is in their eye. These are notoriously inaccurate except in some patients with acute, intermittent secondary glaucomas with wide fluctuations of IOP. Yet, we have been impressed over the decades by how many questions and comments from glaucoma patients that were initially quickly dismissed only later proved to have some merit. We should listen to our glaucoma patients for potential new insights, and although we still may not really believe that patients can sense their IOP (except for perhaps the above acute secondary elevations), it is possible that there is some subgroup or some heretofore unappreciated mechanism for this symptom in certain patients.

What needs also to be emphasized is the obligation of the clinician to take the time to talk to all patients with glaucoma, fully explaining their condition and listening to their concerns, and especially to be sensitive to how their disease and our treatments affect their quality of life. The glaucomas are one of only a few chronic eye conditions that are usually slowly progressive with time, requiring repetitive visits with usually only our nonspecific therapies to offer. Most glaucoma patients bond with their glaucoma practitioner, and such communication is an obligation of our profession. Sometimes, all that can be done for patients is to talk to them and honestly explain their condition. It is humbling how many second opinions are requested by glaucoma patients, in truth only to find a clinician who will take the time to talk to them.

Blackouts

With high levels of IOP in the 50 mm Hg range or greater, whether due to acute or chronic causes, patients may experience blackouts, presumably because the elevated IOP is interfering with vascular perfusion of the optic nerve or retina, or because of obstruction of axoplasmic flow. In patients with more moderate elevation of IOP, blackouts should suggest the possibility of underlying carotid disease, where presumably ocular hypoperfusion is being exacerbated by the elevated IOP. Glaucoma patients with this symptom should have a neuro-ophthalmological evaluation.

SYSTEMIC DISEASES

Epidemiological studies are becoming increasingly important in ophthalmology, and as glaucoma represents a very common progressive chronic disease of the eye, there is a special need for such studies in glaucoma patients. There are tantalizing leads that deserve more extensive evaluation.

How might one explain the relationship between systemic hypertension and trabecular and optic nerve pathology in POAG?[2,3] Perhaps they share aging connective tissue on the one hand, but abnormal vascular structures on the other hand. (Schlemm's canal can be considered a vessel of sorts, perhaps related to venules or lymph channels, with adjacent contractile cells and adventitia).

There is preliminary evidence that thyroid disease may be associated with POAG[4] and anecdotal experience[5] (that we share) that correction of thyroid status may result in lowering of IOP.

Diabetes has sometimes been associated with POAG,[6-8] but the mechanism has not been established.

There are no other recognized common systemic diseases that have been unequivocally associated with POAG, but have we performed the appropriate inquiries?

There are many secondary glaucomas that are associated with systemic disease, and they will be detailed in subsequent chapters, for example, increased episcleral venous pressure due to dural shunts or Sturge-Weber syndrome, cortisone-secreting pituitary tumors, various forms of secondary angle closure from tumors, and neovascular glaucomas from diabetes or carotid ischemic disease. One might suspect that formation of pseudoexfoliation material should be part of some systemic disease. In fact, there is evidence of systemic deposition of similar material,[9,10] and the genetics of pseudoexfoliation are being worked out.[11-16]

ACTIVITIES

There is no evidence that patients with POAG or truly any other form of glaucoma should alter their daily-life activity. Some patients with pigmentary glaucoma (see Chapter 21) episodically liberate pigment into the anterior chamber, sometimes after vigorous exercise of certain types usually involving head movement. In the absence of more specific management, treatment is given like that for POAG to prevent acute damage to the optic nerve from the transient IOP elevation. It is unclear whether it might even be desirable to shed this pigment earlier and acutely rather than later and more chronically.

Exercise both acutely[17] and chronically[18] may actually lower IOP in POAG patients. One should be aware that vigorous exercise by patients just prior to their ophthalmologic visit should be discouraged to avoid spuriously low IOP readings.

Some have claimed that a supine position at night results in spikes of IOP elevation and optic nerve damage. It is true that in both normal and glaucoma patients, the IOP is slightly higher (1 to 2 mm Hg) in the supine position.[19] This likely relates to changes in venous pressure influencing the eye pressure. There are likely compensatory vascular responses. Although this area, like most in glaucoma, deserves further evaluation, it seems quite premature to instruct patients to significantly alter their lifestyle or sleeping postures, without a firm understanding of the implications of this normal postural change in IOP. It is clear, however, that IOP does rise at night and that this is indeed associated with the supine position.[20] One study[21] demonstrated elevated IOP to substantially high levels in patients sleeping prone with firm eye pressure against a pillow. This should also be evaluated further; any change in recommended sleep habits for glaucoma patients seems premature.

A question in all these studies is how long the elevation in IOP is sustained. For example, if one pushes on one's own eye, one can substantially elevate IOP initially, but then changes in ocular vascular volume and enhanced outflow from the eye as in tonography may or may not provide compensation. One might imagine that sustained levels of high IOP might induce pain or some discomfort to either awaken the patient or change head position (which is likely changing spontaneously regardless).

Reading and close work, if anything, by increasing mechanical traction on the scleral spur and TM from contraction of the ciliary muscle, similar to pilocarpine, would be expected to lower IOP in patients with open-angle glaucoma.

Theoretically, close work might be thought to potentially increase relative pupillary block in a patient with a predisposed narrow angle, but if ever a factor, it would be in those patients who had not yet been diagnosed. Those with known angle-closure glaucoma who have had an iridectomy would not be at risk. (Spontaneous angle-closure attacks precipitated by close work must be very rare, perhaps for the same reason that very weak concentrations of pilocarpine similarly do not precipitate such attacks, and more commonly can actually be used to treat an attack—see Chapter 22 for a discussion of vectors involved in acute angle-closure glaucoma due to pupillary block.)

EMOTIONS

Many patients with POAG will inquire whether their emotions affect their IOP, and rarely a patient is encountered whose IOP seems better controlled when tranquilizers are prescribed. (Some patients get apprehensive having their IOP measured, especially at the slit lamp, and may hold their breath or contract their eye muscles to give spurious readings—see subsequent chapters for techniques to avoid such artifacts, eg, use the Perkins handheld applanation tonometer or pneumatonometry.) Yet, there still is a rare patient in whom tranquilizers seem to cause modest, though real, IOP lowering. Except for this rare and seemingly real occurrence, in general, the answer to this question is that there is no such known relationship between IOP in POAG and emotion. One hopes that time will not prove this to be a premature incorrect answer based on insufficient data, similar to past patient queries about such conditions as systemic hypertension.

In contrast, in patients with unsuspected narrow angles, emotion (presumably from sympathetic discharge resulting in pupillary dilatation) can precipitate an attack of angle-closure glaucoma. Numerous cases have been observed where emotion was believed to have been involved. Of course, patients with known angle closure who have had iridectomies will not be at risk (except perhaps for some rare cases of plateau iris [see Chapter 26]). A common situation where emotion-induced glaucoma may occur is in the fellow eye of an eye with acute angle-closure glaucoma (which often from the acute pain, etc, has much emotional effect on the patient), as well as strong emotional events such as death of a close relative or severe physical injury or illness.

FOOD AND DRINK

In the patient's diet, we know of no food that influences glaucoma one way or another, although some transient osmotic influences might be detectable. Large volumes of water consumed rapidly do cause a transient rise in pressure in many glaucomatous eyes, and this is the basis of the so-called water-drinking test. However, the fluid intake in ordinary living, if it has any deleterious effect on glaucoma at all, must be so insignificant in the overall picture that it has not seemed to us necessary to advise a patient with glaucoma to change his or her usual intake of fluid in any way. In the case of tea and coffee, we think the same advice generally applies.

Rarely, very high levels of caffeine intake in patients with POAG have been associated with some IOP elevation, but attempts to study this systematically in POAG patients have commonly yielded negative results.[22] Therefore, it seems that this must be a very rare phenomenon. Regardless, patients with POAG under poor control with vastly excessive caffeine intake (usually from coffee) should prudently be counseled to try to decrease intake for general medical health reasons, if not also for some possible beneficial effect on IOP.

Argemone oil has been an occasional toxic contaminant of edible cooking oils. It has been of interest for many years, principally in India, because it has been suspected of causing epidemic dropsy glaucoma. This glaucoma is described as a reversible, noninflammatory, open-angle glaucoma occurring in epidemics of toxic dropsy. The IOP is raised, and, in the most severe cases, there is glaucomatous damage to the optic nerve. The elevation of IOP is spontaneously reversible, but the damage to the optic nerve is not. Alkaloids that are found in argemone oil, particularly sanguinarine and dihydrosanguinarine, have been suspected to be the active toxic components of argemone oil. A more detailed review of observations on argemone oil was made in 1993 by Grant and Schuman.[23]

Alcoholic beverages need not be avoided by glaucomatous patients. In fact, the IOP is nearly always temporarily lowered by strong alcoholic drinks, and it may be lowered even by wine and beer.[24,25] Patients, however, should be asked not to imbibe on the day of an office visit simply because it may result in a falsely low IOP level that is not sustained. Lowering of pressure by alcohol is slight in normal eyes, but, in glaucomatous eyes, it is occasionally sufficient to cause a transitory decrease from pressure levels of 30 or 40 mm Hg to normal. When the equivalent of 50 mL of ethyl alcohol is consumed rapidly, the IOP may be lowered for several hours,

returning to its previous level in 4 or 5 hours. The condition of the IOP in a so-called hangover has not been investigated. In exceptional instances, before the prolonged lowering of IOP, there has been a brief rise of a few millimeters of IOP a few minutes after drinking whiskey.

The duration of lowering of pressure is longer than we would expect from the theoretical osmotic action of ethyl alcohol, which is known to pass from blood to aqueous humor only a little less rapidly than water. In general, it has been found that alcohol taken in a dilute form, such as beer, can induce essentially the same changes in IOP as an equal amount of alcohol in concentrated form, such as whiskey.

It is most intriguing that the duration of diuresis induced by alcohol is similar to the duration of effect on IOP. Because alcohol is believed to induce diuresis principally through suppression of release of antidiuretic hormone from the hypophysis, it would be interesting to learn whether the change in concentration of the hormone in the circulation is involved in the lowering of IOP.

SYSTEMIC MEDICATIONS

Atropine and many drugs having anticholinergic, atropine-like properties are reputed to be dangerous for patients who have glaucoma. For this reason, a considerable proportion of drugs that have been introduced in recent years, including many psychopharmacologic agents, antihistaminics, antispasmodics, and medications for Parkinsonism, have been labeled with warnings against their use in the presence of glaucoma. Actually, only in eyes that are anatomically predisposed to angle-closure glaucoma do atropine-like drugs present a significant hazard, and these eyes constitute a small proportion of all glaucomatous eyes in the Western hemisphere. In eyes that have the anatomic peculiarity of a very shallow anterior chamber with precarious narrowing in the periphery, the angle can be caused to close, and an attack of acute angle-closure glaucoma can be provoked by dilation of the pupil with atropine-like medicines given systemically. Eyes of this special type are subject to angle-closure glaucoma from many other influences, including sympathomimetic agents and mydriasis in response to darkness.

Ironically, patients who have precariously narrowed angles, in whom an acute attack of angle-closure glaucoma may be precipitated by an atropine-like drug, are rarely aware of any threat of imminent glaucoma in their eyes, whereas patients in whom chronic open-angle glaucoma has been diagnosed and who are under proper treatment stand in little or no danger from systemic use of drugs having atropine-like effects. In other words, the atropine-like drugs pose a threat to people who are unaware of the possibility of glaucoma, whereas these drugs present little or no problem to people in whom glaucoma is already diagnosed and under proper treatment. On the warning labels of drugs having atropine-like effects, it is appropriate to advise that one should be alert to the possibility of precipitating acute glaucoma in patients who have abnormally shallow anterior chambers.

Simple inspection with a flashlight is useful and effective to detect abnormal shallowness of the anterior chamber. With a little practice, every physician can easily learn to identify eyes in which the iris is situated hazardously close to the cornea and to distinguish these from eyes in which there is a relatively safe, wide space separating iris and cornea. Eyes that appear to have abnormally shallow anterior chambers by this simple method of inspection should be examined further with slit-lamp and gonioscope. If the angle then proves to be precariously narrow, one should be prepared to diagnose and treat angle-closure glaucoma, in case it develops. In detecting eyes that are prone to trouble from dilation, simple inspection with a flashlight is more effective than routine tonometry, because in most susceptible eyes the IOP is normal until the angle closes and glaucoma actually develops.

In eyes that have open-angle glaucoma, the dimensions of the anterior chamber are usually near normal, and closure of the angle is not induced by dilation of the pupil; however, paralysis of accommodation in open-angle glaucoma can in some cases cause IOP to rise. If the patient is already under treatment for chronic open-angle glaucoma, the effect of locally applied miotic drugs is expected to outweigh the effect of the relatively small concentration of parasympatholytic, atropine-like compounds that may reach the eye via the systemic circulation.

In patients under treatment for open-angle glaucoma, we have found that the simplest answer to the question of whether it is safe to administer an anticholinergic drug systemically is to go ahead and try it and base the conclusion on a comparison of IOPs measured before and after the drug is administered. As a rule, standard antiglaucoma treatment is adequate to prevent appreciable rise of IOP.

In patients who have open angles of safe width and moderately elevated IOP, but who, because of entirely normal optic discs, are not being treated for glaucoma, the question of whether it is safe to administer an anticholinergic drug systemically can be answered differently. One can test for IOP's tendency to rise by applying 2 drops of cyclopentolate to one eye and measuring the IOP every half hour for 2 hours. If the topical anticholinergic cyclopentolate cycloplegia does not cause IOP to rise, we believe there will also be no rise from a systemic anticholinergic drug. If the topical cyclopentolate does cause a rise, then one needs to test the systemic drug in the same manner as in patients under treatment for open-angle glaucoma. If much of a rise is produced by the systemically administered drug, one should weigh whether to accept this as a justifiable additional risk to the optic disc or whether to start some antiglaucoma treatment to counteract the influence of the drug on the IOP.

Vasodilator drugs administered systemically are safe in both open-angle glaucoma and in eyes with narrow angles, according to our experience and what has been published by others. Inhalation of 10% CO_2 causes a brief, small rise

---

STEROID-INDUCED ELEVATION OF INTRAOCULAR PRESSURE
David L. Epstein, MD, MMM

Although classically believed to require about 6 weeks of topical corticosteroid therapy to produce an IOP elevation in patients predisposed to POAG, this dogma actually reflects one particular dosage regimen of one particular strength of drug. The steroid-induced increase in aqueous outflow resistance is a dose-response phenomenon perhaps in all individuals, with an increased sensitivity in patients predisposed to POAG. Thus, very frequent (eg, hourly) dosages of a strong, topical corticosteroid can cause some IOP elevation within a day or 2 (and, commonly, some contralateral effect). On the other hand, reported weaker topical corticosteroids that supposedly do not usually elevate IOP may still, in fact, do so with longer periods of continued therapy and observation. Systemic corticosteroids, presumably because they yield lower intraocular drug levels than topical preparations, may similarly require a longer time to produce elevation of IOP. By derivation, but also based on some clinical evidence, normal patients without a predisposition to POAG may possibly still show IOP elevation with long enough duration of therapy of high enough dosage.

Thus, the ophthalmologist and the general medical doctor need to understand these dose-response relationships in arranging follow-up for such patients. The bottom line: with long-term use of either systemic or topical corticosteroids, potential IOP effects need to be monitored, even if shorter-term observations fail to detect IOP elevation.

Systemically administered corticosteroids can cause elevation of IOP in patients with POAG, although less so than topical corticosteroids. There is a considerable latency for this action, usually more than several weeks. Therefore, in any urgent situation, corticosteroids can be given to patients with POAG and ophthalmological evaluation routinely scheduled at a later time. Although probably prudent to evaluate such patients initially and after a few weeks of continued systemic corticosteroid therapy, likely the greater risk is after several months (or years) of such treatment, and it is important for the ophthalmologist to arrange such longer term surveillance, even if there is no short-term elevation of IOP.

---

of IOP that disappears in minutes even if the inhalation is continued. We see no reason to withhold systemic vasodilators from glaucoma patients when vasodilators are indicated for systemic disease.

SPECIAL POINTS IN THE PATIENT HISTORY

A complete medical and ocular history including current and past medications should be routine, but the following are points of potential special interest.

Use of Corticosteroids

Sustained periods of corticosteroid use, whether by ocular, systemic, nasal spray,[26,27] or dermatologic use about the eyes, may have caused past periods of elevated IOP and disc cupping, which now may present as an apparent low tension glaucoma-like condition.

Past History of Trauma

Angle recession from trauma may be subtle, but typically leads to glaucoma years to decades later. These past episodes are often forgotten by the patient. (Any truly unilateral case of open-angle glaucoma needs to be explained as something other than POAG.)

Systemic Diseases

There is a known association of POAG with systemic hypertension,[2,3] diabetes,[6-8] and thyroid disease[4,5] (and likely other diseases that have so far been unappreciated but may only be detected by compulsive documentation). Systemic diseases may require use of medications, such as corticosteroids or beta-blockers, with direct relationships to IOP.

It is also very important to probe the patient about cardiovascular disease and especially any respiratory disease that might influence one's choice of antiglaucoma therapy. The presence of respiratory allergies or childhood asthma even though no longer present, should be warning flags against the potential use of topical beta-blockers. It is shocking how it is not rare for topical beta-blockers to precipitate respiratory symptoms only after chronic use, and only then do patients sometimes recall asthmatic symptoms in childhood or adolescence. Topical beta-adrenergic agonists can also have cardiac side effects. Systemic carbonic anhydrase inhibitors are relatively contraindicated in patients with respiratory or renal disease.

Systemic Medications

Corticosteroids have been mentioned. Patients on systemic beta-blockers can show some reduction of IOP (which is quite individually variable), and this can lead to a confusing picture of a seeming low-tension glaucoma equivalent. Calcium channel-blockers are important to document, as some observers have felt they might be protective of the optic nerve in low-tension glaucoma, and it is possible that some preparations may have some IOP-lowering effects.

Family History

There is a genetic component to many of the glaucomas, and in the future, genetic analyses will likely identify different subtypes with different prognoses. However, in general, the presence of family members who are blind from glaucoma or who take medications, have had surgery, or laser for glaucoma, should be a true warning signal to the clinician. Even if the patient in question has elevated IOP with no end organ damage, the presence of a family history of such real glaucoma should serve to make the clinician more aggressive about this patient's disease with regard to closeness of follow-up and the likely need for treatment.

Symptoms of Secondary Disease

Many such symptoms were discussed. However, one always probes for symptoms of past uveitis perhaps associated with systemic disease, but also perhaps just ocular, such as in glaucomatocyclitic crisis. Past episodes of red eyes, photophobia, and corneal epithelial edema are searched for in the history.

Exercise-induced symptoms are routinely queried with particular relevance to pigmentary glaucoma. Neurological queries (headaches, weakness, and ischemic symptoms) should also be routine (glaucoma in the end is an optic neuropathy!). Neurological symptoms in the presence of low-tension glaucoma are an indication for neurological referral. Migraine and Raynaud's phenomenon have been associated with low-tension glaucoma.[28] Dural shunts can cause increased episcleral venous pressure and secondary open-angle glaucoma.

Retinal tears and detachments, often subtle, can cause puzzling forms of glaucoma[29] (Schwartz's syndrome). Histories of seeing flashes or floaters should be solicited. In addition, miotics, usually the stronger ones but also pilocarpine,[30] can cause posterior vitreous detachment and retinal tears.

Sudden Loss of Vision

There are uncommon patients with apparent progressive low-tension glaucoma that both symptomatically and with follow-up seem to behave as if some type of acute, nonprogressive optic nerve event had occurred. This is very uncommon, and because low-tension glaucoma is characteristically slowly progressive, the burden is on the ophthalmologist to be sure such a diagnosis is, in fact, accurate. As mentioned previously, some patients with low-tension glaucoma or myopia notice the sudden onset of a paracentral scotoma close to fixation, but more global loss of vision is unusual and may offer a clue to a possible diagnosis of a past acute event.

Loss of Consciousness and Massive Blood Loss

It has been reported that a history of loss of consciousness and massive blood loss can be associated with a nonprogressive form of low-tension glaucoma.[31] Although there seem to be some rare cases where this is true, the overwhelming majority of cases of low-tension glaucoma even with such a history are, in fact, progressive, and all nonprogressive forms of low-tension glaucoma place an extreme burden on the ophthalmologist for accurate diagnosis.

Recent Myocardial Infarction or Hypotension

Cases have been well-documented where, with seemingly well-controlled open-angle glaucoma, a recent myocardial infarction has led to unexpected disc and field progression. Patients with recent myocardial infarcts deserve special evaluation with this possibility in mind, as do patients with substantial hypotensive episodes from other causes. Unfortunately, such patients can continue to show further progression of their disease without any other (obvious) acute episodes.

References

1. Tuulonen A. Asymptomatic miniocclusions of the optic disc veins in glaucoma. *Arch Ophthalmol.* 1989;107:1475-1480.

2. Wilson MR, Hertzmark E, Walker AM, Childs-Shaw K, Epstein DL. A case control study of risk factors in open angle glaucoma. *Arch Ophthalmol.* 1987;105:1066-1071.

3. Dielemans I, Vingerling JR, Algra D, Hofman A, Grobbee DE, de Jong PTVM. Primary open-angle glaucoma, intraocular pressure, and systemic blood pressure in the general elderly population. *Ophthalmology.* 1995;102:54-60.

4. Smith KD, Arthurs BP, Saheb N. An association between hypothyroidism and primary open angle glaucoma. *Ophthalmology.* 1993;100:1580-1584.

5. Smith KD, Tevaarwerk GJM, Allen LH. Reversal of poorly controlled glaucoma upon diagnosis and treatment of hypothyroidism. *Can J Ophthalmol.* 1992;27:345-347.

6. Becker B. Diabetes mellitus and primary open-angle glaucoma. The XXVII Edward Jackson Memorial Lecture. *Am J Ophthalmol.* 1971;71:1-16.

7. Klein BEK, Klein R, Jensen SC. Open-angle glaucoma and older-onset diabetes. *Ophthalmology.* 1994;101:1173-1177.

8. Tielsch JM, Katz J, Quigley HA, Javitt J, Sommer A. Diabetes, intraocular pressure, and primary open-angle glaucoma in the Baltimore Eye Survey. *Ophthalmology.* 1995;102:48-53.

9. Schlötzer-Schrehardt UM, Koca MR, Naumann GOH, Volkholz H. Pseudoexfoliation syndrome. Ocular manifestation of a systemic disorder? *Arch Ophthalmol.* 1992;110:1752-1756.

10. Streeten BW, Li Z-Y, Wallace RN, Eagle RC, Keshgegian AA. Pseudoexfoliative fibrillopathy in visceral organs of a patient with pseudoexfoliation syndrome. *Arch Ophthalmol.* 1992;110:1757-1762.

11. Thorleifsson G, Magnusson KP, Sulem P, et al. Common sequence variants in the LOXL1 gene confer susceptibility to exfoliation glaucoma. *Science.* 2007;317:1397-1400.

12. Lemmelä S, Forsman E, Onkamo P, et al. Association of LOXL1 gene to Finnish exfoliation syndrome patients. *J Hum Genet.* 2009;54(5):289-297.

13. Yang X, Zabriskie NA, Hau VS, et al. Genetic association of LOXL1 gene variants and exfoliation glaucoma in a Utah cohort. *Cell Cycle.* 2008;7(4):521-524.

14. Challa P, Schmidt S, Liu Y, et al. Analysis of LOXL1 polymorphisms in a United States population with pseudoexfoliation glaucoma. *Mol Vis.* 2008;14:146-149.

15. Fan BJ, Pasquale L, Grosskreutz CL, et al. DNA sequence variants in the LOXL1 gene are associated with pseudoexfoliation glaucoma in a U.S. clinicbased population with broad ethnic diversity. *BMC Med Genet.* 2008;9:5.

16. Hewitt AW, Sharma S, Burdon KP, et al. Ancestral LOXL1 variants are associated with pseudoexfoliation in Caucasian Australians but with markedly lower penetrance than in Nordic people. *Hum Mol Genet.* 2008;17(5):710-716.

17. Harris A, Malinovsky V, Martin B. Correlates of acute exercise-induced ocular hypotension. *Invest Ophthalmol Vis Sci.* 1994;35:3852-3857.

18. Passo MS, Goldberg L, Eliott DL, Van Buskirk EM. Exercise training reduces intraocular pressure among subjects suspected of having glaucoma. *Arch Ophthalmol.* 1991;109:1096-1098.

19. Anderson DR, Grant WM. The influence of position on intraocular pressure. *Invest Ophthalmol.* 1973;12(3):204-212.

20. Liu JH, Zhang X, Kripke DF, Weinreb RN. Twenty-four-hour intraocular pressure pattern associated with early glaucomatous changes. *Invest Ophthalmol Vis Sci.* 2003;44(5):1586-1590.

21. Kornefeld MS, Dueker DK. Occult intraocular pressure elevations and optic cup asymmetry: sleep posture may be a risk factor. *Invest Ophthalmol Vis Sci.* 1994;34(4):994.

22. Higginbotham EJ, Kilimanjaro HA, Wilensky JT, Batenhorst AL, Hermann D. The effect of caffeine on intraocular pressure in glaucoma patients. *Ophthalmology.* 1989;96:624-626.

23. Grant WM, Schuman JS. *Toxicology of the Eye.* 4th ed. Springfield, IL: Thomas; 1993.

24. Peczon JD, Grant WM. Glaucoma, alcohol, and intraocular pressure. *Arch Ophthalmol.* 1965;73:495-501.

25. Houle RE, Grant WM. Alcohol, vasopressin, and intraocular pressure. *Invest Ophthalmol.* 1967;6(2):145-154.

26. Dreyer EB. Inhaled steroid use and glaucoma [letter]. *N Engl J Med.* 1993;329:1822.

27. Opatowsky I, Feldman RM, Gross R, Feldman ST. Intraocular pressure elevation associated with inhalation and nasal corticosteroids. *Ophthalmology.* 1995;102:177-179.

28. Corbett JJ, Phelphs CD, Eslinger P, Montaguet PR. The neurologic evaluation of patients with low tension glaucoma. *Invest Ophthalmol Vis Sci.* 1985;8:1101-1104.

29. Netland PA, Mukai S, Covington HI. Elevated intraocular pressure secondary to rhegmatogenous retinal detachment. *Surv Ophthalmol.* 1994;39:234-240.

30. Schuman JS, Hersh P, Kylstra J. Vitreous hemorrhage associated with pilocarpine. *Am J Ophthalmol.* 1989;108(3):333-334.

31. Drance SM, Morgan RW, Sweeney VP. Shock-induced optic neuropathy: a cause of nonprogressive glaucoma. *N Engl J Med.* 1973;288(8):392-395.

Examination of the Eye

Ian P. Conner, MD, PhD; Joel S. Schuman, MD, FACS;
Malik Y. Kahook, MD; and David L. Epstein, MD, MMM

It is very important to perform a complete ophthalmo-logical examination including dilated slit-lamp examination and peripheral retinal examination, in addition to the specific glaucoma evaluation in all patients with glaucoma. For the most common form of glaucoma, primary open-angle glaucoma (POAG), there are no other apparent ocular signs; therefore, a diagnosis of POAG is really a diagnosis of exclusion. Ophthalmologists should view themselves as diagnostic sleuths, looking for unusual causes and looking for new insights into mechanisms of the disease, including POAG. It is really astounding how little we understand about the various glaucomas. Even more importantly, glaucoma, because it likely involves interconnection of more than one pathogenic mechanism, offers the opportunity to the observant and inquisitive clinician to make important new discoveries about known and new forms of glaucoma. This can only happen as a result of a complete and meticulously documented full ophthalmological examination.

In design of a patient chart, one of us (DLE) recommends that the initial full comprehensive examination be set apart in an easily accessible location for constant reference. One frequently wants to know what the patient's examination showed at baseline.

One should develop a routine for approaching the patient. Obviously, as long as a truly complete ophthalmological examination is performed, the sequence can vary, but one approach is as follows.

REFRACTION

Patients should be refracted first for their best distant and near acuity. As detailed, measurement and assessment of visual acuity (which can be adversely affected by the glaucoma disease process itself) are very important in the glaucoma patient evaluation. The proper refraction should be determined, and

this information should be used for visual field testing, which is best performed before any ocular diagnostic manipulation.

PENLIGHT EXAMINATION

There is a tendency to hone in right away on the slit-lamp examination and optic nerve evaluation, especially in the follow-up of glaucoma patients in continuing care. However, glaucoma patients can develop basal cell carcinomas or neurologic motility abnormalities, as much as any other patient. It is useful, therefore, to first approach the patient with a penlight: examine the lids and conjunctiva grossly. Topical allergies to glaucoma medications and diseases of the conjunctiva are often more apparent on penlight examination than on slit-lamp examination, especially if high magnification for the latter is routinely chosen. Note the position of the upper lids. This can be very important in planning where to perform a laser iridotomy or a filtration procedure in the future, so that the lid will naturally cover the manipulated site (even slight exposure of such sites can produce monocular diplopia and unrelenting patient unhappiness).

Ptosis can develop after filtration or cataract surgery due to uncertain mechanisms (lid or superior rectus surgical trauma or possible filtration surgery fluid movement) and needs to be discriminated from neurological causes.

Next, the pupils should be examined both as to size and reactivity with the penlight. The swinging flashlight test should be performed, looking for an afferent pupillary defect (Marcus-Gunn pupillary phenomenon). The latter is obviously important to potentially diagnose other neuro-ophthalmologic diseases that may be masquerading as glaucoma and also as a baseline for future examinations when, for example, new neurologic symptoms might develop from other causes and complicate the clinical situation and diagnosis. This is also an example of what was mentioned

Kahook MY, Schuman JS, eds.
Chandler and Grant's Glaucoma, Fifth Edition (pp 33-40).
© 2013 SLACK Incorporated.

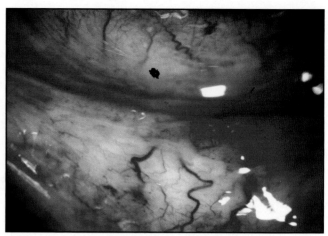

Figure 5-1. Conjunctival follicles from apraclonidine allergy.

SLIT-LAMP EXAMINATION

One should always use at least 2 levels of magnification on slit-lamp examination. Some observations are actually easier to make with lower magnification (eg, conjunctival disease and iris transillumination defects). Start with low power, and examine the lids and conjunctiva. Note whether the punctum is in proper position. Many patients with glaucoma complain of epiphora, which may be a sign of drug allergy, but more commonly results from nonrelated abnormalities of lid position, meibomianitis, punctal stenosis, or dry eyes. Patients with underlying external ocular disease may complain of excessive stinging and irritation (and thus intolerance) of antiglaucoma agents. Initial treatment of a coincident chronic external ocular disease might allow subsequent acceptance of topical antiglaucomatous therapy (or at least a more accurate assessment of the side effects of the latter).

Note palpebral conjunctival injection or follicle formation (Figure 5-1). The latter are common side effects from adrenergic agonists, such as epinephrine and apraclonidine (and more recently brimonidine), and the redness from these agents is often not correctly interpreted by the patient because they are commonly a delayed response (because the initial conjunctival response to the adrenergic agonist may be vasoconstriction, patients often feel these drugs help their red eye, and many patients do not inform their ophthalmologist about their red eye, attributing it to general allergies). Thus, the ophthalmologist may not be the first to correctly identify that there is a problem.

Patients may develop follicles from other causes (eg, benign lymphoid hyperplasia or lymphoma), and such entities are often best appreciated under lower magnification.

Always pull down the lower lid and look for possible early symblepharon formation, which might indicate early pemphigoid-type disease (Figure 5-2). Although uncommon, miotics, especially acetylcholinesterase inhibitors but also direct cholinergic drugs such as pilocarpine, can cause

above about clinician sleuths making new and important observations, even in POAG. It was once believed that a positive swinging flashlight test (Marcus-Gunn pupillary phenomenon) was indicative of nonglaucomatous optic nerve disease, but it is now understood that this can occur as a result of glaucoma alone. Patients with extensive asymmetric glaucomatous damage or, even more importantly, glaucoma patients with field loss close to fixation can demonstrate an afferent pupillary defect (as can patients with unilateral macular disease, demonstrating that the pupillary light reflex is relatively macula driven).

Heterochromia (eg, in Fuchs' heterochromic iridocyclitis) can often be best appreciated on penlight examination (or even better with bright room-light or sunlight).

Binocular eye position (cover test) and extraocular movements should also be routinely evaluated. Although one can correctly argue that these probably relate the least to glaucoma, nevertheless, most patients with glaucoma will bond to one clinician for life, and glaucoma patients may develop other ocular and systemic diseases in the course of their routine glaucoma follow-up. Examples of these include exophorias and tropias in patients who develop unilateral cataracts (not uncommon in patients with previous filtration surgery, especially with long-term follow-up), ocular muscle restrictions following tube shunt-type implants, diabetic nerve palsies, and ocular myasthenia.

Documenting the actual size of the pupils in patients on cholinergic miotic therapy may help the clinician gain insight into issues of medication compliance over time.

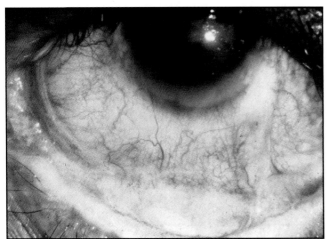

Figure 5-2. Fornix shortening and fibrosis in ocular cicatricial pemphigoid.

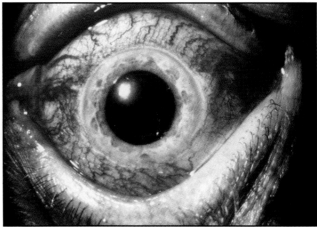

Figure 5-3. Dilated episcleral vessels in a patient with dural sinus fistula.

a pemphigoid-type syndrome,[1] which can be progressive (and indicate the need to discontinue the medication). Here again, one finds extremely useful and important one's baseline, compulsively thorough, comprehensive ophthalmologic examination. Patients with primary ocular pemphigoid can develop POAG as a separate unrelated entity,[2] and the frequent lack of baseline data may obscure a proper interpretation of the exact incidence of miotic-induced (or other antiglaucoma agent) ocular pemphigoid and confuse the choice of appropriate glaucoma therapy.

As a routine, it is useful to test conjunctival mobility superiorly, in case filtration surgery is required in the future. The presence of conjunctival scarring from previous ocular surgery (most commonly cataract surgery, but also perhaps childhood motility surgery that might not be recalled by the patient), from early yet undiagnosed pemphigoid syndromes, or previous inflammatory disease is important for one's therapeutic plan, prognosis, and discussions with the patient.

Look at the episcleral vessels on the bulbar conjunctiva. Increased episcleral venous pressure (see Chapter 46) is not a rare cause of secondary open-angle glaucoma. The prominent, usually dilated episcleral veins are the signature of this entity and can sometimes be missed. In fact, this glaucoma with red eyes is sometimes attributed incorrectly to ocular injection as a side effect of topical medication. The anterior ciliary arteries in the episclera can usually be distinguished from episcleral veins as the arteries extend forward from the recti muscles and usually penetrate deep into the sclera, often in pairs, and disappear a few millimeters from the limbus. (Some have described the anterior ciliary arteries as being more attenuated in eyes with POAG than in normal eyes.) Episcleral veins may be thin and inconspicuous in healthy eyes, but, with increased episcleral venous pressure, they become quite prominent, dilated, and seemingly more numerous (Figure 5-3). The pressure in these episcleral veins can be measured with a special device (see Chapter 46).

If there is any confusion between conjunctival blood vessels that may be dilated due to topical allergy or inflammation and dilated episcleral veins, one should place a drop of a topical vasoconstrictor, such as 2.5% phenylephrine, on the eye. This test will blanch the conjunctival but not the episcleral vessels.

In normal eyes, one can sometimes identify clear channels within a millimeter of the limbus that are carrying aqueous humor to the surface of the eye. These aqueous veins (of Ascher) merge into episcleral veins, and at the junction of the 2, a laminated appearance where aqueous is mixing with blood is sometimes apparent. Curiously, such aqueous veins are only rarely seen in eyes with POAG.

CORNEA

One examines the corneal epithelium looking for corneal edema and the corneal stroma looking for ghost vessels (signaling old interstitial keratitis) or increased thickness (some have reported that abnormal stromal thickness may substantially alter IOP measurements[3]). One routinely examines the corneal endothelium for signs of Fuchs' corneal endothelial dystrophy, which may possibly be associated with POAG, but that also has implications for possible future glaucoma surgery (shallow postoperative chambers create potential additional problems in patients with preexisting corneal endothelial disease—even iris touch can be damaging). In the various iridocorneal endothelial (ICE) syndromes, abnormalities (a beaten metal mini-guttata appearance) occur in the corneal endothelium. Posterior polymorphous dystrophy can also seemingly be associated with open-angle glaucoma (Figure 5-4). One should always look for the presence of peripheral anterior synechiae that extend onto the peripheral cornea (eg, in the ICE syndromes [Figure 5-5] or after a postoperative flat chamber). Various anterior segment cleavage syndromes, such as Rieger syndrome, contain bridging iris processes to

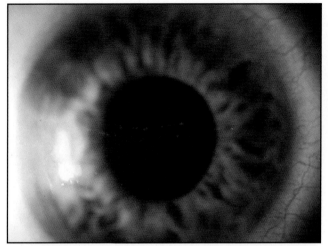

Figure 5-4. Cornea in a patient with posterior polymorphous dystrophy.

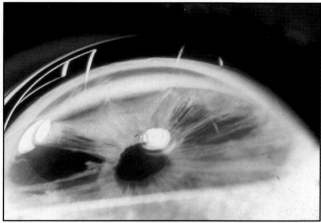

Figure 5-5. Iris changes with synechial angle closure in a patient with essential iris atrophy.

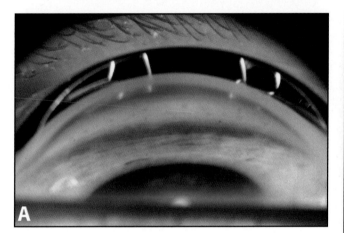

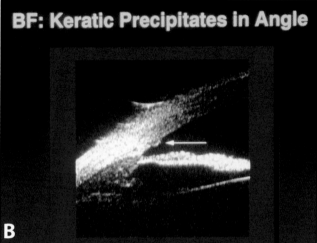

Figure 5-6. (A) Note subtle KP in inferior angle of patient with uveitis. (B) KP in the angle of a patient imaged using ultrasonic biomicroscopy.

a prominent posterior embryotoxon (posterior termination of Descemet's membrane).

In the ICE syndromes, there may also be a peculiar yellow deposit at the level of the corneal endothelium just anterior to the synechiae.

One should critically examine the corneal endothelium, looking for deposits from the aqueous humor. Pigment deposition may not form a true Krukenberg spindle, but might still be a sign of pigmentary dispersion, pseudoexfoliation, iris and ciliary body cysts, or past inflammation. A very small amount of corneal endothelial pigmentation can occur as a normal aging change, perhaps commonly in postpartum women, or can accompany changes of Fuchs' corneal endothelial dystrophy, but pigment on the corneal endothelium always needs to be explained.

Inflammatory deposits on the corneal endothelium (keratic precipitates [KP]) are a sign of ocular inflammatory disease that may explain certain puzzling cases of glaucoma

(Figure 5-6). However, such KP can be subtle, often no more than a single smudge or 2, especially in cases of occult trabeculitis (occult KP in the angle). (Glassy, stellate KP with indiscreet margins is commonly seen in Fuchs' heterochromic iridocyclitis.) One should attempt to explain all corneal endothelial deposits or abnormalities.

ANTERIOR CHAMBER DEPTH

The clinician should routinely record the anterior chamber depth both axially and peripherally in all patients. The easiest way to do this is to estimate the number of corneal thicknesses that one can place between the back of the cornea and the anterior surface of the crystalline lens (axial depth) and between the back of the peripheral cornea and the surface of the peripheral iris (peripheral depth).

In estimating peripheral chamber depth, one needs to construct one's own standard curve and standardize one's

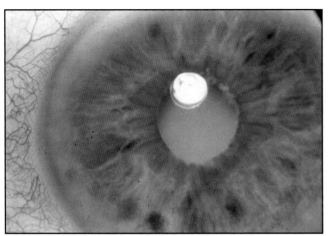

Figure 5-7. Note accumulation of exfoliative material on pupillary margin.

technique on normal patients. Different slit-lamps may give slightly different normal values. In general, one directs the beam 45 to 60 degrees at the far peripheral cornea, and the observation of one-quarter corneal thickness or less for this peripheral anterior chamber depth is suspicious of a narrow, occludable angle (Van Herick's method).

Because of relative pupillary block in most phakic elderly eyes, the pressure is higher in the posterior chamber than in the anterior chamber, and the peripheral iris is ballooned convex forward toward the peripheral cornea (see Chapter 22). (In myopic eyes without this iris convexity and without such relative pupillary block, the peripheral anterior chamber depth may, in contrast, be one full corneal thickness or greater). After laser iridotomy for eyes with narrow angles, with pressure now equalized in the posterior and anterior chambers, peripheral chamber depth should deepen, but usually just to one-quarter to one-half corneal thickness.

Although the peripheral anterior chamber depth deepens after laser iridotomy, the axial depth remains unchanged.

The axial depth reflects the position of the crystalline lens. In hyperopic eyes where the middle segment of the eye is short, the crystalline lens is normally closer to the corneal endothelium than in an emmetropic or myopic eye. Using a similar technique as for measuring peripheral anterior chamber depth, axial anterior chamber depths of 3 corneal thicknesses or less are suggestive of a narrow angle. After iridotomy and alleviation of relative pupillary block, the crystalline lens position does not change; that is, there is no change in the axial anterior chamber depth. In fact, conditions in which the axial anterior chamber depth does change are indicative of other pathological processes, such as postoperative malignant glaucoma or other causes of increased posterior segment volume (see Chapter 29). In these situations, it is very important to appreciate the fact that the crystalline lens has shifted forward in order to diagnose and appropriately treat the disease. For example, with axial anterior chamber depth shallowing associated with elevated IOP after

filtration surgery, the diagnosis must be malignant glaucoma (or suprachoroidal hemorrhage) until proven otherwise. Similarly, in other clinical settings, sequential changes in axial depth are important in the management of the patient. For example, progressive deepening in a postfiltration surgery patient with choroidal detachment may indicate that the condition is spontaneously improving and that surgical drainage may not be required. A patient with normal axial anterior chamber depth but shallow peripheral depth should be suspected of having plateau iris (see Chapter 26). It is thus essential to accurately estimate the depth of both the axial and peripheral anterior chambers. These considerations are further discussed in Chapter 22.

IRIS

Transpupillary iris transillumination should be a routine part of every slit-lamp examination. The slit-lamp beam should be narrowed vertically and placed coaxial with the oculars, and the width should be adjusted to fill the pupil. The transillumination pattern should be viewed under low magnification. Peripupillary defects are frequently observed in exfoliation (and pseudoexfoliation) syndrome and midperipheral radial slits in pigmentary dispersion syndrome (with or without glaucoma). In addition to transpupillary retroillumination, iris transillumination can be performed using a fiberoptic light-source (see Chapter 21).

The pupillary collarette should be carefully examined. Loss of pupillary ruff can occur in exfoliation (Figure 5-7). Rubeosis is often first seen in the pupillary area. Ectropion uveae occurs in neovascular glaucoma. Pupillary sphincter tears are indicative of past blunt trauma. Slight eccentricity of the pupil can be seen in the ICE syndromes. Vertical extension of the pupil postoperatively should suggest iris incarcerated in the surgical wound.

The texture of the iris should be commented on, and nevi should be noted and drawn in the chart. Iris nodules can be seen in certain manifestations of the ICE syndromes, in neurofibromatosis, and with inflammatory deposits in various uveitides.

Sometimes, it is easy to miss mass lesions on the iris (eg, early iris melanoma or juvenile xanthogranuloma), unless iris texture is carefully examined.

Gray areas of iris stromal atrophy are usually indicative of past episodes of angle closure (see Chapter 23), although they can also be observed from severe episodes of past iritis, especially due to herpes zoster. Iris stromal atrophy leading to hole formation can be seen in the ICE syndromes.

Iridoschisis is associated with (usually chronic) angle-closure glaucoma.

Membranes may occur on the surface of the iris or extend into the anterior chamber (eg, in epithelial cysts [Figure 5-8] or, if localized, with fibrous downgrowth). Membranes are also histologically associated with the ICE syndromes, angle recession, and certain postinflammatory conditions.

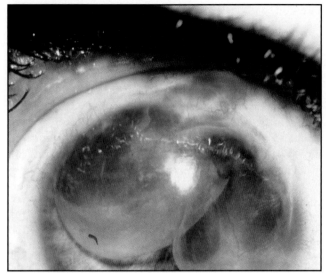

Figure 5-8. Postsurgical epithelial inclusion cyst.

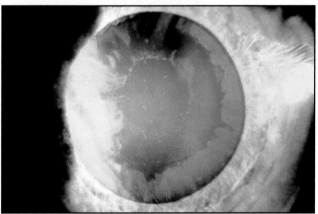

Figure 5-10. Marked exfoliation on anterior lens surface. Exfoliation is often subtle and easily overlooked, especially if the patient is not re-examined at the slit-lamp after dilation.

In neovascular glaucoma, the meandering blood vessels on the iris surface are accompanied histologically by a fibrous membrane that is not apparent clinically except perhaps by a subtle loss of iris surface texture.

Iris pigment epithelial cysts (see Chapter 34) on the posterior surface of the iris cannot be directly visualized, except occasionally after pupillary dilation or if there is an iridectomy (Figure 5-9). However, such cysts often produce a bumpy peripheral iris contour that may be better appreciated on gonioscopy.

Crystalline Lens

The anterior surface of the lens should be examined, looking for changes of exfoliation (Figure 5-10). Through an undilated pupil, the changes of exfoliation can be subtle and easily missed. Most commonly, the central pupillary area of the lens demonstrates a matted, translucent disc of exfoliation. After

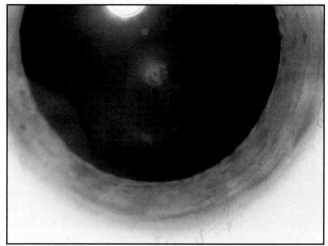

Figure 5-9. Pigmented iris cyst in a patient observed after dilation.

pupillary dilation, slit-lamp examination should be repeated with a drawing of existing lens opacities both by angled-slit view but also retroillumination. Exfoliation or pigment on the zonular fibers, partial subluxation, and other abnormalities should be noted. In exfoliation, there is commonly a clear area on the anterior capsule that separates the central matted disc from more peripheral scallops of white material. In pigmentary dispersion syndrome, there is commonly pigment deposited in a peripheral pocket between the posterior lens surface, zonular fibers, and hyaloid face that can only be appreciated following pupillary dilation. In patients who have had acute angle closure in the past, glaukomflecken may be present within the anterior lens cortex (see Chapter 23).

Vitreous

During the slit-lamp examination, the anterior vitreous should be examined for cells or pigment. Pigment particles in the vitreous may be seen with inflammation but should always raise concern for certain glaucoma syndromes associated with retinal detachment (Schwartz's syndrome). The presence of a posterior vitreous detachment, if present, should be recorded.

Intraocular Pressure

The above has detailed penlight examination and then slit-lamp examination, but has so far not mentioned IOP measurement (see Chapter 6). Although it seems common to perhaps first measure the IOP and then perform the slit-lamp examination, this is not recommended. Slit-lamp examination should be performed first if for no other reason than to rule out infection or corneal epithelial abnormalities. Also, the act of taking the IOP first can cause a fine corneal epithelial irregularity (and fluorescein staining) that can interfere with the clarity of the subsequent examination and also can produce artifacts on visual field measurements. It is recommended, therefore, that visual field testing be performed prior to ocular manipulation.

How Much Visual Acuity Decrease Does the Media Explain?

In all patients with decreased visual acuity, the ophthalmologist must try to explain the reason for this on the basis of the clinical examination. The best way to assess the contribution of ocular media to diminished visual acuity is with the direct ophthalmoscope to compare the patient's visual acuity with the clarity of one's own view of the patient's fundus. If one has a clear view of the disc and posterior pole, then this is a 20/20 view. If the disc can only hazily be seen, then this is commonly a 20/200 view. One quickly learns the range in between. For example, in patients with best-corrected visual acuity of 20/70, one can be very definitive that the media either does or does not explain the visual acuity.

It is best to perform this important evaluation with the direct ophthalmoscope before anesthetic drops are applied to the eye or other examination manipulations occur, such as gonioscopy. Therefore, a usual routine is to perform the penlight and slit-lamp examinations (which also might help orient the clinician as to the cause of the media changes) and then perform direct ophthalmoscopic examination of the posterior pole (drawing the disc cupping) and media through the patient's undilated pupil (this is the aperture through which the patient is looking, so the clinician should look in through the same opening to assess media clarity). Visual acuity and media assessment can be repeated after dilation for supplemental data, but the patient has usually experienced tonometry, gonioscopy, and application of various topical agents that might complicate the interpretation. Always record the estimate of the visual acuity that the patient's media accounts for, along with the examination technique that was used.

With long-term follow-up of glaucoma patients, it is not rare for there to be uncertainty as to whether the vision is decreased on the basis of cataract or glaucoma. For example, a not uncommon scenario is that a patient with 20/60 visual acuity but no documentation as to the cause undergoes possibly successful filtration surgery, but over the years there is further visual acuity decrease. Should the cataract be removed? What visual acuity does the current media explain? What were the findings at the time of filtration surgery? A glaucoma patient with advanced disease may have filtration surgery to save his or her vision, but then with the passage of time and cataract formation, there is a tendency to write off the eye because of severe damage from glaucoma.

The commonly occurring fact that the eye did not see well from the time of filtration surgery (which may have been due to early cataract formation or progression of the pre-existing cataract but was not documented) may thus not be appreciated, and therefore, erroneously, appropriate cataract surgery may not be performed.

Thus, assessing the effect of the media on visual acuity should be a routine part of every glaucoma examination, and it should be performed before there is other manipulation of the eye.

Another clinically important point is that, for an eye with advanced glaucoma field loss close to fixation, lesser amounts of cataract formation may explain a disproportionately larger effect on visual acuity. It is as if with existing scotoma present adjacent to fixation, small amounts of added distortion can produce larger decreases in visual acuity than without such paracentral scotoma. With experience and the routine use of this method of assessing media clarity, the glaucoma clinician learns to appropriately assess such patients.

Optic Nerve Evaluations

It is frequently useful even with an undilated pupil to perform 90-diopter (D) lens evaluation of the optic nerve. As will be commented on in an upcoming chapter, we need to take every opportunity to examine the optic nerve for changes of glaucoma with multiple different techniques of examination (which frequently seem to highlight different aspects of disc cupping). We are critically examining the contour of the remaining rim of tissue of the optic nerve, and our methods are somewhat gross, likely not detecting very early changes, and thus there is merit to multiple methods of examination, including direct ophthalmoscopy.

Obviously, at the time of direct ophthalmoscopy, an assessment and drawing of the optic disc as far as the contour changes of cupping (see Chapter 8) should be made through the undilated pupil, even if the patient will subsequently be dilated (when this should be repeated). In many follow-up visits, the pupil will not be dilated, and therefore it is useful to have this baseline information as viewed through the undilated pupil.

After penlight, slit-lamp, and then direct ophthalmoscopic examination, IOP should next be measured as detailed in Chapter 6. After this, gonioscopy should be performed (see Chapter 7), and then pupillary dilation. (During the latter, the patient should be instructed to keep his or her eyes closed to prevent corneal drying from infrequent blinking, resulting from the use of topical anesthetics for the IOP measurement and gonioscopy.)

Dilated slit-lamp examination with description and drawing of crystalline lens changes should then be made along with examination of the vitreous for pigment and cells, as well as evaluation of the optic nerve with the 60-, 78-, or

90-D lens, as will be detailed later. Then, it is useful to repeat direct ophthalmoscopy of the disc (and macula). Although a nonstereo view, use of parallax in direct ophthalmoscopy can complement contour information from direct stereo methods. The disc cupping and rim contour should be drawn.

Indirect ophthalmoscopy with retinal drawing with attention to the retinal periphery for possible occult tears (that might explain certain unusual secondary glaucomas such as Schwartz's syndrome), or areas of peripheral retinal pathology that might contraindicate miotic therapy, should be performed. The status of the macula (because this also influences visual acuity assessment) should next be evaluated and drawn.

Baseline stereo disc photographs should be performed on all patients with glaucoma or risk of glaucoma for future reference (thus constituting a true baseline standard to assess future change). Such photographs should be repeated every year or 2, depending on disease severity.

The examination is not complete until the impressions are listed with an assessment of the glaucoma status and target IOP, and then the plan of action is laid out in the medical record.

Finally, it is very important to talk to the patient and fully explain the condition, the plan, and the areas of uncertainty. If one can relate the plan to the patient in terms of what one would do if the clinician's own eye were so affected, then this is the highest level of care. Especially for new patients, adequate time to talk to the patient must be scheduled.

REFERENCES

1. Patten JT, Cavanagh HD, Allansmith MR. Induced ocular pseudopemphigoid. *Am J Ophthalmol.* 1976;82:272-276.
2. Tauber J, Melamed S, Foster CS. Glaucoma in patients with ocular cicatricial pemphigoid. *Ophthalmology.* 1989;96:33-37.
3. Johnson M, Kass MA, Moses RA, et al. Increased corneal thickness simulating elevated intraocular pressure. *Arch Ophthalmol.* 1978;95:664-665.

6

Tonometry and Tonography

Jeremy B. Wingard, MD and Joel S. Schuman, MD, FACS

TONOMETRY

The Goldmann applanation tonometer (Haag-Streit, Koeniz, Switzerland) remains a standard of reference in clinical tonometry (Figure 6-1). The principle of applanation tonometry is old. It is based on the physical relationship that applies to the flat end of a piston at rest: The pressure against the piston is calculated from the force applied to the piston divided by the area of the face of the piston. This principle has been used in the Russian Maklakov applanation tonometer since the 19th century, but it was never applied with great precision until the advent of the Goldmann applanation tonometer. In the Goldmann instrument, the force is measured with a sensitive spring or counterpoise balance, and the area is precisely established by an accurate split-field device.

Simple as the principle of applanation tonometry may appear to be, seeming only to require measurements of the applied force and of the resulting flattened area of cornea for determination of the pressure, in actual development of a practical and accurate instrument, a number of additional complicating factors had to be considered. These factors include the effect of capillary attraction between the face of the applanation tonometer and the cornea, the stiffness of the cornea itself, the translation of the force and area on the outer surface of the cornea to intraocular pressure (IOP) at the inner surface of the cornea, the influence of varying corneal curvatures, the influence of corneal astigmatism, the influence of varying amounts of fluid on the cornea, and the influence of varying scleral rigidity. The Goldmann applanation tonometer actually permits measurement of IOP with very little disturbance of this pressure and with insignificant error from variation of scleral rigidity. It also has a well-defined range of insensitivity to the other factors listed.[1]

In the Goldmann applanation tonometer, the endpoint diameter of applanation is fixed by the construction of the plastic prisms within the instrument to be suitable,

especially for the human eye. The diameter of applanation has been selected to give a balance between the capillary attractive force of the tear film and the opposing resistive force of the cornea, while producing essentially the same area of flattening of the endothelial surface of the cornea. For the human eye, the diameter of flattening employed is 3.06 mm. The same diameter is not suitable for use on animal eyes, presumably due to differences in structures of the corneas. For each species, Goldmann found that it is necessary to use a different, specific diameter of flattening, usually larger than that which is best for the human eye.

A portable adaptation of the spring-type Goldmann applanation tonometer, available as the Perkins applanation tonometer (Haag-Streit; Figure 6-2), is well suited to measurements on patients in either the seated or the supine position. The Perkins applanation tonometer is particularly useful in measuring the IOP in young children, permitting accurate measurement without having to position the child at a slit-lamp, which can be both inconvenient and alarming to the child. The Perkins applanation tonometer, in addition to several other devices that are discussed in this chapter, has made tonometry on awake children so much easier than formerly that the need for general anesthesia has been reduced; however, this tonometer is also convenient and well suited for measurements on children in the supine position under general anesthesia.

The Perkins applanation tonometer allows the accurate measurement of IOP in individuals in whom the Goldmann tonometer produces a falsely elevated IOP. The IOP can be measured more accurately with the Perkins than the Goldmann tonometer in people who hold their breath during Goldmann tonometry, obese individuals, extremely large-breasted women, patients with tight collars, or patients with great anxiety at the slit-lamp. By permitting applanation tonometry outside the confines of the slit-lamp, the Perkins tonometer enables precise assessment of the IOP in a more relaxed setting for the patient.

Kahook MY, Schuman JS, eds.
Chandler and Grant's Glaucoma, Fifth Edition (pp 41-50).
© 2013 SLACK Incorporated.

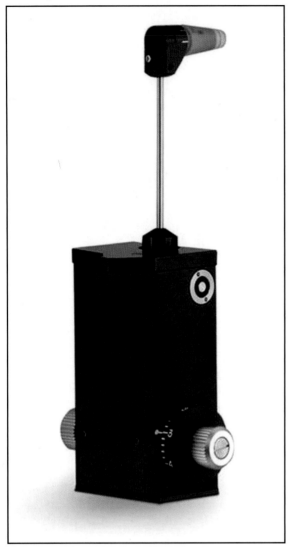

Figure 6-1. The Goldmann applanation tonometer, the gold standard instrument for the measurement of IOP. (Reprinted with permission from Haag-Streit.)

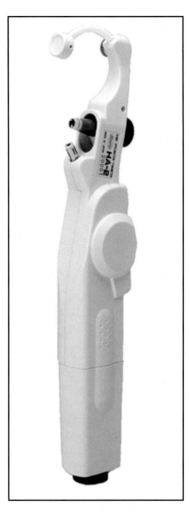

Figure 6-2. The Perkins applanation tonometer is portable and allows accurate IOP measurement without the use of a slit-lamp. It is useful in applanation on children and elderly patients. Occasionally, patients (particularly if they are obese) demonstrate breath holding and presumed increased venous pressure when IOP is measured with the slit-lamp, with false elevation of IOP; these elevations are not confirmed when the Perkins instrument is used. (Reprinted with permission from Haag-Streit.)

For topical anesthesia for Goldmann applanation tonometry, use is made of a drop of a preparation (Fluress, Akorn, Inc, Lake Forest, IL) containing both a topical anesthetic (benoxinate) and 0.25% fluorescein stabilized by polyvinylpyrrolidone, or of proparacaine 0.5% and a fluoresceinated paper strip. The resulting fluorescent tear film is more suitable than a colorless film for observing and measuring flattening of the cornea by the applanation device. To enhance fluorescence, a blue light is used to illuminate the eye and its tear film. Looking with a slit-lamp microscope, one sees at the moment of contact of the tonometer with the eye a bright yellow-green spot that breaks into 2 bright yellow-green semicircular arcs as the tonometer is moved slightly farther forward. The arcs should then be seen in sharp focus. By suitable adjustment of a graduated drum, varying the force applied to the cornea, the arcs can be made to overlap so that the inner edge of the upper can be aligned with the inner edge of the lower. This is the desired endpoint at which a reading is taken from the graduated drum. The numerical reading on the drum indicates grams of force applied by the tonometer and equivalent mm Hg IOP. Thus, number 1 on the drum is equal to 10 mm Hg, and 2 is equal to 20 mm Hg.

The precision with which the inner edges of the overlapping upper and lower arcs can be lined up is limited because of the ocular pulse, causing the edges to swing back and forth. The best that can be done is to adjust the alignment to a mean position in which there is equal swing to either side of the aligned position.

Measurement is made first on one eye and then the other, alternating back and forth, repeating measurements until reasonably constant values are obtained. This is important because, particularly with apprehensive patients, the initial reading may be several mm Hg higher than the readings obtained when the patient has become relaxed and accustomed to the procedure. Usually, 3 measurements on each eye is sufficient, but if the last 2 measurements do not agree within 1 mm Hg, more measurements should be made. Presumably, when initial measurement is higher than the later steady-state measurement, the initial measurement is erroneous.

The significance of readings obtained with the Goldmann applanation tonometer when the patient is relaxed may be generalized as follows: reliable and repeated measurements of 22 or more mm Hg pressure suggest that the eye is abnormal.

In practically all eyes that have a definite pressure of 22 mm Hg or higher, the tonographic P_O/C ratio (steady-state pressure to facility of aqueous outflow) is 100 or higher, indicating possible glaucoma. The higher the pressure, the more definite is the indication. How dangerous a given pressure may be to a given eye depends on many additional factors, such as the nature of the optic nerve head, height and duration of IOP elevation, and possibly blood pressure, all of which are discussed throughout this book.

An IOP of 21 mm Hg by applanation should be regarded as borderline. IOP from 18 to 20 mm Hg does not rule out glaucoma if these are single samplings at a single time of day. It is not uncommon for the IOP in eyes having definite glaucoma to vary during the course of 24 hours from the high-teens to the high 20s, 30s, or even 40s. Thus, a single measurement, be it ever so accurate at the moment, may give a completely misleading impression if by chance it happens to be obtained at the low point of the daily fluctuation.

The Goldmann applanation tonometer can be modified for use on the eyes of infants with small palpebral fissures as well as on eyes of adult patients who have had penetrating keratoplasty and are suspected of developing glaucoma. The end of the cylindrical plastic cone of the tonometer can be reduced in diameter by turning-down in a lathe, leaving just enough of the flat applanating surface to still give accurate pressure measurements.[2,3]

In most of the developed world, the Schiotz tonometer is a seldom-used instrument for estimation of IOP, but it offers a reasonable combination of convenience and reliability. It is subject to more error than the Goldmann applanation tonometer, but the Schiotz tonometer has advantages in portability, availability, ease of use, and lower price.

In the customary manner of using the Schiotz tonometer, the patient is recumbent with gaze vertical and corneas anesthetized by a drop of topical anesthetic. The tonometer is allowed to rest on the patient's cornea, and the extent to which the weighted plunger of the tonometer indents the cornea is shown on a scale by a simple lever-arm indicator. The lever-arm system magnifies the motion of the plunger 20-fold so that a 0.05-mm movement of the plunger is represented by a 1-mm space between units on the tonometer scale. Thus, the scale readings merely indicate the depth to which the plunger indents the eye. The softer the eye, the greater is the depth of the indentation. A reference point is provided by a convex test block resembling the cornea but made of steel, plastic, or glass, that will not indent. On a suitable test block of this sort, the tonometer should give a reading of zero.

A conversion table or graph is required to convert from scale readings obtained when the Schiotz tonometer is resting on the cornea to the corresponding mm Hg IOP. The precision with which the scale reading can be ascertained from the tonometer is limited by oscillation of the indicator needle caused by the ocular pulse and by other physiologic moment-to-moment variations in IOP. The accuracy with which IOP can be estimated is further limited by variability of elastic properties of the eye and by variation in curvature of the cornea. In common clinical practice, the mechanical Schiotz tonometer (Gerhard Biro, Burladingen, Germany) is read to the nearest quarter-scale unit, but it is sometimes difficult to read to the nearest half-scale unit. More precise readings, estimating to the nearest tenth of a scale unit, can be made with electronic Schiotz tonometers (V. Mueller, Chicago, IL), in which the scale of the instrument is expanded by the use of electronic amplification in place of the simple lever arm.

In interpreting the scale readings obtained when the Schiotz tonometer is applied to the patient's eye, it can be said that most normal eyes give readings from 5 to 8 units on the scale and that when readings of 4 or less units on the scale are obtained, the eye should be suspected of being glaucomatous and should be subjected to additional testing.

If the IOPs indicated by the Schiotz tonometer on any type of eye are near borderline between normal and glaucomatous, the IOP should also be measured with the Goldmann applanation tonometer. In the myopic eye in particular, the IOP should be checked by an applanation tonometer, even though it is apparently normal by Schiotz tonometry. There is little need to resort to the applanation tonometer for cases in which the Schiotz tonometer gives measurements well in the glaucoma range in eyes of ordinary size and shape. There is, however, an advantage to comparing the Schiotz and applanation tonometers to determine whether the values indicated by the Schiotz tonometer are accurately applicable to a given eye or whether a correction factor is needed.

Patients with abnormal corneas may present difficulty in measurement of IOP. After penetrating keratoplasty, if irregular mires are observed, Goldmann applanation tonometry should be performed. It is often useful to rotate the applanation prism into more than one meridian to check the reliability of the measurement. If distorted mires are observed due to the presence of an abnormal cornea, a pneumotonometer (Reichert Technologies, Depew, NY; Figure 6-3) or Mackay-Marg tonometer have proven useful in estimating IOP.

The pneumotonometer measures IOP by calculating the force required to flatten an area of cornea using an elastic membrane inflated with gas or air. The current models use compressed air rather than fluorocarbon gas. This device is extremely useful and accurate, especially in the setting of an irregular corneal surface. Additionally, the pneumotonometer can be used against the sclera near the limbus, with IOP results nearly identical to those achieved by contact with the cornea. Pneumotonometry also produces a tracing of the IOP during measurement; this gives the examiner the ability to determine the quality of the examination.

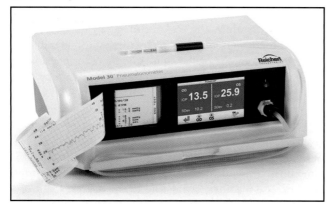

Figure 6-3. The pneumotonometer is useful in measuring IOP in patients with abnormal corneas in whom regular mires with the Goldmann applanation tonometer cannot be obtained, or in children or patients with limited ability to cooperate for Goldmann applanation tonometry. Shown is a newer version with a touch-screen interface. Tonography is also possible with this device. (Reprinted with permission from Reichert Technologies.)

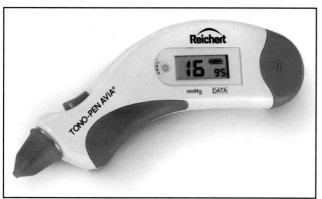

Figure 6-5. This is another, newer version of the Tono-Pen (AVIA), slightly more ergonomic and with longer battery life. (Reprinted with permission from Reichert Technologies.)

A good measurement will produce a flat tracing, with the presence of ocular pulsations evident. During the examination, there is a high-pitched, whining noise. Absence of the pulsations or of this sound indicates an error in measurement. The pneumotonometer handpiece has 2 lines, 1 black and 1 red, on the metal rod, which moves within the handpiece and to which the elastic membrane is attached. For proper measurement, when the handpiece is placed on the cornea, the red line should just be visible, but the black line should be hidden within the housing of the handpiece.

The Tono-Pen (Reichert Technologies) can be used for IOP measurement both as a screening tool and in eyes with irregular surfaces (Figures 6-4 and 6-5).[4-6] This tonometer, however, may overestimate the IOP in eyes with low IOP and underestimate the IOP in eyes with high IOP.[6-8] The Tono-Pen also has poor reproducibility of measurements.[9]

Despite the problems with early models of the instrument, the Tono-Pen has improved over the years and is in frequent use, especially by nonglaucoma specialists. The Tono-Pen's

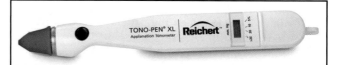

Figure 6-4. The Tono-Pen is a small, portable device that can be used with ease even by technicians. This is an earlier model (Tono-Pen XL) with a linear design, showing a disposable tip cover in place. (Reprinted with permission from Reichert Technologies.)

ease of use and the fact that it can measure IOP even in the presence of corneal irregularity have aided technicians and other support personnel in the evaluation of patients by recording IOP taken with this device. Additionally, its portability allows the use of the Tono-Pen in examination of IOP in remote locations and screenings. Nevertheless, the Goldmann tonometer remains the gold standard and, if available, is preferred to the Tono-Pen in the measurement of IOP.

A relatively new device introduced in the past decade is the dynamic contour tonometer (PASCAL DCT device, Ziemer Ophthalmic Systems AG, Port, Switzerland; Figure 6-6). This instrument measures IOP by inducing conformation of the patient's cornea to the concave instrument tip while applying 1 g of force. A sensor in the instrument tip measures IOP. IOP measurements are similar to Goldmann applanation tonometry, but with less confounding by corneal thickness; however, corneal biomechanical properties still affect IOP assessment with this device.[10]

Noncontact, air-puff tonometers have been used for screening of IOPs, especially in optometry (Figure 6-7). No anesthesia is required for measurement with this device. Unfortunately, reproducibility of measurements is poor.[9] Additionally, a microaerosolized mist of tear film is created on use of air-puff tonometers, introducing the risk of dispersion of infectious material, particularly viral particles.[11]

The Ocular Response Analyzer (ORA; Reichert Technologies; Figure 6-8) is a noncontact tonometer designed to address measurement of corneal biomechanical properties while assessing IOP. The ORA measures corneal hysteresis, or the response of the cornea to bursts of air blown by the device. The change in shape of the cornea and the pressure at which the cornea is flattened by the air jets permit calculation of IOP and corneal biomechanical properties of hysteresis.[12] Variability has been an issue with this device, but future iterations of the technology may permit more accurate and reproducible measurements.

Impact tonometry, also called rebound tonometry, in which a lightweight magnetic probe in an enclosed shaft is propelled toward the cornea and the rebound characteristics of the probe are measured, has shown promise. The first version of this device (Icare TAO1i tonometer, Icare Finland Oy, Helsinki, Finland; Figure 6-9) requires patients to be completely vertical, but as anesthesia is unnecessary due to the very brief impact time of the probe, it has become useful for

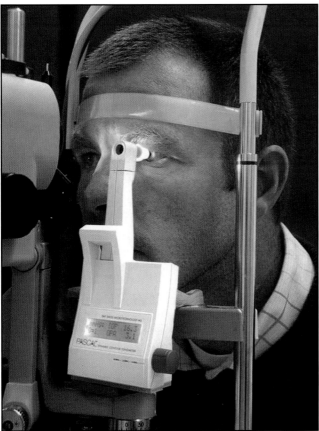

Figure 6-6. PASCAL dynamic contour tonometer applied to a patient's eye. This instrument measures IOP by inducing conformation of the patient's cornea to the concave instrument tip while applying 1 g of force. A sensor in the instrument tip measures the IOP. Correlation with Goldmann applanation is good and with less confounding by corneal thickness. (Reprinted with permission from Ziemer Ophthalmic Systems AG.)

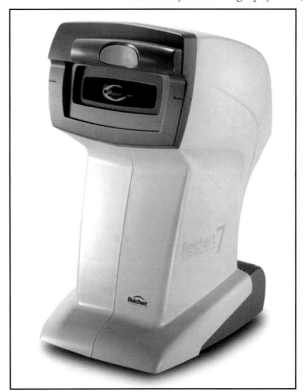

Figure 6-7. The noncontact air-puff tonometer has the advantage of decreasing the risk of transmission of communicable disease, but suffers from lack of accuracy. (Reprinted with permission from Reichert Technologies.)

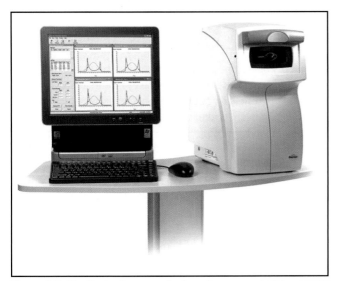

Figure 6-8. The Ocular Response Analyzer is a noncontact tonometer designed to address measurement of corneal biomechanical properties while assessing IOP. (Reprinted with permission from Reichert Technologies.)

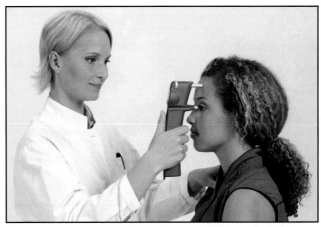

Figure 6-9. Tonometry with the Icare TA01i tonometer rebound tonometer is demonstrated. Rebound, or impact, tonometry employs a lightweight magnetic probe in an enclosed shaft that is propelled toward the cornea. The rebound characteristics of the probe are measured, and IOP is given based on these data. Sterile probes minimize the risk of infectious spread, and a topical anesthetic is not necessary. (Reprinted with permission from Icare Finland.)

pediatric exams in the clinic. Sterile probes are available for each measurement, minimizing the risk of infectious spread. This new technology has been developed for use in humans, large animals, and laboratory rodents.[13]

The estimation of IOP by palpation of the globe is notoriously inaccurate. This technique can be relied on only to determine whether the eye is hard or soft and can be depended on to distinguish an IOP greater than 30 mm Hg.[14]

The following section deals with tonography, a technique by which the actual facility of aqueous outflow is measured in living patients. While it is the only clinical measure of trabecular meshwork (TM) function available to ophthalmologists, it is exceedingly difficult to perform and interpret, requiring the resources of a skilled technician to perform the test and a trained ophthalmologist to interpret it. Additionally, results can be variable, as well as technician dependent. For these reasons, tonography is relegated to the status of research tool. We find that this is a valuable clinical research resource and recognize the difficulty involved in bringing this technology to the community.

TONOGRAPHY

Tonography, in ophthalmology, means recording IOP during several minutes while the eye is subjected to the weight of the Schiotz tonometer, the purpose being to determine how rapidly the pressure drops under this load, and from this to calculate the facility of aqueous outflow.[15,16]

Clinically, the principal reason for resorting to tonography is that tonometry alone may not give enough information about the eye unless it is repeated several times in the course of 24 hours; the IOP may be found normal by tonometry during some portions of the day, even though the facility of aqueous outflow is all the while much less than normal. In eyes with subnormal facility of aqueous outflow, significant elevation of IOP may be detectable by ordinary tonometry only if by chance the tonometry is performed at a time when the pressure happens to be elevated. Although, in most cases, frequent and careful tonometry can make it unnecessary for one to resort to tonography, in some ways tonography is more convenient and, in certain cases, can provide valuable warning of the danger of pressure rise before such a rise is actually detectable by regular tonometry. For example, one might expect that the patient with compromised outflow will experience wider swings in IOP related to variations in aqueous production than the patient with normal outflow facility. This aids the clinician in the assessment of patients, especially those with borderline IOPs in the 24- to 29-mm Hg range, as these patients are likely to experience greater IOPs throughout the day. The clinician sees only a snapshot of the IOP in time; tonography permits extrapolation to the IOPs the patient may experience when not in the office.

Another situation in which tonography can provide a warning of potential rise of IOP before it is detectable by regular tonometry is after operation or after intraocular inflammation, which may be followed by days, weeks, or months of low IOP. If in these conditions the facility of aqueous outflow remains subnormal, eventually, the IOP is likely to rise to glaucomatous levels. Tonography can provide warning of this possibility.

In pure primary open-angle glaucoma (POAG), there is chronically subnormal facility of outflow, with the angle of the anterior chamber open at all times, whereas, in pure angle-closure glaucoma, the facility of outflow is impaired in direct proportion to the extent of closure of the angle and is entirely normal when the angle is open. Tonography in association with gonioscopy has been instrumental in establishing this fundamental difference between open-angle and angle-closure glaucoma.[17,18]

Tonography has been useful not only in evaluating physiologic, pathologic, and surgical influences on the hydrodynamics of the eye, but also has helped in analyzing the mode of action of drugs on the hydrodynamics of the eye. Tonographic measurements have, for instance, shown that drugs related to pilocarpine reduce IOP by enhancing facility of aqueous outflow and have shown that drugs related to acetazolamide reduce IOP by reducing the rate of formation of aqueous humor.

The equipment needed for tonography consists of an electronic Schiotz tonometer and a recorder to make a record of the movement of the plunger of the tonometer. When an electronic Schiotz tonometer is not available, use can be made of a pneumotonometer; the procedure can then be called pneumotonography.[19,20]

The technique of carrying out tonography on patients has been described in detail in the third edition of this book, but in the present edition is only briefly outlined.

With the patient comfortably recumbent, a drop of topical anesthetic is applied to each eye, and the tonometer is allowed to rest on the cornea as in ordinary tonometry. However, instead of the tonometer being applied only momentarily, it is allowed to rest on the cornea of each eye for at least 4 minutes. During this time, the tonometer and recorder will show that the IOP has been gradually falling. The aim is to obtain a smooth tonographic curve with a superimposed ocular pulse. The tonographic curve may be interpreted as follows.

Before the Schiotz tonometer is applied, the eye is in a steady state, with steady IOP, steady rate of formation of aqueous, and steady outflow of aqueous, but when the tonometer is placed on the eye, the IOP is immediately artificially raised, as a result of indentation of the cornea. Raising IOP raises the rate of outflow of aqueous, with little or no influence on formation of aqueous. As soon as aqueous outflow exceeds inflow, the IOP begins to fall, gradually approaching the pressure of the original steady state. In performance of tonography, the recording shows the IOP immediately raised at the start, then gradually falling. The rate of fall depends on the facility of aqueous outflow and the height to which the IOP was initially raised above steady state. Data from the first 4 to 5 minutes of recording are used for calculation of the facility of aqueous outflow (C).

For numerical evaluation of the data supplied by the tonographic curve, the initial tonometer scale reading provides, by way of standard tables, knowledge of the IOP in the steady-state before application of the tonometer, and IOP with the tonometer applied to the eye. (These parameters are known as P_O and P_T [in mm Hg], respectively.) The volume of aqueous humor expressed from the eye in excess of steady-state, or as a function of time, can be obtained from standard tables relating ocular pressure (in mm Hg) to volume (in microliters). A simple nomogram can be used to determine C from scale readings at the initial peak and at 4 minutes. Essentially, the same results can be obtained from tonographic curves more quickly and conveniently by computer.[21-25] The C value is expressed in μL/min/mm Hg of IOP, based on calculations for eyes of supposedly average physical characteristics. We have established by comparison of results from a large number of tonograms that the C value, obtained by means of a nomogram from scale readings at the start and at 4 minutes from a smoothed curve carefully drawn through acceptable recordings, is in good agreement with the value obtainable by more laborious calculation from a great many points on the original recordings.

For clinical detection of glaucoma, the ratio of P_O to C is considerably more useful than either P_O or C individually. In the absence of all forms of treatment, both local and systemic, a P_O/C ratio less than 100 is characteristic of normal eyes, while a P_O/C ratio greater than 100 is characteristic of glaucomatous eyes.

For purposes other than diagnosis, such as for evaluating effectiveness and mechanism of action of medical and surgical treatment for glaucoma, individual variations of P_O and C are interpreted according to the belief that steady-state IOP is governed by only 3 variables: the net rate of flow of aqueous humor through the eye, the facility of aqueous outflow, and the back-pressure in the recipient veins. Because the recipient venous pressure seldom varies, except in unusual conditions, the steady-state IOP is considered to be governed principally by the other 2 variables, the net rate of aqueous flow, and the facility of aqueous outflow. Thus, at levels of IOP above the normal recipient venous pressure of about 10 mm Hg, any lack of correlation between measured variation in P_O and C is blamed on variation in rate of aqueous formation.

However, there has been increasing recognition that variation in uveoscleral outflow needs also to be taken into consideration, particularly in studies of mechanism of action of drugs that influence IOP.[26]

The possibility of error in evaluating P_O and C because of abnormalities of the physical characteristics of individual eyes is quite real when the conversion from Schiotz scale readings to P_O and C values is based on data for average

normal eyes. At present, the most sensitive and reliable means for detecting significant abnormalities in the elastic properties of individual eyes is based on comparison of the P_O value given by the Goldmann applanation tonometer and the P_O value given by the Schiotz tonometer.

Table 6-1 contains typical data derived from tonography measurements to illustrate how the basic parameters of episcleral venous pressure (P_e), flow rate or rate of formation of aqueous humor (F), facility of outflow (C), and IOP relate to one another in various types of eyes. Not included in this table are data for *pseudofacility* (ie, suppression of aqueous formation by IOP). Also not included are data for change in facility of outflow by IOP and data for uveoscleral outflow. However, the data that are presented suffice to illustrate some general conceptual principles concerning the manner in which normal and glaucomatous eyes differ from each other clinically in the behavior of their IOP.

In this table, the episcleral venous pressure (P_e) has been assumed to be constant at 9 mm Hg under all the illustrated clinical circumstances. This is probably a valid approximation according to most of what has been published on the subject, but there are conditions in which P_e is significantly different. These special conditions will be considered elsewhere. This table is intended to illustrate only the most common clinical conditions and concepts.

In the first section of this table, which exemplifies "normal" parameters, a 2-fold change in the rate of aqueous formation can be expected to cause a change in IOP of only 4 mm Hg, and a change in facility of outflow of 0.05 μL/min/mm Hg is expected to produce a change of IOP of only 1 mm Hg in a normal eye.

In the second section of the table, exemplifying glaucoma, the noteworthy differences from the normal include the low facility of outflow and the elevated IOP and, in particular, the fact that a 2-fold change in the rate of aqueous formation can be expected to cause a change in IOP of 20 mm Hg instead of the 4-mm Hg–change seen in the normal eye. Furthermore, in the glaucoma example, a change in facility of outflow of 0.05 μL/min/mm Hg is expected to produce a change in IOP of 15 mm Hg, in contrast to the 1-mm Hg–change seen in the normal eye. The main concept to be derived from this comparison is that glaucomatous eyes have reason to exhibit greater variability of pressure than normal eyes in response to changes in aqueous formation and in facility of outflow. This helps explain to us why a glaucomatous eye (with open angles) can show spontaneous diurnal variations of pressure considerably greater than normal and why various drugs that influence facility of outflow or aqueous formation tend to cause greater changes in pressure in glaucomatous than in normal eyes.

The data presented in the lower half of Table 6-1 exemplify relationships between the extent of closure of the filtration angle (by synechiae or by apposition of the iris to the TM) and the IOP, as influenced also by the underlying characteristics of a given eye when its angle is normally

TABLE 6-1. EXAMPLES OF DIFFERENCE IN THE DEGREE TO WHICH THE INTRAOCULAR PRESSURE (P) IS CALCULATED TO BE AFFECTED BY CHANGES IN FLOW (F) AND FACILITY OF OUTFLOW (C) IN DIFFERENT TYPES OF EYES, ASSUMING CONSTANT EPISCLERAL VENOUS PRESSURE (P$_e$)						
	(mm Hg)		(µL/min)		(µL/min/mm Hg)		(mm Hg)
	P$_e$	+	(F	÷	C)	=	P
Normal =	9		1.5		0.25		1.5
	9		1 to 2		0.25		13 to 17
	9		1.5		0.30		14
Glaucoma =	9		1.5		0.05		39
	9		1 to 2		0.05		29 to 49
	9		1.5		0.10		24
Good normal =	9		1.5		0.30		14
½ angle closed =	9		1.5		0.15		19
¾ angle closed =	9		1.5		0.075		29
Poor normal =	9		1.5		0.15		19
½ angle closed =	9		1.5		0.075		29
¾ angle closed =	9		1.5		0.0375		49

open. It will be noted that, in the lower half of the table, we are concerned with a good-normal eye and a poor-normal eye. This distinction is based on the fact that, among normal human eyes, there is a wide range of normal pressures (eg, 10 to 20 mm Hg) and a range of normal values of facility of outflow (eg, 0.15 to 0.60). Thus, some eyes are naturally far from glaucomatous (for instance, the good-normal eye in the table with facility of outflow of 0.30 µL/min/mm Hg and IOP of 14 mm Hg). Other eyes are not so far from the end of the normal range where it begins to border on glaucomatous, for instance, the poor-normal eye with facility of outflow of 0.15 µL/min/mm Hg and IOP of 19 mm Hg.

The next conceptually and practically important point is to note the effects of obstructing aqueous outflow through the angle of the anterior chamber in either one-half or three-quarters of its circumference (such as by peripheral anterior synechiae [PAS] or by appositional angle closure). Obstruction of half the circumference reduces the facility of outflow by 50%, and obstruction of three-quarters reduces facility of outflow by 75%. The practical clinical consequence of this upon the IOP is different for the good-normal eye with its angle completely open than for the poor-normal eye with its angle open. Closing or otherwise obstructing the filtration angle in half of the circumference raises the pressure in both eyes—only to 19 mm Hg (still within the normal range) in the good-normal eye, but to 29 mm Hg in the poor-normal eye. With closure of three-quarters of the angle, the difference between the eyes in resultant elevation of IOP is still more drastic—29 mm Hg compared to 49 mm Hg.

We conclude from these considerations, derived from our clinical tonographic and gonioscopic observations, that it is useful to take into account the original facility of outflow and IOP of a given eye when attempting to assess how much of a therapeutic problem a given extent of PAS may pose for that eye. This may have a decisive influence on the choice of operation and will be considered further in Chapter 23, where it is pointed-out that angle-closure glaucoma often develops in one eye before the other and that comparing tonographic and gonioscopic data from the eye with closure of part of its angle compared with data from the contralateral eye with its open angle can be utilized to advantage in deciding on the type of treatment.

DIURNAL VARIATIONS

In normal eyes, the IOP varies no more than 2 or 3 mm Hg throughout the day and night. Also, in some glaucomatous eyes, the pressure shows little variation and remains elevated at all times. However, more characteristically in glaucomatous eyes, the pressure varies up and down in a diurnal pattern that seems to be an exaggeration of the slight variation detectable in normal eyes. This variation can be studied best in eyes in which there is a constant obstruction to aqueous outflow, such as in glaucoma due to PAS, traumatic recession of the angle, the innate changes in the aqueous outflow channels in well-established POAG, in open-angle glaucoma associated with pseudoexfoliation, or in pigmentary glaucoma. (One cannot identify the diurnal variation of pressure very well in intermittent angle-closure glaucoma because of additional and confusing variation attributable to opening and closing of the angle.)

From tonographic measurements in eyes having various forms of open-angle glaucoma uncomplicated by intraocular inflammation, the facility of aqueous outflow is usually at almost the same subnormal value at both the high and low points in the diurnal curves of variation of IOP. The pressure in the aqueous veins has been reported to remain essentially constant. Therefore, we conclude that the fluctuation of IOP is attributable mainly to a varying rate of formation of aqueous humor.

Observations on patients having different severity of open-angle glaucoma in the 2 eyes or having one normal and one glaucomatous eye show that the spontaneous diurnal variations of pressure usually run parallel in the 2 eyes but that, in the eye having the greater obstruction to aqueous outflow, the variation in pressure characteristically exceeds the variation in the more nearly normal eye. There may be a striking difference in the 2 eyes in the amplitude of fluctuation, but usually not in the timing. In general, IOP rises at night, and this most likely is associated with the supine position.[27]

The range of diurnal variation of IOP for a given severity of glaucoma varies greatly from patient to patient and seems to be more closely related to some special characteristic of the individual patient than to the absolute degree of obstruction of aqueous outflow. One cannot predict with certainty from the fact that the tonographic facility of outflow is low that there will be significant diurnal fluctuation of IOP, but the likelihood of large fluctuation is slight in eyes with normal or near-normal facility of outflow.

These observations strongly suggest that the variation in the rate of aqueous formation that is manifest in both eyes simultaneously must result from some systemic controlling influence reaching both eyes simultaneously. One can be reasonably sure that this influence does not reach the eyes via the ocular nerves. Clinical observations on patients who have various defective innervations of the eye and experimental studies on animals involving either stimulation or interruption of nerves to the eye have not as yet provided evidence for neural influence on diurnal variation of aqueous formation or IOP of the magnitude that is observed clinically. The only other way that systemic influences might reach the eye would be through variations in composition of the blood or through variations in circulating hormones. Hormonal control seems to us to be the most attractive probability.

When investigating the mechanism of diurnal variation of IOP, it is attractive to attempt to relate this to diurnal variations in other physiologic functions, such as kidney function, and this may ultimately prove fruitful. A peculiarity of the diurnal variation of IOP is that, in most glaucomatous patients, it results in rise of pressure to a maximum early in the morning before the patient gets out of bed, but in another considerable proportion of patients, the maximum occurs at a different time, such as late afternoon or evening.

The reason for these differences is unknown. However, these individual differences may well prove to be a valuable feature when attempts are made to correlate this phenomenon with other systemic variables.

No investigator has provided a greater understanding of aqueous humor flow than Brubaker and colleagues.[28,29] Brubaker[30] has demonstrated through fluorophotometry, a technique that demonstrates aqueous humor production by diffusion of fluorescein into the anterior chamber and then dilution of that fluorescein concentration over time, that the rate of aqueous humor production is lowest during sleep and it increases dramatically just before waking. The cycle of aqueous production corresponds to the diurnal variation in IOP. Further, Brubaker showed that circulating catecholamines, specifically epinephrine, may be responsible for the diurnal variation in aqueous production.[30]

One feature of diurnal IOP variation that deserves particular thought is that the fundamental problem seems not to be to explain the high phase of IOP, but rather to explain the low phase of the IOP. When the IOP is high, it appears from tonographic measurements that aqueous humor is being formed at a normal rate and that, when the IOP decreases spontaneously to a lower level, with facility of outflow still subnormal, this decrease of pressure is attributable to a decrease in aqueous formation to a subnormal rate. An explanation is needed for this decrease in aqueous formation. If we understood it, we might be able to exploit it therapeutically.

Practically, measurement of the IOP at intervals of 2 to 4 hours around the clock is a valuable procedure, not only in establishing the diagnosis of glaucoma, but in the management of cases of established open-angle glaucoma. If IOP is measured in the office at approximately the same time at each visit, we may be measuring IOP at the time of the lowest level of diurnal variation and thus have a false sense of security, whereas if the IOP had been measured at a different time of day, we might have found a considerably elevated IOP and then would have realized that things were not going as well as we had thought. With hospital costs so high, it is impractical in most cases to admit a patient to the hospital for IOP studies around the clock. Furthermore, the necessarily artificial inpatient environment seems in some patients to alter the magnitude of the diurnal variation. A possible alternative is to see the patient in the office at intervals from early morning until late in the afternoon for measurement of IOP. However, the amplitude of the IOP variation from day to day may not be constant, and it may be necessary to make repeated IOP measurements during 3 or more cycles to obtain a fair understanding of the degree and timing of the variation.

Another way is to furnish the patient with a Tono-Pen, Icare rebound device, or other home tonometer and teach a member of the family to measure the IOP at various times during the day and night. We have found this valuable in a number of instances, although this is not suitable for many patients.

REFERENCES

1. Goldmann H. Applanation tonometry. In: *Symposium on Glaucoma. Transactions of the Second Conference.* New York, NY: Josiah Macy Jr Foundation; 1957.

2. Menage MJ, Kaufman PL, Croft MA, et al. Intraocular pressure measurement after penetrating keratoplasty: minified Goldmann applanation tonometer, pneumotonometer, and Tono-Pen versus manometry. *Br J Ophthalmol.* 1994;78:671-676.

3. O'Donoghue E. The minified Goldmann applanation tonometer. *Br J Ophthalmol.* 1994;78:671-676.

4. Christoffersen T, Fors T, Ringberg U, et al. Tonometry in the general practice setting (I): Tono-Pen compared to Goldmann applanation tonometry. *Acta Ophthalmologica.* 1993;71:103-108.

5. Denis P, Normann JP, Bertin V, et al. Evaluation of the Tono-Pen 2 and the X-Pert noncontact tonometers in cataract surgery. *Ophthalmologica.* 1993;207:155-161.

6. Geyer O, Mayron Y, Loewenstein A, et al. Tono-Pen tonometry in normal and in postkeratoplasty eyes. *Br J Ophthalmol.* 1992;76:538-540.

7. Moore CG, Milne ST, Morrison JC. Noninvasive measurement of rat intraocular pressure with the Tono-Pen. *Invest Ophthalmol Vis Sci.* 1993;34:363-369.

8. Zimmerman TJ, Gupte RK, Wall JL. Tonometry comparison: Goldmann versus Tono-Pen. *Ann Ophthalmol.* 1992;24:29-36.

9. Wilson MR, Baker RS, Mohammadi P, et al. Reproducibility of postural changes in intraocular pressure with the Tono-Pen and Pulsair tonometers. *Am J Ophthalmol.* 1993;116:479-483.

10. Kanngiesser HE, Kniestedt C, Robert YC. Dynamic contour tonometry: presentation of a new tonometer. *J Glaucoma.* 2005;14:344-350.

11. Britt JM, Clifton BC, Barnebey HS, et al. Microaerosol formation in noncontact air-puff; tonometry. *Arch Ophthalmol.* 1991;109:225-228.

12. Martinez-de-la-casa JM, Garcia-Feijoo J, Fernandez-Vidal A, et al. Ocular Response Analyzer versus Goldmann applanation tonometry for intraocular pressure measurements. *Invest Ophthalmol Vis Sci.* 2006;47:4410-4414.

13. Kontiola AI, Goldblum D, Mittag T, Danias J. The induction/impact tonometer: a new instrument to measure intraocular pressure in the rat. *Exp Eye Res.* 2001;73(6):781-785.

14. Baum J, Chaturvedi N, Netland PA, et al. Assessment of intraocular pressure by palpation. *Am J Ophthalmol.* 1995;119:650-651.

15. Grant WM. Past, present, and future. *Ophthalmology.* 1978;85:252-258.

16. Grant WM. A tonographic method for measuring the facility and rate of aqueous flow in human eyes. *Arch Ophthalmol.* 1950;44:204-314.

17. Chandler PA. Narrow angle glaucoma. *Arch Ophthalmol.* 1952;47:695-716.

18. Grant WM. Clinical measurements of aqueous outflow. *Arch Ophthalmol.* 1951;46:113-131.

19. Feghali JG, Azar DT, Kaufman PL. Comparative aqueous outflow facility measurements by pneumotonography and Schiotz tonography. *Invest Ophthalmol Vis Sci.* 1986;27:1776-1780.

20. Langham ME, Leydhecker W, Krieglstein G, et al. Pneumotonographic studies on normal and glaucomatous eyes. *Adv Ophthalmol.* 1976;32:108-133.

21. Woodhouse DF. A computer evaluation on tonography. *Exp Eye Res.* 1969:127-142.

22. Dallow RL, Adler A, Weihrer AL, et al. Tonogram reading by digital computer. *Am J Ophthalmol.* 1970;70:922-928.

23. Brennen M. Tonography software and hardware interface. *Ann Ophthalmol.* 1984;16:1133-1135.

24. Eisenberg DL, Schuman JS, Wang N. An ultra-sensitive ocular perfusion system. *Invest Ophthalmol Vis Sci.* 1984;(ARVO suppl).

25. Teitelbaum CS, Podos SM, Lustgarden JS. Comparison of standard and computerized tonography instruments on human eyes. *Am J Ophthalmol.* 1985;99:403-410.

26. Crawford K, Kaufman PL, Gabelt BT. Effects of topical PGF2 alpha on aqueous humor dynamics in cynomolgus monkeys. *Curr Eye Res.* 1987;6:1035-1044.

27. Liu JH, Zhang X, Kripke DF, Weinreb RN. Twenty-four-hour intraocular pressure pattern associated with early glaucomatous changes. *Invest Ophthalmol Vis Sci.* 2003;44(5):1586-1590.

28. Maurice DM. The movement of fluorescein and water in the cornea. *Am J Ophthalmol.* 1960;49:1011-1016.

29. Jones RF, Maurice DM. New methods of measuring the rate of aqueous flow in man with fluorescein. *Exp Eye Res.* 1966;5:208-220.

30. Brubaker RF. Flow of aqueous humor in humans. *Invest Ophthalmol Vis Sci.* 1991;32:3145-3166.

W. Morton Grant, MD, now deceased, was an original author on this chapter.

7

The Angle of the Anterior Chamber

Joel S. Schuman, MD, FACS; Deval Joshi, MD; and Lisa S. Gamell, MD

The angle of the anterior chamber normally provides the main outflow system for aqueous humor. In most of the glaucomas, it is here that aqueous outflow is obstructed. Gonioscopy is our clinical means for looking into the angle and identifying the cause of obstruction in many cases. This chapter offers details regarding the examination of the drainage angle while maintaining much of the historical perspective from the original writings of Dr. W. Morton Grant.

GONIOSCOPY (PROCEDURE)

Gonioscopy is one of the most important tools in the management of glaucoma. Historically, many cases of glaucoma were treated successfully without gonioscopy, but, in many other cases, gonioscopy may be the sole means of arriving at the correct diagnosis, leading to the correct treatment. Inaccurate gonioscopy may not only be unhelpful, it may actually be misleading. Whereas accurate gonioscopy can give the correct diagnosis and point to the most appropriate treatment, an incorrect interpretation of the gonioscopic findings may lead the ophthalmologist far astray. It is certainly worth the time and effort to learn gonioscopy well and to make the best use of it in every case of glaucoma.

In this chapter, we will describe methods that, in our hands, have been most satisfactory for learning gonioscopic anatomy and for performing gonioscopy on patients. Throughout the text, frequent consideration will be given to gonioscopic findings. Peculiarities of the angle in infants and children, as well as congenital abnormalities of the angle, are discussed in Chapter 68.

LEARNING GONIOSCOPY

The most effective and valuable step in learning gonioscopy makes use of enucleated human eyes, such as those used as donors in corneal transplanting procedures. By studying the angle of the anterior chamber with the binocular microscope and by performing simple dissections, one can obtain the best understanding of the identity and anatomical relationship of the structures seen in the eyes of patients.

To obtain the most instructive view of the anatomy of the angle, one makes a cut with a razor blade perpendicularly through the center of the cornea, bisecting the anterior segment, cutting smoothly through the angle structures and the anterior 2 or 3 mm of sclera on both sides. Then, with scissors, half of the bisected anterior segment is removed by cutting the sclera circumferentially, parallel to the limbus. This leaves half the circumference of angle open to direct viewing as in clinical gonioscopy and, at the same time, provides a cross-sectional display of the angle where the structures have been cut by the razor blade at both sides of the hemisphere.

The eyes prepared in this manner can be examined with a slit-lamp microscope or a dissecting microscope; or one can use the handheld gonioscopy microscope and a focal illuminator, as in clinical Koeppe gonioscopy. In this arrangement, there is, of course, no need for a gonioscopic contact lens, as there is no cornea in the line of view.

One should first identify the structures of the cross-sectioned angles, because this will be the most readily recognizable aspect, because it is similar to the cross-sectional type of view that is so familiar in microscopic histology slides used in the study of ocular pathology. One should have no trouble identifying ciliary muscle, ciliary processes, and iris, as well as sclera and cornea. Finer details may require considerable study to recognize, and it is helpful to have a stained microscopic section to refer to for comparison.

In the dissected unstained eye, there is a conspicuous continuous dark brown, almost black, pigmented layer on the back surface of the iris and on the processes and pars plana of the ciliary body, but beneath this pigmented layer the ciliary body and the ciliary muscle are remarkably pale and colorless. In bisected eyes, the ciliary muscle is often

Kahook MY, Schuman JS, eds.
Chandler and Grant's Glaucoma, Fifth Edition (pp 51-80).
© 2013 SLACK Incorporated.

separated from the sclera by an artifactual anterior choroidal separation, except at its most anterior extremity where it attaches like a fine tendon to the scleral spur and corneoscleral trabecular meshwork (TM). Just anterior and close to the scleral spur, a fine slit can be identified as Schlemm's canal, cut in cross section. For easier identification, the lumen of Schlemm's canal may be caused to open slightly by gentle traction applied to the ciliary muscle or to the iris.

Angle structures that are seen in frontal view of the angle can be identified with the same structures in the cross-sectional view, by following each structure from its perpendicularly cut surface to the farthest recess of the open anterior chamber. In this way, one should be able to identify the corneoscleral TM, Schlemm's canal, scleral spur, and ciliary band.

On further study, one can see that the corneoscleral TM and the scleral spur have a special whiteness that is attributable to a background of white sclera. A transition from the white of the scleral spur to the slight gray shade of the ciliary band can be seen. Posterior to the scleral spur, the sclera curves away with a greater radius of curvature so that it is more tangential to the gonioscopic line of view than is the scleral background of the corneoscleral TM and, therefore, reflects the gonioscopic light less efficiently. Furthermore, the anterior end of translucent ciliary muscle is attached to the scleral spur, and this also reduces the amount of light reflected from the sclera posterior to the spur. In White patients, there is little or no pigment in the anterior sclera or ciliary muscle to influence the color of the ciliary band. Only in darkly pigmented patients is pigmentation in these structures sometimes enough to make the ciliary band appear slate gray, with or without distinguishable brown infiltration.

Schlemm's canal and the filtration portion of the TM, just anterior to scleral spur, are often demarcated in eyes of elderly people by a finely granular collection of pigmented particles within the portion of the TM overlying Schlemm's canal. This pigment is visible as a narrow, finely granular, brown band just anterior to the white of scleral spur within that portion of the TM that separates Schlemm's canal and anterior chamber, through which aqueous humor passes to reach Schlemm's canal.

Once the principal anatomical features of the angle have been learned in enucleated eyes, it is easy to proceed to examination of patients, to become familiar with features that are not otherwise readily appreciated, particularly the variable character of anterior chamber depth, contour of iris, distribution and texture of uveal meshwork, and presence of blood vessels in iris and angle. Variations of details in the gonioscopic findings and abnormalities in the angle will be discussed later in this chapter.

CLINICAL PROCEDURE

For clinical gonioscopy, the equipment that proved most satisfactory to us from the 1950s to the 1990s included the following:

- The Koeppe gonioscopy contact lens
- The Barkan handheld focal illuminator or, alternately, a transilluminator or muscle light
- A handheld binocular microscope

In more recent times, other gonioscopic equipment has become more popular, particularly to meet requirements of new procedures, such as laser treatment of the angle.

Modern systems of gonioscopy employ mirrored contact lenses, such as the Goldmann lens (Ocular Instruments, Bellevue, WA) and the slit-lamp biomicroscope, and require the patient to be sitting-up. These lenses provide a reversed image, but the image is not crossed. In other words, if one were looking at the inferior angle through a Goldmann lens, with the goniomirror centered at 12 o'clock, the 7 o'clock angle would be seen at the 11 o'clock position, the 6 o'clock angle at the 12 o'clock position, and the 5 o'clock angle at the 1 o'clock position (Figure 7-1).

The lens and light source must be manipulated to alter the angle of view over peripheral convex iris or to examine successive portions of the circumference. The need for these manipulations may result in a false interpretation of angle depth. For example, in eyes having convex irides, the angle may appear to be partially closed with a mirrored contact lens due to the inability to vary the angle of view so as to look down into the crack between iris and angle wall. We have seen numerous examples in which such angles that were judged to be closed by use of a mirrored lens have in fact been observed to be open to the full width of TM, scleral spur, and, occasionally, even narrow ciliary body band with the use of a Koeppe lens system (Ocular Instruments).

On the other hand, corneal distortion and indentation with the use of a mirrored contact lens can actually open an angle that is appositionally occluded. The angle is opened by posterior displacement of aqueous humor against the iris, consequent to the corneal indentation. This phenomenon is actually put to good use with the Zeiss indentation gonioscopy lens (Zeiss) by Max Forbes,[1] in which such displacement can be used to identify peripheral anterior synechiae (PAS). Because differentiating open-angle from angle-closure glaucoma is perhaps the most important question asked during clinical gonioscopy, we routinely employ the Koeppe system as the first method of gonioscopy, particularly in new patients, because it allows a direct view into the angle over a convex iris without corneal distortion.[2] Additionally, it permits bilateral, simultaneous gonioscopy, as well as examination of the angle by multiple observers without removal and replacement of contact lenses. In cases of suspected angle closure, this can then be followed by indentation gonioscopy with the Zeiss lens to evaluate the angle for the presence of PAS.

We recommend that the beginner learn to perform gonioscopy with the single, simple, universally applicable system of direct examination with the Koeppe lens and then to use the various mirrored indirect lenses (Figure 7-2) For example, the Goldmann gonioscopic lens (Ocular Instruments)

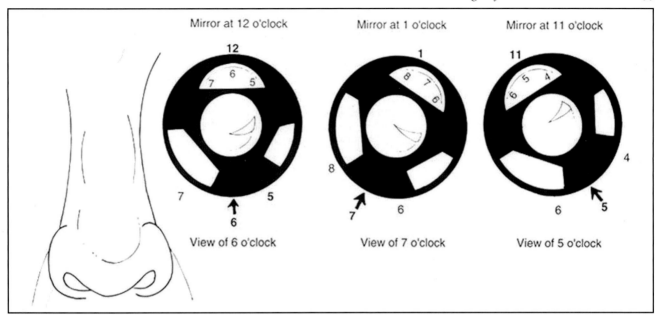

Figure 7-1. The mirrored goniolens does not invert the image of the angle. If the mirror is centered at 12 o'clock, the 12 o'clock position of the mirror represents 6 o'clock, the 11 o'clock position of the mirror represents 7 o'clock, and the 1 o'clock position of the mirror represents 5 o'clock. Knowledge of the position in the angle relative to the image in the mirror is essential, particularly in laser treatment of the angle.

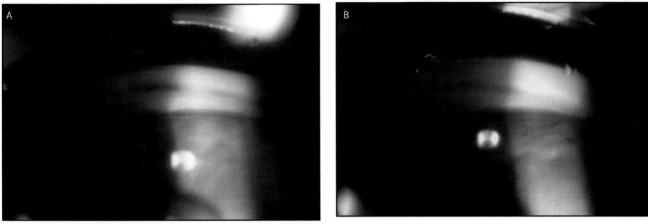

Figure 7-2. Zeiss indentation gonioscopy. (A) Zeiss gonioscopy view of closed angle. (B) Indentation gonioscopy reveals appositional closure, with absence of peripheral anterior synechiae.

provides an excellent high-magnification view of certain angle details, such as new blood vessels, and inflammatory deposits. Use of this gonioscopic lens is required when performing laser treatment to the angle, and it needs to be mastered by the ophthalmologist. The Zeiss indentation gonioscopy lens is invaluable in identifying PAS during indentation and can be used to rapidly view an angle at the slit-lamp in a postoperative patient.

GOLDMANN 3-MIRROR GONIOSCOPY

The Goldmann 3-mirror lens (Ocular Instruments) is an invaluable tool and is the utility player of the gonioscopist's roster. It is useful in quick evaluation of the angle, as well as for intense, high-powered scrutiny, laser trabeculoplasty or gonioplasty, examination of the peripheral retina, or even stereoscopic study of the optic nerve head. The student of gonioscopy must become a master with this lens to succeed at the task, but such mastery is not difficult.

The lens is applied using methylcellulose as a coupling agent. The patient's lids are spread wide, and the lens is fitted into the palpebral fissure by using one edge to push down the lower lid from the bulbar side, then inserting the upper portion of the lens beneath the upper lid, while lifting that lid with the other hand. Performing this procedure gently is essential in order to maintain the patient's confidence.

Once the lens is in place, the angle is studied using the goniomirror, the parabola-shaped mirror of the 3, which reflects the TM and other structures. The slit-lamp biomicroscope is used at high power, and the slit beam is adjusted so as to distinguish the structures in the angle. The slit beam can be narrowed to give the parallelepiped effect, in which the beam reflected from the anterior cornea and that portion reflected from the posterior cornea come together at Schwalbe's line. This can be used in poorly pigmented angles to determine whether the angle is open or not, if the landmarks of the TM are indistinguishable due to pallor. The techniques of gonioscopy are described next, but some mention should be made first of the Zeiss goniolens.

ZEISS 4-MIRROR GONIOSCOPY

The Zeiss 4-mirror goniolens is every gonioscopist's friend, handy for a quick assessment of the angle or for indentation gonioscopy to determine if closure is appositional or synechial. This lens requires only the natural tears for coupling and, of course, topical anesthetic for the patient. While the lens is useful, one can easily be misled with the Zeiss lens, such as by a convex iris in which the angle structures cannot be seen due to a steep approach to the angle (the gonioscopist with a Zeiss lens would call this angle appositionally closed, as the TM can be seen only with indentation, when in reality it can be seen to be open with a narrow inlet by Koeppe gonioscopy). The Zeiss lens can also readily fool the gonioscopist into thinking that an appositionally closed angle is open, due to unintentional pressure placed on the lens, the diameter of which, unlike the Koeppe or Goldmann, is less than that of the cornea, although the radius of curvature is greater than that of the cornea. This diameter and radius of curvature are what allow indentation gonioscopy. The same is true for the Sussman lens (Ocular Instruments), a Zeiss lens without a handle, or the Posner lens (Ocular Instruments), which is a Zeiss lens with a screw-in handle. All of these lenses can cause unintentional compression; however, the gonioscopist has clues that compression is occurring. Folds are seen in Descemet's membrane, and gentle, partial removal of the lens results in lens-iris diaphragm movement anteriorly.

INDENTATION GONIOSCOPY

When indentation gonioscopy is intentionally sought, the Zeiss 4-mirror lens is applied, and the angle is carefully examined using the slit-lamp biomicroscope at high magnification. While observing the angle, the lens is moved slightly posteriorly, indenting the cornea and forcing the lens-iris diaphragm posteriorly in cases of relative pupillary block. The lens-iris diaphragm will not move in the presence of a patent surgical iridectomy, but generally will be forced back even with a patent laser iridectomy, due to its small size. Indentation gonioscopy is useful in evaluating the angle for appositional closure or peripheral anterior synechiae, as well as for iridodialysis or cyclodialysis clefts.

For Koeppe gonioscopy, a handheld microscope can be used, such as is salvageable from old slit-lamp microscopes or is manufactured in lighter weight expressly for gonioscopy by Haag Streit. The size of Koeppe lens suitable for most eyes is 18 mm in diameter (measured from the outer edges of the flange that fits under the lids against the eye); but, occasionally, for eyes having an abnormally small palpebral fissure and for children, a 16-mm diameter lens is useful. This combination of equipment, which is to be used with the patient recumbent, provides a direct panoramic magnified view of the angle in a simple manner, requiring the patient to do nothing but to lie relaxed. This same simple arrangement for direct gonioscopy is practical in the operating room for examination of patients on the operating table, such as for immediate preoperative evaluation of the extent of opening of the angle by intensive medication in angle-closure glaucoma and for examination of infants under general anesthesia, particularly in relation to congenital glaucoma.

Another favorable factor is observed in examination of eyes having convex irides and narrow or possibly closed angles, when it is necessary to vary the angle of view to look down into the crack between iris and angle wall as far as possible to determine whether the filtration portion of the TM is occluded by the periphery of the iris. Using the Koeppe lens and handheld microscope, the examiner can vary his or her direction and angle of view with ease to select the most suitable position for seeing into the slit between convex iris and angle wall, without having to make any change of position of the lens. Also, one can quickly compare one portion of the angle with another, or the angle of one eye with that of the other.

In certain conditions, such as in suspected traumatic recession of the angle and in congenital glaucoma, comparison of one eye with the other is particularly helpful. This is conveniently accomplished with Koeppe lenses on both eyes, alternating the view with the handheld microscope easily back and forth from one eye to the other.

It is convenient to have the examiner's stool or chair freely sliding or rolling on casters so that the examiner can swing around from one side of the recumbent patient to the other to obtain a panoramic view of the whole circumference. If the patient is recumbent in an examining chair, the examiner may conveniently use a typist's chair on casters, with the chair turned backward, so that the examiner sits straddling the back of the chair, using its back for a support for his or her elbows, or he or she may steady his or her arms on the side of the back if the patient's head is lower. In this way, a continuous inspection of the whole angle is easily made as the examiner rolls in an orbit around the head of the patient. Only to examine the 12 o'clock portion of the angle is it necessary to lean forward somewhat over the patient's chest. When the Koeppe gonioscope lens is used, air bubbles can be displaced from the small space between cornea and the back of the lens with a few drops of a suitable solution, such as sterile 0.9% to 1.4% sodium chloride solution. The solution must contain no chlorobutanol preservative, however, because this preservative, when held in contact with the epithelium for several minutes, can produce a keratitis epithelialis that can make the patient uncomfortable for many hours, or until the epithelium heals spontaneously in a day or two. Methylcellulose may also be used to provide an excellent interface between the cornea and contact lens, and its viscosity limits the entry of air bubbles into the field of view.

If a lens is chosen to have a radius of inside curvature of 7.8 to 8.0 mm instead of the more common 7.4 mm, the space between lens and cornea is so small that it can be filled by the patient's tears. However, one should avoid an excessively shallow lens that actually presses on the cornea, because this can distort the cornea, inducing corrugations of the posterior surface of the cornea, interfering with a view of the angle.

The lens should be centered on the cornea and not allowed to become displaced into an eccentric position, because if the rim of the lens encroaches on the cornea excessively in one quadrant, it tends to indent the limbus and to cause artificial narrowing of the angle. This is most likely to occur if the patient's head is elevated on a thick pillow, which causes the neck to be flexed forward. In this position, when the gaze is vertical, as it should be for gonioscopy, the upper lid presses excessively on the Koeppe lens and may make the upper angle appear closed. As a warning sign of this artifact, the gonioscopist may observe that a ridge paralleling the limbus is protruding inward at the periphery of the cornea superiorly and that, on the inner surface of the cornea, there are abnormal rugae or wrinkles running radially over the ridge, due to wrinkling of Descemet's membrane. Correction of this condition is simple. One merely removes the excessively thick pillow or has the patient raise the chin and extend the neck, so that the excess pressure of the upper lid on the lens is relieved. The gonioscopist then sees that the artificial ridge disappears, and what may have been thought to be a sector of closed angle may be seen actually to be open. Unwanted indentation of the limbus due to eccentricity and uneven pressure on the lens can be induced in other quadrants if the head is turned or if one holds the lens forcefully against the eye. With a cooperative patient and proper lens, there is no need for the lens to be malpositioned or to be held by hand.

Modifications that have occasionally been suggested in the direct gonioscopy method consist of suspension of the microscope to lessen its weight and fixation of the light to the microscope to make it a one-handed affair. A simple suspension system consisting of a cord from the handheld binocular microscope going up over a couple of pulleys to a counterweight is simple, practical, and greatly favored by some expert gonioscopists, but is not essential, because one can readily learn to rest the elbows on the examining table, the back of a chair, or on one's knees for support and stability. It is best not to have the light attached to the microscope, in the interests of flexibility and variability of illumination.

GONIOSCOPY DURING OPERATION
Joel S. Schuman, MD, FACS

In certain cases of angle-closure glaucoma (eg, when a laser iridectomy cannot be performed or its patency is uncertain), it is impossible to tell by regular gonioscopy how much of the closure is due to permanent synechial adhesion of iris to corneoscleral TM and how much is due to a simple pressing of the iris against the meshwork without actual attachment. If extensive closure of the angle is present, it is very important in deciding the type of operation that will be most suitable to determine accurately how much of the closure is permanent and how much is functional and reversible. This is most clearly and conclusively accomplished in the operating room as a preliminary to the antiglaucoma operation itself. Under sterile conditions, a corneal paracentesis is performed, and the aqueous is drained completely, allowing sufficient time for emptying of the aqueous from the posterior chamber, through the pupil to the anterior chamber, as well as for evacuation of the anterior chamber. Then, sterile saline solution is injected through the paracentesis wound into the anterior chamber. The iris acts as a check valve against the crystalline lens to prevent saline solution from going behind the iris into the posterior chamber. The result is that the iris is no longer ballooned forward in the periphery by fluid in the posterior chamber, and the angle can become greatly widened as the anterior chamber is filled with saline solution. By gonioscopy under sterile conditions, one sees that the iris becomes closely applied to the entire front of the crystalline lens and dips into a distinct sulcus at the equator of the lens. In portions of the angle in which there are no synechiae, the angle wall is displayed in full width, with all structures clearly identifiable; but where there are peripheral anterior synechiae, the attachment of iris overlying the scleral spur and corneoscleral TM appears distinct and in unmistakable contrast.

It is preferable to hold the microscope in one hand and the light in the other with the 2 hands partially interlocked and the elbows resting on some support. While looking at the angle, it is useful to be able to vary the path of illumination, particularly when the cornea is not clear, and to be able to change from a sharp focal line in the angle to various degrees of indirect illumination by simple small changes in the position of the handheld light.

GONIOSCOPY (FINDINGS)

In this section, we will discuss variations and abnormalities that are found by gonioscopy.

Iris Contour and Character

At the start of the gonioscopic examination, one can decide whether the contour of the iris is to be characterized as slightly convex, very convex, flat, or concave (Table 7-1).

A slight convexity of the iris is seen in the majority of normal adult eyes, due to a pushing forward of the pupillary portion of the iris by the anterior surface of the lens and a slight, physiologic ballooning forward of the periphery of the

TABLE 7-1. Conditions Involving Iris Contour and Character	
Findings	**Conditions**
Slight convexity	Normal, physiologic
Excessive convexity	Hypermetropia
	Angle-closure glaucoma
Plateau iris	Angle-closure glaucoma
Flat iris	Pigmentary glaucoma
	Myopia, aphakia
Concave iris	Cyclitic membrane
	Pigmentary glaucoma
	Peripheral anterior synechiae in aphakia
Irregularity of contour	Dislocation of lens
	Cyst or tumor
	Pupillary block in aphakia
	Segmental atrophy
Segmental atrophy of iris	Previous acute glaucoma
	Herpes zoster
Pigment sprinkling	Exfoliation
	Pigmentary glaucoma
	Malignant melanoma
	Tumors or cysts of iris or ciliary body
Pigmentation abnormality	Nevus
	Heterochromic cyclitis
	Glaucomatocyclitic crises
	Hemangioma
	Neurofibroma
	Siderosis or chalcosis

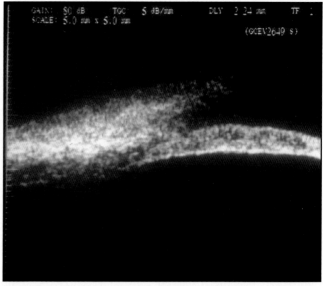

Figure 7-3. Convex iris and narrow angle in a hyperopic patient. Only mid-TM is visible, and the angle is judged to be potentially occludable. Ultrasound biomicrograph of convex iris and narrow angle. Ultrasound biomicroscopy allows high-resolution (20 to 50 μm) imaging of the anterior segment in cross-section, to a depth of approximately 4 mm.

iris caused by a physiologic difference in pressure between posterior chamber and anterior chamber. The pressure in the posterior chamber ordinarily is slightly greater than that in the anterior chamber because of a small resistance that the aqueous encounters in flowing forward through the area of contact of iris and lens en route to the pupil and anterior chamber. We have often noted that the peripheral convexity of the iris in the average eye is lost when a hole is made in the periphery of the iris. This allows aqueous to go freely from posterior to anterior chamber. The convexity also is lost when the pupil is widely dilated or when the crystalline lens is removed. A convex iris contour is seen typically in hypermetropic eyes that have a small anterior segment (Figure 7-3). If the lens is relatively large and positioned

forward, shallowing the anterior chamber axially, the resistance to flow of aqueous forward from posterior to anterior chamber is greater than normal, and this may cause the periphery of the iris to bulge forward so as to narrow or even close the angle (Figure 7-4). Beyond the central convex portion of the iris, in many eyes, a peripheral furrow or sulcus is found. The farther back the root of the iris is attached on the ciliary muscle and the shallower the axial depth of the anterior chamber, the more likely there is to be a peripheral sulcus. The peripheral sulcus develops gradually during childhood and later life, as the lens grows. No sulcus is found in infants' eyes.

A flat iris contour and, in exceptional cases, even a slight concavity, is most characteristically observed in myopia and aphakia. When the iris is flat, one should note where the plane of the iris lies in relation to the structures in the angle. In myopic and aphakic eyes, this plane generally lies well back of the level of the scleral spur. However, in other types of eyes, the plane of the iris is sometimes quite differently situated. Particularly, in the peculiar condition known as plateau iris, the root of the iris is attached close behind the scleral spur, and the plane of the iris is even further forward, sometimes at the level of the anterior TM or Schwalbe's line. This brings the peripheral iris almost against the filtration portion of the TM with little or no assistance from excess pressure of aqueous in the posterior chamber. This is the rare type of eye in which, even after an iridectomy has been performed, dilation of the pupil can cause closure of the angle and glaucoma. In such eyes, the ciliary processes can be abnormally rotated forward, in contact with the back of the iris, seemingly holding the iris forward in the periphery

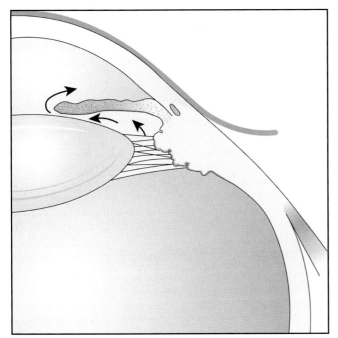

Figure 7-4. Aqueous humor is formed by the ciliary epithelium and moves between posterior iris surface and lens through the pupil and into the anterior chamber. In small hyperopic eyes, some resistance is present to flow through the pupil (relative pupillary block) that results in a slightly greater pressure in the posterior chamber than in the anterior. The result is forward iris convexity.

(Figure 7-5). In normal eyes, the ciliary processes are not in contact with the back surface of the iris.

Most emmetropic eyes demonstrate a slight iris convexity (forward) due to slight relative pupillary block. When a high degree of relative pupillary block is present, angle-closure glaucoma can ensue from the resulting forward movement of the iris into the angle.

Concavity in the iris contour may be associated with pigment dispersion syndrome and pigmentary glaucoma (Figure 7-6); old posterior uveitis, from contraction of inflammatory tissue behind the iris; or peripheral anterior synechiae in aphakic eyes.

Irregularity of iris contour in moderate degree is not necessarily abnormal. Eyes having a coarse or lacy stromal structure are particularly likely to have wave-like billows or prominences at various places in the angle, without pathologic significance or threat of angle closure. However, a large, rounded, mound-like elevation of one portion of the iris can signify a dislocation and forward tilting of the lens in that area or the presence of cyst or benign or malignant tumor of ciliary body or posterior layer of the iris. A cyst may be solitary and present in only one eye, but, more characteristically, cysts are multiple and present in both eyes. If a single isolated cyst is present, it is usually situated temporally. Often, the spaces in the iris stroma over a cyst are slightly spread apart by the stretching over the bulge, so that some of the front surface of the pigment layer can be seen.

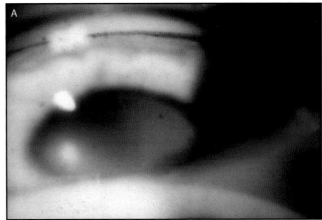

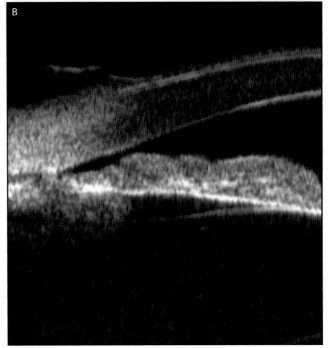

Figure 7-5. Plateau iris configuration. (A) Goniophotograph. (B) Ultrasound biomicrograph. Iris is pushed into angle by anteriorly rotated ciliary processes, causing angle closure with dilation despite the presence of a patent peripheral iridectomy in plateau iris syndrome.

Segmental atrophy of the iris with localized flattening, contrasting with a general convexity of the rest of the iris, is seen most typically in eyes that have suffered an attack of acute glaucoma with high IOP. In this condition, the atrophic, thinned area of iris has a grayish appearance. Previous herpes zoster with iritis can also cause atrophic areas in the iris but with less characteristic segmental character and gray appearance.

Pigment sprinkling on the anterior surface of the iris is recognizable and not uncommon in association with pigmentary glaucoma and exfoliation, also with malignant melanoma and other tumors and cysts of the ciliary body. Pigment sprinkling on the surface of the iris is less definite and less readily noticeable than pigmentation of the angle,

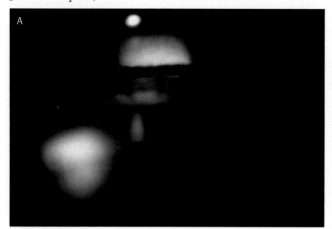

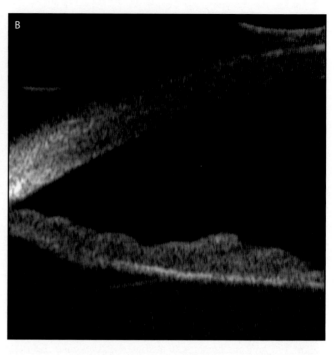

Figure 7-6. Pigmentary glaucoma. (A) Goniophotograph. (B) Ultrasound biomicrograph. Note especially concave iris configuration, particularly evident in ultrasound biomicrograph.

which will be discussed in the section "Pigment in the Angle" later in this chapter.

Abnormal pigmentation of the iris also occurs with nevi and heterochromia. Nevi are not of much significance unless they extend forward over the TM. Heterochromia of the iris is an accompaniment of heterochromic cyclitis, glaucomatocyclitic crises, hemangiomatosis, neurofibromatosis, and discoloration from intraocular copper or iron. Abnormalities of vessels of the iris and adhesions of iris to other structures are discussed in sections "Blood Vessels in the Angle" and "Peripheral Anterior Synechiae," respectively, later in this chapter. Iridodonesis is easily detectable during gonioscopy with the patient recumbent. It is common in myopia, in pigmentary glaucoma, and after rupture of lens zonules.

Angle Width

After noting the contour and character of the iris, one may estimate the width of the angle by examining the distance between Schwalbe's line and the nearest part of the iris. The angle may be described as wide, intermediate, narrow, excessively narrow, or closed (Table 7-2). Simple descriptive words are more explicitly and more widely understood than arbitrary classifications by numbers. The angle tends to be wide in normal, myopic, and aphakic eyes, but narrower in hypermetropic eyes.

The width of the angle normally varies about the circumference, anatomically usually narrowest at the 12 o'clock portion. An uncommon unevenness in width of the angle may be caused by cysts of the posterior layer of the iris or of the ciliary body, by dislocation of the lens, by tumors of the ciliary body (Figure 7-7), or by pupillary block accompanied by extensive posterior adhesions to the lens, to the vitreous, or to membranes in aphakic eyes. One sees excessive narrowing of the angle in eyes subject to angle-closure glaucoma.

Table 7-2. Conditions Reflecting Angle Width	
Findings	**Conditions**
Wide	Normal, myopia and aphakia
Intermediate width	Normal
Narrow	Hypermetropia
Excessively narrow	Angle-closure glaucoma
Closed	Angle-closure glaucoma
Irregular narrowing	Anatomical narrowing superiorly
	Subacute angle-closure glaucoma
	Dislocation of lens
	Cysts
	Posterior adhesions plus pupillary block
Irregular widening	Traumatic recession of angle
	Dislocation of lens
	Cyclodialysis

The angle is uniformly narrowed in eyes subject to severe acute attacks of angle-closure glaucoma, whereas it is narrowed less uniformly in eyes subject to subacute or chronic angle-closure glaucoma. The angle is seen to be closed in the whole circumference in an acute attack and in a part of the circumference in a subacute episode.

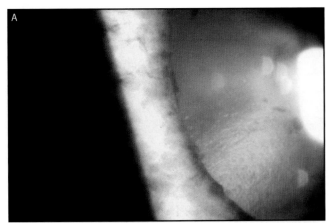
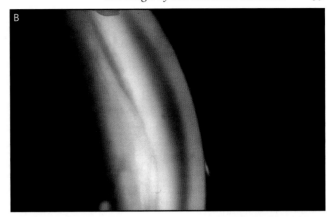

Figure 7-7. Ciliary body adenoma causing focal area of angle closure. Note smooth contour of iris elevation and heavy pigmentation of TM. (A) Slit-lamp photograph. (B) Goniophotograph.

TABLE 7-3. CONDITIONS INVOLVING THE SCLERAL SPUR	
Findings	**Conditions**
Spur all visible	Angle open
Spur hidden	Uveal meshwork
	Excessively narrow angle
	Closed angle
	Synechiae
Spur unusually prominent and white	Inflammatory exudates
	Uveal meshwork torn
	Ciliary muscle torn
	Cyclodialysis cleft

Scleral Spur

After the examiner has formed his or her opinion of the contour of the iris and the width of the angle, he or she should attempt to identify the scleral spur, because this is helpful for orientation in an open angle and also valuable in narrow angles to determine whether the angle is open back beyond the filtration portion of the TM (Table 7-3). In closed or extremely narrow angles, the scleral spur is hidden by the peripheral iris. Even in an open angle, the scleral spur is not always readily visible, for it is often covered and obscured by uveal meshwork. In a wide and open angle, the scleral spur is obscured in this way, most commonly in the nasal quadrant, where the uveal meshwork is usually most abundant. Sometimes, the uveal meshwork is abundant in the whole circumference, but there is almost always some area or portion of the angle in which uveal meshwork is thin enough and the scleral spur is sufficiently distinct so that it can be identified. Once identified, the spur can usually be traced around even in the areas in which uveal meshwork is thickest. When the scleral spur can be seen, it is recognizable as

the posterior edge of the corneoscleral TM. It is of the same whiteness as the TM and whiter than the ciliary band that extends posteriorly from the scleral spur.

If the scleral spur can be positively identified in the whole circumference at a time when the intraocular pressure (IOP) is elevated or the facility of outflow is subnormal, one can be sure that some form of open-angle glaucoma rather than angle-closure is responsible for the obstruction to outflow and elevated pressure. Rarely, the scleral spur inferiorly can be hidden by inflammatory exudates.

An abnormal whiteness, distinctness, and protrusion of the scleral spur may result from disruption of the uveal meshwork and detachment of the ciliary muscle from the scleral spur, such as is caused by blunt trauma to the eye or by surgical cyclodialysis.

Ciliary Band

The ciliary band is composed of the anterior end of the ciliary muscle where it is within gonioscopic view, extending from the root of the iris to the scleral spur, plus a variable layer of uveal meshwork and occasional strands of iris stroma overlying the muscle. The overlying uveal meshwork varies greatly in texture, density, and pigmentation, in some eyes scarcely veiling the muscle, whereas in other eyes completely hiding it behind a dense forest of brown strands. These variations are discussed further under "Uveal Meshwork." Almost always, even with the most abundant uveal meshwork, one can find some chinks or thinner places somewhere in the circumference through which to identify ciliary muscle, provided that the angle is not too narrow and that the iris is not attached abnormally far forward.

When the ciliary muscle can be seen, its color has some racial variations dependent upon the presence or absence of pigment among the muscle fibers (Table 7-4). Characteristically, in White races, with either blue or brown eyes, the ciliary muscle itself is unpigmented and appears only slightly

TABLE 7-4. CONDITIONS INVOLVING THE CILIARY BAND	
Findings	**Conditions**
Very light gray	Normal in White patients
Darker gray, traces of brown	Normal in darkly pigmented patients
Darker, slate gray	Melanoma
Whitish, cobwebby	Tear into the muscle
Scleral whiteness, cleft behind the spur	Tear through the muscle, or cyclodialysis

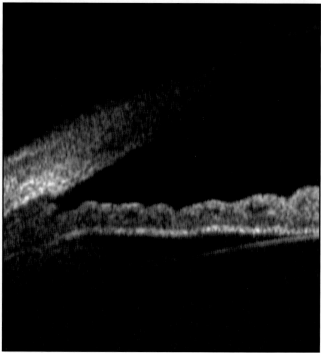

Figure 7-8. Ultrasound biomicrograph of 360-degree angle recession. Posterior displacement of the root of the iris is present with a widening of the ciliary body band. The gray veil-like tissue in the ciliary body band represents a probable previous tear into the ciliary muscle. The round black deposits on the TM represent degenerated blood elements from the original injury.

less white than the corneoscleral TM. In darkly pigmented races, the ciliary muscle usually contains an appreciable amount of melanin and has a gray appearance or may even show traces of brown deep within the tissue.

An abnormal amount of pigment in the ciliary muscle gives the ciliary band a slate-gray or dark-brown appearance that may be a clue to malignant melanoma in the ciliary body. When present in only part of the circumference, the discoloration contrasts with the color of the normal portions.

An abnormally light-gray appearance with a fine, loose, cobwebby texture, lacking the customary structure of uveal meshwork, is characteristic of a tear into the ciliary muscle. The intact muscle is nearly colorless or very slightly gray in White races, and when the muscle has been torn, the lighter appearance is presumably due to the white of sclera showing through the thinned layer of tissue.

A scleral whiteness of the ciliary band results when the full thickness of ciliary muscle has been torn off the scleral spur, exposing the sclera to gonioscopic view. Sclera may be identified not only by its color, but sometimes by the presence of penetrating branches of short anterior ciliary arteries on its inner surface. These vessels emerge from the sclera a variably short distance behind the scleral spur and run directly posteriorly out of sight behind the ciliary body.

Defects in the ciliary band after blunt trauma to the eye (Figure 7-8) often consist of a tearing apart of the ciliary muscle and the overlying uveal meshwork, sometimes associated with tearing or indirect damage to the TM, leading to glaucoma. A defect in the ciliary band is also found after surgical cyclodialysis that leaves a cleft just behind the scleral spur. The cleft following successful cyclodialysis is a bottomless tunnel going back as far as one can see; but when the operation has failed, the cleft can usually be seen to have a definite bottom where the tissues have healed together.

The level of attachment of the periphery of the iris on the ciliary muscle has a wide range of anatomic variation, and this influences the width of the ciliary band. Unusual narrowness of the ciliary band is common in congenital glaucoma. Abnormal synechial attachment of the iris to scleral

spur or to corneoscleral TM can narrow or completely hide the ciliary band. Abnormal widening of the ciliary band is usually caused by tearing of the ciliary muscle by blunt trauma or by surgical cyclodialysis. Irregularity or unevenness in width of the ciliary band that is noted as one scans the whole circumference is often a clue to abnormality, such as a tear, in the ciliary muscle, which can be discerned by close inspection.

Blood vessels and pigment on the ciliary band are discussed later in this chapter under "Blood Vessels in the Angle" and "Pigment in the Angle," and involvement in "Peripheral Anterior Synechiae" is described under that heading.

Uveal Meshwork

The uveal meshwork deserves considerable attention, not because of any known functional significance, but because proper recognition and appreciation of the character of the uveal meshwork helps one to avoid errors in identification of normal structures in the angle and particularly helps to avoid confusion with peripheral anterior synechiae that sometimes look misleadingly similar.

The uveal meshwork lines the angle from peripheral iris over ciliary band, scleral spur, and part of the TM in all eyes, but it varies greatly in thickness, pigmentation, texture, and

TABLE 7-5. CONDITIONS INVOLVING THE UVEAL MESHWORK	
Findings	**Conditions**
Homogeneous, transparent, glittering, unpigmented	Infantile
Network of grayish strands, variable amount	In blue-eyed adults
Network of brown strands, variable amount	In brown-eyed adults
Uneven pigmentation	Corresponding to uneven iris pigmentation and nevi
Greater amount nasally	Common normal finding
Disruption or defects, bearing underlying structures	Result of tear by blunt trauma or cyclodialysis
Separation of sheet or shelf	Result of blunt trauma

extent from patient to patient. It also varies remarkably with age, developing from an inconspicuous and colorless, fine, homogeneous structure in the infant to a coarse, lacy forest of brown strands in some adult eyes or to an unpigmented, fine fibrillar layer in others (Table 7-5).

In addition to the uveal meshwork, which essentially lines the angle, in some eyes, there are occasional separate, distinctive iris processes. The iris processes are long, slender, isolated strands that stand-out away from the uveal meshwork and bridge the angle from the periphery of the iris to the anterior half of the corneoscleral TM. These strands may have a remote relationship to the pectinate ligaments of animal eyes. In adults, the iris processes are pigmented or unpigmented, corresponding to the stroma of the iris. In infants, the iris processes may be present at a time when the uveal meshwork is a homogeneous undifferentiated sheet (by gonioscopy), but iris processes are usually colorless and inconspicuous at that stage. The distribution of iris processes seems to be haphazard from eye to eye and from one part of the circumference to another. The iris processes seem to have little diagnostic or pathologic significance, except that one may note that they are ruptured in association with traumatic recession of the angle, and one might speculate that they could provide the initial bridge for development of the strange iridocorneal adhesions of essential atrophy of the iris. We will say no more about iris processes and, in the rest of this section, will discuss only the uveal meshwork proper.

Incidentally, we avoid using the term *pectinate ligaments* in describing structures of the human angle, because we feel that this term is properly restricted to a specific type of structure characteristically present in the eyes of certain

animals, but not present in any closely related form in human eyes.

A good appreciation of the nature of the uveal meshwork is obtained by considering its development. At birth and during the first few months of life, in normal human eyes, the uveal meshwork can be discerned, by careful focusing of the goniomicroscope, as a smooth, delicate, homogeneous layer extending from iris periphery toward the anterior part of the TM. The infantile uveal meshwork is situated in front of the ciliary band, scleral spur, and filtration portion of the TM, but distinctly separated from them. It comes into focus a little closer to the observer than the other structures of the wall of the angle. The infant's uveal meshwork has a finely granular texture with a surface luster or glitter suggestive of ice or finely ground glass. It has no discernible holes or coarse strands in its structure, but is so delicate and transparent that the anatomical landmarks on the wall of the angle beyond are clearly seen through it. In fact, one can easily fail to notice the uveal meshwork in the infant's eye unless examining with special care.

Toward the end of the first year of life, in eyes having brown irides, there commonly develops a fine fringe of brown strands or tendrils extending from the iris forward on the face of the uveal meshwork. In eyes of darkly pigmented individuals, fine brown strands appear also at a deeper layer, at the level of the ciliary muscle.

During childhood, the uveal meshwork gradually loses its homogeneous sheet-like appearance and changes to a more lacy, open structure that appears to be composed of fibrils or strands. Through childhood, the surface generally maintains a more lustrous, reflective quality than is observed in the adult eye, in which there is much variation in the final form the uveal meshwork develops. In blue eyes, the layer of uveal meshwork that lines the angle, overlying ciliary band, scleral spur, and TM most commonly becomes a delicate grayish or colorless structure of fine strands that interferes little with the visibility of ciliary band, scleral spur, or TM. In brown eyes, it may become much more conspicuous, owing to the development of brown pigmentation of the same color as the iris stroma. The amount of pigmentation and the coarseness and density of the tissue vary even among brown eyes, in some being only a fine lacy brown network overlying the ciliary body, but in others consisting of a dense forest of coarse interlacing brown strands extending from peripheral iris to various levels on the TM, hiding ciliary band, scleral spur, and posterior portion of the TM. Most commonly, in eyes having moderate pigmentation of the iris stroma, the pigmented uveal meshwork consists of a lacy open-textured network of strands extending from iris periphery and terminating on the TM over the filtration area.

Typically, the spaces between strands of uveal meshwork in adults are coarse enough to permit the ciliary band and scleral spur to be discerned behind this meshwork. The most common form of pigmented uveal meshwork might be likened to ivy on a wall. Typically, its anterior edge on the

TM has many fine branching terminations like the tendrils that hold a vine to a wall, often with darker tiny clusters of pigment where the tendrils attach to the wall.

Appreciation of normal variations in uveal meshwork can be obtained occasionally in eyes in which pigmentation is splotchy or in which portions of the iris are blue and portions are pigmented. In such eyes, parts of the angle show the inconspicuous, fine, grayish uveal meshwork characteristic of the blue eye, while adjacent portions of the circumference show the more conspicuous brown pigmented uveal meshwork of brown eyes.

The uveal meshwork is normally avascular at all stages. However, normal vessels of ciliary body and iris are occasionally seen on the ciliary band, and pathologic new vessels sometimes grow over the angle. This is discussed in the section "Blood Vessels in the Angle."

A satisfactory firsthand examination of variations in character of uveal meshwork can be obtained in enucleated human eyes in which a 5- or 6-mm porthole has been cut out of the center of the cornea with a trephine to permit direct inspection of the angle structures. In brown eyes with extensive brown uveal meshwork extending up onto the TM, it is easy by means of a goniotomy knife to peel the uveal meshwork from its forward edge backward toward the iris. The uveal meshwork separates easily and cleanly, leaving the TM and the scleral spur unnaturally distinct. Measurement of facility of aqueous outflow by aqueous perfusion before and after coarse pigmented uveal meshwork has been dissected off the TM has shown no significant influence on facility of outflow.

Also in blue eyes, the uveal meshwork can be dissected-off as a definite, although inconspicuous, veil of tissue, and this, as in brown eyes, makes the corneoscleral TM and its scleral spur appear strikingly white and distinctly contrasting with the off-white shade of the adjacent ciliary muscle. This simulates what one sometimes sees in an eye after blunt trauma has caused tearing apart of uveal meshwork, but little disruption of ciliary muscle.

The greatest practical problem that the uveal meshwork presents is that it often misleads those who are learning gonioscopy into a mistaken diagnosis of peripheral anterior synechiae. We have seen many patients who have been referred with a description of synechiae in the angle, when the angle presented only an unusually abundant or extensive uveal meshwork. It is very important to make the correct identification, because, as will be discussed in more detail under "Peripheral Anterior Synechiae," the presence of synechiae can be a crucial factor in identifying the type of glaucoma and in determining the appropriate treatment. Experience in looking at many angles is the most valuable and effective means of gaining familiarity with the fundamental characteristics and the great variations of the uveal meshwork.

The feature that seems to be most significant in distinguishing normal tissue from acquired synechiae is a difference in apparent solidity of the tissue. The uveal meshwork in normal adult eyes regularly has the lacy, open character of a meshwork made up of many interconnected strands, with spaces and holes between; whereas peripheral anterior synechiae regularly have a more uniform, solid, and imperforate character.

Another feature that can help in distinguishing uveal meshwork from peripheral anterior synechiae is the location of radial iris blood vessels. The radial blood vessels of the iris are normally never attached forward anterior to the scleral spur, but iris vessels may be drawn abnormally forward in formation of synechiae. One must carefully distinguish dragged radial iris vessels from new-formed vessels and from loops or knuckles of large circumferentially arranged blood vessels that are not uncommonly seen on the ciliary band in the uveal meshwork and from certain other vessels to be described under "Blood Vessels in the Angle."

Defects in the uveal meshwork are seen after blunt trauma to the eye, even in cases in which no tear of the ciliary muscle is observable. These defects are noticeable in 2 forms. In one, the ciliary band has an uncommonly blank or bare appearance. If one makes a careful comparison with the other eye, especially by using gonioscopic lenses on both eyes at the same time, or if one compares various portions of the circumference, one may see that, in the damaged portion, there are broken iris processes and that the lacy uveal meshwork has been disrupted and characteristically has contracted into little clumps where its ends have remained attached. The bared ciliary muscle appears unusually pale and clean, and the scleral spur may look white and more prominent than normal. In the other form of defect in uveal meshwork from trauma, the most notable feature is a lamina or shelf of uveal meshwork stretching as a cord across one sector of the angle, with only one free edge detached and separated from the wall of the angle. This lamina may hang down in front of the ciliary band, revealing an unusually white and glistening scleral spur above and beyond it.

Finding defects in the angle that can be attributed to trauma may help to establish the cause of an otherwise puzzling monocular glaucoma or, in cases of bilateral but asymmetrical chronic open-angle glaucoma, may help to explain why the glaucoma has been so much more severe in one eye than in the other.

Trabecular Meshwork

The corneoscleral TM extends from scleral spur to Schwalbe's line. How well it can be seen and identified depends largely on how much uveal meshwork overlies and hides the scleral spur and the posterior portion of the TM (Table 7-6). Identification of the anterior edge of the TM depends upon the distinctness of Schwalbe's line. Identification is easy if scleral spur has little covering and is well-developed and distinct. Also, identification is easy if Schwalbe's line happens to be present as a prominent refractile ridge at the termination of Descemet's membrane. Otherwise, one may recognize a

TABLE 7-6. VARIATIONS IN THE TRABECULAR MESHWORK	
Findings	**Conditions**
Normal variables	Covering by uveal meshwork
	Distinctness of scleral spur
	Distinctness of Schwalbe's line
	Blood in Schlemm's canal
Characteristic feature	Filtration area finely granular, translucent, with or without pigment
Acquired abnormalities	Excessive pigment
	Inflammatory deposits
	Blood vessels
	Synechiae
	Loss of normal texture
	Traumatic rupture
Congenital abnormalities	Posterior embryotoxon
	Iridocorneal malformations

characteristic grayish, finely granular texture or sometimes a narrow band of pigment granules in the filtration portion of the TM, between the middle and posterior thirds, just anterior to the scleral spur. Even when free of pigment, the corneoscleral TM is not as white as its scleral background. It is distinguishable from sclera not only by its characteristic finely granular texture, but by a slightly translucent quality, unlike solid sclera. As an additional aid in identification, during gonioscopy, one occasionally sees blood in Schlemm's canal. One sees it as a red line or band showing through the filtration portion of the TM just anterior to scleral spur, in a part or all of the circumference. The translucent filtration portion of the TM veils the line of blood slightly but does not hide its bright redness. This has such a distinctive appearance that, from it, one can feel sure of one's orientation. Entrance of blood into Schlemm's canal is favored by low IOP and local congestion of the episcleral circulation when the pressure of the rim of the gonioscopic lens is uneven. It is common to see the blood come and go or shift into different quadrants during the examination. So far, little significance has been attached to variations in appearance of blood in the canal, except perhaps in connection with hemangioma of the lid and glaucoma.

Having identified the corneoscleral TM, one examines it particularly to assess the amount of pigment accumulated in it and the presence on it of inflammatory exudates, blood vessels, or synechiae. Each of these is of great significance in the diagnosis of different types of glaucoma, and each often also involves adjacent tissues, in addition to the TM.

However, there is a rule applying specifically to the TM that pigment and peripheral anterior synechiae cause glaucoma only when they obstruct the filtration portion of this tissue. It is, therefore, important in the gonioscopic examination to establish accurately the degree and extent to which the filtration area is involved. As we have already mentioned, the filtration area is just anterior to the scleral spur, overlying Schlemm's canal, and constitutes approximately the middle-third of the TM, appearing normally to have a slightly granular and translucent character by gonioscopic observation. It is through this portion that the aqueous humor passes on its way out. From clinical observations and experiments on enucleated eyes, we believe very little goes through the anterior third of the TM and very little goes through the scleral spur or through the ciliary band. In primary open-angle glaucoma and in glaucoma attributable to abnormal accumulation of pigment filtered out of the aqueous in the filtration portion of the TM, quantitative aqueous perfusion measurements and dissections postmortem have indicated that the principal glaucomatous obstruction lies in the filtration portion of the corneoscleral TM.

Trauma occasionally causes a splitting or circumferential rupture of TM, as though it was ripped by a momentary strong pull by the ciliary muscle on the scleral spur. When fresh, the split in the filtration portion of the TM has sharp or distinct edges, gaping slightly, but, in the course of months, the edges of the tear become rounded and less distinct. Eventually, a small trough-like depression in the meshwork is all that remains (Figure 7-9).

Congenital abnormalities affecting portions of the TM, such as posterior embryotoxon and Rieger's syndrome, are discussed principally elsewhere in this text. However, these abnormalities are also seen in adults. They consist of abnormalities in the development of the periphery of the cornea, sometimes associated with abnormal connections between the iris and cornea. The peripheral rim of Descemet's membrane is particularly involved. This rim forms the so-called Schwalbe's line at the anterior edge of the corneoscleral TM. Occasionally, it is thickened, beaded, and prominent, conspicuous both on gonioscopy and on slit-lamp examination. This condition, known as *posterior embryotoxon*, when it occurs alone, is compatible with normal functioning of the eye. However, when the iris is also involved, glaucoma may result. One finds in glaucoma from Rieger's syndrome that, along with posterior embryotoxon, the peripheral iris may be congenitally irregularly attached in sheets or strands to Schwalbe's line or that coarse ropes of refractile material bridge across the angle from the region of Schwalbe's line to the iris. The angle may in part appear to be obstructed or blanketed by the tissues that extend across the angle, and this could account for the associated glaucoma; but, even in the open portions of the angle, the TM usually does not seem to have normal texture, and the other angle structures are difficult to recognize.

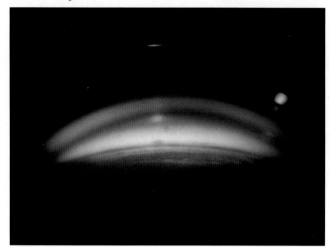

Figure 7-9. Tear in TM, an occasional result of blunt trauma to the globe. Note bright white band, the outer wall of Schlemm's canal, visible through torn TM.

Pupil and Lens

Through the gonioscopic contact lens and microscope, one can occasionally discover abnormalities of the pupil and lens that may be difficult or impossible to see from a frontal view with the slit-lamp biomicroscope.

Exfoliation often can be diagnosed by looking just behind the border of the pupil where the iris touches the lens. Not uncommonly, one can discover the pathognomonic, fine dandruff-like material hidden in this little niche, although none may be evident by frontal view on the anterior edge of the pupillary margin or on the front surface of the lens, unless the pupil is dilated. Discovery of the material of exfoliation can be a great help in establishing what type of glaucoma is present.

Posterior synechiae, between iris and lens, occasionally can be identified more definitely by looking behind the pupillary border through the gonioscopic apparatus than by viewing from in front with the slit-lamp.

Cysts of the iris at the pupillary border, such as are induced by strong miotics, are usually seen as easily by ordinary frontal view as from the gonioscopic viewpoint, because they tend principally to project into the pupil. However, occasionally, the type of cyst that develops spontaneously in the posterior pigment layer of the iris extends from the periphery to close behind the pupillary margin and is seen only with the gonioscopic apparatus. The cysts of ciliary body and posterior layer of iris that are located more peripherally usually elevate the peripheral iris in rounded mounds without disturbing the pupil. To see and positively identify this type of cyst, one must dilate the pupil widely and look in back of the iris. Typically, one or more smooth, rounded, dark-brown masses are seen between iris and lens, holding the iris forward and sometimes indenting the lens. Characteristically, a slightly glistening reflex is evident through the layer of dark-brown

pigment. The relationship of cysts of this type to glaucoma is discussed in Chapter 34.

Atrophy of the pupillary border, both the diffuse patchy-type associated with old age and with exfoliation and the type associated with segmental grey atrophy of the iris from previous very high IOP, is about as well-determined by ordinary slit-lamp biomicroscopic view as by gonioscopic view. In exceptional instances, when there is some difficulty in distinguishing between tiny pale patches of pupillary atrophy and possible exfoliation material, the decision is relatively easy from the gonioscopic view. Also, in those rare instances after a severe attack of acute angle-closure glaucoma in which the pupil is irregularly and permanently dilated in association with segmental grey atrophy of the iris, it is sometimes possible by means of the gonioscopic apparatus to find a space where the iris has actually become lifted away from the lens, providing an unimpeded path for aqueous from posterior to anterior chamber and, thus, making impossible any further attacks of angle closure.

Ectropion of the pupillary margin sometimes is correlated most conveniently during gonioscopic examination with abnormalities in the angle, particularly with peripheral anterior synechiae. Peripheral anterior synechiae and slight ectropion of the pupillary margin in the same sector are observable with all types of peripheral anterior synechiae, most strikingly with those of neovascular glaucoma and essential atrophy of the iris, suggesting that the iris stroma is pulled peripherally to the area of synechia, causing the pupillary margin to roll out slightly in the same direction.

Pigment behind the equator of the lens, where the posterior zonules attach to the lens, is well-seen in many cases of pigmentary glaucoma, if one looks through the pupil and examines this region, making use of the gonioscopic apparatus.

Dislocation of the lens in cases in which the lens has returned to an axial position may be revealed by inspection with the gonioscopic apparatus. A different level or convexity of the iris on one side compared with the other is a clue to tilting of the lens, and this may be noted when the pupil is small. When the pupil is intermediate in size, one may find, in addition, a slight tilting of the pupil and front surface of the lens. If the pupil is dilated, one may look through the pupil behind the iris. On the side on which the lens is tilted backward, one may see a rounded bulge of vitreous herniating anterior to the equator of the lens where zonules and hyaloid have been ruptured. The vitreous may hold the dilated pupil away from the lens without actually reaching the pupil where it would be visible by frontal slit-lamp view.

Ciliary Processes

One can see and examine the ciliary processes by means of gonioscopic equipment in several special conditions (Table 7-7). Sometimes, the tips of the processes can be seen when the pupil is extremely dilated, but they are more readily

TABLE 7-7. CONDITIONS INVOLVING CILIARY PROCESSES	
Findings	**Conditions**
Visible gonioscopically	In extreme mydriasis
	With cyst or tumor behind iris
	With dislocated lens
	In surgical coloboma
	In aniridia
Enlargements	Cysts, tumor
Lateral displacements	By epithelial implantation cysts
	By tumors of ciliary body
Gray covering or discoloration	Exfoliation
	Epithelialization
	Cyclitic membrane
Shrinkage and pallor	Postinflammatory atrophy
Elongated or sheet-like	Buphthalmos
Anteriorly rotated	Plateau iris, angle-closure
	Anterior choroidal separation
	After scleral buckling operation
	From adherence to limbal scar

Cysts originating in the ciliary processes and iris are readily distinguishable from implantation cysts of epithelium introduced by a penetrating traumatic or surgical wound from the outside. Both types may push aside ciliary processes as they grow and may involve the iris extensively, but implantation cysts have thin gray or translucent walls without surface pigmentation. Also, characteristically, inside an implantation cyst, one may see gray particulate debris that is partially suspended and floating about in a fluid, showing a considerable flare in a focused beam of light. Implantation cysts are accompanied by evidence of previous penetrating injury or operation, usually including injury to the lens with loss of all or a large part of the lens.

Tumors such as malignant melanoma of the ciliary body and choroid usually do not involve the ciliary processes primarily, but, by growing and expanding from locations closer to the sclera, may push a row of ciliary processes and the adjacent pars plana inward toward the lens.

Powdery, light-gray material clinging to otherwise normal-appearing ciliary processes is sometimes seen in eyes having exfoliation.

Envelopment of ciliary processes in a grayish, cobwebby cocoon may be seen in epithelialization of the anterior chamber in aphakic eyes. The epithelial membrane can be seen to have spread from a limbal wound over contiguous iris and vitreous face, often extending circumferentially in the posterior chamber on the vitreous behind the pillars of a coloboma in the iris.

Shrinkage and whitening of the ciliary processes can occur as a result of inflammation or cyclodestructive treatment. With protracted iridocyclitis, the ciliary processes may become remarkably shrunken, in extreme cases practically disappearing. At the same time, they may become whitish from a covering of cyclitic membrane. Only a low, whitish ridge may remain with no discernible individual processes. In eyes having this degree of atrophy of the ciliary body, the formation of aqueous humor is far below normal. In some such eyes, even if there is extensive obstruction of the angle by postinflammatory synechiae, the IOP may not be elevated, or, if it is elevated, it is subject to erratic variation because of precarious and uncertain balance between the effects of damage to the mechanisms of both inflow and outflow.

In infants' eyes in which the diameters of the cornea and anterior chamber have greatly enlarged as a result of abnormally high IOP, the ciliary processes tend to become elongated radially, with the rest of the ciliary body extending from them peripherally in a flattened sheet. The lens remains of normal size in buphthalmos, but the ring of ciliary body increases in diameter as the cornea and sclera stretch. Because the ciliary body is attached by the zonules to the lens, it seems that the deformed, drawn-out appearance of the processes is probably a mechanical result of the disproportion between the size of the lens and the size of the anterior segment.

seen when a cyst, tumor, or a dislocated lens holds a portion of the iris forward. They are most easily and most commonly seen through a surgical coloboma of the iris. In congenital aniridia, one sees the full extent of ciliary processes. In general, the ciliary processes have a brown irregular surface, not as dark-brown as the posterior pigment layer of the iris. Normally, the processes are uniform in size and do not hold the periphery of the iris forward.

The abnormalities that may be discovered by means of gonioscopy include cysts, tumors, discoloration, distortion, atrophy, and abnormal positioning.

Cysts of the posterior iris and ciliary body can cause a special variety of angle-closure glaucoma, and these cysts also can be a source of abnormal pigment deposition in the TM. Cysts originating in the iris have a smooth, dark-brown, rounded surface. Cysts involving the ciliary processes at times convert several adjacent processes into grotesquely enlarged structures that may push against and indent the lens, as well as push the iris forward to close the angle. Cysts of the ciliary processes are usually brown, smooth, and slightly glinting, but, in some instances, they may be unpigmented and clear.

Anterior rotation of the ciliary processes is observed infrequently and only in rather special conditions. We have seen certain instances of angle-closure glaucoma in which the iris had a plateau form, instead of the common general convexity. Even after good iridectomies were performed, angle-closure glaucoma recurred spontaneously or under the influence of a mydriatic. These angles could be reopened by miosis induced by light or medication. After iridectomy, the periphery of the iris appeared to be raised in a uniform roll or hump above the central plain of the iris, making the angle precariously narrow. The position of the ciliary processes seen through the surgical coloboma was abnormally rotated forward in a position to hold the periphery of the iris forward. Nothing else was seen to explain the peripheral elevation of the iris. The posterior chamber was otherwise ample, and the equator of the lens was well-separated from ciliary processes and iris. The condition has tended to be binocular and is an anatomical peculiarity. More recently, ultrasound biomicroscopy has confirmed the anatomic position of the ciliary processes in many additional cases of plateau iris configuration (see Figure 7-5).

Anterior rotation of ciliary processes and narrowing or closure of the angle similarly are seen in association with anterior separation of choroid and ciliary body or as a consequence of scleral buckling.

We have reproduced this condition experimentally in enucleated human eyes[3-8] and have determined by quantitative aqueous perfusion that, as the ciliary processes are made to rotate forward, the resistance to aqueous outflow increases. We have found that this effect can be induced without closure of the angle and even after the whole iris has been removed. However, with the iris intact, if the ciliary processes are made to rotate far enough forward to push the iris against the TM, this does produce angle closure with severe obstruction of aqueous outflow.

Forward rotation of the ciliary processes with obstruction of the mid- and posterior TM can have a profound effect on outflow facility, as aqueous is drained primarily through the mid- to posterior TM, with little outflow through the anterior TM. This holds true in primary angle-closure glaucoma as well. If only the anterior TM remains unobstructed, the effect on outflow facility (and IOP) can be nearly as pronounced as if the angle were closed completely.

The influence of inducing forward rotation of ciliary processes on facility of outflow is opposite to that which results when the ciliary processes are forced backward, such as by artificial deepening of the anterior chamber,[3-8] in which case the facility of outflow is increased. We postulate that, in both conditions, the abnormal position of the ciliary body exerts forces on the TM that influence the facility of flow through this tissue. In support of this belief, we find that detachment of the ciliary body from the TM or an incision made from the anterior chamber to Schlemm's canal abolishes the effect of artificial deepening of the anterior chamber.

TABLE 7-8. FINDINGS INVOLVING THE VITREOUS FACE
Findings in phakic eyes:
Rupture of peripheral hyaloid with dislocation of lens
Vitreous in antiglaucoma filtration fistula
Findings in aphakic eyes:
Adhesion of vitreous to cornea underlying bullous keratopathy
Vitreous block of pupil and iridectomy
Adhesion of vitreous to surgical wound
Epithelialization

A local distortion of ciliary processes with adhesion to a surgical scar or an amputation of ciliary processes at the site of operation is a common gonioscopic finding. These have little significance, except in cases in which ciliary processes may be seen to be plugging an intended filtration fistula, which can explain the failure of an antiglaucoma filtration operation.

Vitreous Face

The view that one can obtain of the face of the vitreous with gonioscopic equipment is often much more informative than that obtained from a frontal view with the slit-lamp biomicroscope (Table 7-8). This is so because the most significant portions are often hidden from direct frontal view, in the angle, or behind the iris, or behind an area of corneal edema.

In phakic eyes, rupture of the hyaloid commonly occurs when the eye has been hit hard enough to rupture some of the zonules of the lens. The lens may remain in the pupil, but it is usually tilted. By looking through the gonioscopic lens under the pupillary border of the iris in the space between the back of the iris and the backward-tilted lens, one may identify a rounded, colorless mass of vitreous herniating in front of the equator of the lens, showing the hyaloid, as well as the zonules, to have been ruptured.

Vitreous in an antiglaucoma filtration fistula is found occasionally by gonioscopy in phakic eyes in which the zonules of the lens and the hyaloid were inadvertently injured during surgery. A column of colorless vitreous may be seen extending forward, attached to the surgical fistula on the inside of the eye, sometimes apparently filling the opening.

In aphakic eyes, vitreous block of the pupil and iridectomy can be established only by gonioscopy. Of course, if no iridectomies were performed, the presence of pupillary block can be established by ordinary slit-lamp examination on the basis of complete filling of the pupil by bulging hyaloid associated with shallowing of the anterior chamber. If iridectomies were performed, one can reasonably infer that the iridectomies as well as the pupil are blocked, if, in addition to forward bulging of hyaloid and iris, the IOP is even slightly elevated. If there is any question of pupillary block from findings at slit-lamp examination, a gonioscopic examination is indicated. If complete iridectomy has been performed, one can examine the most peripheral portions of the coloboma and can ascertain whether the hyaloid is in a position to block the whole opening.

Often, a supposedly complete iridectomy can be seen to be not truly basal, but merely an upward enlargement of the pupil. One can see the hyaloid filling the opening completely in contact with the borders of pupil and iridectomy all around, leaving no place for unobstructed flow of aqueous from posterior to anterior chamber and establishing pupillary block.

One can establish that an eye does not have pupillary block if one can see that the vitreous face, although in contact with the lower portion of the pupil, is distinctly separated peripherally from one or both pillars of the coloboma. When one can see that the hyaloid curves normally backward behind the ciliary processes, with a definite space separating the hyaloid from one or both edges of the coloboma in the iris, one can be sure that there is an unobstructed opening for flow of aqueous from the posterior to the anterior chamber. This is what is usually found when iridectomy is truly basal.

If surgical peripheral iridectomy has been performed and vitreous is blocking the iridectomy as well as the pupil, one can identify the slightly glistening hyaloid filling the peripheral hole in the iris, provided that the anterior chamber is not too shallow at the time of examination. Normally, without block, when one examines a peripheral iridectomy, the hole in the iris appears completely unobstructed. If the hole is large enough, one may see normal ciliary processes and may be able to identify the hyaloid further posteriorly.

In aphakic eyes, adhesion of vitreous to the surgical wound may or may not be associated with pupillary block or with edema of the adjacent cornea. Most commonly, a slightly gray and sometimes glistening thin sheet of hyaloid, obviously continuous with the hyaloid in the pupillary portion of a surgical coloboma of the iris, extends forward to where it is caught in the inner lips of the wound. This does not necessarily cause trouble. Exceptionally, one sees a broad sheet of hyaloid and the adjacent pillars of the surgical coloboma of the iris caught and held in the wound, usually because of loss of vitreous at surgery. If the whole pupil and coloboma are sealed by the sheet of hyaloid and there is no patent peripheral iridectomy, pupillary block is almost certain. In these particular circumstances, with pupil and hyaloid updrawn, the anterior chamber may not become so conspicuously shallowed axially as in other forms of pupillary block; but, interiorly, the angle may be seen to be closed, and, as usual, glaucoma results.

Epithelial invasion of the eye is seen advantageously with gonioscopic equipment. With rare exceptions, it occurs in eyes with all or most of the lens missing. Epithelium enters the eye by way of a surgical or traumatic wound, usually in the angle of the anterior chamber. By slit-lamp, the ingrowing epithelium appears as a thin gray membrane resembling ground glass, extending onto the hyaloid and iris and usually onto the back surface of the cornea from the region of the wound. Epithelialization has to be differentiated from the following abnormalities:

- Corneal scar that is stationary
- Remnants of capsule that have a characteristic coiled and refractile appearance
- Corneal edema caused by pupillary block and adhesion of vitreous to cornea that can be identified gonioscopically
- Inflammatory membranes that tend to be more opaque

An epithelial sheet tends to be more homogeneous than other membranes. Confusion with fibrovascular or neovascular membranes is unlikely, because the membrane of epithelialization is avascular.

In epithelialization, the membrane is very thin, translucent, and gray. By transillumination with the slit-lamp, it has a finely granular appearance, resembling ground glass. The advancing edge on the back of the cornea is usually slightly thickened and forms a slight ridge. By gonioscopy, the epithelial sheet may be seen to extend from the wound indiscriminately onto all contiguous structures of the anterior segment. If the hyaloid and iris pillars have been caught in the surgical scar, the epithelial membrane may be observed to grow down, sealing the face of vitreous and iris together and causing pupillary block when the pupil has been sealed completely. On the surface of the iris, the advancing edge of epithelium is less obvious than it is on the hyaloid, but one can distinguish the epithelial membrane on the face of the iris by an appearance of smoothness and slight glistening of the surface not seen in the unaffected normal areas. If hyaloid and iris are not caught in the wound, the pupil is not so readily blocked by spread of the sheet of epithelium, which may develop into a thicker, grayer membrane on iris and hyaloid before it causes glaucoma by obstructing the angle itself. With an open coloboma of the iris, the epithelium may extend posteriorly to form a gray cocoon, enveloping the ciliary processes, with delicate cobwebby gray sheets on the adjacent vitreous face.

Gonioscopic distinction of epithelialization from inflammatory membrane involving remnants of hyaloid or lens remnants presents the greatest difficulty, and one may have to rely upon observing characteristic progressive spread to identify epithelialization. If a leaking fistula in the wound and hypotony are present, these strongly favor the diagnosis of epithelialization.

Blood Vessels in the Angle

Normal vessels in the angle vary greatly from eye to eye in different individuals, but certain characteristics permit one to distinguish the normal from the abnormal with reasonable certainty. To become familiar with the characteristics and identity of the vessels visible by clinical gonioscopy in normal eyes, it is worthwhile to review the anatomy of the blood supply of the anterior segment.

In the human eye, the principal arterial source for the structures of the angle is the arterial circle of the ciliary body. This "circle" is formed by the joining of long posterior ciliary arteries and anterior ciliary arteries, mostly within the ciliary muscle. The long posterior ciliary arteries come forward on the inner surface of the sclera, one nasally and one temporally. These each divide in the anterior segment of the globe into branches that arch and run circumferentially in the ciliary body. The anterior ciliary arteries enter the globe anteriorly from the outer surface. The anterior ciliary arteries have a distinctive, conspicuously sinuous or serpentine form on the outer surface of the sclera, and they typically enter the globe abruptly via small pits in the sclera known misleadingly as emissaries. These entrances are scattered at varying distances from the limbus, usually between 1 and 4 mm. The anterior ciliary arteries penetrate the sclera to the ciliary muscle and join the arching branches of the long posterior ciliary arteries there.

The arterial circle in the ciliary muscle is actually irregular, rarely a true uniform circle. The segments of which the circle is formed are wandering and usually not continuous in the circumference. The nasal and the temporal halves in particular tend to be separate. From this arterial circle and from its tributary posterior and anterior ciliary arteries arise fine branches that supply the ciliary muscle and larger branches, which become the radial arteries of the iris.

The arterial circle of the ciliary body, as a rule, is posterior to the periphery of the iris. The radial arteries of the iris generally extend forward a short distance from their origin in the arterial circle to the peripheral fold or knuckle of the pigment layer of the iris. There, they turn and extend in the stroma of the iris in the direction of the pupil. The radial arteries in the stroma of the iris appear by gonioscopic view much as they do by slit-lamp, their visibility being influenced by the thickness and degree of pigmentation of the stroma. They have a variable corkscrew form, influenced by the size of the pupil. They tend to go directly to the region of the pupil, and the returning veins tend to radiate similarly directly to the periphery, where they turn posteriorly around the peripheral fold or knuckle of the pigment layer of the iris to pass into the ciliary processes and back to choroid and vortex veins.

Normal radial iris vessels can be seen to have a covering of iris stroma and characteristically conform to a radial pattern, with little tendency to branch, anastomose, or wander diagonally. When the eye is inflamed or the IOP is elevated, the normal radial vessels tend to enlarge and become more noticeable.

In the human eye, there is no arterial circle of the iris; and in most eyes, the arterial circle of the ciliary body is not visible by gonioscopy. Occasionally, however, portions of the arterial circle of the ciliary body are situated uncommonly far forward on the surface of the ciliary muscle and may be seen anterior to the root of the iris on the ciliary band. Sometimes, the artery encroaches on the root of the iris at its juncture with the ciliary band.

Characteristically, only short segments of the artery come into gonioscopic view in this way, and these always have an obviously circumferential direction. Typically, such circumferential vessels are seen in profile and suggest in appearance a sea serpent with an undulating form, the anterior portion of some of the loops being in view and the posterior portions out of view below the level of attachment of iris on the ciliary muscle. The extent to which anteriorly wandering loops of circumferential artery are visible gonioscopically is affected in part by the thickness and degree of pigmentation of the uveal meshwork and iris stroma. Vessels of this type tend to be most conspicuous in eyes in which the superficial tissues are thin and unpigmented and are least noticeable when the covering tissues are thick and dark brown.

Normal circumferential vessels on the ciliary band never attach anterior to the scleral spur. However, a knuckle of vessel carrying uveal meshwork or strands of iris stroma occasionally protrudes from the surface of the angle sufficiently far forward in the angle to stand in front of the scleral spur and TM, locally obscuring these from direct gonioscopic view, but not in contact with the TM, as can be determined by viewing the angle slightly tangentially.

In addition to the normal radial vessels of the iris and wandering portions of the circumferential artery of the ciliary body, a third type of vessel is seen occasionally in normal human angles (ie, vertical vessels deep in the ciliary band), probably the anterior ciliary arteries, extending from the interior surface of the sclera, from an emissary passage, to the arterial circle in the ciliary muscle. These deep vertical vessels against the sclera are visible in the ciliary band in eyes that are lightly pigmented and have thin, fairly transparent uveal meshwork. One must look through the uveal meshwork and ciliary muscle to see them. These same vessels are sometimes laid bare to gonioscopic view as a result of traumatic disruption of the overlying uveal meshwork and ciliary muscle, the so-called traumatic recession of the angle. They are not normally bare or near the inner surface of the angle.

In rare instances in normal eyes, we have seen what appeared to be an anterior ciliary artery on the inner surface of the ciliary band extending straight forward, without branching, to disappear abruptly into the sclera, usually just behind the scleral spur, but once or twice into or just anterior to the spur, with no evidence of connection with Schlemm's canal (ie, no blood in the canal).

Two varieties of abnormal, newly formed vessels are distinguishable in the angle:

1. Neovascularization associated with vascular retinopathy secondary to occlusion of the central retinal vein or artery, diabetes, Eales' disease, or extraocular arteriovenous fistula.

2. Neovascularization associated with chronic iridocyclitis or cyclitis, especially with heterochromic cyclitis.

The vessels of neovascularization of the angle that are associated with vascular retinopathy appear to be of the same sort in the several different types of retinopathy, but to differ appreciably from the new vessels of chronic iridocyclitis. In association with the retinal vascular diseases listed above, new vessels grow from the circumferential artery of the ciliary body onto the surface of the iris and onto the surface of the wall of the angle. On the iris, these vessels are seen to take an erratic, meandering course, without either the distinct radial or the circumferential direction that is characteristic of the normal vessels. The new vessels also are distinguished from the normal by the fact that they grow on the surface of the iris, not within the stroma. They usually are not connected with the normal stromal vessels.

Neovascularization of the iris in some cases conspicuously involves the portions of the iris visible by slit-lamp, producing so-called rubeosis. Less frequently, new vessels extend in the form of a fibrovascular membrane onto the pupil itself, onto the surface of the lens, or onto pupillary membranes of other sorts.

In some cases, neovascularization is restricted to the angle, at least at an early stage, and is detectable only by gonioscopy. In the angle, one sees vessels extending from the juncture of iris and ciliary band onto the periphery of the iris and up the wall of the angle. On the wall, the vessels grow vertically forward over the ciliary band and scleral spur onto corneoscleral TM, where they arborize and often appear to dip into the filtration portion of the meshwork as though to Schlemm's canal. Usually, there are multiple arborizing vessels.

Newly formed vessels are readily distinguishable from the rare solitary, unbranching anomalous vessel from ciliary band to TM. New vessels are also different from vessels associated with congenital abnormalities of the angle, which consist of knuckles or hairpin loops of radial iris vessels, tented forward and unbranching.

New blood vessels on the angle wall, and also those on the iris, are accompanied by a transparent sheet of fibrous tissue that cannot be seen by gonioscopy or by slit-lamp biomicroscopy. The fibrous sheet does not noticeably hide underlying angle structures from view, yet, presumably, it is this transparent sheet between the vessels, rather than the slender vessels themselves, which obstructs the filtration portion of the TM and interferes severely with aqueous outflow, causing the disastrous form of glaucoma known as neovascular or hemorrhagic glaucoma. In this type of glaucoma, the IOP can become greatly elevated when nothing is visible by gonioscopy on the TM but the arborizing new vessels. The fibrovascular membrane is demonstrable only histologically.

The neovascularized angle associated with vascular retinopathy usually does not long remain as described above, but tends to go through the following stages. Some of the vertical, newly formed vessel trunks lining the wall of the angle from iris root to TM tend to enlarge and to stand out from the angle wall as stout columns. Along the sides of these vascular columns, the iris appears to be pulled forward until tents of iris stroma reach the TM. From these initial points of attachment, the iris becomes progressively more widely adherent to the TM, both circumferentially and anteriorly, until the whole angle may be closed far forward by peripheral anterior synechiae. The layer of fibrovascular tissue that first grew on the angle wall becomes sandwiched in the adhesion between iris and wall of the angle. At this stage, the vessels on the surface of the iris can be seen to enter and disappear at the point of juncture of iris and angle wall. Later, the membrane on the front of the iris may contract and cause extensive ectropion uveae at the pupil.

The character of vascularization of the angle in neovascular glaucoma associated with retinopathy appears to be the same whether it is associated with diabetic retinopathy or is secondary to occlusion of the central retinal artery or vein or other vascular retinopathy.

The other type of neovascularization of the angle that is associated with heterochromic or other chronic iridocyclitis appears to differ in some fundamental way. Both types of neovascularization cause obstruction of the TM and induce glaucoma that is resistant to medical treatment, owing to formation of a membrane over the TM, but the membrane associated with vascular retinopathy has a great tendency to induce peripheral anterior synechiae or synechial closure of the angle, whereas the membrane associated with neovascularization of chronic iridocyclitis does not. Both types of membranes are transparent and are not ordinarily discernible by gonioscopy, although they are demonstrable histologically. Occasionally, however, in eyes that have a cuticular membrane covering the angle, comparison made with a contralateral normal eye produces the impression that the angle structures have a less distinct appearance in the affected eye than in the normal.

In Fuchs' heterochromic cyclitis, the vessels appear to be finer, fewer, and more solitary and have less tendency to arborize on the TM than vessels associated with neovascular glaucoma secondary to vascular retinopathy. The fine solitary vessels found in the angle in heterochromic cyclitis have a tendency to wander apparently aimlessly over all the angle structures, circumferentially as well as radially, whereas those associated with vascular retinopathy cross the angle only in a direct radial manner. The vessels in heterochromic cyclitis have a characteristic tendency to bleed easily, either spontaneously or as a consequence of abrupt lowering of the IOP by paracentesis or other operation. The amount of bleeding typically is small, detectable by microscopic examination of a sample of aqueous, or visible gonioscopically as a fine line of blood squirting from the vessel on the angle wall to form a tiny hyphema, which may be visible only gonioscopically. In heterochromic cyclitis, abnormal vessels may also be found in eyes that do not develop glaucoma.

In rare instances, in otherwise normal eyes, a solitary vessel is seen extending from the ciliary band forward, crossing the scleral spur, and disappearing into the corneoscleral TM just anterior to the scleral spur. Although the vessel disappears in the region of Schlemm's canal, no blood has been observed in the canal in such eyes. Such vessels may possibly be aberrant anterior ciliary arteries. They have no branchings on the TM or on the ciliary band.

Normally, all vessels in the angle are restricted to the ciliary band and iris and do not go as far forward as the scleral spur or TM.

Congenitally abnormal vessels are seen in cases of congenital glaucoma, in which the iris stroma is abnormally knuckled forward in the periphery. Exceptionally, there is also a forward bend or knuckling of the radial vessels of the iris, which may go anterior to the level of the scleral spur. In cases of embryotoxon and of Axenfeld's syndrome, such vascular loops sometimes extend even as far forward as Schwalbe's line. The arch or loop form of the vessels, which may approximate the shape of a hairpin, and the accompanying iris stroma serve to distinguish these congenital abnormally placed vessels from those of neovascularization. The vessels of neovascularization typically have one end at the root of the iris and the other ending in fine branches on the TM, whereas the congenitally looped vessels have both ends in the iris and do not arborize on the angle wall.

In association with persistent hyperplastic primary vitreous in infants, one may see a vessel taking a bizarre course from behind the iris through the pupil, bending sharply around the pupillary border and extending across the surface of the iris to the ciliary band.

In conclusion, one can make the following generalizations concerning vessels in the angle. No pathologic significance is attached to radial vessels seen within the iris stroma, sea-serpent type circumferential vessels seen in the angle in the periphery of the iris or against the ciliary band, or short, straight vessels seen deep in the ciliary muscle and disappearing below the scleral spur. However, vessels that have an erratic course on the surface of the iris without either distinct radial or circumferential direction and vessels that extend up the angle wall beyond the scleral spur to the TM are, with rare exceptions, pathologic.

Pigment in the Angle

In evaluating pigment in the angle, one must distinguish pigment that is deposited in the angle from the brown uveal meshwork that is normally present in many eyes. This distinction is readily made on the basis of the location, form, and color of the pigment. Brown uveal meshwork typically occurs in the form of strands or a network of strands, often extending across the ciliary band and scleral spur onto the posterior half of the corneoscleral TM. Deposited pigment, which has been carried by the aqueous to the TM, is characteristically located in a band overlying Schlemm's

canal in the filtration portion of the meshwork, roughly in its middle third. Occasionally, pigment may also be indiscriminately scattered on the back of the cornea, on Schwalbe's line, and on other structures, particularly in the lower angle. Deposited pigment, either that in the filtration portion of the TM or that which is indiscriminately scattered, characteristically has a finely granular appearance and is brown or black, like the pigment of the posterior pigment layer of the iris, distinctly darker than the brown of the iris stroma (Table 7-9).

Through infancy and childhood, the TM remains completely clean of pigment deposits, but, during adult life, there is commonly a gradual, slight accumulation of pigment in the TM, faintly delineating the filtration area overlying Schlemm's canal. In advanced years, a distinct, fine, granular brown band of pigment commonly accumulates in the TM. The slender band of deposited pigment in elderly people is usually most evident in the nasal quadrant, where the uveal meshwork also tends to be most pronounced. In some such normal eyes, the faint but definite band extends also into the lower and upper nasal quadrants. However, with rare exceptions, the temporal quadrant remains clean in normal eyes.

Pigment deposition in a solid band in the whole circumference is, in almost all instances, pathologic. The denser and broader the band, the more likely it is to be pathologic. In an elderly patient, when excessive pigment deposition is seen in the angle, the first suspicion is exfoliation, which can readily be looked for under the pupillary border where the gonioscope reveals fine light-gray flecks of material that look like dandruff.

In young individuals, before the age of nuclear sclerosis, excessive pigment in the TM first suggests pigmentary glaucoma, in which there is degeneration of the posterior pigment layer of the iris toward the mid-periphery and no dandruff-like exfoliation. This occurs most commonly in association with myopia in young males and is usually, but not always, accompanied by abnormal deposition of pigment on the back of the cornea. In this condition, transillumination of the globe typically shows abnormal transillumination of the pigment layer of the iris in a patchy annulus in the mid-periphery, with no discernible abnormality of the stroma of the iris.

Although excessive pigment deposition in the TM seems both clinically and experimentally to obstruct aqueous outflow and cause glaucoma, not every eye having excessive pigment in the angle is glaucomatous. One sees occasional instances of Krukenberg spindle pigment on the back of the cornea, with heavy deposition of pigment in the whole angle, with normal pressure and normal facility of outflow. It may be that the size of pigment particles can differ enough and be sufficiently critical to influence significantly the degree of obstruction. We suppose that if the particles are large enough they may stay on the surface rather than penetrate into the deeper portion of the TM and may, therefore, fail to

Pigment in the Angle	Conditions
None	Normal in young
Band nasally and inferiorly	Normal in elderly
Faint band, whole circumference	Normal in elderly
Dense band, whole circumference, both eyes	Exfoliation
	Pigmentary glaucoma
	Pigment dispersion syndrome
Dense band, whole circumference, one eye	Exfoliation
	Malignant melanoma
	Cysts or tumors of iris or ciliary body
Scattered, mostly in lower angle	Previous intraocular surgery
	Previous inflammation
	Previous hyphema
Patchy band, whole circumference	Occasional in open-angle glaucoma
Dense isolated patch	Nevus
Light-brown, very fine pigment	From brown iris stroma
Dark-brown fine granular pigment	From posterior pigment layers
Black, fine and coarse, balls and granules	Old blood

TABLE 7-9. CONDITIONS INVOLVING PIGMENT IN THE ANGLE

plug the channels in the presumably most critical endothelial layer next to Schlemm's canal. Differences in trabecular endothelial cell response to the pigment may also be important. Presumably, phagocytosis of the pigment by trabecular endothelium can unplug the outflow channel. We have perfused homologous pigment into the outflow pathways of living monkeys and produced the expected temporary obstruction to aqueous outflow. Despite repeated pigment perfusions, however, outflow facility always returned to normal values in these monkeys.[9] Thus, it seems that, in pigmentary glaucoma, there must be other abnormalities in addition to pigment particle liberation and that it may be the trabecular cell response to pigment, rather than the pigment itself that results in the reduction of outflow facility.

When excessive pigmentation of the filtration portion of the angle occurs in only one eye of a patient, this suggests exfoliation as a first possibility. The pigmentation in exfoliation tends to be coarser and more of a salt and pepper pattern than the uniform, fine pigmentation seen in pigment dispersion. This may relate to the mechanism of pigment release, with pigment dispersion syndrome typically resulting from ballottement of the posterior iris against the zonules and pigment release in pseudoexfoliation coming from rubbing of the iris against the abnormally roughened anterior lens capsule. Otherwise, asymmetrical pigmentation suggests cysts of iris or ciliary body or malignant melanoma in the ciliary body or iris, which can cause shedding of pigment that comes forward and becomes enmeshed in the TM, sometimes enough to cause glaucoma.

Pigment that is coarser and scattered indiscriminately in tiny clumps of varied sizes in the dependent portion of the angle, concentrated along Schwalbe's line, and rather diffusely dirtying the TM without selective concentration in the filtration portion is a common finding after intraocular surgery or inflammation and does not necessarily produce glaucoma. Similar indiscriminately scattered pigment that is black, varying from fine to coarse, and especially in the form of small balls is characteristic of previous hyphema and presumably consists of the decomposition products of blood (Figure 7-10).

In eyes having open-angle glaucoma, we have occasionally seen a small amount of pigment in the filtration portion of the TM in a conspicuously patchy distribution in the whole circumference, but we have not seen this in completely normal eyes. The appearance suggests to us that, in such eyes, this patchy distribution may be caused by irregular pathologic alteration of the TM. This is possibly a manifestation of increased resistance and less-than-normal flow of aqueous through those areas that are white, with most of the flow restricted to the adjacent areas in which the accumulation of pigment indicates that aqueous has been undergoing filtration. A number of alternate explanations occur to us, but all are conjectural, and not worth detailing at this time.

After laser trabeculoplasty, the TM may take on a variegated appearance, with intermittent areas of pigmentation and whitening. It is not known whether the white areas represent laser-damaged tissue that is no longer filtering or areas stimulated by the laser treatment to be cleared of pigment.

Inflammatory Deposits in the Angle

In association with intraocular infection, inflammation, or rarely, tumor,[10] *hypopyon* is commonly detectable by ordinary examination with a flashlight or slit-lamp, but, occasionally, a hypopyon is so small and so peripherally situated that it is detectable only by gonioscopy. When one inspects a hypopyon with the gonioscope, one sees a blanket of whitish inflammatory exudate extending from peripheral iris over the angle structures, filling in the angle and hiding the angle structures to a variable degree, with considerable resemblance to a snowdrift. A hypopyon characteristically is associated with obvious cellular reaction in the aqueous and most commonly is restricted to the lower quadrant of the angle, as a result of the cells settling to the lowest portion. This is often

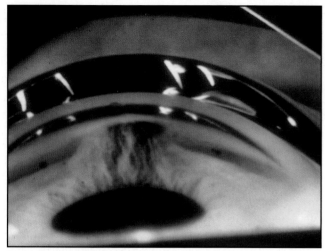

Figure 7-10. Round black balls in angle represent old blood, most likely secondary to blunt trauma.

the case in intraocular infections, more rarely in simplex keratitis, occasionally in spontaneous lysis and leakage of hypermature cataracts, and in cases of retained cortex after extracapsular extraction or traumatic cataract. In such cases, inflammatory cells may be present and demonstrable histologically in the TM in the whole circumference in sufficient quantity to obstruct aqueous outflow and cause glaucoma, yet not of sufficient density to be discernible gonioscopically except in the lower quadrant. However, in rare instances, we have seen a complete blanketing of the angle in the whole circumference by inflammatory exudate accompanied by severe glaucoma. In one patient, who a short time later died of acute pneumococcal septicemia, the angle of each eye was completely blanketed, and IOPs were in the 80s. Histologically, the TM was densely infiltrated, as well as completely covered by inflammatory cells. There were no synechiae.

Inflammatory precipitates on the TM in the form of keratic precipitates (KPs) are far less obvious than hypopyon in the angle and are easily overlooked, unless one has them specifically in mind during examination of the angle. KPs on the TM are apparently the same as KPs on the back of the cornea, consisting of discrete clumps of inflammatory cells, but, in certain cases, KPs are detectable in the angle when none are found on the cornea and when there is no evidence of inflammation by slit-lamp. This condition occurs especially in sarcoidosis. The discovery of KP by careful gonioscopy can provide the most important clue for explaining the basis for a puzzling case of glaucoma.

KPs on the TM are sometimes very inconspicuous. They consist of small gelatinous-looking, colorless mounds, projecting into the anterior chamber from the surface of the TM. They resemble KPs seen on the cornea, but generally are broader and flatter. They may be confluent, making a continuous line of exudate over 2, 3, or 4 hours of the clock. Their presence is most readily revealed by their projection

from the surface, which is notable because, by gonioscopic view, they are seen mainly in profile (Figure 7-11).

Occult KPs in the angle can simulate primary open-angle glaucoma if not properly diagnosed. Proper detection and treatment are essential, as a paradoxical response to treatment can result if KPs on the TM are not suspected. For example, in this setting, pilocarpine can cause a dramatic elevation in IOP, while topical steroid therapy can be curative.

Peripheral Anterior Synechiae

The term *peripheral anterior synechia* (PAS) signifies a condition in which the iris has become attached further forward in the angle than normal. The abnormal forward attachment may extend to anterior portions of the ciliary band, to the scleral spur, to corneoscleral TM, to Schwalbe's line, or, in some instances, even to the cornea. Peripheral anterior synechiae are a complication of many ocular conditions and may develop in various ways (Table 7-10). Their presence and special characteristics are significant in differential diagnosis in certain instances, but their principal importance is that they can interfere with aqueous outflow if they obstruct a significant portion of the TM and can cause IOP to become elevated.

In open-angle glaucoma that is not associated with intraocular inflammation, PAS do not occur, unless the original disease is complicated by some additional disease, such as occlusion of the central retinal vein, or by surgery or laser therapy. Following laser trabeculoplasty, it is not uncommon to see small, irregular PAS to the level of scleral spur and occasionally to posterior TM in the areas of treatment. Rarely, extensive PAS with accompanying significant obstruction to outflow may be observed.

We have seen no exception to the rule that PAS are never found in uncomplicated primary open-angle glaucoma, in open-angle glaucoma associated with exfoliation, or in pigmentary glaucoma (except after laser therapy).

If a definite PAS is seen in a case of supposedly primary open-angle glaucoma, it most commonly is the result of previous surgery or is a manifestation of neovascular glaucoma due to occlusion of the central retinal vein. If a definite PAS is present but there is no supporting evidence of neovascular glaucoma or previous operation, then the diagnosis must be changed to some form of secondary glaucoma, most often due to KP in the angle.

The most common mistake leading to an erroneous diagnosis of PAS is to confuse normal uveal meshwork with acquired synechial attachment of iris to angle wall. Both normal uveal meshwork, pigmented or unpigmented, and peripheral anterior synechiae are found in similar locations, overlying ciliary band, scleral spur, and corneoscleral TM, but uveal meshwork and PAS have definite distinguishing characteristics that one can recognize gonioscopically. As already described in a previous section on "Uveal

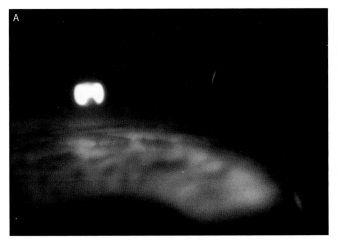
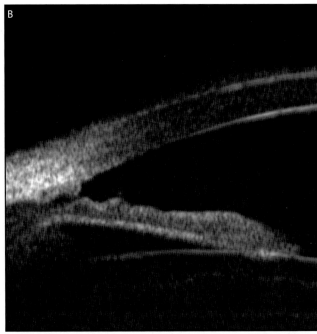

Figure 7-11. Inflammatory precipitates in angle. (A) Goniophotograph. (B) Ultrasound biomicrograph. Precipitates are gelatinous and amorphous in appearance and can be very difficult to distinguish. Ultrasound biomicroscopy enables quantification of precipitate dimensions and facilitates follow-up. Typically, such precipitates are exquisitely sensitive to topical steroid therapy.

TABLE 7-10. Variations in Peripheral Anterior Synechiae	
Conditions	Findings
Primary open-angle glaucoma	Never synechiae in these glaucomas, so long as uncomplicated by other disease or by operation
Exfoliation with glaucoma	
Pigmentary glaucoma	
Heterochromic cyclitis with glaucoma	Synechiae to all levels, but not to cornea, and not bridging angle structures
Angle-closure glaucoma	
Absence or excessive shallowing of the anterior chamber after surgery	Synechiae to all levels, sometimes to cornea, after surgery sometimes bridging angle
Iris bombé in phakic or aphakic eyes	Same as above
Glaucoma secondary to iridocyclitis or KPs on the TM	Typically tents and columns to all levels, but not to cornea
Neovascular glaucoma	Broad synechiae to full width of angle, with new vessels
Essential atrophy of the iris	Synechiae advancing on the cornea, sometimes obstructing TM
Chandler's syndrome of atrophy of stroma of iris with corneal endothelial dystrophy and edema	Synechiae advancing irregularly on corneoscleral meshwork, later to cornea
After laser trabeculoplasty	Small irregular synechiae to scleral spur, occasionally to posterior TM
KPs: keratic precipitates; TM: trabecular meshwork.	

Meshwork," this tissue in adult eyes is present normally in the angle in amounts and densities varying from a thin, delicate, colorless veil in some blue eyes to a thick brown forest of strands in some brown eyes, but it always has a lacy structure composed of a network of strands with discernible openings and is porous in appearance. The strands may extend individually vertically up the wall of the angle, or they may be part of a lacy sheet extending from peripheral iris to the angle wall. Transillumination, with the light turned just to one side or other of the field of view, so that it illuminates the white scleral background and displays pigmented structures in the angle in contrast as dark against the bright background, can be used in some brown eyes to demonstrate the porosity of the uveal meshwork especially well. Not uncommonly in brown eyes, the uveal meshwork presents a network of fine strands that is more extensive where it overlies the mid-portion of the TM than where it crosses the ciliary muscle band. Tiny feet or dots of darker brown are often evident at the anterior edge of a fringe of brown lacy uveal meshwork on the TM.

True PAS differ from uveal meshwork in being more solid and in being definitely composed of iris stroma. Synechiae take numerous characteristic forms, ranging from tiny tent-like adhesions to complete closure of the angle. The type of PAS is related to the variety of disease that has caused the formation of the adhesion. This is worth special attention as an aid in differential diagnosis.

True acquired PAS are seen in the following conditions:

- Angle-closure glaucoma
- After prolonged absence of the anterior chamber after intraocular surgery
- After laser trabeculoplasty
- After iris bombé in both phakic and aphakic eyes
- In certain forms of glaucoma due to intraocular inflammation
- In iridocorneal endothelial (ICE) syndromes
- After injury to the eye

In instances in which PAS are attached to the cornea anterior to Schwalbe's line, as in certain cases of ICE syndrome or after iris bombé either in phakic or aphakic eyes, the PAS may be readily detected by slit-lamp examination. In other cases, the diagnosis must be made by gonioscopy.

One of the most significant features to determine gonioscopically is whether the PAS are in a position to obstruct the filtration portion of the TM, just anterior to the scleral spur, approximately the central third of the TM directly overlying Schlemm's canal, the portion in which pigment particles become trapped as the aqueous is filtered on its way out of the eye. Extension of PAS onto the anterior third of the TM is of little additional significance. Probably very little aqueous goes through the anterior third of the TM.

In angle-closure glaucoma, identification of peripheral anterior synechiae is important. If the angle is examined between attacks and is found to be hazardously narrow, but open, the diagnosis may remain uncertain, but if true residual synechiae are identifiable, this strongly substantiates the diagnosis. However, in angle-closure glaucoma, it may be very difficult to be sure in the unoperated eye whether an area of closure represents simple contact of iris with TM or is actual synechial closure. If, in surveying the angle, one finds an abrupt transition from clearly open angle to adjacent definitely closed angle, there is a strong probability that the closure is synechial, but one cannot be certain. In eyes in which there is no pigment line delineating the filtration portion of the corneoscleral meshwork and the angle is so narrow that the scleral spur cannot be seen, it may be difficult to estimate how much of the filtration area is covered and whether it is by simple contact or by synechiae.

In these situations, use of the Zeiss lens for indentation gonioscopy is most informative. As mentioned previously, simple placement of the Zeiss lens on the cornea commonly indents the cornea and displaces aqueous humor posteriorly; this can be accentuated by deliberate posterior movement of the lens on the cornea. The iris is observed to be bowed posteriorly, and areas of previous iris-angle appositional closure can be observed to open under the influence of the indentation lens. Alternatively, definite peripheral anterior synechiae can be identified as areas of continued adherence of iris to angle wall despite the indentation. However, for the latter, substantial displacement of the iris should be observed during the indentation process. Often, good indentation cannot be performed when the IOP is high. One can be more certain of PAS with this method when there is an abrupt transition from deep open angle to localized synechiae. It is often easier to diagnose the absence rather than the presence of PAS with this technique. The absence of PAS with indentation gonioscopy does not rule out chronic appositional angle-closure glaucoma.

In angle-closure glaucoma, episodes of closure of the angle by contact eventually lead to synechial closure. The duration of closure by contact necessary to cause synechial closure appears to vary greatly from patient to patient. The congested eye appears to form synechiae more quickly than the quiet eye. However, there are exceptions to this rule. Eyes have been observed in which the angle opened completely after an acute attack lasting many days. In other eyes, an acute attack lasting no more than 48 hours has been known to result in extensive synechial closure. One extraordinary patient whom we have seen had a history of repeated attacks of angle closure over a period of 8 years, yet, after peripheral iridectomy, only a small fraction of the angle was found to be closed by PAS.

Primary angle closure typically causes adhesion of the iris to the wall of the angle from its deepest portion forward to various levels on the TM, forming no bridges and sparing no structures in the advance of the iris forward, but never extending anterior to Schwalbe's line. The synechiae characteristically consist of bands of adhesion, rather than narrow tents or columns, such as produced by inflammation. The bands of PAS are often broad and, in the worst cases, involve the whole circumference. How far forward the iris is adherent is important because obstruction to aqueous outflow is caused only by synechiae that cover the filtration portion of the TM, not by attachments posterior to this special area.

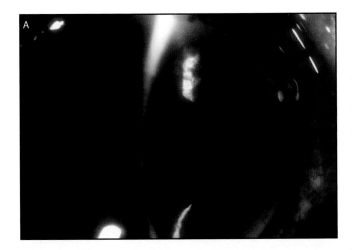
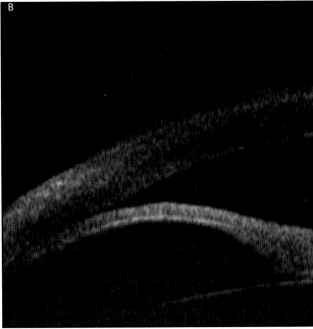

Figure 7-12. Iris bombé and angle-closure glaucoma due to posterior synechiae from chronic uveitis. (A) Slit-lamp photograph. (B) Ultrasound biomicrograph.

Prolonged absence of the anterior chamber after surgery for glaucoma or cataract is also a well-known cause of PAS, usually in the form of broad bands of adhesion of iris to various levels on the angle wall similar to those that occur in primary angle-closure glaucoma. However, sometimes after postoperative flat anterior chamber, a row of fine tent-like synechiae results. More rarely, the iris appears to become adherent anterior to the filtration portion of the TM, forming a bridge, with an open tunnel between the iris and the filtration zone. In such instances, gonioscopy may suggest that there is extensive synechial closure of the angle, but the IOP is much easier to control, and the facility of outflow is much better than one would expect if the angle were actually closed so extensively. On close inspection of the lateral edges of the bands of synechia, one may be able to see the open end of a tunnel running behind the synechia, although it is not possible to say how far. This has to be inferred from measurement of the IOP and the facility of outflow.

When pupillary block develops after surgery for congenital cataract in childhood, it is prone to cause disastrous PAS. In children, the PAS acquired in this way often extend onto clear cornea. Once extensive PAS develop in such cases, treatment becomes very difficult and unsatisfactory.

After filtering operations for glaucoma, absence of the anterior chamber is not unusual and may lead to the formation of PAS. PAS formation is usually not extensive. If one is fortunate enough to obtain an excellent filtering scar, the IOP may be controlled despite extensive PAS, but if the filtering scar is less than adequate or fails to develop entirely, extensive PAS from prolonged absence of the anterior chamber may make the glaucoma much worse than it was before operation.

Iris bombé (Figures 7-12 and 7-13) from posterior synechiae in phakic eyes can quickly lead to PAS that may extend onto the cornea and cause severe glaucoma. The bombé should be relieved as promptly as possible by laser iridectomy with the aim of preventing further formation of PAS.

Acute iritis and uveitis rarely cause PAS and probably do so only in eyes having anatomically narrow angles in which the edematous peripheral iris may actually come in contact with the trabecular wall. However, in a form of chronic iridocyclitis characterized by exudates on the corneoscleral meshwork similar to KP, PAS frequently form. Gonioscopically, one can observe these exudates in all stages of organization forming synechiae.

When a collection of inflammatory cells protrudes far enough from the surface of the TM to touch the periphery of the iris, a junction is formed. The space between the projecting mound of inflammatory cells and the periphery of the iris may be narrowed by inflammatory thickening of the iris and by a layer of inflammatory exudate on the surface of the iris. When the space is bridged and contact is made, the iris adheres, and it may be pulled further forward when KPs organize. A tent of iris then remains fastened by a scar to the TM. Organization of KP on the TM in uveitis most characteristically forms columnar or pyramidal synechiae.

In neovascular glaucoma, after the angle has become lined by a fibrovascular membrane, PAS are formed, as described in the section "Blood Vessels in the Angle." Severe glaucoma is usually present both before and after PAS develop. The formation of PAS in this condition seems to be caused by contracture of the fibrovascular membrane, which can completely close an angle that was formerly wide open. The membrane of new vessels and fibrous tissue grows initially flat on the surface

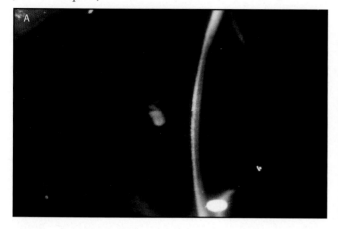
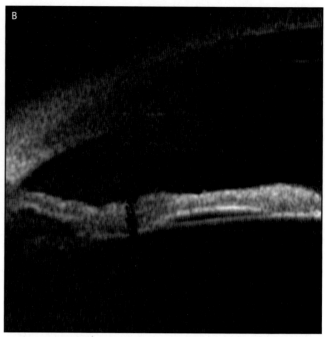

Figure 7-13. Eye following laser peripheral iridectomy. Note resolution of iris bombé, but persistence of posterior synechiae. (A) Slit-lamp photograph. (B) Ultrasound biomicrograph.

of all the angle structures, then, some of the vessels stand out from the surface, bridging from the iris to the corneoscleral meshwork. Contraction of these bridging vessels pulls the iris forward until it is in complete contact with the angle wall as far forward as Schwalbe's line. This process usually goes on in several regions of the angle simultaneously, forming broad columns and bands of PAS that may close the entire angle, sandwiching new vessels and fibrous tissue between iris and angle wall, as far forward as Schwalbe's line.

In ICE syndrome, special types of PAS develop, associated with spread of a transparent cellular and basement membrane. In these conditions, PAS can be observed gonioscopically in all stages of development, without any evidence of inflammation. Typically, in the essential atrophy of the iris form of ICE syndrome, the PAS are gross, and they may extend anterior to Schwalbe's line onto the cornea. A small amount of yellowish amorphous material may be noted at the juncture of synechiae with the cornea. The synechiae tend to spread circumferentially with distortion of the pupil and atrophy and partial disappearance of all layers of the iris. If synechiae obstruct the filtration portion of the corneoscleral meshwork, IOP may rise dangerously. Where the angle wall is visible between synechiae, it may function normally, or it may be obstructed by overgrowth of a membrane.

Synechial attachments of iris, extending farther forward than Schwalbe's line, actually onto the back of the cornea, are found not only in ICE syndrome, but also in the following conditions: after neglected postoperative flat anterior chamber; with epithelialization of the anterior chamber; with iris bombé either in phakic, pseudophakic, or aphakic eyes;

occasionally in neovascular glaucoma; and with pupillary block, especially after congenital cataract operation.

In certain cases of essential atrophy of the iris, a considerable extent of the angle may be hidden by synechiae, but there may be no proportional elevation of IOP, and facility of aqueous outflow may be surprisingly good. This is analogous to the condition occasionally observed when there has been prolonged absence of the anterior chamber after cataract extraction. A large portion of the angle may appear closed on gonioscopic examination, yet the IOP may be readily controlled by medical means. In such cases, the iris root appears actually to bridge the corneoscleral meshwork and attach only to Schwalbe's line and cornea, leaving the filtration portion of the meshwork uninvolved.

Attachments between peripheral iris and Schwalbe's line that bridge the angle, with an open tunnel behind the bridge, may be seen not only with essential atrophy of the iris and following flat anterior chamber after cataract operation, but also as congenital anomalies in association with posterior embryotoxon, in which Schwalbe's line is characteristically abnormally coarse, thickened, and beaded. No such bridging of the meshwork seems to occur in primary angle closure or as a result of intraocular inflammation. In these conditions, the iris becomes firmly attached to all structures beneath, and if the filtration portion of the corneoscleral meshwork is covered, there is a proportionate interference with aqueous outflow.

Treatment of PAS, with the aim of removing obstruction to aqueous outflow, appears to be ineffectual, except in the case of very fresh and tenuous adhesions. Experimental dissection of peripheral anterior synechiae from the TM and evaluation of facility of outflow by perfusion postmortem show that synechialysis is of no benefit once synechiae have become well-established. Microscopy of cross-sections shows disorganization or scarring of the corneoscleral TM in areas underlying old synechiae, and it is understandable that, even with the synechiae freed, the meshwork itself does not function normally. However, it is likely that freeing very recently formed PAS may be of some value. Experimentally, significant improvement in facility of outflow was obtained by synechialysis postmortem in one eye that had very recently formed PAS.

Gonioplasty with the argon laser has proven efficacious in freeing recently formed PAS. With the pupil made miotic with pilocarpine, treating the peripheral iris with large spot diameter, low-energy laser burns through a goniolens can cause prompt lysis of the iris adhesion. We have observed improvement in IOP and tonographic outflow facility in cases treated with iridogonioplasty as long as 6 months after angle closure and formation of PAS.

If gonioplasty is ineffective, it is occasionally valuable to perform the procedure of deepening the anterior chamber and goniosynechiolysis. This is accomplished by paracentesis and release of aqueous, allowing sufficient time for escape of aqueous from the posterior as well as from the anterior chamber, after which saline solution is injected through the paracentesis opening to deepen the anterior chamber at the expense of evacuated posterior chamber, and thus to spread the angle wide and display to direct gonioscopic examination the extent of actual attachment of iris onto the angle wall. Old PAS can be freed surgically with a spatula; however, we have abandoned this procedure because of lack of evidence of benefit to the glaucoma, although others have reported success with this operation.[11]

In practice, the principle stands that the most desirable and effective countermeasures against PAS are those designed to prevent their formation.

Blood in the Angle

When fresh and red, blood in the angle presents no problem in recognition, appearing much as it does by ordinary slit-lamp examination, but in some cases the amount is so small that it is discoverable only by gonioscopy. Old, degenerated blood characteristically consists of black deposits, varying from fine granules to coarse balls, scattered indiscriminately on all angle structures, but most densely in the lower angle. A blood clot that has persisted extraordinarily long in the angle can become fibrosed and produce synechial obstruction of the angle (Table 7-11).

Spontaneous hyphema, without history or evidence of trauma, most often comes from the abnormal new vessels that develop in the angle in association with the vascular retinopathy from diabetes or in association with occlusion of the central retinal vein or artery. Gonioscopic search for

TABLE 7-11. CONDITIONS INVOLVING BLOOD IN THE ANGLE	
Conditions	Findings
Fresh blood	Bright red puddle, sheet, or clot
Old, degenerated blood	Black particles and balls scattered in the angle
Organized persistent clot	Synechiae filling the angle
Spontaneous hyphema	From new vessels in angle or iris associated with neovascular glaucoma
	From microhemangiomas of iris
	From blood in Schlemm's canal
	From vessels on inner surface of the cataract wound
Hyphema from sudden hypotony	In infants: xanthogranuloma
	From new vessels in the angle in heterochromic cyclitis
	From blood in Schlemm's canal
Hyphema from blunt trauma	From rupture of vessels in angle or iris

neovascularization in the angle is necessary to establish the diagnosis, unless rubeosis of the iris is already evident by slit-lamp examination. Glaucoma is usually already present when hyphema develops from neovascularization.

In rare instances, we have seen sudden small spontaneous hemorrhage develop in eyes that have been otherwise normal to all examination, including gonioscopy, and we have not discovered the source. IOP has become moderately elevated within a half hour because of measurable obstruction to outflow, but within a few hours there has been spontaneous improvement. Within a day or two, the blood has gone, and the pressure and facility of outflow have returned to normal. Rarely, we have seen eyes with subtly abnormal iris vascular tufts at the pupillary margin present with this clinical picture.

In rare instances, in normal eyes during gonioscopy, we have seen blood dribble into the angle from some indifferent-looking site in the TM, from blood that has been caused to reflux into Schlemm's canal by the pressure of the rim of the contact lens. This has been transient and of no special significance that we are aware of.

Bleeding in the angle is occasionally induced by a sudden fall of IOP, resulting from the escape of aqueous humor from the eye during diagnostic aspiration of the aqueous. This occurs rarely in normal eyes. However, in eyes that have heterochromic iridocyclitis, acute hypotony characteristically causes slight, inconsequential bleeding into the anterior chamber from the special type of new blood vessels that form in the angle in this disease. (These vessels have been described in the section "Blood Vessels in the Angle.")

Blood rarely refluxes from Schlemm's canal through normal TM into the anterior chamber when the IOP is rapidly lowered, but, after a goniotomy has been performed, blood often refluxes into the anterior chamber while the goniotomy knife is being withdrawn from the eye and the aqueous is escaping from the wound in the cornea. Anatomically, it appears that the junctions between the endothelial cells of the inner wall of Schlemm's canal ordinarily prevent blood reflux back from the canal into the eye,[12] but this can be altered in certain abnormal conditions.

Vascularization of the inner aspect of a cataract wound can cause repeated hyphema. This has been well-described by Swan.[13] Treatment of the abnormal vessels with the argon laser can be effective. Rarely, a similar chronic vascularization process can occur on the inner aspect of a trabeculectomy (scleral flap filter) wound. Occasionally, also in the immediate postoperative situation, hyphema can occur, ostensibly originating from the cut edge of Schlemm's canal. This is rarely a chronic problem, although we have observed recurrent hyphema for as long as 3 weeks after trabeculectomy.

Blunt trauma to the eye is probably the most common cause of hyphema. The blood comes from torn vessels in the angle. Gonioscopy most commonly reveals a tear or disruption of the uveal meshwork and ciliary muscle. Anterior ciliary arteries entering the ciliary muscle from the sclera seem to be in a particularly vulnerable position. Less commonly, dialysis of the iris is found in the periphery; the associated rupture of radial arteries of the iris near their origin from the circumferential ciliary artery is a potential source of bleeding.

Particles in the Angle

In the angle of the anterior chamber, it is not uncommon to see one or more particles that are obviously sitting on the surface of the angle structures and are not a part of them. Particles are most often seen after intraocular surgery or injury. One should distinguish these surface particles from diffusely deposited pigment granules infiltrating the TM and from inflammatory precipitates in the angle, which appear cemented in intimate contact with the TM (Table 7-12).

Brown chunks, strands, or fragments of pigmented tissue in the dependent angle or on the back of the cornea are usually small pieces of iris left in the anterior chamber after operations involving the iris and have no special significance except to be distinguished from pigmented masses, such as nevi and melanomas and from pigmented KPs and PAS.

Black balls in the angle typically are from degenerated blood, as described under "Blood in the Angle." These may remain for many years.

Gray flakes or particles, sometimes fluffy, sometimes resembling dandruff, and usually inconspicuous, are characteristic of exfoliation. Typically, the material is more obvious at or under the pupillary border, and very few flakes are seen

Findings	Conditions
TABLE 7-12. CONDITIONS INVOLVING PARTICLES IN THE ANGLE	
Brown chunks	Tissue remnants from surgery
Black balls	Old blood
Gray flakes or particles	Exfoliation
Refractile scrolls	Descemet's membrane
Refractile solid particles	Glass, plastic
Light gray fibers	Cotton fibers
Bright red specks	Rubber
Silvery particles	Aluminum
Chalk-white particles	Congenital cataract remnants

in the angle. There may or may not be an associated abnormal deposition of pigment in the corneoscleral TM. Usually, there is when glaucoma is present.

Refractile scrolls in the angle, resembling coiled or curved small pieces of thin, shiny, or glassy plastic, are most characteristic of pieces of Descemet's membrane that have been inadvertently torn from the back of the cornea by a knife tip, cyclodialysis spatula, or iris repositor during intraocular surgery or that, in one case we have seen, were blasted off the back of a portion of the cornea by a firecracker. The lens capsule has a similar refractile appearance and could be mistaken for Descemet's membrane if a piece were loose in the angle; but, almost always, when remnants of capsule are left in an eye, they seem to be held in a wound or in a pupillary membrane, rather than being completely detached. In time, pieces of either material may adhere to the iris if they are in contact with it. In themselves, sheets of Descemet's membrane or lens capsule have no tendency to cause glaucoma.

Refractile solid particles that are flat, with sharp irregular edges, and varying thickness, rather than the uniform thickness of sheets of Descemet's membrane or lens capsule, are usually foreign bodies of glass or solid plastic. If these particles are free to move in the anterior chamber, they sometimes injure the corneal endothelium and cause edema, usually in the lower third or half of the cornea. If one is unaware of the foreign body, which frequently can be discovered only by gonioscopy, one may suspect glaucoma to be the cause of the edema, but glaucoma is seldom induced by this type of foreign body, unless the irritation also gives rise to iritis, which, in rare instances, may be accompanied by glaucoma.

Light gray fibers in the angle and on the surface of the iris are ordinarily cotton fibers introduced inadvertently during intraocular surgery. Usually, they are solitary and seem to excite no reaction. Fragments of cellulose microsponges used during intraocular surgery have rarely been observed

Error	Solution
Angle closed	Ensure that view is good, that maximal angle is seen. If using a mirrored lens, have patient look toward mirror to maximize view. Still, if the angle has a narrow approach, but is actually open, a mirrored goniolens, even with the best viewing technique, may give the appearance of angle closure, particularly if the iris is excessively convex. A Koeppe lens is the best solution to this problem; to maximize the view, move into position to obtain best view of the angle.
Angle excessively deep	This problem occurs most commonly with the Zeiss, Posner, or Sussman lens, and is due to the small diameter of the lens allowing the lens to rest on the cornea only, without extending onto the sclera, as the other goniolenses do.
	This property, which permits indentation gonioscopy, can also result in the appearance of an excessively deep angle or can make an appositionally closed angle appear open. The solution is to apply less pressure to the goniolens. A clue that this problem is occurring is the presence of folds in Descemet's membrane.
Angle recession	This can easily be missed, especially if subtle. The optimal solution is to perform bilateral simultaneous Koeppe gonioscopy and to switch back and forth between eyes to compare for asymmetry. Other clues are an abnormally bright whiteness of the scleral spur and absence or tearing of iris processes and uveal meshwork.
Appositional versus synechial angle closure	The Zeiss, Posner, or Sussman lens allows indentation gonioscopy, permitting differentiation between appositional and synechial angle closure.

Table title: **TABLE 7-13. COMMON ERRORS IN GONIOSCOPY** (with column headers Error | Solution)

in the angle, occasionally associated with a mild inflammatory reaction.

Bright red specks, usually with a slightly granular or irregular surface, typically are of red rubber, coming from rubber bulbs used to irrigate the anterior chamber during intraocular surgery. These particles in the angle or on the surface of the iris have not been seen to excite an appreciable reaction and are now rare due to modifications in surgical equipment and technique.

Chalk-white particles in the angle are seen after extracapsular operations for congenital cataract. These particles are characterized particularly by their whiteness and opaque appearance, which is suggestive of calcification. Usually, very few or just a single particle is seen, and the sizes vary widely. They appear to excite no reaction and may persist for 20 or 30 years, or possibly longer, in the angle. Presumably, these are pieces of the original dense white plaques that are seen in some congenitally cataractous lenses and that may be released into the anterior chamber after the capsule is opened. These do not appear to be a cause of glaucoma. We have seen them in one eye of a middle-aged woman who was developing open-angle glaucoma in both eyes many years after uncomplicated operations for congenital cataracts in childhood; no particles were present in the other eye, and we think the glaucoma was the primary hereditary variety, unrelated to the earlier cataracts and surgery.

Common errors in performing gonioscopy are presented in Table 7-13.

REFERENCES

1. Forbes M. Indentation gonioscopy and efficacy of iridectomy in angle-closure glaucoma. *Trans Am Ophthalmol.* 1974;72:488-515.
2. Campbell DG. A comparison of diagnostic techniques in angle-closure glaucoma. *Am J Ophthalmol.* 1979;88:197-204.
3. Rosenquist RC Jr, Melamed S, Epstein DL. Anterior and posterior axial lens displacement and human aqueous outflow facility. *Invest Ophthalmol Vis Sci.* 1988;29:1159-1164.
4. Van Buskirk EM, Grant WM. Lens depression and aqueous outflow in enucleated primate eyes. *Am J Ophthalmol.* 1973;76:632-640.
5. Van Buskirk EM. Changes in the facility of aqueous outflow induced by lens depression and IOP in excised human eyes. *Am J Ophthalmol.* 1976;82:736-740.
6. Van Buskirk EM. Anatomic correlates of changing aqueous outflow facility in excised human eyes. *Invest Ophthalmol Vis Sci.* 1982;22:625-632.
7. Barany E. On the mechanism by which chamber depth affects outflow resistance in excised eyes. *Doc Ophthalmol.* 1959;13:84-89.
8. Grant WM. Experimental aqueous perfusion in enucleated human eyes. *Arch Ophthalmol.* 1963;69:783-801.
9. Epstein DL, Freddo TF, Anderson PJ, et al. Experimental obstruction to aqueous outflow by pigment particles in living monkeys. *Invest Ophthalmol Vis Sci.* 1986;27:387-395.
10. Donaldson DD. *Atlas of External Diseases of the Eye.* St Louis, MO: Mosby, Co; 1966:I-III.
11. Campbell DG, Vela A. Modern goniosynechialysis for the treatment of synechial angle-closure glaucoma. *Ophthalmology.* 1984;91:1052-1060.

12. Raviola G. Effects of a paracentesis on the blood-aqueous barrier: an electron microscope study on Macaca mulatta using horseradish peroxidase as a tracer. *Invest Ophthalmol.* 1974;13:828-858.

13. Swan KC. Late hyphema due to wound vascularization. *Trans Am Acad Ophthalmol Otol.* 1976;81:138-144.

W. Morton Grant, MD, now deceased, was an original author on this chapter.

Examination of the Optic Nerve

Ian P. Conner, MD, PhD; Joel S. Schuman, MD, FACS; and David L. Epstein, MD, MMM

METHODS OF EXAMINATION

The clinician should use all available techniques to examine and draw the optic nerves in patients with glaucoma and repeat these during the examination and after pupillary dilation. It is curious how the cupping contour can look different with different tools, and one is striving to make very subtle, yet anatomically correct drawings and interpretations. Having observed residents in training, one of us (DLE) has concluded that it is only after hundreds of disc evaluations/drawings that one becomes sensitive to the changes in glaucoma to accurately draw.

There are essentially 3 tools for examining the optic nerve: the direct ophthalmoscope, the 90-diopter (D) lens at the slit-lamp, and stereo photographs. As indicated in Chapter 5, even if the patient is being dilated subsequently, one should assess the disc appearance (and the clarity of the media) undilated, for, on the one hand, the patient will not be dilated at every follow-up visit and, therefore, the undilated appearance of the disc is important for future reference, and, on the other hand, comparison of the undilated interpretation with the later dilated appearance will improve the clinician's skills in optic nerve evaluation.

Although the direct ophthalmoscope provides a nonstereo view, the use of parallax and the attention to the bend of small vessels after they cross the disc margin provide remarkably accurate assessment (confirmed by subsequent comparison to stereo disc photographs) of the contour of the rim tissue, which is the key parameter that is being assessed. If one chooses general ophthalmology practice, ophthalmoscopy with the direct ophthalmoscope must be mastered because it is a critical tool. The ophthalmology resident must realize that it is much easier to evaluate optic disc cupping in a referral glaucoma center during training, when the pupils of all patients are dilated (and the diagnosis of a possible glaucoma entity has already been made). In the real world,

the general ophthalmologist must evaluate many patients through undilated pupils and, for the first time, detect possible glaucoma-like changes. The general ophthalmologist must be a true disc sleuth and deserves all of our praise for detecting glaucomatous changes in the optic nerve (usually initially through an undilated pupil).

Unfortunately, many senior clinicians have observed that recent residency graduates are not as skilled with the direct ophthalmoscope as the previous generation; new techniques should supplement but not totally replace previous valid methods. The truth is that we need all the help we can get in this difficult assessment, which unfortunately represents damage to the optic nerve at a later stage than we ultimately aspire to detect it.

The 90-D lens at the slit-lamp is a very important technique to master, in addition to direct ophthalmoscopy. For this technique, the slit beam of the slit-lamp is made coaxial with the oculars, the 90-D lens is placed in front of the patient's eye perpendicular to the beam, and anteropostero movements are made to bring the optic nerve into focus. This technique is easiest to perform with a dilated pupil, but sometimes it is surprising how good the view can be with an undilated pupil. It is important to draw what one sees and later compare this to actual stereo photographs. It is curious how contour changes sometimes are accentuated with the 90-D lens and sometimes not as easily appreciated as with direct ophthalmoscopy. We therefore need to master all techniques in order to properly assess these contour changes.

One should draw (at least once) the appearance of the optic nerve using the above methods, but with the pupil dilated, stereo disc photographs should be obtained and later compared to the drawings. If stereo photographs cannot be obtained, a nonstereo photograph should be obtained, especially for a baseline. Disc drawings are notoriously inaccurate. All subsequent evaluations will be asking the question: has there been

Kahook MY, Schuman JS, eds.
Chandler and Grant's Glaucoma, Fifth Edition (pp 81-94).
© 2013 SLACK Incorporated.

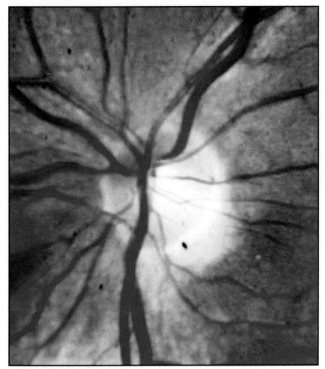

Figure 8-1. Normal optic nerve.

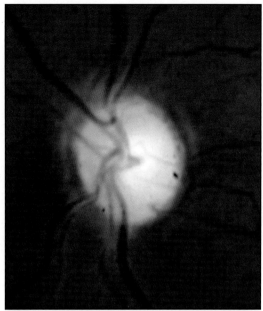

Figure 8-2. Appearance of optic nerve after resolution of acute optic neuritis. Note optic nerve pallor without associated cupping.

progression in the optic nerve cupping and visual field? Evaluation of the visual field alone, which is a subjective technique, is not sufficient. Detailed baseline information, as indicated in Chapter 5, is crucial to optimal patient management.

Some stereo disc cameras do not obtain true simultaneous stereo photographs, and some artifact from the resulting 2 photographic angles is possible. But, it is an imperfect world, and our 90-D drawings and direct ophthalmoscopic views also have their artifacts. This is why it is important to assess the appearance of the optic nerve using all available methods. When one thinks about it, the optic nerve is "staring us in the face" and thus should be available to provide us with objective data about the progress of the glaucomatous process, if we could only design the proper detection instrument. In the future, the evolving optical/computer evaluation techniques should make this possible, but at the present time we must rely on the above 3 clinical methods. When we evaluate cupping, we are looking at the actual signature of the disease process, and we must strive repetitively and compulsively to depict it accurately.

Therefore, stereo or other disc photographs must be reviewed when they become available and compared with the physician's disc drawings. This is a learning process for all clinicians. One of us (DLE) strongly recommends that residents in training have disc drawing rounds.

Indirect ophthalmoscopy provides notoriously inaccurate assessment of the contour changes in glaucoma and should be avoided as a technique for glaucoma evaluation (although it is important in all glaucoma patients to examine the peripheral retina with indirect ophthalmoscopy).

We have found determination of cup/disc ratio to be practically useless in the management of any individual patient. The glaucomatous changes in the contour of the rim tissue rarely are exactly symmetrical and, thus, do not lend themselves to such a general measurement. This term could be used in verbal discussions dealing with generalities, but otherwise should be avoided.

The process of glaucoma affects the contour of the rim tissue between the edge of the physiological cup and the edge of the disc (Figure 8-1). The glaucoma process causes a backward bowing of this rim tissue that may result in a fairly discreet (deep) extension of the cup in one meridian, or a gentler posterior sloping that may be termed *saucerization*. With this loss of substance of the optic nerve, there is a change in color, presumably due to the accompanying loss of small blood vessels. However, the key parameter is the change in the contour of the rim tissue.

In nonglaucomatous optic atrophy, there is loss of color, hence, atrophy, but there is usually no contour change in the rim tissue. For example, after vascular occlusion, the disc is pale, but there is usually no increase in size of the cup (ie, no contour change; Figure 8-2). However, there are certain optic atrophies that can be accompanied by contour changes, and these occasionally present diagnostic puzzles: temporal arteritis, other ischemic optic neuropathies, intracranial neoplasms, methanol intoxication, hereditary optic atrophies, lues, and, of course, optic cup pits or colobomas. These are uncommon (except perhaps for temporal arteritis and certain dominant hereditary optic neuropathies such as

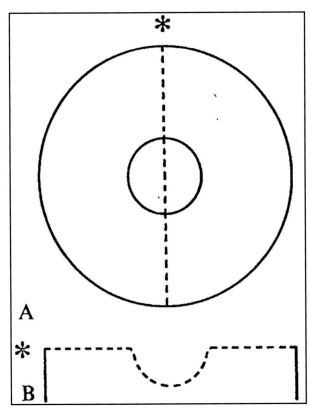

Figure 8-3. (A) Frontal view of central physiologic cup. (B) Cross-sectional view of central physiologic cup.

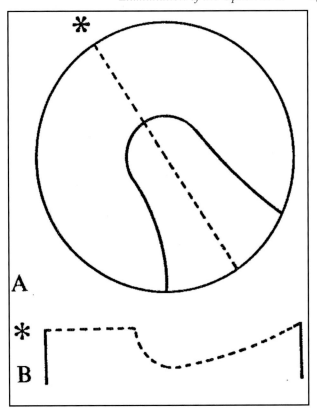

Figure 8-4. (A) Frontal view of cup extending to the margin below and temporally (left eye). (B) Cross-sectional view. The cup is shelving. It is not an excavation. There is no field defect.

Kjer's). Some of these have been called pseudoglaucomatous because of the contour change. What often proves helpful in diagnosing pseudoglaucomatous contour changes is to assess the color of the intact rim tissue in the other quadrants of the disc. In pseudoglaucomatous cases, the color of the intact rim tissue is often pale, unlike glaucoma where normal color is observed.

The assessment of the contour of the remaining optic nerve rim tissue throughout its entire circumference is crucial both to the detection of glaucoma and also its progression. We use all 3 of the above diagnostic evaluation methods, which include true stereo viewing, as well as parallax and clues, such as the course of small vessels that cross the disc margin, to make this crucial assessment.

Figures 8-3 through 8-8 portray the "Chandler and Grant" interpretation of the changes in rim contour that occur in the progression of the glaucomatous process, based on their long-term clinical observations. The cross-sectional views in these figures help clarify what is observed, and we have used these in patient charts. Beginning residents in ophthalmology are encouraged to draw these cross-sectional diagrams.

The key is the detection of the backward bowing and the extent of this in relation to the edge of the disc and the apparent depth of this change. The following terms have been used to characterize the apparent depth of the contour

change: *saucerization* (as in a saucer plate) connoting a mild change in depth, *shelving* an intermediate change in depth, and *excavation* a precipitous change in depth like the edge of the normal central cup. Chandler and Grant intended the term saucerization to indicate an uncommon, more generalized backward bowing like a saucer plate (see Figure 8-8) to contrast this with the more common excavated change of a tea cup, but the term saucerization has evolved to indicate a common subtle change in disc rim contour that appears to be acquired early in the glaucomatous process.

For practical purposes, the terminology is not as important as the detection of the contour change of shallow or deep backward bowing of disc rim tissue. The deeper changes, whether shelving or excavation, are difficult to fully differentiate from each other, but the more subtle posterior bowing of rim tissue commonly called saucerization and its progression to deeper and/or more extensive changes has become an important part of disc sleuthing.

Thus, although the disease process does produce glaucomatous optic atrophy and thereby a color change in the disc, as in other cases of optic atrophy, it is the contour changes that distinguish the changes in glaucoma from these other conditions. The clinician needs to be able to assess and record these contour changes to diagnose and evaluate follow-up in patients with glaucoma.

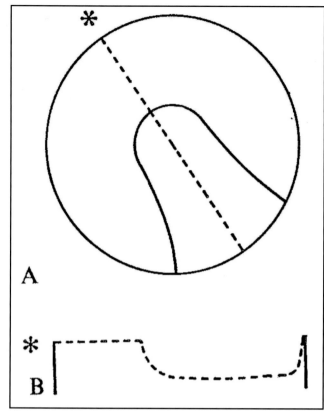

Figure 8-5. (A) Similar frontal view of cup extending to the margin below and temporally (left eye). (B) Cross-sectional view. The cup is now an excavation. There is an upper field defect.

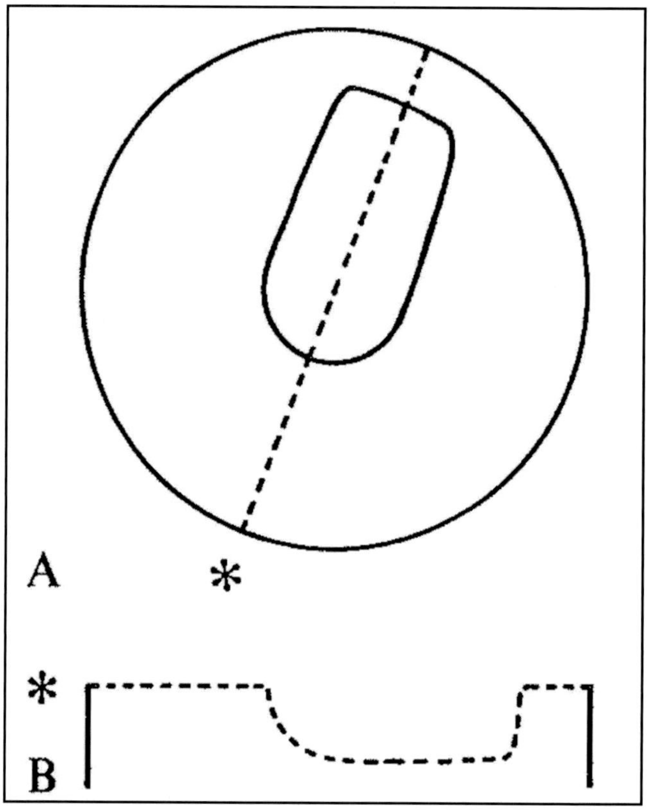

Figure 8-6. (A) Frontal view of enlargement of the cup above and temporally. It does not reach the margin (left eye). (B) Cross-sectional view. The upper border of the cup is an excavation. There is a lower field defect.

In assessing the contour of the rim tissue of the optic nerve, special attention should be placed on the straight temporal portion of the optic disc that receives the papillomacular bundle fibers. In primary open-angle glaucoma (POAG) associated with myopia and in low-tension glaucoma, there can be preferential early cupping in this area with corresponding field loss that can extend into or actually involve central fixation. Therefore, the amount of rim tissue and its healthiness in terms of contour changes in this directly temporal area are important factors in glaucoma decision making.

As will be discussed in Chapters 18 and 19, in patients with advanced disease, it is crucial to know how much margin there is that can be followed further should the target intraocular pressure (IOP) be incorrect. Although this margin can be expressed as the amount of remaining field and the actual sensitivity measurements close to fixation, another factor is the contour condition of the straight temporal optic disc rim tissue that corresponds to these central points in the visual field. For example, sometimes, fixation is split in glaucoma, but in addition to assessing the actual sensitivities in the central field in the remaining half (eg, the inferior field), evaluating the extent of contour changes in the corresponding (superior) portion of the straight temporal rim tissue of the optic nerve provides additional information about how much margin there is left to follow.

The myopic disc is notoriously difficult to evaluate for early glaucomatous changes because of its usual generalized sloping contour. Nevertheless, in POAG associated with myopia, one needs to carefully examine the straight temporal margin of rim tissue for early glaucomatous contour changes because of the possibility that the initial field loss might involve central fixation (see Chapter 18). This uncertainty in detecting the earliest possible disc-cupping change in myopic eyes legitimately suggests the need to potentially treat elevated IOP somewhat more vigorously in these eyes.

Chandler and Grant were excellent observers of the optic nerve and emphasized the importance of asymmetry and verticalization of the cup, as well as the predictive value of the optic nerve changes for visual field changes. They wrote:

> In nearly every type of glaucoma, we are greatly concerned with the condition of the optic disc (optic nerve head). In the diagnosis of glaucoma, the appearance of the optic disc often provides us with valuable clues. In decisions concerning the necessity for and in evaluation of the adequacy of treatment of glaucoma, we can often obtain essential guidance from the appearance of the optic disc and evaluation of the field of vision.

It is true that, in certain varieties of glaucoma, a decision that treatment is urgently needed can be made mainly on the

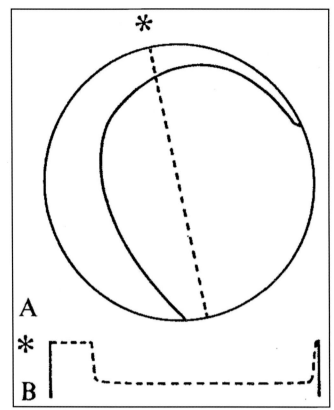

Figure 8-7. (A) Frontal view of cup reaching the margin below and temporally, not quite to the margin above (left eye). (B) Cross-sectional view. There is an excavation both above and below. There is both an upper and a lower field defect.

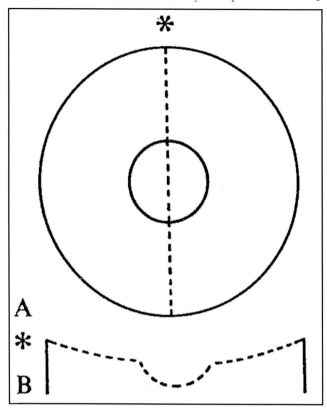

Figure 8-8. (A) Frontal view of a disc with saucerization. The physiologic cup is not enlarged. (B) There is backward bowing of the entire disc, but the physiologic cup is unchanged.

basis of very high IOP, but, in many more cases, the character of both the optic disc and visual field greatly influences the decision.

Change in the optic disc can forewarn of change in the visual field in some cases, and usually the nature of the abnormality of the optic disc can be valuably correlated with abnormality of the visual field to help establish whether a given field defect is correctly attributable to glaucoma or to some other cause.

We will first describe the changes in appearance of the optic disc that are characteristic in glaucoma and their correlation with abnormalities in the visual field.

OPHTHALMOSCOPIC FINDINGS

Nearly all of the observations to be described were made originally with the direct ophthalmoscope, which, though monocular, permits valuable appreciation of depth and contour, confirmed by comparison with stereo photographs. However, considerable practice is required to learn how to make use of a number of monocular clues to depth perception.

Asymmetry of the Optic Cups

A simple enlargement of the physiologic cup in all directions is not infrequently a sign of early glaucoma. Asymmetry of the physiologic cups in the 2 eyes is seldom seen in normal eyes, and, until proven otherwise, must be considered a sign of early glaucoma (Figure 8-9). When the asymmetry of the physiologic cups is first noted, the IOP is usually slightly higher in the eye with the wider cup, but this is not invariably the case. With Paul A. Chandler, an asymmetry of the physiologic cups was first discovered when the IOP was normal and equal in both eyes. It was only after 4 or 5 years that an elevated IOP was found in the eye with the wider cup.

The size of the physiologic cup in normal eyes varies considerably from person to person, and, if the cups are equal in size, one cannot tell from a single examination whether the cups are larger than they were previously. The only way the ophthalmologist can say that the cups are becoming larger (ie, due to bilateral early glaucomatous change) is to compare the results of this examination with previous stereo photographs of the discs or very accurate, previously prepared drawings. The photographs are much to be preferred. Because previous stereo photographs or accurate drawings are seldom available to the practicing ophthalmologist, if the

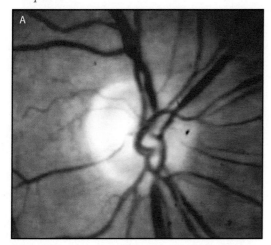 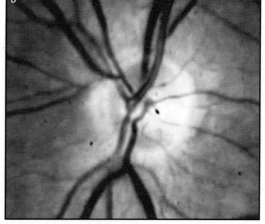

Figure 8-9. Asymmetry of optic nerve cupping with the (A) right eye significantly more cupped than the (B) left eye in this patient. This degree of asymmetry is unusual in the normal population.

cups are symmetric and equal in size, one cannot be sure from the first examination whether the size of the physiologic cups is normal for this individual.

However, if the physiologic cups are asymmetric, that is, if the cup in one eye, although physiologic when considered by itself, is definitely wider than the cup in the fellow eye, this must be considered very likely to be an early glaucomatous change. A difference in the size of the cups in the 2 eyes is a common finding in early glaucoma.

There has been considerable discussion in the ophthalmic literature concerning cup/disc ratio. We know that the size and depth of the physiologic cup vary greatly among different individuals. We feel that the significant factor is not the cup/disc ratio, but the shape of the cup and its comparison to that of the cup in the fellow eye (see Figures 8-3 and 8-4).

Abnormal Cupping

In most patients for whom glaucomatous changes develop in the optic disc, the physiologic cup enlarges to reach the margin downward and temporally. This is a definite glaucomatous change, but at first there may not be a visual field defect with only optic disc shelving (see Figure 8-4).

The shelving of the cup to the lower temporal margin gradually becomes deeper, not yet a real excavation. Gradually, the cup becomes deeper at the margin, and a real excavation becomes evident (see Figure 8-5). It is now usually possible to find an upper field defect—an upper Bjerrum scotoma, nasal step, or both—but there may be none if there is not yet atrophy of nerve fibers. At first, such pathologic cupping extends only to the major inferior vessels, but later may involve the entire lower pole of the disc.

Excavation, as we use the term, indicates that the wall of the cup is precipitous. It does not necessarily imply undermining of the edge or a disappearance of blood vessels from view.

In certain cases, the physiologic cup first enlarges upward. As the disease progresses, the upwardly enlarged cup comes closer to the disc margin and is seen to be excavated at its upper border (see Figure 8-6). At this stage, although the cup still does not quite reach the upper outer margin, there is usually a lower field defect—a lower Bjerrum scotoma, a lower nasal step, or both.

In some cases, the cup may enlarge toward both the upper and lower borders simultaneously (see Figure 8-7), and it is in this type of glaucomatous change that we eventually find both an upper and lower Bjerrum scotoma, isolating a central island of vision, varying in size from patient to patient, with variable degree of loss in the peripheral field.

Eventually, the excavation reaches the margin above as well as below, and the disc may become totally cupped to the margins everywhere; however, in some such cases, there is still a rim of normal tissue on the nasal side.

Not all visual field defects in a patient with elevated IOP are necessarily due to glaucoma. It is important to correlate the optic cup appearance with the visual field. Dense field defects are to be regarded with suspicion if they are not explainable by the optic disc appearance.

We, therefore, emphasize the importance of excavation in determining whether there is a field defect. This seems clear enough when the cupping is lower temporal and the excavation extends to the margin, but it is not so obvious when the cupping extends upward. We have seen that even when the cup has not reached the margin above and temporally, there may be a lower field defect. This may seem surprising, but when we analyze such an upward and temporally enlarged cup, we note that this often represents an excavation rather than a shelving from the very beginning; whereas, when the cup reaches the margin below and temporally, it is for some time commonly a shelving cup, not an excavation, and we may find no field defect. It is only when the lower outer enlargement becomes an excavation that we almost always find a field defect. Thus, we see that the contour of the pathologic cup appears to be the most important factor in determining whether a field defect will be found and where it will be found. With a lower excavation, the excavation may in some cases at first be narrow, and it is not unusual to find a narrow upper Bjerrum scotoma. As the lower excavation becomes broader, the Bjerrum scotoma becomes wider.

In an upper excavation, the excavation is wider from the beginning, and we usually do not find a very narrow lower Bjerrum scotoma similar to the narrow upper scotoma that sometimes is seen superiorly. The lower Bjerrum scotoma, even at an early stage, is wider. This might suggest that, from a clinical standpoint, there is a mechanical (anatomical) factor in the pathologic cupping that causes field defects in glaucoma. We will leave it to others to provide a scientific explanation of these clinical findings.

Saucerization

Uncommonly, the first pathologic change in the disc may be a slight backward bowing in the periphery of a portion of the disc or of the whole disc, in a form that we have called saucerization (see Figure 8-8). The contour of such a disc closely resembles the contour of an ordinary saucer plate, in contrast to an excavation, in which the contour of the disc more closely resembles the contour of a teacup. We do not call the early shelving cup to the lower outer margin saucerization. Saucerization has a different appearance that can be difficult to describe. It involves not less than a quadrant of the disc and may involve any portion of the disc, sometimes even the nasal portion or the entire disc. In some cases, one may see pathologic cupping at one border of the disc and saucerization at the other. Whether the saucerization involves the entire disc or only a portion, it represents a definite glaucomatous change and must be taken into account along with the other signs in the management of the case.

In some cases, there is saucerization of the entire disc, but there still may be no field defect until the saucerization becomes considerably deeper. Eventually, we find loss of field; with advanced saucerization of the whole disc, however, this may not be the typical nerve fiber bundle defect, but rather a concentric contraction of the field. Such cases are much more difficult to follow by perimetry than those characterized by the ordinary type of cupping.

Saucerization of the disc is a relatively rare form of glaucomatous cupping. We find ordinary glaucomatous cupping in 9 out of 10 cases. Its importance seems to be that if we recognize saucerization of a portion or of the whole disc, even if there is no loss of field whatsoever, we can make a positive diagnosis of glaucoma no matter what level of IOP is found at the moment.

In many eyes, we find a crescent all around the disc, sometimes called a halo (Figure 8-10). In such cases, it may be difficult to determine just where the border of the disc is. If we consider the crescent as the disc border, we may conclude that the cup, although large, does not

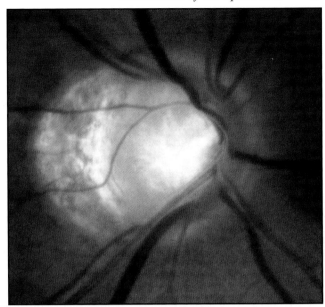

Figure 8-10. Peripapillary crescent in this patient with glaucoma.

reach the margin anywhere; whereas, with a more critical examination, we may conclude that the cup does in fact reach the margin of the disc, which is well inside the borders of the crescent.

Atrophy

Thus far, we have spoken mainly of the changes in contour of the optic disc that occur in glaucoma and have only incidentally mentioned atrophy. We must remember that the ultimate cause of irreversible loss of function in glaucoma is atrophy of nerve fibers, whether or not there is pathologic cupping.

With the exception of cases of high IOP or acute glaucoma in which atrophy and loss of vision may develop with little or no pathologic cupping, and about which we will say more later, in most cases of chronic glaucoma without exceptionally high IOP, the first change in the optic disc is a change in the cupping that conforms to the various patterns described in Figures 8-3 through 8-8. As already stated, abnormal changes in the contour of the optic disc are characteristically recognized before there is an irreversible abnormality in the visual field detectable by ordinary clinical means. It is when atrophy of nerve fibers develops in association with cupping that characteristic changes in the visual field appear, corresponding anatomically to the location of visibly affected portions of the optic disc. In exceptional cases, there may be typical glaucomatous visual field defects that do not correspond to visible changes in the optic disc if the fields are measured when the IOP is considerably elevated, but these are functional changes that are commonly reversible when the IOP is reduced. Reversible field defects can be induced in normal eyes and in glaucomatous eyes by raising the IOP, such as by pressing on the eye.

Our prime concern is with the irreversible loss of visual field, and it is here that ophthalmoscopic recognition of atrophy can be helpful in validating results of visual field testing. When atrophy and field loss are extensive, it is generally easy to recognize the degree of atrophy by the whiteness and lack of fine vessels in the optic disc, but, when atrophy is partial or limited to a small portion of the disc, it may be difficult to be certain. Characteristically, when there is localized pathologic cupping and corresponding field defect, one can appreciate that the affected portion of the disc is atrophic by its relative lack of pink coloring compared with the more normal portions of the disc. The affected area may even appear slightly gray.

One can be misled in evaluating atrophy of the optic disc with the ophthalmoscope and fail to appreciate the characteristic whitening of the disc if the patient's crystalline lens has yellow nuclear sclerosis. This yellow lens can act as a filter, altering the apparent color of the disc. Examination of the lens with the slit-lamp biomicroscope helps to evaluate how much yellowing of the nucleus is present. One can also be misled and fail to appreciate the whiteness of an atrophic optic disc if the incandescent bulb of the ophthalmoscope is operated at subnormal voltage because this can also provide a yellowish light.

In eyes with considerable hyperopia, optic disc atrophy may have a special ophthalmoscopic appearance. Eyes that are very hyperopic tend normally to have rosy-appearing discs, with small physiologic cups. In such eyes, partial optic atrophy may not cause the optic disc to appear white but may only cause it to lose some of its previous pink or rosy appearance.

VIEWING THE DISC THROUGH THE KOEPPE LENS

Ophthalmoscopic examination of the optic disc is extraordinarily difficult in some patients, but there are several circumstances in which the examination can be greatly facilitated by the use of the same type of Koeppe contact lens that is used for gonioscopy.

The Koeppe goniolens can be applied in the same manner as it is for regular gonioscopy, with the patient supine, and the space between lens and cornea can be filled with sterile saline solution. This is particularly convenient if one is planning to perform both gonioscopy and ophthalmoscopy. However, if gonioscopy has been performed at some other time, and one merely wishes to use the lens to facilitate direct ophthalmoscopy, this can be done easily with the patient sitting up, as for ordinary direct ophthalmoscopy. For use sitting up, the concavity of the goniolens is filled with clear goniogel, and the lens is applied to the patient's eye just as though he or she were lying down, with the flange under the upper and lower lids. The lens is best held in place with thumb and forefinger while ophthalmoscopy is carried out in the normal manner.

Looking through the Koeppe goniolens at the central fundus, one needs several more diopters of plus lens in the ophthalmoscope than when one looks at the fundus without the Koeppe lens. The optic disc appears smaller when seen through the Koeppe lens, but it may be seen with striking clarity. One of the advantages of funduscopy through the Koeppe lens is that, when holding the lens against the eye with thumb and forefinger, the examiner can steady the eye during the examination and can easily move the eye to bring the disc or macula conveniently into view.

We have found ophthalmoscopy through the Koeppe goniolens to have real advantages in the following situations:

- In infants and adults with irregularity of the surface of the cornea, either from drying or from epithelial edema, one can usually obtain a clearer view of the fundus by using the lens.

- In children with aniridia and nystagmus, or with nystagmus from other causes, the rubber-flanged Koeppe lens permits one to hold the eye still and to examine the fundus with most of the motion eliminated.

- In older people with small pupils that one cannot dilate or does not wish to dilate, or in people who seem unable to keep their eyes still, application of the Koeppe lens permits easier viewing of the central fundus. Also, in older patients who have immature cataracts, it is sometimes surprising how well the optic disc and central fundus can be seen through the Koeppe lens, even though it can be almost impossible to see them without this aid.

A wider, more panoramic view of the fundus is obtained more easily with the direct ophthalmoscope through a pupil of moderate size when the Koeppe lens is used than by the direct ophthalmoscope unaided.

RELATION OF OPTIC DISC TO VISUAL FIELD

The extent and location of field defects from cupping and atrophy in glaucoma correspond to changes that are visible in the optic disc with the ophthalmoscope. For instance, if the pathologic cupping and atrophy are confined to the lower-outer pole of the disc, as they are in the majority of early glaucomas, the only possible field defect due to glaucoma is an upper nasal step, an upper Bjerrum scotoma, or both.

If, on the other hand, the physiologic cup enlarges upward and the lower pole of the disc is still normal, any glaucomatous field defect will be a lower Bjerrum scotoma, lower nasal step, or both. If the pathologic cupping involves the entire temporal side of the disc, then there may be an upper or lower Bjerrum scotoma, or both. With an inverse-type disc in which the principal vessels leave the disc on the temporal rather than on the nasal side, the first cupping may be nasal and the field defect temporal.

In cases of total cupping and atrophy or excavation to the margin of the temporal half or two-thirds of the disc, one cannot tell from the appearance of the optic disc what the location or the type of field defect may be. Also, in highly myopic eyes, the appearance of the disc is notoriously difficult to interpret from the standpoint of glaucoma.

We believe that, in most eyes (not highly myopic), there can be no field defects due to glaucoma if the disc is normal, unless the IOP is high at the time of the examination or has been high a short time previously. If the IOP is elevated at the time of examination, glaucomatous field defects may be found. Such defects may disappear if IOP is promptly reduced to normal. If such field defects are permanent, then, within a few weeks, atrophy will be evident. In the type of case in which the IOP is high at the time of examination, or has been high in the recent past, treatment is generally planned on the basis of IOP alone. Measurement of the field is of limited value in management of such a case.

In exceptional cases, one may find glaucomatous-type field defects, such as a Bjerrum-type scotoma or a Ronne step, with the IOP and the disc completely normal, but these field defects we know cannot be due to glaucoma. We have seen many patients who had glaucoma and were alleged to be losing field, or who had lost field despite good IOP control, but the appearance of the disc did not correlate with the field defect. The inconsistencies triggered further causative investigation and were resolved by the findings of vascular occlusions, old chorioretinitis, drusen on the optic disc, or neurologic disorders, including brain tumors, retinitis pigmentosa, retinal detachment, or retinoschisis (Figure 8-11).

Local indentations of the peripheral fields that do not correspond to expectation from the appearance of the disc indicate, in particular, a search for retinoschisis or retinal cyst. A dense arcuate scotoma extending from the blind spot can be produced by drusen in the optic nerve head (ONH), by juxtapapillary choroiditis, by occlusion of a macular artery, or by pituitary tumor. A ring scotoma simulating a double Bjerrum scotoma can be produced by retinitis pigmentosa.

Any disparity between the visual field and the character of glaucomatous changes in the optic disc should raise suspicions of nonglaucomatous intraocular or extraocular cause of the defect. Of course, one is most easily misled if the patient does have glaucoma with some correlating cupping, atrophy, and field loss, but also has homonymous hemianopsia from cerebrovascular occlusion or bitemporal constriction from pituitary tumor. These can be detected by their lack of conformity to the types of changes in the optic nerve and visual field produced by glaucoma.

The following case illustrates field loss in a glaucomatous eye that was actually due to retinal detachment.

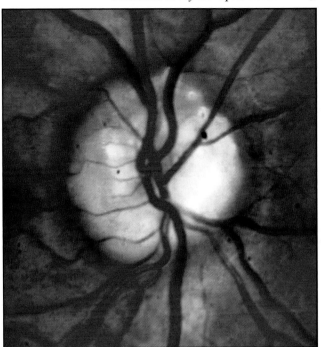

Figure 8-11. Multiple drusen of the optic disc in a patient who has open-angle glaucoma. Such drusen themselves can produce various field defects and should be searched for (among other possibilities) when the disc appearance does not explain the field defect.

Case 8-1

A 56-year-old man was referred with a history of IOP of 41 mm Hg OD and 31 mm Hg OS, but, under pilocarpine, OD and OS 18; corrected vision OD 6/9+, OS 6/6; angles wide and open. The cups were physiologic, but the cup was wider in the left eye than in the right. The fields were full. A year and a half later, he was referred back. IOP was 19 mm Hg OU, and fields were full. One year later, he was referred back because of loss of the entire upper field in the right eye. However, this could not be explained by glaucoma because the discs were unchanged. Examination indicated detachment of approximately the lower half of the right retina. A retinal reattachment operation was performed successfully. Seven years later when last seen, corrected vision was 6/12 OD, 6/6 OS; there were increased reflexes in the macula of the right eye; fields were normal.

INTRAOCULAR PRESSURE AND CHANGES IN THE OPTIC DISC

An important factor in pathologic cupping of the optic disc, regardless of type, might be called susceptibility. It has not been explained to our satisfaction why some eyes develop pathologic cupping and field loss with IOP a little above normal, or even in the normal range, and other eyes

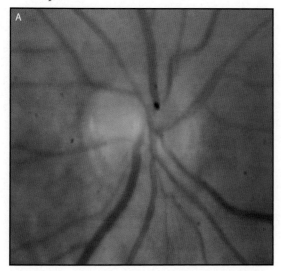

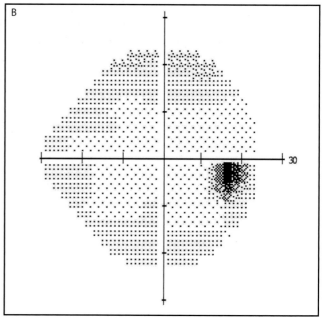

Figure 8-12. (A) Healthy central cup in a patient with elevated IOP. Abundant disc rim tissue between the edge of the cup and the edge of the disc is present. The rim tissue is of normal contour and is on a plane with the retina (compare Figure 8-3). (B) No field loss would be expected with such a disc appearance. The scleral crescent should not be mistaken for the edge of the disc.

sustain a much higher IOP over a long period of time without developing pathologic cupping. It is, however, a commonly described phenomenon. Whatever level of IOP is found, if there is pathologic cupping, we must strive with all the means at our disposal, both medical and surgical, to bring the IOP to a lower level.

The degree of glaucomatous cupping and atrophy of the disc is a particularly important consideration in estimating how low one may need to reduce the IOP in the treatment of individual cases of glaucoma. Thus, if the disc is normal when the diagnosis of glaucoma is first made, one finds that the eye tends to withstand elevated IOP relatively well. In an eye with a completely normal disc, especially if the physiologic cup is small and the color rosy, an IOP as high as 30 mm Hg may cause little or no loss of function over a period of many years (Figure 8-12). Where there is already marked acquired glaucomatous cupping at the initial diagnosis of glaucoma, to prevent further loss of function, a much lower IOP is required than in a case in which the disc shows minimal cupping. If excavation of the disc is severe, an IOP as high as 18 mm Hg typically can cause loss of function over a period of years. In cases of limited cupping, the eye tolerates increased IOP less well than in cases in which the disc is normal, but better than in cases of total cupping. Thus, the greater the extent and depth of glaucomatous cupping, the lower the IOP must be maintained in order to prevent further loss of vision.

The types of cupping, atrophy, and field loss that develop in POAG, progressing in some eyes even after the IOP is reduced to the high normal range and stopping only when a very low IOP is achieved, appear clinically identical with the changes that are found in patients who have never been known to have had abnormally elevated IOP (normal-tension glaucoma). These circumstances, sometimes termed *normal-tension glaucoma equivalent*, are discussed further in Chapter 19.

It has been suspected that the blood pressure and the circulation of the ONH may have significant influence on its vulnerability in these circumstances. This possibility is discussed later in this chapter under the heading "Blood Pressure and the Optic Disc."

When the IOP is elevated, we know that the higher the IOP, the greater is the danger to the optic disc, but we should also be aware that the height of the IOP significantly influences the type of damage that is done to the optic nerve. In fact, highly elevated IOP alone can sometimes acutely enlarge the optic cup, especially in young patients. This change is reversible if the IOP is reduced within a few days or weeks.

A moderate elevation of IOP produces the common varieties of glaucomatous pathologic cupping, followed by atrophy, whereas a high IOP can cause a predominance of atrophy with less pathologic cupping in a shorter period. Thus, an IOP of 40, 50, or 60 mm Hg maintained over several weeks may cause atrophy, with minimal pathologic cupping.

With persistent or repeated IOP of 40 to 50 mm Hg or higher, one should rely more on visual fields than on ophthalmoscopy to warn of increasing damage to the ONH, because, at these pressures, loss of vision may occur before there is appreciable increase in cupping and before atrophy of the optic disc is visible.

In neglected acute angle-closure glaucoma, where the IOP is characteristically very high, the end result may be relatively pure atrophy with virtually no pathologic cupping.

We have called attention to the clinical observation that optic discs with acquired glaucomatous cupping are more susceptible than normal discs to damage by IOP, but clinical observation suggests that atrophy apart from cupping does not make the disc abnormally susceptible to further damage by IOP. It seems that an ONH that has been made pale or whitish by partial optic atrophy with little or no cupping after acute high IOP or due to some other cause is not abnormally susceptible to injury by subsequent moderate pressure elevation. Thus, after acute glaucoma and partial disc atrophy, when IOP has been reduced by surgery and medicine, it seems that, in order to prevent further loss of vision, the control of IOP needs to be no more strict than for other discs that have the same type of cup. However, these clinical situations need further evaluation.

Returning to discussion of differences in vulnerability among optic discs that ostensibly are not yet pathologically cupped and are not atrophic, we also need to consider whether eyes with unusually large physiologic cups are extraordinarily vulnerable.

In some eyes, the physiologic cups are exceptionally wide and deep; in some, the rim of normal tissue at the border of the disc may be no more than the width of 1 or 2 major vessels on the disc. Eyes with such wide and deep cups withstand increased IOP more poorly than eyes in which the physiologic cup is considerably smaller.

There are 2 other important factors in myopic eyes with POAG. It may be difficult to detect early cupping because of the sloped nature of the myopic disc, and such eyes may demonstrate initial field loss due to glaucoma close to or actually involving fixation. Therefore, myopic eyes with POAG require special attention and likely earlier treatment (see Chapter 18).

BLOOD PRESSURE AND THE OPTIC DISC

There is an important and debated question concerning whether the level of the arterial blood pressure influences the susceptibility of the optic disc to damage by IOP. The question is, does elevated arterial blood pressure tend to protect the optic disc from elevated IOP, and, conversely, does low blood pressure render the disc more vulnerable? There are 2 conditions in which this question has great practical relevance. First, in patients who have both glaucoma and systemic hypertension, is there risk of an increase in damage to the optic discs if the systemic hypertension is treated and the blood pressure is reduced? Second, in patients with normal-tension glaucoma, or its equivalent (see Chapter 19), can cupping, atrophy, and loss of vision be caused by subnormal arterial blood pressure while the IOP is within the normal range? The most fundamental question underlying these practical clinical questions is to what extent ischemia is involved in damage of the optic disc in chronic glaucoma. The answer is not yet known, but opinions are not lacking.[1]

We will examine clinical information concerning influences on the optic disc, first from systemic blood pressure and then from arterial occlusive disease affecting the blood supply to the eye.

Systemic Blood Pressure

Clinical comparisons have been made between groups of glaucomatous patients with similar IOPs but different blood pressures, looking for differences in the prevalence of visual field defects. Such studies have led Reese and McGavic,[2] Sachsenweger,[3] Lobstein,[4] Ebner,[5] and Said et al[6] to believe that elevated blood pressure had an unfavorable influence. In similar studies, Fruhauf,[7] Tuovinen et al,[8] and Simonett,[9] found no evidence of influence of arterial blood pressure. There are great difficulties in making meaningful comparisons in this way, because, in addition to the blood pressure, the IOP, the extent of pathologic cupping, and the visual fields at the time of testing, there are many other variables to be taken into consideration.

Some clinicians who have written about the influence of blood pressure seem to have been most impressed with individual case reports in which rapid deterioration of visual field was observed when elevated blood pressure was drastically reduced in patients who had glaucoma that previously had been considered to be adequately regulated. However, there are many patients who have both chronic glaucoma and systemic hypertension, and a large number of these people have been given treatment to reduce their blood pressure. In view of this, the small number of cases of apparent adverse effects actually reported is remarkable. The cases most often cited are those of Harrington,[10] who described 3 patients who had high blood pressure and who had been under treatment with pilocarpine for glaucoma, with IOPs not normalized, but stable visual fields for 3 years, 2 years, and a shorter period, when reserpine, with or without hydralazine, was started. These patients had large decreases in blood pressure and distinct increases in visual field defects within a few days to 4 weeks, without change in IOP or in appearance of the discs. Cessation of systemic medications was followed by partial recovery of lost field in only one case.

McLean[11] mentioned, without further details, one patient who lost visual field after dramatic control of his systemic hypertension.

Francois and Neetens[12] have given brief case reports (with no information on time relationships) of 7 instances of increase in loss of visual field after medical treatment for systemic hypertension while IOP was thought to be adequately controlled.

In these few suggestive case reports, there has been no way to be sure that the changes in visual fields after antihypertensive treatment were caused by reduction of blood pressure or were coincidental. The need is evident for a large-scale prospective clinical study, extending over many years, to ascertain whether elevated systemic blood pressure is in fact protective against the damaging effect of elevated IOP on the optic disc and whether treating systemic hypertension in glaucomatous patients significantly increases the risk of damage to the optic disc.

Kolker and colleagues[13] have used corticosteroids, Heilmann[14] has used acetazolamide and clonidine, and Phelps and Phelps[15] have used phenylephrine in acute experiments to alter relationships between IOP and blood pressure and to examine the influence on visual fields in glaucoma, indicating that reduced blood pressure is disadvantageous. Such short-term experiments on visual fields, however intriguing and suggestive, do leave the question unsettled as to whether there are corresponding long-term relationships and what relationship there may be to the cupping of the optic disc.

There have been several recent reports calling attention to the potential adverse influence of nocturnal hypotension on the course of glaucomatous optic nerve damage.[16-20]

While the role of blood pressure and the mechanism of glaucomatous cupping and atrophy are being investigated in clinical and experimental research centers, it seems reasonable from a practical clinical standpoint that, whenever medication for systemic hypertension is given to a patient who has glaucoma that is not very well-controlled, the frequency of examination of the optic disc and visual fields should be increased. In patients who demonstrate unexpected progression of their glaucoma, the possibility of nocturnal hypotension needs to be contemplated and internal medicine consultation obtained.

ARTERIAL OCCLUSIVE DISEASE

In questioning the possible relationship of blood pressure and vulnerability of the optic disc in glaucoma, it is relevant to note that interference with arterial blood supply by extraocular vasculopathy has not thus far been shown to have significant influence. One would think that there must be many patients who have carotid obstructive disease, often unilateral, as well as glaucoma, and that if a normal arterial supply was critically important for the fate of the optic disc in glaucoma, then we would see evidence of it.

The literature[21-23] on ocular effects associated with occlusion of carotid arteries and with the aortic arch syndrome, or pulseless disease, contains many example in which the influences on IOP and on ocular pulse are described. Acute common and internal carotid occlusions are known to produce a sudden decrease of IOP by a few mm Hg, as repeatedly demonstrated during carotid compression tonography. During chronic occlusion, the ocular pulse, recorded by

---

CLINICAL ASSESSMENT OF THE NERVE FIBER LAYER
Joel S. Schuman, MD, FACS

Examination of the retinal nerve fiber layer (RNFL) is a challenging portion of the ophthalmologic evaluation. It requires patience and practice, and is not easily mastered. The RNFL, because of its structure of parallel tubular fibers, reflects light differently than the remainder of the retina. The absence of these fibers results in decreased reflectance.

The RNFL is most easily visualized using red-free light. It can be examined using a direct ophthalmoscope, but is better appreciated with a dilated pupil and a 78-D lens in stereoscopic biomicroscopy at the slit-lamp. The beam is widened slightly from that used for anterior segment evaluation to provide an adequate field of view, but not so wide as to cause discomfort to the patient. In younger patients with clear media, a gleam can sometimes be seen from the internal limiting membrane. The RNFL appears as a series of striations radiating in an arcuate fashion from (really toward) the optic nerve head (ONH) over and under the macula, not crossing the horizontal meridian. Because the RNFL is thickest at the superior and inferior poles, the reflectance is greatest in these areas, and they appear more white.

When examining the RNFL, one looks for areas of focal loss, which appear as dark bands fanning out from the ONH, with a bright-dark-bright pattern or areas of diffuse loss. Diffuse loss is seen as a decrease in reflection from the tissue, and the underlying vasculature can then be differentiated more easily. In the peripapillary region, less than 1 disc diameter from the ONH, secondary, tertiary, and quaternary vessel branches are poorly seen and do not have sharp borders with a healthy RNFL. As the RNFL thins, the vessels and vessel borders become more distinct. This is most clearly evident in advanced glaucoma, when all vessel branches are easily distinguished.

Documentation of RNFL appearance by photography is probably the best way to examine this structure, but the technique is difficult to perform and requires a willingness on the part of the photographer. Red-free photographs, in black and white, can be studied for RNFL appearance and provide an excellent record to use for future visits.

Several methods have been devised for grading the degree of NFL loss quantitatively, but they are difficult to learn and to use. Simple qualitative assessment of NFL status seems the best option for examination of this tissue, with descriptive terms such as normal, thin, or absent, or a description of which vessels are visible and to what level of branching in a given area.

Because clinical examination of the RNFL is qualitative and difficult, technology is currently under development, with some already available, for actual quantitation of RNFL thickness, as described in Chapter 9. No technology, however, can replace the ophthalmologist's study of the patient's eye, and evaluation of the RNFL clinically is an essential part of that examination.

---

tonography or by measurement of the corneal pulse, and the orbital pulse, recorded by ophthalmodynamography, are reduced, and pressure in the central retinal arteries can be shown by ophthalmodynamometry to be reduced. However, rarely is mention made of influence on cupping or atrophy of the optic disc or changes in the visual field, such as are associated with glaucoma. It might be postulated that the optic nerve may be protected from reduced arterial supply by a simultaneous reduction of IOP. However, only severe reduction of arterial blood supply, such as that produced by bilateral carotid disease or by the aortic arch syndrome, produces much chronic decrease in IOP.

When the arterial supply to the eye is so severely insufficient that it causes marked reduction of IOP, meaningful long-term studies of the influence of the blood supply on the optic disc are practically precluded by degenerative changes in the eye, such as secondary neovascularization of the iris and anterior chamber angle, necrosis of the anterior segment, hypoxic retinopathy, and retinal degeneration.

A long-term study and comparison of the optic discs and visual fields in patients with moderate reduction of blood supply to one eye and constantly, equally elevated IOP in both eyes would be most informative. One eye would serve as a control for the other, the difference in arterial supply being the principal variable. It is remarkable how little information of this sort is available.

Ignoring for the moment cases of temporal or giant cell arteritis because they tend to be complicated by intraocular vascular disease, which would confuse the study of the influence of blood supply alone, there is one report[21] in which patients with normal IOPs but with reduced ocular blood supply due to so-called subclavian steal have had atrophic changes and cupping in the disc, with visual field change in the periphery, sometimes with an upper nasal defect, usually bilaterally. The nature of the cupping and any anatomic relationship to loss of visual field are not described in this study, so it is unclear whether there is significant analogy to the changes in glaucoma or in progressive normal-tension glaucoma.

Another study[22] concerns 13 patients with IOPs in the normal range who had their retinal arterial pressure reduced 20% to 25% in one eye for several years after unilateral carotid ligation. In these patients, the optic nerves and all visual functions remained intact.

Coming closer to the desired controlled study of bilaterally glaucomatous eyes with asymmetric arterial supplies is a report of 5 patients[23] with elevated IOP, but bilateral severe artery disease, who developed no glaucomatous disc or field changes during observation for 3 to 12 years. This is interesting, but the definitive controlled investigation is yet to be done.

The reported effects of temporal or giant cell arteritis on the ONH are mentioned here because they are interesting in their own right, indicating a relationship of intraocular vascular disease to cupping of the optic disc. However, we do not know what relationship this may have to the main topic of blood pressure and the optic disc.

Hayreh[24] and Miller[25] have reported that when ischemic optic neuropathy has developed from occlusion of posterior ciliary arteries in temporal arteritis, there has been loss of central vision with pale edema of the optic disc, followed 2 to 3 months later by cupping and atrophy of the optic disc, becoming deep after 4 to 5 months. This has occurred in eyes that have been thought to have had normal IOP throughout. Hayreh noted relatively slight cupping in eyes with occlusion

of posterior ciliary arteries due to arteriosclerosis. We have observed at least 5 cases of anterior ischemic optic neuropathy secondary to biopsy-proven giant cell arteritis where optic nerve changes indistinguishable from glaucomatous cupping were observed.[26] After nonarteritic ischemic optic neuropathy, we have only rarely observed any suspicious glaucoma-like changes involving the optic nerve.

REFERENCES

1. Maumenee AE. The pathogenesis of visual field loss in glaucoma. In: Brockhurst RJ, Boruchuff SA, Hutchinson BT, Lessell S, eds. *Controversy in Ophthalmology*. Philadelphia, PA: WB Saunders Co; 1977:301-311.
2. Reese AB, McGavic JS. Relation of field contraction to blood pressure in chronic primary glaucoma. *Arch Ophthalmol*. 1942;27:845-850.
3. Sachsenweger R. Der Einluss des Bluthochdruckes auf die Prognose des Glaukoms. *Klin Monatsbl Augenheilkd*. 1963;142:625-633.
4. Lobstein A. Factors affecting the susceptibility of the glaucomatous eye to raised intraocular pressure. In: Sampaolesi R, ed. *Modern Problems in Ophthalmology*. New York, NY: Karger; 1968; 73-93.
5. Ebner R. Die Prognose des Glaukoms im Hinblick auf den arteriellen Blutdruck. *Wien Med Wochenschr*. 1967;117:1024-1026.
6. Said A, Labib MAM, Abboud I, et al. The relationship between systemic hypertension and chronic simple glaucoma. *Bull Ophthalmol Soc Egypt*. 1967;60:71-81.
7. Fruhauf A. Untesuchungen über den Einfluss des arteriellen Blutdrucks auf den Verlauf des Glaucoma simplex. *Dtsch Gesundheitsw*. 1971;26:273-275.
8. Tuovinen E, Jägerroos P, Vänttinen S. Die Bedeutung des arteriellen Blutdruckes für die Prognose des Glaucoma simplex. *Wiss Z Univ Rostock, Math.* 1965;14:131-137.
9. Simonett B. Der Brachialisblutdruck und seine Beziehung zum Verlauf des Glaucoma simplex. *Klin Monatsbl Augenheilkd*. 1959;135:196-205.
10. Harrington DO. The pathogenesis of the glaucoma field. Clinical evidence that circulatory insufficiency in the optic nerve is the primary cause of visual field loss in glaucoma. *Am J Ophthalmol*. 1959;47:177-185.
11. McLean JM. Management of the primary glaucomas. *Am J Ophthalmol*. 1957;44:323-334.
12. Francois J, Neetens A. The deterioration of the visual field in glaucoma and the blood pressure. *Doc Ophthalmol*. 1970;28:70-132.
13. Kolker AE, Becker B, Mills DW. Intraocular pressure and visual fields: Effects of corticosteroids. *Arch Ophthalmol*. 1965;72:772-782.
14. Heilmann K. Augendruck, Blutdruck und Glaukomschaden. *Bucherei des Augenartes*. 1972;61:1-82.
15. Phelps GK, Phelps CD. Blood pressure and pressure amaurosis. *Invest Ophthalmol*. 1975;14:237-240.
16. Kaiser HJ, Flammer J. Systemic hypotension: a risk factor for glaucomatous damage? *Ophthalmologica*. 1994;203:105-108.
17. Hayreh SS, Zimmerman MB, Podhajsky P, et al. Nocturnal arterial hypotension and its role in optic nerve head ischaemic disorders. *Am J Ophthalmol*. 1994;117:603-624.
18. Deokule S, Weinreb RN. Relationships among systemic blood pressure, intraocular pressure, and open-angle glaucoma. *Can J Ophthalmol*. 2008;43(3):302-307.
19. Béchetoille A, Bresson-Dumont H. Diurnal and nocturnal blood pressure drops in patients with focal ischemic glaucoma. *Clin Invest*. 1994;232:675-679.
20. Graham SL, Drance SM, Wijsman K, Douglas GR, Mikelberg FS. Ambulatory blood pressure monitoring in glaucoma, the nocturnal dip. *Ophthalmology*. 1995;102:61-69.
21. Dwyer-Joyce P. The fields in subclavian steal. *Trans Ophthalmol Soc UK*. 1972;92:819-824.

22. Cristiansson J. On the late effect of carotid ligation upon the human eye. *Acta Ophthalmol.* 1962;40:271-280.

23. Jampol LM, Miller NR. Carotid artery disease and glaucoma. *Br J Ophthalmol.* 1978;6:324-326.

24. Hayreh SS. Pathogenesis of cupping of the optic disc. *Br J Ophthalmol.* 1974;58:863-876.

25. Miller S. The enigma of glaucoma simplex. Optic disc cupping in normal eyes. *Trans Ophthalmol Soc UK.* 1972;92:563-584.

26. Sebag J, Thomas JV, Epstein DL, et al. Optic disc cupping in arteritic anterior ischemic optic neuropathy resembles glaucomatous cupping. *Ophthalmology.* 1986;93:357-361.

Imaging of the Optic Nerve Head and Nerve Fiber Layer

Lindsey S. Folio, MS, MBA; Gadi Wollstein, MD; and Joel S. Schuman, MD, FACS

Glaucoma is the second leading cause of blindness worldwide.[1] Currently, there is no cure for this irreversible disease; therefore, it is best treated with early diagnosis and timely medical treatment. Glaucoma presents as an optic neuropathy, accompanied by characteristic vision loss and structural damage. Common methods of clinical glaucoma assessment include optic nerve head (ONH) examination, intraocular pressure (IOP) measurement, and visual field testing. However, these methods are limited because they are subjective and rely heavily on clinical interpretation. Additionally, it has been shown that 40% of nerve fibers could be lost before being detected by these subjective methods.[2,3] Recent advances in imaging technologies have greatly improved the objective evaluation techniques for glaucoma management because they are capable of obtaining quantitative measurements of the ONH and surrounding retinal tissues. Studies have shown that imaging technologies offer a similar or improved glaucoma diagnostic ability to that of clinical evaluation of optic disc photographs.[4-9] Current clinical glaucoma management has, therefore, combined the use of both subjective and quantitative methods for optic disc evaluation and glaucoma diagnosis.

This chapter will present a summary of common methods of optic nerve evaluation in glaucoma including pertinent imaging technologies such as confocal scanning laser ophthalmoscopy (CSLO), scanning laser polarimetry (SLP), and optical coherence tomography (OCT), as well as time domain (TD) and spectral domain (SD) OCT.

HISTORICAL PERSPECTIVE

The first observation of the ONH was documented with the invention of the ophthalmoscope in 1851.[10] Four years later, glaucoma was detailed by von Graefe[11] as consisting of excavation of the optic nerve. Schnabel[12] was the first to relate nerve fiber loss to glaucoma in evaluating tissue cavities. However, it was not until 1922 that Fuchs[13] and Elliot[14] described in great detail the structural changes to the optic nerve caused by glaucoma. Fuchs[13] observed a disappearance of anterior glial fibers, followed by deeper glial fibers, accompanied by backward bending and thinning of the lamina cribrosa. Fuchs noted these changes found in the ONH preceded vision loss and coincided with an increased IOP. Since these observations, the gold standard in glaucoma evaluation has focused on ONH examination, IOP measures, and visual field tests. However, there are many limitations to these 3 nonimaging evaluation techniques. ONH examination can be performed using direct ophthalmoscopy, indirect ophthalmoscopy, and slit-lamp biomicroscopy. The subjectivity associated with ONH visual examination presents as a limitation because the assessment can be inconsistent between visits and has been found to vary between clinicians.[15] IOP is limited because of its wide diurnal variation, absence of IOP abnormality in a substantial percentage of glaucoma patients, namely subjects with normal-tension glaucoma, and because it does not directly assess the degree of damage. Visual field tests are shown to be inconsistent with repeated examination.[16] These limitations created a great need for an objective method of glaucoma assessment, which was recently fulfilled by imaging devices.

The diagnostic techniques of imaging devices have become a complementary part of clinical glaucoma assessment. They remove subjectivity by providing unmatched visualization of ocular structures and by presenting quantitative data to aid in glaucoma diagnostics. As first pointed out by von Graefe[11] and Schnable,[12] glaucomatous damage appears most clearly in the optic nerve and retinal nerve fiber layer (RNFL). Therefore, the methodologies of imaging

Kahook MY, Schuman JS, eds.
Chandler and Grant's Glaucoma, Fifth Edition (pp 95-109).
© 2013 SLACK Incorporated.

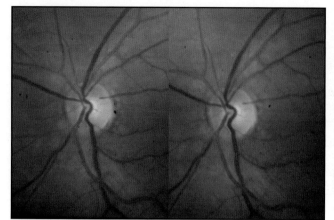

Figure 9-1. Stereoscopic fundus photograph of healthy subject.

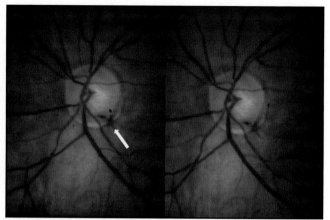

Figure 9-2. Stereoscopic fundus photograph of a glaucoma patient with an optic disc hemorrhage (arrow).

in glaucoma have focused on extracting measurements of tissue morphology from these 2 regions.

ASSESSMENT OF THE OPTIC NERVE HEAD

Precise examination and subsequent documentation of the ONH make up a critical portion of glaucoma evaluation. The ONH is composed mainly of load-bearing connective tissues and neural tissues. The neural tissues are in the form of approximately 1 to 1.2 million retinal ganglion cell (RGC) axons.[17] These axons come together and exit the eye by way of the ONH. Damage that presents as cupping to the ONH is an appropriate indicator of the state of health of the RGCs and connective tissues. Additionally, one of the postulated locations for the initial glaucomatous damage is at the point where the RGC axons intersect the lamina cribrosa mesh-like structure. This reinforces the necessity to accurately assess the optic disc region in glaucoma evaluation. Fundus photography, CSLO, and OCT all provide reliable and reproducible methods to evaluate the health of the ONH.

Stereoscopic Fundus Photography

A fundus camera is a special camera designed with a microscope to effectively capture the inner workings of the eye, including the retina, optic disc, and macula. The benefit of the fundus camera over clinical ONH examination techniques, such as direct ophthalmoscopy, indirect ophthalmoscopy, or slit-lamp biomicroscopy, is that it creates a photograph (Figure 9-1). The stereoscopic feature allows a 3-dimensional fundus image to be captured, giving the clinician a more realistic view to assess cupping of the ONH tissues. Stereoscopic fundus photography's ability to capture images of the ONH greatly aids in increasing the reliability of glaucoma evaluation over time, because the photographs can be directly compared. Glaucoma is a slowly progressing disease, so minor changes to the optic disc can easily go unnoticed until damage reaches a more severe level.

Fundus photography allows better assessment of these minor changes.

Stereoscopic fundus photography also offers visualization of certain traits characteristic of glaucoma that cannot be seen with other imaging methods. The characteristic optic disc pallor, pale-yellow coloring and the ability to document disc hemorrhage (Figure 9-2), a common occurrence in glaucomatous eyes, are examples of important clinical cues that can be documented with this method of imaging. For these reasons, fundus photography will continue to be a crucial component of glaucoma clinical management in the foreseen future.

The major limitation of fundus photography is the subjective component of the image assessment. Studies have shown disagreements between glaucoma experts in glaucoma discrimination determined from stereophotos.[4,18,19] New developments in image processing allow some automated quantification of ONH structures from the photographs.[20,21] Other approaches involve the presentation of the photographs in ways that enhance the ability to detect ONH changes. One example is Matched Flicker (EyeIC, Narberth, PA), which aligns and flickers between 2 sets of photographs to allow detection of small changes.

Confocal Scanning Laser Ophthalmoscopy

CSLO, first described by Webb and colleagues in 1987,[22] is a techniques used to image the ONH. A beam of light is directed at the retinal tissue of interest and is reflected and detected by a sensor. To reach the sensor, the reflected light must pass through a set of 2 conjugated pinholes, located in front of the detector and adjacent to the light source. This method ensures that only light reflected from the focal plane is detected by the sensor.[23] To acquire a 3-dimensional representation of the ONH, the focal plane is adjusted during image acquisition. These images obtained from the multiple parallel focal planes

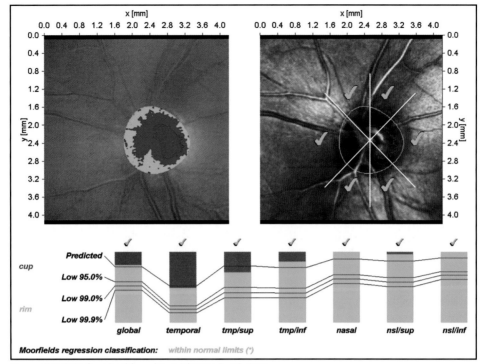

Figure 9-3. MRA for a healthy subject (obtained with HRT).

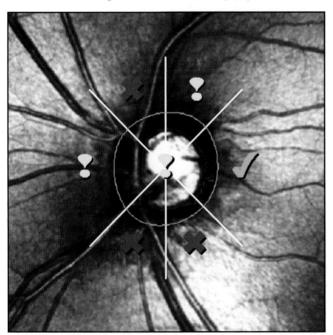

Figure 9-4. GPS for a glaucoma patient appearing outside normal limits inferiorly and superonasally; borderline globally, nasally, and superotemporally; and within normal limits temporally (obtained with HRT).

are then reconstructed to form one image that represents the topography of the ONH.

The most commonly used CSLO device is the Heidelberg Retinal Tomography (HRT; Heidelberg Engineering, Heidelberg, Germany). The current version of the device (HRT3) uses a 670-nm wavelength laser beam to capture between 16 and 64 2-dimensional scans at different focal planes. Each 2-dimensional scan is made up of a grid of 384×384 points from a 15×15 degrees field of view. The device is capable of acquiring scans with 10-mm transverse and 300-mm axial resolutions. To obtain quantitative parameters from the image, the device requires the user to define the ONH margin by marking a contour line surrounding the disc. Parameters abstracted from the image include disc area, rim area, rim volume, cup area, cup volume, and cup/disc ratios.

The HRT includes Moorfields Regression Analysis (MRA) and Glaucoma Probability Score (GPS) assessment software. MRA assesses the likelihood of glaucoma by comparing the predicted rim area, after accounting for the disc area and age, to the measured rim area globally and in 6 predefined sectors. Each sector, as well as the overall disc, is then classified as within normal limits (WNL), borderline, or outside normal limits (ONL) when compared to a normative distribution of the population (Figure 9-3). The bar graph in Figure 9-3 demonstrates the predicted computed rim area as the upper horizontal line with the corresponding cutoff values of abnormalities (low 95%, 99%, and 99.9%) with the colored bar representing the actual measurement. A green bar terminating below the 99.9% cutoff will be marked as abnormal. Alternatively, the GPS software provides an operator-independent method to assess the ONH where there is no need to manually delineate the disc margin (Figure 9-4). This method relies on typical 3-dimensional configuration of the ONH region and automatically determines the probability of glaucomatous changes in this region. GPS quantitative scoring assessment has been found to be consistent with glaucoma discrimination by subjective optic disc assessment.[24]

In addition to advanced evaluation software, CSLO offers benefits such as automatic image registration with previously acquired scans for longitudinal assessment. CSLO has also been shown to be highly reproducible[25] and simple to operate and requires no pupil dilation in most subjects. Nevertheless, CSLO has been found to be more sensitive in discriminating between healthy and glaucomatous eyes than stereoscopic optic disc photographs[5] and has been shown to offer high diagnostic precision in early glaucoma cases.[26]

Another advantage of the CSLO technology is the inclusion of progression analysis software, also known as Topographic Change Analysis (TCA), in the operating system. TCA uses the registration capability of the CSLO images to assess the thinning or thickening of the topography surrounding the ONH over time. This assessment compares a baseline scan to follow-up images and accounts for possible variabilities between scans when reporting change. The variability is defined for each subject based on the first 2 baseline tests, and a consequent change that exceeds this variability will be marked as progression. The topographic change is reported as superpixel clusters on the CSLO image, as shown in Figure 9-5. Quantitative measures abstracted from the analysis include thinning or thickening area and thinning or thickening volume. A plot showing the changes in cluster size over time can also be created from the software to show progression. It should be noted that the superpixels labeled as change from baseline often appear adjacent to blood vessels due to the variability in the timing of data acquisition during the cardiac cycle. This variability is apparent in Figure 9-5 as red and green clusters located on the blood vessels. It has been suggested that the most reliable parameter to detect glaucoma progression is the cluster size within the ONH.[27] Figure 9-5 presents an example of a cluster of neuroretinal rim loss in the temporal inferior region that gradually expands during follow-up. An adjacent retinal wedge defect (red cluster) enlarges in the final 2 visits.

Limitations of CSLO include the operator dependence of the ONH margin's location, the required reference plane to obtain quantitative measurements of the ONH that might vary between visits, and the inclusion of blood vessels as part of the rim, thus overestimating this structure while underestimating cup measurements.

Optical Coherence Tomography

OCT is an imaging technique used to evaluate the ONH, RNFL, and the macula. First described by Huang and colleagues in 1991, OCT is performed similar to B-mode ultrasound except it uses light waves instead of sound waves to create a cross-sectional image.[28] It is a noninvasive, noncontact technique that uses the differences in optical properties of tissue structures to create an image.

The cross-sectional image created by TD-OCT comes from information in backscattered light. OCT uses a broad bandwidth, low coherence light source from a superluminescent diode coupled to a fiberoptic Michelson interferometer. The projected light is divided so that part of it is directed toward a mirror contained in a reference arm and the other to the tissue of interest. When the beams are reflected, the signals recombine at a detector to create an interference pattern that corresponds to the axial reflectivity of the sample. The interference pattern can only be assessed at the detector when the light reflected from the sample and the light reflected from the mirror are within the coherence length of the light. The axial reflectivities recorded represent one A-scan, or depth measurement, of the OCT image. A series of A-scans can be obtained to create a cross-sectional image, otherwise known as an OCT B-scan. Figure 9-6 shows a circumpapillary OCT B-scan obtained by a circle scanning pattern surrounding the ONH.

TD-OCT is capable of obtaining images of 8- to 10-μm axial resolution at 400 A-scans/second. Sampling densities for TD-OCT can be set to 512, 256, and 128 A-scans per B-scan, where scans are generally completed in a line or circular pattern. Once a scan is completed, a fundus image is acquired to verify the placement of the scan (Figure 9-7). Because this fundus image is obtained postscanning, it does not precisely represent where the OCT image was obtained, but provides a close estimation. The TD-OCT's ONH scan employs six 4-mm radial line scans centered on the ONH. One line scan from the ONH scanning pattern is shown in Figure 9-8. To determine quantitative measurements of the ONH, the device uses an algorithm that automatically delineates the disc margin. Quantitative parameters that can be obtained from TD-OCT's ONH scan include rim area, disc area, cup area, disc diameter, cup diameter, vertical integrated rim area (volume), cup/disc vertical ratio, cup/disc horizontal ratio, and cup/disc area ratio.

More recent advances in OCT technology have led to the development of spectral-domain (SD)-OCT or frequency domain OCT. SD-OCT A-scans are recorded in the frequency domain by splitting the interference pattern into its frequency components. Each frequency of light represents a different tissue depth; therefore, each A-scan can be acquired instantaneously. The mirror in the reference arm is stationary, unlike the moving mirror in TD-OCT, which markedly reduces acquisition time. SD-OCT techniques were first reported by Wojtkowski and colleagues[29,30] in 2001. Current SD-OCT systems are capable of recording up to 680,000 A-scans/second[31] and axial resolutions in the range of 4 to 8 μm.[32] The improved image quality achieved with this iteration of the OCT technology compared to TD-OCT is evident in the cross-section shown in Figure 9-9. Moreover, the rapid scan speed of SD-OCT is capable of producing 3-dimensional images, allowing advanced visualization and sophisticated postprocessing.

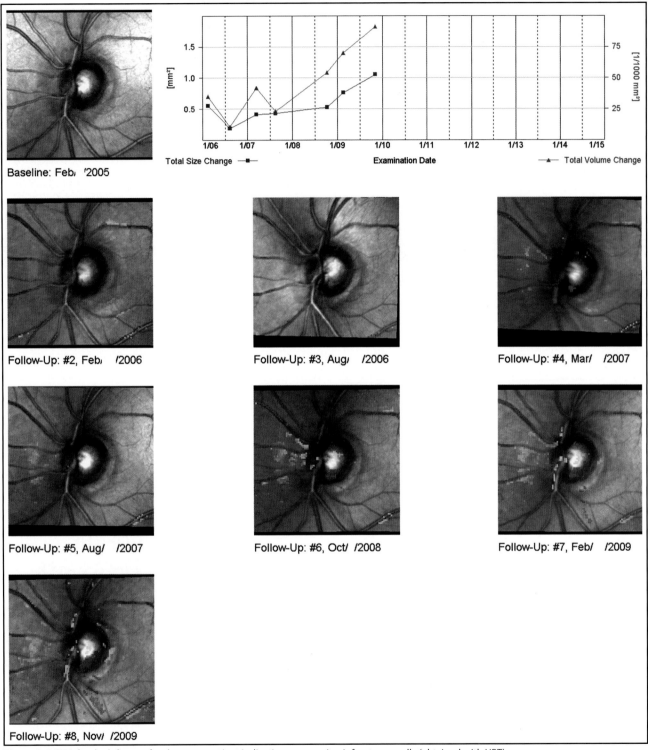

Figure 9-5. TCA for the left eye of a glaucoma patient indicating progression inferotemporally (obtained with HRT).

There are multiple commercially available SD-OCT systems available today with ONH image acquisition and analysis capabilities. SD-OCT is capable of acquiring a 3-dimensional cube of data, making it a useful device to image and assess the ONH. The cube scans (Figure 9-10) are composed of a series of consecutive high-density scans stacked together. In addition to the cube scan, scanning patterns composed of a combination of SD-OCT radial and concentric circle scans can also be used to obtain quantitative measurements of the ONH, as shown by the analysis in Figure 9-11. The disc and cup margins are defined automatically in some SD-OCT devices, while others

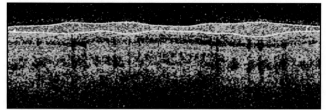

Figure 9-6. Circumpapillary RNFL B-scan for a healthy subject (obtained with Stratus TD-OCT Fast RNFL scanning pattern).

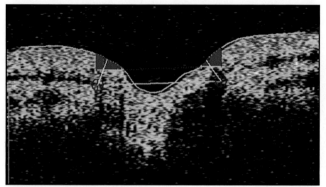

Figure 9-8. ONH B-scan for a healthy subject (obtained with Stratus TD-OCT Fast RNFL scanning pattern).

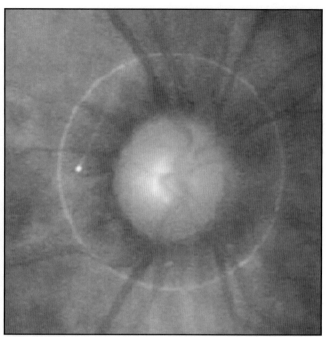

Figure 9-7. Peripapillary RNFL fundus image corresponding to the scan in Figure 9-6 (obtained with Stratus TD-OCT Fast RNFL scanning pattern).

require manual delineation. Quantitative parameters from SD-OCT ONH scans include optic disc area, optic cup area, rim area, nerve head volume, cup volume, rim volume, cup/disc area ratio, and local radial rim and disc measurements.

The benefits of OCT include its ability to provide real-time visualization and quantification of retinal pathologies.[33,34] This function helps remove some subjectivity from previous glaucoma assessment methods. Images and data obtained from OCT have been shown to be reproducible and provide powerful glaucoma discrimination capability.[35-37] Studies[38-40] have also shown that structural damage in OCT images corresponds to visual field (VF) defects and histological retinal assessment. OCT and CSLO have been shown to be highly correlated in ONH assessment.[41]

Limitations of OCT include imaging difficulty when ocular opacities are present and patient movement that can cause errors in data collection. Postacquisition techniques, however, have been able to correct for motion artifact by re-aligning 3-dimensional cubes. In addition to image registration to correct scan alignment, registration techniques can be used to match image locations from visit to visit. This aids in evaluating changes in structural measurements or progression from one clinical visit to the next. Further OCT progression software analysis will be discussed in the RNFL assessment section.

SD-OCT is being offered with a wide range of additional features among the various commercially available devices. Some features include incorporating an eye movement tracking system that corrects for motion artifacts during image acquisition, SLO that is used as a guide for registering retinal features, retinal flow measurements (Doppler),

retinal angiography, fundus photography, and autofluorescence. Figure 9-12 shows a SLO image paired with a B-scan obtained directly across the ONH. The clinical utility of these OCT features has yet to be completely discovered, but for now OCT can provide an excellent method of optical imagery, revealing structural information about glaucoma and other ocular pathologies.

ASSESSMENT OF THE RETINAL NERVE FIBER LAYER

Glaucoma is associated with damage to the RNFL that is conveyed in the axons of the RGCs toward the optic nerve.[42] Quantitatively measuring this structure will, therefore, closely assess the damage to the ganglion cells. RNFL measurements obtained with imaging devices, such as scanning laser polarimetry (SLP) and OCT, have shown glaucoma discrimination ability.[9,43,44] Due to the micron scale resolution and good reproducibility of these devices, they show promise in their ability to monitor structural changes to the RNFL over time.

Scanning Laser Polarimetry

SLP is an imaging method used to assess the RNFL thickness. SLP was first described by Weinreb and colleagues in 1995[45] as a means to compare the RNFL between healthy and glaucomatous patients. SLP uses a confocal scanning laser ophthalmoscope with a polarized laser beam that is directed at retinal tissue. The parallel microtubules of the

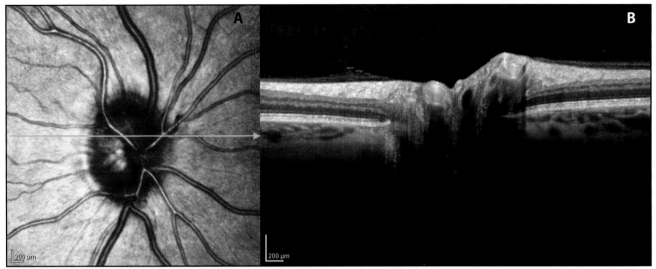

Figure 9-9. (A) SLO image of the ONH. (B) SD-OCT B-scan across the ONH for a healthy subject (obtained with Spectralis HRA+OCT).

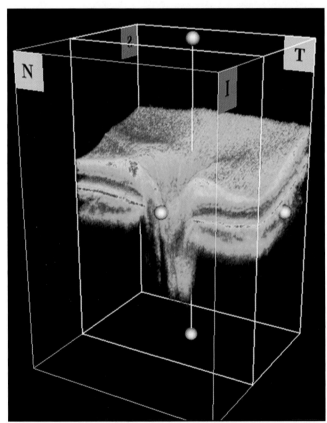

Figure 9-10. ONH 3-dimensional cube scan for a healthy subject (obtained with 3D OCT-1000 3-dimensional cube scan).

RNFL cause a phase shift in the laser beam, known as *retardation*. The state change of the beam caused by the birefringent RNFL correlates directly to the RNFL thickness. SLP uses a light with wavelength 780 nm and scans a 256 × 256 point area on the retina, centered on the ONH, to create a retardation map. The retardation map is used to evaluate the RNFL thickness across the scanned area. The most recently available SLP, GDx by Carl Zeiss Meditec (Dublin, CA), uses an enhanced corneal compensation (ECC) method to relate the birefringence of the tissue to RNFL thickness. Because the cornea and the lens can affect the birefringence, their optical properties must be accounted for to ensure accurate assessment of the RNFL. This is accomplished by initially scanning the macula region to serve as a guide to properly correct for these confounders. In addition to compensating for the anterior segment, the ECC corrects for atypical retardation patterns (ARP) that are commonly seen on SLP RNFL maps.[46] Figure 9-13 shows the RNFL thickness map acquired from the GDx-ECC for a healthy subject, and Figure 9-14 shows the RNFL thickness map acquired for a glaucomatous patient.

The GDx uses the acquired retardation map to sample the RNFL thickness from the circumpapillary region. The circular scan pattern allows sampling of all axons originating from the RGCs for the entire retina on their way to the ONH. GDx measures and reports the average RNFL thickness across all quadrants (temporal, superior, nasal, and inferior temporal [TSNIT]), the RNFL thickness in the superior and inferior quadrants, the standard deviation between measurements, and the inter-eye symmetry. Numerous studies have demonstrated good discrimination ability of the device between healthy and glaucomatous eyes.[47-49] Benefits of imaging with SLP include the device's ease of use and that, in most cases, pupil dilation is not necessary to obtain a good scan. The limitations associated with SLP include the atypical birefringence patterns that still occur in some subjects and lead to inaccurate RNFL thickness measurements.

A new innovation in SLP imaging includes progression analysis software. GDx-guided progression analysis (GPA) software measures the change over time of the global,

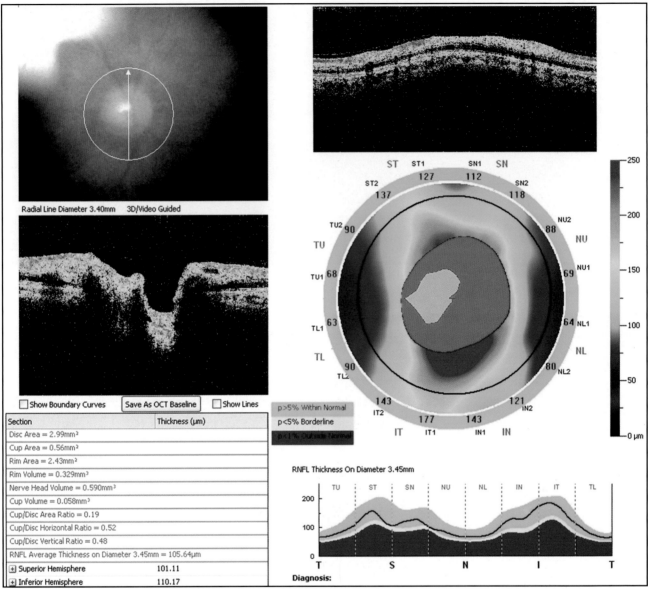

Figure 9-11. ONH scanning analysis (obtained with RTVue-100 ONH scan).

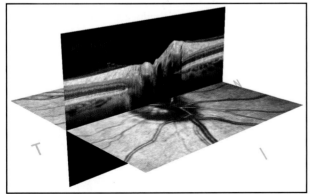

Figure 9-12. OCT B-scan across the ONH and corresponding scanning laser ophthalmoscopy image (obtained with Spectralis HRA+OCT line scan).

inferior quadrant, and superior quadrant RNFL thickness, as shown in Figure 9-15. The analysis includes 3 methods for assessing progression. The image progression map evaluates change from baseline that exceeds the threshold in the entire scanning region. This map is primarily useful for detecting narrow localized progression. The TSNIT progression map assesses change from baseline along the sampled circumpapillary band. This map is mostly useful for broader localized events. The summary parameter charts assess the RNFL globally and in the superior and inferior hemifield for progression over time. This map is useful mostly for broader abnormality and for future prediction of progression. All 3 analyses can be obtained by conducting either the standard or extended modes. The standard mode uses a single test from each time point, and threshold for progression is defined from population-based data. The extended

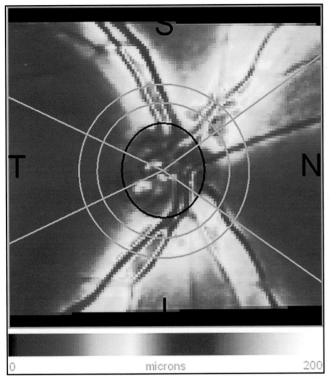

Figure 9-13. RNFL thickness map for a healthy subject (obtained with GDx-ECC).

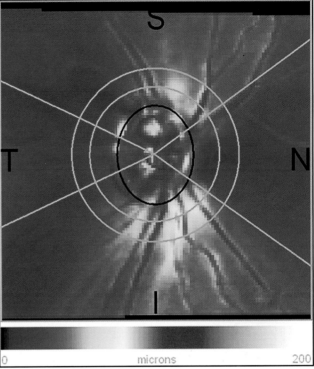

Figure 9-14. RNFL thickness map for glaucoma patient indicating structural damage (obtained with GDx-ECC).

Optical Coherence Tomography

mode uses 3 tests at each visit. The variability between the first 2 sets of tests is used to calculate the variability for each subject and to define the progression threshold accordingly. Several studies demonstrated that the rate of SLP RNFL progression in eyes that were defined by VF as progressors was significantly faster than eyes that were defined as VF nonprogressors.[50,51] Further studies to assess the longitudinal performance of SLP are currently underway.

Both TD-OCT and SD-OCT are capable of obtaining images of the peripapillary region. TD-OCT is limited to obtaining these data along a circle centered on the ONH, while SD-OCT can obtain a 3-dimensional cube of data of this region due to the faster scanning speed. The conventional scan circle diameter is 3.4 mm, which has been shown to provide reproducible RNFL measurements while remaining far enough from the disc margin and peripapillary atrophy region for most subjects. The OCT images are automatically processed using segmentation algorithms to determine the borders of the RNFL. The segmentation algorithms make use of the different reflectancies of the layers of the retina to distinguish one layer from another. The anterior boundary of the RNFL is defined at the vitreoretinal interface, and the posterior boundary is defined at the posterior edge of the RNFL. Figure 9-6 shows RNFL segmentation of a TD-OCT scan.

Figure 9-16 shows white lines segmenting the highly reflective RNFL in a SD-OCT scan. When comparing these 2 scans, the higher resolution of SD-OCT is clearly noticeable.

The acquisition of a 3-dimensional cube of data with SD-OCT allows sophisticated postprocessing, including repositioning of the circle location anywhere within the cube of data. This is especially beneficial when evaluating RNFL thickness measurements over time because the circle location can be registered to match the baseline visit location, thus reducing the inter-visit variability and enabling more exact comparisons. It also allows evaluation of the RNFL thickness within the entire scanned area (and is not bound to the circle), thus improving the ability to detect early wedge defects that might have limited impact at the location of the conventional circle. Figure 9-17 shows a fundus image obtained with SD-OCT where RNFL thickness is compared to population-derived normative measurements. Locations deviating from the normative range are marked with a red (below 1% cutoff of the normal population) or yellow (below 5%) background. The purple line marks the location of the conventional circle.

Global and sectoral RNFL thicknesses are compared to a population-derived normative dataset to enhance the ability to detect abnormality. Each measurement is categorized as within normal limits, borderline (lower 5%), or outside normal limits (lower 1%). Figure 9-18 shows a circumpapillary B-scan and the corresponding quadrant

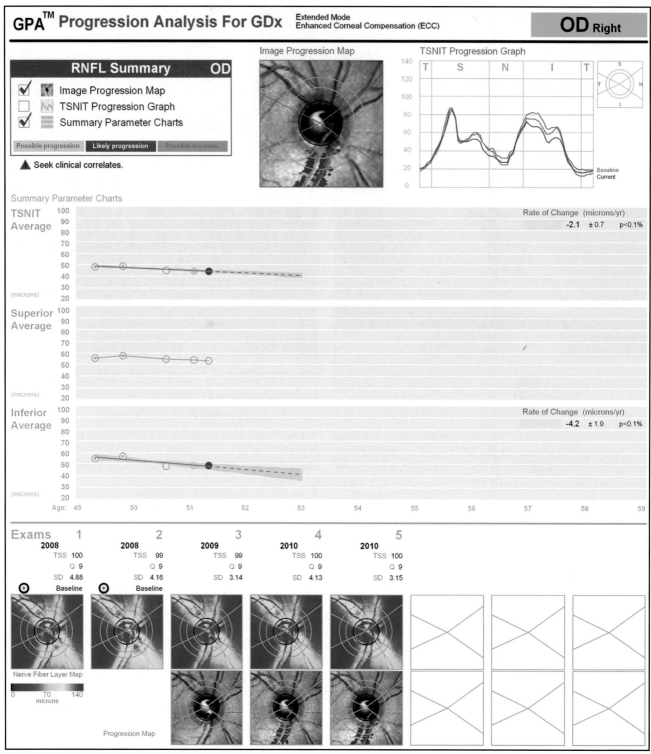

Figure 9-15. Glaucoma progression analysis with SLP showing progression in both the TSNIT and inferior average summary parameter charts and on the image progression map in the temporal inferior region (obtained with GDx-ECC).

and clock-hour RNFL thicknesses, as well as the RNFL thickness distribution from the SD-OCT device. The RNFL thickness values achieved from this scan are color-coded to match the appropriate normative database category to which they belong. Figure 9-18 indicates all measurements are within normal limits of an age-matched normative population. Both TD-OCT and SD-OCT have been shown to provide highly reproducible RNFL measurements and to be powerful diagnostic tools for glaucoma detection.[36,52-55]

Current methods for detecting glaucoma progression with OCT are mostly based on simple comparisons or linear regression analysis of consecutive scans. Figure 9-19

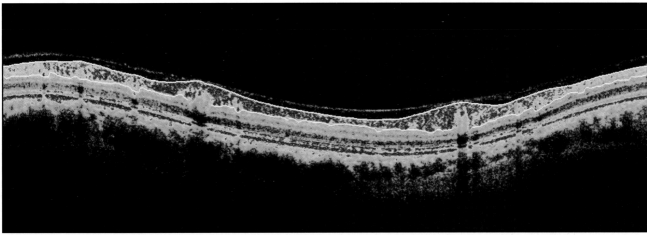

Figure 9-16. Circumpapillary RNFL scan showing segmentation of the RNFL (white lines; obtained with 3D OCT-1000 circle scan).

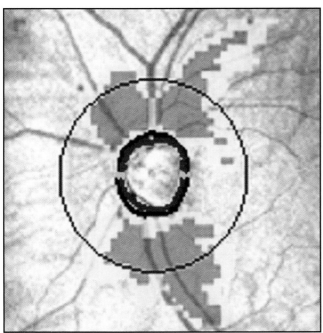

Figure 9-17. OCT fundus image of a glaucoma patient showing the disc margin in black, cup margin in red, 3.4-mm diameter circumpapillary circle in purple, and RFNL thickness measurements that deviate from a normal age-matched population in the red and yellow clusters (obtained with Cirrus HD-OCT Optic Disc Cube 200 × 200 scan).

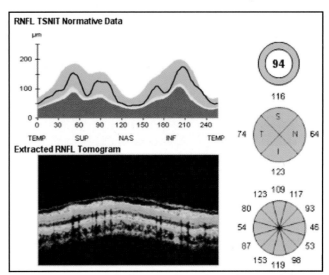

Figure 9-18. (Bottom left) Circumpapillary B-scan where (Top left) RNFL thickness is shown as black line in comparison with the normative distribution. (Right) Global, quadrant, and clock-hour RNFL thickness measurements with color-coded comparison with the normative data (obtained with Cirrus HD-OCT Optic Disc Cube 200 × 200 scan).

shows an SD-OCT RNFL thickness progression analysis for a healthy subject, obtained from the ONH scan. The scanning protocol for this analysis involves 12 3.4-mm radial scans and 6 concentric circle scans varying from 2.5 to 4 mm in diameter. Each radial scan is composed of 452 A-scans, and each circle scan consists of 587 to 775 A-scans. This thickness analysis reports all RNFL thickness measurements to be within normal limits. The graph in the lower left corner also shows the patient is stable, with no changes in RNFL measurements. Figure 9-20 shows the SD-OCT RNFL thickness progression analysis of

a glaucoma subject with superotemporal progression. Of note is the outside normal limits (red) classification in the clock-hour analysis and decrease in the height of the superior hump in the thickness distribution. The mean RNFL thickness compared to time plot displays a slight downward trend, indicative of progression. Figure 9-21 shows a RNFL progression analysis performed using the data from a 200 × 200 optic disc cube scan for a glaucoma patient. The analysis shows likely progression was indicated in the RNFL thickness map and the average RNFL thickness measurement. Possible progression was indicated in the RNFL thickness profile. These printouts represent 2 different examples of progression analysis from an SD-OCT device. Each different manufacturer has its own way of presenting the data for clinical review.

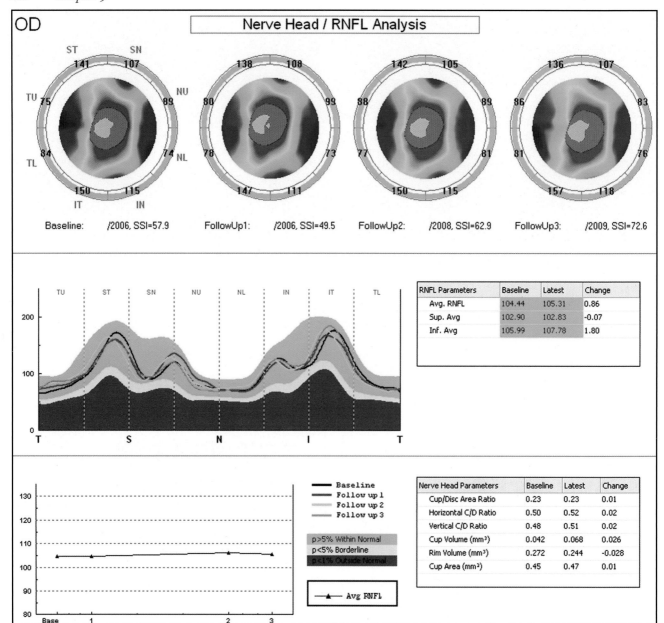

Figure 9-19. RNFL progression analysis for a healthy subject showing minimal variability between visits and less than a micrometer change in overall RNFL thickness (obtained with RTVue-100 ONH scan).

CONCLUSION

Through effective clinical management of glaucoma, ophthalmologists strive for early detection and treatment to increase the amount of vision preserved. The use of the imaging technologies described combined with clinical evaluation and functional testing offers the most complete clinical assessment plan. Imaging technologies have the ability to characterize the ONH and RNFL quantitatively as well as to provide unmatched progression analysis techniques. These developments allow ophthalmologists to identify the presence of glaucoma and glaucoma progression and to initiate treatment before vision loss occurs or becomes worse.

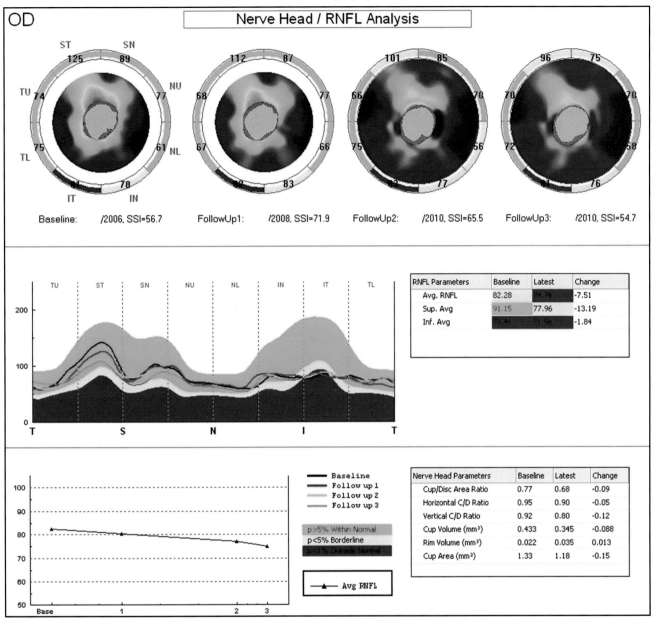

Figure 9-20. RNFL progression analysis for a glaucoma patient showing progression superotemporally (obtained with RTVue-100 ONH scan).

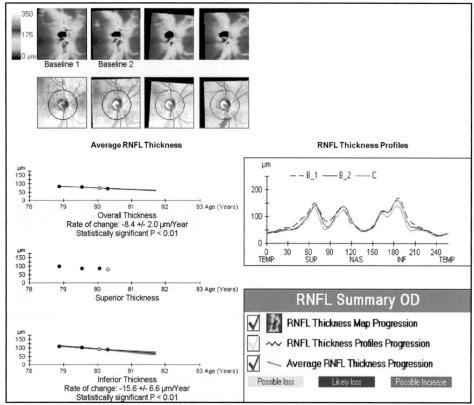

Figure 9-21. RNFL progression analysis for a glaucoma patient showing likely progression (obtained with Cirrus HD-OCT Optic Disc Cube 200 × 200 scan).

REFERENCES

1. Quigley HA, Broman AT. The number of people with glaucoma worldwide in 2010 and 2020. *Br J Ophthalmol.* 2006;90(3):262-267.

2. Quigley HA, Addicks EM, Green WR. Optic nerve damage in human glaucoma. III. Quantitative correlation of nerve fiber loss and visual field defect in glaucoma, ischemic neuropathy, papilledema, and toxic neuropathy. *Arch Ophthalmol.* 1982;100(1):135-146.

3. Quigley HA, Miller NR, George T. Clinical evaluation of nerve fiber layer atrophy as an indicator of glaucomatous optic nerve damage. *Arch Ophthalmol.* 1980;98(9):1564-1571.

4. Reus NJ, Lemij HG, Garway-Heath DF, et al. Clinical assessment of stereoscopic optic disc photographs for glaucoma: the European Optic Disc Assessment Trial. *Ophthalmology.* 2009;117(4):717-723.

5. Wollstein G, Garway-Heath DF, Fontana L, Hitchings RA. Identifying early glaucomatous changes. Comparison between expert clinical assessment of optic disc photographs and confocal scanning ophthalmoscopy. *Ophthalmology.* 2000;107(12):2272-2277.

6. Zangwill LM, Bowd C, Berry CC, et al. Discriminating between normal and glaucomatous eyes using the Heidelberg Retina Tomograph, GDx Nerve Fiber Analyzer, and Optical Coherence Tomograph. *Arch Ophthalmol.* 2001;119(7):985-993.

7. Greaney MJ, Hoffman DC, Garway-Heath DF, Nakla M, Coleman AL, Caprioli J. Comparison of optic nerve imaging methods to distinguish normal eyes from those with glaucoma. *Invest Ophthalmol Vis Sci.* 2002;43(1):140-145.

8. Vessani RM, Moritz R, Batis L, Zagui RB, Bernardoni S, Susanna R. Comparison of quantitative imaging devices and subjective optic nerve head assessment by general ophthalmologists to differentiate normal from glaucomatous eyes. *J Glaucoma.* 2009;18(3):253-261.

9. Deleon-Ortega JE, Arthur SN, McGwin G Jr, Xie A, Monheit BE, Girkin CA. Discrimination between glaucomatous and nonglaucomatous eyes using quantitative imaging devices and subjective optic nerve head assessment. *Invest Ophthalmol Vis Sci.* 2006;47(8):3374-3380.

10. Hemholtz H. *Beschreiburg eines Augenspiegels zur Untersuchung der Netzhaut in lebenden Augi.* Berlin: A Forstner; 1851.

11. Von Graefe A. Ueber die wirkug der iridectomie bei glaucom. *Arch Ophthalmol.* 1857;3:456.

12. Schnabel J. Die Entwicklungsgeschichte der glaukomatösen Exkavation. Zeitschrift für Augenheilkunde. *Ophthalmologica.* 1905;14:1-22.

13. Fuchs W. Uber die Lamina Cribosa. *Graefes Arch Clin Exp Ophthalmol.* 1916;91:435-485.

14. Elliot RU. *Treatise on Glaucoma.* London: Henry Fraude and Hodder & Stroughton LTD; 1922.

15. Tielsch JM, Katz J, Quigley HA, Miller NR, Sommer A. Intraobserver and interobserver agreement in measurement of optic disc characteristics. *Ophthalmology.* 1988;95(3):350-356.

16. Keltner JL, Johnson CA, Quigg JM, Cello KE, Kass MA, Gordon MO. Confirmation of visual field abnormalities in the Ocular Hypertension Treatment Study. Ocular Hypertension Treatment Study Group. *Arch Ophthalmol.* 2000;118(9):1187-1194.

17. Jonas JB, Schmidt AM, Müller-Bergh JA, Schlötzer-Schrehardt UM, Naumann GO. Human optic nerve fiber count and optic disc size. *Invest Ophthalmol Vis Sci.* 1992;33:2012-2018.

18. Azuara-Blanco A, Katz LJ, Spaeth GL, Vernon SA, Spencer F, Lanzl IM. Clinical agreement among glaucoma experts in the detection of glaucomatous changes of the optic disk using simultaneous stereoscopic photographs. *Am J Ophthalmol.* 2003;136(5):949-950.

19. Coleman AL, Sommer A, Enger C, Knopf HL, Stamper RL, Minckler DS. Interobserver and intraobserver variability in the detection of glaucomatous progression of the optic disc. *J Glaucoma.* 1996;5(6):384-389.

20. Xu J, Ishikawa H, Wollstein G, et al. Automated assessment of the optic nerve head on stereo disc photographs. *Invest Ophthalmol Vis Sci.* 2008;49(6):2512-2517.

21. Abramoff MD, Alward WL, Greenlee EC, et al. Automated segmentation of the optic disc from stereo color photographs using physiologically plausible features. *Invest Ophthalmol Vis Sci.* 2007;48(4):1665-1673.

22. Webb RH, Hughes GW, Delori FC. Confocal scanning laser ophthalmoscope. *Applied Optics.* 1987;26(8):1492-1499.

23. Stein DM, Wollstein G, Schuman JS. Imaging in glaucoma. *Ophthalmol Clin North Am.* 2004;17(1):33-52.

24. Alencar LM, Bowd C, Weinreb RN, Zangwill LM, Sample PA, Medeiros FA. Comparison of HRT-3 glaucoma probability score and subjective stereophotograph assessment for prediction of progression in glaucoma. *Invest Ophthalmol Vis Sci.* 2008;49(5):1898-1906.

25. Lin D, Leung CK, Weinreb RN, Cheung CY, Li H, Lam DS. Longitudinal evaluation of optic disc measurement variability with optical coherence tomography and confocal scanning laser ophthalmoscopy. *J Glaucoma.* 2009;18(2):101-106.

26. Badala F, Nouri-Mahdavi K, Raoof DA, et al. Optic disc and nerve fiber layer imaging to detect glaucoma. *Am J Ophthalmol.* 2007;144(5):724-732.

27. Bowd C, Balasubramanian M, Weinreb RN, et al. Performance of confocal scanning laser tomograph Topographic Change Analysis (TCA) for assessing glaucomatous progression. *Invest Ophthalmol Vis Sci.* 2009;50(2):691-701.

28. Huang D, Swanson EA, Lin CP, et al. Optical coherence tomography. *Science.* 1991;254(5035):1178-1181.

29. Wojtkowski M. Phase sensitive interferometry in optical coherence tomography. *Proc SPIE.* 2001:4515.

30. Wojtkowski M, Leitgeb R, Kowalczyk A, Bajraszewski T, Fercher AF. In vivo human retinal imaging by Fourier domain optical coherence tomography. *J Biomed Opt.* 2002;7(3):457-463.

31. Zhang K, Kang JU. Real-time 4D signal processing and visualization using graphics processing unit on a regular nonlinear-k Fourier-domain OCT system. *Opt Express.* 2010;18(11):11772-11784.

32. Drexler W, Fujimoto JG. State-of-the-art retinal optical coherence tomography. *Prog Retin Eye Res.* 2008;27(1):45-88.

33. Fujimoto JG, Brezinski ME, Tearney GJ, et al. Optical biopsy and imaging using optical coherence tomography. *Nat Med.* 1995;1(9):970-972.

34. Fujimoto JG, Pitris C, Boppart SA, Brezinski ME. Optical coherence tomography: an emerging technology for biomedical imaging and optical biopsy. *Neoplasia.* 2000;2(1-2):9-25.

35. Blumenthal EZ, Williams JM, Weinreb RN, Girkin CA, Berry CC, Zangwill LM. Reproducibility of nerve fiber layer thickness measurements by use of optical coherence tomography. *Ophthalmology.* 2000;107(12):2278-2282.

36. Paunescu LA, Schuman JS, Price LL, et al. Reproducibility of nerve fiber thickness, macular thickness, and optic nerve head measurements using Stratus OCT. *Invest Ophthalmol Vis Sci.* 2004;45(6):1716-1724.

37. Anton A, Moreno-Montanes J, Blazquez F, Alvarez A, Martin B, Molina B. Usefulness of optical coherence tomography parameters of the optic disc and the retinal nerve fiber layer to differentiate glaucomatous, ocular hypertensive, and normal eyes. *J Glaucoma.* 2007;16(1):1-8.

38. Badlani V, Shahidi M, Shakoor A, Edward DP, Zelkha R, Wilensky J. Nerve fiber layer thickness in glaucoma patients with asymmetric hemifield visual field loss. *J Glaucoma.* 2006;15(4):275-280.

39. Toth CA, Narayan DG, Boppart SA, et al. A comparison of retinal morphology viewed by optical coherence tomography and by light microscopy. *Arch Ophthalmol.* 1997;115(11):1425-1428.

40. Hood DC, Harizman N, Kanadani FN, et al. Retinal nerve fibre thickness measured with optical coherence tomography accurately detects confirmed glaucomatous damage. *Br J Ophthalmol.* 2007;91(7):905-907.

41. Schuman JS, Wollstein G, Farra T, et al. Comparison of optic nerve head measurements obtained by optical coherence tomography and confocal scanning laser ophthalmoscopy. *Am J Ophthalmol.* 2003;135(4):504-512.

42. Schuman JS. Spectral domain optical coherence tomography for glaucoma (an AOS thesis). *Trans Am Ophthalmol Soc.* 2008;106:426-458.

43. Chen HY, Huang ML. Discrimination between normal and glaucomatous eyes using Stratus optical coherence tomography in Taiwan Chinese subjects. *Graefes Arch Clin Exp Ophthalmol.* 2005;243(9):894-902.

44. Lauande-Pimentel R, Carvalho RA, Oliveira HC, Goncalves DC, Silva LM, Costa VP. Discrimination between normal and glaucomatous eyes with visual field and scanning laser polarimetry measurements. *Br J Ophthalmol.* 2001;85(5):586-591.

45. Weinreb RN, Shakiba S, Zangwill L. Scanning laswer polarimetry to measure the nerve fiber layer of normal and glaucomatous eyes. *Am J Ophthalmol.* 1995;119:627-636.

46. Toth M, Hollo G. Enhanced corneal compensation for scanning laser polarimetry on eyes with atypical polarisation pattern. *Br J Ophthalmol.* 2005;89(9):1139-1142.

47. Weinreb RN, Shakiba S, Zangwill L. Scanning laser polarimetry to measure the nerve fiber layer of normal and glaucomatous eyes. *Am J Ophthalmol.* 1995;119(5):627-636.

48. Weinreb RN, Zangwill L, Berry CC, Bathija R, Sample PA. Detection of glaucoma with scanning laser polarimetry. *Arch Ophthalmol.* 1998;116(12):1583-1589.

49. Choplin NT, Lundy DC, Dreher AW. Differentiating patients with glaucoma from glaucoma suspects and normal subjects by nerve fiber layer assessment with scanning laser polarimetry. *Ophthalmology.* 1998;105(11):2068-2076.

50. Grewal DS, Sehi M, Greenfield DS. Comparing rates of retinal nerve fibre layer loss with GDxECC using different methods of visual-field progression. *Br J Ophthalmol.* 2011;95(8):1122-1127.

51. Alencar LM, Zangwill LM, Weinreb RN, et al. Agreement for detecting glaucoma progression with the GDx guided progression analysis, automated perimetry, and optic disc photography. *Ophthalmology.* 2010;117(3):462-470.

52. Budenz DL, Fredette MJ, Feuer WJ, Anderson DR. Reproducibility of peripapillary retinal nerve fiber thickness measurements with stratus OCT in glaucomatous eyes. *Ophthalmology.* 2008;115(4):661-666.

53. Kim JS, Ishikawa H, Sung KR, et al. Retinal nerve fibre layer thickness measurement reproducibility improved with spectral domain optical coherence tomography. *Br J Ophthalmol.* 2009;93(8):1057-1063.

54. Schuman JS, Hee MR, Arya AV, et al. Optical coherence tomography: a new tool for glaucoma diagnosis. *Curr Opin Ophthalmol.* 1995;6(2):89-95.

55. Schuman JS, Pedut-Kloizman T, Hertzmark E, et al. Reproducibility of nerve fiber layer thickness measurements using optical coherence tomography. *Ophthalmology.* 1996;103(11):1889-1898.

10

Imaging Devices for Angle Assessment

Mina B. Pantcheva, MD and Malik Y. Kahook, MD

During the past 20 years, several advances in technology have enabled the clinician to assess the angle with methods other than traditional direct or indirect visualization. Many of these technologies are evolutionary upgrades to commonly used devices for biometry or imaging of the anterior/posterior segment. Although this chapter is not meant to be exhaustive, it will hopefully show the ability of imaging devices to complement traditional methods of examination.

The 2 major categories that devices fall under are ultrasound (contact) and optical (noncontact). Although the range of ultrasound technology falls into a single category of ultrasound biomicroscopy (UBM), optical devices fall under a broader range of optical coherence tomography (OCT), Scheimpflug imaging, and scanning slit topography (Orbscan, Orbtek Inc, Salt Lake City, UT).

ULTRASOUND BIOMICROSCOPY

Background

Mechanical waves and vibrations are the basic constituents of ultrasound, and the range can be measured by vibrations per second (Hz). The audible spectrum ranges from 10 to 20 kHz. Traditional B-scan ultrasound is in the range of 10 MHz and allows for resolution of 0.2 mm axially and 0.5 mm transversely. The approximate penetration for a traditional 10 MHz ultrasound is 50 mm, which is adequate enough for gross examination of the anterior and posterior segments. Increasing the frequency of the transducer can increase the resolution obtained by ultrasound. In the early 1990s, following the development of higher-frequency transducers for blood vessel imaging, came the development of high-frequency ultrasound for the eye. UBM is performed in a frequency range between 40 and 100 MHz. The increased frequency leads to decreased depth of penetration (for

example, a 60-MHz transducer can penetrate approximately 5 mm). The combination of higher resolution and decreased depth of penetration is ideal for evaluation of the anterior segment. Detailed images of the anterior chamber, drainage angle, and ciliary body can be obtained with an axial resolution of about 25 µm and lateral resolution of about 50 µm (Figure 10-1).[1,2] Polymers such as polyvinylidene difluoride and polyvinylidene difluoride-trifluorethylene have been essential advancements in transducer technology to allow for these higher frequencies. Steps for performing UBM to image the anterior segment are similar to performing an immersion B-scan.

Quantitative Measurements

A commonly described benefit of most new imaging modalities is the ability to quantitatively describe the angle. This brings the hope that interobserver bias becomes reduced and that progression as well as prevention of disease can be reliably monitored. As the utility of these devices continues to be investigated, many new quantitative parameters are described. We will describe a few that are commonplace in UBM and have been translated over to optical devices (Figure 10-2). The principal point of reference in UBM is the identification of the scleral spur. The trabecular meshwork (TM) consistently falls 250 µm anterior from the scleral spur. The anterior aspect of the TM generally falls within 500 µm from the scleral spur. If a line is drawn from either point perpendicular to the TM toward the opposing iris, the length would be described as a very commonly used parameter known as *angle opening distance* (AOD_{250} or AOD_{500}). The trabecular-iris angle (TIA) is defined as the angle measured with the apex in the iris recess and the arms of the angle passing through a point on the TM 500 µm from the scleral spur and the point on the iris perpendicularly opposite to it. The trabecular-ciliary process distance (TCPD) is the length

Kahook MY, Schuman JS, eds.
Chandler and Grant's Glaucoma, Fifth Edition (pp 111-115).
© 2013 SLACK Incorporated.

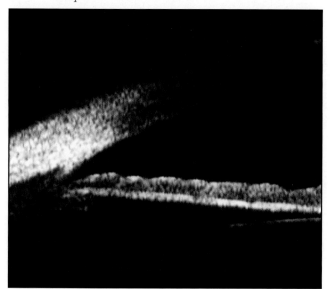

Figure 10-1. A normal UBM of an open angle.

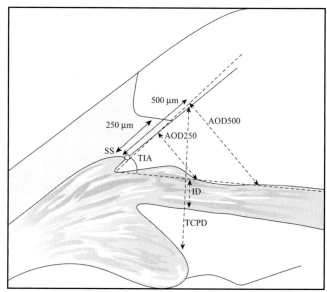

Figure 10-2. The determination of the parameters on the UBM image. Angle-opening distance (AOD_{250} and AOD_{500}) between the posterior corneal surface and the anterior iris surface measured on a line perpendicular to the TM at 250 μm and 500 μm, respectively, from the scleral spur. ID—thickness of the iris; TCPD—trabecular-ciliary process distance; TIA—trabecular-iris angle.

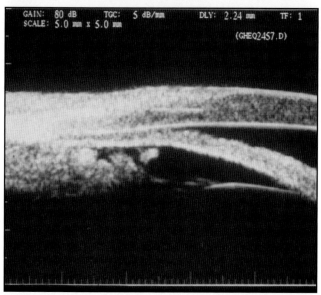

Figure 10-3. UBM of plateau iris configuration. The forward positioned and rotated ciliary processes come in contact with the peripheral portion of the iris and cause closure of the ciliary sulcus, supporting the iris root. The iris root cannot detach from the TM even in the presence of an iridotomy.

of the line extending from the corneal endothelium 500 μm from the scleral spur perpendicularly through the iris to the ciliary process. The angle recess area (ARA) is the area between the AOD and angle recess. If the area posterior to the scleral spur is excluded, the parameter known as trabecular iris space area (TISA) is used.[3-5]

Clinical Applications

Primary Angle-Closure Glaucoma

Quantitative measurements have enabled researchers to investigate the mechanisms of primary angle-closure glaucoma (PACG) and offer theories on why some eyes with narrow angles progress to pupillary block whereas others do not. Classical theories for pupillary block and PACG include the idea that an area of iridolenticular touch causes increased posterior chamber pressure. Dilation is thought to exaggerate this to a point where increased posterior chamber pressure results in pushing the peripheral iris forward to occlude the angle. With UBM, it has been shown that iridolenticular contact is small in pupillary block and actually decreases with dilation. UBM has revealed that angle narrowing or closure occurs quickly (no time was required for aqueous pressure buildup) on pupillary dilation and is thought to be caused by a combination of increased iris thickening and increased anterior bowing as the iris tip moves toward the iris root (light dark paper). Thus, UBM can be used to perform provocative testing in narrow-angle eyes. Similarly, a thicker peripheral iris (as well as a narrower angle or anterior position of the ciliary body) was associated with progressive angle closure in fellow eyes of those with PACG attack.

Plateau Iris

Plateau iris configuration has been defined as a normal-depth anterior chamber, a flat iris plane, and an extremely narrow angle. Plateau iris syndrome is defined when a patient with a plateau iris configuration remains capable of angle closure despite the presence of a patent peripheral iridotomy site (Figure 10-3). This is thought to be caused by anterior ciliary process positioning and ciliary sulcus closure. UBM has become the definitive method in the diagnosis of plateau iris configuration and syndrome. Although diagnostic criteria

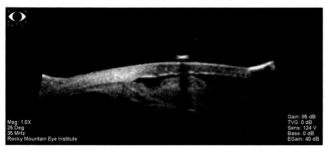

Figure 10-4. UBM of iris melanoma.

vary, plateau iris may be defined by UBM when all of the following criteria are present in 2 or more quadrants:

- Anteriorly directed ciliary processes, supporting the peripheral iris such that it is parallel to the TM
- An iris root with a steep rise from its point of insertion, followed by a downward angulation from the corneoscleral wall
- The presence of a central flat iris plane
- An absent ciliary sulcus
- Irido-angle contact (above the level of the scleral spur) in the same quadrant[6]

Anterior Segment Tumors

UBM can help evaluate tumors of the anterior segment (Figure 10-4). Because of the penetration of UBM, it has the ability to differentiate between cystic structures and solid structures. It allows for delineation of the location, size, and extent of the tumor. Ciliary body cysts appear as clear, echo-free, thin-walled bodies. Reflectivity can help differentiate the nature of solid tumors, such as ciliary body melanoma (low reflectivity), as well as a finding that melanomas show irregularity and convex bowing of the posterior iris plane not seen in nevi.[7]

Cyclodialysis Clefts

Cyclodialysis clefts are readily visible with UBM as well as anterior suprachoroidal effusions, either of which may not be easily detected with conventional exam. Nolan described the advantage of UBM for the detection of cyclodialysis clefts and the value of anterior segment optical coherence tomography as a noncontact examination technique for rapid follow-up after treatment.[8]

OPTICAL

Optical Coherence Tomography

In 1995, optical coherence tomography (OCT) became available for retinal imaging. Low coherence interferometry measures the delay and intensity of backscattered light by comparing it to light that has travelled a known reference path length using a Michelson-type interferometer.[9] It is analogous to ultrasound, but uses light instead of sound. Recent changes in clinically utilized OCT technology principally involve increases in speed and wavelength. A traditional OCT device uses a wavelength of light of ~830 nm, which is close to the visible wavelength and therefore cannot visualize the angle due to scatter of light near the limbus.[10,11] With a scan speed of 100 to 400 axial scans per second, an image of the anterior segment would appear coarse and grainy with possible motion artifact when captured over a full second. Anterior segment OCT uses a wavelength of 1310 nm and a scan speed up to 4000 scans/second, which allows for better penetration and resolution by providing images of the cornea, iris, angle, anterior lens, retro-iris lens, ciliary body, and ciliary sulcus. At 1310 nm, 90% of the signal is lost before reaching retina and currently cannot be used for retinal imaging.[12,13]

There are multiple commercially available systems capable of anterior segment OCT, including the Visante AS-OCT (Carl Zeiss Meditec Inc, Dublin, CA) and Slit Lamp-OCT (SL-OCT) (Heidelberg Engineering, Heidelberg, Germany). The Visante AS-OCT performs up to 2048 axial (A)-scans/second and provides an axial resolution of up to 18 μm and transverse resolution of up to 60 μm. The SL-OCT is an OCT that is incorporated into a modified slit-lamp biomicroscopy system. It has a slower image acquisition speed with an axial resolution of less than 25 μm and transverse resolution between 20 and 100 μm. Furthermore, the SL-OCT requires manual rotation of the scanning beam. Another difference is that the Visante AS-OCT has an internal fixation target to adjust for subjects' refraction. Correction of refractive error is essential to minimize the effect of the variability of pupil size and lens position secondary to accommodation of the eye on measurement of the angle. Similar measurements for biometry, such as AOD, ARA, and TISA, can be performed (SL-OCT includes automated software for such numbers). Comparison studies between Visante AS-OCT and gonioscopy found the AS-OCT detected a higher rate of closed angles than gonioscopy, particularly in the superior and inferior quadrants.[14,15] Using gonioscopy as the reference standard, the sensitivity and specificity of AS-OCT to identify angle closure were 98% and 55.4%, respectively, using a definition of one or more quadrants of nonvisibility of the TM.[14] Several explanations have been suggested for the disparate findings between gonioscopy and AS-OCT. Inadvertent pressure on the globe and too much exposure of the pupil to visible light during gonioscopy may alter the configuration of the angle, leading to spurious widening of the angle. Another reason could be a difference in the definition and description of the landmarks used to define angle closure. On gonioscopy, angle closure was defined as the apposition between the iris and the posterior TM, whereas, on the AS-OCT, it was defined as any contact between the iris and the angle structures anterior to the scleral spur. Sakata and colleagues[16] showed the scleral spur was detected in 72% of the Visante AS-OCT images and that the superior and inferior quadrants were less detectable compared with the nasal and temporal quadrants. In another study comparing angle measurements between Visante AS-OCT and SL-OCT, the inter-observer coefficient of variation ranged between 4.4% and 7.8% and between 4.9% and 7.0%, respectively. Nevertheless, the measurement agreement for the 2 instruments was poor.[17] The spans of 95% limits of agreement of the nasal/temporal angle measurements between the instruments were 437/531 µm, 0.174/0.186 mm², and 25.3/28.0 degrees for AOD, TISA, and TIA, respectively.[17]

RTVue FD-OCT (Optovue, Fremont, CA) is another commercially available device that can take an image of the angle by attaching the cornea-anterior module (CAM). A study[18] comparing Visante time-domain OCT system and the RTVue-100 Fourier-domain corneal anterior module OCT system did not find any significant differences between the instruments. The Cirrus HD-OCT (Carl Zeiss Meditec) also allows anterior segment imaging with the built-in 60-D aspheric lens. The anterior segment five-line raster is the preferred scan protocol for the angle. It is capable of detecting the scleral spur in 78.9% and the Schwalbe's line in 93.3% of quadrants in 45 individuals recruited from a glaucoma clinic.[19]

The swept-source OCT is a form of Fourier-domain OCT. The swept-source OCT uses a monochromatic tunable fast-scanning laser source and a photodetector to detect wavelength-resolved interference signal.[20,21] The CASIA OCT (Tomey, Nagoya, Japan) is a commercially available swept-source OCT designed specifically for anterior segment imaging. The wavelength of the swept-source laser is 1310 nm. The scan dimensions are up to 16 mm (width) × 16 mm (length) × 6 mm (depth). With a scan speed of 30,000 A-scans/second, it is feasible to collect a series of 64 radial scans across the whole anterior chamber in 1.2 sec. With reconstruction of individual image frames, a 3-dimensional display of the iris and the anterior chamber angle can be generated. An advantage of the CASIA OCT is the ability to visualize both the scleral spur and the Schwalbe's line in high-resolution scan mode.[22]

Ultrahigh-speed 1050-nm swept-source Fourier-domain OCT for anterior segment imaging is under development, and imaging at a speed of 100,000 to 400,000 A-scans/second has been recently demonstrated.[23] The development of high-resolution and high-speed OCT imaging systems, angle structures including the scleral spur, Schwalbe's line, and Schlemm's canal can be examined improving detection of angle closure and could provide mechanistic insights into the pathophysiology of acute primary angle-closure and angle-closure glaucoma.

One limitation of OCT is its limited capability to penetrate and delineate tumors to the extent that UBM does, especially with larger, solid, and pigmented tumors.[24,25]

Scheimpflug Imaging

The Scheimpflug principle describes the change in focal plane that occurs when the film plane is tilted, such that the focal, lens, and film planes are not parallel. The shifting of the plane of sharp focus to the intersection point of the film and lens planes allows slit images of the anterior segment of the eye to be obtained. The Topcon SL45 (Topcon Medical Systems Inc, Oakland, NJ) and the Nidek EAS-1000 (Nidek Co, Ltd, Aichi, Japan) are the 2 most widely used in the study of ACA anatomy and anterior chamber depth (ACD) assessment.[26-28]

The Pentacam (Oculus Inc, GmBH, Wetzlar, Germany) uses a rotating Scheimpflug camera (RSC).[29] In total, up to 25,000 height values are detected and processed to a 3-dimensional model of the anterior eye segment. Along with pachymetry, densitometry of the intraocular lens, and corneal topography, the device can measure ACD, angle, and volume. It does not, however, provide direct visualization of the angle. The noncontact device requires good fixation, which may be difficult in children, older patients, or patients with nystagmus. One study[30] has found that angle measurements from Scheimpflug images were less sensitive to changes in illumination compared with those obtained using UBM. Scheimpflug photography was reported[31] to provide insufficient detail of the angle for assessment of angle anatomy, with limited agreement existing between gonioscopy, Scheimpflug photography, and UBM.

Scanning Slit Topography

Scanning slit topography is based on the principle of measuring the dimensions of a slit-scanning beam as it is projected on the cornea. Although it does not provide direct visualization of the angle, it can estimate ACD and the iridocorneal angle in a noncontact fashion with little user experience. It creates true 3-dimensional maps from the anterior segment of the eye using measurements based on the Scheimpflug principle. Therefore, the corneal thickness or ACD can be calculated by measuring the distance in elevation between the anterior and posterior surfaces of the cornea and between the cornea and anterior lens surface, respectively.[32] Studies show that ACD measurements using the Orbscan system are equivalent to common reference measurements.[33-35]

CONCLUSION

There are multiple imaging modalities that allow for the objective assessment of anterior segment structures of the eye and provide valuable information for the diagnosis of disease. Their accuracy and repeatability, advantages and disadvantages, as well as their ease of use are all important to consider when used in clinical practice. Future advances will allow for enhanced reproducibility, improved resolution, as well as automated data interpretation.

REFERENCES

1. Pavlin CJ, Harasiewicz K, Sherar MD, Foster FS. Clinical use of ultrasound biomicroscopy. *Ophthalmology.* 1991;98:287-295.

2. Pavlin CJ, Sherar MD, Foster FS. Subsurface ultrasound microscopic imaging of the intact eye. *Ophthalmology.* 1990;97:244-250.

3. Pavlin CJ, Harasiewicz K, Foster FS. Ultrasound biomicroscopy of anterior segment structures in normal and glaucomatous eyes. *Am J Ophthalmol.* 1992;113:381-389.

4. Ishikawa H, Liebmann JM, Ritch R. Quantitative assessment of the anterior segment using ultrasound biomicroscopy. *Curr Opin Ophthalmol.* 2000;11:133-139.

5. Radhakrishnan S, Goldsmith J, Huang D, et al. Comparison of optical coherence tomography and ultrasound biomicroscopy for detection of narrow anterior chamber angles. *Arch Ophthalmol.* 2005;123(8):1053-1059.

6. Kumar RS, Baskaran M, Chew PT, et al. Prevalence of plateau iris in primary angle closure suspects an ultrasound biomicroscopy study. *Ophthalmology.* 2007;115(3):430-434.

7. Marigo FA, Esaki K, Finger PT, et al. Differential diagnosis of anterior segment cysts by ultrasound biomicroscopy. *Ophthalmology.* 1999;106(11):2131-2135.

8. Nolan W. Anterior segment imaging: ultrasound biomicroscopy and anterior segment optical coherence tomography. *Curr Opin Ophthalmol.* 2008;19:115-121.

9. Brezinski M, Fujimoto J. Optical coherence tomography: high resolution imaging in nontransparent tissue. *IEEE J Select Top Quantum Electron.* 1999;5:1185-1192.

10. Swanson EA, Izatt JA, Hee MR, et al. In vivo retinal imaging by optical coherence tomography. *Opt Lett.* 1993;18:1864-1866.

11. Hee MR, Izatt JA, Swanson EA, et al. Optical coherence tomography of the human retina. *Arch Ophthalmol.* 1995;113:325-332.

12. Izatt JA, Hee MR, Swanson EA, et al. Micrometer-scale resolution imaging of the anterior eye in vivo with optical coherence tomography. *Arch Ophthalmol.* 1994;112:1584-1589.

13. Wirbelauer C, Karandish A, Haberle H, Pham DT. Noncontact goniometry with optical coherence tomography. *Arch Ophthalmol.* 2005;123:179-185.

14. Nolan WP, See JL, Chew PT, et al. Detection of primary angle closure using anterior segment optical coherence tomography in Asian eyes. *Ophthalmology.* 2007;114:33-39.

15. Sakata LM, Lavanya R, Friedman DS, et al. Comparison of gonioscopy and anterior segment ocular coherence tomography in detecting angle closure in different quadrants of the anterior chamber angle. *Ophthalmology.* 2008;115:769-774.

16. Sakata LM, Lavanya R, Friedman DS, et al. Assessment of the scleral spur in anterior segment optical coherence tomography images. *Arch Ophthalmol.* 2008;126:181-185.

17. Leung CK, Li H, Weinreb RN, et al. Anterior chamber angle measurement with anterior segment optical coherence tomography: a comparison between slit lamp OCT and Visante OCT. *Invest Ophthalmol Vis Sci.* 2008;49:3469-3474.

18. Wylegala E, Teper S, Nowińska AK, et al. Anterior segment imaging: Fourier-domain optical coherence tomography versus time-domain optical coherence tomography. *J Cataract Refract Surg.* 2009;35:1410-1414.

19. Wong HT, Lim MC, Sakata LM, et al. High-definition optical coherence tomography imaging of the iridocorneal angle of the eye. *Arch Ophthalmol.* 2009;127:256-260.

20. Yun S, Tearney G, de Boer J, et al. High-speed optical frequency-domain imaging. *Opt Express.* 2003;11:2953-2963.

21. Yasuno Y, Madjarova VD, Makita S, et al. Three-dimensional and high-speed swept-source optical coherence tomography for *in vivo* investigation of human anterior eye segments. *Opt Express.* 2005;13:10652-10664.

22. Leung CK, Weinreb RN. Anterior chamber angle imaging with optical coherence tomography. *Eye (Lond).* 2011;25(3):261-267.

23. Potsaid B, Baumann B, Huang D, et al. Ultrahigh speed 1050nm swept source/Fourier domain OCT retinal and anterior segment imaging at 100000 to 400000 axial scans per second. *Opt Express.* 2010;18:20029-20048.

24. Bianciotto C, Shields CL, Guzman JM, et al. Assessment of anterior segment tumors with ultrasound biomicroscopy versus anterior segment optical coherence tomography in 200 cases. *Ophthalmology.* 2011;118(7):1297-1302.

25. Pavlin CJ, Vásquez LM, Lee R, et al. Anterior segment optical coherence tomography and ultrasound biomicroscopy in the imaging of anterior segment tumors. *Am J Ophthalmol.* 2009;147(2):214-219.

26. Richards DW, Russell SR, Anderson DR. A method for improved biometry of the anterior chamber with a Scheimpflug technique. *Invest Ophthalmol Vis Sci.* 1988;29:1826-1835.

27. Baez KA, Orengo S, Gandham S, et al. Intraobserver and interobserver reproducibility of the Nidek EAS-1000 Anterior Eye Segment Analysis System. *Ophthalmic Surg.* 1992;23:426-428.

28. Lam AK, Chan R, Woo GC, et al. Intra-observer and inter-observer repeatability of anterior eye segment analysis system (EAS-1000) in anterior chamber configuration. *Ophthalmic Physiol Opt.* 2002;22:552-559.

29. Rabsilber TM, Khoramnia R, Auffarth GU. Anterior chamber measurements using Pentacam rotating Scheimpflug camera. *J Cataract Refract Surg.* 2006;32:456-459.

30. Friedman DS, Gazzard G, Foster P, et al. Ultrasonographic biomicroscopy, Scheimpflug photography, and novel provocative tests in contralateral eyes of Chinese patients initially seen with acute angle closure. *Arch Ophthalmol.* 2003;121:633-642.

31. Friedman DS, Gazzard G, Min CB, et al. Age and sex variation in angle findings among normal Chinese subjects: a comparison of UBM, Scheimpflug, and gonioscopic assessment of the anterior chamber angle. *J Glaucoma.* 2008;17:5-10.

32. Rabsilber TM, Becker KA, Frisch IB, et al. Anterior chamber depth in relation to refractive status measured with the Orbscan II Topography System. *J Cataract Refract Surg.* 2003;29:2115-2121.

33. Auffarth GU, Tetz MR, Biazid Y, Völcker HE. Measuring anterior chamber depth with the Orbscan Topography System. *J Cataract Refract Surg.* 1997;23:1351-1355.

34. Vetrugno M, Cardascia N, Cardia L. Anterior chamber depth measured by two methods in myopic and hyperopic phakic IOL implant. *Br J Ophthalmol.* 2000;84:1113-1116.

35. Koranyi G, Lydahl E, Norrby S, Taube M. Anterior chamber depth measurement: A-scan versus optical methods. *J Cataract Refract Surg.* 2002;28:243-247.

11

Visual Fields and
Their Relationship to the Optic Nerve

Joshua D. Stein, MD, MS and R. Rand Allingham, MD

The 2 most important factors to consider when determining whether a patient has glaucoma and the severity of disease are the structural appearance of the optic nerve and the presence of functional damage as detected by visual field testing. Evaluation of the optic disc for glaucomatous damage was covered in detail in Chapter 8. This chapter will describe the methods of checking for functional damage including the different types of visual field tests available, characteristics of normal and glaucomatous visual field loss, and how to correlate structural damage to the optic nerve or nerve fiber layer with functional damage detected on visual field testing. Correlating the information obtained from careful examination of the optic nerve with functional damage detected by perimetric testing is far superior to relying on either piece of information alone.

THE VISUAL FIELD

The Normal Visual Field

The visual field can be defined as that area of vision seen with eyes open. The dimensions of the field of vision are defined relative to central fixation. The normal visual field extends approximately 60 degrees nasal and superior, 70 degrees inferior, and 90 to 100 degrees temporal to fixation. The blind spot in the field of vision corresponds to the area defined by the optic nerve head (ONH) and is typically located 15 degrees temporal to fixation. It varies in size according to optic disc size and extent of peripapillary retinochoroidal atrophy.

Traquair[1] described the visual field in 3 dimensions, as "an island of vision surrounded by a sea of blindness." This important concept reflects the addition of retinal sensitivity to the 2-dimensional area of visual field. The most sensitive region in the normal visual field is the portion of the field detected by the fovea. The retinal sensitivity drops rapidly within 15 degrees of the foveal peak. From this point, there is a gradual reduction in retinal sensitivity that extends to the periphery where it abruptly drops off. In cross-section, the blind spot appears on Traquair's island of vision as a well with steep sides.

The size and contour of the visual field can be influenced by a multitude of factors. In addition to glaucomatous or neuro-ophthalmic conditions, other factors that can affect visual field performance include facial structure, eyelid anatomy, pupil size, ocular media (clarity of the cornea, lens, and vitreous), refractive error, testing artifact, as well as patient experience, cognitive status, reliability, and fatigue.

The Glaucomatous Visual Field

Glaucomatous optic nerve damage produces characteristic changes in the contour and shape of the visual field.

Generalized depression of the visual field is considered the most common change noted in glaucoma.[2] However, this finding is nonspecific and can be produced by a variety of other conditions as well, including cataract, corneal disease, fatigue, and incorrect refractive correction, among others.

Nerve fiber bundle defects as a result of glaucomatous optic nerve damage produce visual field changes that are

Kahook MY, Schuman JS, eds.
Chandler and Grant's Glaucoma, Fifth Edition (pp 117-130).
© 2013 SLACK Incorporated.

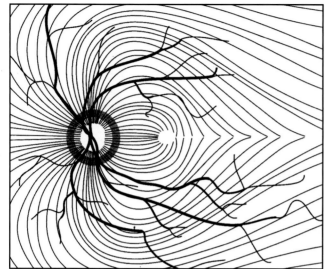

Figure 11-1. Superotemporal and inferotemporal retinal nerve fibers follow an arcuate path around the fovea, meeting at median raphe. Damage to this portion of the nerve fiber layer is responsible for arcuate field defects seen in glaucoma. (Reprinted with permission from Heijl A, Patella VM. *Essential Perimetry: The Field Analyzer Primer.* 3rd ed. Dublin, CA: Carl Zeiss Meditec; 2002:71.)

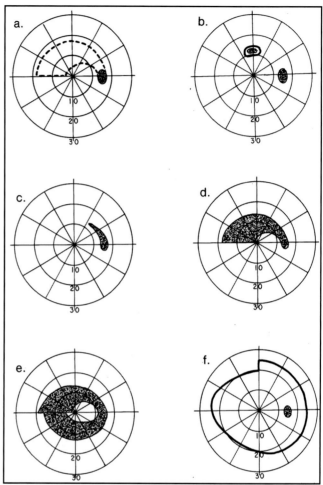

Figure 11-2. Arcuate visual field defects. (A) Bjerrum's region extends from the blind spot to the median raphe in an arcuate path that encompasses 10 degrees to 20 degrees nasally from fixation. (B) Seidel scotoma. (C) Paracentral scotomas. (D) Arcuate or Bjerrum scotoma. (E) Double arcuate scotoma. (F) Temporal wedge defects are produced by damage to the nasal neuroretinal rim and are not arcuate in nature. (Reprinted with permission from Shields MB. *Textbook of Glaucoma.* 3rd ed. Baltimore, MD: Williams & Wilkins; 1992.)

considered to be characteristic of glaucoma. These changes reflect retinal and optic nerve anatomy. Retinal nerve fibers radiate from the ONH and are distributed in an arcuate manner around the foveal region (Figure 11-1). Therefore, glaucomatous damage to the ONH produces visual field defects in the region subserved by the affected nerve fibers. The visual field defects produced from retinal nerve fiber bundle defects include localized paracentral scotomas, arcuate defects, nasal steps, and temporal defects (Figure 11-2). The most common location of visual field defects occur within an arcuate area commonly referred to as Bjerrum's area (or region), which includes that portion of the arcuate region that extends from the blind spot to the median raphe, where it extends 10 to 20 degrees nasally from fixation.[3]

Paracentral scotomas are discrete defects in the visual field caused by localized reduction in retinal sensitivity. These may be relative or absolute and are frequently found in Bjerrum's region.[4] Initially, these may appear intermittently as one or more shallow depressions detected sporadically on repeat examination prior to developing into permanent visual field defects.[6,7] With progression, paracentral scotomas become deeper and larger and may gradually coalesce, forming an arcuate or Bjerrum scotoma.

A nasal step occurs when there is a difference in the rate or location of visual field loss above and below the horizontal raphe nasal to fixation. This produces a distinct step that may occur along any, but not necessarily all, isopters.[8,9]

Temporal visual field defects are produced by damage to the nasal neuroretinal rim. Nerve fibers radiate without deviation from the nasal optic nerve; therefore, wedge defects develop. Temporal defects are usually found as a late manifestation of glaucomatous visual field loss.[10]

Methods of Perimetry

Representation of the Visual Field

Typically, the results of visual field testing are represented in 2 dimensions. The actual features of the field are determined by the method of testing.

Kinetic visual field testing is performed, as the name implies, with a moving test object. The object, usually a light of variable size and intensity projected on an evenly illuminated background, is moved from a nonseeing area toward a seeing area. The location is recorded when the patient is able to see the object. The process is repeated until a boundary of seeing and nonseeing is determined. This boundary line is called an *isopter* (Figure 11-3). Several isopters are usually obtained using test objects of different sizes or intensities.

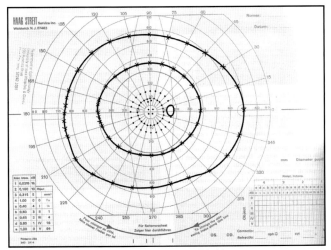

Figure 11-3. Normal kinetic and static visual field.

Static visual field testing involves the use of nonmoving test objects. Test objects are presented to the patient for a short period of time. A record of the patient's response is then made (seen or not seen) at the specific location. There are several different testing strategies for static perimetry. A supra-threshold test uses test objects that have a higher intensity than those that are normally seen at specific locations within the visual field. Threshold testing uses several test objects of increasing or decreasing intensity at each location. Based on patient response to such stimuli, the testing determines the threshold stimulus, or that stimulus that is seen 50% of the time in each location. The result is typically recorded as a symbol, numeric value, or graphically in gray scale (Figure 11-4).

CONFRONTATIONAL VISUAL FIELDS

During the initial evaluation of all new patients, eye-care providers should routinely perform confrontation visual field testing as a first step. A confrontation field can often be performed even with the most uncooperative patient in whom one can quickly identify gross field defects. The confrontation field may be of great value and the only practical method for patients who have limited visual acuity due to dense media opacities, such as cataracts or corneal disease. It is also of considerable practical value in determining the location and approximate size of a small residual field in individuals with advanced glaucoma. In some cases, a visual field has been recorded as a central island in patients in whom visual acuity was less than 6/60, due not to media opacity or macular change, but to glaucoma itself. In these cases, the true temporal location of the field defect can be quickly determined by confrontational visual field testing.

Tangent Screen

This device consists of an evenly illuminated flat black screen with a central fixation target mounted on a wall. The patient is seated 1 or 2 meters away facing the screen. The central 30 degrees of the visual field can be tested using both kinetic and static methods employing test objects of different size or color.

Although infrequently used today, the tangent screen, when used in experienced hands, can be an extremely valuable method to detect the relative size and location of visual field defects in patients with glaucoma and neuro-ophthalmic disorders. However, similar to confrontation fields, a limitation of using the tangent screen in caring for patients with glaucoma is that it is not possible to detect small progressive changes in the visual field, which is essential to the management of the patient with glaucoma.

Manual Perimetry

Manual perimetry (visual field testing) involves the use of a perimetrist, an individual skilled in the science (and art) of performing perimetry, and an instrument used by a perimetrist to perform and usually record the result. Several different instruments are available, although some are primarily of historical interest.

Manual Bowl Perimetry

The prototype instrument for most modern perimetry is the Goldmann perimeter. It consists of an evenly illuminated bowl (31.6 apostilbs) with a radius of approximately 300 mm. A chin rest supports the patient's head. A lens holder is used to provide correct refraction for central visual field testing.

The Goldmann perimeter is used to assess the central and peripheral visual field by employing illuminated test objects of variable size, intensity, and transmission. This instrument can be used for kinetic or static perimetry.

Automated Perimetry

Since the results of manual perimetry can be heavily influenced by the skill and technique of the perimetrist, a great deal of effort has been expended to reduce this variable by automating perimetry. Several computer-driven automated instruments are available.

Most automated perimeters use static targets and employ suprathreshold or threshold strategies. Test targets can be projected onto the bowl or are integrally placed in the bowl as light-emitting diodes (LEDs) or with fiberoptics. Fixation can be monitored with a telescope, verified by periodically testing the blind spot or by monitoring the corneal light reflex. Testing strategies are controlled by a computer, and the results are recorded on a computer printout.

Despite the implication that these units are fully automated, there is still a critical need for skilled technical support before and during visual field testing with these units

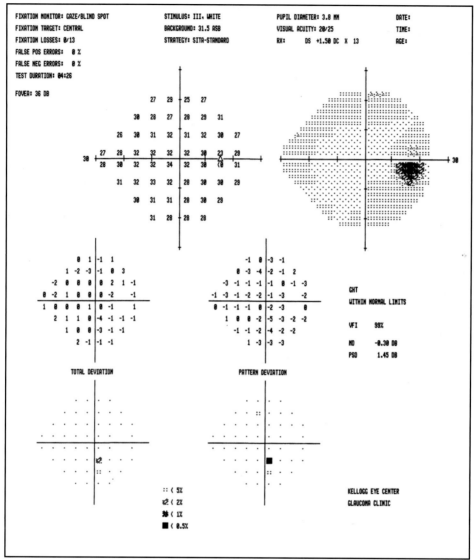

Figure 11-4. Normal (static) automated full-threshold visual field (Humphrey Field Analyzer, Central 24-2).

to maximize patient performance on these tests (Table 11-1). Prior to administering the test, technicians should check the size of the patient's pupils. Although relatively uncommon today, patients who are taking miotics or who have pupils with a diameter less than 3 mm may require dilation prior to perimetric testing to prevent artifactual depression of the visual field. Similarly, it is important to check manifest refraction and correct any refractive error present. Patients should be properly positioned so that they are comfortable during perimetric testing, and to optimize performance, careful instruction regarding the process and rationale of the test should be reviewed with the patient prior to initiating the test. The importance of fixation throughout the test should be emphasized to the patient. Simple encouragement can be very helpful for patients, as these tests are often protracted, tiring, and anxiety provoking. Ultimately, the reliability and usefulness of the test result is very dependent on the manner in which the test is conducted.

Reliability indices help the clinician evaluate patient performance. Those indices most commonly used are short-term fluctuation, false-positive responses, false-negative responses, and fixation losses.

Short-term fluctuation represents intratest variability. During the test, several locations are re-tested, and the differences in threshold values at these locations are determined. Short-term fluctuation is the square root of the variance obtained from the re-test values. Some short-term fluctuation is expected. However, when this value is abnormally high, it may represent a lack of attention or reliability on the part of the patient. Alternatively, high amounts of short-term fluctuation may occur as a result of extensive visual field damage.

TABLE 11-1. COMMON CAUSES OF VISUAL FIELD ARTIFACT

Source	Comment
Refractive error	Check refraction
Improper near correction	Always use full correction according to perimeter manual for patients with pseudophakia, aphakia, and after cycloplegia
Lid artifact	May need to gently elevate lid with tape
Lens rim artifact	Reposition patient or corrective lens
Fatigue or stress	Patient reassurance, rest between visual fields, use SITA-Fast or FASTPAC algorithms, only perform testing on one eye per visit
Patient movement	—
Miotic pupil	—
Cognitive decline or impairment	Reposition patient
Dilate pupil before testing	Frequent reminders during testing, may require testing using manual perimetry

SITA: Swedish interactive thresholding algorithm.

False-positive errors occur when a patient gives a response when no target is presented (though a sound may be made by the machine). False-positives may result from "trigger happy" patients or those who are trying to "help" the test. The anxiety of not seeing stimuli that are infrathreshold can be substantial. Patients may feel that their condition may be getting worse, and their worry may cause them to respond to stimuli that do not exist. Reassuring the patient before and during the test that it is normal not to see some of the targets can reduce this problem.

False-negative errors occur when the patient fails to respond to a stimulus that is of greater intensity than one seen previously in the same location. False-negatives may represent inattentiveness, a shift in head position, or may be a byproduct of searching for targets. Careful reinstruction often remedies this problem.

Fixation losses reduce reliability of visual field testing. Patients may alter fixation as a natural response to stimuli in the peripheral field, a desire to "help" the examiner or, in some cases, due to vision loss when the patient is unable to see the fixation target. Generally, careful instruction during testing will remedy the first 2 of these issues. Some perimeters have a group of fixation targets surrounding central fixation, which help the patient center his or her gaze when loss of central vision is the primary problem. For patients who are unable to suppress their desire to look around during testing, manual perimetry with constant observation by the perimetrist may be required.

TESTING STRATEGIES

Automated perimeters present stimuli randomly within a fixed pattern. This eliminates the patient's ability to anticipate the location of the next stimulus and may help reduce fixation losses from this source. Stimulus intensity is adjusted to "fit" the visual field contour, which helps reduce testing time.

Suprathreshold testing involves the use of stimuli that are of greater intensity than the presumed threshold one should be able to visualize at each location. Some instruments present a second high-intensity stimulus at locations where the first stimulus is not detected to differentiate between relative and absolute visual field defects. Suprathreshold testing may be useful for glaucoma screening; however, this test strategy does not precisely delineate the depth of visual field abnormalities and is therefore not suitable for baseline or follow-up examinations of patients known to have glaucoma.

Full-threshold testing is a strategy that quantifies the patient's retinal threshold for correctly reporting a stimulus 50% of the time. A stimulus is presented at increasing intensity levels of 4 decibels until it crosses the patient's retinal threshold for detection. Next, the stimulus intensity is reduced in 4-decibel increments until it is unable to be visualized. Finally, this process is repeated using 2-decibel intensity increments to further define the threshold value measured. The visual field pattern typically consists of 70 or more test locations distributed within the central 24 to 30 degrees.

FASTPAC is an alternative testing algorithm to full-threshold field testing. Unlike full-threshold testing, the FASTPAC strategy presents stimuli at increasing intensity levels of 3 decibels until it is identified. Once the stimulus is identified, the testing of that particular point is complete. Compared with full-threshold testing, FASTPAC is much quicker to perform. However, comparison of patient performance on both measures demonstrates greater variability in performance with FASTPAC, which may limit the ability to use this test to monitor patients for glaucomatous disease progression.[11]

One of the difficulties of performing visual field testing using the threshold testing strategy is that the test can be quite time consuming for patients and patient fatigue can affect performance. Swedish interactive thresholding algorithm (SITA) was developed as a means of capturing field loss more quickly and efficiently while still maintaining the same level of quality attained by performing threshold testing, a feature that FASTPAC testing could not fully accomplish. SITA determines a threshold value at each test point and estimates the level of certainty of the threshold value obtained. Once the level of certainty surpasses a predetermined level, testing of that particular point stops. With SITA, the threshold and level of certainty of specific points on the field can be influenced by values obtained for adjacent points. Studies have demonstrated that SITA testing generates similar results to those obtained by full-threshold testing,[12] that it has a high sensitivity and specificity for detecting glaucomatous field loss,[13] and that it is much less time consuming as compared with full-threshold testing.[14] There are 2 SITA testing strategies: SITA-Standard and SITA-Fast. SITA-Standard generates results similar to those obtained by full-threshold testing while SITA-FAST generates results similar to those obtained by using FASTPAC.

INTERPRETING VISUAL FIELD TEST RESULTS

Gray Scale

The gray scale on the visual field printout is a graphical representation of the threshold values obtained for each of the points tested. Clinicians can show this graphical display to patients to explain the extent of visual field loss present, and reviewing serial gray scale printouts with patients can show them whether the extent of the visual field loss has been stable over time or whether there has been disease progression.

Global Indices

Automated perimeters have the capability of statistically analyzing the output generated during visual field testing to detect subtle patterns of field loss. These analyses are known as global indices and are often found on the right side of the visual field printout. Common global indices include the mean deviation (MD), the pattern standard deviation (PSD), and the corrected pattern standard deviation (CPSD).

Mean Deviation

The MD is a global measure of a patient's performance on the visual field test relative to the norm. It answers the question of whether the hill of vision recorded for the patient differs significantly from the normal hill of vision. It is an average of all the points in the total deviation plot. The *p*-value accompanying the mean deviation indicates what percentage of the normal population (people without glaucoma) would obtain a value larger than the numeric value generated by the patient performing the test. MD scores can be affected by cataracts, media opacities, uncorrected refractive error, and miotic pupils.

Pattern Standard Deviation

The PSD assesses how different the shape of the patient's hill of vision departs from the expected hill of vision for a "normal" patient of similar age. This test captures localized

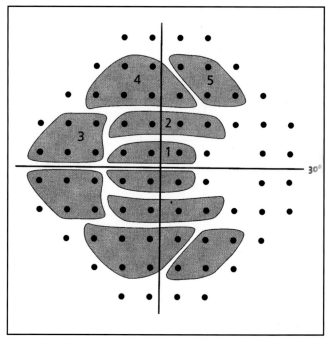

Figure 11-5. Superior visual field zones used in the glaucoma hemifield test. Summated test scores (in decibels) within each zone are compared with the mirror zone below the horizontal meridian.

field loss, which is often caused by glaucoma as opposed to global field loss, which can be attributable to glaucoma, media opacities, or other causes.

Corrected Pattern Standard Deviation

The CPSD takes into account the effect of short-term fluctuation on the field of vision. Once the hill of vision is smoothed out to account for short-term fluctuation, it assesses the shape of the hill of vision and whether it deviates from the normal.

Glaucoma Hemifield Testing

Glaucoma hemifield testing (GHT) is an additional test strategy that involves comparing patient performance on specified regions of the visual field above and below the horizontal midline (Figure 11-5). This approach has a high degree of specificity and sensitivity at detecting glaucoma when compared with other test strategies.[15-17] GHT results are classified as *within normal limits*, *borderline*, or *outside of normal*. The results are displayed on the standard 24- or 30-degree visual field printouts.

Testing Patterns

Automated perimeters offer an array of different testing patterns from which to choose. The 2 most commonly used test patterns involve testing the central 24 or 30 degrees of the visual field around central fixation. These testing patterns assess stimuli at test locations spaced 6 degrees apart from one another. Another testing pattern assesses the

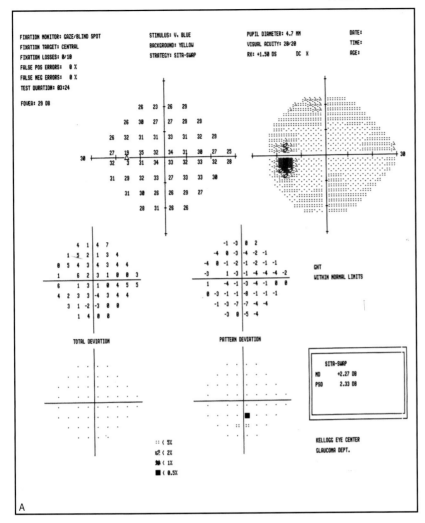

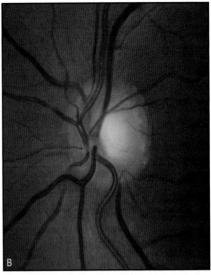

Figure 11-6. (A) Short-wave automated perimetry (SWAP) visual field. (B) Digital photo of patient with normal SWAP.

central 10 degrees of the visual field. The test locations for the central 10 degrees of field are spaced 2 degrees apart from one another. This testing pattern is often used for patients with advanced glaucoma who only have a central island of vision remaining. Finally, there is a 120-point full-field pattern, which can be used for screening purposes.

Blue-on-Yellow Perimetry

The loss of short-wavelength sensitivity is greater in eyes with glaucoma than normal eyes.[18-20] This has led to the development of a form of perimetry that uses a blue stimulus on a yellow background (blue-on-yellow), also known as short-wave-automated-perimetry (SWAP). Because SWAP is selectively testing for damage to the S-cones, and there is less redundancy of those cells relative to others in the retina, this form of perimetry can identify early glaucomatous damage years before such damage becomes detectable by using standard white-on-white perimetry. When comparing standard white-on-white with blue-on-yellow perimetry for identifying patients with glaucomatous field loss, visual field defects can be identified up to 10 years earlier and appear

to be larger and denser with blue-on-yellow perimetry.[21-24] SWAP perimetry can be performed on the Humphrey visual field units (Figure 11-6).

A limitation of original SWAP testing algorithm is that this test can be difficult to perform on patients who have dense cataracts. In addition, blue-yellow perimetric testing can be quite lengthy, taking up to 18 minutes per eye to perform this test. The recent development of SITA SWAP has reduced testing time down to under 4 minutes per eye, making this test much easier to perform on patients.[25,26]

Frequency-Doubling Perimetry

Frequency-doubling perimetry (FDP) is a form of perimetry that uses a stimulus that consists of rapidly alternating (flickering) dark and light stripes. The magnocellular ganglion cells (M-cells), which specialize at motion detection, are stimulated by this flickering stimulus. Studies suggest that M-cells are preferentially affected in patients with early glaucoma.[27] Like SWAP, FDP has a role in identifying individuals with early glaucoma before field loss becomes detectable on standard white-on-white perimetry. Studies

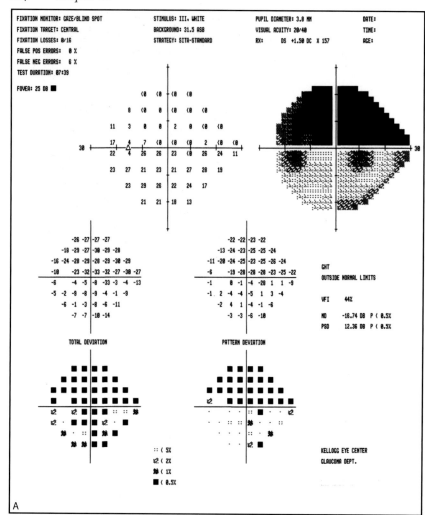

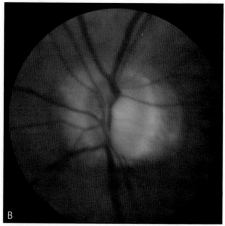

Figure 11-7. (A) Patient with considerable superior visual field loss, corresponding with damage to the inferior rim of the optic nerve. (B) Digital photo with thinning of the inferior rim margin corresponding to dense superior field loss.

comparing FDP with standard perimetry have demonstrated that FDP has good sensitivity and specificity at detecting early glaucoma.[28,29]

There are screening (suprathreshold) and threshold testing strategies for FDP. The newest model of FDP, the Humphrey Matrix, generates comparable output to standard white-on-white perimetry with a gray scale plot, total and pattern deviation plots, and global indices (MD, PSD, and GHT).

CORRELATING THE OPTIC NERVE WITH THE VISUAL FIELD

Change in the optic disc from glaucoma often predates change in the visual field.[30-32] Additionally, the location of the abnormality of the optic disc typically correlates with abnormalities detected on perimetric testing.

In most patients in whom glaucomatous changes in the optic disc develop, the physiologic cup enlarges to reach the disc margin downward and temporally. This is a definite glaucomatous change, but, at first, the cup becomes shelved rather than excavated. A visual field defect may not be present at this early stage. As the cup becomes deeper at the inferior disc margin, a real excavation becomes evident, which may then produce a superior visual field defect (Figure 11-7).

Similarly, in other cases, the physiologic cup may enlarge superiorly. As the disease progresses, the cup comes closer to the superior disc margin and becomes excavated. At this stage, although the cup still does not quite reach the upper outer margin, there is usually a lower field defect—a lower Bjerrum scotoma, a lower nasal step, or both (Figure 11-8).

The cup may enlarge toward both the upper and lower borders simultaneously. It is in this type of glaucomatous change that we eventually find both an upper and lower Bjerrum scotoma, isolating a central island of vision, varying in size from patient to patient, with variable degrees of loss of the peripheral field.

Eventually, the excavation may reach the margin above as well as below, and the disc may become totally cupped to all margins. In these cases, the central visual field may be lost or

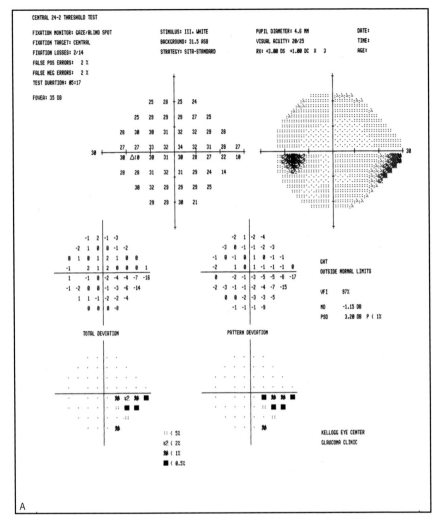

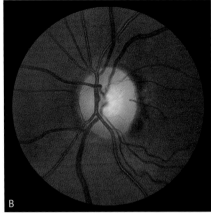

Figure 11-8. (A, B) Patient with an inferior nasal step, corresponding to damage to loss of superior neuroretinal rim tissue.

consist of a small central island. Usually, the nasal neuroretinal rim is the last portion of the nerve to get damaged from glaucoma. Individuals who only have viable tissue at the nasal neuroretinal rim may only possess a temporal island of remaining vision. Ultimately, in the absence of effective intervention, all vision will be lost.

We believe a valuable axiom is that in ordinary eyes (not those which are highly myopic) there can be no field defects due to glaucoma if the disc appearance is normal, unless the intraocular pressure (IOP) is high at the time of the examination or has been high a short time previously. If the IOP is elevated at the time of examination, glaucomatous field defects may be found. Such defects may reverse if the IOP is promptly reduced to normal. If such field defects are permanent, then within a few weeks, evidence of optic atrophy usually becomes evident.

In cases in which glaucoma-like visual field defects occur where the IOP and the disc appear completely normal, another explanation for the field loss should be sought out. We have seen many patients who had glaucoma and were alleged to be losing field or who had field loss despite good IOP control where the appearance of the optic nerve did not correlate with the field defect. In the vast majority of cases, these inconsistencies were explained by the presence of other pathology, such as ONH drusen, retinal vascular occlusions, chorioretinal lesions, retinal degeneration, retinal detachment, retinoschisis, or neurologic disorders, such as brain tumors, stroke, or head trauma (Figure 11-9 and Table 11-2). Poor test performance can also be responsible for field loss that does not correlate with the appearance of the optic nerve. Before initiating an extensive work-up to try to identify an alternative explanation for a field defect, it is advisable to first repeat the visual field to confirm that the field loss is reproducible.

The Visual Field in Normal-Tension Glaucoma

Unlike most forms of glaucoma, which first cause peripheral visual field loss and then, as the disease progresses, affect central vision, patients with normal-tension glaucoma often experience dense visual field loss close

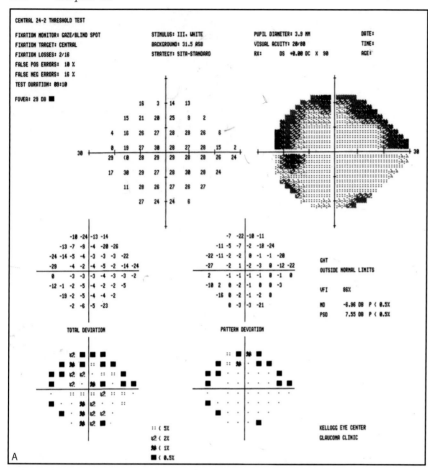

CENTRAL 24-2 THRESHOLD TEST

FIXATION MONITOR: GAZE/BLIND SPOT   STIMULUS: III, WHITE   PUPIL DIAMETER: 3.9 MM   DATE:
FIXATION TARGET: CENTRAL   BACKGROUND: 31.5 ASB   VISUAL ACUITY: 20/80   TIME:
FIXATION LOSSES: 2/16   STRATEGY: SITA-STANDARD   RX: OS +0.00 DC X 90   AGE:
FALSE POS ERRORS: 18 %
FALSE NEG ERRORS: 16 %
TEST DURATION: 09:10

FOVEA: 29 DB ■

TOTAL DEVIATION

PATTERN DEVIATION

GHT   OUTSIDE NORMAL LIMITS

VFI   86%

MD   -6.96 DB P < 0.5%
PSD   7.55 DB P < 0.5%

:: < 5%
⚃ < 2%
⚄ < 1%
■ < 0.5%

KELLOGG EYE CENTER
GLAUCOMA CLINIC

A

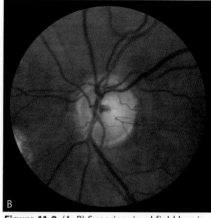

Figure 11-9. (A; B) Superior visual field loss in a patient with proliferative diabetic retinopathy who had previously undergone panretinal photocoagulation. Note that the optic nerve does not exhibit glaucomatous optic nerve damage.

TABLE 11-2. CAUSES OF GLAUCOMA-LIKE VISUAL FIELD DEFECTS	
Eyelid ptosis or dermatochalasis	Optic nerve head lesions
Chorioretinal lesions	Optic nerve head drusen
Chorioretinal scars	Optic nerve coloboma or pit
Retinal vascular occlusions	Chronic papilledema
Retinal detachment	Anterior ischemic optic neuropathy
Retinoschisis	Lesions posterior to optic nerve head
Myelinization of NFL	Chiasmal lesions (eg, pituitary adenoma)
Postsurgical states	Optic foramen or perisellar tumor (eg, meningioma)
Panretinal photocoagulation, cryotherapy, scleral buckle	Cerebrovascular disease
NFL: nerve fiber layer.	

to fixation before the peripheral field is extinguished (Figure 11-10). In these patients, the optic nerve can exhibit focal notching of the optic nerve and nerve fiber layer dropout in the area corresponding to the visual field loss. These patients are also prone to experiencing disc hemorrhages, a sign that the disease may be progressing.

ADVANCED VISUAL FIELD LOSS

Central and Temporal Islands

When glaucoma becomes very advanced to a point where only a small central island of vision remains intact, patients are often able to subjectively tell when this central island is becoming extinguished. Therefore, it is useful during routine follow-up visits to ask such patients whether they notice any changes in their vision. If subjective changes are occurring, the clinician should have a low threshold to intervene and lower the IOP further. In addition to inquiring about subjective changes in vision, clinicians should perform more frequent visual field assessments to objectively monitor for disease progression in patients with advanced disease. If automated perimetry is being used, assessing only the central 10 degrees with a finer grid

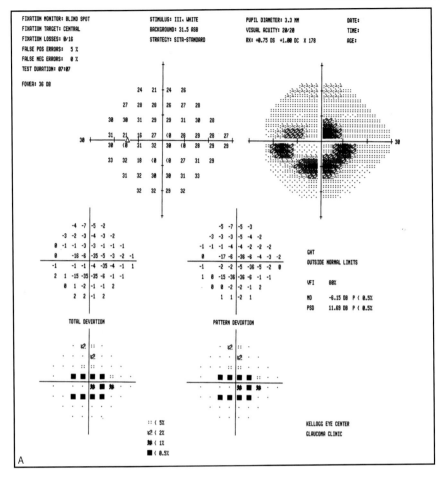

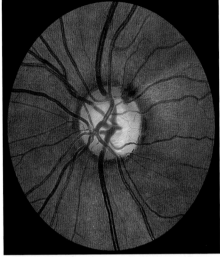

Figure 11-10. (A) A patient with normal-tension glaucoma. Note the superior and inferior paracentral visual field loss, which corresponds with superior and inferior notches in the optic nerve. (B) Digital photo.

pattern can improve resolution of the remaining visual field and reduce test time compared to using the standard 24- or 30-degree field testing (Figure 11-11). The Humphrey Field Analyzer has a 10-2 test that can be used to assess the central field. Not only is this test useful in quantifying field loss in patients with advanced glaucoma, but it is also useful in checking for chloroquine toxicity and other maculopathies that tend to affect central vision.

When there is little or no remaining central vision but only a temporal island of vision left, Goldmann perimetry may be used to follow the residual visual field. When the central field is severely depressed but not completely lost, a larger target size, for example size V, can be substituted for the standard target size (III) to quantify the field in vision in such patients.

FREQUENCY OF VISUAL FIELD TESTING

The baseline visual field will, in most cases, be referred to for comparison after each subsequent visual field. Due to a well-described "learning curve," initial visual field tests should not be relied on as baseline examinations. Two or more examinations may be required before visual field test results are consistent, reliable, and can be used for future reference. These tests should be spaced within a few months of

each other to promote the learning process. As stated above, monitoring patients for glaucoma using perimetric testing should only employ quantitative threshold rather than suprathreshold testing; the latter strategy does not quantitate defects and is only suitable for screening purposes.

In patients who require periodic visual field assessment, testing may be repeated in weeks, months, or years depending on specific clinical circumstances. In cases where IOP, optic nerve status, and visual fields have been stable for years (eg, glaucoma suspects), annual or even biannual visual field assessment may suffice, though ophthalmic examinations may be required more often.

In most cases in which IOP is well controlled, visual fields should be repeated every 9 to 15 months. However, when an interim change is detected in a visual field, a repeat examination should be performed within weeks or months to confirm the findings. Because inter-test (long-term) fluctuation is common, it is wise not to undertake a major therapeutic intervention based on a single examination. In most cases, patients should undergo repeat testing to confirm the newly detected field loss before deciding whether to change patient management.

Relatively frequent visual field assessment (eg, every 2 to 4 months) may be required in cases where there is advanced

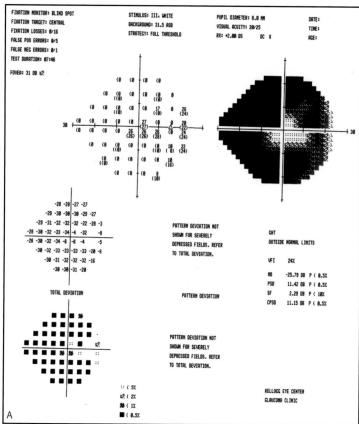

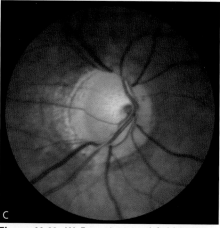

Figure 11-11. (A) Extensive visual field loss in a patient with advanced glaucoma captured on a 24-2 visual field test. (B) A 10-2 visual field of the same patient demonstrating the extent of visual field loss approaching central fixation. (C) Digital photo.

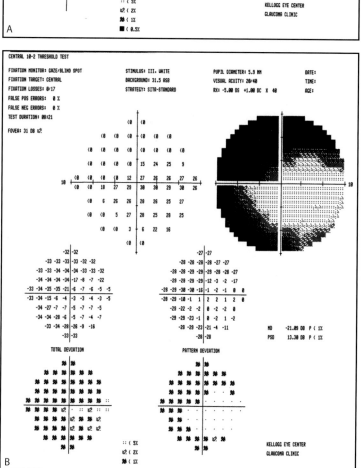

visual field loss. In these situations, surgical intervention may be considered for small degrees of progressive visual field loss.

PROGRESSION OF VISUAL FIELD LOSS

Determining whether visual fields are stable or, in fact, whether progressive visual field loss has occurred can be challenging. A multitude of factors should be considered before one can conclude that glaucomatous visual field progression has taken place.[33]

The process of comparing visual fields is best done in a methodical manner. Comparison of new fields should be made to a reliable and stable baseline examination along with a representative sample (preferably all) of the intervening visual fields. A common error is to compare visual fields to only those obtained most recently, because they are often the most readily located in the medical record. In this manner, small changes can easily be explained away as long-term fluctuation, and the recognition of significant visual field loss may go unnoticed for long periods of time. It is best to have all visual fields for each eye placed sequentially in one location in the medical record for easier reference and comparison.

It is important to consider visual field reliability, which eye was tested first, pupil size, whether eyelids were taped or not during the examination, the perimetrist's comments regarding patient performance, and other factors for each examination. It is advisable to discard early pre-baseline and unreliable visual fields.

The most common patterns of field loss should be considered. Not only is the superior hemifield the region most likely to demonstrate early visual field loss, but it is also the region where loss is most rapidly progressive.[34,35] For this reason, one should be cautious about explaining the cause of superior visual field loss as a droopy eyelid. More often than not, field loss remains confined to one hemifield for extended periods of time.[36,37] Additionally, areas of existing damage are far more likely to demonstrate progressive loss, either by scotomatous enlargement or deepening, than undamaged areas.[37] Therefore, it is useful to examine these areas more carefully when examining a series of visual fields.

It is difficult if not counterproductive to give specific decibel cut-offs for progression versus long-term fluctuation when examining inter-test changes. The more eccentric the test location from fixation, the greater the long-term fluctuation.[38] Additionally, progression may have occurred if 2 or more test locations are depressed versus a single point, especially if these are within or adjacent to a region of previous field loss.

The ability to quickly and easily compare visual fields over time has been greatly enhanced by glaucoma progression analysis (GPA) software. This software compares patient performance on sequential full-threshold, SITA-Standard, or SITA-Fast visual field tests. The first 2 tests a patient takes provide baseline information for which subsequent tests are compared against. The GPA software identifies worsening of test points relative to baseline performance. Different symbols on the GPA printout identify worsening on 1, 2, and 3 consecutive subsequent field tests. The software also classifies whether there is no progression, "possible progression," or "likely progression" of visual field loss.

A new measure that captures glaucoma progression is the Visual Field Index (VFI). The VFI uses regression to offer a trend-based analysis of the speed by which visual field loss is occurring. The VFI generates a score from 0 (complete loss of field) to 100 (completely full field).

Finally, if new visual field loss is suspected, it is necessary to repeat the visual field examination and perform a corroborative optic nerve and fundus evaluation before reaching a firm conclusion or recommending a change in therapy.

REFERENCES

1. Traquair HM. Perimetry in the study of glaucoma. *Trans Ophthalmol UK.* 1931;51:585-599.
2. Anctil JL, Anderson DR. Early foveal involvement and generalized depression of the visual field in glaucoma. *Arch Ophthalmol.* 1984;102:363.
3. Harrington DO. The Bjerrum scotoma. *Am J Ophthalmol.* 1965;59:646.
4. Hart WM, Becker B. The onset and evolution of glaucomatous visual field defects. *Ophthalmology.* 1982;89:268.
5. Harrington DO. The pathogenesis of the glaucomatous visual field. *Am J Ophthalmol.* 1958;47:177.
6. Drance SM. The early field defect in glaucoma. *Invest Ophthalmol.* 1969;8:84.
7. Werner EB, Drance SM. Early visual field disturbances in glaucoma. *Arch Ophthalmol.* 1977;95:1173.
8. LaBlanc RP, Becker B. Peripheral nasal field defects. *Am J Ophthalmol.* 1971;72:415.
9. Drance SM. The glaucomatous visual field. *Br J Ophthalmol.* 1972;56:186.
10. Brais P, Drance SM. The temporal field in chronic simple glaucoma. *Arch Ophthalmol.* 1976;88:518.
11. Barton JJS, Benetar M. *Field of Vision.* Totowa, NJ: Humana Press Inc; 2003.
12. Heijl A, Bengtsson B, Patella VM. Glaucoma follow-up when converting from long to short perimetric threshold tests. *Arch Ophthalmol.* 2000;118:489-493.
13. Sekhar GC, Naduvilath TJ, Lakkai M, et al. Sensitivity of Swedish interactive threshold algorithm compared with standard full threshold algorithm in Humphrey visual field testing. *Ophthalmology.* 2000;107:1303-1308.
14. Sharma AK, Goldberg I, Graham SL, Mohson M. Comparison of the Humphrey Swedish interactive thresholding algorithm (SITA) and full threshold strategies. *J Glaucoma.* 2000;9:20-27.
15. Budenz DL, Rhee P, Feuer WJ, McSoley J, Johnson CA, Anderson DR. Sensitivity and specificity of the Swedish Interactive Threshold Algorithm for glaucomatous visual field defects. *Ophthalmology.* 2002;109:1052-1058.
16. Bengtsson B, Heijl A, Olsson J. Evaluation of a new threshold visual field strategy, SITA, in normal subjects: Swedish Interactive Threshold Algorithm. *Acta Ophthalmol Scand.* 1998;76:165-169.
17. Asman P, Heijl A. Glaucoma hemifield test. Automated visual field evaluation. *Arch Ophthalmol.* 1992;110:812-819.
18. Asman P, Heijl A. Evaluation of methods for automated hemifield analysis in perimetry. *Arch Ophthalmol.* 1992;110:820-826.

19. Asman P. Computer-assisted interpretation of visual fields in glaucoma. *Acta Ophthalmol.* 1992;206(suppl):1-47.
20. Drance SM, Lakowski R, Schulzer M, et al. Acquired color vision changes in glaucoma: use of 100 Hue Test and Pickford anomaloscope as predictors of glaucomatous field change. *Arch Ophthalmol.* 1981;99:829-831.
21. Adams AJ, Rodie R, Husted R, et al. Spectral sensitivity and color discrimination changes in glaucoma and glaucoma-suspects. *Invest Ophthalmol Vis Sci.* 1982;23:516-524.
22. Sample PA, Weinreb RN, Boynton RM. Acquired dyschromatopsia in glaucoma. *Surv Ophthalmol.* 1986;31:54-64.
23. Johnson CA, Adams AJ, Casson EJ, et al. Progression of early glaucomatous visual field loss as detected by blue-on-yellow and standard white-on-white automated perimetry. *Arch Ophthalmol.* 1993;111:651-656.
24. Sample PA, Weinreb RN. Progressive color visual field loss in glaucoma. *Invest Ophthalmol Vis Sci.* 1992;33:2068-2071.
25. Sample PA, Taylor JD, Martinez GA, et al. Short-wavelength color visual fields in glaucoma suspects at risk. *Am J Ophthalmol.* 1993;115:225-233.
26. Johnson CA, Adams AJ, Casson EJ, et al. Blue-on-yellow perimetry can predict the development of glaucomatous visual field loss. *Arch Ophthalmol.* 1993;111:645-650.
27. Turpin A, Johnson CA, Spry PGD. Development of a maximum likelihood procedure for Short Wavelength Automated Perimetry (SWAP). In: Wall M, Mills RP, eds. *Perimetry Update 2000/2001.* The Hague: Kugler Publications; 2001:139-147.
28. Bengtsson B, Heijl A. Normal intersubject threshold variability and normal limits of the SITA SWAP and full threshold SWAP perimetric programs. *Invest Ophthalmol Vis Sci.* 2003;44: 5029-5034.
29. Landers JA, Goldberg I, Graham SL. Detection of early visual field loss in glaucoma using frequency-doubling perimetry and short-wavelength automated perimetry *Arch Ophthalmol.* 2003;121:1705-1710.
30. Cello K. Frequency doubling technology perimetry for detection of glaucomatous visual field loss. *Am J Ophthalmol.* 2000;129(3): 314-322.
31. Bowd C, Zangwill LM, Berry CC, et al. Detecting early glaucoma by assessment of retinal nerve fiber layer thickness and visual function. *Invest Ophthalmol Vis Sci.* 2001;42:1993-2003.
32. Zeyen TG, Caprioli J. Progression of disc and field damage in early glaucoma. *Arch Ophthalmol.* 1993;111:62-65.
33. Pederson JE, Anderson DR. The mode of progressive disc cupping in ocular hypertension and glaucoma. *Arch Ophthalmol.* 1980;98:490-495.
34. Odberg T, Riise D. Early diagnosis of glaucoma: the value of successive stereophotography of the optic disc. *Acta Ophthalmol.* 1985;63:257-263.
35. Zulauf M, Caprioli J. What constitutes progression of glaucomatous visual field defects? *Semin Ophthalmol.* 1992;7:130-146.
36. Heijl A, Lundqvist L. The location of earliest glaucomatous visual field defects documented by automated perimetry. *Doc Ophthalmol Proc Series.* 1983;35:153-158.
37. O'Brien C, Zangwill LM, Berry CC. the visual field in chronic open angle glaucoma: The rate of change in different regions of the field. *Eye.* 1990;4:557-562.
38. Hart WM, Becker B. The onset and evolution of glaucomatous visual field defects. *Am J Ophthalmol.* 1989;89:268-279.

SECTION *II*

MEDICATIONS USED IN GLAUCOMA THERAPY

12

Adrenergic Agents
Blockers and Agonists

Pratap Challa, MD, MS and David L. Epstein, MD, MMM

Topical beta-blockers decrease aqueous humor formation (AHF)[1,2] and are used long-term in the therapy of the chronic open-angle glaucomas and short-term for various acute glaucomas. The introduction of the topical beta-blocker timolol in 1978 was greeted with overwhelming enthusiasm not only because of the remarkable efficacy of beta-blockers, but also because of the relative low frequency of ocular side effects. Before the beta-blockers, the only topical antiglaucoma medications available were the miotics and epinephrine-like compounds, the potential side effects of which will be discussed shortly. In practice, the potential ocular side effects from these latter agents resulted in an appropriate hesitancy for clinicians to treat elevated intraocular pressure (IOP), even if substantial, unless there was obvious end-organ damage (optic nerve) or abnormalities in (pre-automated perimetry) visual fields. The occurrence of these side effects also adversely affected patient compliance when aggressive therapy was required for advanced glaucomatous damage.

In the ensuing years, we have continued to observe that ocular side effects from topical beta-blockers are not common, and, in fact, potential long-term adverse effects of reduced aqueous humor flow on intraocular structural integrity, which some had predicted, have not occurred. However, we have become increasingly aware of the possibility of significant systemic side effects[3] from topical beta-blockers, even in patients with no known systemic predisposition. In fact, systemic side effects are the major limitation to the use of topical beta-blocker therapy.

Although there likely is some absorption through conjunctival blood vessels, a major site for systemic absorption of topical drugs seems to be the nasal mucosa. Therefore, we frequently instruct patients to perform punctal occlusion[4] for a few minutes after eye drop administration: the eye is closed and the index finger exerts firm pressure over

the (lower) punctum, conceptually thus preventing egress of excess medication from the tear film into the nasal mucosa via the occluded punctum (Figure 12-1). Alternatively, gentle eyelid closure for several minutes by itself without punctal occlusion (and without blinking) has been reported by Zimmerman et al[5] to be just as effective as punctal occlusion and likely more patient friendly.

Punctal occlusion or gentle eyelid closure is effective in some but not all patients, especially those with mild or moderate symptoms. However, it is not a panacea, and we have been disappointed in its efficacy in patients with advanced systemic symptoms, which most often requires discontinuation of the medication.

Systemic symptoms from topical ocular beta-blockers can be serious and even life threatening. The most common of these symptoms is systemic beta-blockage involving respiratory and cardiac function. The ophthalmologist needs to be alert for symptoms of bronchospasm and bradycardia. Frequently, the patient is either unaware of or misinterprets the cause of these symptoms, attributing it to primary systemic disease. The diagnosis of a presumed systemic condition is often made by the general physician for the first time only after the patient has been placed on topical beta-blockers. We have not made an effective-enough effort of informing our family medicine and internal medicine colleagues about the occurrence of these systemic symptoms resulting from topical ocular medication.

It is very important to listen to patient breathing at the time of slit-lamp examination; patients will commonly not call symptoms of dyspnea to the attention of their ophthalmologist (because they do not associate eye drops with systemic problems) and often may not themselves be fully cognizant that their breathing has "been a little worse lately," since the topical beta-blocker therapy was initiated. Routinely check the pulse

Kahook MY, Schuman JS, eds.
Chandler and Grant's Glaucoma, Fifth Edition (pp 133-147).
© 2013 SLACK Incorporated.

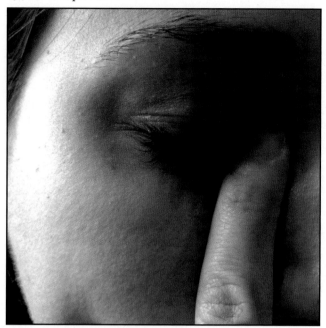

Figure 12-1. Technique of punctal occlusion. The index finger is placed over the lower punctum, and gentle pressure is applied with the eyelid closed. Pressure is then removed, and the eye is opened after 5 minutes.

rate and blood pressure of patients receiving ocular beta-blocker therapy. Patients are often unaware of bradycardia, which may not be fully symptomatic until a threshold level (that occurs subsequently) is passed. Any patient with a cardiac conduction defect or bradycardia should avoid beta-blockers.

Topical beta-blockers should be used with caution in heart failure patients because the beta-1 blocking activity could depress myocardial contractility and theoretically worsen heart failure. However, systemic beta-blockers have been shown to decrease morbidity in heart failure patients and are essentially standard therapy in this disorder. One should realize that systemic beta-blocker therapy is typically started at low dosages and titrated to the highest dose that does not worsen the heart failure. Therefore, patients are likely in a narrow therapeutic range with their current systemic therapy, and the addition of a topical beta-blocker may tip the patient over into worsening heart failure. Therefore, topical beta-blockers should be used in consultation with the patient's cardiologist. Very uncommonly, patients with no apparent heart failure symptoms (but likely pre-existing maximally compensated heart function) can develop heart failure for the first time as a result of topical beta-blocker therapy.

Some patients receiving topical ocular beta-blockers report fatigue, which may not be due to bradycardia or heart failure, but rather might have a central (nervous system) origin. Symptoms of fatigue can occur with systemic beta-blocker therapy[6] and seem to represent a real potential side effect from topical beta-blockers. Such symptoms seem to respond better to punctal occlusion or gentle eyelid closure than those of bradycardia or bronchospasm, the latter 2 of which, it again is stressed, can be life threatening and require discontinuation of the drug.

Depression has also been associated with systemic beta-blocker therapy.[6] However, recent studies have not supported the concept of increased depression among patients receiving topical[7] or systemic[8] beta-blockers.

The true majority of glaucoma patients treated with topical beta-blockers does not develop any systemic side effects, and this class of therapy has been a remarkable advance in our armamentarium. But, the ophthalmologist needs to be vigilant for the possible occurrence of such systemic symptoms, even in patients with no known predisposition. It is this latter group that has sensitized us all to the potential systemic hazard of this form of glaucoma therapy, because the occurrence of these serious systemic symptoms has been so unexpected but also so frequently undetected or misdiagnosed. There is no "free lunch" for either the patient with glaucoma or for us as glaucoma clinicians, and, unfortunately, all of our therapies have benefit/risk considerations. We have not yet developed the "magic bullet" for either the trabecular meshwork or optic nerve in glaucoma, but when we do, such therapy will likely also entail benefit/risk considerations.

Other uncommon systemic side effects, such as sexual dysfunction[9] and rarely Raynaud's disease-type symptoms have occasionally been attributed to topical ocular beta-blocker therapy (as well as to systemic beta-blocker therapy). In our experience, occasional patients do report sexual side effects, and punctal occlusion or gentle eyelid closure can be effective in preventing these side effects. Regarding Raynaud's type symptoms (presumably vasoconstriction of peripheral vessels from unopposed adrenergic input), we have yet to see a patient with this. Moreover, the literature has anecdotal case reports of this phenomenon,[10] and studies[11,12] have not shown adverse effects of beta-blockers in Raynaud's patients. Other rarely reported side effects include masking hypoglycemic symptoms[13] in diabetic patients, masking of symptoms of thyrotoxicosis, enhanced muscle weakness in certain myasthenic syndromes, and interactions in patients on systemic catecholamine-depleting drugs, such as reserpine.

Topical beta-blockers, like almost all topical ocular drugs, have not been proven safe in pregnancy or in breastfeeding mothers and should also be used with caution in pediatric patients. Fetal bradycardia and cardiac arrhythmias have been reported from topical timolol use during pregnancy.[14]

Topical nonselective beta-blockers may cause a small but meaningful adverse effect on blood lipoproteins presumably due to systemic absorption.[15] Topical carteolol, in addition to its nonselective beta-blocking ability and intrinsic sympathomimetic action, has been reported to have less of this effect.[16] The true implications of this observation need further elucidation, and this phenomenon does not, in itself, direct our choice of a beta-blocker for initial therapy.[17] On the other hand, this observation involving systemic lipoproteins might indicate the need to have all patients taking topical beta-blocker therapy perform punctal occlusion or gentle eyelid closure.

Evaluating Clinical Trials

Pratap Challa, MD, MS and David L. Epstein, MD, MMM

When evaluating clinical trials involving glaucoma patients, it should be noted whether the population being studied consists of patients who have never been treated with the specific medication or whether *glaucoma veterans* are studied. The latter type is what one commonly observes in pharmacological studies in the literature, and there is then an important preselection factor that the reader should understand. Not only are the latter veteran glaucoma patients already using the antiglaucoma therapy that is being evaluated in the study and, therefore, more likely to respond with a therapeutic IOP response to the given agent (otherwise, why were they being treated chronically before the study with the given agent?), but they are also preselected to not have developed untoward side effects (yet) to the given medication.

Thus, the use of glaucoma veterans in these clinical trials usually underestimates the frequency of side effects and overestimates the IOP efficacy. Yet, studies using such patients are the "bread and butter" of clinical pharmacological glaucoma research. These patients frequently receive a given therapy for a long time period and then have this therapy discontinued for several weeks (termed a *washout* period). They are then randomized to 1 of 2 agents, which usually includes the previous therapy. Meaningful clinical information can be obtained by such studies, which are often the only way to obtain the large numbers of patients required. However, it should be understood that the clinical relevance to one's practice from such studies is usually framed more appropriately as the question, "If I have a patient on agent X, what is the relative benefit of switching the patient to agent Y?" There may be residual effects lasting even more than a few weeks[1,2] in washing out patients from existing therapy that can complicate the interpretation (eg, when one is dealing with adrenergic agonists and antagonists in the same study).

It follows that for the clinical question, "What antiglaucoma agent should I use in the newly diagnosed patient with glaucoma?" one would prefer a study of *ocular virgins*. But as mentioned, it is harder to find patients for such a protocol. Yet, this real life-type of study is important and can offer important clinical information. The following 2 examples may be appropriate.

When we performed a randomized prospective clinical trial of timolol therapy versus no treatment in ocular virgins with elevated IOP,[3] a surprising and unanticipated substantial incidence of side effects occurred in the timolol group that resulted in cessation of therapy and complicated the statistical analysis (once randomized, always analyzed). Yet, the occurrence of these side effects in patients never treated with timolol before was a clinically relevant important observation in itself. Also, although some have criticized this particular study because the sample size was too small (n = 107) and meaningful conclusions could only thereby be achieved in a larger multicenter study (which creates other problems of standardization and true comparison), it was often forgotten that our sample consisted only of ocular virgins, which is an important clinical group.

In truth, there are weaknesses in most clinical studies in glaucoma, if for no other reason than individual glaucoma classifications likely represent more than one disease, the subclassification of which we have been unable to discriminate. It is one of the challenges but also one of the charms of the field that glaucoma clinicians can thus constantly refine our understanding by performing more than a single study with the same apparent protocol. We seem to spend too much time criticizing studies, especially when they do not conform to our previous dogma, and spend insufficient time trying to gain potentially important clinical insights within the context of the limitations of the data, which are our constant companion.

The second example is another study[4] in which we randomized primary open-angle glaucoma virgins in a different proposed long-term protocol to either treatment with timolol or epinephrine. Although nowadays epinephrine is rarely used to treat glaucoma, this example is still conceptually valid. At the time, our rationale was that epinephrine was the only glaucoma agent that seemingly had been documented to alter the natural history of the disease.[5,6] Hence, we wanted to compare the efficacy of timolol to this standard. We were surprised (and it actually ruined the study) to find out that about one-third of such unselected glaucoma patients did not get a clinically meaningful reduction in IOP from epinephrine.[6] That is, about one-third of new glaucoma patients are nonresponders to epinephrine. "In a newly diagnosed glaucoma patient, should I utilize timolol or epinephrine as initial therapy?" is different from "In glaucoma patients who are both 'epinephrine responders' and 'timolol responded,' which is the better therapy?" If one, as has been common in the literature, chooses patients already receiving chronic epinephrine-like antiglaucoma therapy, and thus are likely epinephrine responders, washes them out, and then randomizes them to timolol or epinephrine, this potentially offers information to this second question, but not the first. The reader should keep this example in mind when reading published drug therapy trials.

References

1. Thomas JV, Epstein DL. Timolol and epinephrine in primary open angle glaucoma: transient additive effect. *Arch Ophthalmol.* 1981;99:91-95.
2. Cyrlin MN, Thomas JV, Epstein DL. Additive effect of epinephrine to timolol therapy in primary open angle glaucoma. *Arch Ophthalmol.* 1982;100:414-418.
3. Epstein DL, Krug Jr JH, Hertzmark E, et al. A long-term clinical trial of timolol therapy versus no treatment in the management of glaucoma suspects. *Ophthalmology.* 1989;96:1460-1767.
4. Alexander DW, Berson FG, Epstein DL. A clinical trial of timolol and epinephrine in the treatment of primary open angle glaucoma. *Ophthalmology.* 1988;95:247-251.
5. Becker B, Morton WR. Topical epinephrine in glaucoma suspects. *Am J Ophthalmol.* 1966;62:272-277.
6. Shin DH, Kolker AE, Kass MA, Kaback MB, Becker B. Long-term epinephrine therapy of ocular hypertension. *Arch Ophthalmol.* 1976;94:2059-2060.

Respiratory side effects with beta-blockers are attributed to beta-2 receptor actions. Thus, one might expect that beta-1 selective blockers might be free from such beta-2 blocking side effects. But the key word is selective, which is a relative rather than an absolute term. For example, Betoptic (betaxolol), a selective beta-1 blocker, was observed in one human study[18] to produce aqueous humor levels sufficient to produce substantial beta-2 blockade. Thus, betaxolol can demonstrate some beta-2 blockade properties, and such terminology, regardless, ignores other important biochemical issues, such as turnover time on the beta-receptor and other important pharmacodynamic issues. Also, because a drug systemically absorbed from ocular administration would pass first to the lung from the right side of the heart (first-pass phenomenon), the lung tissue might experience higher drug levels than those commonly measured in the peripheral venous system. From a practical clinical point of view, a beta-1 selective blocker such as betaxolol is not absolutely safe for glaucoma patients with respiratory disease. In fact, in patients with respiratory disease, a beta-blocker should not be the initial therapy. In patients with respiratory disease that is not severe, a beta-1 blocker can sometimes be used with great caution and close observation, but it is best to do this with the consultation of a pulmonologist. Regardless, the selective advantage of beta-1 blockers, such as betaxolol, is relative.

SYSTEMIC BETA-BLOCKERS AND PSEUDO-LOW-TENSION GLAUCOMA

Systemic beta-blocker therapy can lower IOPs and hence explain certain patients who appear to have low-tension glaucoma. The IOP was higher in the past when nerve damage apparently occurred before the patient was placed on systemic beta-blocker therapy for other systemic disease.

Because both betaxolol, a beta-1 selective blocker, and timolol, a nonselective (beta-1 and beta-2) blocker, both block beta-1 receptors, one would think that both drugs should produce similar degrees of bradycardia (a beta-1 action). But, again, the selectivity of the agent should not be equated with beta-blocker potency. The latter involves issues including drug turnover and bioavailability. In fact, betaxolol seems to produce less bradycardia than timolol,[19] and, sometimes, if one has exhausted other therapeutic options, with internal medicine consultation, one can try betaxolol in glaucoma patients in whom bradycardia has developed while receiving timolol. We have used this several times with success. However, this should never be attempted in patients who develop severe bradycardia or who have pre-existing bradycardia. For such patients, the risks are too great in the long-term, even if it were effective in the short-term.

INTERACTIONS OF TOPICAL BETA-BLOCKER THERAPY WITH SYSTEMIC BETA-BLOCKER THERAPY

Some have reported that topical beta-blockers added to systemic beta-blockers can produce, for the first time, symptoms of systemic beta-blocker side effects. This is very rare and unexpected in our experience, considering the usual fluctuation in blood levels of drugs given systemically compared with those given topically.

A more common question is whether topical beta-blockers are as effective in decreasing IOP in patients already taking systemic beta-blocker therapy. Systemic beta-blockers can produce IOP lowering[20,21] (this observation is what originally initiated the interest in topical beta-blocker therapy

---

TIMOLOL AND ALBINO RABBITS

Pratap Challa, MD, MS and David L. Epstein, MD, MMM

Timolol produces minimal if any IOP reduction in albino rabbits.[1] This is the usual, although questionable, model for glaucoma drug testing and has led many to predict the unsuitability of timolol and other beta-blockers for human glaucoma therapy. The differences between normal, young, healthy rabbits and aged humans with disease are extraordinary, yet the rabbit model for glaucoma drug screening persists. How many other potentially useful antiglaucoma therapies may have been similarly missed due to the lack of a suitable animal model for drug testing?

REFERENCE

1. Bartels SP, Roth HO, Jumblatt MM, et al. Pharmacological effects of topical timolol in the rabbit eye. *Invest Ophthalmol Vis Sci.* 1980; 19:1189-1197.

---

for glaucoma), but the effect is usually small and somewhat variable. In practical terms, if a topical beta-blocker would seem to be the logical first choice of drug, it should still be initiated in glaucoma patients who are receiving oral beta-blocker therapy for systemic disease. In fact, in keeping with the above systemic blood drug level considerations, there likely is a lesser chance for systemic side effects from topical beta-blockers in glaucoma patients who are already taking systemic beta-blocker therapy for other medical purposes.

Why systemic beta-blockers do not produce greater IOP lowering than they do has not been fully clarified, but this is most likely due to insufficient ocular levels of the drug, or possibly bioavailability factors. Beta-blocker receptors in the eye are responsible for decreasing AHF and reside on vascular or ciliary epithelial cell membrane sites. The observed weak IOP-lowering effect of systemic beta-blocker therapy might provide important insight into physiological mechanisms (and perhaps favor the theory of a cellular site of drug action).

OCULAR SIDE EFFECTS

Despite great initial concern about the potential for ocular side effects when the topical beta-blockers were introduced (because of the observation of an idiosyncratic reaction of a pemphigoid-like syndrome with one systemic beta-blocker,[22,23] and also the potential of beta-blockers to induce corneal anesthesia[24]), such ocular side effects have been uncommon. Topical beta-blockers are very well-tolerated topical medications for glaucoma patients. As with any drop, symptoms of stinging, burning, redness, itching, and tearing may occur and be troublesome.

Corneal hypesthesia can definitely occur[25] and can be of concern, but it is uncertain whether a small measured decrease in corneal sensitivity without any clinical symptoms or signs is clinically important. In patients with punctate keratitis, the topical beta-blocker therapy should be suspected. Switching to another topical beta-blocker (if the symptoms and signs are not severe), especially, at least theoretically, one without significant membrane-stabilizing activity (which seems at least theoretically to relate to the hypesthetic potential) should perhaps be tried first and can be surprisingly effective. Furthermore, the benzalkonium preservatives used in many eye drops can produce punctate keratitis as well. If the surface disease is refractory to switching topical drops, then one can consider prescribing preservative-free timolol. Available as Timoptic Ocudose in 0.25% and 0.50% concentrations, these are single-dose vials of timolol prescribed twice daily.

Medications can produce a great variety of side effects, and this needs to be kept in mind with topical beta-blocker therapy. But from a practical point of view, the systemic[26] rather than the ocular side effects have been the major limitation to the use of topical beta-blocker therapy for glaucoma.

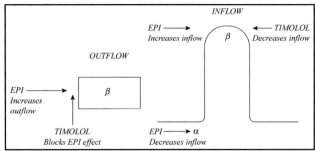

Figure 12-2. Conceptual scheme for explaining IOP effects of epinephrine, timolol, and their combination. (Left) By stimulating beta receptors in the trabecular meshwork, epinephrine improves outflow facility. Timolol blocks this effect of epinephrine, but because no innervative "tone" in the primate meshwork exists, when timolol is used alone, it does not impair outflow facility. (Right) Epinephrine effect on inflow is mixed due to a combined beta effect stimulating inflow and a nonbeta effect (alpha) decreasing inflow. Because there is "tone" to the ciliary body, timolol blocks beta-receptors, and it causes a decrease in inflow.

ESCAPE AND DRIFT IN INTRAOCULAR PRESSURE ON BETA-BLOCKER THERAPY

The first drop of a beta-blocker such as timolol applied to a glaucoma patient's eye produces a greater IOP-lowering effect than the subsequent drops over the next couple days. Some have called this phenomenon *beta-blocker escape*.[27,28] This effect quickly plateaus in a steady-state of sustained, clinically meaningful, IOP reduction for more than 90% of glaucoma patients.[29] This phenomenon was extensively studied by Boger and colleagues,[27,28] who along with Irving Katz, MD, at Merck, deserve a great deal of credit for persisting and advocating continued clinical evaluation of timolol when some thought that the escape phenomenon was equivalent to a tachyphylaxis-type mechanism. (Zimmerman[30] and others were also important advocates and deserve our praise, but Boger and Katz deserve special credit for their elucidation of chronic dosing phenomena.)

Beyond these short-term events of escape, which at a cellular level might possibly relate to changes in the actual receptors themselves, in glaucoma patients who were receiving long-term beta-blocker therapy, there was a slow but real upward *drift* in IOP.[27,28] In our studies of timolol versus no treatment in patients with elevated IOP,[31] we observed this apparent drift in the timolol group. We also observed a similar, comparable phenomenon in the no-treatment group, suggesting to us that timolol (and likely other beta-blockers) does not diminish in ability to decrease the rate of AHF in glaucoma eyes once the patient is beyond the short-term escape phenomenon. Rather, the disease process in the trabecular meshwork in such early glaucoma patients continues to worsen (in both control and timolol-treated patients), which results in the apparent drift upwards of IOP. That is, at the level of the ciliary body, timolol with chronic therapy does not progressively lose its ability to decrease aqueous humor production but rather there is a slow

decrease of trabecular meshwork function due to the underlying disease process.

MECHANISM OF ACTION OF BETA-BLOCKERS: INTERACTIONS WITH ADRENERGIC AGONISTS

Initially, the fact that both beta-blockers and beta-agonists could each lower IOP was confusing (and, in fact, unanticipated from laboratory rabbit data). Combination studies of agonists and antagonists have been fairly consistent in their results and led us to the following concept that has achieved general, although perhaps not universal, acceptance.

The fact that both beta-agonists and antagonists can lower IOP is explainable in part because each is believed to exert its beneficial action at a different site within the eye—the beta-blocker at the ciliary body and the beta-agonist in the outflow pathway (Figure 12-2). As mentioned previously, although beta-agonists are not commonly used for glaucoma management due to their high frequency of side effects, one still needs to understand their mechanism of action and side effects because there is ongoing research into developing new variants of these medications.

Beta-agonist activity is involved in the active secretion of aqueous humor.[32] It is, therefore, likely that either sympathetic nervous system action or endogenous circulating catecholamines are involved in stimulating AHF and are somehow involved in maintaining the usual rate of production. Therefore, beta-blockers block this beta-agonist-driven process involved in AHF and, thus cause a decrease in AHF[1,2] and a reduction in IOP. The beta-2 receptors on the ciliary epithelium are commonly thought to be responsible for this effect, although beta-blockade of the beta-2 receptors on the ciliary arteries may also play a role via vasoconstriction and decreased aqueous production.

Laboratory Glaucoma Models

Pratap Challa, MD, MS and David L. Epstein, MD, MMM

We commonly encounter confusing data from certain laboratory glaucoma studies as far as applicability to humans, because we still do not really have adequate animal or in vitro models for what we want to study. The fact has been mentioned that albino rabbits do not show much if any reduction of IOP in response to topical beta-blockers, and, in truth, there are very substantial differences between rabbits and humans both in terms of ocular anatomy and tissue reactivity. It is sad, therefore, that rabbits continue to be the predominant model for glaucoma drug development. More recently, rodents have been used to study glaucoma medications and outflow physiology. Rodents have a more similar outflow pathway to humans with a visible trabecular meshwork. However, no spontaneous models of primary open-angle glaucoma exist. The rodent models of glaucoma that have been employed consist of damaging the outflow pathway in unnatural ways (sclerosing episcleral vessels/Morrison model) or appear to mimic pigmentary forms of glaucoma (DBA2J mice). However, recent developments in generating transgenic rodent models may hold more promise. These transgenic models can be used to test the effects of altering specific glaucoma genes or even splicing human disease variant genes into the mouse genome. Combined with instruments that measure rodent IOPs, optical coherence tomography of the ganglion cell layers, and facility of outflow measurements, rodent models are becoming very powerful to test new glaucoma hypotheses.

Nonhuman primates offer more similarity to humans, but there are issues of cost, availability, and ethics. Certainly, before drugs are used on humans, it would be more appropriate to use these in nonhuman primates. But for earlier development, we are still lacking appropriate, readily available testing models. One consideration is to use in vitro models[1,2] or certain cell culture assays[3] for high-throughput drug screening. In fact, assays of cell shape and attachment[4] and cell monolayer permeability[5] may be the most efficient and effective means to screen for aqueous humor outflow glaucoma drugs. These models are currently being used to screen for drugs that affect the cytoskeleton of trabecular meshwork cells. By altering their shape—essentially shrinking these cells—a decrease in aqueous outflow resistance can be achieved. Rho and Rho-associated kinase (ROCK) inhibitors are drugs that fall into this category and are currently undergoing human trials (and a version of these will likely be the next glaucoma drug).

There are notable differences between nonhuman and human primates; there seems to be a substantially higher outflow through the nontrabecular unconventional outflow pathway in the nonhuman primate. Further, in anterior chamber perfusion studies, the conventional trabecular outflow pathway in the nonhuman primate is believed to behave physiologically differently than in humans, by demonstrating a progressive decline in outflow resistance (washout effect) with continued perfusion.[6] Further, there are, unfortunately, no animal models for human glaucoma, and diseased, aged human outflow pathway tissues[7] might respond differently from young, normal animal tissue with an anatomically and physiologically different outflow pathway. In one study,[8] the threshold dosage for a drug outflow effect was seemingly 10-fold lower in the human eye than the animal eye. Therefore, in vitro models will likely become even more important in the future of glaucoma drug development.

We need to keep this in mind in our research efforts in glaucoma. There likely is also much more that can be done in direct evaluation of humans with glaucoma. Tonography studies[9] allowed the dissection of beta-1 and beta-2 effects directly in human glaucoma patients and helped clarify what was a confusing clinical situation at the time. Such a study was a source of much satisfaction for the clinicians involved. One thinks also of the work of Richard Brubaker,[10] who by measuring AHF in human subjects, is adding further clarity not only to antiglaucoma drug effects, but also to normal physiological influences.[10]

For clinician scientists, patients with disease are a clinical laboratory from which it is possible to make meaningful observations from "nature's own experiments."

References

1. Erickson-Lamy K, Rohen JW, Grant WM. Outflow facility studies in the perfused human ocular anterior segment. *Exp Eye Res.* 1991;52:723-731.
2. Johnson DH, Tschumper RC. Ethacrynic acid: outflow effects and toxicity in human trabecular meshwork in perfusion organ culture. *Curr Eye Res.* 1993;12:385-396.
3. Erickson-Lamy K, Schroeder A, Epstein DL. Ethacrynic acid induces reversible shape and cytoskeletal changes in cultured cells. *Invest Ophthalmol Vis Sci.* 1992;33:2631-2640.
4. Grewal A, O'Brien ET, Epstein DL. Control of cell shape in the trabecular meshwork. *Invest Ophthalmol Vis Sci.* 1994;35(suppl):2725.
5. Underwood J, Alvarado JA, Murphy CG, et al. Steroid-induced decreases in hydraulic conductivity (HC) were blocked in human trabecular meshwork (TM) cells by an antisense oligonucleotide to ZO-I. *Invest Ophthalmol Vis Sci.* 1994;35(suppl):1847.
6. Erickson-Lamy K, Epstein DL, Schroeder AM, et al. Absence of time-dependent facility increase ("washout") in the perfused enucleated human eye. *Invest Ophthalmol Vis Sci.* 1990;31:2384-2388.
7. de Kater AW, Melamed S, Epstein DL. Patterns of aqueous humor outflow in glaucomatous and nonglaucomatous human eyes. A tracer study using cationized ferritin. *Arch Ophthalmol.* 1989;107:572-576.
8. Liang LL, Epstein DL, de Kater AW, Shahsafaei A, Erickson-Lamy KA. Ethacrynic acid increases facility of outflow in the human eye in vitro. *Arch Ophthalmol.* 1992;10:106-109.
9. Allen RC, Epstein DL. Additive effect of betaxolol and epinephrine in primary open angle glaucoma. *Arch Ophthalmol.* 1986;104:1178-1184.
10. Brubaker RF. Flow of aqueous humor in humans [The Friedenwald Lecture]. *Invest Ophthalmol Vis Sci.* 1991;32:3145-3166.

Furthermore, because beta-blockers can also bind to Ca^{+2} channel receptors and Ca^{+2} blockers have been shown to decrease IOP, this mechanism may also play a role. In particular, this pathway may play a role in betaxolol's effect.[33]

It follows that beta-agonistic drugs might act to increase further the rate of AHF, unless it normally is set at a maximum rate. Epinephrine, which is used in the treatment of glaucoma, can slightly stimulate AHF, likely through such a beta-agonist mechanism.[34] The reason that epinephrine does not have more of a resulting contrary effect as an antiglaucoma agent can be explained by the following: this beta effect to stimulate AHF is small (ie, the normal "machinery" of beta "tone" is set at a near maximal level), the alpha-agonistic effect of epinephrine acts in an opposite way to decrease AHF, and, regardless, the primary effect of epinephrine on IOP is by an enhancement of the outflow process (see Figure 12-2).[35,36]

Beta-agonists act to increase aqueous humor outflow as demonstrated tonographically in humans[35-37] and in perfusion studies in nonhuman primates.[38-42] Concomitant administration of beta-blockers with beta-agonists blocks the latter agonist effect, presumably because, as a class, adrenergic-blocking agents have greater affinity for the appropriate receptor than agonists.[43] Thus, simultaneous administration of timolol and epinephrine results in no improvement in outflow, whereas treatment with epinephrine alone causes an increase in outflow. Because the epinephrine inflow action is a mix of its alpha-effect to decrease inflow and its beta-effect to increase inflow (which is presumably blocked by the concomitant beta-blocker therapy), addition of epinephrine (or dipivefrin) to timolol therapy results in only a small, further decrease in IOP due to this added (unblocked) alpha-agonistic inflow effect. However, the predominant IOP effect of epinephrine to increase outflow is blocked by the beta-blocker (see Figure 12-2).

Although timolol, for example, can block the beta-effect of epinephrine on outflow, by itself timolol does not affect outflow.[35] Presumably, unlike considerations for aqueous humor production, there is no intrinsic beta-driven stimulation of outflow that potentially could be blocked. The process of aqueous humor outflow through the trabecular outflow system is believed to be a passive,[44] pressure-driven seepage-type process, unlike inflow, which is an active, secretory process.

It has been interesting trying to discriminate between beta-1 and beta-2 effects in these inflow and outflow actions. Curiously, more than 90% of the beta receptors in the ciliary epithelium are of the beta-2 class.[45] Thus it is surprising that beta-1 selective blockers, such as betaxolol, work well to decrease aqueous humor production.[46] Therefore, its cross-reactivity with beta-2 receptors and its calcium channel-blocking effects produce its clinical effect. Likely, we will learn more in the future about subclassification of these receptors that will provide better insight. Finally, as discussed, beta-1 selective blockers such as betaxolol are not as potent as the nonselective beta-blockers (eg, timolol) in lowering IOP.[19]

Tonographic studies in humans were actually the first to suggest that the beta sub-type class important for aqueous humor outflow was the beta-2.[37] Timolol was observed to fully block the ability of epinephrine to increase outflow, whereas betaxolol, a beta-1 blocker, did not.[37] Thus, in the latter case, unblocked beta-2 receptors in the presumably trabecular outflow pathway were free to respond to epinephrine. This observation has been subsequently confirmed in perfusion studies of nonhuman primates.[42] Also, predominantly beta-2 receptors have been identified in human trabecular meshwork cells in culture.[47-49] The clinical correlate to these findings is that, although betaxolol alone is not as potent as timolol in decreasing IOP, epinephrine-like drugs have greater additivity to betaxolol (because of this allowed outflow

effect)[37] than timolol. Thus, betaxolol plus epinephrine (dipivefrin) is at least equivalent to timolol plus epinephrine (dipivefrin) with regard to IOP-lowering efficacy.

CHOICE OF BETA-BLOCKER DRUGS

Timolol (Timoptic) was the first topical beta-blocker introduced for treating glaucoma, and thus there is perhaps the greatest experience with it. It is a nonselective (that is, both beta-1 and beta-2) blocker and thereby is fully potent for IOP reduction. Both twice-a-day and once-a-day formulations are available, and Timolol-GFS). Timolol maximally reduces the IOP because of its nonselectivity, but the latter produces the full potential for the systemic side effects mentioned. Betimol is timolol hemihydrate, Timoptic is timolol maleate, and Istalol is a potassium salt, but the 3 salts appear to have approximately equal efficacy (Table 12-1).

Betaxolol is a selective beta-1 blocker and does not produce the same magnitude of IOP-lowering as timolol.[19,50] However, it has a greater systemic safety profile. Both of these phenomena are attributed to its relative beta-1 selectivity, which is not absolute. It should be administered twice a day and behaves in some patients as if there were a sharper 12-hour cut-off for maximal effect than with the nonselective beta-blockers.[51]

Levobunolol (Betagan)[51] is a nonselective beta-blocker that is probably equivalent to timolol in both efficacy and potential for side effects. Occasionally, one observes patients who seem to respond better to timolol than levobunolol.

Metipranolol[52,53] (Optipranolol) is another nonselective beta-blocker. Carteolol[54] (Ocupress) is a nonselective beta-blocker with some intrinsic sympathomimetic activity. The implication of the latter for the ocular effects of the drug has not been defined. As mentioned, carteolol has fewer adverse systemic effects on lipoprotein profiles than other beta-blockers.[16]

Beta-Blocker Strategy

The usual question in initiating antiglaucoma therapy with topical beta-blockers is whether one wants maximal IOP efficacy with a nonselective agent because of the severity of the disease or greater systemic safety at the price of slightly less IOP potency with a selective beta-1 agent. If the patient has severe disease and there is not an obvious contraindication to beta-blocker therapy, we choose a nonselective agent. If there is severe disease but a systemic concern, we choose the selective beta-1 agent, as we do even without known systemic concern if maximal IOP reduction is not necessarily required. For many, but not all, patients, a selective beta-1 agent, such as betaxolol, may produce near maximal (if not equivalent) IOP reduction.

TABLE 12-1. ADRENERGIC AGENTS FOR THE TREATMENT OF GLAUCOMA			
	Trade Name	Dosage	Frequency
Beta-Blockers			
Nonselective			
Timolol	Timoptic, Betimol, Istalol	0.25% to 0.50%	qd-bid
Timolol gel-forming solution	Timoptic XE, Timolol GFS	0.25% to 0.50%	qd
Timolol gel-forming solution	Nyogel	0.10%	qd
Levobunolol	Betagan	0.25% to 0.50%	qd-bid
Carteolol	Ocupress	1.00%	bid
Carteolol gel-forming solution	Arteoptic	1.00% to 2.00%	qd
Metipranolol	Optipranolol	0.30%	bid
Selective			
Betaxolol	Betoptic	0.50%	bid
	Betoptic-S	0.25%	bid
Adrenergic Agonists			
Nonselective			
Epinephrine	Epifrin	0.25% to 2.00%	bid
Dipivalyl-epinephrine	Propine	0.10%	bid
Alpha-2 Selective			
Apraclonidine	Iopidine	0.50% to 1.00%	tid
Brimonidine Tartrate	Alphagan	0.20%	bid-tid
Brimonidine Tartrate with Purite	Alphagan-P	0.10% to 0.15%	bid-tid
Fixed Combination Medications			
Cosopt	Dorzolamide 2%/Timolol 0.5%		bid
Combigan	Brimonidine 0.2%/Timolol 0.5%		bid

The issue of potential submaximal efficacy also relates to 2 other issues involving beta-blockers that are often confusing to the clinician: drug concentration and dosage interval. For example, some beta-blockers are formulated in 2 concentrations: 0.25% and 0.50%. Some have argued that for most patients the 0.25% drug concentration should be the top of the dose-response curve. This is probably true but, in practical terms, it is difficult to be sure of this in any given patient. (Recall the discussion in Chapter 1 about how our IOP office measurements are just one snapshot in time, and we are in need of more extensive IOP data between visits that reflect full diurnal variation.) We suppose that one can choose to do full 24-hour diurnal IOP curves repetitively to determine equivalency between concentrations in any given patient (but remember to allow weeks of washout time between the 2 concentrations tested), but in practical terms, the decision comes down to the same basic question of the need for maximal IOP reduction or not. If maximal IOP reduction is needed, then the higher strength agent should be used. Sometimes one

has no choice, as the presence of borderline side effects on the higher strength will indicate the need to try the lower strength (with punctal occlusion or gentle eyelid closure). With only anecdotal data, maximal IOP reduction is more likely to be achieved with 0.25% of a nonselective beta-blocker than 0.5% of betaxolol, if the potential for systemic side effects allows the clinician this choice.

There are similar considerations to the question of possible once-a-day beta-blocker therapy. Levobunolol was believed by some to be more effective for once-a-day therapy than timolol.[55,56] The issue, though, has become confused. What the clinician commonly desires is a once-a-day dosage that is fully potent for the full 24 hours. It is crucial what the IOP-lowering effect is during the time interval 12 to 24 hours after the once-a-day dosage. In our experience, like others, once-a-day timolol can produce IOP lowering for a full 24 hours,[57] and likely once-a-day levobunolol can do somewhat better, but if we require maximal IOP reduction for the full 24 hours, then a twice-a-day dosage for both timolol and levobunolol is commonly required. Of note, recall that aqueous secretion is reduced during the nocturnal hours (less sympathetic activity). Therefore, the effects of several drugs, including the beta-blockers, are decreased during this part of the diurnal cycle. Therefore, the magnitude of the IOP-lowering effect is less at night but nonetheless a greater effect can be obtained with bid dosing over qd dosing. The discussion in the box, "Clinical and Statistical Significance," addresses the fact that the lack of a statistically significant difference between 2 drugs or regimens does not necessarily mean clinical equivalency. Such issues apply not only to new formulations of once-a-day drugs, but also to new agents that are sometimes marketed with these statistical arguments to imply clinical equivalency. Once-a-day dosing is both more convenient and increases patient compliance. Therefore, several once-a-day beta-blocker formulations have been developed. Most of these involve making a gel solution to increase the corneal residence time of the drug and hence increase delivery of the drug to the anterior chamber (and, as a corollary, decrease systemic delivery). Timolol is available as Timoptic-XE and various generic gel solutions (eg, carteolol [Arteoptic]; Nyogel has the lowest concentration at 0.1%). In general, most of the gel solutions are well-tolerated with patients complaining of mild stinging or short-term blurriness due to the increased viscosity of the drops that makes them stick to the cornea longer. In general, once-a-day medications are preferred due to their increased patient compliance and convenience, but one has to be cognizant that some patients can have submaximal IOP-lowering toward the end of 24 hours. Furthermore, if the patient takes the one-per-day drop every morning, then the peri-awakening IOP spike (see Chapter 3) may also be submaximally suppressed. Therefore, for patients with advanced disease, twice-daily therapy may be the better choice. It should be noted that recent research into 24-hour IOP curves has illustrated a lack of nocturnal efficacy of the beta-blocker timolol (0.5% Timoptic-XE gel) when dosed once in the morning.[58] Data for twice-a-day dosing of the topical beta-blocker drops have shown both diurnal and nocturnal IOP-lowering efficacy, thus conflicting with the data obtained from the timolol gel formulation.[59]

More recently, several fixed combinations of timolol with other drugs, such as carbonic anhydrase inhibitors and alpha-2 adrenergic agents, have become commercially available. Prostaglandin analog-fixed combinations are available in some parts of the world and will be covered separately. The large number of timolol-fixed combination medications demonstrates both the efficacy and additivity of beta-blockers to several other glaucoma medications.

EPINEPHRINE AND DIPIVEFRIN

Epinephrine and dipivefrin act predominantly to increase aqueous humor outflow[35-37,42] through the trabecular outflow pathway or possibly through the unconventional uveal scleral outflow pathway.[60] The mechanism of enhanced outflow is believed to be by a beta-2 mechanism.[37,47-49] Epinephrine-like compounds have a small but mixed effect on aqueous humor inflow with alpha-type actions believed to decrease inflow,[35,36] but beta-mechanisms to actually somewhat increase inflow.[32,34] Epinephrine and dipivefrin may actually show an improved effect on IOP with time[61] (even with combination therapy with nonselective beta-blockers).[36] Therefore, when therapy with these agents is initiated, efficacy should be assessed after several weeks of therapy.

These agents are rarely used because of their side-effect profiles and relative weaker IOP effects than other classes of medications. As many as one-third of patients do not respond to these agents with a clinically meaningful reduction in IOP.[29] The major side effects of these agents are ocular irritation, injection, and palpebral conjunctival follicle formation that necessitates discontinuation of the agent. Patients often incorrectly attribute ocular injection to other therapeutic agents, because, when these adrenergic drugs are placed in the eye, initial vasoconstriction may occur, to be followed only later (usually 1 to 2 hours) by rebound injection.

Dipivefrin[62] is a pro-drug of epinephrine, which was designed to decrease the ocular side effects by theoretically exposing the external ocular tissues to an inactive compound that becomes active only upon entering the corneal stroma. The drug contains 2 pivalyl groups that have been added to the epinephrine molecule. The pivalyl groups are cleaved when the drug passes through the cornea,[63] producing epinephrine. Once activated, the drug can then diffuse into the anterior chamber. Therefore, the decrease in side effects seen by means of this pro-drug approach is due to the lower drug concentration needed for efficacious administration.

Rarely, systemic side effects relating to heart function, such as tachycardia and blood pressure elevation, have been reported with the topical ocular use of these agents. Punctal occlusion or gentle eyelid closure[5] are indicated to decrease these side effects. However, the main reason these compounds need to be discontinued usually relates to ocular rather than systemic side effects. The latter are, in fact, rare in our experience.

These compounds presumably need to be administered twice a day, although when discontinued, residual IOP effects can last for weeks (necessitating several weeks at least for washout periods in clinical pharmacological studies[36]). They can be administered 5 minutes after other ocular drugs. It once seemed theoretically possible that hours of separation between beta-agonist and beta-blocker topical therapy might lessen the ability of the blocker to interfere with the agonist on the receptor site. However, clinical studies demonstrated that such a separation did not provide better IOP-lowering efficacy, thus indicating that, with both

STATISTICAL AND CLINICAL SIGNIFICANCE

Pratap Challa, MD, MS and David L. Epstein, MD, MMM

The lack of a statistically significant difference between 2 drugs or regimens in clinical studies does not necessarily signify clinical equivalency. That is, one can never actually prove a negative hypothesis (ie, that 2 antiglaucoma agents are not different).

A good example of this principle occurred when the selective beta-1-blocker betaxolol was first introduced. Some of the early studies found that the IOP reduction in betaxolol-treated patients was not statistically different from the IOP reduction in timolol-treated patients. This was true, but when one looked at the actual data, in many of these studies, the mean IOP reduction was greater (albeit still not statistically significantly different) in the timolol group. Statistical significance depends on the sample size and the amount of *noise* in the study due to the design (ie, different patients in the 2 groups versus cross-over in the same patient, homogeneity of the patient population, number of IOP determinations, and consistent time of IOP measurement). If there is too much noise or an insufficient sample size, mean (and clinically real) measured differences will not show statistical significance.

In our studies,[1] we did observe statistically significant differences between betaxolol and timolol in IOP reduction. Our study had patients with more severe glaucoma and IOP abnormality who were more homogeneous, and perhaps our design was less "noisy" or perhaps we were fortunate, but our deduction from the study and our continuing clinical impression has been that for patients with severe glaucoma disease in whom maximal IOP reduction is desired, timolol does produce clinically meaningful, greater IOP reduction than betaxolol.

Betaxolol, also in our study, produced substantial IOP reduction, although it was not equivalent to timolol. Therefore, in a new patient, when antiglaucoma therapy is initiated within the previously discussed guidelines, it may be appropriate to choose betaxolol. Our study would support this. It is a different question, however, whether patients currently well-controlled on timolol can be switched to betaxolol with no change in IOP control. Our study predicted what we believe has subsequently proven to be the clinical observation[2] with such a switch. For many patients, there is no clinically meaningful difference after the switch, but for some there is definite loss of IOP control when switched from timolol to betaxolol.

For any individual patient, there can be clinical equivalency, but it is difficult to document this with our snapshots of IOP, and in patients with advanced disease who need maximal IOP control continuously, our uncertainty about equivalency is an important clinical factor to consider.

The latter is also true for the questions of drug concentration equivalency or dosage interval equivalency. One can never prove a negative hypothesis. Specifically, it is not sufficient (for patients with advanced disease) that for the lower concentration or less frequent dosing interval, the IOP reduction is not statistically different from the usual alternative.

The clinician should look closely at the actual mean differences at all the data points in these published studies, as well as critically examine the protocol and adequately assess the noise.

REFERENCES

1. Allen RC, Hertzmark E, Walker AM, et al. A double-masked comparison of betaxolol vs timolol in the treatment of open angle glaucoma. *Am J Ophthalmol.* 1986;101:535-541.
2. Vogel R, Tipping R, Kulaga SF, et al. Changing therapy from timolol to betaxolol. Effect on intraocular pressure in selected patients with glaucoma. Timolol-betaxolol study group. *Arch Ophthalmol.* 1989;107:1303-1307.

---

the blocker and agonist, there is a long residual effect.[36,64] However, beta-adrenergic agonists are at present used infrequently, primarily due to their side effects and diminished potency compared to more modern agents.

In patients with aphakic[65,66] or pseudophakic eyes, epinephrine or dipivefrin can produce cystoid macular edema; therefore, we tend to avoid use of these drugs in these patients. However, not all aphakic eyes did, in fact, develop cystoid macular edema with epinephrine therapy.[67] Furthermore, this propensity is even less in pseudophakic compared with aphakic eyes. Therefore, as a last topical choice for antiglaucoma therapy, dipivefrin can still be considered for use in pseudophakic eyes where all other options have been extinguished. However, the macular status needs to be carefully monitored. If cystoid macular edema is detected early, it is believed to be fully reversible in almost all patients. However, chronic cystoid macular edema may produce permanent macular damage.

Because epinephrine-like compounds are only minimally additive to nonselective beta-blockers,[35-37] we tend to avoid adding these agents to pseudophakic eyes already being treated with these topical beta-blockers (the benefit/risk ratio does not seem appropriate).

Although epinephrine-like compounds are free from accommodative-type side effects, some pupillary dilation may be produced, producing symptoms of visual blurring. This is especially noted when these drugs are used in combination with beta-blockers (presumably because they produce now unopposed alpha-adrenergic activity, although this is speculation).

Adrenachrome breakdown products can occasionally be observed on the palpebral conjunctiva. This is more commonly seen with epinephrine use than dipivefrin.

In summary, the epinephrine-like drugs are rarely used for glaucoma management due to their relatively high incidence of side effects. They also tend to have less hypotensive effects than more modern medications and are generally not additive to nonselective beta-blockers. However, they are unique in that their primary action is to increase aqueous outflow through the conventional pathway.

ALPHA-2 AGONISTS

Adrenergic antagonists and agonists have been used to treat glaucoma for decades. The beta-adrenergic antagonists have already been discussed and now we will discuss the next

Mechanisms of Epinephrine-Induced Cystoid Macular Edema

Pratap Challa, MD, MS and David L. Epstein, MD, MMM

Very rarely, epinephrine-like compounds can produce cystoid macular edema in phakic eyes. Ordinarily, it would seem that the presence of the crystalline lens somehow retards fluid movement from the anterior segment to the posterior segment. We do know, however, that some aqueous humor from the posterior chamber does make its way into the posterior segment and retinal area. In experimental retinal detachment, it is believed that fluid from the vitreous moves into the subretinal space.[1] However, the extreme rarity of phakic cystoid macular edema due to epinephrine-like compounds likely indicates that significant drug levels do not ordinarily develop in the retina.[2] In aphakic eyes, this barrier function of the crystalline lens is obviously lost,[2] but in pseudophakic eyes, one would imagine there to still be some barrier function.

There may be pathways to the posterior segment by avenues other than via the vitreous. For example, in postsurgical or inflamed eyes, fluid potentially carrying topically applied medications may pass via the uveo-vascular-scleral outflow pathway potentially to the posterior segment uvea.

References

1. Pederson JE, Toris CB. Experimental retinal detachment. IX. Aqueous, vitreous, and subretinal protein concentrations. *Arch Ophthalmol.* 1985;103:835-836.
2. Kramer SG. Epinephrine distribution after topical administration to phakic and aphakic eyes. *Trans Am Ophthalmol Soc.* 1980;78:947-982.

class of agents: alpha-adrenergic agonists. Both classes of drugs have the primary action of decreasing aqueous inflow. Clonidine is an alpha-agonist that was originally introduced as a decongestant. However, it was quickly noted to have potent ocular and systemic hypotensive effects. These hypotensive effects are thought to be a combination of both centrally mediated and local effects. Vertebral artery injection of clonidine in cats results in a greater IOP decrease than intravenous administration despite a higher ocular concentration in the latter.[68,69] Therefore, the drug is acting both centrally in the brain and locally in the eye to reduce IOP but appears to have a greater central effect. Topical clonidine, as well as a formulation called Isoglaucon, has been shown to reduce IOPs. However, they are of limited use due to their systemic effects of hypotension and somnolence. Therefore, more specific alpha-2 agonists were developed to limit their central action. Both apraclonidine (Iopidine) and brimonidine (Alphagan) were developed, and both are available as branded and generic products. Iopidine is available as 0.5% and 1% solutions, while brimonidine tartrate is available as a 0.2% solution, all of which use a benzalkonium preservative. Alphagan-P is brimonidine tartrate preserved with Purite (chlorine dioxide) and is available as 0.15% and 0.1% solutions. Brimonidine and apraclonidine are both in the same class of medications and will be discussed together as follows. However, it should be noted that

brimonidine is used far more widely to treat glaucoma due to its better side effect profile.

Apraclonidine was the first widely used alpha-2 agonist that was originally developed to diminish iris bleeding (presumably by inducing iris vasoconstriction) during neodymium:yttrium-aluminum-garnet (Nd:YAG) laser iridectomy, but its most significant effect was IOP lowering.[70] This drug is structurally similar to clonidine but it is much more hydrophilic and has decreased ability to cross the blood-brain barrier (and hence fewer central effects). Of note, apraclonidine is reported to be alpha-2 receptor selective, but it still has some affinity for the alpha-1 receptor (analogous to discussion of betaxolol's relative selectivity in prior sections). This is demonstrated by the alpha-1-mediated side effects of conjunctival blanching and lid retraction that occur with this medication while its ocular hypotensive effects are mediated via the alpha-2 receptor. As will be discussed later, these side effects limited the long-term use of this medication, and hence its primary indication is for short-term use after procedures or in patients who are already using maximally tolerated medical therapy. Subsequently, brimonidine was developed as an agent with more alpha-2 specificity to minimize the alpha-1-mediated side effects. Although brimonidine does have more alpha-2 specificity than apraclonidine, it is also more lipophilic. Therefore, its side effect profile is slightly different (involving more central actions) and will be discussed shortly.

Apraclonidine and brimonidine both primarily act to decrease AHF[71] at the level of the ciliary epithelium. Apraclonidine also appears to have other effects on IOP, such as increased fluorophotometric outflow facility measurements (unclear because tonographic outflow does not increase) and decreased episcleral venous pressure.[72] Brimonidine has similar effects on decreasing aqueous flow as shown in comparison studies. There is some evidence that it may increase uveoscleral outflow as well, but this is not definitively proven. Both appear to reduce IOP and aqueous inflow by around 20% to 25%.[73,74] However, brimonidine has increased lipophilicity and thus leads to more central actions of the drug. Indeed, there is some evidence to postulate this because it has a larger contralateral effect on IOP than apraclonidine. However, as noted in previous sections, elucidating such mechanisms of contralateral drug effects is not easy because there is a real phenomenon of a first-pass effect for topical medications.

Moreover, because one can clinically observe a vascular response to apraclonidine in the iris and conjunctiva (minimal with brimonidine), one might also hypothesize a vascular influence at the level of the ciliary body, contributing to IOP reduction. This vascular constriction of the anterior segment vessels has caused some concern that alpha-agonists may decrease optic nerve blood flow. However, no studies have demonstrated this to date. In fact, there has been considerable interest in the potential neuroprotective effects of brimonidine. In rodent models of nerve crush and elevated

IOP, brimonidine-treated rodents appeared to have less ganglion cell damage than controls. However, the clinical significance of this is not clear, because short-term human studies of anterior ischemic optic neuropathy (AION) and acute angle-closure glaucoma failed to show a neuroprotective effect for brimonidine.[75,76]

Both apraclonidine and brimonidine can be used following laser treatment to decrease the rate of pressure spikes. The mechanism for the IOP increase after laser therapies involves an added obstruction to aqueous outflow, possibly mechanically, due to pigment and capsulotomy or lens debris or protein, and not an increase in AHF (not involved in the mechanism of any type of glaucoma). Thus, there is nothing specific as to the cause of the postlaser IOP spike that these drugs effect. They effectively decrease IOP by reducing aqueous inflow that thus compensates for the obstruction to outflow that actually causes the elevated IOP. Other studies indicate that apraclonidine can blunt the IOP spike after both Nd:YAG[77] and argon iridectomy,[78] Nd:YAG posterior capsulotomy,[79] and laser trabeculoplasty[80] as well as having potential efficacy for certain patients in chronic therapy.[81-83] One study has suggested that apraclonidine is superior to acetazolamide, timolol, dipiverine, and pilocarpine in decreasing the rate of IOP spikes following argon laser trabeculoplasty (ALT).[84] Subsequent studies have shown equivalence of apraclonidine 1% and brimonidine 0.2% in treating IOP spikes from ALT, Nd:YAG capsulotomy, and laser peripheral iridotomy. In clinical practice, either medication can be used to blunt the IOP spikes associated with these procedures.

Apraclonidine when used for either pre- or postlaser treatment is administered in either a 0.5% or 1% strength. In such short-term use, side effects except for lid retraction and conjunctival blanching are uncommon. The drug has been approved in 0.5% strength to be taken 2 to 3 times a day for the chronic treatment of the glaucomas. In some patients, there is substantial efficacy even when 0.5% solution is added to maximally tolerated medical therapy, but curiously, in some patients, there is little to no additive effect. The reason for this difference in clinical response is not readily apparent, but it would be interesting and potentially useful to understand this better. Ongoing studies in pharmacogenomics may someday answer this question. Furthermore, brimonidine can also be used in any of the 3 concentrations to decrease the rate of postlaser IOP spikes. For short-term use, side effects are rarely encountered unless the individual has a pre-existing sensitivity to the drug, or, very rarely, it can cause increased somnolence in the elderly. Additionally, it is approved and frequently used for chronic treatment of the glaucomas.

Apraclonidine has been shown to have the common side effects of lid retraction, conjunctival blanching, dry nose, and dry mouth. The last 2 can be improved significantly with punctal occlusion techniques. Long-term use of apraclonidine adds the signs of ocular allergy or sensitivity and, unfortunately, limits many patients from using this medication. Papillary and follicular reactions can develop with varying degrees of conjunctival injection. Even when the latter is not severe, patients still complain of ocular irritation and require discontinuation of the medication. Thirty percent to 48% of patients have been shown to develop allergic reactions.[81,85,86] Our clinical experience agrees with this in that we see approximately one-third of patients develop such side effects. However, for those patients who have exhausted other therapies and do not develop allergies, we have been able to maintain patients on chronic apraclonidine therapy. Moreover, there is little allergic cross-reactivity between apraclonidine and brimonidine.[87,88] Therefore, one could consider using apraclonidine even after a patient has shown brimonidine sensitivity. Mild mydriasis can also occur with treatment; however, this is not severe enough to preclude its use in acute angle-closure glaucoma.

Similarly, brimonidine can also produce the same immediate and long-term side effects as apraclonidine. However, because brimonidine has less affinity for the alpha-1 receptor, there is little lid retraction and conjunctival blanching. Furthermore, it has a slightly different side effect profile because it can cross the blood-brain barrier. Therefore, it has more central nervous system and systemic side effects.[89] Decreased resting systolic blood pressure and heart rate have been reported, as has increased fatigue and somnolence. Increased susceptibility to these central actions occurs particularly in the very young and elderly and is a relative contraindication for use in the pediatric population. There are numerous reports of hypothermia, hypotension, hypotonia (*floppy baby*), and apnea in children given brimonidine.[90] Furthermore, up to 10% of adults have reported increased fatigue or drowsiness with brimonidine 0.2%,[91] and in our experience, the rate appears to increase with increasing age. As discussed previously, these types of systemic side effects need to be actively elicited by the physician because patients do not always associate systemic symptoms with a topical drop. Regarding use during pregnancy, there are no studies of either medication, and apraclonidine is listed as a category C and brimonidine as a category B1. In general, because their effects are unknown, they should be avoided (because there are no good drug choices for use during pregnancy, if needed, one could consider nonmedication IOP treatment, such as trabeculoplasty).

Another consideration is that, because these drugs (primarily apraclonidine) do have alpha-1-mediated anterior segment vasoconstrictive effects, they should be used with caution in patients with anterior segment ischemia. However, there are no reports to corroborate this, and use of these medications should be based on a risk/benefit discussion with the patient. One contraindication that is frequently reported with alpha-2 agonists is that of concurrent use with monoamine oxidase inhibitors (MAOIs). There is a theoretical risk of severe hypotension, and like the previous concern, there are no reports in the literature of such a drug interaction occurring in a patient. The theoretical risk is as follows:

MAO inhibition increases central levels of norepinephrine (NE), which binds to alpha-2 receptors and produces vasodilation and decreased systolic blood pressure. Because brimonidine can cross the blood-brain barrier, it may have a synergistic effect with NE and potentially produce greater hypotension. However, there are no reports to corroborate this but, because this is specifically listed as a contraindication, use of alpha-agonists in patients with MAOIs should be avoided or done in consultation with an internist.

In addition, there is concern that, with long-term administration (after 2 to 12 months), the efficacy of apraclonidine and brimonidine may diminish due to some form of tolerance (tachyphylaxis). The data in the literature are somewhat conflicting in this regard,[83,92,93] and similar to considerations of beta-blocker drift, this phenomenon possibly may reflect, at least in part, the progressive worsening of the diseases in the trabecular meshwork rather than a diminished efficacy of the drug at the level of the ciliary body.

Brimonidine is available as a 0.2% generic with benzalkonium as a preservative and as a branded drug (Alphagan-P with chlorine dioxide preservative) at 0.15% and 0.1% concentrations. The change in preservative and concentration was done to decrease the side effects and increase the tolerability of the medication. Comparison studies have shown that IOP reductions are relatively equivalent between the different concentrations with decreasing ocular side effects in the lower concentrations. Moreover, the drug was initially approved for 3-times-daily dosing but is frequently used twice daily due to improved patient adherence and convenience. Analogous to the discussion of once-a-day versus twice-a-day beta-blockers, one has to consider whether there is a submaximal effect of decreased frequency and concentration of drugs. Indeed, brimonidine does appear to lose more of its effect at trough times versus timolol, and this is more apparent with the twice-daily dosing.[94] Therefore, with certain patients, if one needs a maximal effect, then 3-times-daily dosing would be preferred. Of course, the higher concentrations and more frequent dosing would need to be tempered based on the occurrence of side effects. (See prior discussion of the fact that the lack of a statistically significant difference between 2 drugs or regimens does not necessarily mean clinical equivalency.)

The alpha-2 agonist effect is additive in most patients to beta-blockers, which also act to decrease aqueous humor flow.[74,82] Therefore, brimonidine is available as a fixed-combination therapy as brimonidine 0.2%/timolol 0.5%. This is marketed as Combigan, dosed twice daily, and, as expected, it lowers IOPs better than either drug used alone.[95] As discussed previously, if a maximal effect is needed in certain patients, then an additional drop of brimonidine alone can be added between the fixed-combination drops.

Alpha-2 agonists for the treatment of glaucoma have perhaps been late to be developed because the prototype compound, clonidine, after topical administration, demonstrated dramatic systemic effects involving decreased blood pressure and other central actions. Both apraclonidine and brimonidine are effective drugs that decrease aqueous inflow. Brimonidine is used more widely due to its better tolerability.

Finally, we need to consider whether there is a maximum amount of reduction in AHF that is either possible or wise to produce. Too much reduction in aqueous flow, which carries nutrition to anterior segment structures, might potentially produce adverse consequences. It is for this reason that we have placed a major emphasis on the development of outflow rather than inflow drugs for glaucoma in the future. Nevertheless, the possibility of more effective aqueous humor suppressants in the adrenergic class should continue to be explored.

REFERENCES

1. Coakes RL, Brubaker RF. The mechanism of timolol in lowering intraocular pressure in the normal eye. *Arch Ophthalmol.* 1978;96:2045-2048.

2. Yablonski ME, Zimmerman TJ, Waltman SR, Becker B. A fluorophotometric study of the effect of topical timolol on aqueous humor dynamics. *Exp Eye Res.* 1978;27:135-142.

3. Frishman WH, Fuksbrumer MS, Tannenbaum M. Topical ophthalmic beta-adrenergic blockade for the treatment of glaucoma and ocular hypertension. *J Clin Pharmacol.* 1994;34:795-803.

4. Zimmerman TJ, Sharir M, Nardin GF, et al. Therapeutic index of pilocarpine, carbachol, and timolol with nasolacrimal occlusion. *Am J Ophthalmol.* 1992;114:1-7.

5. Zimmerman TJ, Kooner KS, Kandarakis AS, et al. Improving the therapeutic index of topically applied ocular drugs. *Arch Ophthalmol.* 1984;102:551-553.

6. Wiklund I. Quality of life and cost-effectiveness in the treatment of hypertension. *J Clin Pharm Ther.* 1994;19:81-87.

7. Kaiserman I, Kaiserman N, Elhayany A, et al. Topical beta-blockers are not associated with an increased risk of treatment for depression. *Ophthalmology.* 2006;113(7):1077-1080.

8. van Melle JP, Verbeek DE, van den Berg MP, et al. Beta-blockers and depression after myocardial infarction: a multicenter prospective study. *J Am Coll Cardiol.* 2006;48(11):2209-2214.

9. Fraunfelder FT, Meyer SM. Sexual dysfunction secondary to topical ophthalmic timolol. *JAMA.* 1985;253:3092.

10. Vinti H, Chichmanian RM, Fournier JP, et al. Systemic complications of beta-blocking eydrops. Apropos of 6 cases [in French]. *Rev Med Interne.* 1989;10(1)41-44.

11. Franssen C, Wollersheim H, de Haan A, et al. The influence of different beta-blocking drugs on the peripheral circulation in Raynaud's phenomenon and in hypertension. *J Clin Pharmacol.* 1992;32(7):652-659.

12. Csiki Z, Garai I, Shemirani AH, et al. The effect of metoprolol alone and combined metoprolol-felodipin on the digital microcirculation of patients with primary Raynaud's syndrome. *Microvasc Res.* 2011;82(1):84-87.

13. Silverstone BZ, Marcus T. Hypoglycemia due to ophthalmic timolol in a diabetic. *Harefuah.* 1990;118:693-694.

14. Wagenvoort AM, van Vugt JM, Sobotka M, et al. Topical timolol therapy in pregnancy: is it safe for the fetus? *Teratology.* 1998;58(6):258-262.

15. Coleman AL, Diehl DL, Jampel HD, Bachonik PS, Quigley HA. Topical timolol decreases plasma high-density lipoprotein cholesterol level. *Arch Ophthalmol.* 1990;108:1260.

16. Freedman SF, Freedman NJ, Shields MD, et al. Effects of ocular carteolol and timolol on plasma high-density lipoprotein cholesterol level. *Am J Ophthalmol.* 1994;16:600-611.

17. Diggory P, Cassels-Brown A, Fernandez C. Topical beta-blockade with intrinsic sympathomimetic activity offers no advantage for the respiratory and cardiovascular function of elderly people. *Age Ageing.* 1996;25(6):424-428.

18. Vuori M, Kaila T, Jisalo E, et al. Concentrations and antagonist activity of topically applied betaxolol in aqueous humour. *Acta Ophthalmol.* 1993;71:677-681.

19. Allen RC, Hertzmark E, Walker AM, et al. A double-masked comparison of betaxolol vs timolol in the treatment of open angle glaucoma. *Am J Ophthalmol.* 1986;101:535-541.

20. Wettrell K, Pandolfi M. Effect of oral administration of various beta blocking agents on the intraocular pressure in healthy volunteers. *Exp Eye Res.* 1975;21:451.

21. Pandolfi M, Ohrstrom A. Treatment of ocular hypertension with oral beta-adrenergic blocking agents. *Acta Ophthalmol.* 1974;52:464.

22. Rahi AHS, Chapman CM, Garner A, et al. Pathology of practolol induced ocular toxicity. *Br J Ophthalmol.* 1976;60(5):312-323.

23. Garner A, Rahi AHS. Practolol and ocular toxicity. Antibodies in serum and tears. *Br J Ophthalmol.* 1976;60(10):684-686.

24. Musini A, Fabbri B, Bergamaschi M, Mandelli V, Shanks RG. Comparison of the effect of propranolol, lignocaine, and other drugs on normal and raised intraocular pressure in man. *Am J Ophthalmol.* 1971;72(4):773-781.

25. Van Buskirk EM. Corneal anesthesia after timolol maleate therapy. *Am J Ophthalmol.* 1979;88:739-743.

26. Van Buskirk EM. Adverse reactions from timolol administration. *Ophthalmology.* 1980;87:447.

27. Boger WP III, Puliafito CA, Steinert RF, et al. Long-term experience with timolol ophthalmic solution in patients with open angle glaucoma. *Ophthalmology.* 1978;85:259-267.

28. Boger WP III. Editorial: Timolol: short term "escape" and long term "drift." *Ann Ophthalmol.* 1979;11:1239-1242.

29. Alexander DW, Berson FG, Epstein DL. A clinical trial of timolol and epinephrine in the treatment of primary open angle glaucoma. *Ophthalmology.* 1988;95:247-251.

30. Zimmerman TJ. Timolol maleate—a new glaucoma medication? *Invest Ophthal Vis Sci.* 1977;16:687.

31. Epstein DL, Krug JH Jr, Hertzmark E, et al. A long-term clinical trial of timolol therapy versus no treatment in the management of glaucoma suspects. *Ophthalmology.* 1989;96:1460-1767.

32. Kacere RD, Dolan JW, Brubaker RF. Intravenous epinephrine stimulates aqueous formation in the human eye. *Invest Ophthalmol Vis Sci.* 1992;33:2861-2865.

33. Hoste AM, Sys SU. Ca^{2+} channel-blocking activity of propranolol and betaxolol in isolated bovine retinal microartery. *J Cardiovasc Pharmacol.* 1998;32(3):390-396.

34. Townsend DJ, Brubaker RF. Immediate effect of epinephrine on aqueous formation in the normal human eye as measured by fluorophotometry. *Invest Ophthalmol Vis Sci.* 1980;19:256-266.

35. Thomas JV, Epstein DL. Timolol and epinephrine in primary open angle glaucoma: transient additive effect. *Arch Ophthalmol.* 1981;99:91-95.

36. Cyrlin MN, Thomas JV, Epstein DL. Addictive effect of epinephrine to timolol therapy in primary open angle glaucoma. *Arch Ophthalmol.* 1982;100:414-418.

37. Allen RC, Epstein DL. Additive effect of betaxolol and epinephrine in primary open angle glaucoma. *Arch Ophthalmol.* 1986;104:1178-1184.

38. Bill A. Early effects of epinephrine on aqueous humor dynamics in vervet monkeys (Cercopithecus ethiops). *Exp Eye Res.* 1969;8:35-43.

39. Bill A. Effects of norepinephrine, isoproterenol and sympathetic stimulation on aqueous humor dynamics in vervet monkeys. *Exp Eye Res.* 1970;10:31-46.

40. Neufeld AH. Influences of cyclic nucleotides on outflow facility in the vervet monkey. *Exp Eye Res.* 1978;27:387-397.

41. Kaufman PL. Epinephrine, norepinephrine, and isoproterenol dose-outflow facility response relationships in cynomolgus monkey eyes with and without ciliary muscle retrodisplacement. *Acta Ophthalmol (Copenh).* 1986;64:356-363.

42. Robinson JC, Kaufman PL. Effects and interactions of epinephrine, norepinephrine, timolol, and betaxolol on outflow facility in the cynomolgus monkey. *Am J Ophthalmol.* 1990;109:189-194.

43. Neufeld AH. Experimental studies on the mechanism of action of timolol. *Surv Ophthalmol.* 1979;23:363-370.

44. Van Buskirk EM, Grant WM. Influence of temperature and the question of involvement of cellular metabolism in aqueous outflow. *Am J Ophthalmol.* 1974;77:565-572.

45. Wax MB, Molinoff PB. Distribution and properties of yS-adrenergic receptors in human iris-ciliary body. *Invest Ophthalmol Vis Sci.* 1987;28:420-430.

46. Gaul GR, Will NJ, Brubaker RF. Comparison of a noncardioselective beta-adrenoceptor blocker and a cardioselective blocker in reducing aqueous flow in humans. *Arch Ophthalmol.* 1989;107:1308-1311.

47. Jampel HD, Lynch MG, Brown RH, Kuhar MJ, De Souza EB. Beta-adrenergic receptors in human trabecular meshwork. Identification and autoradiographic localization. *Invest Ophthalmol Vis Sci.* 1987;28:772-779.

48. Wax MB, Molinoff PB, Alvarado J, et al. Characterization of beta-adrenergic receptors in cultured human trabecular cells and in human trabecular meshwork. *Invest Ophthalmol Vis Sci.* 1989;30:51-57.

49. Polansky J, Friedman Z, Fauss D, Kurtz R, Alvarado J. Effects of betaxolol/timolol on epinephrine stimulated cyclic-AMP levels in human trabecular meshwork cells. *Int Ophthalmol.* 1989;13:95-97.

50. Vogel R, Tipping R, Kulaga SF, et al. Changing therapy from timolol to betaxolol. Effect on intraocular pressure in selected patients with glaucoma. Timolol-betaxolol study group. *Arch Ophthalmol.* 1989;107:1303-1307.

51. Long DA, Johns GE, Mullen RS, et al. Levobunolol and betaxolol. A double-masked controlled comparison of efficacy and safety in patients with elevated intraocular pressure. *Ophthalmology.* 1988;95:735.

52. Hickey-Dwyer M, Campbell SH, Harding S. Doubled-masked 3-period crossover investigation of metipranolol in control of raised intraocular pressure. *J Ocular Pharmacol.* 1991;7:277-283.

53. Serle JB, Lustgarten JS, Podos SM. A clinical trial of metipranolol, a noncardioselective beta-adrenergic antagonist, in ocular hypertension. *Am J Ophthalmol.* 1991;112:302-307.

54. Flammer J, Kitazawa Y, Bonomi L, et al. Influence of carteolol and timolol on IOP and visual fields in glaucoma: a multi-center, double-masked, prospective study. *Eur J Ophthalmol.* 1992;2:169-174.

55. Wandel T, Fishman D, Novack GD, Kelley E, Chen KK. Ocular hypotensive efficacy of 0.25% levobunolol instilled once daily. *Ophthalmology.* 1988;95:252-254.

56. Derick RJ, Robin AL, Tielsch J, et al. Once-daily versus twice-daily levobunolol (0.5%) therapy. A crossover study. *Ophthalmology.* 1992;99:424-429.

57. Silverstone D, Zimmerman T, Choplin N, et al. Evaluation of once-daily levobunolol 0.25% and timolol 0.25% therapy for increased intraocular pressure. *Am J Ophthalmol.* 1991;112:56-60.

58. Liu JH, Kripke DF, Weinreb RN. Comparison of the nocturnal effects of once-daily timolol and latanoprost on intraocular pressure. *Am J Ophthalmol.* 2004;138(3):389-395.

59. Quaranta L, Katsanos A, Floriani I, Riva I, Russo A, Konstas AG. Circadian intraocular pressure and blood pressure reduction with timolol 0.5% solution and timogel 0.1% in patients with primary open-angle glaucoma. *J Clin Pharmacol.* 2012;52:1552-1557.

60. Higgins RG, Brubaker RF. Acute effect of epinephrine on aqueous humor formation in the timolol treated normal eye as measured by fluorophotometry. *Invest Ophthalmol Vis Sci.* 1980;19:420-423.

61. Ballintine EJ, Garner LL. Improvement of the coefficient of outflow in glaucomatous eyes. *Arch Ophthalmol.* 1961;66:314-317.

62. Albracht DC, LeBlanc RP, Cruz AM, et al. A double-masked comparison of betaxolol and dipivefrin for the treatment of increased intraocular pressure. *Am J Ophthalmol.* 1993;116:307-313.

63. Nakamura M, Shirasawa E, Hikida M. Characterization of esterases involved in the hydrolysis of dipivefrin hydrochloride. *Ophthalmic Res.* 1993;25:46-51.

64. Tsoy EA, Meekins BB, Shields MD. Comparison of 2 treatment schedules for combined timolol and dipivefrin therapy. *Am J Ophthalmol.* 1986;102:320-324.

65. Kolker AE, Becker B. Epinephrine maculopathy. *Arch Ophthalmol.* 1968;79:552-562.

66. Obstbaum SA, Galin MA, Poole TA. Topical epinephrine and cystoid macular edema. *Ann Ophthalmol.* 1976;8:455-458.

67. Thomas JV, Gragoudas ES, Blair NP, et al. Correlation of epinephrine use and macular edema in aphakic glaucomatous eyes. *Arch Ophthalmol.* 1978;96:625-628.

68. Innemee HC, van Zwieten PA. The distribution in the eye and the effect on intraocular pressure of clonidine. *Albrecht Von Graefes Arch Klin Exp Ophthalmol.* 1979;209(3):189-198.

69. Innemee HC, van Zwieten PA. The central ocular hypotensive effect of clonidine. *Albrecht Von Graefes Arch Klin Exp Ophthalmol.* 1979;210(2):93-102.

70. Robin AL, Pollack IP. Uses of ALO 2145 in anterior segment glaucoma laser surgery. In: Shields MB, Pollack IP, Kolker AE, eds. *Perspectives in Glaucoma.* Thorofare, NJ: SLACK Incorporated; 1988.

71. Gharagozloo NZ, Relf SJ, Brubaker RF. Aqueous flow is reduced by the alpha-adrenergic agonist, apraclonidine hydrochloride (ALO 21 45). *Ophthalmology.* 1988;95:1217-1220.

72. Toris CB, Tafoya ME, Camras CB, et al. Effects of apraclonidine on aqueous humor dynamics in human eyes. *Ophthalmology.* 1995;102(3):456-461.

73. Maus TL, Nau C, Brubaker RF. Comparison of the early effects of brimonidine and apraclonidine as topical ocular hypotensive agents. *Arch Ophthalmol.* 1999;117(5):586-591.

74. Schadlu R, Maus TL, Nau CB, Brubaker RF. Comparison of the efficacy of apraclonidine and brimonidine as aqueous suppressants in humans. *Arch Ophthalmol.* 1998;116(11):1441-1444.

75. Wilhelm B, Lüdtke H, Wilhelm H; BRAION Study Group. Efficacy and tolerability of 0.2% brimonidine tartrate for the treatment of acute nonarteritic anterior ischemic optic neuropathy (NAION): a 3-month, double-masked, randomised, placebo-controlled trial. *Graefes Arch Clin Exp Ophthalmol.* 2006;244(5):551-558.

76. Aung T, Oen FT, Wong HT, et al. Randomised controlled trial comparing the effect of brimonidine and timolol on visual field loss after acute primary angle closure. *Br J Ophthalmol.* 2004;88(1):88-94.

77. Kitazawa Y, Taniguchi T, Sugiyama K. Use of apraclonidine to reduce acute intraocular pressure rise following Q-switched Nd:YAG laser iridotomy. *Ophthalmic Surg.* 1989;20:49-52.

78. Robin A, Pollack I, deFaller J. Effects of topical ALO 2145 (p-aminoclonidine hydrochloride) on the acute intraocular pressure rise after argon laser iridotomy. *Arch Ophthalmol.* 1987;105:1208-1211.

79. Pollack IP, Brown RH, Crandall AS, Robin AL, Stewart RH, White GL. Prevention of the rise in intraocular pressure following neodymium-YAG posterior capsulotomy using topical 1% apraclonidine. *Arch Ophthalmol.* 1988;106:754-757.

80. Robin A, Pollack I, House B, et al. Effects of ALO 2 1 45 on intraocular pressure following argon laser trabeculoplasty. *Arch Ophthalmol.* 1987;105:646-650.

81. Nagasubramanian S, Hitchings RA, Demailly P, et al. Comparison of apraclonidine and timolol in chronic open angle glaucoma. A 3 month study. *Ophthalmology.* 1993;100:1318-1323.

82. Morrison J, Robin A. Adjunctive glaucoma therapy: a comparison of apraclonidine to dipivefrin when added to timolol maleate. *Ophthalmology.* 1989;96:3-7.

82. Lish A, Camras C, Podos S. Effect of apraclonidine on intraocular pressure in glaucoma patients receiving maximally tolerated medications. *J Glaucoma.* 1992;1:19-22.

84. Robin AL. Argon laser trabeculoplasty medical therapy to prevent the intraocular pressure rise associated with argon laser trabeculoplasty. *Ophthalmic Surg.* 1991;22(1):31-37.

85. Wilkerson M, Lewis RA, Shields MB. Follicular conjunctivitis associated with apraclonidine [letter]. *Am J Ophthalmol.* 1991;111:105-106.

86. Butler P, Mannschreck M, Lin S, et al. The efficacy of apraclonidine as an adjunct to timolol therapy. *Arch Ophthalmol.* 1995;113:293-296.

87. Gordon RN, Liebmann JM, Greenfield DS, et al. Lack of cross-reactive allergic response to brimonidine in patients with known apraclonidine allergy. *Eye (Lond).* 1998;12(pt 4):697-700.

88. Williams GC, Orengo-Nania S, Gross RL. Incidence of brimonidine allergy in patients previously allergic to apraclonidine. *J Glaucoma.* 2000;9(3):235-238.

89. Nordlund JR, Pasquale LR, Robin AL, et al. The cardiovascular, pulmonary, and ocular hypotensive effects of 0.2% brimonidine. *Arch Ophthalmol.* 1995;113:77-83.

90. Enyedi LB, Freedman SF. Safety and efficacy of brimonidine in children with glaucoma. *J AAPOS.* 2001;5(5):281-284.

91. Derick RJ, Robin AL, Walters TR, et al. Brimonidine tartrate: a one-month dose response study. *Ophthalmology.* 1997;104(1):131-136.

92. Stewart WC, Ritch R, Shin DH, Lehmann RP, Shrader CE, van Buskirk EM. The efficacy of apraclonidine as an adjunct to timolol therapy. *Arch Ophthalmol.* 1995;113(3):287-292.

93. Cardakli F, Smythe BA, Eisele FR, Kaufman PL, Perkins TW. Effect of chronic apraclonidine treatment on intraocular pressure in advanced glaucoma. *J Glaucoma.* 1994;2:271-278.

94. Cantor LB. The evolving pharmacotherapeutic profile of brimonidine, an alpha 2-adrenergic agonist, after four years of continuous use. *Expert Opin Pharmacother.* 2000;1(4):815-834.

95. Craven ER, Walters TR, Williams R, Combigan Study Group. Brimonidine and timolol fixed-combination therapy versus monotherapy: a 3-month randomized trial in patients with glaucoma or ocular hypertension. *J Ocul Pharmacol Ther.* 2005;21(4):337-348.

13

The Miotics

Pratap Challa, MD, MS and David L. Epstein, MD, MMM

Miotics, or more appropriately termed *muscarinic (cholinergic-acting) agonists*, have been used in the treatment of the glaucomas for more than 100 years. This is the first class of medications used to treat glaucoma, and they remain an important glaucoma therapy for both open-angle and angle-closure glaucomas. It is noteworthy that our understanding and discrimination between open-angle and angle-closure glaucomas has been widely recognized for only the past 60 or 70 years (Paul Chandler was an important voice in teaching this differentiation). Cholinergic-acting agonists are miotics, but this effect on the pupil is of significance only in the acute treatment of angle-closure glaucoma due to pupillary block. For the chronic treatment of primary open-angle glaucoma (POAG), the side effects of pupillary miosis and accommodation can be bothersome for many patients and can lead to discontinuation of these medications. Some of the discussion in this chapter is of more historical than clinical relevance because the practice patterns of medical care have shifted over time. It is intrinsic, however, to understand the history of miotics as it relates to glaucoma therapy and to recognize the continuing role that this group of medications has in patient care.

Miotics are classified as weak (eg, pilocarpine or carbachol) or strong (eg, echothiophate iodide). The former refers to direct-acting acetylcholine-mimicking drugs that bind directly to the receptor site, whereas the latter refer to indirect-acting (acetylcholinesterase) enzyme inhibitor drugs that allow the endogenous normal transmitter, acetylcholine, to accumulate at the receptor site.

In acute angle-closure glaucoma, the miotic effect of pilocarpine, the most commonly used agent, may decrease pupillary block at the level of the pupil by this miotic action on the usually semidilated pupil. But probably just as important is the drug acting to constrict the iris out of the angle and to increase iris tension that in turn helps resist the increased pressure in the posterior chamber found in pupillary block.

At the level of the pupil, these cholinergic drugs may increase pupillary block if there is excessive miosis (the pupil is more closely apposed to the convex forward crystalline lens) and if the cholinergic effect on the ciliary muscle results in ciliary muscle contraction and release of zonular tension that can allow the crystalline lens to move forward to the pupil and thus actually increase pupillary block. On occasion, patients with underlying POAG thus can develop a superimposed angle-closure component from the use of miotic therapy. Hence, gonioscopy should be repeated in patients who have POAG and are taking miotic therapy.

In patients with POAG or with chronic forms of (noninflammatory) secondary open-angle glaucoma, such as exfoliation, the mechanism of intraocular pressure (IOP) lowering by miotics has nothing to do with the pupillary effect. It is due to the contraction of the longitudinal portion of the ciliary muscle that inserts on the scleral spur. The latter is adjacent to, and receives also the insertion of, the trabecular meshwork (TM). The IOP-lowering effect of miotics is due almost exclusively to the outflow effect produced by mechanical traction by the longitudinal ciliary muscle onto the scleral spur and thus the non-seeing. Anatomically, cholinergic therapy alters the spaces within the TM and makes them more open or wide and increases the number of pores in the inner wall of Schlemm's canal.[1] Experimentally, when the ciliary muscle is disinserted from the scleral spur, cholinergic drugs do not improve outflow.[2] (The latter observation also might have potential relevance to the clinical conditions of cyclodialysis or angle recession, although likely the overall circumferential extent of these conditions might be an important determinant of cholinergic drug efficacy.)

Some have described small effects of cholinergic-acting drugs on reducing aqueous humor formation or a potential direct effect on the TM. These proposed alternative actions deserve further evaluation, but the existing data strongly

Kahook MY, Schuman JS, eds.
Chandler and Grant's Glaucoma, Fifth Edition (pp 149-157).
© 2013 SLACK Incorporated.

indicate that the effects of these muscarinic drugs on outflow are mainly mechanical from longitudinal ciliary muscle contraction. The latter action likely produces few adverse effects, except perhaps for the risk of mechanical traction on attachments to the ora serrata potentially leading to detachment of the retina. Macular hole formation has also been associated with cholinergic therapy, and, therefore, all patients should have a careful retinal examination both before and after initiation of these medications. Unfortunately, it is not (yet) possible to have drugs that exert cholinergic effects on only this longitudinal portion of the ciliary muscle (although some have argued that aceclidine exerts a preferential effect on the longitudinal muscle).[3] Furthermore, the necessary accompanying contraction of the circular and other portions of the ciliary muscle from cholinergic-acting drugs leads to relaxation of zonular tension, increased axial lens diameter, and forward movement of the lens iris diaphragm. This then produces accommodation and the commonly unacceptable symptoms of visual blurring and myopia. In young patients, myopia-producing effects are frequently intolerable.

On the other hand, many presbyopic patients achieve a re-establishment of their near point, and if the accompanying miosis does not adversely affect their visual function (by cutting down light entering the eye, especially at night) and there are not excessive problems with the required frequency of drug administration or ocular irritation, many patients accept this therapy. Like miosis, the effect on accommodation is not part of the IOP-lowering mechanism (and, therefore, is not necessary for efficacy). The therapeutic efficacy is due to the contraction of the longitudinal portion of the ciliary muscle, which is mechanically connected to the TM via the scleral spur.

Another effect of this class of medications is that contraction of the ciliary muscle may obliterate some of the extracellular spaces available for uveoscleral outflow and thus cause a decrease in outflow by this unconventional outflow pathway.[4,5] In general, this effect is of little importance when treating glaucoma in most patients, except in rare individuals who are primarily dependent on the unconventional outflow pathway. Such individuals have exhibited a paradoxical rise in IOP.[6] However, pilocarpine does not appear to inhibit the increased uveoscleral outflow effects produced by prostaglandin analogs (PGAs), suggesting that the biochemical changes induced by PGAs are not affected by the mechanical effects of miotics.[7]

Considering the effect of miotics on anterior chamber depth and its mechanism of action, it does not come as a surprise that there are several forms of glaucoma that are not amenable to miotic therapy or are worsened by it (Table 13-1). Forms of angle-closure glaucoma in which axial shallowing, such as malignant glaucoma or that following an acute central retinal vein occlusion, are worsened by miotics. Additionally, neovascular and inflammatory forms of secondary angle-closure glaucoma are not amenable to miotic treatment.

TABLE 13-1. CONTRAINDICATIONS FOR MIOTICS	
Contraindication	Comment
Secondary angle-closure glaucomas	Worsens angle closure by shallowing anterior chamber (miotics produce forward movement of lens-iris diaphragm)
Malignant glaucoma	
Status postvitreoretinal surgery	
Status post-PRP or retinal cryopexy	
Status post-CRVO (acute)	
Secondary to sulfa drugs	
Associated with ciliary body swelling	
Uveitic glaucoma	Increases inflammation, may paradoxically increase IOP
Neovascular glaucoma	Increases inflammation, may produce hyphema, ineffective
Trauma (recent, with inflammation)	Increases inflammation, increases ciliary spasm and pain
CRVO: central retinal vein occlusion; PRP: panretinal photocoagulation.	

Miotics have many ocular side effects that should be considered before and after initiating therapy (Table 13-2).

VISUAL SIDE EFFECTS OF MIOTICS

In patients with early cataractous lens changes, especially those close to the visual axis, miotic therapy can be visually disabling. In such patients who are well-controlled on miotic therapy but have visual disability, the substitution by other medications or laser trabeculoplasty should be considered. The patient's objective and subjective vision should be assessed when miotic therapy has been stopped for a few days, if possible. Less desirable is to assess this after pupillary dilatation (which unfortunately itself, likely due to light scattering and spherical aberration, may make cataract symptoms worse). It is useful to ask patients about their visual function in the morning before putting their miotic drops in, for this may offer a clue as to the role of the miotics in the visual disability. In patients with early cataract formation, a substitution strategy for miotic therapy is often effective in delaying the need for cataract surgery and thus allowing longer time for the glaucoma status to be evaluated (for example, time often can help answer the question whether cataract surgery alone or, in fact, combined cataract and filtration surgery is required).

Adverse Effect	Cause	Comment
Dimmed vision	Miosis	Reduce concentration of miotic
	Pre-existing cataract	Trial of "slow release" miotic (Ocusert or pilocarpine gel)
		Strong miotics may induce cataract formation and should not be used in phakic patients
Brow ache	Ciliary muscle spasm	Symptoms usually transient if mild, reassure patient
		Always initiate miotic therapy with 0.5% to 1% pilocarpine (or carbachol equivalent)
		Strong miotics should only be started after pilocarpine treatment and at a low initial dose (0.03% to 0.06% echothiophate iodide)
Reduced visual acuity	Induced myopia	Refract patient
Floaters	Cataract	Young patients (< 40 years) prone to induced myopia
Change in visual field	Vitreous detachment	Trial low concentration miotic (0.5% pilocarpine), Ocusert, or pilocarpine gel
	Retinal detachment	Strong miotics should not be used in phakic patients (cataractogenic)
		Dilated exam of lens, vitreous (pigment/RBCs), and retina (rule out retinal detachment)
Increased IOP (paradoxical response to therapy)	Occult ocular inflammation	Slit-lamp exam for anterior segment inflammation
	Induced angle closure	Gonioscopy to establish angle open or closed and examine for KPs or PAS
Ocular irritation or epiphora	Drug allergy or toxicity	Examine lids, conjunctiva and cornea (punctal occlusion, follicles, corneal epithelial changes, and fornices for evidence of ocular cicatricial pemphigoid)
		Rule out keratitis sicca

TABLE 13-2. ADVERSE EFFECTS OF MIOTICS

KPs: keratic precipitates; PAS: peripheral anterior synechiae; RBCs: red blood cells.

OCULAR SIDE EFFECTS OF MIOTICS

In addition to the effects of miosis and accommodation (which by allowing the crystalline lens to move forward might have adverse effects beyond the visual, eg, pupillary block and susceptibility to malignant glaucoma-type syndromes), cholinergic-acting drugs appear to increase vascular permeability and perhaps thereby induce some type of pro-inflammatory predisposition in certain eyes. These drugs should not be used in inflammatory glaucoma and, in fact, may cause paradoxical effects on IOP. One of the rules discussed previously is that if a patient with presumed POAG is placed on a miotic and demonstrates an increase in IOP, gonioscopy should be repeated (as always when there is an increase in IOP) with the suspicion of an induced angle-closure component or an accentuated occult inflammatory trabeculitis. Furthermore, chronic miotic therapy can influence surgical considerations by creating small pupil problems and suspected increased

iris rigidity. These eyes are also more injected and frequently have a greater propensity for postoperative inflammation and sustained breakdown of the blood-aqueous barrier. Filtration surgery patients often have greater subconjunctival inflammation and potential scarring at the filtration site. Thus, there is this clinical sense, that perhaps has been somewhat overstated, that chronic miotic therapy is not good for the eye.

The authors share this gestalt. It also must be stated that glaucoma itself is probably not good for the eye and that nearly all medications (and their preservatives) increase ocular injection. If miotics can reasonably control the IOP in patients with various forms of open-angle glaucoma, then the risk/benefit considerations indicate that this therapy should not be avoided. We are dealing again with the humbling realization that all of our treatments for glaucoma are nonspecific and have potential downsides. Many patients appreciate the induced near point visual side effects and the pinhole effect on overall visual acuity from the miosis (except at night). Yet, there is legitimacy to the dissatisfaction that clinicians feel with the use of long-term cholinergic therapy.

Systemic Side Effects

Systemic side effects from cholinergic agents (except for the use of cholinesterase inhibitors [see the following section "Cholinesterase Inhibitors"]) are uncommon. The most frequently seen systemic side effects are gastrointestinal, which seem to be a direct cholinergic effect and likely result from drug reaching the alimentary channels directly through luminal connections from the throat. The latter derives from the topical drug reaching the nasolacrimal duct. Often, this symptom responds well to punctal occlusion (or gentle eyelid closure). Theoretically, this cholinergic symptom could result also from systemic absorption (that would obviously not be responsive to punctal occlusion strategies), and despite the efficacy of punctal occlusion diminishing this symptom, such systemic absorption might be more involved than first appreciated. Rarely, cholinergic bladder symptoms have been observed from topical miotic therapy and cerebral influences that are frequently viewed positively by the rare patient who believes that they are so affected. The latter has been observed more with the use of cholinesterase inhibitors than with short-acting miotics in our experience. Certain cholinergic therapies may positively slightly influence mental function in Alzheimer's disease.[8] Regardless, the bottom line for the clinician is that one should be alert to the possibility of systemic cholinergic symptoms in patients on topical cholinergic therapy to the eye, especially the cholinesterase inhibitors, although these are decidedly uncommon.

CHOLINESTERASE INHIBITORS

The short-acting miotics are cholinergic-acting drugs that mimic and theoretically might compete at the receptor with endogenously released acetylcholine, which is the usual transmitter at cholinergic sites in the eye. Such potential competition of cholinergic drugs with acetylcholine for the receptor, while theoretically possible, does not occur from a practical clinical point of view. Cholinesterase inhibitors and cholinergic drugs are not negatively interactive on IOP[9]; in fact, in some small minority of patients, there is slight additivity.

Significant systemic absorption of a topical ocular drug can occur. Therefore, it is not surprising that this happens also with cholinesterase inhibitors. The clinician should be alert to the potential for gastrointestinal, urological, or cerebral cholinergic side effects, although these are uncommon. However, what is common with the use of topical acetylcholinesterase inhibitors is the inhibition of cholinesterase activity in the blood.[10] For some forms of general anesthesia, certain agents such as succinylcholine are used and require the blood enzyme for inactivation. Therefore, anesthesiology consultation should be obtained preoperatively, and the

anesthesiologist should be informed ahead of time to flag the chart as to the use of topical cholinesterase inhibitors. It may require several months of cessation of such ocular therapy for blood levels of cholinesterase to return to normal. Fortunately, many alternatives exist in the choice of general anesthesia, but the anesthesiologist needs to know ahead of time about the use of this type of medication in patients who have glaucoma.

Potential Retinal Complications

Presumably because the ciliary muscle sends extensions of its tendon to the ora serrata, there is the potential for retinal complications with use of these cholinergic agents as a result of mechanical tension from the muscle's contraction.

As part of the routine of a full ophthalmologic evaluation of the glaucoma patient, indirect ophthalmoscopy should be performed, with special attention to the retinal periphery looking for pre-existing retinal pathology that might be adversely affected by the mechanical actions of miotics. As part of the routine follow-up of patients with glaucoma, the pupil is periodically dilated not only to examine the optic nerve head but also to re-examine the retina.

Patients receiving miotics are told of potential symptoms including flashes, floaters, and curtains. Although rare, retinal tears can occur with weak miotic therapy (eg,

---

ACETYLCHOLINESTERASE
David L. Epstein, MD, MMM

Acetylcholine, which is commonly released at cholinergic nerve terminals in the eye, is normally inactivated by the enzyme acetylcholinesterase. Inhibitors of the latter enzyme allow acetylcholine to accumulate at the receptor site and thus produce a cholinergic miotic effect of long duration. Such acetylcholinesterase enzyme inhibitors have been used as systemic nerve gases or insecticides (where presumably they are lethal as a result of sustained cholinergic stimulation).[1] It is remarkable that such agents in dilute concentrations have found use topically as antiglaucoma agents. With respect for the ocular cholinergic side effects, such cholinesterase inhibitor therapy can be very effective, particularly in pseudophakic or aphakic eyes. This observation, on the one hand, makes one wonder whether all of our current glaucoma therapy is not, in fact, applied toxicology, but on the other hand teaches us the importance of dose-response relationships and therapeutic indexes in the development of all new glaucoma medications (or for any disease). Any drug at a high enough dosage can have substantial side effects. When we screen for new drugs, we commonly use high concentrations, looking for large effects because they are easier to detect initially.

One wonders how many potentially useful drugs may have been missed because of such screening techniques. The first attempts to study topical cholinesterase inhibitor therapy to the eyes of rabbits produced a lethal result!

REFERENCE
1. Rengstorff RH. Vision and ocular changes following accidental exposure to organophosphates. *J Appl Toxicol.* 1994;14:115-118.

pilocarpine).[11] In fact, posterior vitreous detachment may occur more commonly after even weak miotic therapy than is often appreciated. It would make sense, and clinically seems to be the case, that the risk goes up with increasing concentration of miotic and, therefore, with use of the stronger miotics (ie, cholinesterase inhibitors).

The potential for such rare side effects is perhaps another reason why the miotics are no longer the drug of first choice for POAG. But, as discussed, even with these general cholinergic effects on the eye, these agents are still effective medications. As with all glaucoma medications, they have risk/benefit considerations that need to be appreciated by the clinician and discussed with the patient ahead of time.

Whether patients with previous retinal detachment and successful repair should be treated with strong miotics is an interesting question that requires retinal specialist consultation. Retina specialists have given their approval provided they are satisfied with the result of the retinal surgery. Thus, although these strong miotics should still be a drug of last resort, we have used them effectively in such patients. Such patients need continuing evaluation by a retina colleague.

For patients with a predisposition to retinal detachment, whether due to significant myopia or identified retinal thinning, avoid these stronger miotics unless absolutely necessary. Again, retinal consultation is strongly advised, and only the weakest effective solution should be used.

STRATEGIES IN CHOICE/USE OF MIOTICS

Weak Miotics

Pilocarpine is the usual first choice of cholinergic eye drop therapy. Several preparations differ only in the choice of salt, buffer, preservatives, or other constituents added for comfort. Strengths of pilocarpine range from 0.5% to 6%. Some glaucoma clinicians have argued that the maximally effective concentration may occur at concentrations less than 4%, whereas others have argued that 6% is probably the top of the dose-response curve. There is individual variability but we believe that for most patients, except those with heavily pigmented irides, 4% is likely the clinically meaningful top of the dose-response curve and that lesser concentrations are not. Also, although 6% concentration may be slightly more effective in certain heavily pigmented non-White eyes, for practical purposes, 4% pilocarpine is still the highest concentration used, except perhaps for individuals with severe glaucoma.

Even in patients in whom it is anticipated that higher strengths of pilocarpine will be required, one should still start with low strengths of 0.5% or 1% to allow the patient to adapt to the anticipated initial ciliary spasm. Headaches and brow-aches due to miotics are common, and the clinician should spend time explaining this to the patient (eg,

the drug makes the muscle next to the drain contract and open the spaces, and like any muscle that has not been used fully, some initial cramping ["Charlie horse"] is to be anticipated). These symptoms should abate after the first few days. The patient should be told to call if they do not or if there are any other symptoms, such as flashes and floaters.

It is also very useful for the clinician to assess the IOP-lowering efficacy of 1% pilocarpine. Sometimes, there is a surprisingly large IOP effect. In fact, many years ago, a pilocarpine drop test for glaucoma was described in which a large decrease in IOP was anticipated in patients with true glaucoma. It is not certain in the era of this pilocarpine drop test whether all forms of chronic angle closure were well-differentiated from open-angle glaucoma, and there is likely great individual variability, regardless, in IOP reduction in POAG patients from miotics. The clinical point is that some patients with POAG are very responsive to lower strengths of pilocarpine. It is not possible to predict what strength of pilocarpine will be required in the individual patient. In some cases of POAG, perhaps just a slight mechanical widening of whatever the critical space is in the outflow pathway is enough,[1] at least initially, to substantially improve the outflow of aqueous humor from the eye. One of the major problems with pilocarpine and short-acting cholinergic-acting agonists is the short duration of drug effect. This necessitates a need for frequent instillation, usually 4 times a day for pilocarpine that represents medication every 6 hours. Patients do not have to wake up at night after 6 hours of sleep to instill the drop, but it is surprising how many patients, in fact, do this due to inadequate initial instruction! However, while the patient is awake, the drops should be spaced as far apart as possible, approximately every 6 hours. There is the possibility of an IOP spike after 6 hours of sleep. Patients should administer the morning drop soon after awakening.

Clinically, some patients behave as if the maximum IOP effect from pilocarpine lasts only 4 hours, and we have seen some clinicians with good documentation therefore prescribe pilocarpine drops 6 times a day! We as clinicians need to appreciate how disruptive frequent drop regimens are to a patient's lifestyle. In fact, most patients do not adhere to a 4-times-daily dosage regimen.[12,13] For such patients with an apparent shorter time of clinical efficacy from cholinergic therapy, one should consider a higher strength of the drug—up to 6%, or perhaps, more reasonably, the use of pilocarpine ointment at night supplemented with pilocarpine drops during the day.

The need for such frequent dosing with miotics is because, pharmacodynamically, active drug is cleared from the effector site after this time interval. The other side of this issue is that very high concentrations of the drug, therefore, are applied to the eye initially because of this rapid decay. Unfortunately, this likely leads to some of the general side effects.

Drug Therapy Compliance

David L. Epstein, MD, MMM

Compliance is a real issue for the frequent dosing regimen required with weak miotic therapy. Kass and others have documented the surprising magnitude of this problem in glaucoma therapy with the use of a special electronic monitoring eye bottle.[1-4] But the clinician, by simple means, can also sometimes gain insight into this issue in patients who are using miotics. Examination and recording of pupil size is an important part of the eye examination. For example, although the degree of miosis induced by these agents may be variable among different individuals, it should be consistent within the same patient. One often finds that the pupil is somewhat larger at a subsequent visit, and it takes specific physician probing to uncover the fact that the patient (who usually wants to actually please the glaucoma clinician) failed to take the medication, at least on the day of the visit. One patient told us that she did not want to hurt her physician's feelings by telling him that she could not take her medication routinely! It goes without saying that, given the short duration of IOP effect from such therapy, failure to take the medication on the day of examination will cause an unexpectedly higher IOP. Some patients, unless counseled otherwise, routinely will omit their drops on the day of examination for a variety of reasons that reflect miscommunication (eg, "the doctor puts in his own drops at the visit" or "it interferes with the examination").

Patients on miotic therapy (truly, all glaucoma patients) need specific instructions about these issues and about inquiry into actual medication usage. Poor compliance is a common cause of fluctuating IOP. We are aware of cases in which the clinician prescribed a miotic, but the patient, due to confusion, did not take it, and this was not picked up by the office personnel until a referral consultation was arranged, at which time it was observed that the pupil was not miotic! Thus, the recording of the pupil size is an important part of the glaucoma examination.

References

1. Kass MA, Meltzer DW, Gordon M, Cooper D, Goldberg J. Compliance with topical pilocarpine treatment. *Am J Ophthalmol.* 1986;101:515-523.
2. Kass MA, Gordon M, Meltzer DW. Can ophthalmologists correctly identify patients defaulting from pilocarpine therapy? *Am J Ophthalmol.* 1986;101:524-530.
3. Kass MA, Gordon M, Morley RE Jr, Meltzer DW, Goldberg JJ. Compliance with topical timolol treatment. *Am J Ophthalmol.* 1987;103:188-193.
4. Budenz DL. A clinician's guide to the assessment and management of nonadherence in glaucoma. *Ophthalmology.* 2009;116(suppl 11):S43-S47.

This rapid decay phenomenon of pilocarpine may be amenable to therapeutic innovation, and there have been several attempts. Carbachol needs to be given only every 8 hours.[14] Three percent carbachol is equivalent to 4% pilocarpine. Carbachol may not penetrate the cornea as well as pilocarpine in certain patients, and, therefore, the IOP-lowering efficacy as well as dosing frequency needs also to be established for the individual patient.[15] However, for some patients, carbachol 3 times a day can be an effective and acceptable regimen. Carbachol can also be used for those

TABLE 13-3. ANTICIPATED INTRAOCULAR PRESSURE RESPONSE IN ADDING MIOTICS TO OTHER COMMONLY USED GLAUCOMA MEDICATIONS

Miotic added to	Beneficial
Topical and oral CAIs	Yes
Beta-blocker	Yes
Alpha-adrenergic agonists	Yes
Prostaglandin F2α analogs	Yes
CAI: carbonic anhydrase inhibitors.	

who are allergic to pilocarpine. Miotics are generally additive to most classes of glaucoma medications (Table 13-3).

Pilocarpine Ocusert Therapy

The Ocusert (Alza Pharmaceuticals, Palo Alto, CA),[16] no longer commercially available, is a continuous delivery device in which a low level of pilocarpine is constantly released into the tear film over the period of 1 week. Because of the low (but steady) concentration of pilocarpine in the eye at any one time, effects on miosis and accommodation were minimized (and stable), but IOP-lowering effects are maintained. In most patients, the pilo-40 Ocusert was equivalent to 2% to 4% pilocarpine, although, in some patients, the IOP-lowering efficacy was less. For young patients with glaucoma (eg, those with pigmentary glaucoma), this treatment seemed almost a miracle if the patient previously had experienced the induced visual problems with pilocarpine drops. But because most patients with glaucoma are elderly and have problems with insertion and retention of this one-size-fits-all device, they were deemed not very successful with this regimen, unless they were highly motivated and possessed good hand-eye coordination. Some patients were very adept at using this device but as newer, less frequently administered medications became available (prostaglandin analogs), the use of this device became relatively rare.

Pilocarpine Gel

Another potential solution to this problem of required frequent dosing with the shorter-acting miotics has been the development of 4% pilocarpine gel (Pilopine), which was designed to be administered once a day at bedtime and provide 24-hour IOP lowering.[17] In truth, this does represent an important delivery system, which has both efficacy and reasonable patient acceptance. Some patients do not like putting a gel (ointment) in their eye even at bedtime because of visual blurring later at night, which can persist into the morning. Clinically, there is considerable individual variability among patients in the liquefaction of the gel by the normal tear production. Some patients complain that no matter how little gel[18] they put in at night, there is constant blurring the next day. On the other hand, many patients tolerate the regimen without any complaint. However, the complaint of ocular blurring is probably a major contributor to the limited development of an ointment delivery system for glaucoma medications.

When pilocarpine gel was first introduced, a fine corneal haze was observed in several patients that was initially a cause for concern.[19] There was no effect on vision, and there have been no reported long-term sequelae.[20]

Strong Miotics

The stronger-acting miotics, which for practical clinical purposes are restricted now to the acetylcholinesterase inhibitors echothiophate iodide (Phospholine Iodide) and demecarium bromide (Humorsol), require less frequent instillation, usually only once a day but occasionally twice a day. However, the potential for side effects is much greater with these agents than with the weaker miotics. In phakic eyes, these cholinesterase inhibitors are definitely cataractogenic, and, therefore, these agents are avoided in phakic eyes.[21,22] However, for pseudophakic or aphakic eyes, acetylcholinesterase inhibitors can be dramatically effective and actually patient friendly in terms of the frequency of instillation and ocular tolerance. These agents provide greater IOP reduction than the shorter-acting miotics such as pilocarpine.[23] In pseudophakic or aphakic eyes, these agents should be used (at least in a weak strength) after other topical medications are used, before consideration of filtration surgery. (It is equivocal whether laser trabeculoplasty with a more guarded prognosis for efficacy in such eyes should be tried before or after a trial of such strong miotic therapy, although most clinicians would probably proceed with laser trabeculoplasty first.)

Because these strong miotics produce greater and more sustained ciliary muscle contraction, and thereby presumably greater mechanical traction on the retina, there seems to be a greater risk of retinal detachment than with the use of the weaker miotics. The need for a detailed retinal examination on all glaucoma patients has already been mentioned. In addition, this issue of potential retinal complications needs to be specifically discussed with the patient, who is advised about warning signs and symptoms. Nevertheless, the risk/benefit considerations are such that, although the risk of retinal detachment is real (although small), it certainly is appropriate to try these agents before filtration surgery, with full informed consent.

In phakic eyes, anticholinesterase agents are not used, even before filtration surgery, except with a poor surgical prognosis. Because the cataractogenic effect is dose related, the weakest strength possible of the medication should be used first in such eyes for IOP control.

LIMITED DURATION OF ACTIVITY OF PHOSPHOLINE IODIDE

David L. Epstein, MD, MMM

The limited duration of activity of Phospholine Iodide once prepared has important implications for glaucoma patient management. For example, in patients who, over a prolonged period, seem well controlled on Phospholine Iodide therapy, but then suddenly appear with otherwise unexplained elevation of IOP, among other issues, inactive drug should also be suspected, and prior to other maneuvers, the patient should be treated with a fresh new bottle of Phospholine Iodide, after other ocular causes for the IOP elevation have been ruled out. This strategy has quite commonly (but not always) re-established the previous steady state. This phenomenon especially seems to occur during periods of the summer when patients carry their medication with them. Phospholine Iodide should normally be refrigerated, and with the potential for once-a-day dosage, this should not greatly inconvenience the patient. It is useful always to ask the patient how much of the bottle has been used and how long ago was the prescription filled. This is particularly important because there is currently only one manufacturer of the drug and some patients attempt to stockpile a supply of this medication.

Humorsol is slightly less potent than Phospholine Iodide. It probably needs to be given twice a day, but a potential advantage is that the solutions are more stable than Phospholine Iodide, which must be refrigerated, and can be carried at all times by the patient. Humorsol is prepared in 0.125% and 0.25% strengths.

Phospholine Iodide must be prepared fresh from powder, has a limited length of activity, and should be refrigerated. It is probably the most potent miotic and probably needs to be administered only once a day, at higher dosages (0.125% and 0.25%). However, this needs to be established for the individual patient by assessing IOP in the trough period at a time greater than 12 hours after dosage. Because it is an iodide, there is the potential for greater ocular sensitivity and the possible rare occurrence of a pemphigoid-like ocular syndrome,[24,25] which exists for all miotics but seems slightly greater for Phospholine Iodide. This has been hypothesized by W. M. Grant possibly to be due to this iodide content.

Phospholine Iodide is prepared in solution strengths from 0.03% to 0.25%. The 0.06% strength should be evaluated initially, although we have the distinct clinical impression that 0.25% represents maximum potency.

It is important to state again that, even if it is extremely likely that a drug such as Phospholine Iodide will be required for miotic therapy, patients should still start with weaker and then subsequent greater strengths of pilocarpine or equivalent to allow adaptation to the ciliary muscle contraction. Placing a drug such as Phospholine Iodide on the eye that has not been previously treated with miotics usually causes acute ciliary spasm and severe pain that is almost always intolerable to the patient.

As mentioned, because cholinesterase inhibitors such as Phospholine Iodide act pharmacologically to allow endogenously produced acetylcholine to accumulate and act at the receptor, one might have anticipated that a muscarinic drug such as pilocarpine would compete for the same receptor and interfere with the Phospholine Iodide IOP-lowering action. This does not in fact happen,[10] and occasionally there seems to be a slight additivity that might be meaningful in a patient with severe disease. Therefore, a strategy that one of us (DLE) sometimes uses in advanced glaucoma cases is simply to add Phospholine Iodide at bedtime (once a day) to the continued pilocarpine regimen. On the one hand, this might result in some additivity, but on the other, should the Phospholine Iodide decay toward the end of the bottle, the patient still maintains a cholinergic drug effect from the pilocarpine.

Strong miotics may produce cysts at the pupillary margin, which may be innocuous or produce visual symptoms. These are less common with weaker strengths of drug and perhaps with Humorsol. They can be successfully treated with weak solutions of phenylephrine if the patient needs to be maintained on the strong miotic.

Ocular Irritation/Sensitivity From Miotics: Pemphigoid-Like Syndrome

All of the miotics may, in certain individuals, produce ocular allergy or sensitivity that is usually characterized by injection, but also papillary and follicular conjunctival reactions that may mimic and be misinterpreted as an allergy to an epinephrine-like compound, such as dipivefrin hydrochloride (Propine). Corneal abnormalities including rare keratinization-type reactions have been observed. In previous times, an atypical band keratopathy[2-4] was observed in glaucoma patients on one particular brand of pilocarpine that was due to a phenylmercuric nitrate preservative. Nevertheless, true allergies to pilocarpine itself do exist, and if the miotic is efficacious for IOP (see above), carbachol should be tried and usually demonstrates little cross-sensitivity (although the patient may be still intolerant of the usual miotic visual effects that are not a drug sensitivity).

The iodide in Phospholine Iodide may be sensitizing in some patients. We and others have observed the occurrence of an ocular pemphigoid-like syndrome in patients on Phospholine Iodide therapy, which seems likely drug-related (eg, unilateral cases with unilateral drug treatment).[24] The exact incidence of this is unknown because many patients with primary ocular pemphigoid may develop POAG.[25] Likely, this drug-induced pemphigoid syndrome is rare, but this is another reason why such strong agents are drugs of last resort. On the other hand, this pemphigoid syndrome has also been reported after pilocarpine therapy (although our impression is much less commonly than with Phospholine Iodide), suggesting that it may represent a rare cholinergic effect. Laboratory experiments suggest that cholinergic drugs can stimulate conjunctival and corneal epithelial cell proliferation.[26]

An important clinical point is that, as part of one's routine ophthalmological examination, retraction of the lower lid with examination for early symblepharon formation should be performed in all glaucoma patients (not just those on miotics—other occurrences may thus for the first time be noted by the clinician).

In discussing glaucoma drug sensitivity, Chandler and Grant wrote:

> Drug sensitivity not infrequently develops in patients under various forms of treatment for glaucoma. The most common manifestation of drug sensitivity is dermatitis of the lids, with drying and wrinkling of the skin of the lids, particularly the lower lid. In other cases, there is no involvement of the skin of the lids but there is a beefy, fiery redness of the conjunctiva, especially in the lower fornix, usually with enlargement of conjunctival follicles. These sensitivity reactions disappear shortly after the offending drug is discontinued.

> A rare reaction that we have seen in only 2 patients developed after long-term use of pilocarpine. It consisted of a haziness of the corneal epithelium with superficial vascularization extending onto the cornea from all sides and causing marked reduction of vision. In these 2 cases, there were no other specific signs of drug sensitivity, except that the eyes were generally red. Improvement could be noted within 48 hours when pilocarpine was stopped. The following is a description of one of these 2 cases.

> *Case:* A 77-year-old patient had been receiving treatment with pilocarpine for 8 years. IOP was right and left 17, the field in the right eye was almost full with a 10-mm test object, but there was considerable loss of field in the left eye. Fundi could not be seen. Vision was right 15/200, left 120/200. The eyes were red with enlarged follicles in the lower fornices. The conjunctiva had a sort of opaque milky appearance. The entire cornea was hazy in both eyes due to an epithelial disturbance. With a flashlight, the surface of each cornea presented a fine ground-glass appearance. Superficial vessels came in from all sides almost to the border of a 2-mm pupil. Drops were discontinued, and, within 48 hours, there was considerable subjective improvement. One week later, vision was right and left 6/18. A fine haze persisted in the central area of the corneas, but the blood vessels became bloodless "ghost" vessels. When the corneas cleared sufficiently, it could be seen that both discs had pathologic cupping, but most of the persisting reduction of vision was due to nuclear lens opacity rather than glaucoma. Even without further treatment, the IOP ranged only from 15 to 19 mm Hg, and the patient maintained useful vision for several remaining years of his life.

> In this case, whether the corneal and conjunctival reaction was due to the pilocarpine itself or to the chlorobutanol preservative was not determined.

REFERENCES

1. Grierson I, Lee WR, Abraham S. The effects of topical pilocarpine on the morphology of the outflow apparatus of the baboon (Papio cynocephalus). *Invest Ophthal Vis Sci.* 1979;18:346-355.

2. Kaufman PL, Barany EH. Loss of acute pilocarpine effect on outflow facility following surgical disinsertion and retrodisplacement of the ciliary muscle from the scleral spur in the cynomolgus monkey. *Invest Ophthalmol Vis Sci.* 1976;15:793-807.

3. Erickson-Lamy K, Schroeder A. Dissociation between the effect of aceclidine on outflow facility and accommodation. *Exp Eye Res.* 1990;50:143-147.

4. Bill A. The effects of pilocarpine on the dynamics of aqueous humor in a primate (Macaca irus). *Invest Ophthalmol Vis Sci.* 1966;5:170-175.

5. Bill A. Effect of atropine and pilocarpine on aqueous humour dynamics in cynomolgus monkeys (Macaca irus). *Exp Eye Res.* 1967;6:120-125.

6. Bleiman BS, Schwartz AL. Paradoxical intraocular pressure response to pilocarpine. A proposed mechanism and treatment. *Arch Ophthalmol.* 1979;97:1305-1306.

7. Toris CB, Zhan GL, Zhao J, Camras CB, Yablonski ME. Potential mechanism for the additivity of pilocarpine and latanoprost. *Am J Ophthalmol.* 2001;131:722-728.

8. Gray JA, Enz A, Spiegel R. Muscarinic agonists for senile dementia: past experience and future trends. *Trends Pharmacol Sci.* 1989;Dec(suppl):85-88.

9. Kini MM, Dahl AA, Roberts CR, Lehwalder LW, Grant WM. Echothiophate, pilocarpine, and open angle glaucoma. *Arch Ophthalmol.* 1973;89:190-192.

10. Ellis PP, Esterdahl M. Echothiophate iodide therapy in children. Effect upon blood cholinesterase levels. *Arch Ophthalmol.* 1967;77:598.

11. Puustjarvi T. Retinal detachment during glaucoma therapy. Review. A case report of an occurrence of retinal detachment after using membranous pilocarpine delivery system [Pilokarpin lameller (Ocusert) 11 mg]. *Ophthalmologica.* 1985;190:40-44.

12. Kass MA, Meltzer DW, Gordon M, Cooper D, Goldberg J. Compliance with topical pilocarpine treatment. *Am J Ophthalmol.* 1986;101:515-523.

13. Kass MA, Gordon M, Meltzer DW. Can ophthalmologists correctly identify patients defaulting from pilocarpine therapy? *Am J Ophthalmol.* 1986;101:524-530.

14. O'Brien CS, Swan KC. Carbarninoylcholine chloride in the treatment of glaucoma simplex. *Arch Ophthalmol.* 1942;27:253.

15. Smolen VF, Clevenger JM, Williams EJ, et al. Biophasic availability of ophthalmic carbachol I: mechanisms of cationic polymer- and surfactant-promoted miotic activity. *J Pharm Sci.* 1973;62:958-961.

16. Quigley HA, Pollack IP, Harbin RS Jr. Pilocarpine ocuserts. Long-term clinical trials and selected pharmacodynamics. *Arch Ophthalmol.* 1975;93:771-775.

17. Johnson DH, Epstein DL, Allen RC, et al. A one year multicenter clinical trial of pilocarpine gel. *Am J Ophthalmol.* 1984;97:723-729.

18. Fechtner RD, Piltz JR, Starita RJ. A technique for accurate application of pilocarpine gel. *Ophthalmic Surg.* 1988;19:823.

19. Johnson DH, Kenyon KR, Epstein DL, et al. Corneal changes during pilocarpine gel therapy. *Am J Ophthalmol.* 1986;10:13-15.

20. Nagasubramanian S, Stewart RH, Hitchings RA. Long term effects of glaucoma therapy with 4% pilocarpine gel on corneal clarity and endothelial cell density. *Int Ophthalmol.* 1994;18:5-8.

21. Axelsson U, Holmberg A. The frequency of cataract after miotic therapy. *Acta Ophthalmol.* 1966;44:421-429.

22. Thoft RA. Incidence of lens changes in patients treated with echothiophate iodide. *Arch Ophthalmol.* 1968;80:317-320.

23. Reichert RW, Shields MB. Intraocular pressure response to the replacement of pilocarpine or carbachol with echothiophate. *Graefes Arch Clin Exp Ophthalmol.* 1991;229:252-253.

24. Patten JT, Cavanagh HD, Allansmith MR. Induced ocular pseudopemphigoid. *Am J Ophthalmol.* 1976;82:272-276.

25. Tauber J, Melamed S, Foster CS. Glaucoma in patients with ocular cicatricial pemphigoid. *Ophthalmology.* 1989;96:33-37.

26. Cavanagh HD, Colley AM. Cholinergic, adrenergic, and PGE1 effects on cyclic nucleotides and growth in cultured corneal epithelium. *Metab Pediatr Syst Ophthalmol.* 1982;6:63-74.

14

Carbonic Anhydrase Inhibitors
Systemic Use

Pratap Challa, MD, MS and David L. Epstein, MD, MMM

Carbonic anhydrase inhibitors (CAIs) can be useful in the treatment of all the glaucomas by virtue of their ability to reduce aqueous secretion and thus lower intraocular pressure (IOP)[1] regardless of the nature or extent of obstruction to outflow. Their mechanism of action appears to be the inhibition of CA isoenzymes that result in decreased bicarbonate ion secretion into the posterior chamber by the nonpigmented ciliary epithelium.[2] These enzymes are among the fastest known enzymes, and they catalyze the conversion of carbon dioxide and water into bicarbonate and hydrogen ions. Bicarbonate ions are actively secreted into the aqueous humor, resulting in a passive diffusion of water. Therefore, inhibition of bicarbonate formation decreases aqueous formation.

The first agents in this class that were effective in treating glaucoma were given systemically, but now topical agents are available and are frequently used to treat a wide variety of the glaucomas. Topical therapy will be discussed further in the next chapter; however, a brief mention of it in comparison to systemic medications is warranted. Although the site of action for glaucoma therapy is the nonpigmented ciliary epithelium (isoenzymes type II and IV), other ocular structures also express CA, and their inhibition can lead to unintended side effects. Isoenzyme types I and II are important for the corneal endothelial pump function,[3] and the topical application of such drugs will continuously and progressively bathe the corneal endothelium with this enzyme inhibitor as the drug passes into the anterior chamber. Moreover, due to the high efficiency of this enzyme class, nearly total (99.9%) inhibition is needed to achieve pressure lowering. Hence, topical therapies need to cross the cornea and diffuse to the ciliary epithelium in sufficient drug concentrations for therapeutic effect. Topical delivery can thus result in direct exposure of the cornea and result in decreased endothelial

pump function and increased corneal edema. Both reversible and irreversible corneal decompensation has been rarely reported with topical CAI use.[4,5] Oral CAI agents have generally not been reported to have endothelial side effects as strong as topical agents.[6] Because oral agents diffuse through the bloodstream to reach their site of action, avascular structures such as the corneal endothelium have relatively less drug exposure. Therefore, if no other alternative therapies exist, oral agents may be considered in patients at risk for corneal compromise.

Another issue is whether the topical CAI drugs produce maximal IOP lowering, equivalent to that of systemic agents. In general, the authors feel that one oral agent, acetazolamide (Diamox), results in a slightly better pressure-lowering effect than topical agents alone.[7,8] This has been shown to be true in a small case series of patients that compared acetazolamide to topical dorzolamide. Acetazolamide reduces aqueous flow by 29% compared to dorzolamide's 17%.[9] This effect did not appear to be due to the metabolic acidosis induced by systemic CAIs,[10] but rather to their nonselective action on both the CA II and IV isoenzymes of the ciliary epithelium. Of note, topical CAIs have a preferential affinity for the CA II isoenzyme,[11] and thus concomitant topical and systemic CAI therapy is not justified. The readers should also keep in mind that a comparison of 2 different delivery routes is always problematic because equivalent drug levels may or may not reach the site of action. Therefore, bioavailability of a drug plays a major role in efficacy.

The following discussion relates to the oral use of CAI agents with which we have had broad experience and which likely will still continue to be used for the foreseeable future. In general, oral CAIs can be added to most classes of glaucoma medications (Table 14-1).

Kahook MY, Schuman JS, eds.
Chandler and Grant's Glaucoma, Fifth Edition (pp 159-164).
© 2013 SLACK Incorporated.

TABLE 14-1. ANTICIPATED INTRAOCULAR PRESSURE RESPONSE IN ADDING ORAL CARBONIC ANHYDRASE INHIBITORS TO OTHER COMMONLY USED GLAUCOMA MEDICATIONS

Oral CAI Added to	Beneficial
Pilocarpine	Yes
Beta-blocker	Yes
Alpha-adrenergic agonists	Yes
Prostaglandin F2α analogs	Yes
Topical CAIs	No
CAI: carbonic anhydrase inhibitors.	

Oral CAIs are potent antiglaucoma agents that are truly the drug of last resort in most patients because of the potential for serious, even life-threatening systemic side effects.[12] Therefore, topical therapies and even strong miotics, in pseudophakic eyes, despite all their limitations and concerns, are usually preferred to the oral CAIs. In general, laser trabeculoplasty should be performed before use of oral CAIs when possible. Also, for unilateral uncontrolled glaucoma (assuming a good fellow eye), other options should be fully explored first. Yet, oral CAIs are responsible for the prevention of blindness in many patients with glaucoma. Due to the effects of the drug on the renal tubule, patients need to be informed that CAIs do at first cause an acute diuresis, but this is short lasting.[13]

The CAIs are useful in certain secondary glaucomas to protect the eye from damage by the glaucoma until the underlying cause of the glaucoma is removed. Special considerations are involved in use of these drugs in angle-closure glaucoma, and this is further detailed in the chapter dealing with angle-closure glaucoma. In all cases of progressive adult open-angle glaucoma, we currently use topical (and frequently oral) CAI treatment in addition to standard maximal topical antiglaucoma drugs prior to considering surgery. What is written here concerns principally the use of CAI agents in the management of chronic glaucoma when various agents are to be considered. It does not include treatment of acute glaucoma, for which acetazolamide, in addition to topical beta-blockers and alpha-adrenergic agents, is often utilized because of its rapid action (within 30 minutes) and because the course of treatment is so brief that problems of side effects are relatively few.

Some glaucoma patients tolerate oral CAI therapy well and can be maintained on long-term therapy. However, 30% to 50% of patients are unable to take CAI medications for prolonged periods because of unpleasant and sometimes debilitating side effects. The most common side effect that results in discontinuation of long-term oral CAI therapy is a symptom-complex of malaise, fatigue, weight loss, anorexia, depression, and often loss of libido. Patients who have this malaise symptom complex often state that they feel "awful," "do not care whether they live or die," or that "they would rather go blind than continue with this type of drug." We have seen such patients unnecessarily hospitalized for extensive evaluation for occult malignancy or other disease suspected because of severe loss of weight and appetite. The occurrence of such malaise-type symptoms is often associated with the development of systemic metabolic acidosis. All patients undergoing chronic oral CAI therapy develop systemic acidosis, but the patients with these symptoms are generally more acidotic than other patients.[10] Sometimes, in stoic patients on long-term oral CAI therapy, the degree of metabolic acidosis is alarming and may lead to hospitalization in a medical ward.

Some patients on chronic CAI therapy develop symptoms of abdominal distress: cramping, epigastric burning, nausea, irritation, and diarrhea. These gastrointestinal side effects, unlike the malaise symptom-complex, seem to be unrelated to the degree of metabolic acidosis. These gastrointestinal disturbances seem to be local irritative phenomena and have often responded to a simple change in regimen, such as administering the CAI with food, changing to a slow-release oral CAI preparation, or adding alkaline antacid therapy. Patients with a history of gastrointestinal disease who are on CAI therapy sometimes develop symptoms that are refractory to all attempts at relief. It is curious that CAI therapy may be expected to reduce secretion of hydrochloric acid in patients with peptic ulcer, yet such patients may not tolerate CAI therapy because of aggravation of their abdominal symptoms.

The systemic administration of CAIs has also exhibited the rare but potentially lethal side effect of bone marrow suppression. Thrombocytopenia, aplastic anemia, agranulocytosis, and pancytopenia have been reported and can be either idiosyncratic or dose related.[14,15] Of note, topical CAIs have also been reported to result in rare (but reversible) case reports of thrombocytopenia.[16]

Many conflicting statements have been made concerning potassium supplementation in patients on long-term oral CAI therapy. We have found that patients receiving CAI treatment tend to have only small decreases in serum potassium, and the decrease in patients who have the malaise-type side effects is no different from that in patients who do not. However, patients who are concurrently taking oral CAI agents for glaucoma and a thiazide diuretic for systemic hypertension often develop a large decrease in serum potassium and frequently require potassium supplementation. Such patients should have their potassium levels monitored, because hypokalemia can become a life-threatening cardiac situation. In general, we have found that most patients who are taking only CAI and no thiazides do not have an appreciable benefit from potassium supplementation, and thus we just monitor their potassium levels.

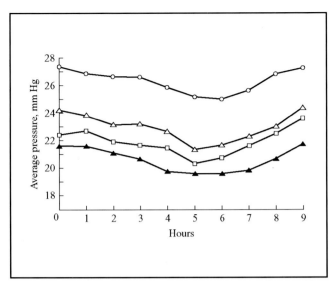

Figure 14-1. Effect of methazolamide dosage 3 times a day on IOP in patients who have glaucoma. Note an increasing effect with increasing dosage. Open circles—baseline; open triangles—25 mg; open squares—50 mg; closed triangles—100 mg. (We subsequently learned that methazolamide only needs to be given twice a day.) (Reprinted with permission from Dahlen K, Epstein DL, Grant WM, et al. A repeated dose response study of methazolamide in glaucoma. *Arch Ophthalmol.* 1978;96:2214-2218. Copyright © 1978. American Medical Association. All rights reserved.)

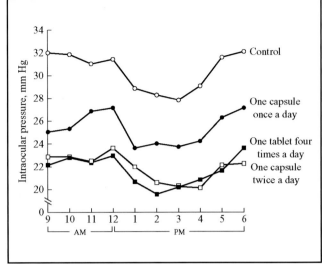

Figure 14-2. Comparison of different dosage regimens of acetazolamide in patients who have glaucoma. For one sequel a day therapy, measurements are 14 to 23 hours after that dosage. For such, a once-a-day 500 mg sequel therapy, a 23-hour IOP lowering occurs that is submaximal during the second 12 hours. Two 500-mg sequels a day are equivalent to four 250-mg tablets. (Reprinted with permission from Berson FG, Epstein DL, Grant WM, et al. Acetazolamide dosage forms in the treatment of glaucoma. *Arch Ophthalmol.* 1980;98:1051-1054. Copyright © 1978. American Medical Association. All rights reserved.)

Paresthesias, headaches, and taste alterations often occur during oral CAI therapy, but these are usually tolerable and only rarely are a cause for discontinuation of CAI agents.

Therapeutic Regimens

The following are currently popular dosages of oral CAI: acetazolamide tablets, 250 mg qid; acetazolamide slow-release capsules, 500 mg bid; and methazolamide tablets, 50 mg bid to tid. Dichlorphenamide is a rarely used glaucoma agent that is dosed 50 mg bid to tid.

Methazolamide has a longer duration of action and probably needs to be administered only twice a day,[17] but it is slower in onset of action than acetazolamide. Accordingly, in acute glaucoma, oral acetazolamide rather than methazolamide is usually employed. Only acetazolamide is available in a form for intravenous administration.

Some ophthalmologists have the impression that methazolamide less often causes side effects than does acetazolamide, but in terms of regulating the patients glaucoma, it may be that currently employed dosages of methazolamide correspond to less than the maximum customary dosage of acetazolamide.[17,18]

We have demonstrated that, for maximal lowering of IOP, a dosage of methazolamide of at least 75 to 100 mg bid is required.[17] This, unfortunately, produces a significant increase in side effects. It is not yet clear whether methazolamide has an advantage over acetazolamide with respect to severity of side effects when dosages that have truly equivalent influences on IOP are employed. On the other hand, methazolamide produces less metabolic acidosis than does acetazolamide, even at therapeutically equivalent dosages.

There are reports in the literature pointing to the effectiveness of low dosages of oral CAI agents in glaucoma therapy. Although it is true that IOP can be reduced somewhat by low dosages, such as 25 mg of methazolamide twice a day, it is incorrect to believe that such low dosages result in maximal lowering of IOP. A dosage of methazolamide of at least 75 to 100 mg bid is required for maximal lowering of IOP (Figure 14-1). Of course, in starting treatment for chronic glaucoma with this drug, it is reasonable to place the patient on only 25 to 50 mg methazolamide bid and observe the effect. If the glaucoma is not too advanced and IOP not too high, then a satisfactory lowering of pressure may be obtained with such a low dosage. If greater pressure lowering is then required, the dosage should be increased unless side effects are excessive.

One acetazolamide slow-release capsule daily (which may be better tolerated in the individual patient) produces a significant lowering of IOP that lasts 24 hours (Figure 14-2), although the magnitude of the pressure lowering during the second 12 hours is often less than with twice-a-day slow-release capsule dosage.[19] Nevertheless, such a single daily slow-release capsule dosage may produce an IOP effect in the second 12 hours equivalent to that of methazolamide 50 mg bid. Therefore, it is often useful to initiate therapy with once-a-day dosage of slow-release capsule and assess pressure lowering 12 to 24 hours following a dose.[19,20] One acetazolamide slow-release capsule taken orally bid appears as effective as acetazolamide 250 mg tablets taken qid.[19]

PRECAUTIONS AND SIDE EFFECTS

CAIs should be given with caution and probably in lower dosages to patients with chronic respiratory acidosis. Such patients with chronic emphysema or bronchitis normally develop a compensatory metabolic alkalosis. As mentioned previously, CAIs produce a metabolic acidosis[20] that can interfere with these compensatory mechanisms.

Occasionally, patients who are receiving standard dosages of CAIs agents develop extraordinarily high serum levels of the agent.[10,18,21] These patients are particularly prone to disabling malaise-type symptoms. In some such patients, a decrease in dosage has resulted in a reduction of side effects, and there has been no apparent worsening of IOP.[10,18]

The frequency with which serum levels higher than needed are to be found in patients with malaise-type symptoms is not yet known, but we think that excessive serum levels probably account for only a minor proportion of these symptoms. Appropriate serum levels need to be better defined. Without sufficient knowledge of the serum levels, it seems reasonable in all patients with side effects to make an arbitrary trial of reducing the oral CAI dosage, but in the majority of such patients the effectiveness of regulation of the glaucoma can be expected to suffer.

Special considerations should be given to the perinatal use of both oral and topical CAIs. Although CAIs have been reported to have teratogenic effects in rodents,[22] to date, no reports have been confirmed in humans. However, none of the drugs have been studied adequately in these patients, and thus there is a relative contraindication to using these medications in such patients. Both topical and oral CAIs can result in inhibition of red blood cell CA type II activity,[23] and although this has little effect in adults, newborns have more fetal hemoglobin that can make them more susceptible to acidosis.[24] Lactating women should also avoid the use of CAIs for the same reason because it can be excreted in milk.[25] Use of this class of medications in the above patients should be done with obstetrics and/or pediatric medicine consultation.

An extraordinarily high serum level of acetazolamide can occur occasionally in patients who are receiving standard dosage and have renal impairment, due presumably to the fact that acetazolamide is entirely excreted in the urine and is not metabolized. This is especially important in diabetic patients with retinopathy and neovascular glaucoma. These patients should be given lower than standard dosages of oral CAI agents. When methazolamide is used, renal function is of less obvious concern, because only 25% of methazolamide is known to be excreted unchanged in the urine. The fate of the remaining 75% is unknown, but presumably it is metabolized.[26]

Some patients without renal impairment, as indicated by normal serum creatinine levels, also develop extraordinarily high serum levels of CAI, with no obvious cause. The elderly may be especially prone to this occurrence.[21] The relationship between dosage and serum level may vary strikingly from patient to patient. Lehmann has observed that as much as a 6-fold difference in acetazolamide dosage may be required to achieve a given plasma level in different patients.[27]

Despite topical CAIs, there are still glaucoma patients for whom the benefits and risks of chronic oral CAI therapy are a preferable alternative to those of filtration surgery. In managing patients with disabling malaise-type CAI side effects, we find the following serum chemical analyses sometimes useful: creatinine, potassium, CAI level, CO_2-combining power, and chloride.[10,18] Serum creatinine identifies patients with impaired renal function who should be given lower than standard dosages of oral CAI. Serum potassium helps identify those patients who are on concurrent diuretic therapy and may require potassium supplementation. The CAI level identifies those patients with apparently higher-than-needed serum levels of the medication, in which a reduction in dosage is indicated. (Unfortunately, facilities for CAI serum assays are available in very few laboratories.) Serum CO_2-combining power and chloride identify possible excessive acidosis as a cause of the side effects.

In excessively acidotic patients with normal serum CAI levels, preliminary studies indicate some effectiveness of additive alkali (sodium acetate) therapy in relieving symptoms.[10,18,28] However, such alkali therapy potentially can lead to other symptoms, such as renal stones or possibly gout, and we therefore have not pursued this strategy further, except for the very rare patient with no other therapeutic options.

Severe metabolic acidosis has been reported in some patients taking CAI and salicylates.[29]

There remain significant numbers of patients who are unable to tolerate long-term oral CAI therapy. We are also intrigued by the fact that there are certain glaucoma patients who do not respond to CAI therapy with a significant lowering of IOP despite proven serum levels of the CAI agent that are therapeutically effective for other patients.[17] Naturally, once it is established that a patient's IOP is not reduced, despite a serum level that should be adequate, there is no point in pursuing this form of treatment.

Kidney stones develop occasionally during oral CAI therapy and are believed to be a result of calcium precipitation secondary to decrease of citrate[30] and/or magnesium excretion in the urine. The decrease of urinary citrate is thought to be a direct consequence of drug-induced metabolic acidosis. Ophthalmologists have had the impression that the incidence of kidney stones is lower with methazolamide than with acetazolamide, and, in fact, recent studies have documented less reduction of urinary citrate by methazolamide (at low dosages) than by acetazolamide.[17]

Management of patients with kidney stones involves use of methazolamide in as low dosages as the severity of the glaucoma permits, restriction of dietary calcium, and use of concomitant chlorothiazide diuretics to alter the calcium/magnesium ratio in the urine. Several of our patients who have developed kidney stones on CAI therapy have been proved to have idiopathic hypercalciuria and have responded well to dietary calcium restriction. Nephrologic consultation and measurements of urinary pH, calcium, and citrate should be obtained in those patients who develop renal stones on CAIs.

A review of more uncommon side effects of CAI medications is available.[12] One of the most worrisome is that of bone marrow suppression that can be fatal and that can occur with methazolamide as well as acetazolamide.[31-33] This may result from either dose-related or idiosyncratic type of reactions. It is currently controversial whether complete blood count profiles should routinely be performed in patients on oral CAI therapy.[32] Patients need to be informed about these potential rare complications and, at a minimum, to report quickly any sores or lesions that do not heal or easy bruisability. The issues are the cost-effectiveness of routine blood profiles for this rare occurrence and the ability to detect it by testing,[32] because many cases are idiosyncratic in origin. At the current time, there is no clear answer to this question except for the clinician to do as if he or she were the patient (ie, treat the patient as one would want oneself to be treated). As mentioned previously, topical CAI therapy has been associated with a milder and reversible form of thrombocytopenia,[16] and similar patient considerations are warranted.

Efficacy of Carbonic Anhydrase Inhibitors in Patients on Beta-Blocker Therapy

Because both CAIs and timolol decrease aqueous humor secretion, it is reasonable to ask whether these effects are fully or only partially additive. We have observed that, when timolol and oral CAI are used together, there is greater IOP lowering than with either agent used alone, but the apparent effects are not fully additive, suggesting some interrelationship of CA and beta-adrenergic mechanisms in aqueous humor secretion.[34-36]

References

1. Brubaker RF. Flow of aqueous humor in humans. *Invest Ophthalmol Vis Sci.* 1991;32:3145-3166.
2. Maren TH. The rates of movement of Na4 , Cl-, and HCO- from plasma to posterior chamber: effect of acetazolamide and relation to the treatment of glaucoma. *Invest Ophthalmol.* 1976;15:356-364.
3. Bonanno JA. Bicarbonate transport under nominally bicarbonate-free conditions in bovine corneal endothelium. *Exp Eye Res.* 1994;58:115-421.
4. Konowal A, Morrison JC, Brown SV, et al. Irreversible corneal decompensation in patients treated with topical dorzolamide. *Am J Ophthalmol.* 1999;127:403-406.
5. Zhao JC, Chen T. Brinzolamide induced reversible corneal decompensation. *Br J Ophthalmol.* 2005;89:389-390.
6. Nielsen CB. The effect of carbonic anhydrase inhibition on central corneal thickness after cataract extraction. *Acta Ophthalmol (Copenh).* 1980;58:985-990.
7. Portellos M, Buckley EG, Freedman SF. Topical versus oral carbonic anhydrase inhibitor therapy for pediatric glaucoma. *J AAPOS.* 1998;2:43-47.
8. Al-Barrag A, Al-Shaer M, Al-Matary N, et al. Oral versus topical carbonic anhydrase inhibitors in ocular hypertension after scleral tunnel cataract surgery. *Clin Ophthalmol.* 2009;3:357-362.
9. Larsson LI, Alm A. Aqueous humor flow in human eyes treated with dorzolamide and different doses of acetazolamide. *Arch Ophthalmol.* 1998;116:19-24.
10. Epstein DL, Grant WM. Carbonic anhydrase inhibitor side effects. Serum chemical analysis. *Arch Ophthalmol.* 1977;95:1378-1382.
11. Sugrue MF. Pharmacological and ocular hypotensive properties of topical carbonic anhydrase inhibitors. *Prog Retin Eye Res.* 2000;19:87-112.
12. Grant WM. Antiglaucoma drugs: Problems with carbonic anhydrase inhibitors. In: Leopold IH, ed. *Symposium on Ocular Therapy.* St Louis, MO: CV Mosby; 1973.
13. Greger R, Lohrmann E, Schlatter E. Action of diuretics at the cellular level. *Clin Nephrol.* 1992;30(suppl 1):S64-S68.
14. Kodjikian L, Durand B, Burillon C, et al. Acetazolamide-induced thrombocytopenia. *Arch Ophthalmol.* 2004;122:1543-1544.
15. Fraunfelder FT, Bagby GC. Monitoring patients taking oral carbonic anhydrase inhibitors. *Am J Ophthalmol.* 2000;130:221-223.
16. Martin XD, Danese M. Dorzolamide-induced immune thrombocytopenia: a case report and literature review. *J Glaucoma.* 2001;102:133-135.
17. Dahlen K, Epstein DL, Granr WM, et al. A repeated dose response study of methazolamide in glaucoma. *Arch Ophthalmol.* 1978;96:2214-2218.
18. Epstein DL, Grant WM. Management of carbonic anhydrase inhibitors side effects. In: Leopold IH, Burns RP, eds. *Symposium on Ocular Drug Therapy.* New York, NY: John Wiley and Sons; 1979:51-64.
19. Berson FG, Epstein DL, Grant WM, et al. Acetazolamide dosage forms in the treatment of glaucoma. *Arch Ophthalmol.* 1980; 98:1051-1054.
20. Berson FG, Epstein DL. Carbonic anhydrase inhibitors. *Perspect Ophthalmol.* 1980;4:91-95.
21. Charpron DJ, Gomolin JH, Sweeney KR. Acetazolamide blood concentrations are excessive in the elderly: propensity for cidosis and relationship to renal function. *J Clin Pharmacol.* 1989;29:348-353.
22. Shepard TH. *Catalog of Teratogenic Agents.* 6th ed. Baltimore, MD: Johns Hopkins University Press; 1989:56.
23. Wilkerson M, Cyrlin M, Lippa EA, et al. Four-week safety and efficacy study of dorzolamide, a novel, active topical carbonic anhydrase inhibitor. *Arch Ophthalmol.* 1993;111:1343-1350.
24. Morris S, Geh V, Nischal KK, et al. Topical dorzolamide and metabolic acidosis in a neonate. *Br J Ophthalmol.* 2003;87:1052-1053.
25. Soderman P, Hartvig P, Fagerlund C. Acetazolamide excretion into human breast milk. *Br J Clin Pharmacol.* 1984;17:59960.
26. Maren TH, Haywood JR, Chapman SK, et al. The pharmacology of methazolamide in relation to the treatment of glaucoma. *Invest Ophthalmol.* 1977;16:730-742.
27. Lehmann B, Linner E, Wistrand PJ. The pharmacokinetics of acetazolamide in relation to its use in the treatment of glaucoma and to its effects as an inhibitor of carbonic anhydrases. In: Raspe G, ed. *Schering Workshop in Pharmacokinetics.* Oxford: Pergamon Press; 1969.

28. Arrigg CA, Giovanoni R, Epstein DL, et al. The influence of supplemental sodium acetate on carbonic anhydrase inhibitor-induced side effects. *Arch Ophthalmol.* 1981;99:1969-1972.

29. Cowan RA, Hartnell GG, Lowdell CP, et al. Metabolic acidosis induced by carbonic anhydrase inhibitors and salicylates in patients with normal renal function. *Br Med J (Clin Res Ed).* 1984;289:347-348.

30. Higashihara E, Nutahara K, Takeuchi T, et al. Calcium metabolism in acidotic patients induced by carbonic anhydrase inhibitors: responses to citrate. *J Urol.* 1991;145:942-948.

31. Werblin TP, Pollack IP, Liss RA. Blood dyscrasias in patients using methazolamide (Neptazane) for glaucoma. *Ophthalmology.* 1980;87:350-354.

32. Mogk LG, Cyrlin MN. Blood dyscrasias and carbonic anhydrase inhibitors. *Ophthalmology.* 1988;95:768-771.

33. Cohen AM, Prialnik M, Ben-Nissan DS, et al. Methazolamide-associated temporary leukopenia and thrombocytopenia. *DICP.* 1989;23:58-59.

34. Berson FG, Epstein DL. Additive effect of timolol and acetazolamide in the treatment of open-angle glaucoma. *Arch Ophthalmol.* 1981;92:788-791.

35. Dailey RA, Brubaker RF, Bourne WM. The effects of timolol maleate and acetazolamide on the rate of aqueous formation in normal human subjects. *Am J Ophthalmol.* 1982;93:232-237.

36. McCannel CA, Heinrich SR, Brubaker RF. Acetazolamide but not timolol lowers aqueous humor flow in sleeping humans. *Graefes Arch Clin Exp Ophthalmol.* 1992;230:518-520.

15

Topical Carbonic Anhydrase Inhibitors

Pratap Challa, MD, MS and Joel S. Schuman, MD, FACS

Carbonic anhydrase inhibitors (CAIs) have been used for glaucoma therapy since 1954, following the description of their efficacy by Becker[1] and Grant et al.[2] Despite the fact that these agents reduce intraocular pressure (IOP), their systemic use has been limited by side effects[3] such as malaise, fatigue, weight loss, depression, anorexia, paresthesias, loss of libido, abdominal cramping, gastric burning and irritation, nausea, diarrhea, kidney stones, bone marrow depression, and even potentially fatal side effects such as aplastic anemia. To reduce the adverse effects associated with these agents, creative use has been made of alkalinizing agents, such as bicarbonate or sodium acetate, to decrease the symptom complex related to the metabolic acidosis induced by CAIs.[3-5] Even with this adjunctive therapy, however, oral CAIs have found limited use in the chronic treatment of glaucoma, primarily because they are poorly tolerated by a significant proportion of patients.

As an attempt to capture the beneficial IOP-lowering action of CAIs, while minimizing their adverse effects, topical CAIs that could decrease IOP without producing the harmful consequences of the oral agents underwent considerable investigation. The quest for such a preparation extends back to Grant's initial publication on acetazolamide, when he found that topical or subconjunctival application of the drug was ineffective in reducing IOP.[2] Over the ensuing years, several compounds were investigated for this purpose, with little success. Some of the more successful agents include dichlorphenamide, which reduced IOP in rabbits,[6] ethoxzolamide analogs,[7-11] ethoxzolamide gel and suspension,[10-13] methazolamide, and benzolamide analogs.[8,9] Each of these agents was investigated thoroughly, but was found to be ineffective, hazardous, or too irritating for topical use. Many of these investigations involved Thomas Maren, who also played a key role in the development of CAIs for systemic use.

In 1988, a breakthrough occurred with the introduction of MK-927, a new topical agent specifically formulated for the eye produced by Merck, Sharp, and Dohme Research Laboratories.[14] This agent proved to be effective in humans and to be well tolerated.[14-16] Double-masked, randomized, placebo-controlled, multicenter studies on this drug demonstrated efficacy and safety, with a peak effect approximately 2 hours after topical administration.[15,17-19]

Laboratory investigation showed that this agent entered the eye not only through the cornea, but primarily via a nonaqueous, trans-scleral route at the limbal region.[20,21] Although many of the other agents investigated for this purpose did not penetrate the eye well, topically administered MK-927 resulted in permeation of the drug to the corneal stroma, aqueous, and ciliary processes.[16] Ocular penetration was most likely related to the property of the drug as an ampholyte, capable of ionizing into anionic and cationic forms. Furthermore, a major advantage to topical administration was that the systemic distribution was decreased over oral agents. The plasma concentration of the drug after a single topical ocular administration was less than 1 µM in rabbits, while at least 2 to 10 µM plasma concentration would be required for physiological side effects. This indicated that systemic toxicity should be minimal or absent,[16,22] which has been confirmed in further human studies.[23,24] Therefore, topical CAIs are preferable over systemic agents due to their decreased systemic side effect profiles.

The first commercially available topical CAI was MK-507 or dorzolamide (Figure 15-1), and it was approved by the United States Food and Drug Administration (FDA) in December 1994. Marketed under the trade name Trusopt, it is also an ampholyte like MK-927.[14,24] One property of the dorzolamide molecule is that it requires an acidic pH (5.6) for solubilization and favorable ocular bioavailability. The acidic nature of this solution results in the frequent ocular complaints of stinging and burning upon drop instillation. In our experience, patients with dry eyes complain the most with this medication, and the use of artificial tears 5 to

Kahook MY, Schuman JS, eds.
Chandler and Grant's Glaucoma, Fifth Edition (pp 165-169).
© 2013 SLACK Incorporated.

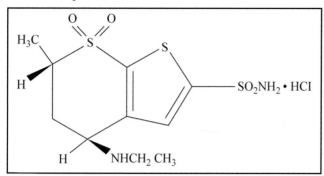

Figure 15-1. The chemical structure of dorzolamide.

10 minutes prior to using dorzolamide can make the drop more tolerable.

A second topical CAI was approved by the FDA in April 1998. It was named brinzolamide and is marketed as Azopt.[25,26] This drug has lipophilic properties that improve its corneal penetration but also make it relatively insoluble in solution. The insolubility problem was addressed by making it into a viscous carbomer suspension with a near-physiological pH (7.5). This prolongs the corneal contact time of the drug and thus increases the drug's bioavailability. However, this also results in the common complaint of blurred vision after drop instillation.

As discussed in the chapter on systemic CAI medications, the site of action of all CAIs is in the nonpigmented ciliary epithelium where they block CA isoenzymes. The topical CAIs have a much greater affinity for CA II over that of I or IV.[27,28] This is in contrast to acetazolamide, which non-selectively inhibits both types II and IV (both found in the nonpigmented ciliary epithelium) and may be responsible for its slightly greater pressure effect.[29]

Both dorzolamide and brinzolamide have proven efficacy in reducing aqueous production and IOP in clinical trials.[24,25,30-33] Both of them appear to have similar effects on IOP, and, as monotherapy (dosed tid), their peak effect occurs at 2 to 3 hours postinstillation and results in a 16% to 24% IOP reduction. Their trough activity is also similar with a 13% to 18% pressure reduction at 12 hours.[24-26,30,33,34] Their activity appears to be comparable to other drugs that decrease aqueous production such as betaxolol[35-37] and brimonidine,[38,39] although the nonselective beta-blocker timolol appears to have a small (5% to 10%) advantage in IOP lowering.[37] They are not as effective as the prostaglandin analogs,[37] and so they are typically used as adjunctive agents after other medications have been initiated. When added to timolol 0.5% or to maximal medical therapy, twice-daily dorzolamide and brinzolamide provide an additional reduction in IOP of 11% to 20% and 11% to 16% at peak and trough, respectively.[40-42] Therefore, fixed combinations of these medications have been developed and are marketed as Cosopt (dorzolamide/timolol) in the United States and Azarga (brinzolamide/timolol) in Europe. The IOP effect of the 2 fixed combinations is similar to each other as well as to concomitant administration of each individual medication.[43,44]

DOSING

The topical CAIs are useful in treating nearly all of the glaucomas. They have been approved for 3-times-daily dosing but, due to patient compliance issues, many practitioners use them twice a day. In their fixed combination formulations, they are dosed twice daily to avoid excessive beta-blocker dosing. For most patients, twice-daily dosing is reasonable with the understanding that there may be slightly less trough IOP control with dorzolamide.[45,46] With brinzolamide, there does not appear to be any statistically significant difference between twice-daily and 3-times-daily dosing.[26,47] Therefore, it is reasonable to use these medications twice daily, but, in those patients who need the flattest diurnal pressure curve possible, we use dorzolamide 3 times daily. For such patients on Cosopt, we sometimes ask them to take an additional dorzolamide drop at mid-day between their Cosopt dosing.

OCULAR HEMODYNAMIC EFFECTS OF THE TOPICAL CARBONIC ANHYDRASE INHIBITORS

The topical (and oral) CAIs have been shown in some studies to alter ocular hemodynamics. They can increase the ocular pulse amplitude,[48] shorten the arteriovenous passage (AVP) time (AVP appears to be increased in glaucoma patients),[49] increase end diastolic velocity of the short posterior ciliary arteries, and increase retinal oxygen saturation.[50,51] Another study has shown no change in retrobulbar hemodynamics.[49] It should be noted that these are difficult parameters to measure with current instruments, but if these changes are further validated, then these drugs could potentially have beneficial effects on ganglion cell function. Increased contrast sensitivity has been reported in low-tension glaucoma patients[52] as has decreased visual field progression in primary open-angle glaucoma (POAG).[51] However, it is difficult to tease out whether these beneficial effects are due to the lowering of IOP versus the hemodynamic effects of these medications. Therefore, the clinical significance of these studies is unclear at present, and they warrant further study.

TOXICITY

As with any glaucoma therapy, CAI agents need to be continuously evaluated by the clinician for both safety and efficacy. These are sulfonamide derivatives so they are contraindicated in patients with known sulfa allergies or hypersensitivities. Sensitivities can also develop over time and can manifest as an allergic conjunctivitis or a periocular contact dermatitis. If these findings develop, then the medication should be immediately discontinued.

TABLE 15-1. ANTICIPATED INTRAOCULAR PRESSURE RESPONSE IN ADDING TOPICAL CARBONIC ANHYDRASE INHIBITORS TO OTHER COMMONLY USED GLAUCOMA MEDICATIONS

Topical CAI Added to	Beneficial
Pilocarpine	Yes
Beta-blocker	Yes
Alpha-2 agonists	Yes
Prostaglandin F2α analogs	Yes
Systemic CAIs	No
CAI: carbonic anhydrase inhibitors.	

complaints include burning, stinging, blurred vision, pruritis, and irritation.[34,47] Ocular irritation is more common with dorzolamide due to the acidic pH of the solution, and blurriness is more common with brinzolamide due to the suspension's viscous nature. In general, brinzolamide has been reported to be somewhat better tolerated.[41,47]

The development of topical CAIs has led to a much better-tolerated glaucoma therapy compared to their oral counterparts. In general, they are less effective than prostaglandin analogs and the nonselective beta-blocker timolol but have similar potency to betaxolol and brimonidine.[37] They also provide relatively stable diurnal pressure control without the tachyphylaxis seen with beta-blockers. Therefore, they are typically used as second-line or adjunctive therapies and can be used to treat nearly all of the glaucomas (Table 15-1).

Although the primary site of action for this drug class is at the ciliary epithelium, one must keep in mind that other ocular structures also express CA and that their inhibition can lead to unintended side effects. The CA isoenzyme types I and II are important for corneal endothelial pump function,[53-55] and, as mentioned before, the topical CAIs are particularly active against type II. This is especially important because these drugs have been optimized for corneal permeation to allow for diffusion to the ciliary body. Moreover, these drugs need to be quite potent due to the high efficiency of this enzyme class; nearly total (99.9%) inhibition is needed to achieve pressure-lowering. Hence, topical delivery can result in direct exposure of the cornea with the potential to affect endothelial pump function. This does not appear to be a problem in ocular hypertensive and open-angle glaucoma patients who have normal endothelial cell counts.[56] However, increased central corneal thickness measurements have been reported in individuals with known corneal guttata[57,58] and even in patients immediately after yttrium-aluminum-garnet (YAG) casulotomy.[59] Furthermore, both reversible and irreversible corneal decompensation has been rarely reported with topical CAI use.[60,61] Therefore, topical CAIs should be used with caution in patients with Fuchs' corneal dystrophy and other endotheliopathies.

The topical CAIs exhibit much fewer systemic side effects compared to oral CAIs. However, serious systemic side effects have been rarely reported with topical CAIs. This includes nephrolithiasis[62] and thrombocytopenia.[63] These drugs should be used with caution in pregnant and lactating women because they have not been sufficiently studied in these groups. Likewise, no formal studies in children have been performed, but retrospective studies suggest that they are well-tolerated.[64] However, one area of concern is that premature and newborn infants may be susceptible to acidosis with these medications.[65]

Less serious side effects, such as abnormal taste, fatigue, headaches, paresthesias, decreased appetite, and malaise, have been reported with topical CAIs, and associated ocular

REFERENCES

1. Becker B. Decrease in intraocular pressure in man by a carbonic anhydrase inhibitor, diamox; a preliminary report. *Am J Ophthalmol.* 1954;37(1):13-15.
2. Grant WM, Trotter RR. Diamox (acetazolamide) in treatment of glaucoma. *AMA Arch Ophthalmol.* 1954;51(6):735-739.
3. Epstein DL, Grant WM. Carbonic anhydrase inhibitor side effects. Serum chemical analysis. *Arch Ophthalmol.* 1977;95(8):1378-1382.
4. Arrigg CA, Epstein DL, Giovanoni R, Grant WM. The influence of supplemental sodium acetate on carbonic anhydrase inhibitor-induced side effects. *Arch Ophthalmol.* 1981;99(11):1969-1972.
5. Epstein DL, Grant WM. Management of carbonic anhydrase inhibitor side effects. In: Leopold IH, Burns RP, eds. *Symposium on Ocular Therapy.* New York, NY: John Wiley & Sons, Inc; 1979.
6. Lotti VJ, Schmitt CJ, Gautheron PD. Topical ocular hypotensive activity and ocular penetration of dichlorphenamide sodium in rabbits. *Graefes Arch Clin Exp Ophthalmol.* 1984;222(1):13-19.
7. Schoenwald RD, Eller MG, Dixson JA, Barfknecht CF. Topical carbonic anhydrase inhibitors. *J Med Chem.* 1984;27(6):810-812.
8. Maren TH, Jankowska L. Ocular pharmacology of sulfonamides: the cornea as barrier and depot. *Curr Eye Res.* 1985;4(4):399-408.
9. Maren TH, Bar-Ilan A, Caster KC, Katritzky AR. Ocular pharmacology of methazolamide analogs: distribution in the eye and effects on pressure after topical application. *J Pharmacol Exp Ther.* 1987;241(1):56-63.
10. Lewis RA, Schoenwald RD, Eller MG, et al. Ethoxzolamide analogue gel. A topical carbonic anhydrase inhibitor. *Arch Ophthalmol.* 1984;102(12):1821-1824.
11. Kalina PH, Shetlar DJ, Lewis RA, et al. 6-amino-2-benzothiazole-sulfonamide. The effect of a topical carbonic anhydrase inhibitor on aqueous humor formation in the normal human eye. *Ophthalmology.* 1988;95(6):772-777.
12. Lewis RA, Schoenwald RD, Barfknecht CF, Phelps CD. Aminozolamide gel. A trial of a topical carbonic anhydrase inhibitor in ocular hypertension. *Arch Ophthalmol.* 1986;104(6):842-844.
13. Lewis RA, Schoenwald RD, Barfknecht CF. Aminozolamide suspension: the role of the vehicle in a topical carbonic anhydrase inhibitor. *J Ocul Pharmacol.* 1988;4(3):215-219.
14. Lippa EA, von Denffer HA, Hofmann HM, Brunner-Ferber FL. Local tolerance and activity of MK-927, a novel topical carbonic anhydrase inhibitor. *Arch Ophthalmol.* 1988;106(12):1694-1696.

15. Bron AM, Lippa EA, Hofmann HM, et al. MK-927: a topically effective carbonic anhydrase inhibitor in patients. *Arch Ophthalmol.* 1989;107(8):1143-1146.

16. Maren TH, Bar-Ilan A, Conroy CW, Brechue WF. Chemical and pharmacological properties of MK-927, a sulfonamide carbonic anhydrase inhibitor that lowers intraocular pressure by the topical route. *Exp Eye Res.* 1990;50(1):27-36.

17. Higginbotham EJ, Kass MA, Lippa EA, et al. MK-927: a topical carbonic anhydrase inhibitor. Dose response and duration of action. *Arch Ophthalmol.* 1990;108(1):65-68.

18. Pfeiffer N, Hennekes R, Lippa EA, et al. A single dose of the topical carbonic anhydrase inhibitor MK-927 decreases IOP in patients. *Br J Ophthalmol.* 1990;74(7):405-408.

19. Serle JB, Lustgarten JS, Lippa EA, et al. MK-927, a topical carbonic anhydrase inhibitor. Dose response and reproducibility. *Arch Ophthalmol.* 1990;108(6):838-841.

20. Michelson SR SH, Baldwin JJ, et al. Topically instilled MK-927: Lack of correlation between corneal penetration rate constant and ocular hypotensive activity in rabbits. *Invest Ophthalmol Vis Sci.* 1989;30(suppl):24.

21. Brechue WF MT. Correlation of drug accession with IOP reduction following local and intravenous carbonic anhydrase inhibitors (CAI). *Invest Ophthalmol Vis Sci.* 1991;32(suppl):1256.

22. Maren TH, Conroy CW, Wynns GC, Levy NS. Ocular absorption, blood levels, and excretion of dorzolamide, a topically active carbonic anhydrase inhibitor. *J Ocul Pharmacol Ther.* 1997;13(1): 23-30.

23. Buclin T, Biollaz J, Lippa EA, et al. Absence of metabolic effects of the novel topically active carbonic anhydrase inhibitor MK-927 and its s isomer during a 2-week ocular administration. *Eur J Clin Pharmacol.* 1989;36:46.

24. Wilkerson M, Cyrlin M, Lippa EA, et al. Four-week safety and efficacy study of dorzolamide, a novel, active topical carbonic anhydrase inhibitor. *Arch Ophthalmol.* 1993;111(10):1343-1350.

25. Silver LH. Clinical efficacy and safety of brinzolamide (Azopt), a new topical carbonic anhydrase inhibitor for primary open-angle glaucoma and ocular hypertension. Brinzolamide Primary Therapy Study Group. *Am J Ophthalmol.* 1998;126(3): 400-408.

26. Silver LH. Dose-response evaluation of the ocular hypotensive effect of brinzolamide ophthalmic suspension (Azopt). Brinzolamide Dose-Response Study Group. *Surv Ophthalmol.* 2000;44(suppl 2):S147-S153.

27. Stams T, Chen Y, Boriack-Sjodin PA, et al. Structures of murine carbonic anhydrase IV and human carbonic anhydrase II complexed with brinzolamide: molecular basis of isozyme-drug discrimination. *Protein Sci.* 1998;7(3):556-563.

28. Sugrue MF. Pharmacological and ocular hypotensive properties of topical carbonic anhydrase inhibitors. *Prog Retin Eye Res.* 2000;19(1):87-112.

29. Larsson LI, Alm A. Aqueous humor flow in human eyes treated with dorzolamide and different doses of acetazolamide. *Arch Ophthalmol.* 1998;116(1):19-24.

30. Long-term glaucoma treatment with MK-507, dorzolamide, a topical carbonic anhydrase inhibitor. *J Glaucoma.* 1995;4(1):6-10.

31. Maus TL, Larsson LI, McLaren JW, Brubaker RF. Comparison of dorzolamide and acetazolamide as suppressors of aqueous humor flow in humans. *Arch Ophthalmol.* 1997;115(1):45-49.

32. Ingram CJ, Brubaker RF. Effect of brinzolamide and dorzolamide on aqueous humor flow in human eyes. *Am J Ophthalmol.* 1999;128(3):292-296.

33. Sall K. The efficacy and safety of brinzolamide 1% ophthalmic suspension (Azopt) as a primary therapy in patients with open-angle glaucoma or ocular hypertension. Brinzolamide Primary Therapy Study Group. *Surv Ophthalmol.* 2000;44(suppl 2):S155-S162.

34. Strahlman E, Tipping R, Vogel R. A six-week dose-response study of the ocular hypotensive effect of dorzolamide with a one-year extension. Dorzolamide Dose-Response Study Group. *Am J Ophthalmol.* 1996;122(2):183-194.

35. Kass MA LR, Lippa EA, et al. Comparative activity of 3% MK-507, a topical CAI, with betaxolol. *Invest Ophthalmol Vis Sci.* 1991;578(suppl 1):989.

36. Strahlman E, Tipping R, Vogel R. A double-masked, randomized 1-year study comparing dorzolamide (Trusopt), timolol, and betaxolol. International Dorzolamide Study Group. *Arch Ophthalmol.* 1995;113(8):1009-1016.

37. van der Valk R, Webers CA, Schouten JS, et al. Intraocular pressure-lowering effects of all commonly used glaucoma drugs: a meta-analysis of randomized clinical trials. *Ophthalmology.* 2005;112(7):1177-1185.

38. Whitson JT, Henry C, Hughes B, et al. Comparison of the safety and efficacy of dorzolamide 2% and brimonidine 0.2% in patients with glaucoma or ocular hypertension. *J Glaucoma.* 2004;13(2):168-173.

39. Sharpe ED, Day DG, Beischel CJ, et al. Brimonidine purite 0.15% versus dorzolamide 2% each given twice daily to reduce intraocular pressure in subjects with open angle glaucoma or ocular hypertension. *Br J Ophthalmol.* 2004;88(7):953-956.

40. Nardin G LR, Lippa EA. Activity of the topical CAI MK-507 bid when added to timolol bid. *Invest Ophthalmol Vis Sci.* 1991;579 (suppl 1):989.

41. Michaud JE, Friren B. Comparison of topical brinzolamide 1% and dorzolamide 2% eye drops given twice daily in addition to timolol 0.5% in patients with primary open-angle glaucoma or ocular hypertension. *Am J Ophthalmol.* 2001;132(2):235-243.

42. Strohmaier K, Snyder E, DuBiner H, Adamsons I. The efficacy and safety of the dorzolamide-timolol combination versus the concomitant administration of its components. Dorzolamide-Timolol Study Group. *Ophthalmology.* 1998;105(10):1936-1944.

43. Hollo G, Bozkurt B, Irkec M. Brinzolamide/timolol fixed combination: a new ocular suspension for the treatment of open-angle glaucoma and ocular hypertension. *Expert Opin Pharmacother.* 2009;10(12):2015-2024.

44. Hutzelmann J, Owens S, Shedden A, et al. Comparison of the safety and efficacy of the fixed combination of dorzolamide/timolol and the concomitant administration of dorzolamide and timolol: a clinical equivalence study. International Clinical Equivalence Study Group. *Br J Ophthalmol.* 1998;82(11):1249-1253.

45. Lippa EA, Carlson LE, Ehinger B, et al. Dose response and duration of action of dorzolamide, a topical carbonic anhydrase inhibitor. *Arch Ophthalmol.* 1992;110(4):495-499.

46. Lupinacci AP, Netland PA, Fung KH, et al. Comparison of twice-daily and 3-times-daily dosing of dorzolamide in ocular hypertension and primary open-angle glaucoma patients treated with latanoprost. *Adv Ther.* 2008;25(3):231-239.

47. March WF, Ochsner KI. The long-term safety and efficacy of brinzolamide 1.0% (Azopt) in patients with primary open-angle glaucoma or ocular hypertension. The Brinzolamide Long-Term Therapy Study Group. *Am J Ophthalmol.* 2000;129(2): 136-143.

48. Costa VP, Harris A, Stefansson E, et al. The effects of antiglaucoma and systemic medications on ocular blood flow. *Prog Retin Eye Res.* 2003;22(6):769-805.

49. Kaup M, Plange N, Niegel M, et al. Effects of brinzolamide on ocular haemodynamics in healthy volunteers. *Br J Ophthalmol.* 2004;88(2):257-262.

50. Siesky B, Harris A, Cantor LB, et al. A comparative study of the effects of brinzolamide and dorzolamide on retinal oxygen saturation and ocular microcirculation in patients with primary open-angle glaucoma. *Br J Ophthalmol.* 2008;92(4):500-504.

51. Martinez A, Sanchez M. Effects of dorzolamide 2% added to timolol maleate 0.5% on intraocular pressure, retrobulbar blood flow, and the progression of visual field damage in patients with primary open-angle glaucoma: a single-center, 4-year, open-label study. *Clin Ther.* 2008;30(6):1120-1134.

52. Harris A, Arend O, Kagemann L, et al. Dorzolamide, visual function and ocular hemodynamics in normal-tension glaucoma. *J Ocul Pharmacol Ther.* 1999;15(3):189-197.

53. Bonanno JA. Bicarbonate transport under nominally bicarbonate-free conditions in bovine corneal endothelium. *Exp Eye Res.* 1994;58(4):415-421.

54. Wistrand PJ, Schenholm M, Lonnerholm G. Carbonic anhydrase isoenzymes CA I and CA II in the human eye. *Invest Ophthalmol Vis Sci.* 1986;27(3):419-428.

55. Holthofer H, Siegel GJ, Tarkkanen A, Tervo T. Immunocytochemical localization of carbonic anhydrase, NaK-ATPase and the bicarbonate chloride exchanger in the anterior segment of the human eye. *Acta Ophthalmol (Copenh).* 1991;69(2):149-154.

56. Lass JH, Khosrof SA, Laurence JK, et al. A double-masked, randomized, 1-year study comparing the corneal effects of dorzolamide, timolol, and betaxolol. Dorzolamide Corneal Effects Study Group. *Arch Ophthalmol.* 1998;116(8):1003-1010.

57. Wirtitsch MG, Findl O, Kiss B, et al. Short-term effect of dorzolamide hydrochloride on central corneal thickness in humans with cornea guttata. *Arch Ophthalmol.* 2003;121(5):621-625.

58. Wirtitsch MG, Findl O, Heinzl H, Drexler W. Effect of dorzolamide hydrochloride on central corneal thickness in humans with cornea guttata. *Arch Ophthalmol.* 2007;125(10):1345-1350.

59. Ornek K, Gullu R, Ogurel T, Ergin A. Short-term effect of topical brinzolamide on human central corneal thickness. *Eur J Ophthalmol.* 2008;18(3):338-340.

60. Konowal A, Morrison JC, Brown SV, et al. Irreversible corneal decompensation in patients treated with topical dorzolamide. *Am J Ophthalmol.* 1999;127(4):403-406.

61. Zhao JC, Chen T. Brinzolamide induced reversible corneal decompensation. *Br J Ophthalmol.* 2005;89(3):389-390.

62. Carlsen J, Durcan J, Zabriskie N, et al. Nephrolithiasis with dorzolamide. *Arch Ophthalmol.* 1999;117(8):1087-1088.

63. Martin XD, Danese M. Dorzolamide-induced immune thrombocytopenia: a case report and literature review. *J Glaucoma.* 2001;10(2):133-135.

64. Portellos M, Buckley EG, Freedman SF. Topical versus oral carbonic anhydrase inhibitor therapy for pediatric glaucoma. *J AAPOS.* 1998;2(1):43-47.

65. Morris S, Geh V, Nischal KK, et al. Topical dorzolamide and metabolic acidosis in a neonate. *Br J Ophthalmol.* 2003;87(8):1052-1053.

16

Prostaglandin Analogs

Angela V. Turalba, MD and Douglas J. Rhee, MD

Unoprostone was the first commercially available prostaglandin analog and was introduced in the mid-1990s. Latanoprost, bimatoprost, and travoprost were released soon after. Because of their favorable balance of intraocular pressure (IOP)-lowering effect and systemic safety, prostaglandin analogs (PGAs) are very popular agents for the medical management of glaucoma.

Prostaglandins and thromboxanes belong to a family of compounds called *prostanoids*, which are defined as cyclooxygenase products derived from C-20 unsaturated fatty acids (namely, arachidonic acid). In the 1930s, Euler isolated a highly active, lipid-soluble compound from sheep vesicular glands and named it *prostaglandin*.[1] Euler's substance was later determined to represent a family of prostaglandins. Bergstrom and Sjovall were the first to characterize the prostaglandin family with the identification of PGE_2 and $PGF_{2\alpha}$ in the 1950s.[2] Ocular prostaglandins (initially called *irin*) were first extracted from a homogenate of iris in 1955.[3] PGE_2 and $PGF_{2\alpha}$ were later identified as the active components of irin in 1966.[4] The ocular hypotensive effect (preceded by an initial hypertensive phase in rabbits) of intracameral prostaglandins was noted in 1971.[5] Camras et al[6] showed a similar effect from topically applied prostaglandins in 1977. In rabbits, the initial hypertensive phase was related to the high doses, induced miosis, breakdown of the blood aqueous barrier, and protein leakage.[7] Further studies[8,9] in the early 1980s revealed that there is a sustained lowering of IOP without a significant hypertensive phase in other species.

MOLECULAR PHARMACOLOGY

PGAs increase aqueous drainage, primarily by enhancing uveoscleral outflow up to 60%.[7,10-12] Additionally, bimatoprost, latanoprost, and travoprost all have some effect on trabecular outflow.[13] PGAs are chemical derivatives of prostaglandin F_2 and agonists of the prostanoid FP_A and FP_B receptors. Latanoprost and travoprost are ester prodrugs, while bimatoprost is an amide prodrug. These prodrugs are hydrolyzed by esterases in the cornea into free acids that are the active compounds that bind the FP receptors. A study[14] using knockout mice have shown that the IOP-lowering effect of PGAs is dependent on the presence of intact FP receptors. FP receptors have been detected in the iris, trabecular meshwork, ciliary muscle, and sclera of the human eye.[15-17] Cloning and sequence analysis of prostaglandin receptors have indicated that prostaglandin receptors are G-protein coupled receptors, which, when activated, initiate a transduction cascade involving protein kinase C and the induction of nuclear transcription factors, specifically c-Fos and C-Jun.[18,19] In trabecular meshwork (TM) cells, stimulation with $PGF_{2\alpha}$ causes an increase in intracellular calcium and inositol phosphate. In ciliary body smooth muscle (CBSM) cells, $PGF_{2\alpha}$ does not change IP3 production, but does increase cyclic AMP (cAMP) levels.[20] The effect of PGAs may be mediated by cAMP production, but $PGF_{2\alpha}$ has the least ability to do so in cultured CBSM cells.[20,21] $PGF_{2\alpha}$ may also mediate its effects through stimulation of phospholipase A_2 causing the release of arachidonic acid for PG synthesis and the endogenous release of PGE_2, PGD_2, $PGF_{2\alpha}$.[22] PGE_2 and PGD_2 are much more potent activators of the adenylate cyclase system.[20,21] In vitro, TM cells produce PGE_2, $PGF_{2\alpha}$, and 6KF1a.[23] The eventual induction of transcription factors resulting from these signaling pathways initiates alterations in gene expression, including the dose-dependent upregulation of matrix metalloproteinases (MMPs) in ocular tissues, including CBSM cells.[19,24,25]

There are 22 unique MMPs, to date.[26] MMPs are zinc-dependent endopeptidases that are collectively capable of degrading all extracellular matrix (ECM) components.[27] As with any enzyme, MMPs can be regulated at

Kahook MY, Schuman JS, eds.
Chandler and Grant's Glaucoma, Fifth Edition (pp 171-176).
© 2013 SLACK Incorporated.

transcription, activation, and kinetics. For most MMPs, with the notable exception of MMP-2, transcriptional regulation is more important. For MMP-2, activation and kinetic inhibition seem to be more important.[26,28,29] Many MMP promoters (MMP-1,-3,-7,-9,-10,-12,-13)[26] contain AP-1 (interacts with Fos and Jun transcription factors) and PEA-3 (interacts with ETS transcription factors) binding sites. MMPs-1 and -3 also contain an additional platelet-derived growth factor-responsive *cis*-acting element.[30,31] Other factors, such as growth factors, hormones, cytokines, and cell-cell and cell-ECM contact, can alter MMP gene expression.[27] Generally, TGFβ, retinoic acids, and glucocorticoids suppress MMP gene expression.[32] Mitogen-activated protein kinases are important to transcription regulation in tumor cells.[27] Activation of pro-MMPs can be performed by soluble enzymes (eg, plasmin), membrane-bound enzymes (eg, MT1-MMP), and autocatalytic activity (eg, MMP-3).[32-34] Enzymatic activity can be inhibited by the tissue inhibitors of metalloproteinases (TIMPs) through direct competitive binding at the catalytic site of the MMP. To date, 4 human TIMPs (TIMPs-1 through -4) have been identified. MMPs with numeric designations higher than 9 and MT-MMPs are not well studied in the trabecular meshwork (with the exception of MT-MMP-1/MMP-14). Plasmin, an activator of MMP activity, is upregulated in response to latanoprost.[35]

On the molecular level, PGAs cause a change in the balance of MMPs and their kinetic inhibitors, TIMPs in both trabecular meshwork and ciliary body smooth muscle cells.[36-38] Although this alteration of MMPs and TIMPs occurs in both cell types, the balance of MMPs and TIMPs is shifted to a larger degree in the ciliary body.[38] Furthermore, PGAs affect the downstream tissues in the uveoscleral pathway, increasing scleral permeability by altering the balance of MMPs and TIMPs in scleral fibroblasts.[39-41]

On a cellular level, the PGA-induced shift in MMPs and TIMPs causes a decrease in ECM around CBSM cells after 4 to 8 days of treatment.[42,43] This finding corresponds to the clinical observation that a larger IOP reduction is observed after 4 to 5 days of daily dosing.[44,45] Chronic PGA use causes a decrease in ECM and alterations of cellular attachments in the juxtacanalicular (JXT) region of trabecular meshwork. In the ciliary body, latanoprost has been found to decrease collagen types I, II, III, IV, and VI, as well as fibronectin, laminin, and hyaluronan.[35,46-48]

From indirect evidence demonstrating the blunting of the $PGF_{2\alpha}$-induced hypotension by pilocarpine, there is some suggestion that CBSM tone may also be partially responsible for the hypotensive effects.[7,49] In vitro experiments with cultured CBSM cells show that there is a dose-dependent increase of calcium efflux (which would cause smooth muscle cell contraction) at high concentrations of $PGF_{2\alpha}$ (10^{-8} to 10^{-6} mol/L). With concentrations lower than 10^{-8} mol/L, there was little change in calcium.[50] Physiologic measurements of contractile

forces of bovine TM and ciliary muscle cells do not show any significant effect from $PGF_{2\alpha}$ agonists.[51]

CLINICAL EFFICACY

There are several prospective clinical trials that demonstrate the efficacy of PGAs to lower IOP in patients with ocular hypertension and open-angle glaucoma. Latanoprost, travoprost, and bimatoprost dosed once daily are at least equally or more effective than timolol in lowering mean diurnal IOP when used as monotherapy.[52-54] Pooled data showed that latanoprost reduces mean diurnal IOP on average by approximately 30%, with a similar degree of IOP lowering seen with bimatoprost and travoprost.[52,55,56] PGAs are also equally or more effective in lowering IOP compared to pilocarpine, brimonidine, dorzolamide, and combination timolol-dorzolamide.[52,57-59] The IOP-lowering effect of PGAs has been demonstrated in various ethnic groups including White, Asian, African, and Hispanic populations.[55] PGAs are not as effective in children compared with adults, though they can significantly reduce IOP in select cases including juvenile open-angle glaucoma and older children.[60-62] Young animals and people have a higher proportion of their outflow through the uveoscleral pathway.[63,64] It is possible that this reduced effectiveness of PGAs in children may be related to a maximal amount of outflow through the uveoscleral pathway.

Except for unoprostone, which is dosed twice daily, the recommended dosage for latanoprost, travoprost, and bimatoprost is once daily in the evening. The evening dosing is thought to block the early morning diurnal IOP spike seen in some patients.[65] Dosage is an important factor that influences the effect of PGAs, and more frequent dosing has been shown to decrease the IOP-lowering effect.[6,54,66] Studies on long-term treatment with PGAs have shown no loss of effect over 1 to 5 years.[53,67,68]

PGAs can produce a substantial additional reduction in IOP when added to other ocular hypotensive agents presumably because they act on different pathways compared to other glaucoma medications. When used with timolol, latanoprost and travoprost produce further reductions in IOP.[69-71] The addition of dorzolamide or brimonidine to a patient taking latanoprost results in additional IOP reduction.[71] Initially, based on data from primate experimental models, pilocarpine was believed to inhibit prostaglandin-induced enhancement of uveoscleral outflow.[49-72] However, in humans, fluorophotometry data suggest that pilocarpine does not inhibit the uveoscleral outflow enhancement of prostaglandins.[73-75] Although more effective combinations exist, prostaglandins and pilocarpine may be effective in lowering IOP when used together.[75] The use of 2 different PGAs in combination has not been demonstrated to have increased efficacy in IOP lowering when compared to the use of a single PGA.[76,77]

SIDE EFFECTS

PGAs are often better tolerated than other topical glaucoma medications, because they have few systemic side effects.[65,78] The active form of latanoprost is metabolized primarily by the liver and has a half-life of 17 minutes. It is measurable in human plasma within the first hour after administration.[79] PGAs are classified as category C medications, and there are no epidemiologic studies on these drugs used during pregnancy. A small observational study found no adverse effects of latanoprost used in pregnant women, though caution is advised in the use of these drugs during pregnancy because of the potential oxytocic effect of all PGAs.[80] PGAs are also well-tolerated in children, although they may be less efficacious than when used in adults.[61,62]

Conjunctival hyperemia is one of the more common side effects of PGAs, especially because prostaglandins have powerful effects on vasculature. The conjunctival hyperemia noted in the large clinical trials is generally mild and does not represent a true allergy.[81] It can occur in about half (47% to 69%) of patients on PGAs, and the degree of hyperemia remains consistent during the first few months of treatment.[56] Compared to bimatoprost and travoprost, latanoprost is associated with less frequent conjunctival hyperemia.[56,82,83]

Irreversible darkening of the iris is another known side effect of topical PGAs. Though most commonly reported with latanoprost, iris darkening has also been associated with travoprost, bimatoprost, and unoprostone.[53,66,81,84] The risk of developing iris changes is dependent on iris color. Hazel irides with mixed coloring are at highest risk of iris darkening with PGAs, with approximately one-third of these patients developing iris changes.[65] In the Japanese population, the incidence of latanoprost-induced iris darkening was reported to be 58% at 12 months.[81] A 5-year safety trial with latanoprost showed that these iris changes typically occur within the first 8 months of use and do not occur after 3 years of treatment.[67] Histologically, the pigment changes are associated with increased melanin production with no significant changes in melanocyte proliferation.[85,86]

Topical PGAs have been shown to increase the length, pigmentation, and thickness of eyelashes.[87] Trichiasis that may require treatment has also been reported with topical prostaglandins.[88] Eyelash changes are seen more frequently with bimatoprost and travoprost compared to latanoprost.[53,56,68,69]

PGAs have also been associated with changes in the periorbital skin and tissues. Periocular skin darkening is a relatively uncommon side effect with a reported incidence of 1.5% to 2.9% at 12 weeks.[56] Unlike induced iris darkening, eyelid skin darkening due to topical prostaglandins is reversible.[89] These skin changes can manifest within months to years after starting treatment.[90,91] The mechanism of these changes is believed to be due to increased melanogenesis

without inflammation or significant increase in melanocyte proliferation.[92] Orbital tissue changes resulting in the deepening of the eyelid sulcus and enophthalmos have also been reported with bimatoprost.[93,94] The periorbital changes appear to be reversible, but the mechanism underlying this side effect has yet to be elucidated.[93]

There have been numerous reports of cystoid macular edema (CME) occurring after the administration of topical PGAs. Case reports documenting the occurrence of CME in patients who were in the recent postoperative period following cataract removal[95,96] along with reports of CME occurring spontaneously in nonoperated eyes raised concerns about PGA use in the postoperative period following cataract removal.[97-99] In general, more cases have been reported in pseudophakic or aphakic eyes. The mechanism of action is likely an alteration of the blood-eye barrier due to the intrinsic pro-inflammatory properties of prostaglandins.[95-100] There has been some conjecture and associative evidence that the preservative benzalkonium chloride (BAC) may have a contributory role.[101,102] However, numerous possible confounding variables, such as chronic medication use and greater uveal manipulation during cataract surgery, may predispose to the development of CME. Additionally, CME following the use of a BAC-free PGA lends evidence to the mechanism being likely due to an intrinsic property of the drug rather than the preservative.[103]

Discontinuation of a PGA prior to cataract surgery remains controversial. The rate of CME in nondiabetics is approximately 2.1%.[104] A randomized controlled trial has not been performed comparing a PGA versus non-PGA following cataract removal; however, preoperative use of a PGA significantly increases the risk (OR 12.45; $p < 0.04$) of postoperative CME in a large case series.[104] PGAs do not appear to affect macular thickness when CME is not present.[105]

There have been several reports of PGAs inducing or reactivating herpetic keratitis and periocular skin dermatitis.[106-108] In rabbits, there is experimental evidence that PGAs exacerbate herpetic keratitis and recurrence.[109-111] In a very rare group of patients, PGAs may increase the risk of reactivation of herpetic keratitis. However, the prevalence of herpes simplex virus (HSV) I is more than 90% in adult glaucoma patients. If PGAs were a significant inciting risk factor for HSV keratitis, this complication would likely be much more common.

Because of the reports of PGA use causing spontaneous nongranulomatous anterior uveitis, there is concern over their use in patients with established uveitic glaucoma. A recent report of PGA use in 84 patients demonstrated that PGAs were effective in lowering IOP, and there was no difference in the frequency of anterior uveitis or rates of CME.[112]

CONCLUSION

Overall, topical PGAs are a valuable option in the medical management of glaucoma. They are a unique class of medications that are effective in lowering IOP by primarily enhancing uveoscleral outflow. Additionally, they are well-tolerated and are associated with mainly localized side effects. The additive IOP-lowering effects of PGAs when used with other classes of hypotensive agents support the development of combination agents containing PGAs.

REFERENCES

1. von Euler U. Zur kenntis der pharmakoligischen wirkungen von nativsekreten und extrakten mannlichter accessorischer geschlechtsdrusen. *Nauyn Schniedebergs Arch Exp Pathol Pharmacol.* 1934;175:78-84.

2. Bergstrom S, Eliasson R, von Euler U, Sjovall J. Some biological effects of two crystalline prostaglandin factors. *Acta Physiol Scan.* 1959;45:133-144.

3. Ambache N. Irin, a smooth-muscle contracting substance present in rabbit iris. *J Physiol.* 1955;129(3):65-69.

4. Ambache NB, Rose JG, Whiting J. Thin-layer chromatography of spasmogenic unsaturated hydroxy-acids from various tissues. *J Physiol.* 1966;135:77-78.

5. Starr MS. Further studies on the effect of prostaglandin on intraocular pressure in the rabbit. *Exp Eye Res.* 1971;11(2):170-177.

6. Camras CB, Bito LZ, Eakins KE. Reduction of intraocular pressure by prostaglandins applied topically to the eyes of conscious rabbits. *Invest Ophthalmol Vis Sci.* 1977;16(12):1125-1134.

7. Lee PY, Podos SM, Severin C. Effect of prostaglandin F2 alpha on aqueous humor dynamics of rabbit, cat, and monkey. *Invest Ophthalmol Vis Sci.* 1984;25(9):1087-1093.

8. Camras CB, Bito LZ. Reduction of intraocular pressure in normal and glaucomatous primate (Aotus trivirgatus) eyes by topically applied prostaglandin F2 alpha. *Curr Eye Res.* 1981;1(4):205-209.

9. Stern FA, Bito LZ. Comparison of the hypotensive and other ocular effects of prostaglandins E2 and F2 alpha on cat and rhesus monkey eyes. *Invest Ophthalmol Vis Sci.* 1982;22(5):588-598.

10. Nilsson SF, Samuelsson M, Bill A, Stjernschantz J. Increased uveoscleral outflow as a possible mechanism of ocular hypotension caused by prostaglandin F2 alpha-1-isopropylester in the cynomolgus monkey. *Exp Eye Res.* 1989;48(5):707-716.

11. Stjernschantz JS, Ocklind G, Resul A. Effects of latanoprost and related prostaglandin analogues. In: Alm AW, ed. *Uveoscleral Outflow. Biology and Clinical Aspects.* London: Mosby-Wolfe Medical Communications; 1998:57-72.

12. Stjernschantz J, Selén G, Sjöquist B, Resul B. Preclinical pharmacology of latanoprost, a phenyl-substituted PGF2 alpha analogue. *Adv Prostaglandin Thromboxane Leukot Res.* 1995;23:513-518.

13. Lim KS, Nau CB, O'Byrne MM, et al. Mechanism of action of bimatoprost, latanoprost, and travoprost in healthy subjects. A crossover study. *Ophthalmology.* 2008;115(5):790-795 e4.

14. Ota T, Aihara M, Narumiya S, Araie M. The effects of prostaglandin analogues on IOP in prostanoid FP-receptor-deficient mice. *Invest Ophthalmol Vis Sci.* 2005;46(11):4159-4163.

15. Ocklind A, Lake S, Wentzel P, Nistér M, Stjernschantz J. Localization of the prostaglandin F2 alpha receptor messenger RNA and protein in the cynomolgus monkey eye. *Invest Ophthalmol Vis Sci.* 1996;37(5):716-726.

16. Anthony TL, Pierce KL, Stamer WD, Regan JW. Prostaglandin F2 alpha receptors in the human trabecular meshwork. *Invest Ophthalmol Vis Sci.* 1998;39(2):315-321.

17. Mukhopadhyay P, Bian L, Yin H, Bhattacherjee P, Paterson C. Localization of EP(1) and FP receptors in human ocular tissues by in situ hybridization. *Invest Ophthalmol Vis Sci.* 2001;42(2):424-428.

18. Narumiya S, Sugimoto Y, Ushikubi F. Prostanoid receptors: structures, properties, and functions. *Physiol Rev.* 1999;79(4):1193-1226.

19. Lindsey JD, To HD, Weinreb RN. Induction of c-fos by prostaglandin F2 alpha in human ciliary smooth muscle cells. *Invest Ophthalmol Vis Sci.* 1994;35(1):242-250.

20. Yousufzai SY, Zheng P, Abdel-Latif AA. Muscarinic stimulation of arachidonic acid release and prostaglandin synthesis in bovine ciliary muscle: prostaglandins induce cyclic AMP formation and muscle relaxation. *Exp Eye Res.* 1994;58(5):513-522.

21. Zhan GL, Camras CB, Opere C, Tang L, Ohia SE. Effect of prostaglandins on cyclic AMP production in cultured human ciliary muscle cells. *J Ocul Pharmacol Ther.* 1998;14(1):45-55.

22. Yousufzai SY, Ye Z, Abdel-Latif AA. Prostaglandin F2 alpha and its analogs induce release of endogenous prostaglandins in iris and ciliary muscles isolated from cat and other mammalian species. *Exp Eye Res.* 1996;63(3):305-310.

23. Weinreb RN, Mitchell MD, Polansky JR. Prostaglandin production by human trabecular cells: in vitro inhibition by dexamethasone. *Invest Ophthalmol Vis Sci.* 1983;24(12):1541-1545.

24. Lindsey JW, Weinreb RN. Effects of prostaglandins on uveoscleral outflow. In: Alm AW, ed. *Uveosceral Outflow: Biology and Clinical Aspects.* London: Mosby-Wolfe; 1998:41-56.

25. Weinreb RN, Lindsey JD. Metalloproteinase gene transcription in human ciliary muscle cells with latanoprost. *Invest Ophthalmol Vis Sci.* 2002;43(3):716-722.

26. Ye S. Polymorphism in matrix metalloproteinase gene promoters: implication in regulation of gene expression and susceptibility of various diseases. *Matrix Biol.* 2000;19(7):623-629.

27. Westermarck J, Kahari VM. Regulation of matrix metalloproteinase expression in tumor invasion. *FASEB J.* 1999;13(8):781-792.

28. Matrisian LM. Metalloproteinases and their inhibitors in matrix remodeling. *Trends Genet.* 1990;6(4):121-125.

29. Fini MC, Mohan JR, Brinckerhoff R. Regulation of matrix metalloproteinase gene expression. In: Parks WCM, ed. *Matrix Metalloproteinases.* San Diego, CA: Academic Press; 1998:300-356.

30. Kirstein M, Sanz L, Quiñones S, Moscat J, Diaz-Meco MT, Saus J. Cross-talk between different enhancer elements during mitogenic induction of the human stromelysin-1 gene. *J Biol Chem.* 1996;271(30):18231-18236.

31. Benbow U, Rutter JL, Lowrey CH, Brinckerhoff CE. Transcriptional repression of the human collagenase-1 (MMP-1) gene in MDA231 breast cancer cells by all-trans-retinoic acid requires distal regions of the promoter. *Br J Cancer.* 1999;79(2):221-228.

32. Nagase H, Woessner JF Jr. Matrix metalloproteinases. *J Biol Chem.* 1999;274(31):21491-21494.

33. Sato H, Takino T, Okada Y, et al. A matrix metalloproteinase expressed on the surface of invasive tumour cells. *Nature.* 1994;370(6484):61-65.

34. Nagase H. Stromelysins 1 and 2. In: Parks WCM, ed. *Matrix Metalloproteinases.* San Diego, CA: Academic Press; 1998:43-84.

35. Ocklind A. Effect of latanoprost on the extracellular matrix of the ciliary muscle. A study on cultured cells and tissue sections. *Exp Eye Res.* 1998;67(2):179-191.

36. Oh DJ, Martin JL, Williams AJ, et al. Analysis of expression of matrix metalloproteinases and tissue inhibitors of metalloproteinases in human ciliary body after latanoprost. *Invest Ophthalmol Vis Sci.* 2006;47(3):953-963.

37. Oh DJ, Martin JL, Williams AJ, Russell P, Birk DE, Rhee DJ. Effect of latanoprost on the expression of matrix metalloproteinases and their tissue inhibitors in human trabecular meshwork cells. *Invest Ophthalmol Vis Sci.* 2006;47(9):3887-3895.

38. Ooi YH, Oh DJ, Rhee DJ. Effect of bimatoprost, latanoprost, and unoprostone on matrix metalloproteinases and their inhibitors in human ciliary body smooth muscle cells. *Invest Ophthalmol Vis Sci.* 2009;50(11):5259-5265.

39. Lindsey JD, Crowston JG, Tran A, Morris C, Weinreb RN. Direct matrix metalloproteinase enhancement of transscleral permeability. *Invest Ophthalmol Vis Sci.* 2007;48(2):752-755.

40. Weinreb RN, Lindsey JD, Marchenko G, Marchenko N, Angert M, Strongin A. Prostaglandin FP agonists alter metalloproteinase gene expression in sclera. *Invest Ophthalmol Vis Sci.* 2004;45(12):4368-4377.

41. Kim JW, Lindsey JD, Wang N, Weinreb RN. Increased human scleral permeability with prostaglandin exposure. *Invest Ophthalmol Vis Sci.* 2001;42(7):1514-1521.

42. Lutjen-Drecoll E, Tamm E. Morphological study of the anterior segment of cynomolgus monkey eyes following treatment with prostaglandin F2 alpha. *Exp Eye Res.* 1988;47(5):761-769.

43. Lutjen-Drecoll ET. The effects of ocular hypotensive doses of PGF F2 α-1-isopropylester on anterior segment morphology. In: Bito LZ, Stjernschantz J, eds. *Progress in Clinical and Biological Research.* New York, NY: AR Liss; 1989:xvi.

44. Camras CB, Podos SM, Rosenthal JS, Lee PY, Severin CH. Multiple dosing of prostaglandin F2 alpha or epinephrine on cynomolgus monkey eyes. I. Aqueous humor dynamics. *Invest Ophthalmol Vis Sci.* 1987;28(3):463-469.

45. Crawford K, Kaufman PL, Gabelt BT. Effects of topical PGF2 alpha on aqueous humor dynamics in cynomolgus monkeys. *Curr Eye Res.* 1987;6(8):1035-1044.

46. Weinreb RN, Kashiwagi K, Kashiwagi F, Tsukahara S, Lindsey JD. Prostaglandins increase matrix metalloproteinase release from human ciliary smooth muscle cells. *Invest Ophthalmol Vis Sci.* 1997;38(13):2772-2780.

47. Lindsey JD, Kashiwagi K, Kashiwagi F, Weinreb RN. Prostaglandin action on ciliary smooth muscle extracellular matrix metabolism: implications for uveoscleral outflow. *Surv Ophthalmol.* 1997;41(suppl 2):S53-S59.

48. Sagara T, Gaton DD, Lindsey JD, Gabelt BT, Kaufman PL, Weinreb RN. Topical prostaglandin F2alpha treatment reduces collagen types I, III, and IV in the monkey uveoscleral outflow pathway. *Arch Ophthalmol.* 1999;117(6):794-801.

49. Crawford K, Kaufman PL. Pilocarpine antagonizes prostaglandin F2 alpha-induced ocular hypotension in monkeys. Evidence for enhancement of uveoscleral outflow by prostaglandin F2 alpha. *Arch Ophthalmol.* 1987;105(8):1112-1116.

50. Weinreb RN, Kim DM, Lindsey JD. Propagation of ciliary smooth muscle cells in vitro and effects of prostaglandin F2 alpha on calcium efflux. *Invest Ophthalmol Vis Sci.* 1992;33(9):2679-2686.

51. Krauss AH, Wiederholt M, Sturm A, Woodward DF. Prostaglandin effects on the contractility of bovine trabecular meshwork and ciliary muscle. *Exp Eye Res.* 1997;64(3):447-453.

52. van der Valk R, Webers CA, Schouten JS, Zeegers MP, Hendrikse F, Prins MH. Intraocular pressure-lowering effects of all commonly used glaucoma drugs: a meta-analysis of randomized clinical trials. *Ophthalmology.* 2005;112(7):1177-1185.

53. Netland PA, Landry T, Sullivan EK, et al. Travoprost compared with latanoprost and timolol in patients with open-angle glaucoma or ocular hypertension. *Am J Ophthalmol.* 2001;132(4):472-484.

54. Eisenberg DL, Toris CB, Camras CB. Bimatoprost and travoprost: a review of recent studies of 2 new glaucoma drugs. *Surv Ophthalmol.* 2002;47(suppl 1):S105-S115.

55. Hedman K, Watson PG, Alm A. The effect of latanoprost on intraocular pressure during 2 years of treatment. *Surv Ophthalmol.* 2002;47(suppl 1):S65-S76.

56. Parrish RK, Palmberg P, Sheu WP. A comparison of latanoprost, bimatoprost, and travoprost in patients with elevated intraocular pressure: a 12-week, randomized, masked-evaluator multicenter study. *Am J Ophthalmol.* 2003;135(5):688-703.

57. Camras CB, Sheu WP. Latanoprost or brimonidine as treatment for elevated intraocular pressure: multicenter trial in the United States. *J Glaucoma.* 2005;14(2):161-167.

58. Day DG, Sharpe ED, Beischel CJ, Jenkins JN, Stewart JA, Stewart WC. Safety and efficacy of bimatoprost 0.03% versus timolol maleate 0.5%/dorzolamide 2% fixed combination. *Eur J Ophthalmol.* 2005;15(3):336-342.

59. O'Donoghue EP. A comparison of latanoprost and dorzolamide in patients with glaucoma and ocular hypertension: a 3 month, randomised study. Ireland Latanoprost Study Group. *Br J Ophthalmol.* 2000;84(6):579-582.

60. Enyedi LB, Freedman SF. Latanoprost for the treatment of pediatric glaucoma. *Surv Ophthalmol.* 2002;47(suppl 1):S129-S132.

61. Black AC, Jones S, Yanovitch TL, Enyedi LB, Stinnett SS, Freedman SF. Latanoprost in pediatric glaucoma–pediatric exposure over a decade. *J AAPOS.* 2009;13(6):558-562.

62. Yanovitch TL, Enyedi LB, Schotthoeffer EO, Freedman SF. Travoprost in children: adverse effects and intraocular pressure response. *J AAPOS.* 2009;13(1):91-93.

63. Townsend DJ, Brubaker RF. Immediate effect of epinephrine on aqueous formation in the normal human eye as measured by fluorophotometry. *Invest Ophthalmol Vis Sci.* 1980;19(3):256-266.

64. Toris CB, Yablonski ME, Wang YL, Camras CB. Aqueous humor dynamics in the aging human eye. *Am J Ophthalmol.* 1999;127(4):407-412.

65. Alm A, Stjernschantz J. Effects on intraocular pressure and side effects of 0.005% latanoprost applied once daily, evening or morning. A comparison with timolol. Scandinavian Latanoprost Study Group. *Ophthalmology.* 1995;102(12):1743-1752.

66. Sherwood M, Brandt J. Six-month comparison of bimatoprost once-daily and twice-daily with timolol twice-daily in patients with elevated intraocular pressure. *Surv Ophthalmol.* 2001;45(suppl 4):S361-S368.

67. Alm A, Schoenfelder J, McDermott J. A 5-year, multicenter, open-label, safety study of adjunctive latanoprost therapy for glaucoma. *Arch Ophthalmol.* 2004;122(7):957-965.

68. Cohen JS, Gross RL, Cheetham JK, VanDenburgh AM, Bernstein P, Whitcup SM. Two-year double-masked comparison of bimatoprost with timolol in patients with glaucoma or ocular hypertension. *Surv Ophthalmol.* 2004;49(suppl 1):S45-S52.

69. Higginbotham EJ, Diestelhorst M, Pfeiffer N, Rouland JF, Alm A. The efficacy and safety of unfixed and fixed combinations of latanoprost and other antiglaucoma medications. *Surv Ophthalmol.* 2002;47(suppl 1):S133-S140.

70. Orengo-Nania S, Landry T, Von Tress M, et al. Evaluation of travoprost as adjunctive therapy in patients with uncontrolled intraocular pressure while using timolol 0.5%. *Am J Ophthalmol.* 2001;132(6):860-868.

71. O'Connor DJ, Martone JF, Mead A. Additive intraocular pressure lowering effect of various medications with latanoprost. *Am J Ophthalmol.* 2002;133(6):836-837.

72. Bill A. Effects of atropine and pilocarpine on aqueous humour dynamics in cynomolgus monkeys (Macaca irus). *Exp Eye Res.* 1967;6(2):120-125.

73. Kent AR, Vroman DT, Thomas TJ, Hebert RL, Crosson CE. Interaction of pilocarpine with latanoprost in patients with glaucoma and ocular hypertension. *J Glaucoma.* 1999;8(4):257-262.

74. Toris CB, Zhan GL, Zhao J, Camras CB, Yablonski ME. Potential mechanism for the additivity of pilocarpine and latanoprost. *Am J Ophthalmol.* 2001;131(6):722-728.

75. Toris CB, Alm A, Camras CB. Latanoprost and cholinergic agonists in combination. *Surv Ophthalmol.* 2002;47(suppl 1):S141-S147.

76. Herndon LW, Asrani SG, Williams GH, Challa P, Lee PP. Paradoxical intraocular pressure elevation after combined therapy with latanoprost and bimatoprost. *Arch Ophthalmol.* 2002;120(6):847-849.

77. Saito M, Takano R, Shirato S. Effects of latanoprost and unoprostone when used alone or in combination for open-angle glaucoma. *Am J Ophthalmol.* 2001;132(4):485-489.

78. Fung AT, Reid SE, Jones MP, Healey PR, McCluskey PJ, Craig JC. Meta-analysis of randomised controlled trials comparing latanoprost with brimonidine in the treatment of open-angle glaucoma, ocular hypertension or normal-tension glaucoma. *Br J Ophthalmol.* 2007;91(1):62-68.

79. Hejkal TC. Prostaglandin analogs. In: Netland PA, ed. *Glaucoma Medical Therapy: Principles and Management.* Oxford: Oxford University Press; 2008:33-53.

80. De Santis M, Lucchese A, Carducci B, et al. Latanoprost exposure in pregnancy. *Am J Ophthalmol.* 2004;138(2):305-306.

81. Alm A, Grierson I, Shields MB. Side effects associated with prostaglandin analog therapy. *Surv Ophthalmol.* 2008;53(suppl 1):S93-S105.

82. Konstas AG, Katsimbris JM, Lallos N, Boukaras GP, Jenkins JN, Stewart WC. Latanoprost 0.005% versus bimatoprost 0.03% in primary open-angle glaucoma patients. *Ophthalmology.* 2005; 112(2):262-266.

83. Li N, Chen XM, Zhou Y, Wei ML, Yao X. Travoprost compared with other prostaglandin analogues or timolol in patients with open-angle glaucoma or ocular hypertension: meta-analysis of randomized controlled trials. *Clin Experiment Ophthalmol.* 2006;34(8):755-764.

84. Yamamoto T, Kitazawa Y. Iris-color change developed after topical isopropyl unoprostone treatment. *J Glaucoma.* 1997;6(6):430-432.

85. Albert DM, Gangnon RE, Zimbric ML, et al. A study of iridectomy histopathologic features of latanoprost- and nonlatanoprost-treated patients. *Arch Ophthalmol.* 2004;122(11):1680-1685.

86. Stjernschantz JW, Albert DM, Hu DN, Drago F, Wistrand PJ. Mechanism and clinical significance of prostaglandin-induced iris pigmentation. *Surv Ophthalmol.* 2002;47(suppl 1):S162-S175.

87. Johnstone MA. Hypertrichosis and increased pigmentation of eyelashes and adjacent hair in the region of the ipsilateral eyelids of patients treated with unilateral topical latanoprost. *Am J Ophthalmol.* 1997;124(4):544-547.

88. Bearden W, Anderson R. Trichiasis associated with prostaglandin analog use. *Ophthal Plast Reconstr Surg.* 2004;20(4):320-322.

89. Doshi M, Edward DP, Osmanovic S. Clinical course of bimatoprost-induced periocular skin changes in Whites. *Ophthalmology.* 2006;113(11):1961-1967.

90. Herndon LW, Robert D Williams, Wand M, Asrani S. Increased periocular pigmentation with ocular hypotensive lipid use in African Americans. *Am J Ophthalmol.* 2003;135(5):713-715.

91. Wand M, Ritch R, Isbey EK Jr, Zimmerman TJ. Latanoprost and periocular skin color changes. *Arch Ophthalmol.* 2001;119(4):614-615.

92. Kapur R, Osmanovic S, Toyran S, Edward DP. Bimatoprost-induced periocular skin hyperpigmentation: histopathological study. *Arch Ophthalmol.* 2005;123(11):1541-1546.

93. Filippopoulos T, Paula JS, Torun N, Hatton MP, Pasquale LR, Grosskreutz CL. Periorbital changes associated with topical bimatoprost. *Ophthal Plast Reconstr Surg.* 2008;24(4):302-307.

94. Peplinski LS, Albani Smith K. Deepening of lid sulcus from topical bimatoprost therapy. *Optom Vis Sci.* 2004;81(8):574-577.

95. Miyake K, Ota I, Maekubo K, Ichihashi S, Miyake S. Latanoprost accelerates disruption of the blood-aqueous barrier and the incidence of angiographic cystoid macular edema in early postoperative pseudophakias. *Arch Ophthalmol.* 1999;117(1):34-40.

96. Yeh PC, Ramanathan S. Latanoprost and clinically significant cystoid macular edema after uneventful phacoemulsification with intraocular lens implantation. *J Cataract Refract Surg.* 2002;28(10):1814-1818.

97. Ayyala RS, Cruz DA, Margo CE, et al. Cystoid macular edema associated with latanoprost in aphakic and pseudophakic eyes. *Am J Ophthalmol.* 1998;126(4):602-604.

98. Warwar RE, Bullock JD, Ballal D. Cystoid macular edema and anterior uveitis associated with latanoprost use. Experience and incidence in a retrospective review of 94 patients. *Ophthalmology.* 1998;105(2):263-268.

99. Altintas O, Yüksel N, Karabas VL, Demirci G. Cystoid macular edema associated with latanoprost after uncomplicated cataract surgery. *Eur J Ophthalmol.* 2005;15(1):158-161.

100. Arcieri ES, Santana A, Rocha FN, Guapo GL, Costa VP. Blood-aqueous barrier changes after the use of prostaglandin analogues in patients with pseudophakia and aphakia: a 6-month randomized trial. *Arch Ophthalmol.* 2005;123(2):186-192.

101. Miyake K, Ibaraki N, Goto Y, et al. ESCRS Binkhorst lecture 2002: Pseudophakic preservative maculopathy. *J Cataract Refract Surg.* 2003;29(9):1800-1810.

102. Miyake K, Ota I, Ibaraki N, et al. Enhanced disruption of the blood-aqueous barrier and the incidence of angiographic cystoid macular edema by topical timolol and its preservative in early postoperative pseudophakia. *Arch Ophthalmol.* 2001;119(3):387-394.

103. Esquenazi S. Cystoid macular edema in a pseudophakic patient after switching from latanoprost to BAK-free travoprost. *J Ocul Pharmacol Ther.* 2007;23(6):567-570.

104. Henderson BA, Kim JY, Ament CS, Ferrufino-Ponce ZK, Grabowska A, Cremers SL. Clinical pseudophakic cystoid macular edema. Risk factors for development and duration after treatment. *J Cataract Refract Surg.* 2007;33(9):1550-1558.

105. Yeom HY, Hong S, Kim SS, Kim CY, Seong GJ. Influence of topical bimatoprost on macular thickness and volume in glaucoma patients with phakic eyes. *Can J Ophthalmol.* 2008;43(5):563-566.

106. Wand M, Gilbert CM, Liesegang TJ. Latanoprost and herpes simplex keratitis. *Am J Ophthalmol.* 1999;127(5):602-604.

107. Morales J, Shihab ZM, Brown SM, Hodges MR. Herpes simplex virus dermatitis in patients using latanoprost. *Am J Ophthalmol.* 2001;132(1):114-116.

108. Kothari MT, Mehta BK, Asher NS, Kothari KJ. Recurrence of bilateral herpes simplex virus keratitis following bimatoprost use. *Indian J Ophthalmol.* 2006;54(1):47-48.

109. Kaufman HE, Varnell ED, Toshida H, Kanai A, Thompson HW, Bazan NG. Effects of topical unoprostone and latanoprost on acute and recurrent herpetic keratitis in the rabbit. *Am J Ophthalmol.* 2001;131(5):643-646.

110. Birkle DL, Sanitato JJ, Kaufman HE, Bazan NG. Arachidonic acid metabolism to eicosanoids in herpes virus-infected rabbit cornea. *Invest Ophthalmol Vis Sci.* 1986;27(10):1443-1446.

111. Kaufman HE, Varnell ED, Thompson HW. Latanoprost increases the severity and recurrence of herpetic keratitis in the rabbit. *Am J Ophthalmol.* 1999;127(5):531-536.

112. Chang JH, McCluskey P, Missotten T, Ferrante P, Jalaludin B, Lightman S. Use of ocular hypotensive prostaglandin analogues in patients with uveitis: does their use increase anterior uveitis and cystoid macular oedema? *Br J Ophthalmol.* 2008;92(7):916-921.

17

Management of Highly Elevated Intraocular Pressure

Joshua D. Stein, MD, MS; R. Rand Allingham, MD; and Pratap Challa, MD, MS

The patient with acutely elevated intraocular pressure (IOP) is usually symptomatic, whereas IOP that has gradually increased, even to relatively high levels, usually does not produce symptoms. Common symptoms from acutely elevated IOP include headache, usually dull or aching, blurred vision, perception of colored haloes, and nausea or vomiting. These symptoms of acutely elevated IOP may be accompanied by signs including conjunctival injection, microcystic corneal edema, pupillary abnormalities, and absence of central retinal arterial or venous pulsations. Although glaucomatous optic nerve damage or visual field loss may not be present in cases of acutely elevated IOP, we still refer to these as forms of glaucoma.

Most forms of glaucoma can cause extremely elevated IOP (Table 17-1). Of these, angle-closure glaucoma, either primary or secondary, is a common cause of acute symptomatic IOP elevation. Acute angle-closure crisis often produces the entire constellation of signs and symptoms of this group of disorders. Secondary angle-closure glaucoma, particularly neovascular glaucoma, is frequently encountered in practice. Secondary open-angle glaucomas, including angle recession, exfoliation, pigment dispersion, Posner-Schlossman syndrome, and steroid-induced glaucoma, occasionally cause a sudden, marked IOP increase. Juvenile open-angle glaucoma, although rare, is the most likely primary open-angle glaucoma to produce symptomatic highly elevated IOP.

DIAGNOSIS

History

A thorough medical history and ocular exam frequently provide diagnostic clues to the cause of highly elevated IOP. Often, the cause is obvious, for example, after laser or incisional surgery. In other cases, there may be no apparent cause. An asymptomatic patient usually has had a gradual increase in IOP, which suggests chronic angle-closure glaucoma or a form of open-angle glaucoma. Patients who have had recent eye surgeries and those with histories of ocular inflammation, trauma, or chronic inflammatory medical conditions (eg, asthma or rheumatoid arthritis) should be questioned about the use of topical or systemic corticosteroids. Histories of ocular trauma are often found in patients with angle-recession glaucoma.

Episodic pain or blurred vision occurring over months or years is more commonly observed with intermittent angle-closure glaucoma, whereas the sudden onset of severe unrelenting pain and blurred vision, particularly in a hyperopic patient, is most commonly seen with acute angle-closure crisis. A history of painless loss of vision in the affected eye can occur with a central retinal vein occlusion (CRVO), or a history of diabetes mellitus would suggest neovascular glaucoma as the cause of the IOP elevation.

IOP spikes can occur during the immediate postoperative period following incisional surgical procedures. Reasons for immediate postsurgical IOP spikes include excessive postoperative inflammation, retained viscoelastic, or debris (vitreous, blood, fibrin, iris tissue) obstructing the outflow pathway. Postsurgical pressure spikes can also be attributable to pupillary block caused by implantation of an anterior chamber intraocular lens or a malpositioned posterior chamber intraocular lens or the use of an intraocular gas bubble during Descemet's stripping automated endothelial keratoplasty (DSAEK) surgery. Less common causes of increased IOP following intraocular surgery include aqueous misdirection or the development of a suprachoroidal hemorrhage. Causes of spikes in IOP that occur weeks to months following incisional intraocular

Kahook MY, Schuman JS, eds.
Chandler and Grant's Glaucoma, Fifth Edition (pp 177-182).
© 2013 SLACK Incorporated.

TABLE 17-1. CAUSES OF ACUTE OR HIGHLY ELEVATED INTRAOCULAR PRESSURE

Angle-closure glaucomas

Primary (pupillary block) angle-closure glaucoma

Acute angle-closure crisis

Chronic angle closure

Intermittent angle closure

Secondary angle-closure glaucoma

Development of anterior or posterior synechiae due to inflammation

Neovascularization

Open-angle glaucomas

Exfoliation syndrome

Pigment dispersion syndrome

Juvenile open-angle glaucoma

Primary open-angle glaucoma (rarely)

Steroid-induced glaucoma

Uveitic glaucoma

Angle-recession glaucoma

Postoperative glaucomas

Status postcataract surgery

Status postvitreoretinal surgery

Status postglaucoma surgery

Status postpenetrating keratoplasty or DSAEK

Status postlaser procedures

Posterior capsulotomy

Iridectomy

Gonioplasty

Trabeculoplasty

Panretinal photocoagulation

Malignant glaucoma

Suprachoroidal hemorrhage

DSAEK: Descemet's stripping automated endothelial keratoplasty.

surgery may be due to the formation of peripheral anterior synechiae and chronic angle closure or from the persistent use of corticosteroids.

In addition to information that may lead to a diagnosis, the general medical history provides essential information that is needed before initiating acute medical treatment. A history of asthma or chronic obstructive pulmonary disease precludes use of beta-blockers. In patients with metabolic acidosis (eg, uncontrolled diabetes mellitus) or chronic renal insufficiency, systemic carbonic anhydrase inhibitors (CAIs) should not be used. Hyperosmotic agents should not be administered if severe renal or heart failure is present.

Examination

Careful examination is often rewarded with an accurate diagnosis in these patients. Because the mechanism of IOP elevation differs among this group of disorders, so does the initial medical management.

Obtaining the patient's refractive error is useful. Myopic patients are prone to pigment dispersion syndrome or retinal detachment (Schwartz's syndrome), whereas hyperopic patients are predisposed to angle-closure glaucoma.

Visual acuity may be reduced secondary to corneal edema, media opacity, or posterior segment pathology. Good visual acuity argues against the diagnosis of ischemic CRVO in a patient with neovascular glaucoma.

The presence of a relative afferent pupillary defect (either consensual or reverse) suggests significant retinal or optic nerve damage, which may be secondary to CRVO, central retinal artery occlusion (CRAO), ocular ischemia, or long-standing glaucoma.

Slit-Lamp Examination

Conjunctival injection is common in patients with acute glaucoma; however, prominent chemosis or proptosis of the globe, coupled with conjunctival injection, would suggest the presence of an arteriovenous fistula.

The cornea should be carefully examined for pigment (Krukenberg spindles), endothelial abnormalities (eg, iridocorneal endothelial [ICE] syndrome), or keratic precipitates in cases of uveitis. In some cases, like Posner-Schlossman syndrome, signs of uveitis such as keratic precipitates may not be evident for days after acute IOP has brought the patient to medical attention.

The anterior chamber may contain flare or cells from ocular ischemia secondary to high IOP. However, more than a few cells would suggest a uveitic or infectious etiology, whereas red cells may indicate bleeding from ischemic tissue, trauma, neoplastic disorders, or vitreous hemorrhage (eg, ghost cell glaucoma). The anterior chamber depth both axially and peripherally should be noted. A peripherally shallow anterior chamber suggests glaucoma secondary to relative pupillary block and subsequent angle closure or plateau iris syndrome, whereas a centrally shallow anterior chamber suggests lens displacement or enlargement, posterior segment pathology, or malignant glaucoma.

The iris should be carefully examined for neovascularization. Iris neovascularization often develops first at the pupil margin. Neovascularization can be missed when IOP is extremely high because abnormal vessels may be difficult to see due both to a reduction in vessel caliber as well as corneal

Medication	Acutely Elevated IOP Marked Symptoms	Markedly Elevated IOP Mild Symptoms
Beta-blockers	q 10 min x 2, then q 12 hrs	q 10 min x 2, then q 12 hrs
Alpha-2 agonists	q 10 min x 2, then q 12 hrs	q 10 min x 2, then q 12 hrs
Miotics (for pupillary block or open-angle glaucoma without inflammation or angle recession)	Pilocarpine 1% to 2% (1 to 2 hrs after aqueous suppressants)	Pilocarpine 1% to 2% (1 to 2 hrs after aqueous suppressants)
Carbonic anhydrase inhibitors	Acetazolamide 500 mg IV or po, topical dorzolamide 2% or brinzolamide 2% q 10 min x 2, then q 8 hrs	Acetazolamide 500 mg (tablets) po *or* topical dorzolamide 2% or brinzolamide q 10 min x 2, then q 8 hours
Osmotics	Mannitol 1 to 2 g/kg IV	Oral glycerol or isosorbide 1 to 1.5 g/kg po on ice

TABLE 17-2. MEDICAL TREATMENT OF DANGEROUSLY ELEVATED INTRAOCULAR PRESSURE

edema or in patients with dark-brown irides. The presence of iris transillumination defects may be a sign of pigment dispersion syndrome, exfoliation glaucoma, uveitic glaucoma, occult tumor, or evidence of prior trauma. Iridodialysis or sphincter tears indicate past trauma.

Although rare, a dislocated or hypermature lens can cause acute glaucoma (pupillary block or phacolytic glaucoma). The anterior lens capsule should be examined for the presence of exfoliation material.

Gonioscopy

Gonioscopy is of vital importance in these cases to determine a rational medical (or surgical) treatment strategy. In cases in which there is significant microcystic corneal edema, topical glycerin will often provide an adequate view of the iris and angle structures to assess whether the angle is open or closed. Alternatively, when the view is compromised due to corneal edema, a paracentesis can be performed to temporarily lower the IOP, permitting improved visualization of the angle structures.[1] Compression gonioscopy can be performed to determine which portions of the angle are appositionally versus synechially closed. If gonioscopy is not possible due to corneal opacity, ultrasound biomicroscopy or anterior segment optical coherence tomography can be used to establish the anatomy of the anterior segment.

Fundus

If possible, the fundus should be examined acutely for evidence of CRVO, CRAO, proliferative diabetic retinopathy, retinal detachment or dialysis (Schwartz's syndrome), and optic nerve damage. In patients with suspected acute angle-closure crisis, dilation should be deferred. In those cases in which a view of the fundus is not possible due to media opacity, B-scan ultrasonography should be strongly considered. Posterior segment tumors (eg, melanoma) and chronic retinal detachment can both present with neovascular glaucoma.

TREATMENT STRATEGY

The goal of treatment in these cases is to reduce the IOP as quickly as possible to a safe level for the optic nerve. After this has been accomplished, one can proceed with additional diagnostic tests and therapies. The approach to extremely elevated IOP can be broken down into a simple paradigm, depending on the diagnosis (Table 17-2). As stated, the treatment approach must be modified according to the patient's medical and allergy history.

IOP can be reduced by increasing outflow or reducing inflow. Inflow drugs include beta-blockers, alpha-2 agonists, CAIs, and osmotic agents. Although not strictly inflow drugs, osmotic agents reduce IOP by dehydrating the vitreous and other ocular structures and are effective in the presence of a functionally closed angle. Miotics primarily increase conventional outflow through action on the trabecular meshwork and can open the angle in pupillary block glaucoma. However, because strong miotics can shift the lens-iris diaphragm forward and worsen pupillary block, these agents should be used with caution.

Beta-Blockers and Alpha-2 Agonists

There is considerable overlap in the mechanism in which these agents reduce aqueous inflow. The IOP-lowering effect of the alpha-2 agonist apraclonidine is partially additive to timolol, when these agents are administered chronically.[2] However, apraclonidine is not additive to timolol if both agents are given simultaneously.[3] In other words, apraclonidine appears to restore the full potency of chronically administered timolol, but is no more potent than timolol when it is given acutely. This may also be true for all nonselective beta-blockers. Therefore, either apraclonidine or nonselective beta-blocker therapy is adequate as initial treatment for patients on no previous glaucoma therapy. Apraclonidine would be the agent of choice in cases in which there is a contraindication to using a beta-blocker. The clinician should not be faulted for using alpha-agonists and beta-blockers concomitantly in patients with acutely elevated IOP. Beta-blockers should be given every 12 hours. Apraclonidine is given every 8 hours. There is no therapeutic benefit in treating more frequently.

Miotics

Direct-acting miotics like pilocarpine are useful in the treatment of glaucoma secondary to angle closure resulting from pupillary block, in addition to open-angle glaucomas in which there is no associated anterior segment inflammation. Indirect-acting agents (eg, echothiophate iodide) are long lasting, difficult to reverse, more likely to increase anterior segment inflammation, and frequently cause severe pain when administered acutely. Therefore, indirect-acting miotics should not be used in treating acute glaucomas.

Pilocarpine (1% to 2%) should be given 1 to 2 hours after aqueous suppressants have been administered. Miotics are frequently ineffective in the presence of extremely high IOP due to secondary ischemia of the iris dilator muscles. Generally, 1 or 2 applications are sufficient. More frequent administration is ineffective and can produce serious gastrointestinal and respiratory side effects.[4]

Miotics are contraindicated when the angle is structurally closed by synechia or neovascularization, mechanically closed from a posterior pushing mechanism (eg, acute angle-closure after panretinal photocoagulation or malignant glaucoma), functionally closed by inflammatory debris (uveitis), or when elevated IOP has produced anterior segment ischemia and the iris sphincter is nonfunctional. In the latter case, delaying the addition of miotics for 1 or 2 hours until the IOP has been reduced by aqueous suppressants, hyperosmotics, or paracentesis is often more effective than starting miotic treatment initially.[5]

Miotics should be used judiciously in patients with acutely elevated IOP. If there is a question as to whether miotics should be used, withhold use until the effect of aqueous suppressant and osmotic therapy can be assessed.

Cycloplegic Agents

Whereas cycloplegics such as tropicamide or cyclopentolate are not used to directly reduce IOP, they are indicated for the treatment of secondary angle-closure glaucomas produced by swelling or rotation of the ciliary body and forward movement of the lens-iris diaphragm, such as malignant glaucoma or acute glaucoma after CRVO. These cases are worsened by miotic treatment. Cycloplegics may also help stabilize the blood-ocular barrier in patients with neovascularization of the iris or angle and in patients with hyphemas.[6]

Carbonic Anhydrase Inhibitors

CAIs, such as acetazolamide and methazolamide, reduce aqueous inflow in a manner that is partially additive to both beta-blockers and alpha-2 agonists. Methazolamide, 50 to 100 mg every 8 hours, or acetazolamide, 250 mg every 4 to 6 hours, should be given orally to adult patients. When using acetazolamide in the setting of acute high IOP, 2 250-mg tablets should be given rather than acetazolamide (Diamox Sequels), a 500-mg sustained release formulation, as the tablet formulation is more rapidly absorbed than the sustained-release preparation. Acetazolamide (500 mg) can be given intravenously for patients who have nausea.

When given systemically, CAIs produce metabolic acidosis and should be used with caution in patients with severe liver disease, renal impairment, or pulmonary insufficiency (see Chapter 14).

Although not as potent as the oral form, the topical CAIs dorzolamide and brinzolamide are available for selected patients (see Chapter 15).[7] For example, they may be useful for treating acute glaucoma when nausea is present or an intravenous line cannot be placed.

Osmotics

Osmotic agents, such as mannitol, isosorbide, and glycerol, are thought to reduce IOP by decreasing the vitreous volume.[8] There may be some effect mediated through the interaction of the central nervous system and optic nerve, although this remains poorly understood.[9] These agents can be given orally or intravenously and are used for emergent control of dangerously elevated IOP. They should not be given chronically and can cause serious side effects.[10]

Glycerol (or glycerin) is administered orally as a 50% solution. The dose is 11.5 g/kg lean body weight. Glycerol is metabolized as a carbohydrate and, if given repeatedly, can cause serious metabolic disturbances in patients with diabetes.[11] Peak IOP reduction after glycerol administration is reached in approximately 30 minutes and lasts for 5 hours.[12]

Isosorbide is also an oral hyperosmotic agent. The dose is 11.5 g/kg lean body weight. Because it is excreted largely unmetabolized in the urine, it is safer for patients with diabetes than glycerin. The peak IOP reduction of isosorbide is reached 1 to 2 hours after administration and lasts for 3 to 5 hours.[13]

Mannitol is a potent osmotic agent that is administered intravenously. It is rapidly excreted unmetabolized in the urine. The recommended dose is 12 g/kg administered in a 20% solution over 20 to 30 minutes.[14] The onset of action occurs within an hour and lasts for up to 6 hours. Due to the rapid infusion of a large volume of fluid, intravenous osmotic agents can precipitate renal or congestive heart failure, and consultation with an internist or family practitioner should be considered before administering mannitol to patients with significant cardiac or renal disease.[15,16]

In general, due to concern about potentially severe systemic side effects, hyperosmotic agents are rarely used in practice today for the management of acutely elevated IOP.

Corticosteroids

If markedly increased IOP is due to ocular inflammation from uveitis in the presence of an open angle on gonioscopy, cautious use of topical corticosteroids may effectively lower the IOP in some cases.

Prostaglandin Analogs

Although prostaglandin analogs are the most commonly used first-line agents for lowering IOP in patients with open-angle glaucoma, there is little role for the use of these agents in patients who require acute IOP lowering. These agents often take 10 to 14 hours before they exert their peak effect on IOP. Furthermore, because they are pro-inflammatory, they can exacerbate inflammation caused by uveitis or acute angle-closure crisis.

MEDICAL MANAGEMENT

After the patient with extremely elevated IOP is examined, an initial working diagnosis is made. Patients can usually be placed into 1 of 2 groups: acutely elevated IOP with marked symptoms or acutely elevated IOP with few or mild symptoms. Treatment can be devised accordingly (see Table 17-2).

All patient groups benefit from maximal aqueous suppressant therapy. Topical beta-blockers, apraclonidine, and CAIs should all be used when the patient's medical condition permits.

Miotics should only be used when the patient has pupillary block glaucoma or open-angle glaucoma without associated inflammation or angle recession. In all other cases, miotics should be deferred until the effect of aqueous suppressant therapy has been determined.

In the patient who is markedly symptomatic, especially one with acute angle-closure crisis in which nausea and vomiting are pronounced, promptly administering acetazolamide can produce a rapid reduction in IOP. Once IOP has been reduced to safer levels, definitive management of the underlying cause is pursued.

SURGICAL MANAGEMENT

Preparing for Surgery

When IOP cannot be lowered by using medications alone, in the acute setting, occasionally it is necessary to intervene surgically. In circumstances when surgery is necessary, administrating IOP-lowering medications prior to and at the time of surgery can minimize the risks of intraoperative bleeding, which may occur when operating on an eye that has markedly elevated IOP.

Depending on the cause of the IOP elevation, there are other interventions that can be administered that can reduce the risks associated with surgery. For example, for patients who have neovascular glaucoma, injecting anti-vascular endothelial growth factor (VEGF) agents such as bevacizumab or ranibizumab into the vitreous cavity or anterior chamber prior to surgical intervention can be beneficial.[16] Occasionally, the use of these agents can cause regression of the angle neovascularization re-establishing outflow of aqueous from the eye. When neovascularization of the angle is long-standing and permanent synechiae have developed, anti-VEGF agents are often ineffective at re-establishing outflow through the trabecular meshwork. However, there is still a role for the use of these agents to help cause regression of the iris neovascularization, which can limit the risk of intraoperative or postoperative bleeding. When possible, it is helpful to administer these agents 24 to 48 hours prior to performing incisional surgery. Patients with neovascular glaucoma may also benefit from topical corticosteroids and cycloplegics prior to surgery.

Surgical Interventions

Peripheral Iridotomy

The definitive treatment for pupillary block angle closure is the creation of a peripheral iridotomy. In most cases, this is accomplished using an argon or yttrium-aluminum-garnet (YAG) laser. Rarely, it may be necessary to perform a surgical iridectomy. Most commonly, this occurs in cases where laser is not possible, for example where media opacity or other anterior segment issues preclude adequate laser treatment. Less commonly, surgical intervention may be necessary where the patient is unable to cooperate for laser treatment or has nystagmus. Whenever possible, it is best to try to break the attack of acute angle-closure crisis using medications and wait a few days until the inflammation has decreased and the corneal edema has cleared before performing this procedure. However, in circumstances when the IOP cannot be reduced using medications alone or it is unsafe to use IOP-lowering medications, it may be necessary to intervene surgically in the setting of markedly elevated IOP.

It can be challenging to perform laser or incisional surgical interventions on patients with markedly elevated IOP because often these patients are very uncomfortable. Judicious use of analgesics and antiemetics can help reduce patient discomfort. A retrobulbar block can also help alleviate the discomfort associated with marked IOP elevation so that the clinician can more easily perform laser or surgical iridectomy.

The recommended technique for laser peripheral iridotomy and surgical iridectomy is described in Chapter 55. Chapter 57 describes how to perform laser iridoplasty, a technique that can be effective at acutely opening the angle when visualization of the iris to perform laser peripheral iridotomy is impaired.

Challenges associated with performing these procedures when the IOP is acutely elevated include reduced visualization of the iris and other structures in the anterior chamber, the need for increased laser energy to penetrate through a thickened inflamed iris, and the increased risk of intraoperative or postoperative bleeding. To improve visualization, a paracentesis can be performed to lower the IOP prior to performing the iridotomy.[1]

Trabeculectomy/Glaucoma Drainage Device Insertion

In settings when the IOP is acutely elevated as a result of mechanisms other than pupillary-block angle closure, it may be warranted to perform a trabeculectomy or implant a glaucoma drainage device. While it is beyond the scope of this chapter to discuss how to perform these procedures, this section will describe techniques that can improve the safety and effectiveness of these procedures in the setting of markedly elevated IOP.

When performing filtering surgery or implanting a glaucoma drainage device in a patient with markedly elevated IOP, it is often useful to gradually rather than abruptly lower the IOP during the surgery. This can be achieved through the use of intravenous acetazolamide or IV mannitol prior to surgery. Another effective strategy is to perform a paracentesis at the start of the procedure, creating a pathway for aqueous to gradually drain through over the course of the procedure. During trabeculectomy, once the sclerostomy is created, the IOP will abruptly drop, and the surgeon can control the IOP by adjusting the tension of the partial-thickness flap sutures. During glaucoma drainage device surgery, when using flow-restrictive devices, the IOP will normalize once the sclerostomy is created and the tube is inserted into the anterior chamber. Because nonflow-restrictive devices are usually tied-off until a capsule has formed around the plate of the implant, the IOP will remain elevated. There are several options for acutely lowering IOP when using nonflow-restrictive implants, such as the Baerveldt or Molteno devices. One option is to include the creation of venting slits (small punctures in the lumen of the tube that allow aqueous to percolate through) in the implant. Other options include creation of an orphan trabeculectomy at the same time as implanting the nonvalved device or the simultaneous insertion of a flow-restricted device such

as an Ahmed S3. The orphan trabeculectomy or Ahmed S3 will function to control the IOP for a few weeks until a capsule has formed around the flow-restricted device.

Cyclophotocoagulation

In eyes that have poor visual potential, an effective option for acutely lowering the IOP and helping reduce discomfort is the use of trans-scleral diode cyclophotocoagulation. Chapter 56 describes the preferred technique for performing this procedure.

REFERENCES

1. Lam D, Chua J, Tham, C, et al. Efficacy and safety of immediate anterior chamber paracentesis in the treatment of acute primary angle-closure glaucoma: a pilot study. *Ophthalmology*. 2002;109:(1):64-70.
2. Gharagozloo NZ, Brubaker RF. Effect of apraclonidine in long-term timolol users. *Ophthalmology*. 1991;98:1543-1546.
3. Koskela T, Brubaker RF. Apraclonidine and timolol. Combined effects in previously untreated normal subjects. *Arch Ophthalmol*. 1991;109:804-806.
4. Greco JJ, Kelman CD. Systemic pilocarpine toxicity in the treatment of angle closure glaucoma. *Ann Ophthalmol*. 1973;5:57-59.
5. Airaksinen PJ, Saari KM, Tiainen TJ, et al. Management of acute closed angle glaucoma with miotics and timolol. *Br J Ophthalmol*. 1979;63:822.
6. Bartlett JD, Jaanus SD. *Clinical Ocular Pharmacology*. 5th ed. Philadelphia, PA: Elsevier Health Sciences; 2008:128.
7. Lippa EA, Carlson LE, Ehinger B, et al. Dose response and duration of action of dorzolamide, a topical carbonic anhydrase inhibitor. *Arch Ophthalmol*. 1992;110:495-499.
8. Robbins R, Galin MA. Effect of osmotic agents on the vitreous body. *Arch Ophthalmol*. 1969;82:694-699.
9. Podos SM, Krupin T, Becker B. Effect of small-dose hyperosmotic injections on intraocular pressure of small animals and man when optic nerves are transected and intact. *Am J Ophthalmol*. 1971;71:898-903.
10. Grabie MT, Gipstein RM, Adams DA, et al. Contraindications for mannitol in aphakic glaucoma. *Am J Ophthalmol*. 1981;91:265-267.
11. Oakley DE, Ellis PP. Glycerol and hyperosmolar nonketotic coma. *Am J Ophthalmol*. 1976;81:469-472.
12. Virno M, Cantore P, Bietti C, et al. Oral glycerol in ophthalmology. A valuable new method for the reduction of intraocular pressure. *Am J Ophthalmol*. 1963;55:1133-1142.
13. Mehra KS, Singh R. Lowering of intraocular pressure by isosorbide. Effects of different doses of drug. *Arch Ophthalmol*. 1971;86(6):623-625.
14. Smith EW, Drance SM. Reduction of human intraocular pressure with intravenous mannitol. *Arch Ophthalmol*. 1962;68:734-737.
15. Havener WH. *Ocular Pharmacology*. 4th ed. St Louis, MO: CV Mosby; 1978:440.
16. Chalam KV, Gupta SK, Grover S, Brar VS, Agarwal S. Intracameral Avastin dramatically resolves iris neovascularization and reverses neovascular glaucoma. *Eur J Ophthalmol*. 2008;18(2):255-262.

18

Primary Open-Angle Glaucoma

Kimberly V. Miller, MD; Joel S. Schuman, MD, FACS; and David L. Epstein, MD, MMM

GENERAL CONSIDERATIONS

Primary Versus Secondary

The overriding fundamental distinction is between open-angle and angle-closure glaucomas. These are all often called primary when there is no apparent ocular or systemic cause and secondary when there is an identifiable initiating ocular or systemic mechanism. Because there is likely more than one mechanism of primary open-angle glaucoma (POAG), the disease entity should likely be termed the POAGs. (Similarly, primary angle-closure glaucoma is usually due to pupillary block, but plateau iris, an uncommon condition, is also often called a form of primary angle-closure glaucoma.) In some ways, these terms are not that important except for clinical categorization, because they reflect that we understand some mechanisms, but not others. For example, it is not uncommon for a patient with apparent POAG to later be discovered to have pseudoexfoliation, at which time the diagnosis is changed to that of a secondary open-angle glaucoma (because we believe we now understand the mechanism of that glaucoma; see Chapter 20).

Also, by analogy, secondary forms of angle-closure glaucoma can involve the same mechanism for iris occlusion of the trabecular meshwork (TM) as primary causes. For example, an increase in posterior segment volume (eg, acute central retinal vein occlusion) may move the crystalline lens forward and result in pupillary block by this means. Thus, there are common final mechanisms for all the glaucomas, whether primary or secondary.

POAG is so called because it occurs spontaneously, without evident antecedent or related disease and with no known basis other than genetic or hereditary predisposition. This is the most common variety of glaucoma in some parts of the world.

Other types of open-angle glaucoma differ from the so-called primary type by the fact that they characteristically occur in conjunction with specific abnormalities or diseases of the eye that can be considered causative of the associated glaucoma. Such types of secondary open-angle glaucoma include pseudoexfoliation with open-angle glaucoma, amyloidosis with open-angle glaucoma, pigmentary glaucoma, and in special instances, glaucoma after trauma and glaucoma due to intraocular inflammation. These glaucomas are discussed in detail under separate headings in this chapter. However, much of what is to be said concerning the treatment of POAG can be applied equally well to other open-angle glaucomas, except those involving active intraocular inflammation.

POAG itself is a clinically well-defined disease, having moderate variation in its characteristics. A small proportion of cases is extraordinary and fall into subcategories.

PRIMARY OPEN-ANGLE GLAUCOMA IS REALLY A DISEASE OF EXCLUSION (OF SECONDARY CAUSES)

POAG is a diagnosis of exclusion. In all cases, no matter how deep the anterior chamber looks on slit-lamp examination, gonioscopy must be performed. One may be surprised by the observation of heretofore unsuspected angle recession; pigment dispersion or exfoliation; fine, new blood vessels in the angle; partial angle closure; or inflammatory precipitates. In diabetes, neovascularization can occur in the angle before the iris is involved. Any abnormal pigment in the angle needs to be explained (eg, pigmentary glaucoma, exfoliation, iris or ciliary body cysts, or melanoma). Chronic silent angle-closure glaucoma may masquerade as POAG.

We make special mention of the entity of occult inflammatory precipitates in the angle. Chandler termed this form of trabeculitis *occult keratic precipitates (KP) in the angle* and stressed how it could mimic POAG. The eyes are notoriously

Kahook MY, Schuman, JS, eds.
Chandler and Grant's Glaucoma, Fifth Edition (pp 185-206).
© 2013 SLACK Incorporated.

white and quiet with absent to very rare cells in the anterior chamber or precipitates on the corneal endothelium. In fact, a subtle solitary smudge on the corneal endothelium is often all that is visible. Thus, this diagnosis is often missed unless careful gonioscopy is performed. Patients do not have obvious uveitis. Another characteristic of this entity is the fact that patients do not respond well to intraocular pressure (IOP)-lowering medications, especially miotics. If patients are placed on standard antiglaucoma therapy and do not show a therapeutic response, gonioscopy should be repeated looking for this entity (as well as other causes, such as previously unsuspected angle closure and neovascularization). Patients with occult KP in the angle commonly need to be maintained on chronic low-dose steroid therapy indefinitely to control the glaucoma.

Paul Chandler, MD, followed several patients with occult KP in the angle. Commonly, intervals may occur when the trabeculitis would slightly worsen, necessitating more intensive steroid therapy. Dr. Chandler would send the patient to the emergency room and instruct the patient not to tell the resident his or her diagnosis, but to have the resident call him. He would then ask the resident what the diagnosis was and what was seen with the *jewel* (gonioscopy lens). (Thus, Dr. Chandler evaluated his residents!)

The presence of KP on the TM can be subtle, mainly because, in their earliest stage, they are clear, and it is easy to look right through them at the angle. One of us (DLE) recalls the first time Dr. Grant called him down to the Glaucoma Clinic to see such a patient. DLE was a pre-resident fellow at the time, eager to learn from his mentor. However, upon looking into the angle, DLE was unable to discern the KP until, after some time with the illuminator becoming hot in his hand, his hand began to slightly tremble and the light subsequently caught the scleral spur adjacent to a KP and retroilluminated it. The KP jumped out at DLE, and it was stunning that he had somehow previously missed it (he wondered what else he had missed). By using this trick of scleral spur retroillumination, almost a dozen KPs were then identified in the entire angle circumference. This experience has been repeated (more subtly) many more times. If one suspects occult KP in the angle, one can view 360 degrees of the angle and perhaps see a questionable area, but as one repeats the circumferential process, multiple trabecular precipitates can often be detected. (DLE always remembers that this angle sleuthing was how Dr. Chandler evaluated the quality of his residents.)

CLINICAL CHARACTERISTICS

In POAG, the angle of the anterior chamber may be wide or narrow, but it remains open at all times, whether the disease is early or advanced and whether IOP is normal or elevated. Even in eyes that have been blind for many years from this type of glaucoma, the angle remains open, unless neovascular glaucoma has become superimposed. The gonioscopic appearance of the angle of the anterior chamber in most cases of POAG is no different from that in normal individuals. Open-angle glaucoma cannot be cured by presently available means, but it can often be controlled by various medical and surgical measures.

In POAG, the facility of aqueous outflow from the anterior chamber is constantly subnormal, whereas the IOP may vary in the course of a day from normal to significantly elevated pressures. This decreased facility of outflow persists throughout the rest of the patient's life and tends to worsen with the passage of time.

The clinical manifestations of POAG vary considerably. In most cases, the glaucoma develops in middle life or later, and the onset is usually gradual and asymptomatic. In the early stages, IOP may be only slightly elevated, but it is higher when the disease is more advanced.

When open-angle glaucoma develops in patients younger than 50 years of age, especially in the 20s and 30s, the onset of elevated IOP in many cases appears to be more abrupt. In this younger group, symptoms of transient blurring of vision and seeing colored haloes around lights are not uncommon. At the first examination, in some younger patients, one may find an IOP of 40 to 70 mm Hg, despite the presence of a normal optic disc and full visual fields. These findings suggest that elevated IOP, especially to such a high level, has not been present for long. A history of transient blurred vision and seeing colored haloes is perfectly consistent in a young individual with a diagnosis of POAG. These symptoms are an indication that there is a considerable and probably rapid increase of IOP, but do not mean that an emergency has arisen and that the glaucoma cannot be controlled medically.

These symptoms occur also in angle-closure glaucoma, and the type of glaucoma must be positively identified. In angle-closure glaucoma, the symptoms of blurring and haloes have an entirely different significance, indicating closure of a considerable portion of the angle and calling for urgent vigorous treatment (eg, laser iridotomy).

Not all of the younger patients have a rapid onset of open-angle glaucoma. In some, the onset is gradual and asymptomatic, as it characteristically is in the older patients.

Whatever the mode of onset of open-angle glaucoma, the disease tends to progress steadily with time. Whatever the cause of the impairment of outflow from the anterior chamber, the outflow tends to become further impaired as time passes. This may not mean in all cases that the IOP steadily rises, for in some older patients with marked obstruction to outflow, the IOP remains, or becomes in time, relatively low due to a lowered rate of aqueous formation.

DIAGNOSIS

The diagnosis of POAG is usually made by routine tonometry and by inspection of the optic nerve heads. The importance of the latter cannot be overemphasized. The IOP at a given examination may be in a normal phase, but if the disc is abnormal, suspicion should be immediately aroused.

If the disc is normal and routine tonometry reveals an IOP at the upper limit of normal, various tests may be used, such as visual field testing, scanning laser polarimetry, confocal scanning laser topography, or optical coherence tomography (OCT; see Chapter 9). Once the ophthalmologist's suspicion is aroused, he or she is bound to keep the patient under close observation. If the patient does in fact have early glaucoma, it will become apparent sooner or later in subsequent examinations.

An IOP of 22 mm Hg or more with the Goldmann applanation tonometer (Haag-Streit, Mason, OH) should arouse suspicion of glaucoma. Screening of all close relatives of a patient with glaucoma will reveal a higher incidence of glaucoma than in the general population.

Many cases of apparent POAG can be diagnosed by inspection of the optic disc. If the optic disc shows changes suggesting glaucoma, even if IOP at the time is normal, further investigation will usually lead to a definite diagnosis. One learns in time to recognize the earliest glaucomatous appearance of the optic disc (see Chapter 8), so that even if the IOP is well within normal limits, one may be sufficiently suspicious to go on to additional subsequent examinations to detect the presence of POAG (or other forms of open-angle glaucoma, eg, normal-tension glaucoma).

Asymmetry of the physiologic cup between the 2 eyes is a significant finding in early detection of open-angle glaucoma. Even though individually each cup appears physiologic and does not reach the disc margin anywhere, if the cup in one eye is definitely different from the cup in the other eye, one's suspicions should always be aroused. Even if at first the IOP is equal in the 2 eyes and well within the normal limits, if the cup is definitely larger in one eye than in the other, the patient should be followed as a glaucoma suspect. In a large number of patients who we have seen and followed, asymmetry of the physiologic cups has been a finding in early open-angle glaucoma.

As a personal illustration, when the son of Dr. Grant was in medical school and was practicing on his father with the ophthalmoscope, he remarked that the optic disc in one eye looked different from that in the other. Dr. Grant confirmed the fact that the physiologic cup was a little wider in the left eye than in the right. IOP was 18 mm Hg in both eyes. Facility of outflow was normal and equal in the 2 eyes on several occasions, but 5 years later, obstruction to outflow became measurable in the eye with the larger cup, and the IOP elevated to a glaucomatous level.

Other early changes in the cup of the optic disc, apart from asymmetry that suggest glaucoma, are as follows:

- A cup that reaches the disc margin at any point, but most commonly inferiorly
- A slight bending of all vessels at the margin
- An appearance (difficult to describe) of little or no bending of vessels at the margin, but gives the impression that the whole disc has a shallow saucer-like depression to the margins, which might be called saucerization of the disc (see Figures 8-8 and 8-12)

Many times we have suspected glaucoma from a slight bending of the vessels at the margin of the disc, or this appearance of saucerization, and the diagnosis has later been confirmed. In normal eyes, the neuroretinal rim generally obeys the ISNT rule. That is, the inferior (I) rim of the optic nerve is the thickest, followed sequentially by the superior (S) rim, nasal (N) rim, and temporal (T) rim. Deviation from this pattern should arouse additional suspicion of glaucomatous damage. One must practice looking at optic discs very critically, and eventually, one will become expert at picking out those that should arouse suspicion of early glaucoma. While the instrumentation described in Chapter 9 helps the clinician with the diagnosis, such optic nerve sleuthing is not obsolete, and the clinician is still obliged to identify even the most subtle disc abnormalities.

The characteristic progressive changes in the discs in glaucoma are described in greater detail, with diagrams, in Chapter 8.

An exception to be remembered is that, in high myopia, it may be extremely difficult to diagnose early glaucoma by the appearance of the optic disc, whereas it is easier to diagnose it in the average eye. In trying to determine whether glaucoma is present in a case of considerable myopia, special care is necessary.

Another special condition of the optic nerve head that is suggestive of glaucoma is occlusion of the central retinal vein in one eye. In such a case, both eyes should be studied carefully for open-angle glaucoma (especially pseudoexfoliation) because a high percentage of patients having occlusion of the central vein in one eye turn out to have open-angle glaucoma in both eyes, either frankly present then or diagnosed later. After occlusion of the central retinal vein, the fellow eye is usually the better eye for vision, so it should receive special attention and early treatment for elevated IOP.

PROVOCATIVE AND CONFIRMATORY TESTS

Tonography

In the past, when suspicion of glaucoma had been aroused by a borderline IOP or a suggestive disc, tonography was used to reveal an impaired facility of outflow that led to a definite diagnosis on the basis of the IOP divided by outflow facility (Po/C).

Water-Drinking Test

An increase in IOP of 8 to 10 mm Hg after rapid ingestion of a quart of water strongly suggests glaucoma, but a negative test does not rule it out. Tonography plus a water-drinking test may reveal an abnormality in cases in which either test alone is inconclusive. Although theoretically useful, we have, in truth, only rarely performed a water-drinking test in recent years and do not recommend it for routine use. On the other hand, some investigators recently have found this test to be of use.[1]

Time

Once glaucoma is suspected, either on the basis of IOP or a suggestive disc, the patient should be kept under observation indefinitely. If glaucoma is developing, eventually, one will find definite elevation of IOP or definite glaucomatous changes in the disc. Stereo disc photographs as well as visual field testing and structural imaging are important bits of the baseline information.

One keeps seeing the patient several times a year. If the patient does have glaucoma, sooner or later, unequivocally elevated IOP and/or optic disc changes are found. Of course, during this time, close watch is kept on the optic nerve appearance and visual fields to be sure that no appreciable change is occurring. Such a leisurely approach is justified only in patients in whom the optic nerve heads have no more than physiologic cupping. If there is pathologic cupping, atrophy, or field loss with initial equivocal IOP measurements, one must examine the problem more intensively and not wait unduly to initiate antiglaucoma therapy. The IOP might be in a normal phase of diurnal fluctuation, or the patient might have a form of normal-tension glaucoma (see Chapter 19).

DIFFERENTIAL DIAGNOSIS

If IOP is definitely elevated or the disc shows definite changes characteristic of glaucoma, one must determine whether the glaucoma is POAG, angle-closure glaucoma, or some form of secondary glaucoma.

If gonioscopy is carried out when IOP is elevated and the angle is seen to be open throughout, angle-closure glaucoma is ruled out, even if the angle is narrow. If the IOP is normal because the patient is already under treatment when gonioscopy is carried out, the finding of a narrow but open angle is inconclusive. Treatment must then be discontinued to allow the IOP to increase, and gonioscopy is repeated. If the angle is still open throughout, the diagnosis is open-angle glaucoma. On the other hand, if one finds closure of the angle consistent with the degree of elevation of IOP (see Chapters 22 and 24), the diagnosis is angle-closure glaucoma. Sometimes, it is difficult to be sure whether a portion of the angle is closed or almost closed, and repeated examination may be necessary, especially in cases in which the IOP without treatment is only moderately elevated. Ultrasound biomicroscopy or anterior segment OCT can be helpful to discern whether or not the angle is closed in these cases. If IOP without treatment increases above 35 mm Hg, in cases under investigation to determine whether one is dealing with open-angle glaucoma with a narrow angle or angle-closure

glaucoma, it is usually not difficult to determine whether there is sufficient closure to account for the elevated IOP. If IOP without treatment increases only to 28 or 30 mm Hg, little of the angle needs to be closed to account for such a moderate elevation of the IOP. It is particularly in these cases that the differential diagnosis between open-angle glaucoma with a narrow angle and angle-closure glaucoma is most difficult.

Beta-blockers, alpha-2 agonists, and carbonic anhydrase inhibitors (CAIs), due to their suppression of aqueous formation, cause some widening of the angle. One may be deceived as to the true width of the angle. In cases in which the angle appears narrow but open while the patient is using these drugs, it may appear narrower or partially closed after the drugs are discontinued.

One must always rule out secondary glaucoma before deciding on a diagnosis of POAG. The possibility that the glaucoma may be secondary to some other abnormality of the eye is one of the many good reasons why one should never omit gonioscopy in any case of glaucoma, no matter if it seems obvious from the appearance at slit-lamp examination that the angle must be wide and open. Findings in the angle that may not be suspected from slit-lamp examination, but that are revealed by gonioscopic examination, and that indicate that the glaucoma is secondary and not primary are peripheral anterior synechia, abnormal vessels, abnormal pigmentation, exudates (KP) on the uveal or corneoscleral meshwork, tumors in the angle, and disruption of the angle from trauma. These abnormal findings in the angle are discussed more fully in chapters on the individual secondary glaucomas.

Finding glaucoma in only one eye while the other eye is completely normal is strongly discordant with a diagnosis of POAG and indicates that one is probably dealing with some other type of glaucoma. However, it is not unusual to have POAG advanced to a more severe stage in one eye than in the other eye, and one must have good tonographic measurements or IOP curves to be sure whether an eye in question is normal. Differential diagnosis of glaucoma restricted to one eye is discussed in Chapter 40.

NORMAL VERSUS ABNORMAL INTRAOCULAR PRESSURE

By general convention, IOPs above 22 mm Hg are considered to be either abnormal or suspicious of being abnormal. This arose originally from population studies in which the mean IOP of normal individuals was determined, and thereby IOPs greater than 2 or 3 standard deviations from this normal mean were defined as being abnormal. However, there are several flaws in the logic of these definitions.

In population studies, patients with frank glaucomatous optic nerve changes and field loss may have a normal IOP, especially if only one measurement is made.[2-5] As mentioned in Chapter 1, our clinical methods of detecting early optic nerve damage or unequivocal visual field loss from glaucoma are not very sensitive. Even with the most sophisticated imaging techniques available today, it can be difficult to discriminate very early glaucoma damage. Therefore, it may be difficult to categorize people as "normal." Finally, the same logic, if applied to systemic hypertension, would result in patients at risk not receiving what is regarded as necessary therapy; with age, systemic hypertension increases in prevalence to seemingly affect as many as one-third of the elderly population (with risk of future end-organ damage).[6-9] Yet, if one surveyed an elderly population and calculated the mean blood pressure and only considered abnormality as being a certain number of standard deviations from the mean, one would mislabel many patients who have systemic hypertension as being normal. Statistical methods of identifying normality are useful only for establishing general guidelines rather than distinct criteria, especially when it is usual or normal for a disease to have a higher prevalence in a certain population.

In many ways, the glaucomas share characteristics with other diseases of aging. Although it may be normal to age, as physicians, we want to intervene to stabilize and prevent further development of aging processes. (Death itself can be considered normal for a certain age group!)

We also know that progressive low-tension glaucoma (LTG; normal-tension glaucoma) is a real entity that in the vast majority of patients has some IOP-sensitive component (see Chapter 19). In LTG, there is something substantially wrong with the optic nerve that we do not fully understand. Ultimately, we need to develop intervention remedies that correct or treat this susceptibility of the optic nerve to glaucomatous damage. However, there is a large body of clinical evidence obtained over long periods that substantiates the clinical impression that decreasing IOP, especially to a very low level, does alter the natural history of this disease in a favorable way. Perhaps, controlled clinical trials may alter this opinion, but at the present time the available clinical information strongly suggests the need to decrease IOP in LTG, which is constituted by more than one entity.[10] The clinical implications of this are that IOP below 22 mm Hg, even if repeatable, may not be normal and, therefore, still can encompass glaucomatous disease.

Further, the original Chandler–Grant tenet[11] that an optic nerve damaged by glaucoma commonly requires a lower-than-normal IOP has now achieved generally wide acceptance. Therefore, for patients with known glaucoma, an IOP simply in the normal range is not necessarily adequate to prevent further progression of the disease.[12]

What then is the clinician to do with the IOP data? What is an abnormal IOP? The diseases of glaucoma behave clinically as if individual eyes (or pairs of eyes) have an individual susceptibility to a given level of IOP that can only be determined for that patient by long-term follow-up. A significant goal in the clinical practice of glaucoma is to

better understand the reasons for this individual susceptibility. We have some guidelines, but the key to the detection of glaucoma is not simply the measurement of IOP but also the simultaneous evaluation of the optic nerve and visual field (the methods for which have their own uncertainties in sensitivity and accuracy).

Glaucoma screenings should therefore involve not only IOP measurements but also ophthalmoscopic evaluation of the optic nerve appearance, and preferably structural imaging and functional testing as well. In any suspect patient, we should obtain stereo disc photographs because, in the progression of glaucoma, the appearance of the cup of the optic nerve will change. Structural imaging will provide an objective, quantitative measure that can be compared to the healthy population and followed for change. In the long-term care of patients with glaucoma or suspicion of glaucoma, it is remarkable how often we wish we had baseline photographs and quantitative imaging data from previous years to assist our clinical judgment. It is excellent ophthalmologic care to obtain stereo disc photographs and structural imaging on any patient with a suspicion of glaucoma or a future risk of developing glaucoma.

ELEVATED INTRAOCULAR PRESSURE ABOVE 22 MM HG

We have so far dealt with the clinical fact that a statistically normal IOP does not by itself indicate the absence of glaucoma. How about the opposite question: Does the presence of an IOP above 22 mm Hg indicate an abnormal condition, that is, the presence of glaucoma?

For this question also, there is surprising uncertainty and varying opinions that have changed over time. Clinically, a great number of patients exist whose optic nerves (and visual fields) seem to tolerate IOPs in the mid- to upper-20s without apparent damage. However, the key word is "seem." Our clinical methods to detect early axonal death in the optic nerve are not very sensitive, but are improving. Structural imaging provides a more sensitive and quantitative, objective measure than simple optic disc examination alone. Glaucoma for the ophthalmologist is truly the "curse" of long-term follow-up, and such observations have led many to realize that elevated IOP is not as benign as once thought. Studies[13-15] have indicated that there is a protective effect of lowering IOP in patients who initially had no apparent end-organ damage. Probably (although not with certainty until our methods can truly detect early damage), there are individuals with IOP elevated into the 20s who will never suffer clinically detectable optic nerve damage, but prospectively it is impossible to identify all such individuals.

One can view this in terms of relative risk. There are risk factors[16] that increase the chances for optic nerve damage, such as the degree of IOP elevation, having large or asymmetrical cups, thin retinal nerve fiber layer, abnormal tonographic outflow,[13] the presence of myopia,[17] a strong family history, African American race,[18] the presence of disc hemorrhages, or below-average central corneal thickness.[19] However, we know that, by treating even patients not considered clinically to be at excessive risk, the risk of developing end-organ damage is reduced.[13-15] In the Boston study,[13] it was clinically sobering to realize that such a protective effect was not apparent at 2 years of follow-up, but only after longer time periods. In the Ocular Hypertension Treatment Study (OHTS),[20] it was clear that the protective effect of treatment increased over time. In those whose treatment was withheld and then started years later, while they developed a parallel risk of developing glaucoma compared to those treated at the outset, they always had a higher risk of manifesting the disease.[20] Early treatment is key, even in glaucoma suspects.

There are strong analogies to a similar clinical question in the treatment of asymptomatic mild-systemic hypertension, where controlled studies have indicated the protective effect of early treatment,[21] and therefore the clinical implication has been to treat all patients with mild elevation of blood pressure, even those without additional risk factors. Yet, a critical examination of the data on which this is based indicates that internists have chosen to treat perhaps a majority of such patients who seemingly will not develop end-organ damage to protect a minority who will, because they cannot prospectively identify those individuals who will develop clinical disease.

We face the same question and dilemma in treating (or not) asymptomatic elevation of IOP. (Glaucoma and systemic hypertension are not totally unrelated diseases from an epidemiologic point of view [see Chapter 4][22]). Although perhaps it could be argued to wait to treat elevated IOP until clinical damage is detected, we also know (from long-term clinical observations) that once a disc is damaged, it commonly requires a progressively lower IOP to prevent further damage. IOP elevation results in damage not only to axons, but to the supporting structures of the optic nerve itself, the cells of the lamina cribrosa, and the extracellular matrix.[23,24] One could hypothesize that a disc damaged by elevated pressure is more susceptible to further damage due to the changes in the substance of the optic nerve head. The implication of this is that earlier preventative treatment could make the subsequent glaucoma less difficult to treat. (Although this latter statement has never been proven, it is the logical deduction from the clinical observation that a disc, once damaged, requires a lower-than-usual IOP for stability.)

We return again to this problem in glaucoma of individual susceptibility of the optic nerve of a given patient, in which general rules or statistical considerations are probably not as meaningful as the detailed clinical observation of the individual patient, using all the clinical means that we have available to document what is present, so that we can accurately detect future change. This individual susceptibility and variability is what makes it impossible to precisely define a normal or abnormal IOP (except for very high IOP levels). However, it is curious how this was defined

25 years ago as IOP in the 40s, where now it is regarded as IOP in the 30s).

A further complicating factor was mentioned in Chapter 1: although the measurement of IOP is usually (but not always) an accurate data point, it is just a snapshot in time. Due to diurnal and seasonal fluctuation in IOP, we are not yet able to determine the true representative (eg, mean, median, or time integrated) IOP of any given patient.

WHEN TO TREAT (WHEN THERE IS NO OBVIOUS END-ORGAN DAMAGE)

A few decades ago, the prevailing clinical opinion was that IOPs below a certain cut-off, usually in the 30- to 33-mm Hg range, did not require antiglaucoma therapy unless there was evidence of optic nerve damage or visual field loss (for which the IOP would be vigorously treated!). There was a belief among some that elevated IOP (to even higher levels than the low-30s) could be a benign separate condition that was sometimes labeled *ocular hypertension*. Regardless, probably most glaucoma clinicians did have an IOP cut-off in the 30-mm Hg range. Today, there is probably general consensus that a separate benign condition of ocular hypertension does not exist (or at least cannot be prospectively distinguished from early POAG), and the cut-off for treating asymptomatic (clinical signs) elevated IOP has been lowered for most clinicians to somewhere in the 20s.

What has been historically curious all along is that when the IOP was elevated from some secondary cause, the threshold of IOP for treatment was in many cases lower than for POAG. We practiced as if elevated IOP in POAG was somehow less damaging than in secondary causes. There is no reason to believe this is true.

The early prospective randomized clinical studies of Epstein et al[13] and Kass et al[14] had different protocols but reached the same conclusion (based on surprisingly similar unexpectedly high rates of clinical failure): lowering the IOP (with a beta-blocker) is protective against end-organ damage. More recently, in a landmark study, the OHTS[15] found that using topical medical therapy to reduce IOP 20% significantly decreased the risk of developing glaucomatous visual field or optic nerve damage.

All clinical studies should be judged by this criterion: does it change the way one practices? A related question involves treating one's patients as one would want his or her own eyes to be treated. The OHTS and earlier studies[13,14] indeed changed clinical practice for many physicians, and, therefore, it seems appropriate to list the following clinical conclusions from OHTS:

- In patients with "elevated" IOP (24 to 32 mm Hg) and no obvious end-organ damage (optic nerve or abnormalities in the visual field), lowering the IOP by a mean of 22.5% is protective against developing end-organ damage as measured by a reproducible visual field defect or reproducible optic disc deterioration attributable to POAG.

- The overall risk of developing progression to glaucoma decreased from 9.5% in the observation group to 4.4% in the treatment group.

- The highest risk of conversion to glaucoma occurred in patients with higher IOP measurements and thinner central corneal thickness measurements.

- Patients with larger vertical cup/disc ratios were more likely to convert to glaucoma than those with smaller cup/disc ratios.

The Boston study,[13] OHTS,[15] the earlier study by Kass et al,[14] and further clinical observation (which is now entering the fifth decade for DLE) have convinced us that moderate elevation of IOP is not as benign a condition as formerly thought. Although exact cut-offs await further studies, we do generally treat patients (except perhaps the elderly) with IOPs of 25 mm Hg or higher with significant risk factors for development of glaucoma, but without identifiable disc or visual field damage. If there are large (even deemed physiological) cups; slight asymmetry of the cups or IOP; thin corneas; severely impaired outflow facility; if the patient is myopic or has a strong family history of POAG; or is an African American treatment for IOPs of 23 mm Hg or higher may be initiated. Obviously, this is modified by individual factors for individual patients, such as their age (because these studies show that damage occurs over years, elevated IOP is therefore a greater risk to younger patients) and side effects from medications (without obvious end-organ damage, such protective therapy, that may not truly be required for all should not disable the patient; if medications cannot be tolerated, the balance of benefits to risks can switch to laser trabeculoplasty or a strategy of close observation). An additional factor to be considered in myopic eyes with POAG is the possibility for the initial field loss to extend close to or actually involve central fixation.

What if the patient without apparent end-organ damage is on therapy, but the IOP exceeds these guidelines? For the patient on maximally tolerated medical therapy already, a decision for surgical intervention usually should require (in the absence of evidence of end-organ damage) very high IOPs (eg, upper-30s or greater). What is known and what is not known should be discussed with the patient who should have input with his or her philosophical wishes (eg, therapeutic activism versus nihilism).

General Principles in Treatment

The goal of treatment in POAG is to prevent loss of visual function. If we prevent loss of function, our treatment is adequate. All of our treatment is designed to lower the IOP, either by increasing the facility of outflow, by suppressing formation of aqueous humor, or both. It is humbling to realize that we have no specific treatment for the outflow abnormality of POAG because the cause is still largely unknown.

There is no absolute level of IOP that must be obtained to ensure successful treatment in all cases. In some eyes with normal optic nerves, if treatment maintains IOP at a level in the mid- or low-20s, no loss of function occurs, and the treatment may be considered successful. On the other hand, in cases of advanced glaucoma, IOP must usually be maintained at much lower levels to prevent continued loss of function.[12] In far advanced glaucoma, IOP in the low teens or lower is required (see next section). The intensity of treatment required may therefore be considerably influenced by the stage of the disease, as evidenced by the condition of the optic nerve and the visual field.

A patient with extensive cupping and considerable field loss, having an initial IOP of 20 mm Hg, should be treated just as vigorously as a patient with a normal disc and IOP in the 40s. Occasionally, one sees a patient of this sort whose IOP is 20 to 22 mm Hg and in whom the IOP can be reduced to less than 15 mm Hg by intensive treatment. Thus, the mere fact that an occasional patient with advanced cupping and field loss does not have a very high IOP does not mean that one should treat him or her with only single-agent antiglaucoma therapy.

A high initial IOP, such as the 40s to the 50s, in patients with little or no field change indicates that the patient has an extremely poor facility of outflow. In such cases, we expect large fluctuations in IOP, often a considerable elevation during a particular portion of the day or night. A slight change in the rate of formation of aqueous humor in such an eye is reflected in a large change in IOP.

Initiating (and Advancing) Treatment With End-Organ Damage

Steps in medical management and laser trabeculoplasty perhaps leading to surgical intervention will be detailed in a subsequent chapter (and also are listed as general guidelines in Table 18-1). However, in terms of general principles, whatever the level of presenting IOP, it is obviously too high, and therefore medical intervention is required to substantially lower the IOP, with an initial goal of 20% to 30% below baseline. Because of the varying susceptibility of an individual's optic nerve to glaucomatous damage (cupping), there is unfortunately no single normal IOP that can be guaranteed to prevent further progression. As always, individual glaucoma patients require individual meticulous follow-up of the optic nerve (with photographic documentation), structural imaging, and visual field, even if the above target for IOP reduction is met. In other words, there are no guarantees of disease stabilization in glaucoma,

TABLE 18-1. GENERAL STRATEGY: STEPS IN MANAGEMENT

1. Prostaglandin analog or laser trabeculoplasty
2. Add others from number 1
3. Beta-blocker
4. Combination agent (beta-blocker plus brimonidine or beta-blocker plus dorzolamide)
5. Add fourth agent (topical CAI or brimonidine)
6. Oral CAI
7. Filtration surgery
CAI: carbonic anhydrase inhibitor.

PRIMARY OPEN-ANGLE GLAUCOMA AND MYOPIA

David L. Epstein, MD, MMM

The reader needs to be aware of an unusual, although not at all rare, syndrome that can occur with POAG and myopia[1]: In myopic eyes, the earliest field loss can extend directly into fixation and can involve central visual acuity. This possibility influences one's threshold IOP for treatment when POAG is associated with myopia. Careful inspection of the directly temporal margin of the disc is important in the assessment of all glaucoma patients, but especially those who are myopic. The normal tilt of the myopic disc makes such analysis very difficult. It is particularly troublesome when one can detect early contour changes. Thus, one usually chooses a lower threshold of IOP elevation to initiate antiglaucoma therapy in such eyes.

REFERENCE

1. Fong DS, Epstein DL, Allingham RR. Glaucoma and myopia: are they related? *Int Ophthalmol Clin.* 1990;30:215-218.

even with initially satisfactory IOP lowering to the arbitrary goal. (Once again, it needs to be mentioned that it would truly revolutionize the field if we could determine accurately what the representative IOP really was, rather than obtain snapshot data points.)

Once an optic nerve is damaged, clinical experience indicates that a lower than merely normal IOP is required. This clinical fact has come from observation of many patients. Clinical appraisal influences the magnitude of the decrease in IOP that is aimed for with antiglaucoma therapy. A damaged optic nerve usually requires an IOP below 18 mm Hg for stability (Figure 18-1). However, a severely damaged optic nerve may require an IOP in the low teens or even lower (depending also on the IOP at which damage occurred) (Table 18-2 and Figures 18-2 and 18-3).

Central visual field testing (24 degrees in most cases, 10 degrees in advanced disease, and probably best if automated so that actual sensitivities close to fixation are measured) is very helpful to identify how much visual field margin there is left to follow. That is, if one achieves significant IOP reduction to the targeted value, but follow-up proves that the target IOP was still too high and that some progression has occurred, if the latter involves increased density of existing scotomata or a new isolated defect away from fixation, then this likely will be of little functional significance in itself, but antiglaucoma therapy can be further escalated. On the other hand, if there is total cupping and the sensitivity close to fixation is already substantially reduced, then an incorrect assessment of acceptable lowering of IOP can lead to progression of loss of field and substantial functional visual loss, including loss of central acuity. In such cases with so little margin to follow, unless there is dramatic lowering of IOP to below levels usually achievable with glaucoma filtration surgery (eg, below 12 mm Hg), it is often wise to proceed rapidly to fistulizing surgery. (IOPs in the upper-single numbers usually confer stability for such patients).

In progressive normal-tension glaucoma (NTG), there is an IOP-sensitive component in most cases, although

unfortunately this is not the entire story. One needs to conceptualize that the statistically normal level of IOP has resulted in damage to the susceptible (due to unknown causes) optic nerve, and therefore the IOP needs to be reduced by at least 20%. Starting with normal IOPs, such a target for IOP reduction is sometimes difficult to achieve in NTG except by fistulizing surgery, but the usual steps should be applied, unless there is no margin to follow (in which case fistulizing surgery should be promptly performed).

For every patient, a target for desired IOP should be set prospectively and written in the chart. This is not an exact science, and sometimes due to other considerations of age, side effects from medications, or the patient's own input after full discussion, one may modify this. (Except for advanced disease with no margin to follow, the decisions for use of oral CAIs or incisional glaucoma surgery require documented disease progression because of their inherent increased risks.) However, glaucoma charts tend to get cluttered, and setting such a target pressure in writing assists clarity of thought and effective patient management.

General guidelines for target IOP are presented in Table 18-2. These are not set in stone and are modifiable, depending on many of the factors discussed above, including information about the level of IOP at which damage occurred. For lesser amounts of glaucomatous damage, the target IOP in the table represents a reasonable goal for IOP, at which, if further progression were to occur due to individual susceptibility, there is sufficient margin to be able to assess this without the patient experiencing any (further) functional impairment. For greater amounts of glaucomatous damage indicated in the table, the target IOP chosen reflects the fact that there is progressively less "margin" available to follow the patient further without the risk of progressive functional impairment. As indicated previously, in the extreme, if field loss involves central fixation, then one is justified to proceed rapidly to incisional surgery to achieve the very low IOP levels required (Table 18-3).

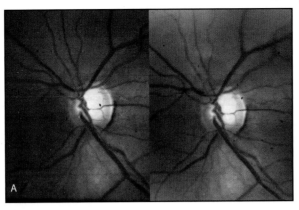

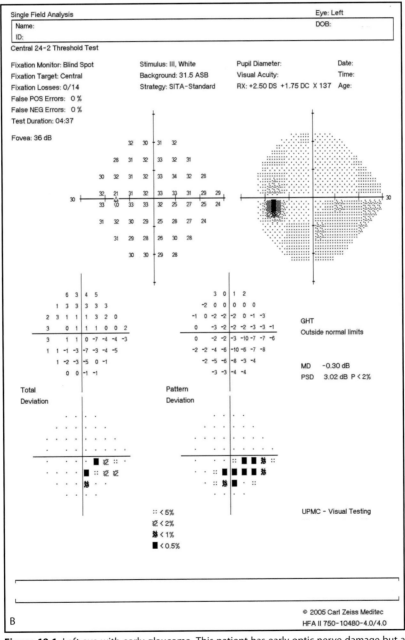

Figure 18-1. Left eye with early glaucoma. This patient has early optic nerve damage but a full visual field. Target IOP is 18 mm Hg (previous IOP mid-20s). (A) Stereoscopic optic disc photography. (B) Humphrey 24-2 visual field. (C) OCT. (D) Confocal scanning laser ophthalmoscopy. (E) Scanning laser polarimetry.

PAGE 194 Chapter 18

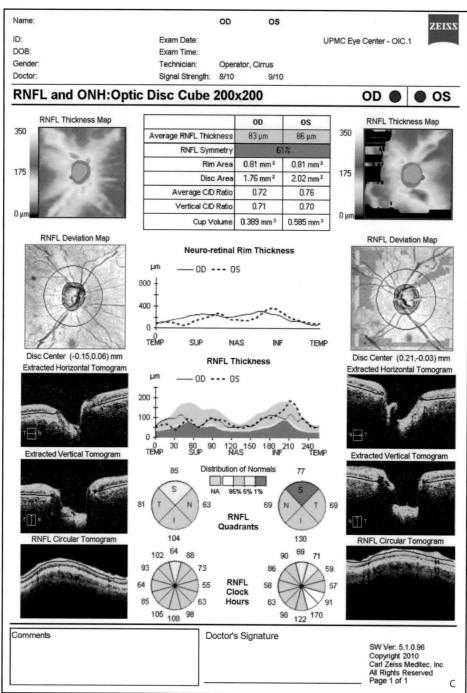

Figure 18-1. *(Continued)* Left eye with early glaucoma. This patient has early optic nerve damage but a full visual field. Target IOP is 18 mm Hg (previous IOP mid-20s). (A) Stereoscopic optic disc photography, (B) Humphrey 24-2 visual field. (C) OCT. (D) Confocal scanning laser ophthalmoscopy. (E) Scanning laser polarimetry.

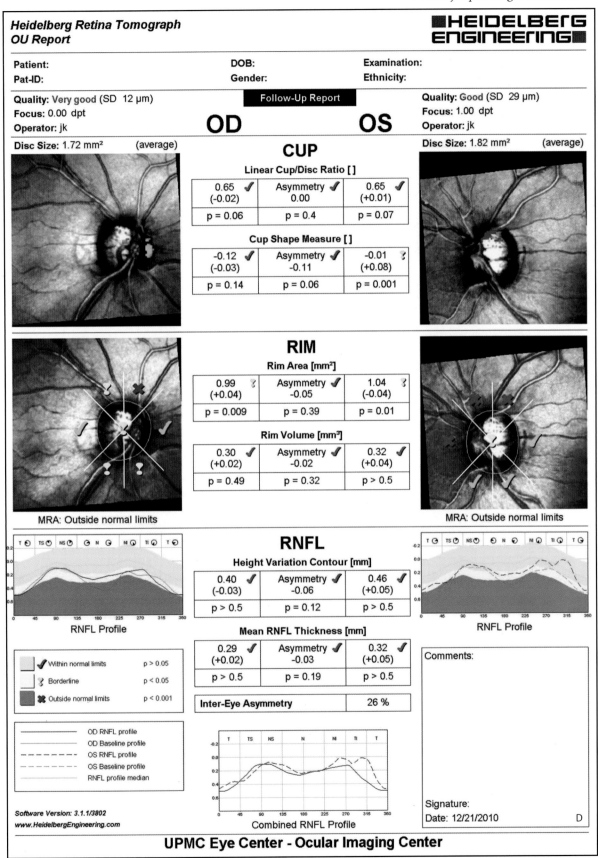

Figure 18-1. *(Continued)* Left eye with early glaucoma. This patient has early optic nerve damage but a full visual field. Target IOP is 18 mm Hg (previous IOP mid-20s). (A) Stereoscopic optic disc photography. (B) Humphrey 24-2 visual field. (C) OCT. (D) Confocal scanning laser ophthalmoscopy. (E) Scanning laser polarimetry.

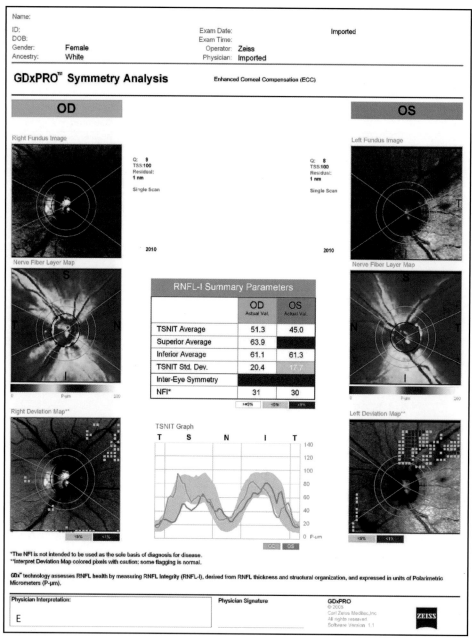

Figure 18-1. *(Continued)* Left eye with early glaucoma. This patient has early optic nerve damage but a full visual field. Target IOP is 18 mm Hg (previous IOP mid-20s). (A) Stereoscopic optic disc photography. (B) Humphrey 24-2 visual field. (D) Confocal scanning laser ophthalmoscopy. (E) Scanning laser polarimetry.

TABLE 18-2. GENERAL GUIDELINES FOR TARGET INTRAOCULAR PRESSURE*	
Findings	**Target IOP (mm Hg)**
Suspicious-appearing optic nerves; no definite field loss	21
Early glaucomatous disc damage and field loss (see Figure 18-1)	18
Moderate to advanced disc damage and field loss superiorly and inferiorly (see Figure 18-2)	15
Advanced disc damage and field loss involving areas close to fixation (see Figure 18-3)	12
Glaucoma damage with central fixation threatened	9

* Modified by IOP level at which damage occurred (see text).

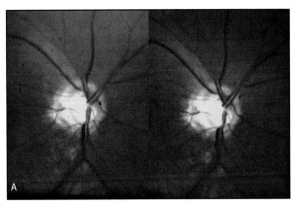

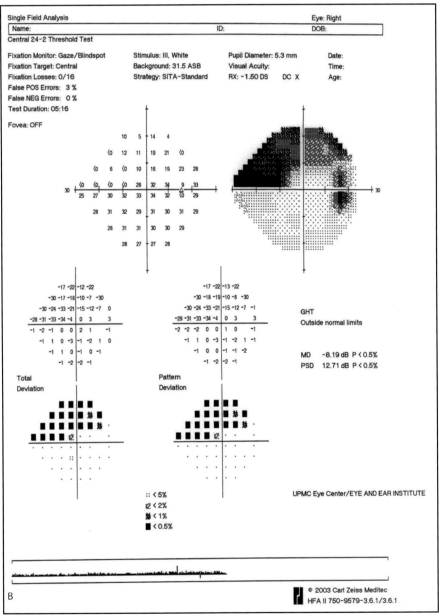

Figure 18-2. Right eye with moderate to advanced glaucoma. There is more disc damage and field loss than seen in Figure 18-1, with a dense superior scotoma splitting fixation and loss of the corresponding neuroretinal rim. Target IOP is 15 mm Hg (or slightly higher). (A) Stereoscopic optic disc photography. (B) Humphrey 24-2 visual field. (C) OCT. (D) Confocal scanning laser ophthalmoscopy. (E) Scanning laser polarimetry.

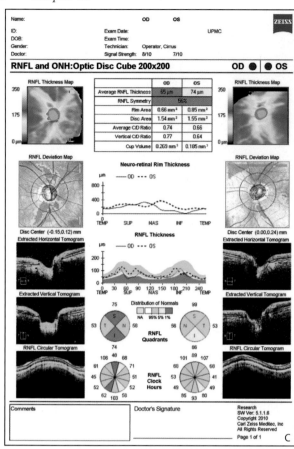

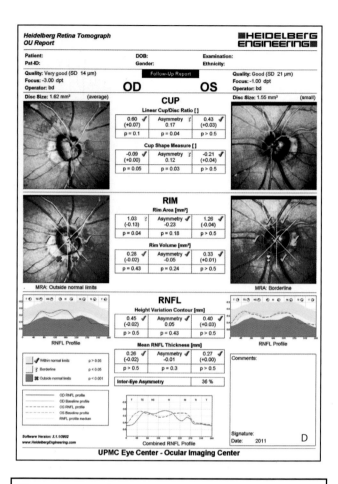

Figure 18-2. *(Continued)* Right eye with moderate to advanced glaucoma. There is more disc damage and field loss than seen in Figure 18-1, with a dense superior scotoma splitting fixation and loss of the corresponding neuroretinal rim. Target IOP is 15 mm Hg (or slightly higher). (A) Stereoscopic optic disc photography. (B) Humphrey 24-2 visual field. (C) OCT. (D) Confocal scanning laser ophthalmoscopy. (E) Scanning laser polarimetry.

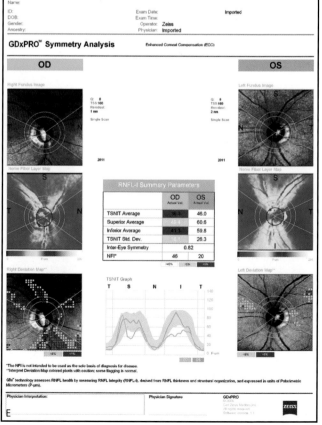

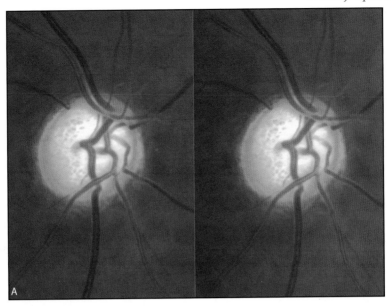

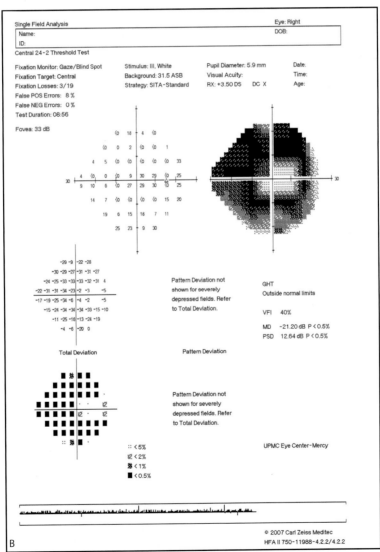

Figure 18-3. Right eye with advanced glaucoma and loss of visual field both above and below the horizontal meridian. Such an eye requires an IOP below 11 mm Hg. (A) Stereoscopic optic disc photography. (B) Humphrey 24-2 visual field. (C) OCT. (D) Confocal scanning laser ophthalmoscopy. (E) Scanning laser polarimetry.

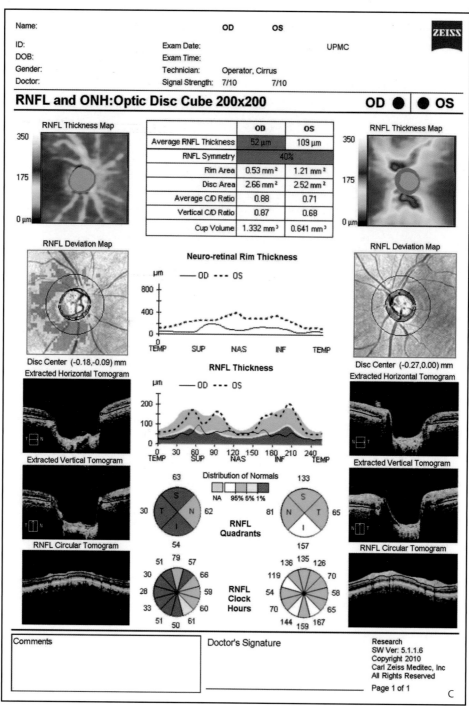

Figure 18-3. *(Continued)* Right eye with advanced glaucoma and loss of visual field both above and below the horizontal meridian. Such an eye requires an IOP below 11 mm Hg. (A) Stereoscopic optic disc photography. (B) Humphrey 24-2 visual field. (C) OCT. (D) Confocal scanning laser ophthalmoscopy. (E) Scanning laser polarimetry.

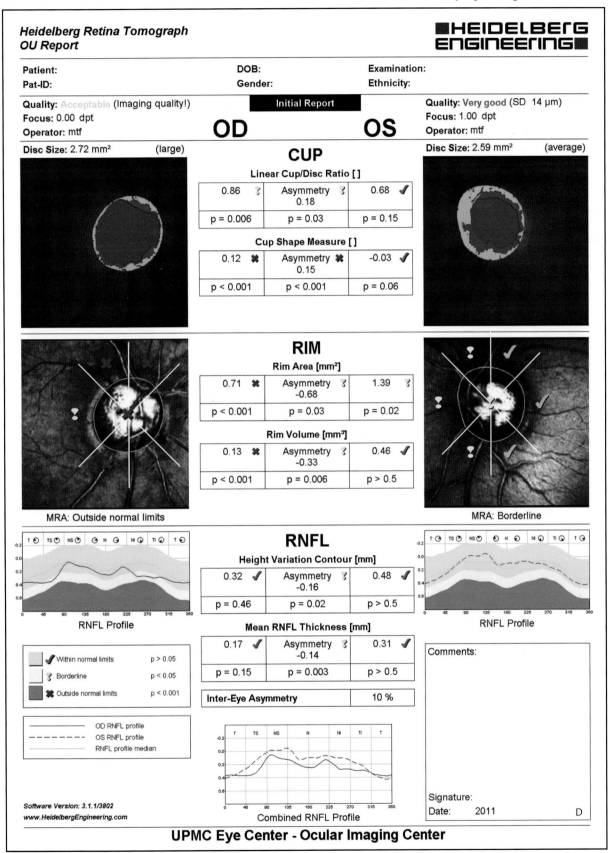

Figure 18-3. *(Continued)* Right eye with advanced glaucoma and loss of visual field both above and below the horizontal meridian. Such an eye requires an IOP below 11 mm Hg. (A) Stereoscopic optic disc photography. (B) Humphrey 24-2 visual field. (C) OCT. (D) Confocal scanning laser ophthalmoscopy. (E) Scanning laser polarimetry.

Name:

ID: Exam Date: UPMC Eye Center
DOB: Exam Time:
Gender: Operator: **Zeiss**
Ancestry: Physician: **admin**

GDxPRO™ Symmetry Analysis   Enhanced Corneal Compensation (ECC)

OD   ### OS

Right Fundus Image   Left Fundus Image

Q: 9   Q: 8
TSS:100   TSS:100
Residual: Residual:
1 nm   1 nm

Single Scan   Single Scan

2011   2011

Nerve Fiber Layer Map   Nerve Fiber Layer Map

RNFL-I Summary Parameters	OD Actual Val.	OS Actual Val.
TSNIT Average	23.5	52.4
Superior Average	22.5	57.1
Inferior Average	28.2	74.1
TSNIT Std. Dev.	7.1	28.0
Inter-Eye Symmetry	0.50	
NFI*	98	12

>=5%   <5%   <1%

Right Deviation Map**   Left Deviation Map**

TSNIT Graph
T   S   N   I   T
140
120
100
80
60
40
20
0 P-μm

OD   OS

<5%   <1%   <5%   <1%

*The NFI is not intended to be used as the sole basis of diagnosis for disease.
**Interpret Deviation Map colored pixels with caution; some flagging is normal.

GDx™ technology assesses RNFL health by measuring RNFL Integrity (RNFL-I), derived from RNFL thickness and structural organization, and expressed in units of Polarimetric Micrometers (P-μm).

Physician Interpretation:	Physician Signature	GDxPRO
		© 2008
		Carl Zeiss Meditec,Inc
		All rights reserved.
		Software Version 1.1

ZEISS   E

Figure 18-3. *(Continued)* Right eye with advanced glaucoma and loss of visual field both above and below the horizontal meridian. Such an eye requires an IOP below 11 mm Hg. (A) Stereoscopic optic disc photography. (B) Humphrey 24-2 visual field. (C) OCT. (D) Confocal scanning laser ophthalmoscopy. (E) Scanning laser polarimetry.

COMMON MISTAKES IN GLAUCOMA MANAGEMENT
David L. Epstein, MD, MMM
INCORRECT DIAGNOSIS

POAG is a diagnosis of exclusion. In addition to gonioscopy, a careful external slit-lamp biomicroscope (including dilated slit-lamp) and fundus examination are important to rule-out secondary causes, such as increased episcleral venous pressure, occult inflammation, silent angle closure, exfoliation, or retinal detachment (Schwartz's syndrome). The 2 most common masqueraders of POAG are chronic silent angle closure and occult TM inflammation (trabeculitis).

Note that when a patient with presumed POAG returns for examination and the IOP is elevated, always perform repeat gonioscopy (look for unsuspected chronic angle closure or occult inflammation). Misinterpreting chronic angle closure as POAG is perhaps the most common diagnostic error in glaucoma.

UNDERTREATING PATIENTS WITH ADVANCED DISC CUPPING AND FIELD LOSS

These patients often require a low normal IOP to prevent further progression (not simply an IOP in the high teens). Depending also on the IOP level at which damage occurred, if there is severe field loss in both the superior and inferior field, a target IOP of 12 mm Hg or lower is commonly set. If field loss encroaches on fixation, a target IOP below 10 mm Hg is set. Central 10-degree fields should be performed to indicate how much margin is left to follow should the target IOP be incorrect or not realized.

OVERTREATING EARLY PRIMARY OPEN-ANGLE GLAUCOMA

Although, as indicated in the text, we truly believe that elevated IOP is not as benign as once thought, it is nevertheless an error to disable patients with antiglaucoma regimens, especially without evidence of end-organ damage. For example, in such patients, if a single medication decreases the IOP from the upper-20s to the lower-20s, and it would be desired to lower the IOP even further, but such medication is disabling to the patient, the risk/benefit (toxicity) ratio shifts such that it is prudent to follow the patient on the regimen with careful monitoring of the optic nerve and visual field. Obviously, the presence of risk factors for optic nerve susceptibility to IOP would make one push more toward increased therapy, but the entire picture of the patient and his or her life needs should also be evaluated. In the absence of end-organ damage, with margin that can be followed, and in the presence of a dedicated patient to whom the benefits, risks, and options have all been fully explained, it is permissible to closely monitor the patient on the suboptimal regimen.

TALK TO THE PATIENT WITH GLAUCOMA

Explain all the options, and have the patient participate in all decisions. Be sensitive to the potential for glaucoma medications to disable the patient. It is useful for the clinician or the office assistant to list all the medications and times of dosage on a medication card, which would include information such as drug name, cap color, treated eye, dosage, and time for dosing. This enhances patient compliance, but also may obviously indicate the disruption in the patient's lifestyle that some therapeutic regimens are causing.

TABLE 18-3. INDICATIONS FOR INCISIONAL SURGERY IN PRIMARY OPEN-ANGLE GLAUCOMA

1. Progressive field loss and/or disc cupping and/or RNFL thinning despite maximal medical therapy

2. Sustained high IOP (eg, consistently in the 40s)

3. Markedly advanced field loss, encroaching on central fixation (no margin left to follow), with IOP at levels higher than can be achieved with filtration surgery

IOP: intraocular pressure; RNFL: retinal nerve fiber layer.

MECHANISM OF THE DISEASE

What are the underlying tissue abnormalities in the TM and optic nerve that are responsible for POAG? Possible vascular and mechanical factors involved in optic disc cupping have been alluded to in Chapter 8. We truly do not know whether the progressive cupping of the optic nerve and death of axons is a result of direct mechanical pressure on the axons at the level of the disc, or perhaps represents a vascular effect that may also involve mechanical pressure (ie, the mechanical theory versus the vascular theory). We do know that all the features of typical glaucomatous cupping of the optic nerve can be produced in previously normal monkeys by induced elevation of IOP[25] and that certain features of such cupping can be correlated with anatomical structural aspects of the lamina cribrosa.[26] Yet, this does not explain the variable susceptibility of the optic nerve to IOP that patients with POAG typically demonstrate, which would seem therefore to involve, in addition to (but not excluding) IOP, some other systemic or local optic nerve factor. An understanding, which is not yet available, of the factors truly involved in glaucomatous cupping and atrophy—whether mechanical, vascular, constitutive, or environmental—has the potential to radically re-direct and improve glaucoma therapy.[27]

In the TM, many different and sometimes conflicting histopathological correlates have been reported in POAG. Denudation of the trabecular beams with collapse of the structure and disorganization are likely only end-stage phenomena. The 2 observations now most readily accepted by most (but not all) investigators as earlier events include the following:

- A decreased cellularity in the trabecular outflow pathway[28]
- The presence of extracellular plaque material in the juxtacanalicular meshwork[29,30]

The latter finding was discussed in another chapter in terms of potential novel trabecular drug therapy that

Trabecular Glaucoma Versus Optic Nerve Glaucoma

David L. Epstein, MD, MMM

As indicated in Chapter 1, the sometimes "either/or" approach to these subjects has led to confusion and suboptimal patient management on occasion. Almost all glaucomas have a hydrodynamic component involving IOP, and it is useful to frame one's thinking from the perspective of the TM for this component of the disease. But the end organ, which is damaged by the trabecular glaucoma is the optic nerve, which has a varying susceptibility to IOP due to unknown factors that we strive to understand. Glaucoma thus is an optic neuropathy, but this does not mean we should ignore the role of IOP, which is the one factor we can identify and the only factor that we can directly manipulate.

It is often very useful to approach the patient with glaucoma from the perspective of both the TM and the optic nerve. Why is the IOP now elevated in this patient? What is the reason for this worsening of the trabecular glaucoma? (Repeat gonioscopy may uncover new findings, including pseudoexfoliation, occult inflammatory precipitates, and partial angle closure) Why is the optic nerve showing progressive damage at this IOP? (Has the IOP been higher in the interval? What is the state of the trabecular glaucoma?) Why is this optic nerve so vulnerable? What are the systemic or ocular factors that lead to this vulnerability?

Although the last question currently has no definite answers, we are confident that by framing thought processes in this way, the astute clinician will eventually hypothesize possible answers. But perhaps even more importantly, by framing thoughts this way to separate hydrodynamic disease from varying end-organ damage, it allows more effective patient management. Patients with melting susceptible discs are thus clearly identified, and more vigorous hydrodynamic IOP-lowering therapy is initiated, without specific regard for the state of the trabecular disease. On the other hand, patients with severe trabecular disease are identified as having real disease (rather than some statistical variant of normal) that is very likely, given enough time, to result in end-organ damage.

We seem to be on the threshold of new specific drugs targeted at the TM that might restore normal function. Obviously, these agents will treat trabecular glaucoma and offer nothing, except by chance, for the susceptibility factors involved in optic nerve glaucoma. Yet, if one can eliminate trabecular glaucoma, it might greatly simplify the elucidation of these factors. Regardless, we need clear thinking about separate disease processes in both the TM and optic nerve for this discovery and for optimal patient management.

Tonography

David L. Epstein, MD, MMM

It is unfortunate that tonography is so patient and physician unfriendly. Tonography (see Chapter 6) provides the only estimate of outflow function and facility that we have. As the reader may surmise, we have had a special interest in "what is going on in the TM," "why," and especially "what is the severity of the trabecular disease?" In the past, we routinely obtained tonography on all new patients and found that about one-third of the time it did provide clinically important information. We used a qualitative approach to tonography: Was outflow severely impaired, moderately abnormal, or within or close to normal? If patients had severe impairment of outflow ("almost a flat line"), these patients were believed to have serious disease and all other factors being equal were more vigorously treated hydrodynamically. For example, if outflow was severely impaired, one could logically, and with some historical validation, presume that there was the potential for more diurnal variation in IOP with small changes in aqueous humor formation. This might then indicate the need to treat rather than observe a patient with IOPs in the 20s or to presume a significant IOP-related pathophysiological mechanism between visits for patients with progressive field loss but reasonable IOP at the snapshot that occurred at the time of the office visit.

But tonography is also very useful in answering the question: Is the TM function normal in patients with angle recession, pigmentary dispersion syndrome, pseudoexfoliation, uveitis, or puzzling apparent unilateral glaucoma? Because of potential influences on aqueous humor formation in diseased eyes or the normal diurnal variation in aqueous production, a single snapshot IOP measurement might be misleading, especially at knowing (in an increasingly cost-obsessed environment) how closely to follow the patient.

Regardless, the reader is urged to always ask the following 2 questions in the care of glaucoma patients: What is going on in the TM? What is going on in the optic nerve?

In the end, we may discover that there are certain common pathogenetic mechanisms involved in both tissues (eg, at the connective tissue level, but we need to include both tissues in our clinical disease framework for analysis).

might allow this material to be removed from the outflow pathway. Some have argued that the amount of this extracellular plaque material is not sufficient, in and of itself, to mechanically obstruct the pathway for flow,[31] and others have indicated that there may be other proteinaceous materials obstructing the outflow channels.[32-34] Regardless, it is not known whether these extracellular accumulations are a primary or secondary process. Hypotheses concerning the former include proposed direct oxidation of extracellular proteins in the outflow pathway from oxidative species

present in the aqueous humor,[35,36] while those concerning the latter have involved a postulated primary trabecular cell dysfunction[37] that may also relate to the observed reduced cellularity in the TM.[28] But, it is not clear (even in the various hypotheses!) whether the initiating pathological event for the observed increase in outflow resistance in POAG might be a direct mechanical obstruction of the spaces in the extracellular outflow pathway or a cellular defect in fluid movement (thus resulting in a secondary accumulation of extracellular proteinaceous material). Another theory conceptualizes the TM and Schlemm's canal complex as a mechanical pump responsive to IOP.[38] Finally, one of us (JSS) has shown that there is activation of a tissue-specific nonlethal stress-response pathway in glaucomatous TM, involving interleukin-1, NF-kB and ELAM-1. This study[39] suggests that proinflammatory cytokines are constitutively activated in the TM in glaucoma, perhaps as a response to stress (oxidative or otherwise) or perhaps as a component of the disease process. Such understanding has important future therapeutic implications,[27] and it seems likely that future trabecular cellular glaucoma drug therapy may target and prove effective in treating these underlying mechanisms.

Our research has suggested an additional hypothesis concerning the possible underlying defect in the TM in POAG: a dynamic abnormality in cell function. Histopathological studies that have been in some conflict are a static "picture frozen in time" of the outflow pathway tissue (that is also chemically fixed for preservation). What if the trabecular cells are normally much more dynamic than these frozen pictures would suggest? That is, we do know that the morphology of the outflow pathway cells can change dramatically and acutely in response to different IOP conditions.[40,41] We know that these cells are capable of contracting and changing their cell shape and attachment in response to pharmacological agents.[42-46] Could these cells be constantly sensing their microenvironment and responding with dynamic cellular changes involving their cytoskeleton? Could such dynamic changes underlie the normal self-regulation of outflow that many have suspected to exist in the TM itself (because there are no innervation or feedback vascular loops in this tissue)? Could such dynamic trabecular cellular events be abnormal in POAG? Could such defective dynamic cellular processes in the trabecular outflow tissue also explain the poor ability of POAG trabecular cells to grow out in tissue culture monolayers (the process of which requires normal cytoskeletal function)? These are intriguing possibilities, not only because they might direct glaucoma therapy in new directions, but because it is now possible to study these dynamic cytoskeletal processes in living glaucomatous TM cells (without the need for a continuous monolayer).[47]

This novel, unproven hypothesis developed as a converse from the trabecular drug studies that identified the cytoskeleton of the TM cells as the cellular target that was associated with the improved fluid outflow.[42] This led to considerations that the cytoskeleton might be involved not only in such pharmacological targeting, but in normal outflow function as well.[43] The corollary of this then might be that abnormalities in such dynamic cytoskeletal function are likely involved in POAG, and such dynamic abnormalities would have been missed with past methods of study (hence, the lack of clarity concerning the true, early histopathological correlate of POAG). One of us (DLE) has proposed this hypothesis in the 16th Annual Robert N. Shaffer Lecture at the American Academy of Ophthalmology, "The Glaucomas: Lessons for a Clinician-Scientist," to both honor Dr. Shaffer, who was a long-standing colleague of Drs. Chandler and Grant, but also to underscore the collective wisdom of these mentors who emphasized that future progress in glaucoma requires clinician-scientists[48] to creatively build upon their foundation of past (clinical and laboratory) observations.

REFERENCES

1. De Moraes CG, Furlanetto RL, Reis AS, et al. Agreement between stress intraocular pressure and long-term intraocular pressure measurements in primary open angle glaucoma. *Clin Experiment Ophthalmol.* 2009;37(3):270-274.
2. Hollows FC, Graham PA. Intra-ocular pressure, glaucoma, and glaucoma suspects in a defined population. *Br J Ophthalmol.* 1966;50(10):570-586.
3. Bengtsson B. The prevalence of glaucoma. *Br J Ophthalmol.* 1981;65(1):46-49.
4. Sommer A, Tielsch JM, Katz J, et al. Relationship between intraocular pressure and primary open angle glaucoma among white and black Americans. The Baltimore Eye Survey. *Arch Ophthalmol.* 1991;109(8):1090-1095.
5. Dielemans I, Vingerling JR, Wolfs RC, et al. The prevalence of primary open-angle glaucoma in a population-based study in The Netherlands. The Rotterdam Study. *Ophthalmology.* 1994;101(11):1851-1855.
6. Schoenberger JA. Epidemiology of systolic and diastolic systemic blood pressure elevation in the elderly. *Am J Cardiol.* 1986;57(5):45C-51C.
7. Davidson RA, Hale WE, Moore MT, et al. Incidence of hypertension in an ambulatory elderly population. *J Am Geriatr Soc.* 1989;37(9):861-866.
8. Strulov A, Epstein L, Harth A, et al. Blood pressure and hypertension in an elderly population. *Eur J Epidemiol.* 1990;6(2):160-165.
9. Hajjar I, Kotchen JM, Kotchen TA. Hypertension: trends in prevalence, incidence, and control. *Annu Rev Public Health.* 2006;27:465-490.
10. Anderson DR, Drance SM, Schulzer M. Factors that predict the benefit of lowering intraocular pressure in normal tension glaucoma. *Am J Ophthalmol.* 2003;136(5):820-829.
11. Chandler PA, Grant WM. *Lectures on Glaucoma.* Philadelphia, PA: Lea & Febiger; 1965.
12. Grant WM, Burke JF Jr. Why do some people go blind from glaucoma? *Ophthalmology.* 1982;89(9):991-998.
13. Epstein DL, Krug JH Jr, Hertzmark E, et al. A long-term clinical trial of timolol therapy versus no treatment in the management of glaucoma suspects. *Ophthalmology.* 1989;96(10):1460-1467.
14. Kass MA, Gordon MO, Hoff MR, et al. Topical timolol administration reduces the incidence of glaucomatous damage in ocular hypertensive individuals. A randomized, double-masked, long-term clinical trial. *Arch Ophthalmol.* 1989;107(11):1590-1598.
15. Kass MA, Heuer DK, Higginbotham EJ, et al. The Ocular Hypertension Treatment Study: a randomized trial determines that topical ocular hypotensive medication delays or prevents the onset of primary open-angle glaucoma. *Arch Ophthalmol.* 2002;120(6):701-713; discussion 829-830.
16. American Academy of Ophthalmology Quality of Care Committee Glaucoma Panel. *Preferred Practice Patterns: Primary Open Angle Glaucoma.* San Francisco, CA: The Academy; 1992.
17. Fong DS, Epstein DL, Allingham RR. Glaucoma and myopia: are they related? *Int Ophthalmol Clin.* 1990;30(3):215-218.
18. Tielsch JM, Sommer A, Katz J, et al. Racial variations in the prevalence of primary open-angle glaucoma. The Baltimore Eye Survey. *JAMA.* 1991;266(3):369-374.
19. Gordon MO, Beiser JA, Brandt JD, et al. The Ocular Hypertension Treatment Study: baseline factors that predict the onset of primary open-angle glaucoma. *Arch Ophthalmol.* 2002;120(6):714-720; discussion 829-830.
20. Kass MA, Gordon MO, Gao F, et al. Delaying treatment of ocular hypertension: the Ocular Hypertension Treatment Study. *Arch Ophthalmol.* 2010;128(3):276-287.

21. Gifford RW Jr. Review of the long-term controlled trials of usefulness of therapy for systemic hypertension. *Am J Cardiol.* 1989;63(4):8B-16B.

22. Wilson MR, Hertzmark E, Walker AM, et al. A case-control study of risk factors in open angle glaucoma. *Arch Ophthalmol.* 1987;105(8):1066-1071.

23. Hernandez MR, Ye H. Glaucoma: changes in extracellular matrix in the optic nerve head. *Ann Med.* 1993;25(4):309-315.

24. Yang JL, Neufeld AH, Zorn MB, et al. Collagen type I mRNA levels in cultured human lamina cribrosa cells: effects of elevated hydrostatic pressure. *Exp Eye Res.* 1993;56(5):567-574.

25. Varma R, Quigley HA, Pease ME. Changes in optic disk characteristics and number of nerve fibers in experimental glaucoma. *Am J Ophthalmol.* 1992;114(5):554-559.

26. Dandona L, Quigley HA, Brown AE, et al. Quantitative regional structure of the normal human lamina cribrosa. A racial comparison. *Arch Ophthalmol.* 1990;108(3):393-398.

27. Epstein DL. Will there be a remedy to reverse the changes in the trabecular meshwork and the optic nerve? A personal point of view on glaucoma therapy. *J Glaucoma.* 1993;2(2):138-139.

28. Alvarado J, Murphy C, Juster R. Trabecular meshwork cellularity in primary open-angle glaucoma and nonglaucomatous normals. *Ophthalmology.* 1984;91(6):564-579.

29. Lutjen-Drecoll E, Futa R, Rohen JW. Ultrahistochemical studies on tangential sections of the trabecular meshwork in normal and glaucomatous eyes. *Invest Ophthalmol Vis Sci.* 1981;21(4):563-573.

30. Rohen JW. Why is intraocular pressure elevated in chronic simple glaucoma? Anatomical considerations. *Ophthalmology.* 1983;90(7):758-765.

31. Alvarado JA, Yun AJ, Murphy CG. Juxtacanalicular tissue in primary open angle glaucoma and in nonglaucomatous normals. *Arch Ophthalmol.* 1986;104(10):1517-1528.

32. Russell P, Koretz J, Epstein DL. Is primary open angle glaucoma caused by small proteins? *Med Hypotheses.* 1993;41(5):455-458.

33. Epstein DL, Hashimoto JM, Grant WM. Serum obstruction of aqueous outflow in enucleated eyes. *Am J Ophthalmol.* 1978;86(1):101-105.

34. Johnson M, Gong H, Freddo TF, et al. Serum proteins and aqueous outflow resistance in bovine eyes. *Invest Ophthalmol Vis Sci.* 1993;34(13):3549-3557.

35. Nguyen KP, Chung ML, Anderson PJ, et al. Hydrogen peroxide removal by the calf aqueous outflow pathway. *Invest Ophthalmol Vis Sci.* 1988;29(6):976-981.

36. Russell P, Garland D, Epstein DL. Analysis of the proteins of calf and cow trabecular meshwork: development of a model system to study aging effects and glaucoma. *Exp Eye Res.* 1989;48(2):251-260.

37. Epstein DL. Open angle glaucoma. Why not a cure? *Arch Ophthalmol.* 1987;105(9):1187-1188.

38. Johnstone MA. The aqueous outflow system as a mechanical pump: evidence from examination of tissue and aqueous movement in human and nonhuman primates. *J Glaucoma.* 2004;13(5):421-438.

39. Wang N, Chintala SK, Fini ME, et al. Activation of a tissue-specific stress response in the aqueous outflow pathway of the eye defines the glaucoma disease phenotype. *Nat Med.* 2001;7(3):304-309.

40. Johnstone MA, Grant WG. Pressure-dependent changes in structures of the aqueous outflow system of human and monkey eyes. *Am J Ophthalmol.* 1973;75(3):365-383.

41. Johnstone MA. Pressure-dependent changes in nuclei and the process origins of the endothelial cells lining Schlemm's canal. *Invest Ophthalmol Vis Sci.* 1979;18(1):44-51.

42. Erickson-Lamy K, Schroeder A, Epstein DL. Ethacrynic acid induces reversible shape and cytoskeletal changes in cultured cells. *Invest Ophthalmol Vis Sci.* 1992;33(9):2631-2640.

43. Epstein DL, de Kater AW, Erickson-Lamy K. The search for a sulfhydryl drug for glaucoma: from chemistry to cytoskeleton. In: Lutjen-Drecoll E, ed. *Basic Aspects of Glaucoma Research III.* Stuttgart-New York: Schattauer; 1993:345-353.

44. Grewal A, O'Brien ET, Epstein DL. Control of cell shape in the trabecular meshwork. *Invest Ophthalmol Vis Sci.* 1994;35(ARVO suppl):2725.

45. Opperman AD, O'Brien ET, Roberts BC. Can a rise in intracellular calcium (CA) explain the cellular effects of ethacrynic acid? *Invest Ophthalmol Vis Sci.* 1994;35(ARVO suppl):3709.

46. Gills JP, Roberts BC, Epstein DL. Microtubule disruption leads to active cellular contraction in human trabecular meshwork cells. *Invest Ophthalmol Vis Sci.* 1996;37(ARVO suppl):3801.

47. O'Brien ET, Epstein DL. Observation of living glaucoma cells by video DIC microscopy. *Invest Ophthalmol Vis Sci.* 1996;37(ARVO suppl):4146.

48. Epstein DL. Is the ophthalmologist as a clinician-scientist still viable? *Arch Ophthalmol.* 1991;109(11):1523-1524.

19

Low-Tension Glaucoma

Ian P. Conner, MD, PhD; Kimberly V. Miller, MD;
Joel S. Schuman, MD, FACS; and David L. Epstein, MD, MMM

DEFINITION

Unfortunately, there is tremendous confusion about low-tension glaucoma (LTG; normal-pressure glaucoma) regarding terminology, inclusion and exclusion criteria, possible different forms and pathophysiological mechanisms, and therapy. This confusion is especially nefarious because LTG is not uncommon (perhaps even increasing in prevalence as the population is aging), is easily missed in its earliest stages (because the intraocular pressure [IOP] is not elevated), can affect central visual function early, and is difficult to treat, with less clear guidelines for the IOP treatment goals (because the IOP is not elevated at baseline). This is among the most difficult of glaucomas for the physician to manage because, unfortunately, this is a potentially blinding, most often progressive disease. In fact, as will be discussed, we believe nonprogressive forms of this entity to be so uncommon that we use the term *LTG* synonymously with the older term *progressive LTG*. LTG is surprisingly common in Japan,[1] but we may be underappreciating its frequency in the United States.

It is useful conceptually to first take a step back and consider optic nerve cupping in response to elevated IOP in the usual forms of (high-pressure) primary open-angle glaucoma (POAG). As previously discussed, elevated IOP is probably not as benign as once thought for many patients, but there is an individual susceptibility of the optic nerve to cupping that exists in response to a given IOP. For example, one patient may show progressive optic nerve damage with IOPs in the low 20s, and another patient, with ostensibly similar IOPs, may show no obvious optic nerve change. What explains the increased susceptibility of the optic nerve to IOP in the first patient? We really do not know, although there has been much discussion about various possible mechanical or vascular factors[2-5] that may lead more readily to cupping. In high-pressure glaucoma, an optic disc that has been damaged may continue to show progressive damage at normal pressures. We term this

LTG equivalent. This entity is further documentation of the phenomenon of individual susceptibility of the optic nerve to cupping in response to a given IOP.

Allowing that there is this variable susceptibility of the optic nerve to cupping at a given level of IOP in the POAG patient, is it not then logical that cases of apparent LTG represent this same phenomenon, but at a more extreme point of the spectrum with respect to IOP? Just because it is logical does not make it true, but this also can be said in criticism of the school of thought that might consider LTG logically to be a separate disease. This book deals with the practical clinical care of the patient with glaucoma and builds on long-term clinical experience with such patients. Our clinical experience strongly indicates that almost all patients with LTG have an IOP-sensitive component and that adequately lowering the IOP improves the natural history of the disease. In addition, it has been shown in a multicenter randomized controlled trial that lowering IOP by 30% or more reduced visual field progression in LTG patients.[6] IOP appears not to be the entire answer, and, in this disease, there is an extreme susceptibility of the optic nerve to cupping (that, if we could only understand, might provide important insight into mechanisms for cupping in higher IOP forms of glaucoma as well).

This lumping rather than splitting truly fits with our clinical experience, and although there likely will prove to be some exceptions as we better define glaucomas in the future, this concept actually simplifies and results in more effective patient management. In LTG, which in the overwhelming majority of patients is a progressive disease that can lead to blindness, there is an IOP-sensitive component combined with extreme optic nerve susceptibility. This concept indicates the need to substantially decrease the IOP below baseline in all patients with apparent LTG.

Nonprogressive forms[7] of LTG are rare in our experience, and the burden is, therefore, on the ophthalmologist when he or she makes this rare diagnosis and chooses no therapy.

Kahook MY, Schuman JS, eds.
Chandler and Grant's Glaucoma, Fifth Edition (pp 207-216).
© 2013 SLACK Incorporated.

However, there remains the "curse" of long-term follow-up, and unfortunately, as one follows such patients, it frequently becomes apparent that this is a progressive, potentially blinding disease for most patients.

For those who might have trouble with this concept, perhaps it is useful to consider this in another way: let us suppose that the etiology of cupping in POAG (so-called high-pressure glaucoma) actually involves a vascular mechanism. Suppose that elevated IOP results in some type of ischemia from pressure directly on the small vessels supplying the optic nerve. The varying susceptibility of the optic nerve to cupping in high-pressure glaucoma might then be due to the presence of small vessel disease in the optic nerve, independent of IOP. In LTG, this small vessel disease in the optic nerve might be extreme, such that normal levels of IOP are additive pathophysiologically. Lowering the IOP does not treat or eliminate the extreme small vessel disease, but it eliminates this additive noxious element of compromise to the vascular supply. Lowering the IOP, therefore, improves the natural history of the disease. This small vessel disease in the optic nerve might, by itself, produce damage to the optic nerve, independent of the additive noxious IOP effect.

One might argue in this construct that the patient will still ultimately go blind (from small vessel disease), but if one can achieve an IOP in the single digits, our clinical experience is that stability is commonly achieved. In many cases of (high-pressure) POAG, our treatments may also only be palliative, but we are striving to delay blindness past the time of natural (whole body) death. As suggested, patients with high-pressure POAG likely share this mechanism of optic nerve susceptibility (hence the variable susceptibility to a given level of IOP in different patients), and, therefore, lowering the IOP in POAG patients may also not be sufficient to prevent progression. Yet, because the IOP is elevated in POAG, we treat it, and if progression occurs, we treat it more aggressively and lower the IOP even further. This strategy is usually, but not always, effective, with similar considerations in LTG.

This discussion suggests that, because there are likely similar phenomena in these 2 forms of glaucoma, there could also be similar mechanisms of pathophysiology that may more obviously be part of the same spectrum.

This discussion of the palliative nature of our treatments for both POAG and LTG implies that, as the population ages and life expectancy increases, there is also the potential for blindness to increase in prevalence. The implication also arises that if and when the curative drug for the optic nerve is developed, it may have effectiveness for both POAG and LTG.

Some have used the term *normal-pressure glaucoma* rather than LTG. For practical purposes, the 2 are interchangeable, leaving the terminology a matter of preference. However, the reader should be reminded that it is difficult to know what normal IOP truly is, and therefore the term *low tension* may indeed be more accurate.

This discussion and construct helps in understanding the spectrum of LTG patients and moves one away from rigid inclusion and exclusion criteria. The key to this enterprise is the concept of the susceptible optic nerve. There is often much effort and controversy created in patients with suspected LTG to determine whether there is ever an elevated IOP measurement above normal, even if it occurs only once among multiple measurements. For example, some have sent suspected LTG patients home with various tonometers to do diurnal curves, and if one IOP above normal is detected, the patient is then reclassified as POAG. What does this observation really mean in the context of IOP measurement accuracy, and what, exactly, constitutes a normal IOP?

Suppose that in an accurate diurnal IOP curve of a patient with progressive LTG there is one elevated IOP measurement and 20 normal IOPs. Does this really mean that this patient with progressive field loss has POAG, when we know that there are patients who have 20 out of 20 elevated IOPs and do not have apparent optic nerve damage? We would argue that this patient unequivocally has a susceptible optic nerve but phenotypically fits in our construct of LTG. If the one elevated IOP measurement would indicate to some readers that the patient has POAG and that only by this diagnosis needs treatment, then how does one know in other patients with apparent LTG when one has performed enough IOP measurements to rule out a single IOP spike?

As one carries this argument further, it is easy to see how clinical presentations may create further confusion, unless one remembers the unifying concept of the susceptible optic nerve combined with some IOP-sensitive component. Clearly, as one part of the spectrum, there are patients with IOPs in the low teens, which never leave this range (and by use of tonography have normal outflow facilities, which would imply the nonoccurrence of abnormally elevated IOPs, [ie, no IOPs in the 20s]), and yet nevertheless demonstrate progressive cupping and field loss. These are indeed the most difficult LTG patients to treat because IOP must be reduced into the single digits in order to achieve clinical stability. Conversely, there are similar patients who present with IOPs in the mid to upper teens (with correspondingly borderline abnormal tonographic outflow facilities). One can waste a lot of time looking for that one elevated IOP measurement, or one can conceptualize that, regardless, this patient fits into the spectrum of the susceptible optic nerve with an accompanying IOP-sensitive component and, therefore, needs an IOP lowered below baseline, even if one considers the baseline normal.

Finally, there is one last clinical example of the spectrum of this disease that involves as the key unifying concept that of varying optic nerve susceptibility to IOP. Suppose a patient with a former diagnosis of high-pressure glaucoma presents with consistent documented IOP in the upper teens, but with nevertheless progressive visual field loss. Before treatment, the patient was documented to have consistent IOPs in the mid-20s. A common example of this phenomenon is a patient with pseudoexfoliation glaucoma or POAG with a good response to laser trabeculoplasty (and again here tonography can document nearly normal outflow facility and implied stability of IOP) who, nevertheless, subsequently demonstrates progressive disc cupping and field loss despite these good IOPs. One can call such patients whatever one wishes as long as it is clinically obvious that treatment must be advanced, but we have used the term *LTG equivalent* to indicate the enhanced susceptibility of the optic nerve to these now reasonable (normal) levels of IOP. Regardless of terminology, these patients should be treated similarly to those with LTG, with more intensive therapy to further lower the IOP. Consider if one did not have the history of elevated IOP in such a patient? What would one then call such a patient? It does not really matter, as long as it is clear that the current level of IOP in the face of clinical progression is too high and, therefore, one needs to lower the IOP further.

For patients with both LTG and LTG equivalent, this strategy is usually successful. The authors are unaware of any data clearly showing that, for a given level of presenting baseline IOP, the prognosis is any different with respect to the efficacy of further reduction of IOP in LTG versus LTG equivalent (which some would call POAG, etc). This further suggests that these conditions likely share unifying features of both enhanced optic nerve susceptibility and IOP susceptibility. Almost all clinicians would advance treatment for LTG equivalent with a history of previously high IOP. Yet, this confusion about LTG has led some to withhold treatment. In the previous example, if one did not or could not know the history of elevated IOP, the patient might not be distinguishable from other cases of LTG.

Thus, there seems little merit to trying to subcategorize apparent cases of LTG. One needs to spend most efforts vigorously lowering the IOP and following the optic nerve appearance and the visual field closely.

The following are at least 3 general rules for the practicing ophthalmologist when a suspicion of LTG is entertained:

1. Obtain a visual field in the presence of a suspicious optic nerve.

2. Obtain structural imaging tests to further elucidate the extent and location of ganglion cell layer damage.

3. Photograph any suspicious disc.

The first and second points are obvious, but the third is often not emphasized enough. Drawings, even in the hands of glaucoma experts are frequently unreliable, and because the detection of disc and field progression is paramount, a baseline photograph for future comparison is essential in order to achieve confidence in one's conclusions. True stereographic disc photographs are preferred, but, if unavailable, a nonstereo baseline disc photograph can enhance patient care in the future. Perhaps the most common question asked in a referral glaucoma practice is: what did the optic disc look like at a previous point in time?

LOW-TENSION GLAUCOMA AND THE GENERAL OPHTHALMOLOGIST
David L. Epstein, MD, MMM

The general ophthalmologist is an unsung but true hero in the detection of patients with LTG. Consider in a busy general practice a patient whose IOP is normal, where in the absence of any visual field data the general ophthalmologist is suspicious about LTG on the basis of his or her evaluation of the optic nerve. This ophthalmologist is a true disc sleuth. Recall the previously described techniques of evaluation of the optic nerve in glaucoma by assessing disc contour (see Chapter 8), as well as optic nerve and nerve fiber layer imaging (see Chapter 9). The goal is to detect LTG before there is clinically significant optic nerve damage, and especially before the patient notices the presence of subjective scotomata, which notoriously can involve points close to central fixation in LTG. Because this disease may be increasing in prevalence in our aging population, the disc sleuthing general ophthalmologist truly deserves our praise.

Disc sleuthing, especially in an elderly population, is challenging. In addition to other features of the aged eye such as a miotic pupil and the frequent presence of lenticular nuclear sclerosis that can falsely give the appearance of a disc having a healthy pink color (but remember it is contour rather than color that is the key parameter to be evaluated), there often is a senile sloping contour to the aged disc. Thus, one should expect to over-read suspect discs in the elderly, but visual fields, structural imaging, and disc photographs help document normal limits in the former and stability in the latter.

SYMPTOMS

Most patients with LTG are asymptomatic and are detected by the ophthalmologist on a routine examination based on the optic nerve appearance. Occasionally, patients present with a subjective scotoma near fixation. Sometimes, there does appear to be a credible history of sudden onset. Of course, one must rule out an acute episode of ischemic optic neuropathy in such patients, but they typically progress as other patients with LTG with no further sudden episodes. From a pathophysiological point-of-view, this symptomatology would seem important to understand, but may simply represent a discovery phenomenon when suddenly forced to use monocular rather than binocular vision.

Patients should be asked about any neurological symptoms, such as weakness in extremities, dizziness, headaches, loss of consciousness, diplopia, etc. If a patient has any such symptoms, except for typical migraine headaches, a neuro-ophthalmological evaluation is indicated. Migraine has sometimes been associated with LTG,[8,9] which again raises the possibility of vascular factors involved in pathogenesis. However, additional studies have failed to elucidate this association.[10,11] Therefore, migraine is not an indication for neurological referral unless atypical.

TABLE 19-1. Differential Diagnosis of Low-Tension Glaucoma	
Disorder	**Comment**
Temporal arteritis	Usually acute severe unilateral vision loss, optic disc swelling, increased disc cupping occurs after acute event, systemic symptoms (myalgias, headache), elevated ESR
Anterior ischemic optic neuropathy	Usually acute unilateral vision loss, disc swollen initially then pale, increase in disc cupping unusual, altitudinal VF loss may mimic glaucoma
Pituitary or intracranial tumors	VF usually bilateral, VF loss rarely appears glaucomatous, early loss of visual acuity and color vision, optic nerve pallor without abnormal disc cupping
Methanol intoxication	History of drinking moonshine, acute severe bilateral vision loss, early disc swelling followed by optic nerve pallor and disc cupping
Kjer's hereditary optic neuropathy	Positive family history, usually bilateral with pallor and excavation affecting temporal disc in a young patient
Congenital optic pit or coloboma	Deeply excavated optic nerve, often unilateral, visual fields stable in absence of serous retinal detachment
Syphilitic (tertiary) optic neuropathy	Optic pallor with abnormal cupping, positive serology (FTA antibody and RPR), other evidence of tertiary syphilis
History of past elevated IOP	Resolved steroid-induced, uveitic, or trauma-induced glaucoma in the past can mimic LTG

ESR: erythrocyte sedimentation rate; FTA: fluorescent treponemal antibody; IOP: intraocular pressure; LTG: low-tension glaucoma; RPR: rapid plasma regain; VF: visual field.

Raynaud's phenomenon has been associated with LTG, and there is some evidence that immunological disease may also be associated with LTG.[12,13]

Systemic factors are likely involved in the pathogenesis of LTG that, once understood, will explain the extreme susceptibility of the optic nerve discussed. Blood pressure is one systemic association that has been hypothesized, specifically the relationship between systemic nocturnal hypotension and glaucoma progression or ischemia perhaps related to microangiopathy and decreased ocular blood flow. However, studies so far have been inconclusive.[14]

The presence of any neurological symptom indicates the need for a neuro-ophthalmological evaluation to rule out neurological disease that might masquerade as LTG. Although the signature of glaucoma is contour changes of the optic nerve (see Chapter 8) and that of neurological disease is pallor of the optic nerve, certain nonglaucomatous conditions can uncommonly cause contour changes as well. The suggestion of accompanying systemic disease, with the exception of migraine, in a patient with LTG would indicate the need for a medical evaluation as part of the global care of the whole patient, which we routinely advocate.

Differential Diagnosis

Certain nonglaucomatous conditions can uncommonly result in contour changes in the optic nerve that might be misinterpreted as LTG (Table 19-1).

Contour changes may occur in approximately one-third or more of patients with a history of temporal (giant cell) arteritis. Usually, there is severe visual field and acuity loss cases that have these glaucoma-like contour disc changes,[15] which usually are first detected a few weeks after the acute event, after the acute disc swelling has subsided. The characteristic history of rapid loss of vision and reduction in central visual acuity are helpful differentiating features. Other forms of ischemic optic neuropathy can rarely produce contour changes that are usually more localized on the disc.

Visible disc cupping is rarely present with pituitary and other intracranial tumors, but thinning of the retinal nerve fiber layer (RNFL) frequently occurs in these circumstances. The RNFL damage is often detectable by optical coherence tomography (OCT), confocal scanning laser ophthalmoscopy, or scanning laser polarimetry. The presence of nonglaucomatous visual field loss, substantial asymmetry of the 2 optic nerves, thin RNFL that corresponds to nonglaucomatous visual field defects, or any unexpected neurological symptoms indicates the need for neuro-ophthalmological evaluation. If in doubt, it is best to refer such a patient for neurological evaluation. It is advisable not to miss an intracranial tumor, even though this is a rare masquerade.

Methanol intoxication is usually detectable by history if one remembers to ask about consumption of moonshine (bootleg liquor) that is probably the most common clinical situation for methanol exposure. There should be a history of acute vision loss accompanied by disc edema (typically bilaterally), which is later followed by atrophy of the optic nerve and occasionally contour changes as well. The rapid loss of vision and usual substantial reduction in central visual acuity that is sustained can also be helpful in differentiation.

The family history (for many reasons should routinely be obtained in all patients with glaucoma) should assist with the diagnosis of Kjer's and other hereditary optic neuropathies, which classically have onset at a young age (younger than 20 years of age).

Lues (tertiary syphilis) has been reported to cause a pseudoglaucomatous disc appearance, but the authors have never observed this occurrence and believe the presentation as a LTG masquerade must be rare.

Colobomas and pits can sometimes create confusion, but usually the deep, focal excavation on careful examination helps establish the diagnosis. Field defects should be nonprogressive, unless serous macular detachment occurs. The widespread use of OCT can be especially helpful in establishing these diagnoses.

In eyes with prior giant cell arteritis, the disc can appear glaucomatously cupped. However, remember that the severe vision loss and usually unilateral condition suggests a diagnosis other than LTG. When the other conditions mentioned cause contour changes on the disc, there is usually some subjective atypical character to the cupping. Most commonly, the atypical finding is the color of the rim tissue not involved in the contour change. This is usually pale (ie, demonstrating optic atrophy) in these pseudoglaucomatous conditions, unlike typical cases of glaucoma in which the unaffected disc tissue seemingly appears normal in color. However, this can be a difficult discrimination, and there do seem to be true, rare cases of intracranial tumors that appear to have more glaucomatous optic nerve changes. Not to miss this rare patient with an intracranial tumor that might be confused with LTG is important, but routine CT or MRI scans in patients with typical LTG is not prudent. On the other hand, one needs to remain alert for possibly atypical (for glaucoma) visual field changes and the presence of unilaterality or substantial asymmetry between the 2 eyes, especially in the presence of any neurological symptoms, and obtain neurological evaluation in all such patients.

Be aware that some patients with nonglaucomatous optic neuropathy can and will develop elevated IOP and glaucoma as a separate clinical disease. One of us (DLE) has seen patients with past methanol intoxication, Kjer's hereditary

TABLE 19-2. WHEN TO PURSUE NEUROLOGICAL WORK-UP IN A PATIENT WITH SUSPECTED LOW-TENSION GLAUCOMA
• Monocular optic nerve involvement or marked asymmetry
• Unexplained reduction in visual acuity
• Color vision loss without advanced visual field loss
• Visual field loss out of proportion to optic nerve damage
• Nonglaucomatous or atypical neurological symptoms
• Optic nerve pallor instead of cupping

optic atrophy, and a corticotrophin-secreting pituitary tumor (that caused elevated IOP reversed after surgical resection) with subsequent development of glaucoma. In addition to other considerations, these patients are a challenge to manage because of their pre-existing optic nerve changes.

In the differential diagnosis of LTG, one must include causes of past elevation of IOP that resulted in optic nerve damage, but are no longer present. Examples include previous steroid usage, uveitis, or trauma-related glaucoma. Such secondary glaucoma may not have been appreciated at the time of occurrence.

WHEN TO OBTAIN NEUROLOGICAL TESTING IN A PATIENT WITH LOW-TENSION GLAUCOMA

LTG is unfortunately not an uncommon disease. Many years ago, we stopped obtaining routine neurological evaluation. Routine scans are not performed, but if there is anything atypical, then at the slightest suggestion, a full neuro-ophthalmological evaluation is obtained (Table 19-2).

We would frame this as the concept of *LTG plus*. If the patient has any neurological symptom as discussed, atypical visual field changes (for glaucoma), a unilateral or highly asymmetric condition between the 2 eyes, or if there is something atypical about the cupping, especially the presence of atrophy in the noncontour-affected portion of the disc rim, then this constitutes the plus component and indicates the need for full neurological evaluation. There is no such entity as unilateral LTG, and substantial asymmetry is very uncommon. All such patients need neurological evaluation. Again, the one diagnosis to not miss is an intracranial tumor, but such an apparent "masquerader" is rare and would be expected to be suspected on the basis of these plus-factors.

Ocular Effects of Calcium-Channel Blockers: Past Promise

Peter A. Netland, MD, PhD

Calcium-channel antagonists block cell membrane-bound calcium channels and inhibit calcium influx, which can have a profound effect on cellular metabolism and function. In blood vessels, these drugs cause relaxation of smooth muscle cells in vascular walls, decrease vascular resistance, and improve blood flow. The ocular effects of calcium-channel blockers were once thought to be of great interest in relation to glaucoma, but much of the previous expectations have not been realized.[1]

Historical studies revealed that the vascular effects of calcium-channel blockers could inhibit vasospasm or enhance ocular blood flow,[2,3] which could then theoretically prove beneficial in glaucoma patients. In "vasospastic" patients and low-tension glaucoma patients, systemic administration of calcium-channel blockers was shown to be associated with improvements in visual field testing.[4,5] Some clinicians believe that improvement or stabilization of visual fields in low-tension glaucoma patients could be significant after treatment with systemic calcium-channel blockers. These beliefs are not substantiated by rigorous studies. In the past, we evaluated serial stereoscopic optic nerve photographs and visual fields for evidence of glaucomatous progression in low-tension glaucoma patients who were concurrently taking calcium-channel blockers compared with controls.[6] In this retrospective study, the use of systemic calcium-channel blockers was associated with a slowed progression of low-tension glaucoma. We have postulated that this apparent beneficial effect may be related to the inhibition of vasospasm or enhancement of optic nerve blood flow caused by these drugs.

The effect of calcium-channel blockers on IOP may also be of significance. Systemic administration of verapamil or nifedipine in rabbits sometimes caused a decrease in IOP.[7,8] In humans, either no effect or sometimes a decrease in IOP after systemic administration of verapamil, nifedipine, nitrendipine, or diltiazem has been observed.[9-12] However, a more pronounced effect was observed in ocular hypertensives or established glaucoma patients, who demonstrated elevated IOP at baseline.[9]

Topical administration of verapamil causes a significant reduction of IOP in ocular hypertensive human subjects.[13] This effect was sustained after topical administration of verapamil 3 times daily for 2 weeks.[14] Significant reduction of IOP has also been observed in normal human subjects after treatment with topical verapamil.[2] Experimental studies in rabbits have shown either no effect[8] or a reduction[15] of IOP after treatment with topical calcium-channel blockers. Topical administration of higher doses of calcium-channel blockers (1.5% to 5%) resulted in transient elevation of IOP,[16] suggesting a dose-dependent, biphasic response at higher doses of these drugs, perhaps due to other nonspecific effects besides calcium-channel blockade.[1] Topical treatment with the calcium ionophores A23187 and X573A have been observed to increase IOP in rabbits.[17] These agents would be expected to demonstrate an opposite action to calcium-channel blockers.

Topical administration of the calcium-channel blocker verapamil, therefore, usually causes a reduction of IOP. The more consistent effect on IOP of topical compared with systemic treatment may be due to higher drug levels reached after topical instillation of verapamil.[18] The mechanism of action may be due to enhancement of outflow facility.[19,20] These studies suggested a future possible role for topical therapy in the management of glaucoma. However, translation of this treatment modality to clinical practice from the preclinical setting and early rudimentary human studies was unsuccessful and the previous hope for this class of therapy was not realized. Association with systemic adverse events was a significant reason for lack of wide use in glaucoma patients.[21,22]

Much of what has been presented in this section is of historical relevance but is still of great value to those developing new therapies for glaucoma. Early promise does not always translate into wide clinical use. However, we learn from every experience and even failures can lead to bigger breakthroughs that will allow us to better treat our patients.

References

1. Netland PA, Erickson KA. Calcium channel blockers in glaucoma management. *Ophthalmol Clin North Am.* 1993;116:778-780.
2. Netland PA, Grosskreutz CL, Feke GT, et al. Color Doppler ultrasound analysis of ocular circulation after topical calcium channel blocker. *Am J Ophthalmol.* 1995;119:694-700.
3. Harino S, Riva CE, Petrig BL. Intravenous nicardipine in cats increases optic nerve head but not retinal blood flow. *Invest Ophthalmol Vis Sci.* 1992;33:2885.
4. Gasser P, Flammer J. Influence of vasospasm on visual function. *Doc Ophthalmol.* 1987;66:3.
5. Kitazawa Y, Shirai H, Go FJ. The effect of Ca2+-antagonist on visual field in low-tension glaucoma. *Graefes Arch Clin Exp Ophthalmol.* 1989;227:408.
6. Netland PA, Chaturvedi N, Dreyer EB. Calcium channel blockers in the management of low-tension and open-angle glaucoma. *Am J Ophthalmol.* 1993;115:608.
7. Green K, Kim K. Papaverine and verapamil interaction with prostaglandin E2 and 9-tetrahydrocannabinol in the eye. *Exp Eye Res.* 1977;24:207.
8. Payne LJ, Slagle TM, Cheeks LT, et al. Effect of calcium channel blockers on intraocular pressure. *Ophthalmic Res.* 1990;22:337.
9. Schnell D. Response of intraocular pressure in normal subjects and glaucoma patients to single and repeated doses of the coronary drug adalat. In: Lochner W, Engel HJ, Lichtlen PR, eds. *Second International Adalat Symposium.* Berlin: Springer Verlag; 1975:290.
10. Monica ML, Hesse RJ, Messerli FH. The effect of a calcium-channel blocking agent on intraocular pressure. *Am J Ophthalmol.* 1983;96:814.
11. Kelly SP, Walley TJ. Effect of the calcium antagonist nifedipine on intraocular pressure in normal subjects. *Br J Ophthalmol.* 1988;72:216.
12. Suzuki R, Hanada M, Fujii H, et al. Effects of orally administered alpha-2-adrenergic blockers and calcium-channel blockers on the intraocular pressure of patients with treated hypertension. *Ann Ophthalmol.* 1992;24:220.
13. Abelson MB, Gilbert CM, Smith LM. Sustained reduction of intraocular pressure in humans with the calcium channel blocker verapamil. *Am J Ophthalmol.* 1988;105:155.
14. Goyal JK, Khilnani G, Sharma DP, et al. The hypotensive effect of verapamil eye drops on ocular hypertension. *Ind J Ophthalmol.* 1989;37:176.
15. Segarra J, Santafe J, Garrido M, et al. The topical application of verapamil and nifedipine lowers intraocular pressure in conscious rabbits. *Gen Pharmacol.* 1993;24:1163.
16. Beatty JF, Krupin T, Nichols PF, et al. Elevation of intraocular pressure by calcium channel blockers. *Arch Ophthalmol.* 1984;102:1072.
17. Podos SM. The effect of cation ionophores on intraocular pressure. *Invest Ophthalmol.* 1976;15:851.
18. Ettl A, Daxer A, Hofmann U. Calcium channel blockers in the management of low-tension and open-angle glaucoma. *Am J Ophthalmol.* 1993;116:778.
19. Erickson KA, Schroeder A, Netland PA. Verapamil increases outflow facility in the human eye. *Exp Eye Res.* 1995;61:565-567.
20. Schuman JS, Beaton MA, Erickson KA, Schroeder A. Effects of topical verapamil on intraocular pressure, aqueous flow, and outflow facility in humans. *Invest Ophthalmol Vis Sci.* 1994;35(suppl):1483.
21. Sinclair NL, Benzie JL. Timolol eye drops and verapamil—a dangerous combination. *Med J Australia.* 1983;1:548.
22. Pringle SD, MacEwen CJ. Severe bradycardia due to interaction of timolol eye drops and verapamil. *Br Med J.* 1987;294:155.

THERAPY

Although there must be some systemic influence in LTG, there is no proven systemic therapy for this condition. There have been conflicting data[16,17] about calcium-channel blockers, which underscores our lack of understanding. It is not certain whether their proposed benefit might result from a vascular or direct axonal effect. Different blockers have different cellular mechanisms, and because we do not understand the mechanism for the optic nerve susceptibility in this condition (is it vascular or mechanical?), it seems quite premature to place LTG patients on such therapy. We would not recommend calcium-channel blocker therapy.

Because in most, if not all, patients with LTG we believe there to be an IOP-sensitive component,[18-20] therapy consists of lowering the IOP. This is all we have to offer, acknowledging that this disease involves a sick optic nerve involving some etiology that we do not fully understand. Documentation of the patient's baseline or representative IOP is critically important. One aims to decrease IOP by 20% to 25% as a first step. Much depends on the margin that is left to follow in the visual field, especially if scotomata are close to central fixation. In following such patients, central 10-degree visual field measurement is useful to supplement the usual 24-degree fields. If there is little margin to follow around fixation, one must be very aggressive in order to obtain IOPs in the single digits. Patients with such advanced field loss should be monitored closely, (eg, at least 3 times a year). Treatment for LTG follows the same protocol as POAG.

Because outflow facility through the TM is usually not substantially impaired in LTG, aqueous suppressants are typically more useful than outflow-enhancing drugs; however, our usual first choice is still the prostaglandin analogs. There are some data about possible adverse influences of certain nonselective beta-blockers on blood flow in the posterior segment,[21] but this class remains useful in the treatment of LTG. Because nonselective beta-blockers usually have a greater potency for IOP reduction than selective beta-blockers (see Chapter 12), and in this condition one starts with "normal" levels of IOP, the clinician usually desires full potency and chooses, if there is no systemic contraindication, a nonselective beta-blocker. In LTG, "every millimeter of mercury" is important, and one is therefore striving to lower the already "low IOP" as much as possible.

Therefore, one typically begins with a prostaglandin analog and progresses to a beta-blocker, nonselective if full potency is required, and advances therapy with alpha-2 agonists, followed by topical carbonic anhydrase inhibitors (CAIs) (or combination preparations for patient convenience and decreased ocular surface toxicity). Laser trabeculoplasty may also be performed as a first-line treatment in patients where compliance or convenience merit. Fistulization surgery, as for other forms of glaucoma, may become necessary when the maximum tolerated medical or laser therapy fails to control the IOP at a level low enough to prevent progressive damage.

As with high-pressure forms of POAG, it is important to establish a target pressure to guide your management. If there is margin to follow and a single drop achieves 20% to 25% IOP reduction, then one can stop here but closely follow the patient for progression. Baseline stereo disc photographs and 24-degree visual fields are important for baseline documentation and need to be re-evaluated as frequently as every 4 to 6 months. Structural imaging of the optic nerve and RNFL is helpful as well.

If there is advanced field loss at presentation and little margin to follow, a greater than 25% reduction in IOP may be required and the therapy advanced quickly. The bottom line is that many patients with LTG require an IOP in the single numbers that can only be obtained with fistulization surgery. Surprisingly, however, laser trabeculoplasty with or without concomitant medical therapy can be often be effective[22] to achieve an IOP around 10 mm Hg.

Many patients with progressive LTG that is not far advanced respond to a 20% reduction in IOP with apparent stability. The key is whether or not there is sufficient margin in the visual field that can be safely and accurately followed. If there is no margin to follow around central fixation, it can be justifiable to proceed rapidly to fistulizing surgery without the requirement of field progression (which in such a situation would likely affect central visual acuity).

NONPROGRESSIVE LOW-TENSION GLAUCOMA

Although much has been written about the entity in which purported acute hemodynamic crises[23] have produced a nonprogressive form of LTG, we believe this condition to be quite rare. The burden is on the ophthalmologist to prove that this apparent LTG does not in fact progress over the years. We would recommend treating all patients with apparent LTG, at least initially, unless there is good documentation for a single nonprogressive (eg, vascular) event in the past, with documented stability over many years. Certainly, in all newly diagnosed cases of LTG, it should be assumed that this will behave as a progressive disease, and therapy should be initiated. It is possible (but uncommon) that one might be treating some patients who will prove to have a nonprogressive disease, but just as likely that one will treat some patients with POAG who will not progress during any given observation period (see Chapter 18). One can rarely discriminate such patients at baseline, and the consequences of not treating axonal ischemia and death are usually greater than the risks of treating. Especially in LTG, in which progression commonly involves functionally important parts of the visual field close to fixation, the benefits of treatment almost always outweigh the risks. One can never prove the negative hypothesis (and therefore prove that a patient will never progress). With increased life expectancy of the population, it likely will prove true that nonprogressive LTG is an extremely uncommon entity.

Low-Tension Glaucoma Equivalent

Chapter 17 presented the concept that an eye with POAG with glaucomatous damage and a history of elevated IOP likely required an IOP of 18 mm Hg or lower in order to prevent further glaucomatous damage. Depending on the extent of the glaucomatous optic nerve and visual field changes, an IOP in the low teens or even single digits might be required for stability. In this discussion, we have termed this common clinical entity *LTG equivalent* because, without the known history of elevated IOP, this condition is indistinguishable from true LTG, and, in fact, it requires the same clinical management considerations and treatment.

We will comment (see Chapter 20) that patients with pseudoexfoliation glaucoma will often develop such LTG equivalent features. It is interesting to speculate whether exfoliation material deposits, even possibly in the optic nerve, might play a role in this phenomenon (see Chapter 1). Regardless, exfoliation glaucoma patients need to be followed with this possibility of LTG equivalent in mind, even if, as often occurs, there is reasonably normal IOP after laser trabeculoplasty or other treatment.

Does sustained previously elevated IOP affect an anatomical weakening on the optic disc structure that results in LTG equivalent?

This is yet another way to conceptualize this entity. From a practical point of view, it does not change the imperative to treat the patient in the same way as primary progressive LTG. In other words, if the current IOP is too high (even if it is "normal" from a statistical population point of view), then therapy needs to be advanced in order to further lower the IOP.

The corollary of this consideration might be that sustained IOP elevation, which, in the short-term, may not produce objective evidence for end-organ damage, can, in the long-term, produce a susceptible optic nerve, which requires a lower than statistically normal IOP in order to prevent progression. Or, as simply taught by Chandler and Grant: a disc once damaged commonly requires a lower-than-normal IOP to prevent further progression.

Chandler[24] wrote:

Progressive LTG is not a rare condition. Once the diagnosis has been established by inspection of the optic disc, repeated IOP measurement, and repeated measurement of the visual field, various medical measures are tried in an attempt to bring the IOP to lower levels. If medical treatment fails to lower the IOP significantly, and if repeated measurement of the field demonstrates progressive loss, we must come to a decision as to the future management of the case. If the patient is of advanced age, we may decide to continue with medical treatment (rather than proceeding with filtration surgery) in the hope of preserving some vision during the patient's lifetime. This is a difficult decision, for our patient might live to an advanced age and eventually become totally blind. When the situation is explained to the patient, he may help us in making a decision.

For many patients with progressive LTG, medical treatment alone will not lower the IOP sufficiently to prevent progressive loss. Therefore, for many such patients, a fistulizing operation has proven to be the best policy, and success in lowering IOP is usually effective in minimizing further loss of vision and field.

The following cases of Chandler are of interest. We consider them to be instances of progressive LTG or LTG equivalent in which cupping, atrophy, and field loss progressed with IOP in the normal range, and in which progression was arrested or conspicuously slowed when IOPs were reduced surgically to low levels.

Case 19-1

A 65-year-old man, previously described by us at an earlier stage, was first seen in 1952 with IOP right 17 mm Hg, left 22 mm Hg, with cupping and field loss that during 3 years progressed seriously threatening total blindness, despite medical maintenance of IOPs in the range of 15 to 20. In 1958 at age 71, each eye was trephined. Thereafter, IOPs remained 10 or below, and to at least age 89, the patient has been able to read and to carry on his profession as a lawyer.

Case 19-2

This man was always myopic and had been seen for refraction up to the age of 15 years. He was next seen at age 45 because his ophthalmologist had found some pathologic cupping of the disc. When seen here, corrected vision was 6/6 in each eye, IOP was right 20 mm Hg and left 17 mm Hg, the angles were wide open, and there appeared to be pathologic cupping of the discs, greater in the left eye. There was a double Bjerrum scotoma in the left eye with a good peripheral field, and in the right eye, the field was full except for a little nasal constriction. Tonography showed a C value of 0.26 right, 0.18 left, both in the normal range. He was next seen almost 1 year later, and there had been considerable loss of field and an increase in the cupping. The cup was now almost total in the left eye, came very close to the margin above and temporally in the right eye. IOP was right 20 and left 17. A trephining was done on both eyes. During the following 14 years, IOP has ranged from 12 to 17. There has been an excellent bleb in the left eye, not so good in the right eye. For several years, he has been pressing on the eyes 4 times a day to encourage the functioning of the blebs, and the IOP is temporarily reduced to a level of 10 or less after this pressure. His lenses are still clear, corrected vision is 6/5, and there has been no significant change in the visual field during the past 14 years.

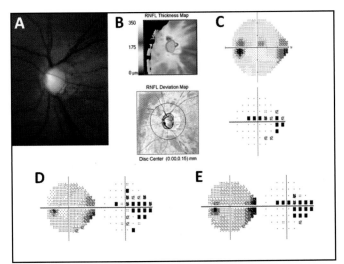

Figure 19-1. This 48-year-old Japanese man was referred to glaucoma service with a 14-year history of glaucoma. His highest recorded IOP was in the high teens in each eye, noted at the time of diagnosis. His IOP upon presentation was measured as 9 OD and 10 OS, using latanoprost and timolol with good adherence. He did not have prior laser trabeculoplasty or incisional surgery. Examination showed tilted myopic nerves with peripapillary atrophy, moderate cupping OD but a very thin rim inferiorly and superotemporal notch OS (A), which corresponded to a RNFL defect on OCT (B) and a superior paracentral and inferonasal step scotoma on Humphrey visual field (C). Follow-up over the next 2 years was concerning for progression OS (D), with inadequate IOP control ranging in the mid-teens, so therapy was advanced to include brimonidine OS. At the most recent follow-up, testing appeared to stabilize with IOP now measuring in the single digits OS (E). Unfortunately, many LTG patients continue to progress despite apparently adequate IOP control and often need surgical intervention to have the best chance at stabilization.

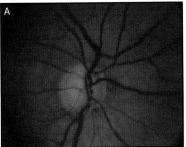
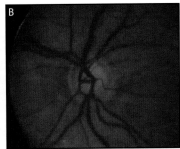
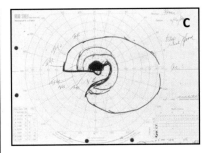

Figure 19-2. A 72-year-old woman with a history of migraine and a family history of glaucoma presented with IOP in the mid-teens OU (outflow facility = 0.15 OU) with severe field loss and disc cupping OD (A). There was a Marcus Gunn pupillary phenomenon OD. The left eye demonstrated advanced disc cupping (B) with earlier field loss. On maximal medical therapy including laser trabeculoplasty, IOP was decreased to 12 OD but there was further field loss 18 months later (C). Filtration surgery was performed OD with resulting IOP 8 to 9 mm Hg and stable visual fields and visual acuity = 20/25 for the subsequent 6 years. In the left eye, despite IOP between 11 and 13 mm Hg, there was further field progression and disc cupping. Laser trabeculoplasty was performed OS with resulting IOP 9 to 11 mm Hg, and the fields have been stable for the subsequent 4 years.

This appeared to be a case of progressive LTG. Before operation, IOP in the upper part of the normal range was evidently too high for his eyes, and the filtering operations appear to have been of real value in slowing up the process.

The following cases (Figures 19-1 through 19-3) illustrate several features of LTG or LTG equivalent. Patients with progressive LTG do not form a uniform group. In some, we believe that IOP, if diurnally measured, would never exceed normal limits (as defined in population studies). We believe that the optic nerves of such patients must have an abnormal susceptibility to their given level of IOP because lowering the IOP medically or surgically can stabilize their disease process. It is not unreasonable for such a varying susceptibility to exist among different people. In other patients with progressive LTG equivalent as defined, the condition represents progressive damage to the optic nerve at normal IOP in patients with initial damage at elevated IOP. Although some of these may represent diurnal fluctuations in our sampling of IOP at office visits or compliance variation in

patient medication, some represent the clinical reality that a damaged optic nerve will often develop progressive damage with a high normal level of IOP. As discussed, what unites all these cases is the apparent increased vulnerability of the optic nerve to IOP.

REFERENCES

1. Shiose Y, Kitazawa Y, Tsukahara S, et al. Epidemiology of glaucoma in Japan—a nationwide glaucoma survey. *Jpn J Ophthalmol.* 1991;35(2):133-155.
2. Usui T, Iwata K. Finger blood flow in patients with low tension glaucoma and primary open-angle glaucoma. *Br J Ophthalmol.* 1992;76(1):2-4.
3. Harris A, Sergott RC, Spaeth GL, et al. Color Doppler analysis of ocular vessel blood velocity in normal-tension glaucoma. *Am J Ophthalmol.* 1994;118(5):642-649.
4. Rader J, Feuer WJ, Anderson DR. Peripapillary vasoconstriction in the glaucomas and the anterior ischemic optic neuropathies. *Am J Ophthalmol.* 1994;117(1):72-80.
5. Stroman GA, Stewart WC, Golnik KC, et al. Magnetic resonance imaging in patients with low-tension glaucoma. *Arch Ophthalmol.* 1995;113(2):168-172.

Figure 19-3. A 63-year-old woman had a history of "nonprogressive LTG" after a hemodynamic crisis 5 years previously. During this interval, there was reported to be a stable optic nerve (A, OD; B, OS) appearance and visual field, which was normal except for an inferior nasal step OS (C). The patient was on no antiglaucoma therapy. IOP was 16 OU (outflow values 0.20 OD and 0.17 OS). However, 4 years later, there was increased cupping OU (D, OS) and field loss OS (E). Antiglaucoma therapy was initiated.

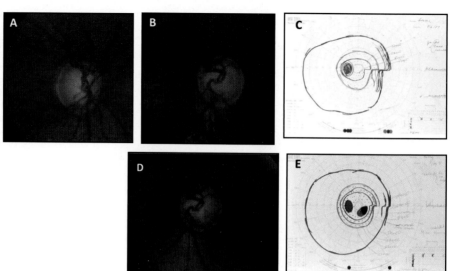

6. The effectiveness of intraocular pressure reduction in the treatment of normal-tension glaucoma. Collaborative Normal-Tension Glaucoma Study Group. *Am J Ophthalmol.* 1998;126(4):498-505.

7. Drance SM. Some factors in the production of low tension glaucoma. *Br J Ophthalmol.* 1972;56(3):229-242.

8. Phelps CD, Corbett JJ. Migraine and low-tension glaucoma. A case-control study. *Invest Ophthalmol Vis Sci.* 1985;26(8):1105-1108.

9. Usui T, Iwata K, Shirakashi M, et al. Prevalence of migraine in low-tension glaucoma and primary open-angle glaucoma in Japanese. *Br J Ophthalmol.* 1991;75(4):224-226.

10. Klein BE, Klein R, Meuer SM, et al. Migraine headache and its association with open-angle glaucoma: the Beaver Dam Eye Study. *Invest Ophthalmol Vis Sci.* 1993;34(10):3024-3027.

11. Krupin T, Liebmann JM, Greenfield DS, et al. The Low-pressure Glaucoma Treatment Study (LoGTS) study design and baseline characteristics of enrolled patients. *Ophthalmology.* 2005;112(3):376-385.

12. Cartwright MJ, Grajewski AL, Friedberg ML, et al. Immune-related disease and normal-tension glaucoma. A case-control study. *Arch Ophthalmol.* 1992;110(4):500-502.

13. Wax MB, Barrett DA, Pestronk A. Increased incidence of paraproteinemia and autoantibodies in patients with normal-pressure glaucoma. *Am J Ophthalmol.* 1994;117(5):561-568.

14. Caprioli J, Coleman AL. Blood pressure, perfusion pressure, and glaucoma. *Am J Ophthalmol.* 2010;149(5):704-712.

15. Sebag J, Thomas JV, Epstein DL, et al. Optic disc cupping in arteritic anterior ischemic optic neuropathy resembles glaucomatous cupping. *Ophthalmology.* 1986;93(3):357-361.

16. Lumme P, Tuulonen A, Airaksinen PJ, et al. Neuroretinal rim area in low tension glaucoma: effect of nifedipine and acetazolamide compared to no treatment. *Acta Ophthalmol (Copenh).* 1991;69(3):293-298.

17. Netland PA, Chaturvedi N, Dreyer EB. Calcium channel blockers in the management of low-tension and open-angle glaucoma. *Am J Ophthalmol.* 1993;115(5):608-613.

18. Abedin S, Simmons RJ, Grant WM. Progressive low-tension glaucoma: treatment to stop glaucomatous cupping and field loss when these progress despite normal intraocular pressure. *Ophthalmology.* 1982;89(1):1-6.

19. Cartwright MJ, Anderson DR. Correlation of asymmetric damage with asymmetric intraocular pressure in normal-tension glaucoma (low-tension glaucoma). *Arch Ophthalmol.* 1988;106(7):898-900.

20. Araie M, Sekine M, Suzuki Y, et al. Factors contributing to the progression of visual field damage in eyes with normal-tension glaucoma. *Ophthalmology.* 1994;101(8):1440-1444.

21. Drance SM, Crichton A, Mills RP. Comparison of the effect of latanoprost 0.005% and timolol 0.5% on the calculated ocular perfusion pressure in patients with normal-tension glaucoma. *Am J Ophthalmol.* 1998;125(5):585-592.

22. Schulzer M. Intraocular pressure reduction in normal-tension glaucoma patients. The Normal Tension Glaucoma Study Group. *Ophthalmology.* 1992;99(9):1468-1470.

23. Drance SM, Morgan RW, Sweeney VP. Shock-induced optic neuropathy: a cause of nonprogressive glaucoma. *N Engl J Med.* 1973;288(8):392-395.

24. Chandler PA, Grant WM. *Lectures on Glaucoma.* Philadelphia, PA: Lea & Febiger; 1965.

Pseudoexfoliation Syndrome and Open-Angle Glaucoma

Pratap Challa, MD, MS and David L. Epstein, MD, MMM

Once thought to be an unusual form of open-angle glaucoma primarily associated with Scandinavian ancestry, we now know that exfoliation (or pseudoexfoliation) glaucoma constitutes a significant portion of most glaucoma practices in the world. This is an age-related systemic disorder that was initially described by Lindberg in 1917[1] when he observed small flecks of bluish-gray material on the pupillary border of many patients with chronic glaucoma. In 1925, Vogt[2] further characterized this disorder and felt that the particles were produced by the lens and was a form of capsular glaucoma. Dvorak-Theobald[3] introduced the nomenclature of pseudoexfoliation of the lens to differentiate this disorder from the rare true exfoliation that occurs from infrared damage in glassblowers (and in recent times, in some welders who do not wear eye protection). Therefore, both pseudoexfoliation and exfoliation usually refer to the same disorder. The presence of glaucoma distinguishes pseudoexfoliation glaucoma from pseudoexfoliation syndrome. In many locations, initial reports indicated that pseudoexfoliation was rare, but then, with more focused detection methods, a higher prevalence was subsequently observed. Several points are worth emphasizing: pseudoexfoliation open-angle glaucoma mimics primary open-angle glaucoma in most, but not all, features and therefore may be under-detected or misdiagnosed. Recognition involves meticulous observation that includes the following (see Chapter 5):

- Careful attention to the crystalline lens on dilated slit-lamp examination
- The need to explain increased pigmentation observed on gonioscopy
- The observation of white flecks in the angle, on the lens, or on the zonules or ciliary processes (when visualized)
- The need to explain peripupillary iris transillumination defects

This is an important disorder that is the most common form of secondary open-angle glaucoma worldwide, accounting for 20% to 25% of open-angle glaucoma.[4]

DISEASE PREVALENCE

Pseudoexfoliation syndrome is a systemic disorder in which a poorly characterized, fibrillar substance is produced in abnormally high concentrations within ocular tissues. The incidence of pseudoexfoliation varies among ethnic groups,[5] with incidences of 20% to 25% in the Scandinavian countries of Iceland and Finland[6] to no reported cases among Greenland Eskimos.[7] The Framingham Eye Study (United States)[8] revealed an age-related increase among nonglaucoma individuals of 0.6% in individuals aged 52 to 64 years that rose to 5.0% for individuals aged 75 to 85 years. A relatively high incidence of pseudoexfoliation has been reported among Navajo Indians attending an eye clinic in New Mexico where 38% of elderly individuals had manifestations of pseudoexfoliation.[9,10] White individuals older than 60 years in the United States have a prevalence of pseudoexfoliation between 1.6% and 3%, and African American individuals are lower at approximately 0.4%.[11,12]

Both Lindberg[1] and Vogt[2] noted pseudoexfoliation's association with glaucoma and increasing age. Pseudoexfoliation is associated with 20% to 60% of open-angle glaucoma in various regions of the world including the Scandinavian countries, Greece, Russia, Iran, Nepal, Ethiopia, and South Africa.[5,13,14] High incidences are reported from Ireland[15] and Sweden[16] where pseudoexfoliation glaucoma is present in up to two-thirds of individuals with open-angle glaucoma. Reported prevalence ranges from 0.4% to 28% of open-angle glaucoma in the United States.[12,17-19] All prevalence rates are complicated by high variability between examiners. This may be due to the difficulty with diagnosing typical deposits

Kahook MY, Schuman JS, eds.
Chandler and Grant's Glaucoma, Fifth Edition (pp 217-225).
© 2013 SLACK Incorporated.

on the lens surface or other intraocular tissues due to both a missed diagnosis and that the deposits can become manifest over time after an initial diagnosis of primary open-angle glaucoma (POAG) or ocular hypertension (OHT).[19,20] Moreover, typical deposits are hard to see unless a postdilation examination of the anterior lens surface is performed. Some individuals have been shown on conjunctival biopsy specimens to have pseudoexfoliation syndrome before the typical slit-lamp findings were present.[21] The authors have observed that some patients who were initially diagnosed with POAG were later found to develop the typical fibrillar deposits on the lens (visible after dilation) and/or pupillary border and hence convert to a diagnosis of pseudoexfoliation glaucoma.

Pseudoexfoliation is a disease of basement membranes of the eye and other systemic tissues.[22,23] As discussed in Chapter 2, the base of the nonpigmented ciliary epithelial cell (head-to-head with the sclerad pigmented ciliary epithelial cell) faces the posterior chamber as does the base of the posterior iris pigment epithelial cell and the base of the lens epithelial cell, which constitutes the lens capsule. The base of all 3 of these cells, which line the posterior chamber, extrude pseudoexfoliation material onto their surface where presumably the material can enter the aqueous humor as well as lead to lens instability by weakening and disinserting zonular attachments.[24-27] Pseudoexfoliation has also been reported to develop locally separate from this, within the trabecular meshwork (TM), around Schlemm's canal,[28] and also in other intraocular sites, such as the corneal endothelium.[29] Pseudoexfoliation has also been reported to develop locally in the palpebral conjunctiva[28,30,31] and at systemic sites[23,32] and is believed to be a systemic abnormality,[23,32] although it is curious that it seems to cause clinical disease only within the eye.

The origin of pseudoexfoliation from multiple basement membrane sites within the eye is also believed to explain certain clinical features, such as the development of glaucoma and weakness of the zonules and/or lens capsule at the time of extracapsular cataract surgery.[33,34] Transmission electron microscopy of the outflow system in patients with pseudoexfoliation glaucoma reveals the presence of an abundance of pseudoexfoliation particles within the juxtacanalicular (JXT) layer with minimal to no material in the uveoscleral and corneoscleral layers of the TM. This favors the concept of local production of the material with possible secondary accumulation of material produced elsewhere in the eye (ie, material produced elsewhere may be floating into the aqueous humor and due to normal aqueous flow it reaches the TM). The accumulation of the pseudoexfoliation material in the JXT leads to compression and even focal collapse of Schlemm's canal (Figure 20-1). This disruption of normal Schlemm's canal architecture then leads to elevated intraocular pressures (IOPs) with associated optic nerve damage[35] and makes this form of glaucoma relatively more resistant to medical therapy. This also has implications for recent surgical techniques focused on Schlemm's canal, such

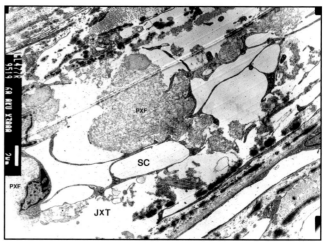

Figure 20-1. Transmission electron microscopy of the JXT region of the TM in a patient with pseudoexfoliation glaucoma. The accumulation of pseudoexfoliation material leads to disorganization and focal collapse of Schlemm's canal. JXT: juxtacanalicular region; PXF: pseudoexfoliation material; SC: Schlemm's canal.

as canaloplasty and trabectome surgery. The authors have found it more difficult to perform these procedures in pseudoexfoliation compared to POAG patients presumably due to focal collapse of Schlemm's canal.

Local production of the material by the lens epithelium and presumably by the ciliary epithelium can lead to zonular weakness and even disinsertion at their attachments to their respective structures. Electron microscopy studies of affected lens tissue demonstrates that the pseudoexfoliation material can aggregate into clumps that appear to work their way through the lens capsule onto the surface of the lens. If they come through the capsule at regions of zonular attachments, they can weaken or even disrupt the zonular insertions.[27,36,37] This process likely accounts for the increased rate of both intraoperative surgical complications and later-onset pseudophakic lens dislocations.[38] Another clinical feature is the loss of pigment from the posterior iris epithelium.[39-41] This appears as transillumination defects in the iris sphincter region and may be due to mechanical rubbing of the iris against the lens surface. Furthermore, pseudoexfoliation patients frequently demonstrate poor pupillary dilation. Histology demonstrates that the pseudoexfoliation material is also produced by the iris vascular endothelium.[42-44] However, iris angiography studies have not established iris ischemia as the causative mechanism for pigment loss and poor pupillary dilation.[45] This may be due to a limitation of this investigative technique, and the authors suspect that a low-grade and progressive iris ischemia may play a partial role in both pigment release and poor dilation.

DISEASE MECHANISM

Until recently, considerable discussion occurred over whether pseudoexfoliation might be only an incidental finding and whether affected patients with glaucoma might actually have simply POAG instead. Current thinking and genetic studies would not support such a tenet. Although it is true that patients can have pseudoexfoliation with no elevation of IOP (and totally normal outflow facility by tonography), there have been important studies, many from Scandinavia, that have documented the increasing risk of development of glaucoma in such patients with time.[46-51] As with pigmentary dispersion syndrome, there may be patients with the distinct syndrome who do not have, and perhaps may never develop, trabecular dysfunction. These diseases may require some trabecular abnormality in addition to either the pseudoexfoliation material or pigment, but it is naive to assume that this is the same trabecular defect that is present in POAG. For example, the latter may not require an insult such as deposited debris or pigment. However, POAG, itself, likely has more than one pathophysiological mechanism and constitutes more than one entity. It appears that the presumed basement membrane abnormality (and accumulation of typical material) within the TM and Schlemm's canal, itself, in pseudoexfoliation is the key to the presence or absence of abnormal outflow function.

There are also sometimes subtle but important clinical differences between pseudoexfoliation and POAG: the frequent substantial asymmetry or unilaterality,[51] the potential for rapid escalation of IOP and refractoriness to antiglaucoma therapy,[52] the more favorable early response to argon laser trabeculoplasty,[53,54] and the lesser incidence of "corticosteroid responsiveness" in pseudoexfoliation.[30,55]

Finally, important histopathological differences occur in the outflow pathway in pseudoexfoliation glaucoma compared with POAG. In the latter, the specific pathological finding is not unequivocal (see Chapter 18), but increased extracellular "plaque material,"[56] decreased cellularity,[57] and a disorganized trabecular beam structure have been observed. In contrast, in pseudoexfoliation glaucoma, the cellularity of the outflow pathway appears generally "normal," except for the presence of the extracellular pseudoexfoliation material.[24,58] However, in more advanced cases, changes in Schlemm's canal architecture can be seen. Thus, we believe that pseudoexfoliation is a secondary open-angle glaucoma due to the locally produced pseudoexfoliation material in the TM.

What contributed in the past to this uncertain discrimination between pseudoexfoliation and POAG was the common occurrence of cases of apparent unilateral pseudoexfoliation but bilateral glaucoma. However, we now know from the work of Mizuno and Muroi[59] that most such cases have occult pseudoexfoliation in the seemingly unaffected fellow eye. We have learned that one of the earliest sites for pseudoexfoliation to be observed is on the ciliary processes rather than the more easily viewed anterior crystalline lens surface.[59] (Of course, a current critical question is: Are we missing detecting even earlier sites because of the limitations of our observation techniques?)

The potential for multiple ocular and systemic sites of production of pseudoexfoliation material raises another consideration that was mentioned in Chapter 19 and may oversimply be stated as follows: there is a strong clinical sense that patients with pseudoexfoliation glaucoma who have had high IOP in the past may demonstrate optic nerves that are still susceptible to further damage despite normalization of the IOP that has been stabilized by medications and/or laser trabeculoplasty. Could local production of pseudoexfoliation or some related fundamental cellular abnormality within the optic nerve and especially its connective tissues explain this susceptibility? (Is there a potential unifying thread of a similar and possibly biochemically related phenomenon with amyloidosis?[60] [see Chapters 1 and 48]) Of note, pseudoexfoliation deposits are present within the optic nerve sheath but what role they play in the pathogenesis of glaucoma is unclear. We do not have an answer to this question, but it deserves attention not only from the clinical management point-of-view, but also because it might lend insight into other causes for low-tension glaucoma-like optic nerve susceptibility. Regardless, the clinical point is that, in patients with pseudoexfoliation open-angle glaucoma, the clinician must pay special attention to the possibility of a low-tension glaucoma equivalent condition (see Chapter 19).

GENETIC STUDIES

Pseudoexfoliation syndrome is a late-onset inherited condition in which pedigrees have demonstrated autosomal dominant, autosomal recessive, and maternal inheritance patterns. A recent genome association study by Thorleifsson and colleagues[61] has demonstrated 3 single nucleotide polymorphisms (SNPs) of the lysyl oxidase-like 1 (LOXL1) gene as strong genetic risk factors for pseudoexfoliation and pseudoexfoliation glaucoma in Icelandic and Swedish populations. LOXL1 is located on chromosome 15q24.1 and is part of a family of 5 lysyl oxidase enzymes (LOX, LOXL1, LOXL2, LOXL3, and LOXL4) that collectively play a key role in cross-linking between collagen and elastin in connective tissues.[62] Individually, LOXL1 catalyzes tropoelastin cross-linking and regulates elastin fiber formation and remodeling.[63] Therefore, perturbations in the function of LOXL1 may be another cause of the zonular instability seen with this disorder. Moreover, a growing body of molecular and biochemical evidence indicates that pseudoexfoliation arises from a stress-induced elastic microfibrillopathy. Although the exact pathogenesis of XFS remains unknown, it is believed to involve inadequate breakdown and/or excessive production of elastic fiber components.[64,65]

Subsequent studies performed in the United States,[66-70] Australia,[71] and Europe[72] have confirmed that 2 nonsynonymous coding SNPs (rs3825942 and rs1048661) and one intronic SNP (rs2165241) from the LOXL1 gene are strong genetic susceptibility factors for pseudoexfoliation and pseudoexfoliation glaucoma. In Indian,[73] Japanese,[74-79] and Chinese[80,81]

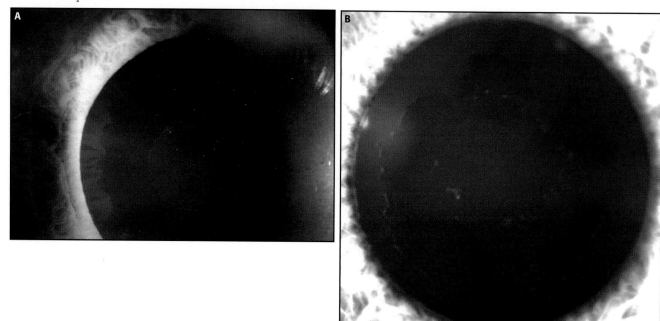

Figure 20-2. (A, B) Two examples of exfoliation of the anterior lens capsule.

cohorts, the association with rs3825942 confirmed that this is the strongest risk allele across different ethnicities and is present in 94% to 100% of affected individuals. However, the causative nature of these SNPs is unclear because other studies have shown inverse relationships for the reported risk alleles of rs3825942 (G), rs1048661 (G), and rs2165241 (T). The rs3825942 has an inverse relationship among individuals from South Africa,[82] while rs1048661 and rs2165241 are inversely related among Japanese[74-79] and Chinese[81] cohorts. This inverse relationship implies that the allele that is associated with the disease in most populations is actually the protective allele in these populations. Furthermore, there is early evidence that the expression of LOXL1 decreases in patients with pseudoexfoliation glaucoma.[83] However, the functional significance of the LOXL1 gene in the pathogenesis of pseudoexfoliation syndrome is unclear at present. Moreover, the disease SNPs are present in a large proportion of the control (unaffected) group—anywhere from 50% to 92% of these individuals—and despite extensive sequencing, the exact gene mutation has not been identified. Therefore, the presence of the LOXL1 SNPs cannot be the only cause of the development of pseudoexfoliation syndrome or glaucoma, and there must be other genes or environmental factors that play a role. Current and future studies may eventually elucidate the exact mechanisms that lead to this disorder.

CLINICAL FINDINGS

Although in many respects this type of glaucoma closely resembles POAG, there are some important differences. In addition, in open-angle glaucoma associated with pseudoexfoliation, we have found in most cases an abnormal accumulation of pigment in the filtration portion of the corneoscleral TM, usually involving the whole circumference, and distinctly more than is found in normal eyes of patients of the same age or in patients who have POAG. Pseudoexfoliation is often monocular, and the associated excessive pigmentation of the TM and the open-angle glaucoma are also commonly limited to the eye showing the pseudoexfoliation. However, sometimes in patients with bilateral pseudoexfoliation glaucoma, the severity of the glaucoma may actually be worse in the eye with lesser trabecular pigmentation (more commonly, however, the more heavily pigmented angle is associated with the more severe glaucoma).

POAG differs in that it almost always affects both eyes, although one eye may be affected more severely than the other, and in that the primary form of open-angle glaucoma usually is not associated with excessive pigmentation of the TM. As mentioned, there is a widely held opinion, which we share, that glaucoma associated with pseudoexfoliation tends to be less responsive to medical treatment than POAG.[30,48,52]

Pseudoexfoliation material is most commonly detected during slit-lamp examination when the pupillary border and face of the lens are examined (Figures 20-2 and 20-3). Fine light-gray amorphous flakes resembling dandruff may be noted at the pupillary margin, or a matte gray membrane with curled edges on the anterior surface of the lens. If the pupil is small, the pseudoexfoliation material may be hidden behind the pupillary margin and may be detected only when, using gonioscopy, one looks just under the pupillary margin. If the pupil is dilated, one may see on the anterior surface of the crystalline lens an area of lusterless gray that is smooth and homogeneous in the pupillary area, but ends in a series of scallops peripherally (see Figure 20-2), with

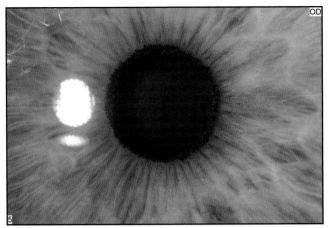

Figure 20-3. Photo demonstrating pseudoexfoliation material at the pupillary border of an affected individual. The material appears as whitish flecks at the pupillary border.

the most peripheral portion of the lens capsule appearing uncoated and normally lustrous. The edges of the coating on the lens sometimes appear rolled as though a portion of the anterior capsule were being exfoliated. If there is a coloboma of the iris, one may see that the amorphous coating on the lens extends further peripherally than in the areas where the iris is intact. Examination through the gonioscope lens and examination of enucleated eyes have established that material having the same gray amorphous appearance is also present on the zonules of the lens, on the ciliary processes, and on the posterior surface of the iris. It may also be occasionally deposited on the corneal endothelium.

When the material on the posterior surface of the iris is lightly brushed experimentally in an enucleated eye, particles of pigment from the pigment epithelium of the iris are released. Also, when patients with pseudoexfoliation material have their pupils dilated, a cloud of pigment particles released into the anterior chamber may be seen by slit-lamp.[84] Transillumination of the iris from behind or through the pupil commonly demonstrates a patchy loss of pigment from the posterior pigment layer adjoining the pupil, but there is no clear indication of loss from peripheral portions of the iris like those seen in pigment dispersion syndrome. Pseudoexfoliation may be associated with cataractous lens changes,[85] especially nuclear sclerosis. Presumably, this relates to the basement membrane changes of the lens epithelium, which might be responsible for fluid movement changes in the crystalline lens over time.

The prevalence of pseudoexfoliation varies according to the criteria of different examiners. As mentioned, at one time, pseudoexfoliation was thought to be rare outside of the Scandinavian countries, but increasing thoroughness in examination has shown it to be common worldwide, with little relation to race or geography. As a rule, it is found with increasing frequency with age. Often it occurs to a much greater degree or much earlier in one eye than the other. A sizable minority of people who have

pseudoexfoliation develop glaucoma, but many others with conspicuous amounts of exfoliation material in their eyes apparently do not get glaucoma during observation for many years. Careful examination of patients with open-angle glaucoma in various parts of the world has disclosed that about 10% to 30% may have pseudoexfoliation material, the proportion increasing with age. From small series of tests that have been done so far, it appears that in most patients with open-angle glaucoma associated with pseudoexfoliation material, corticosteroids do not evoke an elevation of IOP of the degree or the frequency that is encountered in patients with ordinary POAG.[30,55] This is further indication that these are fundamentally different types of glaucomas.

When open-angle glaucoma is encountered with considerably elevated IOP, cupping, atrophy, and field loss in one eye, but with no evidence of glaucoma in the other eye, the most common finding is pseudoexfoliation material in the glaucomatous eye. As described, a ring of pigment is commonly found in the TM of the glaucomatous eye, and not in the other, but this is not an essential feature. In exceptional cases, there are all the features mentioned except the excess pigment, and this naturally makes it seem that pigment in the TM may be much less important in obstructing aqueous outflow than some other factor in glaucoma associated with pseudoexfoliation. The only other known factor is the pseudoexfoliation material itself. This is recognizable by electron microscopy as a peculiar fibrillar material, and it has been identified in the TM of many specimens excised during surgery on eyes with glaucoma too severe to be controlled medically.[30,86,87]

Though the glaucoma associated with pseudoexfoliation material often appears monocularly as just described, when the apparently normal contralateral eye is kept under observation, usually after some years, a little pseudoexfoliation material begins to make its appearance, and IOP slowly begins to rise in that eye also. Mizuno and Muroi[59] have demonstrated with ciliary body indentation the presence of occult pseudoexfoliation in ciliary processes in fellow eyes of patients with apparent unilateral pseudoexfoliation.[19,59] Such occult pseudoexfoliation in the fellow eye does then likely explain the presence of bilateral glaucoma in some patients with apparent unilateral pseudoexfoliation.[19]

ASSOCIATION WITH NARROW ANGLES

Another issue is that it is not unusual for patients with pseudoexfoliation to have narrow angles.[88] This is important, separate from any considerations of acute angle closure, for the following reason: patients with diagnosed pseudoexfoliation open-angle glaucoma might develop a superimposed angle-closure component with the passage of years. Thus, this clinical worsening of the disease might be amenable to improvement with laser iridectomy. This emphasizes again the importance of the rule: if the IOP is elevated on a follow-up visit, always re-gonioscope the patient.

In contrast, however, there may be patients presenting with narrow angles and elevated IOP (see Chapter 22) who did not, in fact, have functional angle closure, but rather open-angle glaucoma due to occult pseudoexfoliation. Not only might laser iridectomy not improve the IOP, but with the existing trabecular dysfunction due to pseudoexfoliation, there is the potential for a substantial acute IOP spike. The rule here is that, in eyes with narrow angles, the clinician, dedicated to the rule of 5% (see Chapter 5) looks diligently and routinely for signs of occult pseudoexfoliation.

CLINICAL COURSE

A rule of 5% clinical point that is not rare is as follows: in patients who have had high IOP due to pseudoexfoliation but a dramatic lowering of IOP following laser trabeculoplasty, the clinician should be alert in his or her further follow-up to the first signs that the IOP, although perhaps still at an acceptable level, is creeping-up a few millimeters of mercury. One may find that, if the next visit after this is scheduled, as is routine, 4 months ahead, the patient returns then with very high IOP again and sometimes further unexpected disc and field damage. We have learned that, although there are more early time period successes with laser trabeculoplasty in pseudoexfoliation glaucoma compared to POAG, there are unfortunately more longer-term failures (such that the survival curves meet and may even slightly cross).[54] Regardless, the clinical point is that the trabecular abnormality present in pseudoexfoliation open-angle glaucoma can dramatically worsen between routine visits, and the clinician needs to be alert to this not only following laser trabeculoplasty, but in the routine system follow-up of pseudoexfoliation patients in general.

A borderline IOP in a pseudoexfoliation glaucoma patient thus is a cause for concern and indicates, at a minimum, the need for closer follow-up. Another corollary of this phenomenon is that, in a borderline situation, it is prudent to be somewhat more aggressive with one's antiglaucomatous therapy or strategy in a patient with pseudoexfoliation glaucoma and glaucomatous end-organ damage (disc cupping and field loss).

It should also be mentioned that it is not rare to see patients with pseudoexfoliation presenting with a central (or branch) retinal vein occlusion. Although, as indicated above, there possibly might be pseudoexfoliation processes intrinsic to the optic nerve, we have regularly explained this clinical finding as being due to the high IOPs found in pseudoexfoliation. Thus, a central retinal vein occlusion may be the first presentation of pseudoexfoliation glaucoma (and, of course, when one clinically encounters such unilateral cases, one needs to look carefully for the presumed underlying pseudoexfoliation open-angle glaucoma and distinguish this unilateral pseudoexfoliation glaucoma from a secondary neovascular or angle-closure disease due to the vein

occlusion). Another corollary of this phenomenon is that, in known pseudoexfoliation patients, the clinician needs to be alert to the occurrence of acute vascular events (including glaucomatous optic nerve damage) due to elevated IOP between clinical visits. The clinical point that needs to be stressed in all this is that, in pseudoexfoliation glaucoma, there is the definite potential for worsening of the glaucoma (both IOP and optic nerve damage) between routine visits.

TREATMENT

The treatment of open-angle glaucoma associated with pseudoexfoliation material is the same as for POAG except that medical treatment tends to be less effective.[30,52,89]

Pseudoexfoliation glaucoma seems to respond better in the short-term than other forms of glaucoma to laser trabeculoplasty (LTP). In view of our observations concerning the pathogenesis of pseudoexfoliation glaucoma,[24] one wonders whether the mechanism of LTP may be biologic[90-92] (eg, inducing phagocytosis of pseudoexfoliation material in the outflow channels or inducing increased trabecular beam cell repopulation[93]). Despite the often dramatic IOP lowering achieved with argon LTP in pseudoexfoliation glaucoma eyes, late failures are unfortunately quite common,[54] as indicated above. This may be due to new deposition of pseudoexfoliation material in the outflow pathway leading to decreasing aqueous outflow. Selective LTP has also been shown to be effective in patients with pseudoexfoliation glaucoma; however, the authors' clinical impression is that, in patients with advanced disease, it has less efficacy.[94] On the other hand, as discussed in earlier chapters, it is likely true that, as

---

TONOGRAPHY IN PSEUDOEXFOLIATION

Pratap Challa, MD, MS and David L. Epstein, MD, MMM

In cases of pseudoexfoliation, the authors have found tonography clinically useful not only to properly assess the status of the fellow eye, but also to detect the presence of severe impairment of outflow (*flat curves*). An important clinical point in dealing with pseudoexfoliation glaucoma, in contrast to most (but not all) patients with POAG, is the potential for galloping open-angle glaucoma. That is, pseudoexfoliation glaucoma patients have the potential for dramatic further escalation of elevation of IOP between routine 3- to 4-month interval visits. Especially given the possible increased susceptibility of the optic nerve to glaucomatous damage in this condition, the clinician must be alert to this possibility. On the other hand, most patients with pseudoexfoliation glaucoma demonstrate the slow gradual worsening course seen in primary open-angle glaucoma.

What is the strategy for not missing such galloping patients? The patient's past history of IOP fluctuation is a guide, but, in general, pseudoexfoliation patients should be followed somewhat more closely, perhaps four times a year rather than 3. In addition, if tonography demonstrated flat outflow, there is the potential, at least, for more rapid escalation, and, therefore, such patients should be followed even more closely.

with all our current glaucoma therapies, none of which are cures,[95] we are aiming mainly to slow the "rate of decay" of the disease process by usage of laser trabeculoplasty in pseudoexfoliation glaucoma. Eventually, the biochemical changes that LTP produces[96] are overwhelmed by the progressive deposition of pseudoexfoliative material and, hence, limit the effectiveness of repeat LTP treatments.

Incisional glaucoma surgery is commonly required in pseudoexfoliation glaucoma. Fortunately, surgical success in pseudoexfoliation appears similar to that seen in POAG.

FURTHER QUESTIONS

The most intriguing questions about pseudoexfoliation glaucoma include the following:

- What is the pseudoexfoliation material?
- Where exactly does the material in the TM come from?
- What is its exact role in aqueous outflow obstruction?
- How do LOXL1 polymorphisms lead to disease?
- What other genes or environmental factors play a role?

No complete answers are yet available. The chemical nature has been guessed at from results of histologic staining, electron microscopy, and proteomic analysis.[97] However, the molecular basis of this disorder has not been elucidated. Of all the different forms of glaucoma, this one appears to be most amenable to direct therapeutic intervention. A majority of pseudoexfoliation glaucoma could likely be cured if a therapy were developed that simply decreased the production of the pseudoexfoliation material in the eye.

At this time, we look on open-angle glaucoma associated with pseudoexfoliation as a secondary type of glaucoma, and we believe there is good reason to try to get at its cause or causes, hoping ultimately to retard or prevent its development. This type of glaucoma represents such a significant fraction of the glaucomas of older people—and one that is relatively refractory to medical treatment—that a means of prevention would have great overall value.

REFERENCES

1. Tarkkanen A, Kivela T. John G. Lindberg and the discovery of exfoliation syndrome. *Acta Ophthalmol Scand.* 2002;80(2):151-154.
2. Vogt A. Ein neues Spaltlampenbild des Pupillengebietes: Hellblauer Pupillensaumfilz mit Hautchenbildung auf der Linsenvorderkapsel. *Klin Monatsabl Augenheilkd.* 1925;75:1-12.
3. Dvorak-Theobald G. Pseudo-exfoliation of the lens capsule: relation to true exfoliation of the lens capsule as reported in the literature and role in the production of glaucoma capsulocuticulare. *Am J Ophthalmol.* 1954;37(1):1-12.
4. Ritch R. Exfoliation syndrome-the most common identifiable cause of open-angle glaucoma. *J Glaucoma.* 1994;3(2):176-177.
5. Forsius H. Exfoliation syndrome in various ethnic populations. *Acta Ophthalmol.* 1988;184(suppl):71-85.
6. Forsius H. Prevalence of pseudoexfoliation of the lens in Finns, Lapps, Icelanders, Eskimos, and Russians. *Trans Ophthalmol Soc U K.* 1979;99(2):296-298.
7. Lantukh VV, Piatin MM. [Features of ocular pathology among the indigenous inhabitants of Chukotka]. *Vestn Oftalmol.* 1982;(4):18-20.
8. Liebowitz HM, Maunder LR. The Framingham eye study monograph. *Surv Ophthalmol.* 1980;24(suppl):335-610.
9. Faulkner HW. Pseudo-exfoliation of the lens among the Navajo Indians. *Am J Ophthalmol.* 1971;72(1):206-207.
10. Friederich R. Eye disease in the Navajo indians. *Ann Ophthalmol.* 1982;14(1):38-40.
11. Mitchell P, Wang JJ, Hourihan F. The relationship between glaucoma and pseudoexfoliation: the Blue Mountains Eye Study. *Arch Ophthalmol.* 1999;117(10):1319-1324.
12. Cashwell LF Jr, Shields MB. Exfoliation syndrome. Prevalence in a southeastern United States population. *Arch Ophthalmol.* 1988;106(3):335-336.
13. Ringvold A. Epidemiology of glaucoma in northern Europe. *Eur J Ophthalmol.* 1996;6(1):26-29.
14. Tarkkanen AH. Exfoliation syndrome. *Trans Ophthalmol Soc U K.* 1986;105(pt 2):233-236.
15. Madden JG, Crowley MJ. Factors in the exfoliation syndrome. *Br J Ophthalmol.* 1982;66(7):432-437.
16. Lindblom B, Thorburn W. Observed incidence of glaucoma in Halsingland, Sweden. *Acta Ophthalmol (Copenh).* 1984;62(2): 217-222.
17. Ball SF. Exfoliation syndrome prevalence in the glaucoma population of South Louisiana. *Acta Ophthalmol.* 1988;184(suppl):93-98.
18. Ritch R. Exfoliation syndrome: The most common identifiable cause of open-angle glaucoma. *J Glaucoma.* 1994;3:176-178.
19. Roth M, Epstein DL. Exfoliation syndrome. *Am J Ophthalmol.* 1980;89(4):477-481.
20. Crittendon JJ, Shields MB. Exfoliation syndrome in the southeastern United States. II. Characteristics of patient population and clinical course. *Acta Ophthalmol.* 1988;184(suppl):103-106.
21. Schlotzer-Schredhardt U, Kuchle M, Dorfler S, Naumann GO. Pseudoexfoliative material in the eyelid skin of pseudoexfoliation-suspect patients: a clinico-histopathological correlation. *Ger J Ophthalmol.* 1993;2(1):51-60.
22. Eagle RC Jr, Font RL, Fine BS. The basement membrane exfoliation syndrome. *Arch Ophthalmol.* 1979;97(3):510-515.
23. Schlotzer-Schrehardt UM, Koca MR, Naumann GO, Volkholz H. Pseudoexfoliation syndrome. Ocular manifestation of a systemic disorder? *Arch Ophthalmol.* 1992;110(12):1752-1756.
24. Richardson TM, Epstein DL. Exfoliation glaucoma: a quantitative perfusion and ultrastructural study. *Ophthalmology.* 1981;88(9):968-980.
25. Schlotzer-Schrehardt U, Naumann GO. A histopathologic study of zonular instability in pseudoexfoliation syndrome. *Am J Ophthalmol.* 1994;118(6):730-743.
26. Assia EI, Apple DJ, Morgan RC, et al. The relationship between the stretching capability of the anterior capsule and zonules. *Invest Ophthalmol Vis Sci.* 1991;32(10):2835-2839.
27. Ritch R, Schlotzer-Schrehardt U. Exfoliation syndrome. *Surv Ophthalmol.* 2001;45(4):265-315.
28. Ringvold A. Electron microscopy of the limbal conjunctiva in eyes with pseudo-exfoliation syndrome (PE syndrome). *Virchows Arch A Pathol Pathol Anat.* 1972;355(3):275-283.
29. Schlotzer-Schrehardt UM, Dorfler S, Naumann GO. Corneal endothelial involvement in pseudoexfoliation syndrome. *Arch Ophthalmol.* 1993;111(5):666-674.
30. Layden WE, Shaffer RN. Exfoliation syndrome. *Am J Ophthalmol.* 1974;78(5):835-841.
31. Streeten BW, Bookman L, Ritch R, et al. Pseudoexfoliative fibrillopathy in the conjunctiva. A relation to elastic fibers and elastosis. *Ophthalmology.* 1987;94(11):1439-1449.
32. Streeten BW, Li ZY, Wallace RN, et al. Pseudoexfoliative fibrillopathy in visceral organs of a patient with pseudoexfoliation syndrome. *Arch Ophthalmol.* 1992;110(12):1757-1762.
33. Lumme P, Laatikainen L. Exfoliation syndrome and cataract extraction. *Am J Ophthalmol.* 1993;116(1):51-55.

34. Lumme P, Laatikainen LT. Risk factors for intraoperative and early postoperative complications in extracapsular cataract surgery. *Eur J Ophthalmol.* 1994;4(3):151-158.

35. Gottanka J, Flugel-Koch C, Martus P, et al. Correlation of pseudo-exfoliative material and optic nerve damage in pseudoexfoliation syndrome. *Invest Ophthalmol Vis Sci.* 1997;38(12):2435-2446.

36. Chijiwa T, Araki H, Ishibashi T, Inomata H. Degeneration of zonular fibrils in a case of exfoliation glaucoma. *Ophthalmologica.* 1989;199(1):16-23.

37. Dark AJ, Streeten BW, Cornwall CC. Pseudoexfoliative disease of the lens: a study in electron microscopy and histochemistry. *Br J Ophthalmol.* 1977;61(7):462-472.

38. Bartholomew RS. Phakodonesis. A sign of incipient lens displacement. *Br J Ophthalmol.* 1970;54(10):663-666.

39. Deodati F, Labro JB, Poitevin B. [Fluorescence angiography of the anterior chamber in capsular pseudo-exfoliation]. *Bull Soc Ophtalmol Fr.* 1975;75(1):107-111.

40. Ghosh M, Speakman JS. The iris in senile exfoliation of the lens. *Can J Ophthalmol.* 1974;9(3):289-297.

41. Konstas AG, Marshall GE, Cameron SA, Lee WR. Morphology of iris vasculopathy in exfoliation glaucoma. *Acta Ophthalmol (Copenh).* 1993;71(6):751-759.

42. Ringvold A. The distribution of the exfoliation material in the iris from eyes with exfoliation syndrome (pseudoexfoliation of the lens capsule). *Virchows Arch A Pathol Pathol Anat.* 1970;351(2):168-178.

43. Ringvold A. Light and electron microscopy of the wall of iris vessels in eyes with and without exfoliation syndrome (pseudoexfoliation of the lens capsule). *Virchows Arch A Pathol Pathol Anat.* 1970;349(1):1-9.

44. Spinelli D, de Felice GP, Vigasio F, Coggi G. The iris vessels in the exfoliation syndrome: ultrastructural changes. *Exp Eye Res.* 1985;41(4):449-455.

45. Parodi MB, Bondel E, Saviano S, Ravalico G. Iris fluorescein angiography and iris indocyanine green videoangiography in pseudo-exfoliation syndrome. *Eur J Ophthalmol.* 1999;9(4):284-290.

46. Hansen E, Sellevold OJ. Pseudoexfoliation of the lens capsule. I. Clinical evaluation with special regard to the presence of glaucoma. *Acta Ophthalmol (Copenh).* 1968;46(6):1095-1104.

47. Odland M, Aasved H. Follow-up of initially nonglaucomatous patients with fibrillopathia epitheliocapsularis (so-called senile exfoliation of the anterior lens capsule). *Acta Ophthalmol.* 1973;120(suppl):77-81.

48. Aasved H. Intraocular pressure in eyes with and without fibrillopathia epitheliocapsularis (so-called senile exfoliation or pseudoexfoliation). *Acta Ophthalmol (Copenh).* 1971;49(4):601-610.

49. Kozart DM, Yanoff M. Intraocular pressure status in 100 consecutive patients with exfoliation syndrome. *Ophthalmology.* 1982;89(3):214-218.

50. Henry JC, Krupin T, Schmitt M, et al. Long-term follow-up of pseudoexfoliation and the development of elevated intraocular pressure. *Ophthalmology.* 1987;94(5):545-552.

51. Hansen E, Sellevold OJ. Pseudoexfoliation of the lens capsule. II. Development of the exfoliation syndrome. *Acta Ophthalmol (Copenh).* 1969;47(1):161-173.

52. Konstas AG, Jay JL, Marshall GE, Lee WR. Prevalence, diagnostic features, and response to trabeculectomy in exfoliation glaucoma. *Ophthalmology.* 1993;100(5):619-627.

53. Psilas K, Prevezas D, Petroutsos G, et al. Comparative study of argon laser trabeculoplasty in primary open-angle and pseudoexfoliation glaucoma. *Ophthalmologica.* 1989;198(2):57-63.

54. Threlkeld AB, Hertzmark E, Sturm RT, et al. Comparative study of the efficacy of argon laser trabeculoplasty for exfoliation and primary open-angle glaucoma. *J Glaucoma.* 1996;5(5):311-316.

55. Gillies WE. Corticosteroid-induced ocular hypertension in pseudo-exfoliation of lens capsule. *Am J Ophthalmol.* 1970;70(1):90-95.

56. Rohen JW. Why is intraocular pressure elevated in chronic simple glaucoma? Anatomical considerations. *Ophthalmology.* 1983;90(7):758-765.

57. Alvarado J, Murphy C, Juster R. Trabecular meshwork cellularity in primary open-angle glaucoma and nonglaucomatous normals. *Ophthalmology.* 1984;91(6):564-579.

58. Lutjen-Drecoll E, Shimizu T, Rohrbach M, Rohen JW. Quantitative analysis of plaque material in the inner- and outer wall of Schlemm's canal in normal- and glaucomatous eyes. *Exp Eye Res.* 1986;42(5):443-455.

59. Mizuno K, Muroi S. Cycloscopy of pseudoexfoliation. *Am J Ophthalmol.* 1979;87(4):513-518.

60. Kivela T, Tarkkanen A, Frangione B, et al. Ocular amyloid deposition in familial amyloidosis, Finnish: an analysis of native and variant gelsolin in Meretoja's syndrome. *Invest Ophthalmol Vis Sci.* 1994;35(10):3759-3769.

61. Thorleifsson G, Magnusson KP, Sulem P, et al. Common sequence variants in the LOXL1 gene confer susceptibility to exfoliation glaucoma. *Science.* 2007;317(5843):1397-1400.

62. Lucero HA, Kagan HM. Lysyl oxidase: an oxidative enzyme and effector of cell function. *Cell Mol Life Sci.* 2006;63(19-20):2304-2316.

63. Liu X, Zhao Y, Gao J, et al. Elastic fiber homeostasis requires lysyl oxidase-like 1 protein. *Nat Genet.* 2004;36(2):178-182.

64. Zenkel M, Kruse FE, Junemann AG, et al. Clusterin deficiency in eyes with pseudoexfoliation syndrome may be implicated in the aggregation and deposition of pseudoexfoliative material. *Invest Ophthalmol Vis Sci.* 2006;47(5):1982-1990.

65. Zenkel M, Kruse FE, Naumann GO, Schlotzer-Schrehardt U. Impaired cytoprotective mechanisms in eyes with pseudoexfoliation syndrome/glaucoma. *Invest Ophthalmol Vis Sci.* 2007;48(12):5558-5566.

66. Aragon-Martin JA, Ritch R, Liebmann J, et al. Evaluation of LOXL1 gene polymorphisms in exfoliation syndrome and exfoliation glaucoma. *Mol Vis.* 2008;14:533-541.

67. Challa P, Schmidt S, Liu Y, et al. Analysis of LOXL1 polymorphisms in a United States population with pseudoexfoliation glaucoma. *Mol Vis.* 2008;14:146-149.

68. Fan BJ, Pasquale L, Grosskreutz CL, et al. DNA sequence variants in the LOXL1 gene are associated with pseudoexfoliation glaucoma in a U.S. clinic-based population with broad ethnic diversity. *BMC Med Genet.* 2008;9:5.

69. Fingert JH, Alward WL, Kwon YH, et al. LOXL1 mutations are associated with exfoliation syndrome in patients from the Midwestern United States. *Am J Ophthalmol.* 2007;144(6):974-975.

70. Yang X, Zabriskie NA, Hau VS, et al. Genetic association of LOXL1 gene variants and exfoliation glaucoma in a Utah cohort. *Cell Cycle.* 2008;7(4):521-524.

71. Hewitt AW, Sharma S, Burdon KP, et al. Ancestral LOXL1 variants are associated with pseudoexfoliation in White Australians but with markedly lower penetrance than in Nordic people. *Hum Mol Genet.* 2008;17(5):710-716.

72. Pasutto F, Krumbiegel M, Mardin CY, et al. Association of LOXL1 common sequence variants in German and Italian patients with pseudoexfoliation syndrome and pseudoexfoliation glaucoma. *Invest Ophthalmol Vis Sci.* 2008;49(4):1459-1463.

73. Ramprasad VL, George R, Soumittra N, et al. Association of nonsynonymous single nucleotide polymorphisms in the LOXL1 gene with pseudoexfoliation syndrome in India. *Mol Vis.* 2008;14:318-322.

74. Hayashi H, Gotoh N, Ueda Y, et al. Lysyl oxidase-like 1 polymorphisms and exfoliation syndrome in the Japanese population. *Am J Ophthalmol.* 2008;145(3):582-585.

75. Mori K, Imai K, Matsuda A, et al. LOXL1 genetic polymorphisms are associated with exfoliation glaucoma in the Japanese population. *Mol Vis.* 2008;14:1037-1040.

76. Ozaki M, Lee KY, Vithana EN, et al. Association of LOXL1 gene polymorphisms with pseudoexfoliation in the Japanese. *Invest Ophthalmol Vis Sci.* 2008;49(9):3976-3980.

77. Fuse N, Miyazawa A, Nakazawa T, et al. Evaluation of LOXL1 polymorphisms in eyes with exfoliation glaucoma in Japanese. *Mol Vis.* 2008;14:1338-1343.

78. Mabuchi F, Sakurada Y, Kashiwagi K, et al. Lysyl oxidase-like 1 gene polymorphisms in Japanese patients with primary open angle glaucoma and exfoliation syndrome. *Mol Vis.* 2008;14:1303-1308.

79. Tanito M, Minami M, Akahori M, et al. LOXL1 variants in elderly Japanese patients with exfoliation syndrome/glaucoma, primary open-angle glaucoma, normal tension glaucoma, and cataract. *Mol Vis.* 2008;14:1898-1905.

80. Lee KY, Ho SL, Thalamuthu A, et al. Association of LOXL1 polymorphisms with pseudoexfoliation in the Chinese. *Mol Vis.* 2009;15:1120-1126.

81. Chen L, Jia L, Wang N, et al. Evaluation of LOXL1 polymorphisms in exfoliation syndrome in a Chinese population. *Mol Vis.* 2009;15:2349-2357.

82. Williams SE, Whigham BT, Liu Y, et al. Major LOXL1 risk allele is reversed in exfoliation glaucoma in a black South African population. *Mol Vis.* 2010;16:705-712.

83. Khan TT, Li G, Navarro ID, et al. LOXL1 expression in lens capsule tissue specimens from individuals with pseudoexfoliation syndrome and glaucoma. *Mol Vis.* 2010;16:2236-2241.

84. Krause U, Helve J, Forsius H. Pseudoexfoliation of the lens capsule and liberation of iris pigment. *Acta Ophthalmol (Copenh).* 1973;51(1):39-46.

85. Puska P. Lens opacity in unilateral exfoliation syndrome with or without glaucoma. *Acta Ophthalmol (Copenh).* 1994;72(3):290-296.

86. Rodrigues MM, Spaeth GL, Sivalingam E, Weinreb S. Histopathology of 150 trabeculectomy specimens in glaucoma. *Trans Ophthalmol Soc U K.* 1976;96(2):245-255.

87. Toriyama K, Maezawa N. [Electron microscopic study on the trabecular tissues in glaucoma capsulare (author's trans)]. *Nihon Ganka Gakkai Zasshi.* 1976;80(9):780-789.

88. Gross FJ, Tingey D, Epstein DL. Increased prevalence of occludable angles and angle-closure glaucoma in patients with pseudoexfoliation. *Am J Ophthalmol.* 1994;117(3):333-336.

89. Aasved H. The frequency of optic nerve damage and surgical treatment in chronic simple glaucoma and capsular glaucoma. *Acta Ophthalmol (Copenh).* 1971;49(4):589-600.

90. Van Buskirk EM, Pond V, Rosenquist RC, Acott TS. Argon laser trabeculoplasty. Studies of mechanism of action. *Ophthalmology.* 1984;91(9):1005-1010.

91. Melamed S, Epstein DL. Alterations of aqueous humour outflow following argon laser trabeculoplasty in monkeys. *Br J Ophthalmol.* 1987;71(10):776-781.

92. Stein JD, Challa P. Mechanisms of action and efficacy of argon laser trabeculoplasty and selective laser trabeculoplasty. *Curr Opin Ophthalmol.* 2007;18(2):140-145.

93. Acott TS, Samples JR, Bradley JM, et al. Trabecular repopulation by anterior trabecular meshwork cells after laser trabeculoplasty. *Am J Ophthalmol.* 1989;107(1):1-6.

94. Song J, Lee PP, Epstein DL, et al. High failure rate associated with 180 degrees selective laser trabeculoplasty. *J Glaucoma.* 2005;14(5):400-408.

95. Epstein DL. Will there be a remedy to reverse the changes in the trabecular meshwork and the optic nerve? A personal point of view on glaucoma therapy. *J Glaucoma.* 1993;2(2):138-139.

96. Melamed S, Pei J, Epstein DL. Delayed response to argon laser trabeculoplasty in monkeys. Morphological and morphometric analysis. *Arch Ophthalmol.* 1986;104(7):1078-1083.

97. Ovodenko B, Rostagno A, Neubert TA, et al. Proteomic analysis of exfoliation deposits. *Invest Ophthalmol Vis Sci.* 2007;48(4):1447-1457.

21

Pigment Dispersion and Pigmentary Glaucoma

Ian P. Conner, MD, PhD; Kimberly V. Miller, MD;
Joel S. Schuman, MD, FACS; and David L. Epstein, MD, MMM

DIAGNOSIS

Pigment dispersion syndrome (PDS) is characterized by loss of pigment from the posterior surface of the iris in the mid-periphery in both eyes and an attendant deposition of pigment on intraocular structures, such as the back of the cornea, the trabecular meshwork (TM), the iris, and the lens. PDS can occur with or without the pigmentary glaucoma (PG) that was first described as an entity by Sugar and Barbour[1] and Sugar.[2]

We have observed the full dispersion syndrome without glaucoma in routine eye examinations, probably as frequently as actual PG. Many pigment dispersion patients have been kept under observation for years and have not developed elevated intraocular pressure (IOP). Patients with PG who we have seen have almost always already had this condition or at least some abnormality in aqueous outflow when first seen by us.

PDS typically occurs in people between the ages of 20 and 45 years, but it has been found in rare instances in teenagers and in the elderly. It is more common in men than women. Women seem to develop PG at a slightly older age than men. A family history of PG is seldom obtained, but PG has been reported in brothers,[3] and we have found it in young female twins and in a father and daughter. Sometimes, there is a family history of primary open-angle glaucoma.

The onset of PG in some cases appears to be rapid, with elevated IOP, fine corneal edema, and symptoms of blurring of vision or seeing of haloes. These symptoms usually make the patient realize that there is a problem, though in most instances there is no pain. In a considerable proportion of cases, the diagnosis can be made before there has been much damage to the optic nerve head. However, the circumstances of onset are not always as fortunate as this. Some young men who we have seen with this type of glaucoma had developed severe cupping and atrophy of their optic discs and loss of visual field before they became aware that anything was wrong, as in the following case.

Case 21-1

A 30-year-old White man presented with a 1-year history of intermittent haloes. A diagnosis of PG had been made in Argentina. He was 6 diopters (D) myopic in both eyes. He had fine pigment deposition on the corneal endothelium and extensive, mid-peripheral iris transillumination. Both lenses showed fine pigment dusting on the anterior capsule and pigmentation of the posterior surface peripherally. Gonioscopy revealed dense pigment bands covering the TM, with fine uveal meshwork ("iris processes") from iris to ciliary body band and scleral spur. IOPs were 30 right and left. There was marked glaucomatous cupping of both discs extending superiorly to the rim with extensive inferior field loss in both eyes.

Treatment was rapidly advanced to maximal tolerated medical therapy. There was evidence of worsening field loss in the right eye. On this basis, a filtering operation was performed on this eye. Although the bleb seemed to fail, with resumption of medical therapy, including use of pilocarpine, Ocusert (Alza Pharmaceuticals, Palo Alto, CA; no longer clinically available at the time of this writing), and later timolol, IOPs were well-controlled in the operated eye. The patient has refused operation on the left eye, but fortunately the IOP in this eye has been sufficiently controlled by topical timolol, and the field has remained stable.

This case also illustrates the fact that eyes with PG (eg, the left eye of this patient) can show spontaneous improvement

Kahook MY, Schuman JS, eds.
Chandler and Grant's Glaucoma, Fifth Edition (pp 227-236).
© 2013 SLACK Incorporated.

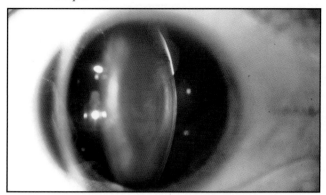

Figure 21-1. Slit-beam photograph of a patient with PDS. This amount of pigment on the corneal endothelial surface (Krukenberg spindle) is exceptional, but illustrates the concept well.

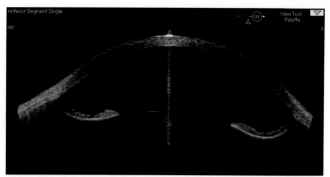

Figure 21-2. Anterior segment OCT demonstrating posterior iris bowing in a patient with PDS (also commonly termed *reverse pupillary block*).

in IOP control with time, even with minimal or conservative treatment.

In some instances, glaucoma without symptoms, but with IOP in the 40s, has been detected on routine examination in young men and occasionally in women, who have sought attention merely for myopic refraction.

Unfortunately, it is not rare for patients with PG to present with reduced vision in one eye,[4] which may have been attributed to optic neuritis in the past. We have wondered, in such patients, whether the commonly observed fluctuating high IOP may have caused a previous acute optic nerve vascular insult.

Most patients with PDS have deep anterior chambers and are usually, but not always, myopic. The first clue to the disease may be found during slit-lamp examination when pigment is seen on the posterior surface of the cornea, occasionally forming a Krukenberg spindle, but this is not seen in every case (Figure 21-1). Some have little or no pigment on the back of the cornea. The reason for the variable pigment deposition on the corneal endothelium is unclear. Aqueous convection currents deposit the pigment on the posterior surface of the corneal endothelium, which may later engulf the pigment. Curiously, the pigment does not typically cause corneal endothelial decompensation.[5] Most commonly, one can observe a sprinkling of pigment on the anterior surface of the iris stroma and on the back of the cornea.

The PDS (with or without PG) is not associated with any external or internal sign of intraocular inflammation, such as synechiae or inflammatory cells in the aqueous humor or on the back of the cornea, but we have seen cases in which pigment particles circulating in the aqueous humor have been mistaken for inflammatory cells and the glaucoma was erroneously attributed to uveitis (eg, glaucomatocyclitic crisis). Attention to the brown color of the particles helps prevent this mistake. (An intriguing untested hypothesis is that there may be something else in addition to pigment particles [melanosomes] that may be released from the back of the iris that might actually be producing the glaucoma in this

condition.[6] Perhaps, in the future, this might be amenable to some type of novel "antipigment" therapy.)

GONIOSCOPY

Gonioscopy in PDS (with or without PG) typically demonstrates in each eye a deep anterior chamber, with a flat and often slightly tremulous iris. A concave (posterior) iris contour is frequently observed (Figure 21-2).[7,8] (This sometimes is more readily apparent on Koeppe gonioscopy [Ocular Instruments, Bellevue, WA] than on mirrored slit-lamp gonioscopy.) The iris stroma appears normal, except for pigment that may be deposited on its anterior surface. The angle is wide and open in all quadrants. The ciliary band is often broad, but sometimes it is not. The most essential feature in the angle is a band of dark-brown, almost black, homogeneous, velvety pigment that may strikingly delineate the filtration portion of the TM in the whole circumference (Figure 21-3). The pigment often covers not only the filtration portion, but the whole width of the TM in the entire circumference, including Schwalbe's line (where it can form a Sampaolesi's line, similar to what is seen in exfoliation syndrome). Pigment may also be deposited on the ciliary body band. During gonioscopy, if one looks through the pupil toward the equator of the crystalline lens, when there is pigment dissemination, one can also see an accumulation of pigment at the posterior surface of the lens (Scheie stripe or Zentmayer line) where zonules or hyaloid face reach the lens and form a sort of pocket. Similarly, in cases with heavy pigment dispersion, there may be pigment deposition on the anterior lens surface as well.

Although a dark, dense, wide band of pigment filling the filtration portion of the TM is the rule in PDS, with or without glaucoma, in rare cases, we have seen the density of the pigment band diminish with age, as described by Lichter and Shaffer.[9] However, we are not convinced that this is necessarily accompanied by an improvement in IOP control. This same phenomenon of decreasing trabecular pigment band density was demonstrated in an experimental monkey model of PDS without producing chronic glaucoma.[6]

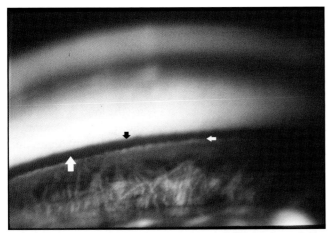

Figure 21-3. Patient with PG demonstrates angle landmarks well. The aqueous humor drains through the posterior aspect of the TM in which the pigment band lies (large white arrow). Anterior TM contains much less pigment. Schwalbe's line (black arrow) and the scleral spur (small white arrow) are easily defined.

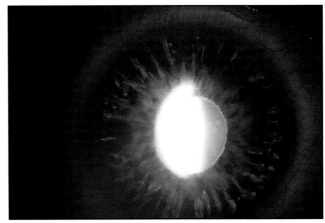

Figure 21-4. Marked loss of posterior iris pigment in a patient with PDS.

In other cases, we have seen patients at a single stage with a typical transillumination pattern of the iris, but with a pigment band in the angle of only moderate density. In such cases, when the typical iris transillumination pattern has been present, we have postulated that some of the trabecular pigment may have washed out through the outflow channels or been carried away by phagocytes. The latter has also been implicated in the experimentally produced model.[6]

IRIS TRANSILLUMINATION

The presence of a typical iris transillumination pattern (Figure 21-4) is considered essential to the diagnosis of the PDS. When the examiner has dark adapted for several minutes and employs a fiberoptic transilluminator in a darkened room, one sees the typical, mid-peripheral iris transillumination pattern that is initially radial and slit or wedge-like, but later may become confluent. In advanced conditions, these abnormal iris transillumination defects can extend into the central third of the iris.

To test for loss of pigment from the posterior layer of the iris, transillumination of the iris is performed by holding a shielded fiberoptic transilluminator against the lower lid temporally or against the sclera temporally, in such a way that light passing through the sclera glows bright and pink from the pupil when one looks directly at the eye. This must be done in a darkened room. In normal eyes, the light does not shine through the iris in the manner characteristic of PDS, but in genuine cases of the syndrome, the iris transilluminates in a striking patchy ring in the mid-periphery. This is due to loss of pigment from this particular portion of the posterior pigment layer. Elsewhere, either near the pupil (except at advanced stages) or in the periphery adjacent to the ciliary body band, the pigment layer appears to remain intact. The selective loss of pigment in the mid-portion of

the iris can sometimes be appreciated better if one performs the transillumination while viewing the iris through the Koeppe gonioscopy lens. Alternatively, at the slit-lamp, the beam may be narrowed and placed coaxial to the observer in the patient's pupil, in order to search for transillumination defects. This maneuver should be a routine part of one's slit-lamp examination.

In the absence of a characteristic iris transillumination pattern, it is difficult to make a definitive diagnosis of the PDS, although there are rare patients (usually with dark irides) who demonstrate all other aspects of the syndrome but in whom the iris does not transilluminate and who have no known source for pigment dissemination other than the iris (ie, exfoliation, iris or ciliary body cysts, or melanoma[10-12] were ruled out). Dr. Grant saw one patient in whom a typical transillumination pattern disappeared, as though from new pigment formation; this patient had gradual disappearance of a pigment band from the angle several years after successful filtration surgery (in retrospect, it is possible that this may have been due to the peripheral iridectomy performed as part of the surgery).

Case 21-2

A 29-year-old man was aware of some aching around his left eye. His ophthalmologist found IOPs of 40 mm Hg in both eyes, with pathologic cupping of both discs, worse on the left, with a Bjerrum scotoma in this eye. When seen here, without treatment, the IOP was 60 with tonographic C values of 0.05 in each eye. Both discs had deep broad cups with central vessels displaced far nasally, a thin layer of tissue preserved within the rim in most of the circumference of the right disc, but excavation to the rim lower temporally in the left. The anterior chambers were deep. By gonioscopy, the irides appeared almost concave, attaching just posterior to the scleral spur in the whole circumference. A dense blackish pigment band covered the filtration portion of the TM in the whole circumference in both eyes. Transillumination showed a striking moth-eaten type of defect of the posterior pigment layer of each iris in a ring peripherally, characteristic of PG in both eyes. Response to treatment with pilocarpine and epinephrine was inadequate. A filtration operation was performed on the left eye, and 3 months later on the right. A better bleb was obtained on the right eye than the left. For several months, the IOP was close to 7 mm Hg in the right and in the mid-20s in the left. Frequent digital pressure on the left globe was employed to try to improve the function of the bleb. A little more than a year after the operation, both eyes had excellent blebs and IOPs of 9 without treatment other than periodic digital pressure. The degree of cupping became notably less in each eye than when first seen, and by 8 years after the bilateral operation, the degree of cupping of both discs had decreased remarkably, though the principal vessels remained far to the nasal side of the right disc and the left was still as pale as it had been at the first observation. By that time, the amount of pigment in the angles appeared to be decreasing, and the transillumination of the irides also appeared less than when the patient was first seen. At nearly 10 years after the operation, the blebs were not quite as good as formerly. IOPs reached the high teens, and epinephrine drops were started in each eye.

At 14 years after surgery, the IOPs were 15 in both eyes under treatment with epinephrine and digital pressure several times a day. Corrected vision was 20/25 right, 20/50 left. The Bjerrum scotoma in the left eye remained unchanged. The pigment in the angles had changed from a dense, almost black pigment band covering the filtration portion of the TM in the whole circumference to a thin line of a distinctly lighter brown color. The filtration blebs contained no pigment. Transillumination of the irides showed no abnormal transillumination of any portion of either iris, except for the surgical iridectomies, in contrast to the striking moth-eaten appearance of pigment loss from the posterior layer of the iris seen peripherally in the initial examinations performed in the same manner. There had been remarkable thinning of the pigment in the angle and disappearance of the transillumination of the irides. (Unfortunately, the glaucoma was actually still slowly worsening with time.)

PATHOGENESIS OF THE IRIS TRANSILLUMINATION DEFECTS AND THE PIGMENT DISPERSION

There is still clinical uncertainty in PG, mainly due to important clinical observations made by observant clinicians. (Glaucoma remains a specialty where important new insights can be made by the clinician who carefully and meticulously [see Chapter 5] examines patients and is an inquisitive observer). Karickhoff[13,14] and Campbell[15] observed that the normally concave iris contour present in PG reverts to a planar configuration after laser iridotomy. This has been confirmed by ultrasound.[7,16] Previously,

Campbell had hypothesized that rubbing of the posterior iris surface against the zonule was responsible for the pigment dispersion from the posterior iris surface.[17] Thus, laser iridotomy, by preventing this rubbing, might have applicability in the treatment of patients with PG.

Nevertheless, it is not yet appropriate[18] to apply laser iridotomy as a potential cure for PG for the following reasons. Clinical studies to date have not shown laser iridotomy to have a clinical benefit in PG.[19] The fundamental question in this disease, whether the pigment loss from the posterior iris surface represents a primary iris pigment epithelial degeneration or abiotrophy (a kind of pre-senile tissue degeneration that may be genetically predetermined)[18,20] or is, in fact, a mechanical disease due to zonular rubbing[17] has still not been totally resolved.[21] The concept of zonular rubbing was ingenious and intriguing but has not, despite its ready popularity, been unequivocally established. The hypothesis was based on studies of enucleated eyes that were fixed in a usual postmortem hypotonous state in which it is difficult to orient zonular packets with the posterior iris defects as they might appear in a normal living eye. Further, in advanced PG, the iris transillumination defects may extend well into the central third of the iris where the zonule is not believed to extend. Also, the posterior surface of the iris folds on itself with pupillary dilation (T. Kuwabara, unpublished observations), such that small segments should be protected from a to-and-fro rubbing, as originally proposed. The peripheral iris transillumination streaks should therefore contain small segments of less dense transillumination. (Actually, a careful clinical examination does indicate that some transillumination defects in PG show this uncommonly.) Of course, this to-and-fro rubbing may not be what is happening mechanically in the living eye, but rather a ballottement of the posterior iris surface against the zonule with eye movement as a consequence of the typical iris concavity in these usually larger myopic eyes. This could then mechanically explain the observed, usually continuous iris transillumination streak.

Even more importantly, there are patients who have the full PDS including iris concavity, typical transillumination defects, and angle pigmentation who do not have elevated IOP or any abnormality in outflow dynamics. There is a strong clinical impression with some limited data that such patients will never, in fact, develop PG. Except for the normal IOP and absence of glaucomatous optic nerve changes, such pigmentary dispersion patients cannot be distinguished from those with PG. In such patients, the same mechanical factors that lead to loss of iris pigment in PG must also be present, and yet there is no glaucoma. There must then be more to PG than pigment dispersion alone. In fact, experimental studies in living monkeys have confirmed that one cannot, in previously normal monkeys, cause PG despite instilling vast quantities of pigment into the anterior chamber and producing TM pigment bands.[6,22] That is, experimentally, one can produce pigmentary dispersion but not PG.

Most likely, there is some trabecular cellular abnormality that is required in addition to the pigment dispersion for the glaucoma to occur.[6] It could be argued that the pigment release is a stress to the TM in such individuals and that, by diminishing this (eg, with laser iridotomy), it might improve the clinical condition. A retrospective study did not show benefit with this approach[19]; however, a prospective randomized trial did indicate less risk of elevated IOP after laser iridotomy in PDS.[23] These trials should be further performed in patients with existing PG (ideally with symmetric disease so that only one eye can be treated, creating an internal control) and not in patients with PDS without glaucoma, who, as indicated, have a very low probability of developing abnormal outflow function.

What also should give one pause is the observation that, as patients with PG age, there is commonly a remarkable decrease in angle pigmentation, producing an increase in relative pupillary block.[17] However, we have not been impressed that the glaucoma status (except perhaps now for the absence of attacks of high IOP associated with pigment storms in the anterior chamber that, regardless, may decrease with the passage of time) has actually concomitantly improved. One might argue in rebuttal that it is too late in the disease process for this to occur, but this still should not be used as justification to treat patients with pigmentary dispersion who have no IOP elevation with prophylactic laser iridectomy.

The loss of iris concavity after laser iridectomy that was originally observed by Karickhoff[13,14] and Campbell[15] has been confirmed,[7,16] but still has no definitive explanation. Some have proposed sudden bursts of aqueous humor flow through the pupil with reverse pupillary block temporarily ensuing—a ball valve effect of the lens and iris.[8,13,15] An alternative that needs evaluation derives from the fact that there is normally protein leakage into the anterior chamber at the base of the iris that explains the higher protein content of pretrabecular aqueous humor compared to that in the central anterior chamber.[24,25] It is conceivable that, in the larger typically myopic eye involved in pigmentary dispersion, the iris may be thinner at the root (in addition to other abiotrophic features of such eyes), and thus there is flow of aqueous humor into the anterior chamber at this site. The latter phenomenon then could explain a slightly higher pressure occurring in the anterior chamber than the posterior chamber and, hence, the resulting iris concavity. Alternatively, abnormalities in the iris dilator muscle have been described in PDS,[20] and perhaps these contribute directly to the observed iris concavity. Possibly the laser-produced hole in the iris mechanically interferes with the underlying structural mechanism (eg, interfering with circumferentially oriented iris tone). When the pupil is dilated with a sympathomimetic agent, the concavity of the peripheral iris of a patient with PDS commonly disappears, presumably due to the contraction of the iris dilator muscle. Perhaps mechanical considerations might also explain the change in iris contour with accommodation[26] that sometimes seems to occur in this condition. These are only speculations, but the effect of laser iridotomy on iris contour does not, in itself, prove that zonular rubbing or ballottement is the cause of pigment release, nor that there will be less pigment release from the posterior iris surface after the procedure. Many myopic eyes show a concave iris contour without any signs of pigment dispersion, and there may be cases of PDS where laser iridectomy does not alter iris concavity.[27]

Despite these reservations, new observations based on detailed clinical examination of patients with this condition (that was available to all of us but not fully appreciated in past years) offer much fresh information for further investigation and clarification. It has been shown in a randomized prospective trial that the chance of elevated IOP in PDS eyes was decreased by laser iridotomy over a period of 10 years.[23] However, there is no definite evidence to support laser iridotomy in eyes with PG, due to the fact that the TM may be already damaged, and laser iridotomy by its nature increases the amount of pigment released into the anterior chamber. Certainly, the time is appropriate for a randomized prospective clinical trial involving one eye of a precisely defined population of patients with symmetric PG. Finally, it would not seem outside the spectrum of acceptable practice, as a last attempt to control PG prior to fistulizing surgery, to offer a laser iridotomy to one eye after a full discussion of the benefits and risks with the affected patient. However, the clinician must keep the limits of our understanding firmly in mind as he or she seeks to determine whether the course of the glaucoma is truly altered, or simply the iris concavity.

Pathogenesis of the Trabecular Glaucoma

The pathogenesis of the chronic impairment in outflow function in PG is still far from clear. There is both clinical[28] and laboratory[6,29] evidence that iris pigment can acutely obstruct outflow of aqueous humor. This seems reasonable but leaves completely unexplained how another group of patients who appear to have the same amount of pigment in their angles have no obstruction of outflow, either by IOP measurement or tonography. Perhaps differences in the response of the trabecular endothelial cells to the pigment may be important in determining whether aqueous outflow is obstructed. Richardson et al reported electron micrographic evidence of trabecular sclerosis in PG,[30] but this is likely a late phenomenon. Alvarado's group has reported abnormalities in the cell-lined outflow pathway in PG.[31,32] Further electron microscopic examination of the PDS without glaucoma, as reported by Fine et al,[18] is needed for comparison with all these studies. Pigment alone does not appear to be obstructing the extracellular outflow pathway in chronic PG.[32]

We produced a model of PDS in living monkeys that has provided some insight to this condition.[6] Homologous uveal pigment was perfused into the anterior chamber of these monkeys. Acutely, there was a substantial lowering of outflow facility, and experimental glaucoma resulted. However, in these otherwise normal monkeys, there was rapid recovery, and despite repetitive perfusions of pigment, outflow facility returned to normal. The monkeys developed trabecular pigment bands, which often decreased in density with time. Morphologic examination indicated that the structure of the TM remained normal despite pigment phagocytosis and possible migration of trabecular endothelial cells. A few animals were observed for several additional years, with once again normal aqueous humor dynamics and TM morphology including cellularity.[22] Our study also raised the issue of whether the loss observed of TM pigment with time was due to wandering macrophages rather than trabecular cell migration. We concluded that factors in addition to iris pigment shedding (eg, underlying trabecular cell abnormalities) are involved in the development of chronic PG.

Some observers have interpreted PG as a congenital mesodermal angle anomaly, or simply as a variant of primary open-angle glaucoma, though tests in patients with PG have indicated a different reactivity to corticosteroids than is found in primary open-angle glaucoma.[33] We often do observe dense or prominent uveal meshwork (so-called iris processes) in patients with PDS, both with and without glaucoma, but we doubt that this type of anatomy is more common in PDS than in similarly myopic eyes that have wide angles without excessive pigment.

DIFFERENTIAL DIAGNOSIS

In the differential diagnosis of PG, one should keep in mind open-angle glaucoma associated with exfoliation (see Chapter 20), in which a smaller amount of pigment is usually seen in the TM, but in which transillumination shows no loss of pigment from the portion of the iris affected in "pigmentary" glaucoma, rather only a loss near the pupil. Rarely, a pigment ring in the angle is seen in amyloidosis with glaucoma (see Chapter 48). Pigment in various amounts is commonly found in the angle in elderly people either without glaucoma or with primary open-angle glaucoma, and some pigment may be found in the angle in association with uveitis (see Chapter 42), with cysts of the iris and ciliary body (see Chapter 34), and after operation, traumatic angle recession, or attacks of acute angle-closure glaucoma. However, the pigment in most of these conditions rarely forms a uniform band in the entire circumference. In the exfoliation syndrome with glaucoma, pigment is seen in the entire circumference, but it is often narrower, coarser, and less dense than in PG. In none of these conditions does the pigment layer of the iris transilluminate abnormally in the mid-periphery as it does in PG. The clinician should always

seek to explain the presence of abnormal pigmentation observed on gonioscopy.

PDS nearly always affects both eyes of an individual, although it may be asymmetric. In rare instances, it occurs only in one eye, but before accepting such a diagnosis, one should be able to identify the iris transillumination pattern and to rule out other causes of monocular pigment dissemination, especially melanoma[12] of the anterior uveal tract (see Chapter 41) causing melanomalytic glaucoma.[10,11]

PIGMENTARY DISPERSION WITHOUT GLAUCOMA

It is strange but true that the PDS can occur with or without glaucoma. Pigment dispersion with consistently normal IOPs can easily escape recognition, because transillumination is not commonly performed routinely, and a Krukenberg spindle may be overlooked or may not be present. We have discovered a number of cases of PDS without glaucoma by doing a screening type of transillumination during routine slit-lamp examination by narrowing the slit beam to fit into the pupil, making the beam coaxial with the microscope, and observing the iris for transillumination with low magnification. The following case is an example.

Case 21-3

A 60-year-old man presented to the emergency room with a corneal abrasion. Bilateral Krukenberg spindles were noted. The past eye history was negative except for conjunctivitis. The family history was negative for glaucoma.

Several areas of abnormal iris transillumination in the mid-periphery were noted, and gonioscopy revealed a heavy trabecular pigment band in both eyes. The discs were normal, and the fields were full. Applanation IOPs were 16 OU, and tonographic C values were 0.23 right and 0.25 left. No exfoliation was seen. During 10 years of follow-up, the IOPs remained in the teens.

This man with PDS without glaucoma is being followed as a PG suspect, but at his age and with his good outflow facility, it is unlikely that he will ever develop PG.

Recognizing that PDS without glaucoma is a real and not-so-rare entity raises the important question of whether these patients will eventually develop PG. It has been observed that the risk of conversion from PDS to PG is 10% in 5 years and 15% in 15 years.[34] Clearly, this means that a large portion of patients may never convert or it may take many years. Sugar has observed the onset of glaucoma 12 to 20 years after pigmentary dispersion was first detected.[2] In our longest follow-up, we can say that a patient with pigmentary dispersion can go for 20 years without developing glaucoma. This occurred in the following case.

Case 21-4

A 76-year-old White man was diagnosed as having pigment dispersion without glaucoma in the emergency room where he sought treatment for blepharitis. According to records of his private ophthalmologist, he had been followed for the previous 20 years for heavy Krukenberg spindles in both eyes, always with normal IOPs and with no treatment. In addition to broad Krukenberg spindles, in both eyes, there were occasional pigment particles present spontaneously in the aqueous humor and moderate pigment deposition on the anterior iris surface. No exfoliation was found. The anterior chambers were deep, and marked iridodonesis was present. Striking spoke-like mid-peripheral iris transillumination was present in all quadrants in both eyes. Applanation IOP was 19 mm Hg in each eye. Gonioscopy revealed wide open angles with dense continuous pigment bands and dense but not abnormal uveal meshwork. Both optic discs had physiologic cups, and the visual fields were full. Tonographic C values were 0.33 right and 0.38 left. Phenylephrine provocative testing of the right eye produced a conspicuous increase in the amount of pigment particles in the aqueous humor, but no change in IOP.

How often should one re-evaluate patients who have typical pigment dispersion but apparently normal IOP? If initially several pressure determinations at different times of the day are normal, or if tonography indicates good facility of outflow, and the discs are normal, we would be content to see the patient every 6 to 12 months, depending on the "healthiness" of the optic nerve heads. We suspect that the majority of such patients with pigmentary dispersion will never develop glaucoma.

ACUTE INTRAOCULAR PRESSURE ELEVATIONS IN PATIENTS WITH PIGMENTARY GLAUCOMA

Pigment particles in the aqueous humor are often seen in eyes with PDS, usually without relation to the level of IOP. In a few cases, the number of pigment particles in the aqueous humor has been observed to increase rapidly, sometimes spontaneously, or as a result of exercise.[35-37] The increase in suspended pigment has in some instances been associated with a marked rise in IOP, as exemplified in the following cases.

Case 21-5

A 30-year-old White male noticed blurring of vision and haloes on several occasions after playing basketball, greater in the right eye than in the left. IOP in each eye was found to be in the 40s on one such occasion. PG was diagnosed. The patient was in good health, with no family history of glaucoma.

Re-examination several days later, without treatment but now asymptomatic, showed diffuse deposits of pigment on the back surface of both corneas. The anterior chambers were abnormally deep with an occasional speck of pigment circulating in the aqueous. A shadow of pigment in the angle could be demonstrated by retroillumination of the sclera at the limbus. Gonioscopy revealed an almost concave iris contour, with a dense black band of pigment in the whole circumference of the TM and pigment behind the equator of both lenses. The irides transilluminated in the mid-periphery. The discs had small physiologic cups. Applanation tensions were then 20 OD and 19 OS. Tonographic C value was 0.09 on the right, not measured on the left.

The patient agreed to go jogging to try to provoke his symptoms. After jogging, the applanation tensions were 31 OD and 22 OS. There were diffuse, fine clouds of pigment in the aqueous, greater on the right than the left. Tonographic C values after exercise were 0.02 right and 0.05 left. The patient stated that activity in which he "jiggled" his head, such as basketball, caused more symptoms than simple running.

Seven months later, the patient returned with recurrent symptoms of haloes. IOPs were 38 OD and 22 OS, with a great amount of circulating pigment in the right anterior chamber, considerably less in the left.

Subsequently, when the increased IOP had spontaneously subsided, phenylephrine provocative testing was done, but it produced only an occasional pigment speck in the aqueous humor and no significant change in IOP. There was a small increase in facility of outflow.

During the next 3 years, the patient had a few minor episodes of exercise-induced visual symptoms. IOP has generally remained below 21 mm Hg in each eye without any treatment, and the discs have remained normal.

Case 21-6

In 1968, a 30-year-old White man with PG gave a history of attacks of pain, haloes, and blurred vision lasting 3 to 4 hours, sometimes in one eye and sometimes in the other. He associated these attacks with dim illumination and occasionally with emotionally upsetting circumstances, but not with exercise. When he was asymptomatic, IOPs were in the low 20s OD and low 30s OS. The angles were open, of safe width, with dense pigment bands on the TM, but no pigment particles in the aqueous humor. Darkroom testing was negative. The discs had small physiologic cups. The left eye was treated with epinephrine and pilocarpine for several years.

In 1976, he had a spontaneous attack in the right eye that occurred while he was working outside in dim light at night. During the attack, the IOP was 55 OD and 22 OS. There were many pigment particles of various sizes in the aqueous humor in the right eye, but only occasional particles in the left. Both angles were open, with dense pigment bands. The patient was treated with acetazolamide, and, with pressure reduced, he was asymptomatic the following morning.

These patients and other similar cases[36,37] seem to support the concept that pigment particles under certain circumstances temporarily obstruct the aqueous outflow channels,[6,29] although it is possible that the IOP elevation and pigment liberation are both secondary to some other process.

Patients with PG should be routinely queried about exercise-induced or spontaneous symptoms of blurred vision and seeing colored haloes. It is remarkable how often the patient initially denies such symptoms, but after being informed about their possible occurrence, returns at a subsequent visit now relating such symptoms in the past. These symptoms are then subsequently documented to be associated with episodic elevations of IOP.

In a few cases, a pigment shower and a transitory increase of IOP have been induced by phenylephrine eye drops, and one might therefore expect this to provide the basis for a provocative test for PG. However, in systematic testing, we have found the amount of pigment liberated is so varied, and the IOP increases so infrequent, that we conclude that phenylephrine testing is not useful for identifying latent glaucoma in patients with PDS.[35] Furthermore, phenylephrine occasionally produces pigment liberation and IOP elevation in patients with primarily open-angle glaucoma and in patients with exfoliation syndrome.[35] It is also noteworthy that the extent of iris transillumination does not correlate with the grade of phenylephrine-induced pigment liberation.

OTHER ASSOCIATIONS

Strangely, diabetes has never to our knowledge been a cause of PG, although diabetes causes the pigment epithelium of the iris to store excessive glycogen and renders these cells so fragile that they can release great showers of pigment during intraocular surgery. PDS has been rarely associated with inner ear deafness (pigment cells), congenital megalocornea, and perhaps pregnancy. The iridodonesis and possibly a higher-than-normal prevalence of retinal detachment are believed to result from the association of myopia with pigmentary dispersion.

TREATMENT

The IOP in PG seems to be subject to large spontaneous fluctuations, particularly in young people. In some cases, this is attributed to release of pigment particles into the anterior chamber with exercise that temporarily obstructs aqueous outflow, but in other cases the cause of this IOP fluctuation is not certain. In evaluation of the response of the IOP to medical treatment, this tendency to spontaneous fluctuation has to be kept in mind.

The principles of treatment of PG are fundamentally the same as those that we have described for primary open-angle glaucoma (see Chapter 18). Prostaglandin analogs can be very effective in PG. Topical beta-blockers, alpha-agonists, and carbonic anhydrase inhibitors (CAIs) are also effective (see Table 18-1). Because the patients are usually young and are often myopic, the use of miotic eye drops may present a considerable problem because of spasm of accommodation and blurring of vision. When it was clinically available, pilocarpine Ocusert (an extended-release zero-order kinetics pilocarpine delivery system) therapy (see Chapter 13) was often tolerated and effective in young patients with PG. Several young myopic patients with PG have been described by Brachet and Chermet[38] as having peripheral chorioretinal degeneration and retinal detachment, which may argue for a relative contraindication of the use of miotics in these patients.

Argon laser trabeculoplasty (ALT) can often produce dramatic IOP lowering in PG, but the results are less uniform than with exfoliation glaucoma, and occasional patients with PG demonstrate substantial IOP elevation, both acute and sustained, after laser trabeculoplasty (ALT or selective laser trabeculoplasty [SLT]). This possibility must, therefore, be discussed with the patient before proceeding with laser trabeculoplasty, and generally lower energy laser settings should be used to mitigate this risk.

CLINICAL COURSE

As mentioned, remarkable fluctuation of IOP may occur in PG. Some patients seem to have periods of "crisis" of elevated IOP and then return to more normal levels. During such crises, symptoms may be acute, with corneal edema and haloes, but usually no pain. In some patients, these crises of pressure elevation seem related to excessive liberation of pigment granules into the anterior segment (see Cases 21-5 and 21-6) that may be associated with exercise, but in others we have recognized no associated factor. In rare cases of PG, we have even seen the IOP return to normal within a few years, almost as if a remission of the glaucoma is occurring, and medication can be reduced or discontinued (see Case 21-5).

Because of the tendency to transitory elevation of pressure and the possibility of some degree of remission, we are much less influenced by the height of the IOP at a given time than by the character of the optic discs and visual fields in deciding when to recommend fistulizing surgery in PG.

The severity of PG and the length of time it can be controlled medically vary considerably from patient to patient. We have a vague impression that the earlier the onset, the more likely the glaucoma will become too severe for medical control and will require surgery. If adequate control cannot be obtained medically, then fistulizing surgery should be undertaken. Fortunately, standard filtration operations are as effective for this condition as ordinary open-angle glaucoma. We have seen no tendency for filtration blebs to become obstructed by particles of pigment, perhaps because of the iridectomy usually performed at the time of filtering surgery.

CONCLUSION

Laser iridotomy has an uncertain role in potentially interrupting one component in the disease mechanism in this condition by changing iris contour. A major area of uncertainty is the factors that are responsible for the disease occurring in only some individuals with PDS. Likely, there are TM processes that contribute, but this remains unclear at this time. It seems most consistent that pigment release due to either intrinsic or mechanical iris factors serves as a stressor to a TM that is at least latently abnormal in this disease. More information is needed on how pigment trapped in the TM intercellularly, and intracellularly, can slowly be disposed of by some natural mechanism. This may involve wandering macrophages, rather than migration of trabecular cells. One might also speculate that clearance of the pigment particles could be favored by enlarging the spaces within the TM by means of newer trabecular drugs, laser trabeculoplasty, or miotics.

More information is also needed on the extent to which pigment that is lost from the posterior layer of the iris early in the disease can apparently be regenerated later, as has been observed in a number of patients.

Campbell[17] has hypothesized that zonular contact and rubbing is responsible for the pigment liberation from the posterior iris surface in this syndrome, and this has been discussed. Most likely, this involves anteroposterior iris ballottement movements against the zonule, rather than a to-and-fro friction. Campbell[17] has also suggested that chronic miotic therapy might decrease this zonular rubbing. Unfortunately, most patients with PG, due to their relatively young age, do not tolerate standard miotics other than Ocuserts, and, therefore, it remains difficult to fully evaluate this possibility. Alpha-blockers with pupillary effects are available but do not appear to have an effect on pigment release. However, recent observations about iris contour change after laser iridotomy will likely lead to a more definitive evaluation of this hypothesis, if proper prospective randomized studies of one of 2 symmetrical eyes with PG are performed. Although intriguing, this hypothesis still leaves unexplained the nature of the trabecular abnormality present in only

certain patients with PDS, which presumably differentiates those who will develop PG from those who will not.

The occurrence of the full PDS without glaucoma (or without even any abnormality in aqueous outflow function) underscores our lack of understanding of the basic mechanisms for a particular glaucoma.[39] The implications of the spontaneous or exercise-induced occurrence of pigment particle floater release into the anterior chamber, the apparent crises of acute pressure elevation, and the frequent usefulness of adrenergic therapy in this condition are unclear. Further careful, detailed, long-term serial observation of all the many parameters[40] are required to increase our understanding of this fascinating syndrome.

REFERENCES

1. Sugar HS, Barbour FA. PG; a rare clinical entity. *Am J Ophthalmol.* 1949;32(1):90-92.
2. Sugar HS. PG. A 25-year review. *Am J Ophthalmol.* 1966;62(3):499-507.
3. Mauksch H. Uber idiopathischen Zerfall des retinalen Pigmentblattes der Iris bei zwei Bruden. *Z Augenheilkd.* 1925;57:262-268.
4. Pickett JE, Terry SA, O'Connor PS, et al. Early loss of central visual acuity in glaucoma. *Ophthalmology.* 1985;92(7):891-896.
5. Lehto I, Ruusuvaara P, Setala K. Corneal endothelium in PG and PDS. *Acta Ophthalmol (Copenh).* 1990;68(6):703-709.
6. Epstein DL, Freddo TF, Anderson PJ, et al. Experimental obstruction to aqueous outflow by pigment particles in living monkeys. *Invest Ophthalmol Vis Sci.* 1986;27(3):387-395.
7. Potash SD, Tello C, Liebmann J, et al. Ultrasound biomicroscopy in PDS. *Ophthalmology.* 1994;101(2):332-339.
8. Liebmann JM, Tello C, Chew SJ, et al. Prevention of blinking alters iris configuration in PDS and in normal eyes. *Ophthalmology.* 1995;102(3):446-455.
9. Lichter PR, Shaffer RN. Diagnostic and prognostic signs in PG. *Trans Am Acad Ophthalmol Otolaryngol.* 1970;74(5):984-998.
10. Van Buskirk EM, Leure-duPree AE. Pathophysiology and electron microscopy of melanomalytic glaucoma. *Am J Ophthalmol.* 1978;85(2):160-166.
11. Yanoff M, Scheie HG. Melanomalytic glaucoma. Report of a case. *Arch Ophthalmol.* 1970;84(4):471-473.
12. Omulecki W, Pruszczynski M, Borowski J. Ring melanoma of the iris and ciliary body. *Br J Ophthalmol.* 1985;69(7):514-518.
13. Karickhoff JR. PDS and PG: a new mechanism concept, a new treatment, and a new technique. *Ophthalmic Surg.* 1992;23(4):269-277.
14. Karickhoff JR. Reverse pupillary block in PG: follow up and new developments. *Ophthalmic Surg.* 1993;24(8):562-563.
15. Campbell DG. Iridotomy, blinking, and PG. *Invest Ophthalmol Vis Sci.* 1993;34(ARVO suppl):993.
16. Carassa RG, Bettin P, Fiori M, et al. Nd:YAG laser iridotomy in PDS: an ultrasound biomicroscopic study. *Br J Ophthalmol.* 1998;82(2):150-153.
17. Campbell DG. Pigmentary dispersion and glaucoma. A new theory. *Arch Ophthalmol.* 1979;97(9):1667-1672.
18. Fine BS, Yanoff M, Scheie HG. Pigmentary "glaucoma." A histologic study. *Trans Am Acad Ophthalmol Otolaryngol.* 1974;78(2):OP314-OP325.
19. Reistad CE, Shields MB, Campbell DG, et al. The influence of peripheral iridotomy on the intraocular pressure course in patients with PG. *J Glaucoma.* 2005;14(4):255-259.
20. Kupfer C, Kuwabara T, Kaiser-Kupfer M. The histopathology of PDS with glaucoma. *Am J Ophthalmol.* 1975;80(5):857-862.

21. Krupin T, Rosenberg LF, Weinreb RN. PG: facts versus fiction. *J Glaucoma.* 1994;3(4):273-274.

22. Epstein DL, de Kater AW, Schroeder A. Long-term observation of living monkeys with experimental pigmentary dispersion. *Invest Ophthalmol Vis Sci.* 1992;33(ARVO suppl):731.

23. Gandolfi SA, Vecchi M. Effect of a YAG laser iridotomy on intraocular pressure in PDS. *Ophthalmology.* 1996;103(10):1693-1695.

24. Barsotti MF, Bartels SP, Freddo TF, et al. The source of protein in the aqueous humor of the normal monkey eye. *Invest Ophthalmol Vis Sci.* 1992;33(3):581-595.

25. Johnson M, Gong H, Freddo TF, et al. Serum proteins and aqueous outflow resistance in bovine eyes. *Invest Ophthalmol Vis Sci.* 1993;34(13):3549-3557.

26. Pavlin CJ, Macken P, Trope G, et al. Ultrasound biomicroscopic features of PG. *Can J Ophthalmol.* 1994;29(4):187-192.

27. Jampel HD. Lack of effect of peripheral laser iridotomy in PDS. *Arch Ophthalmol.* 1993;111(12):1606.

28. Petersen HP. Can pigmentary deposits on the trabecular meshwork increase the resistance of the aqueous outflow? *Acta Ophthalmol (Copenh).* 1969;47(3):743-749.

29. Grant WM. Experimental aqueous perfusion in enucleated human eyes. *Arch Ophthalmol.* 1963;69:783-801.

30. Richardson TM, Hutchinson BT, Grant WM. The outflow tract in PG: a light and electron microscopic study. *Arch Ophthalmol.* 1977;95(6):1015-1025.

31. Alvarado JA, Murphy CG. Outflow obstruction in pigmentary and primary open angle glaucoma. *Arch Ophthalmol.* 1992;110(12):1769-1778.

32. Murphy CG, Johnson M, Alvarado JA. Juxtacanalicular tissue in pigmentary and primary open angle glaucoma. The hydrodynamic role of pigment and other constituents. *Arch Ophthalmol.* 1992;110(12):1779-1785.

33. Zink HA, Palmberg PF, Sugar A, et al. Comparison of in vitro corticosteroid response in PG and primary open-angle glaucoma. *Am J Ophthalmol.* 1975;80(3 pt 1):478-484.

34. Siddiqui Y, Ten Hulzen RD, Cameron JD, et al. What is the risk of developing PG from PDS? *Am J Ophthalmol.* 2003;135(6):794-799.

35. Epstein DL, Boger WP 3rd, Grant WM. Phenylephrine provocative testing in the PDS. *Am J Ophthalmol.* 1978;85(1):43-50.

36. Schenker HI, Luntz MH, Kels B, et al. Exercise-induced increase of intraocular pressure in the PDS. *Am J Ophthalmol.* 1980;89(4):598-600.

37. Haynes WL, Johnson AT, Alward WL. Effects of jogging exercise on patients with the PDS and PG. *Ophthalmology.* 1992;99(7):1096-1103.

38. Brachet A, Chermet M. Association glaucome pigmentaire et decollement de retine. *Ann Oculist (Paris).* 1974;207:451-457.

39. Epstein DL. Will there be a remedy to reverse the changes in the trabecular meshwork and the optic nerve? A personal point of view on glaucoma therapy. *J Glaucoma.* 1993;2(2):138-139.

40. Richter CU, Richardson TM, Grant WM. PDS and PG. A prospective study of the natural history. *Arch Ophthalmol.* 1986;104(2):211-215.

ANGLE-CLOSURE GLAUCOMA

Principles of
Primary Angle-Closure Glaucoma

George Ulrich, MD, FACS and David L. Epstein, MD, MMM

GENERAL CONSIDERATIONS

The classic teachings about the diagnosis and management of primary angle-closure glaucoma remain relevant. Nevertheless, our understanding of angle closure continues to evolve most notably with the introduction of new diagnostic techniques other than gonioscopy that aid significantly in the evaluation of the chamber angle and the angle's potential to become occluded. These technologies include anterior segment optical coherence tomography (AS-OCT) and ultrasound biomicroscopy (UBM).

Because of the affordability and wide availability and utility of gonioscopy, primary angle-closure glaucoma will be discussed extensively in the context of gonioscopy. Throughout the chapter, AS-OCT and UBM will also be considered and demonstrated by illustration to show their respective contribution to understanding the angle-closure glaucomas. While relatively costly, and therefore not universally available, these imaging modalities are important adjuncts in understanding the dynamics of angle closure.

In the various forms of angle-closure glaucoma, the trabecular meshwork (TM) may have intrinsically normal function, but the position of the peripheral iris in front of the TM blocks access of aqueous humor to the outflow pathway. Because there is very limited circumferential flow of aqueous humor once in Schlemm's canal,[1] each portion of the TM circumference functions as if it were a relatively independent outflow segment. Thus, the full blockage of a limited segment of the TM circumference by the peripheral iris results in a proportional decrease in outflow facility.[2,3]

Aqueous humor normally exits through the posterior half of the TM, closest to the scleral spur. This is illustrated by the common observation of relatively increased pigmentation of this posterior half of the TM. Thus, when only the anterior half of the TM is visualized by gonioscopy, and if the unseen posterior half of TM is blocked by iris apposition, there may be limited aqueous outflow occurring through this segment of the angle circumference. This observation may be misinterpreted by beginning gonioscopists who report that they "see some TM." Stated another way, the full width of the TM needs to be visualized to the scleral spur, without indentation, to know that the angle is functionally open. Thus, the term *partial angle closure* does not mean that part of the TM is visible in one area. Rather, the term refers to the fact that the angle is functionally closed by iris apposed to at least the posterior half of the TM in a portion of the 12-clock-hour angle circumference (Figure 22-1).

The peripheral iris that functionally blocks access to the draining posterior-half of the TM either for a limited number of clock-hours or for the full circumference may be apposed without permanent adhesion or alternately with some semi-permanent adhesion. The semi-permanent adhesion is called a peripheral anterior synechia. The terms *chronic appositional angle closure* and *chronic synechial angle closure* are sometimes, respectively, used to describe these 2 clinical situations. In the former situation, in which there is no permanent adhesion, relief of the factors causing the movement of the peripheral iris over the TM can theoretically restore normal outflow. Nevertheless, even in this circumstance of nonpermanent adhesion, some have argued that chronic iris touch can cause permanent TM dysfunction without apparent synechia formation.

In contrast, in the latter situation where peripheral anterior synechiae have formed, altering in some way the factors causing movement of the peripheral iris over the TM will not by itself restore normal TM function. However, it may still be possible to diminish the "permanent" synechiae by means of a technique called argon laser gonioplasty.

Kahook MY, Schuman JS, eds.
Chandler and Grant's Glaucoma, Fifth Edition (pp 239-253).
© 2013 SLACK Incorporated.

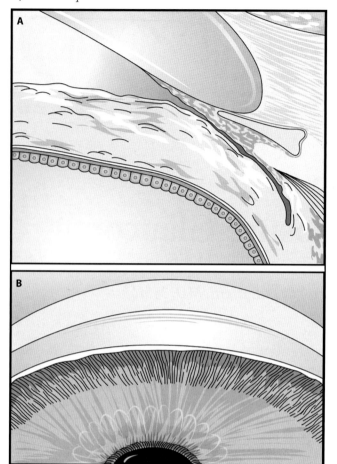

Figure 22-1. Iris apposed to posterior half of TM occludes outflow, despite anterior TM (which is nonfiltering) being visible. (A) Appearance in cross-section. (B) Appearance in gonioscopy.

When the angle is closed in only a part of the circumference, intraocular pressure (IOP) may or may not rise in proportion to the extent of closure. With the angle closed in only a portion of the circumference, the level of IOP may vary in different eyes depending not only on the amount of angle closed, but also on the efficiency of the remaining open angle. Thus, in an eye that has an unusually good facility of outflow, such as 0.40 μL/min/mm Hg, when the angle is entirely open, closure of half the angle may still allow a normal or near-normal IOP. The facility of outflow may still be within the normal range (eg, 0.20 μL/min/mm Hg). In another eye, starting with a borderline facility of outflow of 0.16 μL/min/mm Hg when the angle is open, closure of half of this angle results in a facility of outflow well below normal (eg, 0.08 μL/min/mm Hg), causing a considerable elevation in IOP.

A lack of proportion between the extent of closure and the level of IOP in some eyes may also be caused by a temporary diminution in the rate of aqueous production. This might happen after a severe attack of acute angle-closure glaucoma. In this case, the angle closure may have resolved spontaneously, but there still may be residual permanent outflow obstruction. Yet, because of temporarily reduced

aqueous production, IOP may still be normal or even subnormal for hours or several days, or even as long as weeks despite extensive residual synechial closure of the angle and reduced outflow. However, sooner or later, as the eye recovers from the acute insult, aqueous production resumes. The IOP again rises to a level consistent with the extent of residual closure.

The onset and course of angle-closure glaucoma in most cases is episodic. When the angle closes rapidly in an acute episode, the IOP rises rapidly, causing symptoms of blurred vision, pain, and sometimes an appearance of colored haloes around lights. In subacute angle-closure glaucoma, however, there may be a rapid rise in IOP but not to such a level as in the acute form, because, generally, only a part of the angle is involved in subacute closure. Nevertheless, during an episode of partial or subacute closure, the patient may still note blurring of vision and seeing haloes around lights. In chronic angle-closure glaucoma, the closure is gradual, and the patient may be asymptomatic until the glaucoma is in an advanced state with significant permanent visual field loss. This mimics primary open-angle glaucoma (POAG) and is often misdiagnosed as such.

In its early stages, angle-closure glaucoma is reversible and curable. If the angle reopens throughout the full circumference either spontaneously or as a result of pharmacologic intervention, the eye again has a narrow but open angle, but remains predisposed to further attacks of closure. Repeated episodes of closure usually occur and result eventually in permanent synechial closure.

The tendency toward synechial closure varies greatly in different eyes. In some eyes, a single severe episode of closure of the angle, especially if prolonged, may result in extensive synechia formation. In other eyes, repeated episodes of closure over a period of a year or more may cause little or no formation of synechia. With treatment by laser iridotomy, such an angle may still be capable of opening throughout its circumference. The degree of vascular congestion of an eye probably has some influence on the tendency to form peripheral anterior synechiae during an episode of closure. There may be other factors that influence synechia formation.

NARROW-ANGLED EYES: EVALUATING THE STATUS AND THE RISK FOR GLAUCOMA

In narrow-angled eyes, there are 2 common clinical situations. Each of these 2 situations has different questions that must be addressed to understand the condition and how it should be approached and treated.

Situation 1

The angle is narrow but the IOP is normal. The question is whether the angle is sufficiently narrow such that there is a significant risk of spontaneous (or perhaps pharmacologically induced) angle closure. This situation is referred to as the *occludable angle*.

Situation 2

The angle is narrow, and the IOP is elevated. In this case, the question is different: Is there sufficient functional angle closure around the circumference to explain the IOP elevation? That is, is the IOP elevation due to a form of angle-closure glaucoma with or without synechia formation, or does the patient really have POAG but with a narrow yet functionally open angle? In fact, it may be some degree of both. The angle may be narrow, yet remain functionally open in some portion of the circumference, contributing to an elevated pressure by an open-angle mechanism. At the same time, the angle may be apposed either with or without synechia formation in other areas.

Both processes may be at play. Such a condition is often referred to as *mixed mechanism* glaucoma. The need for such discrimination is not rare in clinical practice. For example, exfoliative eyes (a form of open-angle glaucoma) commonly have narrow angles as well[4] and may have an angle-closure component. There are cases in clinical practice where it is challenging to recognize the contribution of each of these 2 different mechanisms. The approach to doing so will be discussed.

TERMINOLOGY

Angle-closure glaucoma may be acute, wherein there are symptoms of pain and blurred vision with signs of ocular injection and a fixed mid-dilated pupil. The angle in most, if not all, of the circumference has gone suddenly from a narrow but open and functional status to that of dramatic appositional closure.

Angle-closure glaucoma may be termed *subacute* with milder symptoms and signs because only a portion of the 360-degree circumference is functionally closed. This happens intermittently and repetitively. Individual episodes resolve with or without permanent peripheral anterior synechia formation.

Finally, angle closure may be termed *chronic*. This usually implies an asymptomatic long-term condition that mimics POAG. In fact, misinterpreting and erroneously treating chronic angle-closure glaucoma as POAG is among the most common diagnostic errors in glaucoma.

In most patients with such chronic angle-closure glaucoma, there is progressive though gradual increase in the extent of the circumference of the angle involved and progressive synechial closure. This usually begins in the superior angle. Because of the gradual nature of this process, the IOP slowly elevates, and no acute or subacute-type symptoms occur. The term *chronic silent angle closure* is probably more appropriate for this condition.

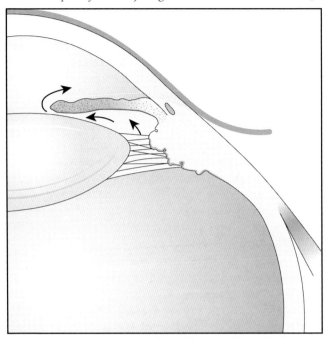

Figure 22-2. Aqueous humor is formed by the ciliary epithelium and moves across the posterior chamber between the posterior iris surface and lens, through the pupil, and into the anterior chamber. Especially in the smaller hyperopic eye, some resistance is present to flow through the pupil (relative pupillary block) that results in a slightly greater pressure in the posterior chamber than in the anterior. The result is forward iris convexity. Most emmetropic eyes demonstrate a slight iris convexity (forward) due to slight relative pupillary block. When a high degree of relative pupillary block is present, angle-closure glaucoma can ensue from the resulting forward movement of the iris into the angle.

THE CONCEPT OF PUPILLARY BLOCK

Aqueous humor is an ultrafiltrate of plasma produced by the ciliary body. Aqueous is secreted into the posterior chamber behind the iris and then flows forward through the pupil into the anterior chamber (Figure 22-2). In most eyes, there is some resistance to flow through the pupillary space due to the close proximity of the pupil to the anterior surface of the crystalline lens. This phenomenon is termed *relative pupillary block*.

The iris functions in some ways as a valve between the posterior and anterior chambers. The iris contour, whether convex toward the cornea, planar, or concave away from the cornea, reflects the pressure differential between the posterior chamber and anterior chamber. In normal eyes, the iris is in contact with the crystalline lens only in the immediate vicinity of the pupillary border, hence the normal slight iris convexity due to a small amount of relative pupillary block. In most clinical situations, it is believed that the pressure differential that results from relative pupillary block is small in magnitude, probably less than 1 mm.

Relative pupillary block is, in general, more marked in hyperopic eyes, which conceptually are smaller eyes with less room in the middle segment for structures such as the lens. Because of this relatively crowded anatomy, there is more potential for pupillary block. The iris may be pushed forward by the lens. In addition, there is a greater-than-usual area of contact between the iris and the anterior surface of the lens. This produces a relatively increased resistance to forward flow of aqueous through the pupil. The relatively greater pressure in the posterior chamber produces a forward convexity in iris contour.

Forward iris convexity is also a very common occurrence in aged eyes and may or may not by itself produce a functionally narrow angle. A functionally narrow angle depends on additional factors and vectors that will be described. Thus, iris convexity by itself is not an indication for iridotomy to prevent angle closure. Rather, the status of the angle is the indication for laser iridotomy.

In young emmetropic eyes, the iris position valve is commonly planar, indicating an absence of relative pupillary block and free flow of aqueous through the pupil. Interestingly, in some myopic eyes and in many eyes with pigment dispersion syndrome, the iris contour is concave, indicating a higher pressure in the anterior chamber relative to the posterior chamber. Aqueous humor still flows forward from the posterior chamber to the anterior chamber in the conventional manner in such eyes. How this paradoxical and hypothetical pressure differential exists is a subject of debate. One hypothesis is that in such eyes, in addition to conventional aqueous flow from the ciliary body into the posterior chamber and then through the pupil to the anterior chamber, there is also movement of fluid into the peripheral anterior chamber directly through the base of the iris. Such a phenomenon has been noted in the study of aqueous dynamics in certain primates.[5] This might be accentuated in myopic human eyes in which there is thinness of the base of the iris.

It is also a matter of debate whether iris concavity is fairly specific for the pigment dispersion syndrome or whether it is related more to myopic anatomy. Regardless, one must keep in mind that the iris contour relates very directly to the relative pressure differential across the iris surface. An interesting corollary is that, when there is posterior segment pathology such as retinal tears with egress of fluid posteriorly through the retinal break,[6] the iris contour may assume a somewhat concave or retracted contour (iris retraction syndrome), especially when there is a condition of pupil sequestration.[7,8]

As the eye ages, the crystalline lens increases in size and thickness, producing some iris convexity, even when there was no pre-existing hyperopia. This iris convexity is due to relative pupillary block. With increasing lens size, there is greater contact with the posterior iris surface. Thus, some relative pupillary block is a normal finding in older eyes and does not, by itself, require intervention. The word *relative* is stressed because normally with iris convexity, there continues to be fluid movement through the pupil into the anterior chamber. There is mildly increased resistance to

transpupillary flow at the level of the pupil that results in only a slightly higher pressure in the posterior chamber.

The pupil in acute angle-closure glaucoma may move into a position where there is presumably total or near total pupillary block (ie, no movement of aqueous into the anterior chamber). The iris bows forward from a build-up of pressure in the posterior chamber to the extent that peripheral iris obstructs the outflow mechanism. The presentation is usually dramatic with an iris bombé configuration.

An alternate presentation of pupillary block occurs when there are 360 degrees of posterior synechiae between the iris and the anterior surface of the lens from uveitis. In this scenario, pupillary block does not occur because of physiologic movement of the pupil into a mid-dilated position. Rather, there is a total adhesion between the border of the pupil and the lens. This condition of total circumferential adhesion is referred to as *pupillary seclusion* or *total pupillary block*. It is usually the sequela of inflammation.

Relative pupillary block causes forward iris convexity that results in the movement of the peripheral iris toward the TM. This narrows the approach to the angle. If the approach to the angle becomes sufficiently narrow, progressive forward movement of the peripheral iris may occlude the TM or a portion of the TM. This might happen spontaneously as the pupil changes in diameter in response to illumination. Relative pupillary block is maximized at one particular size of the pupil—usually mid-dilated. The same dynamic might be precipitated pharmacologically.

Laser iridotomy is the definitive treatment for pupillary block. This intervention will equalize the pressure differential between the posterior chamber and the anterior chamber. The iris may fall back away from the TM and assume a less convex contour. The iridotomy allows free communication of fluid between the 2 chambers without requiring flow through the pupil. The iridotomy opening must be large enough (50 to 60 µm is sufficient) to allow free flow of aqueous across the iris from the posterior to the anterior chamber. The opening must also be full-thickness through the substance of the iris.

It should be noted that any convex iris caused by relative pupillary block can be converted to a planar contour by creating an iridotomy. This physical change is based on the equalization of pressure between the anterior and posterior chambers. Nevertheless, the loss of iris convexity does not, by itself, indicate that iridotomy was justified. The indication for iridotomy depends strictly on the assessment of the angle, not iris contour alone. Most elderly eyes have iris convexity, but only a minority have a corresponding angle narrow enough to warrant prophylactic iridotomy.

If there is relative pupillary block and iris convexity to the extent that the peripheral iris comes forward to appose the TM, there is limited access of aqueous humor to the TM face. Depending on the extent of nonfunctional angle thus created, the IOP will increase. One should keep in mind that

IRIS RETRACTION SYNDROME

David L. Epstein, MD, MMM

An appreciation of vectors affecting iris contour helps in understanding a peculiar condition, termed by Campbell[1] as *iris retraction syndrome*. From a clinical point of view, the presence of this iris retraction syndrome[1,2] should suggest an occult rhegmatogenous retinal detachment. In this syndrome, which is usually associated with pupillary seclusion, the peripheral iris demonstrates a retracted appearance. Some have termed this the iris suck sign. Because of the pupillary seclusion, the patients initially might present in pupillary block associated with iris bombè, but after initiation of aqueous humor suppressant therapy, the peripheral iris surprisingly demonstrates this retracted appearance.

The explanation for this phenomenon is that aqueous humor is exiting the eye posteriorly through the retinal hole, presumably by the pumping mechanism of the retinal pigment epithelium. With reduced rates of aqueous humor formation that may be due to uveitis combined with the effect of aqueous humor suppressants, the rate of aqueous humor production might become less than the posterior outflow rate through the retinal hole. Further, the retinal pigment epithelial pump may be stimulated by the use of carbonic anhydrase inhibitors.[3] The net posterior movement of fluid results in the retracted appearance of the peripheral iris. In this unusual condition, the secluded pupil acts to keep aqueous humor in the posterior chamber from moving into the anterior chamber.

It must also be remembered that, in the normal physiological state, there is some portion of aqueous humor fluid moving posteriorly through the vitreous chamber and likely being pumped[3,4] out of the eye by the retinal pigment epithelium. In fact, interference with such pumping is one possible explanation for the sudden vitreous expansion that may occur in malignant glaucoma.

REFERENCES

1. Campbell DG. Iris retraction associated with rhegmatogenous retinal detachment syndrome and hypotony. A new explanation. *Arch Ophthalmol.* 1984;102:1457-1463.
2. Greenfield DS, Bellows AR, Asdourian GK, et al. Iris retraction syndrome after intraocular surgery. *Ophthalmology.* 1995;102:98-100.
3. Kawano S, Marmor MF. Metabolic influences on the absorption of serous subretinal fluid. *Invest Ophthalmol Vis Sci.* 1988;29(8):1255-1257.
4. Tsuboi S, Pederson JE. Volume flow across the isolated retinal pigment epithelium of cynomolgus monkey eyes. *Invest Ophthalmol Vis Sci.* 1988;29:1652-1655.

outflow facility and the rate of aqueous production are separate terms in the Goldmann equation that determine IOP. Accordingly, the magnitude of the IOP increase, whether subclinical (ie, still in the normal range under 22 mm) or abnormally higher, depends not only on the extent of the closure but also on the inherent filterability (outflow facility) of the part of the angle that remains open. It should be kept in mind that the IOP also remains affected by the rate of aqueous humor production.

In the presence of functional angle closure, an iridotomy relieves the pressure differential that had caused the iris movement over the TM. The iris contour becomes planar after the iridotomy. Whether there is a beneficial effect on IOP depends on whether the previous angle-closure configuration was simply appositional or if it was synechial.

Prior to intervention, indentation gonioscopy of a narrow-angle eye may differentiate potentially reversible apposition from synechial closure. In the former case, the angle opens with pressure applied to the contact gonio lens. In the latter case, the angle may open, revealing the presence of synechiae. This assessment of the angle is more predictive of the benefit of iridotomy than is assessment of the iris contour.

FACTORS THAT MAY INCREASE RELATIVE PUPILLARY BLOCK OR MAY OTHERWISE INFLUENCE THE OCCURRENCE OF ANGLE CLOSURE

Why do some narrow angles close and others do not? Why do some eyes develop chronic angle closure in only a portion of the circumference? Although there is still much that we do not know about angle closure, we do have knowledge of some factors that influence the process. Mapstone[9] has described factors that are involved using the concept of vector forces (Table 22-1). Each of these factors is discussed individually below.

The Pupil

The size of the pupil can influence pupillary block. In mid-dilation, relative pupillary block increases due to greater contact between the posterior surface of the iris and the anterior surface of the lens. This results in a relative increase in pressure in the posterior chamber and increase in iris convexity (Figure 22-3). Progressively, there may be apposition of the peripheral iris over the TM face and sudden ballooning of the peripheral iris over the angle.

This is classic acute angle-closure glaucoma. The pupil is observed to be fixed in a mid-dilated position, presumably from the ischemia of the iris sphincter that results from very high IOP elevation and impairment of blood flow within the iris. In addition to dilation of the pupil to 5 or 6 mm, the peripheral iris may lose rigidity to the extent that the pressure in the posterior chamber can more easily push the iris forward. The iris is pushed forward a critical amount needed to close the angle.

This event of angle closure was initiated by the normal physiologic movement of the pupil. The individual experiences illumination conditions that result in a mid-dilated position (eg, classically, for example, going into a darkened movie theater). The resulting ischemia from high IOP and impaired blood flow then fixes the pupil in this position.

Physiologic dilation of the pupil is probably the factor most often responsible in instances of angle-closure glaucoma. Onset is associated with dim light or darkness,

TABLE 22-1. POTENTIAL VECTORS INVOLVED IN RELATIVE PUPILLARY BLOCK
• Size of the pupil: maximum dilation eliminates pupillary block; mid-dilation increases pupillary block; extreme miosis increases pupillary block
• Position of the crystalline lens
• Rate of aqueous humor formation: force acting on posterior iris surface
• Rigidity of the Iris
• Potential forward position of the ciliary body

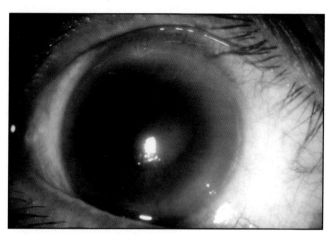

Figure 22-3. Acute angle closure. Note the pupil in classic, mid-dilated position.

emotional disturbances, shock, physical illness, or stress experienced in an accident. Angle-closure glaucoma may also be precipitated in anatomically predisposed eyes by systemic medications, such as gastrointestinal or muscle relaxants, antihistamines, or sedatives. Such drugs have atropine-like, anticholinergic properties and induce a slight mydriasis, predisposing to pupillary block.

Direct sympathomimetic medications, such as those used to treat asthma or respiratory insufficiency, have less frequently been implicated in precipitating acute angle-closure glaucoma. Although such agents contract the iris dilator muscle and create a relatively dilated pupil, at the same time, they increase peripheral iris rigidity, obviating forward iris movement.

Extreme dilation of the pupil is less likely to precipitate closure of the angle than is moderate dilation. Wide dilation lessens iris-lens apposition, altering the dynamics necessary for pupillary block. As will be discussed in Chapter 23, pharmacologic intervention with mydriatic/cycloplegic agents to induce wide dilation may relieve pupillary block and resolve an episode of acute angle closure.

Pilocarpine therapy for acute angle closure theoretically lessens relative pupillary block by inducing miosis and decreasing lens-iris apposition. In addition, the action of miotics of pulling the iris out of the angle is also said to play a role in resolving acute angle closure.

Nevertheless, the situation with pilocarpine intervention is actually more complicated and confounding. Pilocarpine is infrequently applied as an initial treatment to break an attack. The accompanying release of zonular tension by this agent may allow the crystalline lens to move forward and thereby may increase relative pupillary block, making the situation worse. In addition, extreme miosis, as may be achieved with stronger miotics such as 4% pilocarpine and especially with cholinesterase inhibitors, may in some cases increase relative pupillary block by inducing a smaller pupil. In practice, due to iris sphincter ischemia, weaker strengths of pilocarpine do not produce much miosis and do not contribute much to breaking an attack of angle closure.

The use of aqueous suppressants to lower the IOP should be included in initial management of acute angle closure. Aqueous suppressants may positively influence posterior chamber vectors, to be described in this chapter.

The Crystalline Lens

The position of the crystalline lens influences relative pupillary block. If the crystalline lens moves forward toward the pupil, as under the influence of cholinergic drugs or secondarily from some posterior segment phenomenon, relative pupillary block is increased. If the lens moves posteriorly, contact with the iris is reduced, and pupillary block is alleviated. For this reason, because cycloplegic drugs not only cause changes in lens shape but also cause posterior movement of the lens, these drugs have been used successfully to treat acute angle-closure glaucoma. Obviously, if the pupil can be dilated beyond the edge of the crystalline lens equator, this will, in itself, alleviate pupillary block. The potential posterior movement of the crystalline lens is an additional potentially beneficial factor.

Treatment of acute angle closure with mydriatic-cycloplegic drugs is not always successful and can occasionally confound the problem. It is possible that such therapy will not induce the pupil to maximally dilate beyond the lens equator, and dilation may stop at a mid-dilated position, thereby actually increasing relative pupillary block and worsening the acute angle-closure glaucoma situation.

Mydriatic-cycloplegic drugs are not the definitive treatment for acute angle closure; laser iridotomy is the definitive treatment. In addition, if an angle closure eye has been dilated to temporarily alleviate pupillary block, it is more difficult to perform a laser iridotomy. The iris is bunched up peripherally and thickened. There is also the potential for placing the iridotomy in a less peripheral location than desired.

There are other aspects to the position of the crystalline lens that have implications for angle closure and its treatment. For example, the use of osmotics may be effective in addressing acute angle-closure glaucoma, because osmotics produce some posterior movement of the crystalline lens by their dehydrating action on vitreous volume.

A not uncommon clinical situation with the potential for misdiagnosis is the following: in the fellow eye, under the influence of systemic osmotics, posterior movement of the crystalline lens may result in deepening of the angle in both eyes and the misinterpretation that the index eye has presented with a form of unilateral angle-closure glaucoma.

A similar misdiagnosis on the fellow eye can also result from the use of systemic aqueous suppressants, such as carbonic anhydrase inhibitors (CAIs). These systemically administered agents reduce aqueous production in both eyes and decrease the pressure vector in the posterior chamber by reducing aqueous production, again leading to misinterpretation that the anterior chamber is deep and open in the fellow eye. The clinician must remember to repeat gonioscopy on the patient at a later time, when not under the influence of systemic CAIs.

The Rate of Aqueous Humor Formation

Aqueous humor flowing into the posterior chamber from the ciliary body epithelium is the force acting on the posterior surface of the iris. It acts to balloon the iris forward in a convex manner. If the amount of aqueous humor formation is reduced, either by topical or systemic drugs, the vector acting on the posterior surface of the iris is reduced. This has important diagnostic and therapeutic utility. For example, unless pupillary block is total, such as in the case of total seclusion of the pupil, decreasing the aqueous humor "force" in the posterior chamber might allow enough posterior movement of the peripheral iris to functionally open some of the angle. At the same time, it might also allow restoration of the equilibrium between the amount of aqueous humor produced and the amount that is able to seep through the pupil in the existing relative pupillary block state. This net anterior flow of aqueous into the anterior chamber would also tend to decrease the forces ballooning the peripheral iris forward. Thus, in addition to the direct IOP-lowering effect of decreasing aqueous production, by reducing vector forces in the posterior chamber, aqueous suppressant therapy might contribute to reduced iris convexity and reduced obstruction

PSEUDO-UNILATERAL ANGLE CLOSURE

David L. Epstein, MD, MMM

Understanding forces or vectors has important clinical diagnostic implications. In the 1970s, when I was an ophthalmology resident, the following scenario was common: A patient presented to the emergency department with acute angle-closure glaucoma in one eye. The first-year resident initiated treatment with pilocarpine (usually at a 4% strength), as well as treatment with systemic osmotics and systemic carbonic anhydrase inhibitors. When the supervising senior resident subsequently came to see the patient, gonioscopy of the fellow eye indicated a noncloseable angle! Attention was then erroneously directed at causes of unilateral angle-closure glaucoma. This led to an erroneous diagnosis of acute neovascular glaucoma. Confusion increased if the affected eye with angle closure did not respond to the therapy (we now know better the possible contrary influence of stronger miotics on the crystalline lens position and on reduction of zonular tension).

Such patients, according to practice standards, were hospitalized for a surgical peripheral iridectomy. Postoperatively, the index eye might be treated with dilating drops for examination of the posterior segment. It was not a rare occurrence for an attack of acute angle-closure glaucoma to subsequently develop in this fellow eye that had initially been judged to have a nonoccludable angle.

of the TM. Therefore, aqueous humor suppressants play a role in the initial treatment of acute angle-closure glaucoma.

Iris Rigidity (Tension)

Another factor that influences these processes is iris rigidity or, perhaps more correctly, iris tension. Mapstone[10] suggested that iris vectors do influence the process of angle-closure glaucoma. The iris contains 2 muscles: the iris dilator and iris sphincter. The contraction of these muscles influences this tension. It has been mentioned that an action of initial intervention with pilocarpine in acute angle-closure glaucoma is pulling the iris out of the angle and also increasing iris tension to resist pressure from the posterior chamber.

It would seem that contraction of the iris dilator muscle that would occur with the application of a pure sympathomimetic drug would act similarly to increase iris tension. In fact, when sympatholytic drugs, such as the α-blocker thymoxamine or dapiprazole, have been used to produce miosis, precipitation of angle-closure glaucoma has rarely occurred, presumably due to the induced "flaccidity" of the peripheral iris.

Anticholinergic drugs (cycloplegics) exert a positive influence on these processes by altering the crystalline lens position and zonular tension. But at the same time, they act at the level of the iris in a negative way by inducing loss of iris tone. Nevertheless, the positive effects of mydriatic/cycloplegic agents generally outweigh the negative effects, and they have some genuine efficacy.

Iris tension and rigidity is also influenced by the thickness of the iris tissue. Iris rigidity may be involved in explaining the clinical observation that full-blown primary acute angle-closure glaucoma is rare in African Americans, who often have thick, brown irides. In contrast, chronic or subacute forms are commonly seen.[11] Iris texture is thicker and/or more rigid in these individuals. It may be that the rigidity of the iris offers more resistance to hydrostatic forces from the posterior chamber, such as occurs in pupillary block.

On the other hand, acute angle-closure glaucoma is common among Asians, such as Japanese, Chinese, and individuals from Southeast Asia, despite also having thick, brown irides.

The Superior Angle

In general, the narrowest portion of the angle is the superior portion. Whether this results because the "middle segment" of the eye is simply anatomically smaller superiorly or whether it results from some of the vector forces noted above is not definitively known. Curiously, after iridotomy, such a regional difference commonly disappears, suggesting it is a result of vector forces and not purely anatomically based.

PUPILLARY BLOCK VERSUS OTHER FORMS OF PRIMARY AND SECONDARY ANGLE-CLOSURE GLAUCOMA

The terms *primary* and *secondary* can be confusing when applied to angle-closure glaucoma. Nevertheless, the distinctions may not always be clinically relevant. Pupillary block is involved as the mechanism for almost all cases of primary angle-closure glaucoma, and at least to some extent in many cases of secondary angle closure.

In primary angle closure, which occurs spontaneously, there is usually a small and crowded middle segment of the eye with a relative disproportion in size of the crystalline lens. The lens, as in all eyes, continues to grow with advancing age. Over time, this leads to increased relative pupillary block with resulting movement of the peripheral iris over the angle. In such an eye, if an iridotomy is performed at an early enough stage where there are not secondary changes in the TM from synechiae or chronic touch, the procedure is expected to be curative and definitive. The procedure and the resultant hole in the peripheral iris equalizes pressure between the posterior and anterior chambers and thus eliminates pupillary block.

Therefore, pupillary block should be the presumptive diagnosis in almost all forms of spontaneous angle-closure glaucoma. Pupillary block should be treated first and, thereby, eliminated as a contributing mechanism in almost all forms of complicated angle-closure glaucoma. Unless clearly not involved in the mechanism, pupillary block should always be suspected and treated as a first maneuver at the earliest indication in any angle-closure glaucoma, either primary or secondary.

By mechanical posterior pressure moving the crystalline lens forward to the pupil, an additional pupillary block condition may have been created in an eye not otherwise predisposed to primary angle-closure glaucoma. Many senior clinicians have learned the hard way to always suspect a pupillary block mechanism as a component of angle closure, even in these secondary forms of angle closure. Because pupillary block may play some role, addressing this component in complex cases by iridotomy may alleviate the glaucoma to at least some degree.

Another common example is in the secondary angle-closure glaucoma that occurs as a direct result of retinal detachment surgery. It is often debated whether the angle closure is due to direct mechanical factors of the operation and constriction of venous return because of the scleral buckle. There may also be the presence of suprachoroidal fluid and forward pressure from effusion. Thus, it may be that pupillary block is involved, at least as a component. Most of the time, a pupillary block mechanism is at least partially involved, as evidenced from the fact that patients do obtain some benefit from laser iridotomy. Pupillary block may also occur when the posterior segment has been filled with silicone oil, and the pupil may be blocked by silicone fluid. Relief of such block is often obtained by placing a laser iridotomy inferiorly in the iris, below the fluid-silicone interface. Two such inferiorly placed iridotomies are generally recommended.

PLATEAU IRIS

Plateau iris is a rare form of angle closure.[12,13] Because it occurs spontaneously it is also defined among the primary angle-closure glaucomas. In true plateau iris, the mechanism for the glaucoma is the direct crowding of the peripheral iris into the angle without pupillary block. The condition behaves as if the base of the iris is hinged too far anteriorly. With pupillary dilation, as the iris thickens, it obliterates access to the surface of the TM. In plateau iris, maximum pupillary dilation results in maximum crowding of the angle, unlike in pupillary block where maximum dilation tends to relieve pupillary block as the pupil clears the crystalline lens equator. UBM and anterior AS-OCT studies have demonstrated an anterior position of the ciliary processes in plateau iris (Figure 22-4). This acts as a factor responsible for the forward displacement of the peripheral iris base.[13]

True plateau iris is also called plateau iris syndrome. The syndrome then consists of the characteristic plateau iris configuration and the associated propensity for the pressure to elevate as the iris bunches against the face of the TM in dilation even in the presence of a patent peripheral iridotomy. This is distinct from what is termed *plateau iris configuration*, in which the iris may have this anatomic configuration but is not associated with iris bunching on

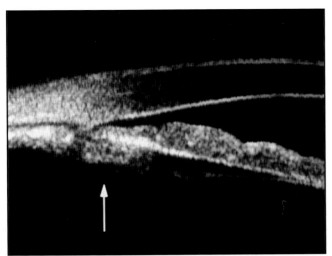

Figure 22-4. Plateau iris with UBM. Note the flat iris plane, the narrowness of the angle, with a steep approach, and the position of the ciliary processes, which are rotated anteriorly and pushing the peripheral iris into the angle.

dilation and elevation of IOP by this mechanism. Plateau iris configuration alone is much more common than plateau iris syndrome.

Plateau iris syndrome can often be treated successfully with weak miotics to prevent spontaneous, physiologic pupillary dilatation. Failing this, it can be treated by gonioplasty—application of argon laser energy to the iris periphery altering the iris tissue properties and inhibiting bunching with dilation.[14]

Plateau iris is initially suspected based on the slit-lamp examination. Unlike primary angle closure due to pupillary block, there is good axial depth to the anterior chamber. This is because, in plateau iris, there is not the relative disproportion between the size of the crystalline lens and the "middle segment" of the eye that there is in primary pupillary block.

However, similar to angle closure from pupillary block, the peripheral anterior chamber depth in plateau iris is narrow. This can be seen with Van Herick's[15] technique for visualizing the peripheral anterior chamber with the slit beam.

This axial/peripheral anterior chamber depth disparity is the first clue to the presence of plateau iris. Even more definitive are the gonioscopic findings where, instead of a convex surface iris contour, the iris is flatter. The examiner finds himself looking "across a plateau" into a narrow angle where only anterior structures are seen. There is a sense of a peripheral trough, which, in the nondilated state, allows the presence of functional open angle just below one's view.

This gonioscopic appearance, which is more easily appreciated with direct forms of gonioscopy such as the Koeppe technique, is characteristic, but is still subject to interpretation. In fact, most cases of suspected plateau iris syndrome,

with TM occlusion and elevated pressure, turn out to be due to pupillary block and not the dynamics of iris bunching against the TM. These cases are cured by peripheral laser iridotomy. Thus, it is common to employ peripheral laser iridotomy in eyes with plateau iris configuration.

Of great clinical relevance, in order to diagnose a true plateau iris (plateau iris syndrome), an iridotomy needs to be performed first, and then the patient undergoes provocative pupillary dilation to discern whether there is still pressure elevation with dilation. If the pressure then rises with dilation, this defines true plateau iris/plateau iris syndrome. Peripheral iris iridoplasty or appropriate pharmacologic intervention may then be employed.

HOW TO DIAGNOSE AN OCCLUDABLE ANGLE

In the era prior to laser iridotomy, surgical peripheral iridectomy was required for treatment. Rigorous diagnostic protocols were applied before subjecting a patient to the surgical procedure. Although surgical iridectomy was largely a successful operation, it had a notoriously long list of possible complications. The advent of laser iridotomy has reduced the overall risk and has certainly loosened the indications for its use.

Prior to the era of the laser, provocative tests such as the darkroom prone test or pharmacological mydriatic tests were commonly performed to identify eyes at risk. Presently, such provocative tests are uncommonly performed. Judgment based on the gonioscopic findings is the usual criterion for considering iridotomy. This may be supplemented by utilizing UBM or AS-OCT imaging when available.

In equivocal situations where there is a strong suspicion of a pupillary block mechanism, the risk/benefit considerations are such that it is justifiable to perform laser iridotomy. The patient is informed of the nature of the procedure, the rationale for the procedure, the likelihood that there will be a benefit, and the degree and type of risk involved. Informed consent includes the patient in the decision-making process, and informed consent guides the decision.

Proximate complications of laser iridotomy include acute IOP elevation after applying energy and inducing inflammation and possible diplopia or ghost image from the iridotomy. It is said that placing the iridotomy superiorly may create more of a problem with ghost imaging due to the prismatic effect of the upper lid tear meniscus, even though the iridotomy may be covered by the lid. For this reason, many advocate temporal placement of the iridotomy.

Besides these proximate complications, there are certain long-term risks to laser iridotomy. These long-term consequences have been anticipated by clinical experience with surgical peripheral iridectomy. Most significantly, there is a long-term risk of accelerated cataract formation,[16] usually nuclear sclerosis. It occurs at an increased frequency even after a technically perfect surgical peripheral iridectomy where the operation on the iris was truly performed outside of the eye with no intraocular manipulation. Accelerated nuclear sclerotic cataract formation is not likely a result of the surgical technique. It is a consequence of the fact that aqueous humor is no longer flowing across the posterior chamber and through the pupil to nourish the anterior surface of the crystalline lens. Instead, it is now "short-circuiting" its way through the iridectomy.

The observation of the development of nuclear sclerosis rather than the development of superior cortical opacity following surgical peripheral iridectomy is consistent with such a mechanism for cataract formation. Although the laser opening in the iris is smaller with laser iridotomy than the opening created by surgical iridectomy, similar short-circuiting of the aqueous flow pathway is still occurring, and there is a definite clinical observation of acceleration of nuclear sclerotic lens change over time as a result of laser iridotomy.

There is another long-term potential complication more common after laser iridotomy than after surgical peripheral iridectomy. This is the manifestation of residual open-angle glaucoma. There are unequivocally more cases of residual open-angle glaucoma in patients who have undergone laser iridotomy for angle-closure glaucoma than there should be based on the prevalence of POAG in the same-aged population.

It is possible that this is partially due to incorrect diagnosis. The ease of performing laser iridotomy has probably loosened the criteria for diagnosis and lessened the requirement for clinical acumen in selecting patients for the procedure. It is also possible that, even though the angle may open after iridotomy, chronic iris touch of the TM during the time when there was apposition may cause residual open-angle glaucoma. Still, the prevalence of POAG after iridotomy is more common than it was after surgical peripheral iridectomy.

A potential explanation for this phenomenon is that the pigment and debris as well as the inflammatory mediators that egress through the TM[17] after technically perfect laser iridotomy may take a toll on the ultimate function of this conventional outflow pathway in certain individuals. With surgical iridectomy, these substances exit the eye through the incision site rather than transiting through the TM, sparing the TM of toxicity and damage.

Thus, one wants to have clear guidelines for performing laser iridotomy and should not perform the procedure indiscriminately. "Above all else, do no harm," and use the "golden rule" in all clinical decision making.

How does one then discern an occludable angle? First of all, it needs to be re-stated for emphasis that the indication for intervention depends on the appearance of the angle, not simply on the presence of iris convexity. A convex iris can always be "cured" (ie, flattened with laser iridotomy), but a convex iris itself does not define risk of angle closure. Risk of angle closure is based on angle appearance on gonioscopy.

General principles and indications for laser peripheral iridotomy include the following:

- If properly performed gonioscopy reveals hardly any visible angle structure
- If only the most anterior portion of the TM can be seen
- If the angle changes in front of one's eyes so that intermittently almost no angle structures are seen

On the other extreme, if despite high iris convexity, the full-width of TM to the level of scleral spur can be seen throughout most of the circumference, this is not an occludable angle and does not require iridotomy.

When the angle is intermediate between these extremes, risk of occludability is less certain. An example would be when only mid-TM is visualized. In the past, provocative testing has been advocated. The darkroom prone test is preferred because it is deemed more physiologic, and there is some clinical impression that a negative test indicates that the risk of acute angle closure is small over the subsequent 6 months.

Pharmacological provocative dilating tests are not routinely performed because they are not physiologic, and they may pharmacologically alter the iris vectors discussed above. In addition, intense pharmacologic pupillary dilation may move the pupil rapidly past the point of greatest danger, mid-dilatation, during initial mydriasis and only later result in angle closure (after the patient has left the office) when the pupil recovers slowly to a smaller mid-dilated size. Although it is possible to keep the patient in the office all day, all this is cumbersome and does not relate to the fundamental question of the patient's risk of spontaneous acute angle closure under normal living conditions. Even though the darkroom prone test is more physiologic than pharmacological testing, there are variables that contribute to inaccuracy, including artificiality to the testing conditions and problems with immediate posttesting IOP measurement.

A more definitive ascertainment of occludability may be obtained with UBM or AS-OCT, if such technology is available to the clinician. The imaging can be conducted in a lit room and then with the room darkened. This may demonstrate iris apposition in dim light or lack thereof in cases that are equivocal by gonioscopy. It also demonstrates the issue that light introduced during gonioscopy may artificially open the angle by inducing contraction of the pupillary sphincter, opening of the angle, and resulting in misdiagnosis.

In these equivocal situations, the assessment should take into account the whole patient. For example, if the patient is young, the problem will not likely improve over time. In fact, it will tend to get worse as the lens ages and enlarges. Also, one must consider the access the patient would have to care if he or she were to experience a spontaneous angle-closure attack. Informed consent requires a discussion with the patient about the findings and the uncertainties in interpretation. If one has access to UBM or AS-OCT, the uncertainties are reduced. In any case, the patient should participate in the decision about laser iridotomy. Having done all this, and if the situation is still truly equivocal, a decision to perform laser iridotomy is reasonable.

When the IOP is normal but there is a question of the risk of angle closure and the need for prophylactic treatment, examination should include compression gonioscopy. This may identify a site of peripheral anterior synechiae formation. Peripheral anterior synechiae, by itself, unless explained by other events such as previous inflammation or penetrating injury, is an indication for laser iridotomy.

To visualize the presence and extent of peripheral anterior synechiae, there must be optimal compression whereby the area on either side of the synechiae is adequately compressed posteriorly. Inadequate compression may relate to improper technique or to other factors, such as the level of the IOP and the resulting resistance to indentation.

The presence of peripheral anterior synechiae in a narrow angled eye "ups the ante" and obviates a strategy of further observation. It indicates that the narrowness of the angle is leading to peripheral anterior synechiae and that there is a potential for future long-term irreversible harm with permanent loss of functioning angle circumference. This is a strong indication for intervention. Whether the IOP is normal or elevated, the defined presence of peripheral anterior synechiae when seen on compression gonioscopy is an indication for laser iridotomy.

In the early stages of chronic apposition and peripheral anterior synechiae formation, the inherent outflow of the remainder of the angle may be intact, and no obvious IOP elevation may be observed. Why some patients with iris apposition to the TM readily form synechiae despite the presence of a quiet eye while others do not is not understood.

Another relevant point in regard to clinical diagnosis is worth making. In narrow angled eyes that presumably do not have a pre-existing form of latent open-angle glaucoma, one would not expect more than 2 mm Hg of IOP asymmetry between the 2 eyes. If there is such a difference in IOP between the 2 eyes, an area of functional angle closure in the eye with the higher pressure is a possible explanation for this small IOP asymmetry. This should be considered while performing careful gonioscopy and should be factored into a decision about intervention.

HOW TO DIAGNOSE A (CHRONIC, SILENT) ANGLE CLOSURE COMPONENT WHEN INTRAOCULAR PRESSURE IS ELEVATED

Chronic, silent, angle-closure glaucoma masquerading as open-angle glaucoma is one of the most common misdiagnoses in clinical glaucoma practice. Contributing to this problem is the use of aqueous humor suppressants. These decrease the vector force in the posterior chamber and may erroneously, for a time, alter the appearance of the angle as observed on gonioscopy, making it appear deeper than otherwise expected and contributing to the perpetuation of the misdiagnosis. This possibility must be kept in mind when evaluating patients on aqueous suppressants. The clinician should perform repeat gonioscopy at various intervals, and certainly in all cases when the IOP has increased between visits.

The first question to be addressed is, "What is the correlation of the angle appearance with the degree of IOP elevation?" This question is relevant whether the patient is on pressure-lowering medications or not.

If the full width of TM to the scleral spur can be visualized, then no matter how narrow the inlet, the angle is functionally open and pressure elevation is from an open-angle mechanism. Intervention to alter the chamber depth with laser iridotomy will not be expected to alter the course. It must be stressed that this consideration applies to the appearance of the undisturbed condition of the angle—the appearance of the angle without compression.

If on the other hand, the full width of the TM to the scleral spur cannot be seen, the overall goal is to correlate the uncompressed angle appearance with the IOP. Consider the following: in 2 separate patients, nondynamic (noncompression) gonioscopy yields similar findings—no angle structures can be seen (Figure 22-5). In the first patient, the IOP is 14 mm Hg. In the second patient, the IOP is 40 mm Hg. What explains the different IOP in the setting of 2 similar gonioscopic appearances? Obviously, in the first patient, although the angle appears closed, it is truly functionally open. This means that in the undisturbed state, if we could only get down there and actually view it, such as can be done with UBM or AS-OCT, there is some space for access of the aqueous humor to the TM. In the second patient, the angle is, in fact, functionally closed. (As an aside, it is still theoretically possible that the patient's angle access in the second patient's angle is open, as it is the first patient, but that the second patient has occult open-angle glaucoma. While this theoretical concern should be kept in mind, especially in eyes with exfoliation, it is a separate issue, and the glaucoma is managed differently.)

Compression gonioscopy can indicate that an angle is openable. So, the next question to be addressed in these cases of chronic angle closure is, what is the correlation of the measured IOP elevation with the angle appearance? Compression gonioscopy simply identifies the presence of peripheral anterior synechiae by its dynamic, mechanical action of pushing the iris posteriorly. In the absence of synechiae, compression gonioscopy does not help resolve whether the undisturbed IOP elevation can be explained by an appositional angle closure alone.

Therefore, in patients with a suspected chronic, silent, angle-closure component to their IOP elevation, the first

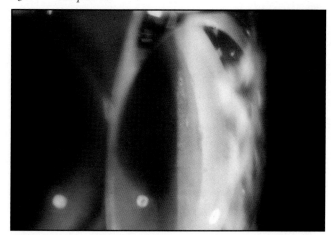

Figure 22-5. No angle structures seen on gonioscopy.

question is whether there is enough of the angle circumference that appears closed to explain the IOP elevation. Only a few hours of apparent functional angle closure cannot by itself explain an elevation of IOP. For example, if the IOP is 30 mm Hg and by gonioscopy, only 90 degrees of the angle appear functionally closed, angle closure by itself cannot explain this degree of IOP elevation.

In such a patient, the clinician performs compression gonioscopy to rule out synechia formation in the affected 90 degrees. The presence of peripheral anterior synechiae would be an indication for laser iridotomy not because this would address the pressure elevation, but rather because it would reduce the risk of further progressive synechial angle closure.

In the absence of synechiae, clinical judgment comes into play. Reasoning that this is most likely open-angle glaucoma accounting for the IOP of 30 mm Hg, albeit with some limited degree of apposition, antiglaucoma therapy for open-angle glaucoma is initiated, and the angle appearance would continue to be monitored. Monitoring is important because aqueous suppressant antiglaucoma therapy for open-angle glaucoma when there is actually silent, chronic progressive angle closure may actually deepen the angle and give a false sense of security.

If over time, the patient's IOP control and angle appearance remain stable and there are no peripheral anterior synechiae, one may be suspicious that the affected 90 degrees that continue to appear narrow are in fact functionally open. If, over time, there is a slow creep upward in the IOP, this might be correlated with a changing angle appearance. Angle closure progressed beyond 90 degrees could now be in play and would explain the progressive rise in pressure. If this is the case, the risk/benefit considerations shift in favor of laser iridotomy.

Unfortunately, such a clinical situation is not rare and does not always have a crystal-clear presentation and course. We most often must depend on clinical judgment.

One might ask, why not simply have performed laser iridotomy from the beginning? In addition to any long-term

considerations such as accelerated cataract formation,[17] patients who have a narrow but largely functional angle, with an underlying open-angle glaucoma mechanism and an IOP of 30 mm Hg, would not be expected to obtain any beneficial IOP lowering from iridotomy. The basic mechanism for the elevated IOP is by an open-angle mechanism.

In fact, superimposing the potential acute IOP spike seen commonly after iridotomy on an outflow system already compromised by open-angle glaucoma might have put the patient at risk for acute adverse events including pressure spike with laser intervention. A good approach in this case would involve establishing initial medical treatment for the underlying open-angle glaucoma and reducing the IOP with medication. This would make subsequent laser iridotomy safer.

By reassessing the angle with gonioscopy in the setting of initial medical therapy, the patient could be spared a procedure that might not be necessary. With residual open-angle glaucoma syndrome following laser iridotomy, the patient might actually be made worse, and pressure might become more difficult to control.

What is clinically most important is understanding whether an angle that appears narrow or closed in a small portion of the circumference is really functionally closed. It might actually be functionally open as in the case of the first patient. Imaging the anterior segment with UBM or AS-OCT can be helpful in verifying this. Regardless, there is no substitute for attempting to make the correct diagnosis initially and understanding the etiology of the IOP elevation (whether open angle or angle closure). Then, one may proceed logically one step at a time. Such an approach allows one to communicate accurately and effectively with the patient about the risk versus the benefit of laser iridotomy intervention.

Suppose in another patient, there is good correlation between the degree of IOP elevation and the amount of the angle circumference that appears apposed and closed. Is there any way to determine whether the seemingly closed portion of the angle is truly functionally closed?

Of historical interest, it has been proposed that producing meiosis using thymoxamine, a pure alpha-1 sympatholytic drug, might be a useful test to address this question. Thymoxamine is free from direct effects on the outflow pathway.[18,19] Pupillary constriction occurs by blockage of alpha-1 receptors. If a patient had a functionally closed portion of angle, thymoxamine would presumably open that portion by reducing sympathetic tone and promoting meiosis, pulling the peripheral iris away from the angle. IOP would be reduced. For many years, the thymoxamine test was performed at the Massachusetts Eye and Ear Infirmary Glaucoma Service. It provided much important clinical information. In addition to the positive and negative tests, there were also equivocal cases where neither the IOP nor the angle appearance changed. Additionally, there were a few cases where application of thymoxamine resulted in acute elevation of IOP from enhancement of the angle closure mechanism presumably by decreasing iris tone.

Currently, it is difficult to obtain thymoxamine. Another alpha-1 blocking sympatholytic drug, dapiprazole, has been developed. This drug too is no longer commercially available. Because of lack of availability of these alpha-1 blockers, provocative tests to determine whether functional angle closure is contributing to IOP elevation are no longer performed. High-resolution anterior segment imaging with UBM and OCT can provide more insight into the anatomy of an angle and the degree of apposition. In addition, the wide availability and relative ease of performing laser iridotomy has decreased the use of sympatholytic provocative testing.

It is important to understand the etiology of the patient's condition ahead of planned intervention. In this way, the patient can be fully apprised of risk. These risks include the potential anticipated magnitude of an IOP spike and the chance of "residual open-angle glaucoma" following the procedure.

In cases of silent chronic angle closure, the patient should not have the expectation that laser iridotomy will cure the glaucoma. Patients should be aware of the possibility that there is an additional open-angle mechanism at play. Similarly, it is important for the clinician to be aware of the possibility that one may be dealing with an open-angle glaucoma process, and prophylactic iridotomy is being accomplished for future considerations of progressive chronic angle closure rather than for proximate IOP control.

Thus in practice, the clinician may apply laser iridotomy to settle this issue and must maintain full awareness of the risk/benefit considerations. With this awareness in an equivocal situation, it is reasonable to perform laser iridotomy.

It would certainly be more satisfying if one could more accurately assess this difficult question of whether there may be a functional angle-closure component in a patient with elevated IOP prior to applying any laser intervention. A classic case with such a concern would be an eye with exfoliative glaucoma. While these eyes have an open-angle mechanism, they also commonly demonstrate narrow angles.[4] The angle narrowing in these cases may progress with the years. It would be ideal to refrain from insulting the diseased TM with debris and pigment from laser iridotomy unless certain improvement in IOP control could be predicted from the elimination of a true superimposed angle-closure component. Even UBM, which reveals the anatomy of the angle with a resolution of 50 μm and which can reveal the presence of appositional or synechial closure and demonstrate aqueous space between the iris and TM, cannot in practice fully address the question of functional closure. High-resolution AS-OCT, on the other hand, may be able to better demonstrate the anatomy.

All patients on antiglaucoma therapy for presumed POAG as well as patients with open-angle glaucoma not under treatment should undergo periodic repeat gonioscopy. This should also be performed when there is an increase in baseline IOP at the current visit. Gonioscopy should be applied to ascertain any changes from baseline that may correlate with elevation of IOP and that may have occurred slowly over time, related to progressive silent angle closure.

Some patients who are seen for the first time are already on antiglaucoma therapy. If such patients also have a narrow angle on presentation, it is worthwhile to try to reassess the patient off current antiglaucoma therapy, specifically aqueous suppressants. Withholding glaucoma medication should be done with close monitoring, taking into consideration the risk to the optic nerve from pressure elevation that may occur when withholding therapy for a brief time. Nevertheless, for the long-term benefit of the patient, it is essential to know the fundamental disease process one is dealing with.

In summary, this entire section has dealt with narrow angled eyes presenting with elevated pressure. It required addressing the question: Is there an angle-closure component to the manifest IOP elevation? On gonioscopy, there may be no appositional or synechial closure. Aqueous has access to the TM, albeit through a narrow passage. In this case, the pressure elevation is caused by an open-angle mechanism, and iridotomy would not be expected to alter the IOP. Nevertheless, even though there is no appositional closure or synechial closure, if the angle appearance is truly dangerously narrow (ie, the angle is occludable), the patient should undergo laser iridotomy.

It is very important to know exactly what type of glaucoma one is dealing with, and it is important to explain to the patient and oneself the exact reasons why some action is being initiated. In this latest example of the potentially occludable angle, the patient should not have the expectation that iridotomy will lower pressure. The patient should understand that the iridotomy would be intended to prevent further worsening of the glaucoma by preventing future angle closure that would likely occur without laser intervention. While indicated as an appropriate treatment for their glaucoma, the procedure itself will not correct the current IOP situation. Even with the iridotomy, he or she will still require the appropriate treatment for open-angle glaucoma.

ANGLE-CLOSURE GLAUCOMA IN MYOPIA

Angle-closure glaucoma is rare in myopic eyes[20] because these usually tend to be large eyes with wide-open angles. However, in rare instances in which myopia is due to an unusually high index of refraction of the crystalline lens or a pronounced curvature of the cornea, the eyeball may not, in fact, be long and large, and angle-closure glaucoma due to a pupillary block type mechanism can occur. These eyes respond in the usual way to laser iridotomy.

Eyes with previous retinopathy of prematurity, sometimes with minimal posterior pole involvement, are often myopic and can develop a progressive secondary angle-closure glaucoma that may or may not respond to laser iridotomy. In these cases, presumed tractional processes involving the ciliary body might cause angle closure from direct local effects on the peripheral iris or from a change in crystalline lens position, thus causing a secondary pupillary block.

NANOPHTHALMOS

Nanophthalmos[21-26] represents a special condition of high hyperopia in which there is an abnormally small (dwarfed) eyeball containing a crystalline lens of disproportionately normal size. Suspicion of this condition should be raised by the presence of hyperopia of 8 D or more, abnormally small corneas, and shallow anterior chambers with chronic angle-closure glaucoma. Nanophthalmos has some unique features that create challenges in management. The sclera may be more than twice as thick as normal, and there is a strong tendency to uveal effusion.[21-23] This predisposes to detachment of the choroid and retina after surgery. In suspected cases, ultrasonography is helpful in establishing the diagnosis by revealing that the globe as abnormally short and the sclera as abnormally thick but that the lens is of normal size. Ultrasonography may also be used preoperatively to detect uveal effusion or thickening of the choroid. Diagnosis and treatment of nanophthalmos are discussed elsewhere in this text.

THE ROLE OF VASCULAR CONGESTION

In eyes with very narrow angles, engorgement of intraocular vessels, such as those in the ciliary body, has been suggested as a mechanism involved in angle closure. Congestion could conceivably contribute to angle closure by pushing the iris forward. There is little evidence for this, however. In cases of shallowing of the anterior chamber or closure of the angle after central retinal vein occlusion or panretinal photocoagulation, the crystalline lens temporarily moves forward as if there is an increased volume behind it, but it is unknown whether this is from intravascular congestion or extravascular edema. The fact that the uveal tract becomes congested after a violent attack of angle-closure glaucoma is well established, but congestion before a spontaneous attack and leading to that attack has not been proven.

The idea that vascular congestion is a factor in development of acute glaucoma is an old one, presumably suggested by the conspicuous shallowness of the anterior chamber and the considerable engorgement of episcleral and conjunctival blood vessels evident after a violent attack has become well-established.

One can demonstrate experimentally in enucleated human eyes that a rapid increase in volume of the vascular bed, by injection into the posterior ciliary arteries, can cause the lens and iris to move forward and shallow the anterior chamber. In living patients who have threatening narrow angles, no vasodilating drug or provocative test based on vasodilation has been found to precipitate an attack of angle closure.

TREATMENT OF ANGLE-CLOSURE GLAUCOMA WHEN ASSOCIATED WITH CATARACT

In eyes with a shallow anterior chamber and cataract, angle-closure glaucoma may occur spontaneously, just as in an eye without cataract. In certain cases, angle closure may be precipitated by a change in the size of the lens associated with the development of cataract. During the stage of intumescence or during an early stage of hypermaturity, the lens may swell sufficiently to cause closure of the angle and induce acute glaucoma by pupillary block. The mechanism for such angle-closure glaucoma associated with cataract is called *phakomorphic glaucoma.*

Treatment in cases of hypermature cataract in which angle-closure glaucoma has occurred from pupillary block may consist of removal of the lens after the IOP has been reduced by aqueous humor suppressants and intravenous or oral hypertonic solutions, as needed. However, because cataract surgery requires a pharmacologically dilated pupil, it may be prudent to perform laser iridotomy prior to cataract surgery.

When acute angle closure occurs spontaneously in an eye that happens to have an immature cataract—without swelling of the lens—the glaucoma can be relieved by peripheral laser iridotomy just as it can in anatomically predisposed eyes with clear lenses. These cases are believed to involve pupillary block. Whether the crystalline lens itself can force the iris into the angle, independent of a pupillary block mechanism, is discussed in Chapter 28.

SECONDARY ANGLE-CLOSURE GLAUCOMAS

Angle-closure glaucoma that occurs spontaneously and can be attributed to anatomic, pharmacologic, and/or physiologic factors is defined as primary. This is distinct from the other category of angle-closure glaucoma in which some pre-existing pathologic condition of the eye causes the angle to close. Such glaucoma is defined as secondary.

This category of secondary angle-closure glaucoma, in which antecedent pathologic factors are responsible for closure of the angles, is encountered in the following conditions:

- After scleral-buckling operation for detached retina
- From multiple cysts of the iris and ciliary body
- Secondary to occlusion of the central retinal vein
- Secondary to drug-induced acute transitory myopia
- From contusion (with dislocation of the lens)
- Associated with spontaneous dislocation of the lens
- Due to pupillary block in aphakia
- Due to intraocular inflammation (with iris bombé)

- Associated with malignant intraocular tumors
- After operation for congenital cataract (with pupillary block)

REFERENCES

1. Van Buskirk EM, Grant WM. Lens depression and aqueous outflow in enucleated primate eyes. *Am J Ophthalmol.* 1973;76:632-640.
2. Grant WM. Experimental aqueous perfusion in enucleated human eyes. *Arch Ophthalmol.* 1963;69:783-801.
3. Rohen JW. Why is intraocular pressure elevated in chronic simple glaucoma? *Ophthalmology.* 1983;90:758-765.
4. Gross FJ, Tingey D, Epstein DL. Increased prevalence of occludable angles and angle-closure glaucoma in patients with pseudoexfoliation. *Am J Ophthalmol.* 1993;117:333-336.
5. Barsotti M, Bartels SP, Freddo TF, et al. The source of proteins in the aqueous humor of the normal monkey eye. *Invest Ophthalmol Vis Sci.* 1992;33:581-595.
6. Pederson JE, Toris CB. Experimental retinal detachment. IX. Aqueous, vitreous, and subretinal protein concentrations. *Arch Ophthalmol.* 1985;103:835-836.
7. Campbell DG. Iris retraction associated with rhegmatogenous retinal detachment syndrome and hypotony. A new explanation. *Arch Ophthalmol.* 1984;102:1457-1463.
8. Greenfield DS, Bellows AR, Asdourian GK, et al. Iris retraction syndrome after intraocular surgery. *Ophthalmology.* 1995;102:98-100.
9. Mapstone R. The syndrome of closed-angle glaucoma. *Br J Ophthalmol.* 1976;60:120-123.
10. Mapstone R. Closed-angle glaucoma. Experimental results [Review]. *Br J Ophthalmol.* 1974;58:41-45.
11. Salmon JF. Presenting features of primary angle-closure glaucoma in patients of mixed ethnic background. *South Africa Med J.* 1993;83:594-597.
12. Wand M, Grant WM, Simmons RJ, et al. Plateau iris syndrome. *Trans Am Acad Ophthalmol Otolaryngol.* 1977;83:122-130.
13. Pavlin CJ, Ritch R, Foster FS. Ultrasound biomicroscopy in plateau iris syndrome. *Am J Ophthalmol.* 1992;113:390-395.
14. Sassani JW, Ritch R, McCormick S, et al. Histopathology of argon laser peripheral iridoplasty. *Ophthalmic Surg.* 1993;24:740-745.
15. Van Herick W, Shaffer RN, Schwartz A. Estimation of width of angle of anterior chamber. Incidence and significance of the narrow angle. *Am J Ophthalmol.* 1969;68:626-629.
16. Godel V, Regenbogen L. Cataractogenic factors in patients with primary angle-closure glaucoma after peripheral iridectomy. *Am J Ophthalmol.* 1977;83:180-184.
17. Robin AL, Pollack IP, Quigley HA, D'Anna S, Addicks EM. Histologic studies of angle structures after laser iridotomy in primates. *Arch Ophthalmol.* 1982;100:1665-1670.
18. Wand M, Grant WM. The thymoxamine test: A test to differentiate angle-closure glaucoma from open-angle glaucoma with narrow angles. *Arch Ophthalmol.* 1978;96:1009-1011.
19. Wand M, Grant WM. Thymoxamine hydrochloride: Effects on the facility of outflow and intraocular pressure. *Invest Ophthalmol.* 1976;15:400-403.
20. Hagan JC, Lederer CM. Primary angle closure glaucoma in a myopic kinship. *Arch Ophthalmol.* 1985;103:363-365.
21. Brockhurst RJ. Vortex vein decompression for a nanophthalmic uveal effusion. *Arch Ophthalmol.* 1980;98:1987-1990.
22. Singh OS, Simmons RJ, Brockhurst RJ, et al. Nanophthalmos: a perspective on identification and therapy. *Ophthalmology.* 1982;89:1006-1012.
23. Jin JC, Anderson DR. Laser and unsutured sclerotomy in nanophthalmos. *Am J Ophthalmol.* 1990;109:575-580.
24. Trelstad RL, Silbermann NN, Brockhurst RJ. Nanophthalmic sclera. Ultrastructural, histochemical, and biochemical observations. *Arch Ophthalmol.* 1982;100:1935-1938.
25. Yue BY, Duvall J, Goldberg MF, Puck A, Tso MO, Sugar J. Nanophthalmic sclera. Morphologic and tissue culture studies. *Ophthalmology.* 1986;93:534-541.
26. Stewart DH 3rd, Streeten BW, Brockhurst RJ, Anderson DR, Hirose T, Gass DM. Abnormal scleral collagen in nanophthalmos. An ultrastructural study. *Arch Ophthalmol.* 1991;109:1017-1025.

23

Acute Angle-Closure Glaucoma
Diagnosis and Treatment

George Ulrich, MD, FACS; Joel S. Schuman, MD, FACS;
David L. Epstein, MD, MMM; and Ian P. Conner, MD, PhD

Angle-closure glaucoma that occurs spontaneously may be acute or subacute (see Chapter 24). In both types, the sole cause of rise in pressure is closure of the angle, but the clinical manifestations are somewhat different. In acute angle-closure glaucoma, symptoms appear suddenly and dramatically. In subacute angle closure, symptoms are less intense and dramatic and tend to resolve spontaneously. With recurrence of episodes, permanent areas of synechial closure may develop. Hence, in the sense that episodes tend to recur and angle changes tend to evolve without intervention, there is some chronicity to the condition.

Distinct chronic angle-closure glaucoma, also referred to as silent chronic angle closure (see Chapter 22), is a separate entity. It develops silently without symptoms. The process may be due to sustained yet potentially reversible appositional closure or to synechial closure.

This chapter will discuss acute angle-closure glaucoma, although many of the same considerations apply to subacute and related chronic angle-closure glaucoma.

DIAGNOSIS

In acute angle-closure glaucoma, the angle is predisposed to the dramatic event of angle closure by being extremely narrow in the whole circumference even before closure occurs (Figure 23-1). During an attack, all or most of the angle closes. Intraocular pressure (IOP) can reach extremely high levels. Acute angle closure represents a small fraction of all the glaucomas, but it is an important variety because it represents one of the true ophthalmic emergencies. If not diagnosed and treated promptly and properly, it can result in blindness in a matter of days. The diagnosis is usually not difficult to make, but certain points deserve emphasis.

Acute Onset

An attack of acute angle closure has the most precipitous onset of any disorder involving the anterior segment. A quiet eye may change from a normal functioning state to a state of violent glaucoma in 30 to 60 minutes. No other disorder involving the anterior segment comes on with such rapidity.

By obtaining an accurate history of acute onset, there is a strong presumption, even before the patient is examined, that the diagnosis will prove to be acute angle-closure glaucoma. A careful history frequently discloses that weeks or months before the severe acute attack, there were premonitory, self-limited episodes of aching and visual blurring, each lasting a few hours and occurring with increasing frequency until the sudden development of the latest, most severe attack.

Dilation of the Pupil

In acute angle-closure glaucoma, there is most often a degree of intermediate dilation of the pupil. The diameter of the pupil can range from 3 to 8 mm. Reaction of the pupil to light is usually minimal or absent.

Shallow Anterior Chamber

In most cases of acute angle-closure glaucoma, the anterior chamber is very shallow axially. In exceptional cases, the axial depth of the anterior chamber may be normal (plateau iris configuration; see Chapter 26). However, the peripheral anterior chamber depth is always shallow.

Kahook MY, Schuman JS, eds.
Chandler and Grant's Glaucoma, Fifth Edition (pp 255-268).
© 2013 SLACK Incorporated.

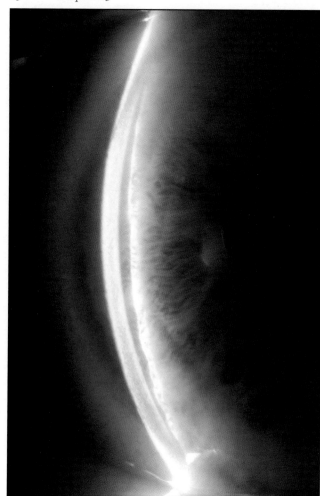

Figure 23-1. Convex iris and narrow angle in a hyperopic patient. Only mid-TM was visible on gonioscopy, and the angle was judged to be potentially occludable.

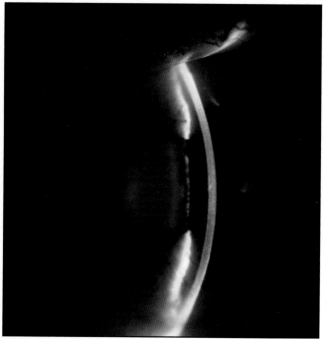

Figure 23-2. Numerous glaukomflecken were observed subsequent to a prolonged attack of acute angle-closure glaucoma.

Gray Atrophy of the Iris Stroma

After an attack of acute glaucoma, patchy gray atrophy of the iris stroma may develop, sometimes in just one quadrant or one small sector of the iris, and other times affecting the iris extensively. Such atrophy is not seen during the acute phase of an initial attack, becoming evident only after a few weeks. Acute angle-closure glaucoma is one of the few conditions that will produce this type of atrophy of the iris stroma. The other possible conditions that have been seen are cases of very high IOP after retinal detachment surgery and cases of hyphema with high IOP after contusion of the globe. If there is typical gray atrophy of the iris stroma, one can usually infer that the patient has experienced a past attack of acute glaucoma, especially when the characteristic atrophy is accompanied by *glaukomflecken*, as will be described in the next section.

The appearance of iris atrophy caused by acute glaucoma is quite distinctive. Other forms of atrophy of the iris, as caused by uveitis, herpes zoster, or essential atrophy of the iris, differ sufficiently in appearance from that caused by acute glaucoma.

The Glaukomflecken of Vogt

Glaukomflecken (Figure 23-2) consist of small white spots immediately in or beneath the anterior capsule of the lens in the pupillary zone, visibly demonstrating necrosis of lens epithelium associated with acutely high IOP. Glaukomflecken are sometimes confluent and form sheet-like opacities. These are a positive sign of a previous attack of acute glaucoma. Although not seen in all cases of acute angle-closure glaucoma, they are also not uncommon.

Glaukomflecken may occasionally be caused by an episode of very high IOP after a surgical procedure for retinal detachment, after hyphema, or from high IOP from blunt trauma to the globe. The opacities are permanent. As time passes and new lens fibers are laid-down, the opacities gradually move deeper into the anterior cortex. This progressive movement to deeper layers happens more rapidly in younger people.

In most cases, the presence of glaukomflecken means there is high potential for another attack of acute angle closure unless the situation is recognized and addressed. Recognition of glaukomflecken may serve as a valuable clue, as illustrated by the following case from the era prior to laser iridotomy.

Case 23-1

A 35-year-old woman had a typical attack of acute angle-closure glaucoma in the left eye several months previously and had undergone a peripheral iridectomy in that eye. The

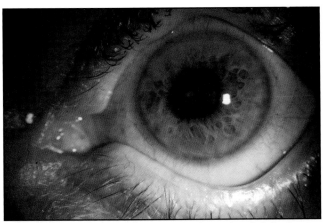

Figure 23-3. Fine corneal haze (epithelial edema) that slightly obscures iris details, caused by sudden elevation of IOP. Patient observed colored haloes around lights.

an indication of a pathologic process other than acute angle-closure glaucoma.

Corneal Edema

The corneal epithelium at first develops edema of a fine ground-glass character, giving the cornea a steamy appearance and causing the patient to see colored haloes around lights (Figure 23-3). Later in the course of a severe attack, at the stage where many cells appear in the aqueous and the eye becomes hyperemic, the whole thickness of the cornea may become swollen with wrinkling of the posterior surface. Wrinkling of the cornea is often prominent after IOP has dropped to normal levels, either spontaneously or as a result of treatment. As a rule, wrinkling of the posterior surface is not seen at the time the IOP is high.

Gonioscopy

If the cornea is sufficiently clear to permit examination of the angle, then extensive closure will be found during an attack. If the cornea is too cloudy to permit accurate gonioscopy in the affected eye, then gonioscopy of the fellow eye will usually reveal a convex iris and a very narrow angle. This finding in the contralateral eye is often very helpful in adding presumptive evidence for the diagnosis.

If the fellow eye is found to have an anterior chamber that is distinctly less shallow and an iris that is less convex than the glaucomatous eye, then one should look at the patient's glasses or refraction record to see if the fellow eye is less hyperopic than the glaucomatous eye. If not, then one should suspect a secondary form of angle-closure glaucoma that can be more often unilateral (see Chapter 40).

If the patient has been treated for acute elevation of pressure with systemic aqueous suppressants and/or osmotics, then this may potentially contribute to opening the angle of the fellow eye and make the findings in this eye equivocal. This medication effect should be taken into account when using the findings in the fellow eye to help establish the diagnosis (see Chapter 22).

Intraocular Pressure

In the midst of an attack of acute angle closure, one may find an IOP of 40 to 100 mm Hg. However, shortly after spontaneous recovery from an attack, IOP may temporarily become subnormal or lower than the fellow eye because of temporary dysfunction of the ciliary body and reduced aqueous.

SPONTANEOUS RECOVERY AND MISDIAGNOSIS

The following are 2 circumstances in which the findings after spontaneous recovery from an acute angle-closure attack might lead to the wrong diagnosis:

referring ophthalmologist had never found an elevated IOP in the opposite eye. Corrected vision was 6/6 OD and 6/6 OS. The IOP was 17 OD and 32 OS. There was atrophy of the stroma of the iris in both eyes and glaukomflecken in both eyes. In the right eye, most of the angle appeared to be open though excessively narrow.

Although the patient had presented with left eye complaints, the appearance of iris stromal atrophy and glaukomflecken were considered evidence that the patient had experienced an attack of acute angle closure in the right eye at some point in the past. The patient at first denied any trouble with the right eye. However, on close questioning, she admitted that for the whole day after the iridectomy operation on the left eye, she had had severe pain in the right eye. It was concluded that she had experienced an attack of acute angle-closure glaucoma in the right eye that subsided spontaneously, leaving the tell-tale residue of atrophy of the iris stroma and glaukomflecken.

A peripheral iridectomy was advised for this eye. This was subsequently accomplished by her ophthalmologist with the result that IOP remained normal without further treatment.

Cells in the Aqueous

In acute angle-closure glaucoma, cells in the aqueous are common. This may sometimes be confused with anterior uveitis. If the patient is seen early in the course of an attack of angle closure, one may see only a few cells or none at all. However, if the attack has been going on for hours or days, and especially if the eye shows considerable redness from vasodilation, the aqueous may contain many cells, as well as fibrin. In neglected cases, the formation of one or more posterior synechiae is not uncommon.

Considerable cellular debris may be seen on the back surface of the cornea, but typically, one does not see true keratic precipitates (KPs). The presence of typical mutton-fat KP is

1. A patient presents a day or 2 after the onset of symptoms in one eye. The history reveals having experienced an acute onset of pain and blurred vision. Within an hour after the onset of symptoms, the patient developed severe pain and blurring of vision. He took some aspirin and went to bed. Overnight, the symptoms became less severe. The vision was much improved though still a little blurred, and there was no longer any discomfort.

   Examination reveals a slightly congested eye, or an eye that may be white and quiet. The pupil is somewhat dilated and reacts sluggishly. There are folds in the posterior surface of the cornea and cells in the aqueous. There may be one or more posterior synechiae. Glaukomflecken may or may not be present. IOP is lower than in the fellow eye. If the cornea is clear enough, on gonioscopy, the angle can be seen to be extremely narrow or closed. The angle in the fellow eye is also found to be extremely narrow.

   The finding of folds in the cornea and of cells in the aqueous along with posterior synechiae in conjunction with a normal or subnormal IOP may point the clinician toward a diagnosis of iritis. However, the history of a typically monocular disorder with acute onset, the dilation of the pupil, and the gonioscopic examination of the angle of the affected eye and of the fellow eye should lead to the correct diagnosis of spontaneous recovery from an attack of acute angle-closure glaucoma.

   It is not at all uncommon in this type of case for a misdiagnosis of iritis to be made and for topical steroids and cycloplegics to be prescribed. In response, the IOP may remain normal, and the eye may promptly resolve its inflammatory appearance. Anterior chamber cells may disappear. Nevertheless, the patient may show up the next week or sometime thereafter with recurrence of an attack of typical acute angle-closure glaucoma.

2. A patient presents with a history of acute onset of pain and blurred vision 1 or more days previously, with partial recovery of vision and disappearance of pain. Examination reveals little or no congestion of the eye. There may be cells in the aqueous or folds in the cornea. IOP is normal or subnormal. Examination of the fundus reveals disc swelling and many retinal hemorrhages throughout the posterior pole. Vision is fairly good.

   At first glance, one might consider a diagnosis of optic neuritis or venous occlusion, but the history of a very acute onset of symptoms, with pain and blurred vision, would be inconsistent with such a diagnosis. Also, the subsequent rapid visual recovery to near normal would not be consistent with occlusion of the central retinal vein or with optic neuritis. Gonioscopic examination reveals the most important clue—an extremely narrow angle that may or may not show areas of closure. The angle in the fellow eye is also found to be extremely narrow.

   Now the correct diagnosis is made. The patient has had spontaneous recovery from an attack of acute angle closure, resulting in temporary hypotony, swelling of the disc, and hemorrhages in the fundus. If the diagnosis was missed, one could expect a recurrence of acute angle closure a few weeks later with a very high IOP and all the characteristic findings.

   The following case represents an instance in which the diagnosis of acute angle-closure glaucoma was not made in the beginning. Dr. Chandler wrote, "This case illustrates the fact that 40 years ago Dr. Chandler still had a lot to learn about glaucoma."

Case 23-2

A 46-year-old woman, seen 40 years previously, gave a history of having developed iritis in the right eye while on a cruise and having been given atropine ointment. When she returned home, her local ophthalmologist continued this treatment. Finally, the eye became completely quiet and she was referred for consultation. Corrected vision was 6/5 in each eye. The media were clear. Discs were normal. Visual fields were full. The anterior chambers were shallow. The right pupil was 4 by 5 mm and displaced slightly temporally, and the left pupil was 3 mm, round, and central. Atrophy of the iris was noted temporally in the right eye. On slit-lamp examination, there were some whitish flecks that seemed to be just beneath the anterior lens capsule. IOP was not measured. Gonioscopy was not done in those days.

There was no further trouble until 8 years later, when she developed acute glaucoma in the same eye. After miotic treatment, an iridectomy was performed. Later, prophylactic iridectomy was performed on the opposite eye at the patient's request. IOP remained normal thereafter in both eyes.

Here is a classic picture of an eye that had acute angle-closure glaucoma. The iritis was undoubtedly sequelae from acute angle-closure glaucoma, and the initial treatment by mydriasis, as sometimes occurs, broke the first attack.

DIFFERENTIAL DIAGNOSES

A number of disorders can produce symptoms and signs of acute angle-closure glaucoma (Table 23-1). Glaucomatocyclitic crisis, neovascular glaucoma, and glaucoma secondary to anterior uveitis must all be considered in the differential diagnosis.

In glaucomatocyclitic crisis, there may be an acute onset of blurring and haloes and often some pain, but the angle is always open during an attack. Usually, one or several KPs are seen.

TABLE 23-1. DIFFERENTIAL DIAGNOSIS OF ACUTE ANGLE-CLOSURE GLAUCOMA	
Disorder	**Comment**
Primary open-angle glaucoma with narrow angle on gonioscopy	Regardless of how narrow the angle, if posterior trabecular meshwork is visible for 360 using Goldmann or Koeppe gonioscopy in a patient with high IOP, diagnosis is usually open-angle glaucoma; however, laser iridotomy may still be required in either case in order to prevent future angle closure.
Neovascular glaucoma	Iris and angle neovascularization may not be apparent with high IOP or corneal edema, requiring re-examination after IOP has been reduced; topical glycerin useful; angle of fellow eye usually open.
Uveitis	Anterior chamber inflammation may be present in both disorders with or without elevated IOP, but true KPs are not seen in angle closure; angle of affected and fellow eye are usually open by gonioscopy in uveitis, though focal PAS may be present; glaucomatocyclitic crisis most likely to confuse clinician.
Nanophthalmos	Patients with nanophthalmos have high hyperopia and short axial length (≤ 20 mm) bilaterally.
Secondary angle-closure glaucoma caused by PRP (acute uveal effusion) Central retinal vein occlusion (acute uveal effusion) Medication induced (eg, sulfonamide allergy) Malignant glaucoma Postvitreoretinal surgery Posterior segment tumors	Complete ocular history and examination will often help identify patients with secondary angle closure; fellow eye may also be narrow in patients with malignant glaucoma and those status postvitreoretinal buckling surgery; B-scan to rule out posterior segment pathology is indicated in all cases where there is a poor view of the fundus and incisional surgery is being contemplated.
IOP: intraocular pressure; KPs: keratic precipitates; PAS: peripheral anterior synechaie; PRP: panretinal photocoagulation.	

In neovascular glaucoma associated with prior occlusion of the central retinal vein, or diabetic retinopathy, and various other ischemic conditions that lead to anterior segment neovascularization, pain may develop acutely with corneal edema.

At first glance, this might be mistaken for angle-closure glaucoma. However, there is no great difficulty in differential diagnosis. If the slit lamp does not reveal rubeosis of the iris (Figure 23-4), gonioscopy may show characteristic neovascularization in the angle (Figure 23-5).

Secondary glaucoma due to iritis or uveitis should likewise present no great difficulty in differential diagnosis. For one thing, the pupil is never dilated. Generally, it is constricted or irregularly shaped from posterior synechiae. Examination of the angle sheds further light on the situation. In primary angle-closure glaucoma, the angle is closed either by apposition or by synechiae. In anterior uveitis, the angle is typically open. Nevertheless, prolonged anterior uveitis may be accompanied by eventual peripheral anterior synechiae formation.

TREATMENT

Medical therapy is usually applied prior to laser iridotomy. This is to decrease IOP and improve the clarity of the media for the laser procedure (Table 23-2). Sometimes, pupillary block can be broken mechanically by vigorous indentation gonioscopy and opening a segment of the angle. Similar indentation may be accomplished by applying pressure against the cornea with the blunt side of a muscle hook.[1] In any case, laser iridotomy with or without laser gonioplasty should be performed promptly.

Medical Treatment

It is recognized that, in the present era of ophthalmology, yttrium-aluminum-garnet (YAG), argon, or diode lasers are usually readily available. If the media is clear, then one should proceed with the laser iridotomy to break the attack.

In the absence of immediate access to an appropriate laser, the following sequence of medical therapy can be used to try to break an attack of acute angle-closure glaucoma.

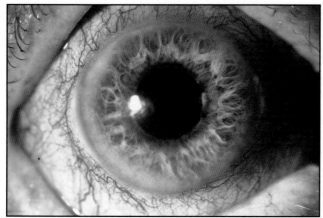

Figure 23-4. Neovascularization of the iris. Note the fine lacy vessels present at the pupillary margin.

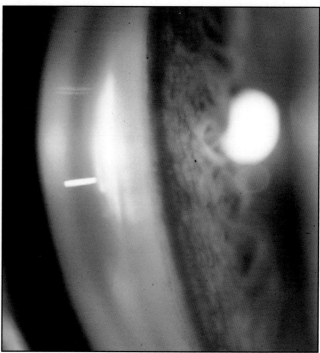

Figure 23-5. Neovascularization of the angle. Note arborization of vessels. Glaucoma can be present with the angle still open at this stage before synechial formation occurs.

However, all efforts should be made to obtain access to a laser for definitive treatment, even as medical treatment is initiated.

No matter how obviously firm the eye is to palpation, IOP should be accurately measured with a tonometer in order to provide an objective point of reference. In this way, IOP can later be used in the course of treatment to determine whether the condition has changed either for the better or for the worse.

Initial medical therapy consists of aqueous suppressants and sometimes weak miotics (Table 23-3). If miotics are elected, then lower concentrations (eg, 1% to 2% pilocarpine) are preferred. Higher concentrations can occasionally worsen pupillary block (see Chapter 22), by allowing greater forward lens movement. Higher concentrations can also cause more pain and discomfort.

Topical beta-blocking agents, alpha-2 agonists, and topical carbonic anhydrase inhibitors (CAIs) decrease aqueous humor production and thereby decrease IOP and hydrostatic pressure against the posterior side of the iris. This may lessen the tendency for the iris to bow forward and occlude the trabecular meshwork (TM). Unless there are contraindications, systemic CAIs and osmotics may also be given. If the patient is not nauseated, 500 mg of acetazolamide (Diamox) in the nonsustained release form and glycerin 1.5 g/kg, mixed with an equal volume of cold water or fruit juice (over ice), may be given by mouth. Acetazolamide is contraindicated if the patient is allergic to sulfa compounds.

If the patient is nauseated and not able to ingest or retain acetazolamide and glycerin, acetazolamide can be administered intravenously. At the same time, mannitol 1 g/kg can also be administered intravenously. Intravenous osmotics should not be applied if the patient has a history of congestive heart failure, as osmotic agents can displace a significant volume of third space fluid into the intravascular space and place additional stress on the heart. Intravenous administration should be administered with

monitoring and under appropriate medical supervision (ie, in the emergency department, typically not in the eye clinic).

Because of the potential for increased inflammation, prostaglandin analogs are not indicated for the initial medical treatment of acute angle-closure glaucoma.

In most patients treated this way, there is a decrease in IOP within 2 hours. The miotic may be continued every 4 hours after the first two doses. IOP may gradually decrease over the next several hours to normal or even subnormal levels as the angle closure resolves.

On the other hand, even with intensive medical treatment, IOP may not only fail to become lower, but may actually become higher. In this situation, access to a laser in order to perform iridotomy becomes paramount. If iridotomy cannot be performed because of a cloudy cornea, then one may still be able to perform gonioplasty[2-4] with the argon laser. Laser energy applied in this way to the peripheral iris may open a segment of the angle and break the attack.

The urgency of early laser intervention in cases in which the IOP is not responding to intensive medical treatment is influenced to a considerable extent by the visual acuity. Some patients at the height of an attack will still have vision as good as 20/40. Other patients may have vision reduced to hand motion or counting fingers at a few feet. The fact that vision is very low is indicative of a very vulnerable eye. In such a case, it is imperative that IOP be lowered as quickly as possible. If IOP in such an eye is allowed to remain very high for an additional 6 hours, then there may be irreparable

TABLE 23-2. OVERALL TREATMENT STRATEGY FOR ACUTE ANGLE-CLOSURE GLAUCOMA	
Treatment	**Comment**
Examination of both eyes (including gonioscopy of fellow eye) prior to treatment	Aqueous suppressants and osmotics alone can dramatically deepen the anterior chamber and widen the angle of both eyes, potentially confounding and delaying definitive treatment of the occludable fellow eye.
Indentation gonioscopy with a small-diameter goniolens or by central corneal indentation with a cotton swab or muscle hook	Sometimes, an attack of acute angle closure can be broken by central corneal compression, which deepens the angle and can break pupillary block.
Medical treatment (see Table 23-3)	Usually, it is best to reduce IOP prior to laser iridotomy; this allows corneal clearing, reduces patient discomfort, and gives time for the pupil to decrease in size, making laser treatment technically easier.
Laser iridotomy	Neodymium:yttrium-aluminum-garnet (Nd:YAG) is preferred for light-colored irides (5 to 7 mJ, 1 to 2 bursts per pulse); for dark brown irides, a chipping technique with short pulse argon laser treatment followed by Nd:YAG is recommended (see Chapter 54).
Peripheral laser gonioplasty	To open synechially closed angle remaining after laser iridotomy or in some cases to break an attack of angle closure (see Chapter 56).
Surgical iridectomy Anterior chamber deepening Trabeculectomy	In some cases, glaucoma is not controlled after laser iridotomy, or it is not possible to perform laser iridotomy; in these instances, multiple surgical options may be considered (see text).

TABLE 23-3. MEDICAL TREATMENT OPTIONS FOR ACUTE ANGLE-CLOSURE GLAUCOMA	
Treatment	**Comment**
Miotics: pilocarpine 1% to 2% q 15 minutes × 2, then q4h	Delayed miotic treatment for 2 to 3 hours (until after IOP has been reduced by aqueous suppressants and osmotics) is as effective as immediate treatment. One percent to 2% pilocarpine is as effective as higher doses and is less likely to cause additional pain and possible forward movement of the crystalline lens.
Topical aqueous suppressants: Beta-blockers q12h Brimonidine q8h Dorzolamide/brinzolamide q8h	Prior to treatment, check medical history for asthma, pulmonary disease, history of heart failure, or bradycardia; if present, do not use beta-blockers.
Systemic carbonic anhydrase inhibitors: Acetazolamide 250 mg PO q6h Methazolamide 50 to 100 mg PO q8h	Check for sulfa allergy (also for dorzolamide above). In nauseated patient, one can use acetazolamide 500 mg intravenously initially.
Osmotics: Glycerin solution (1 to 1.5 g/kg PO) Isosorbide solution (1.5 g/kg PO) Mannitol solution (1 to 2 g/kg IV) (note: dosage calculated for lean body weight)	Patients with severe heart or lung disease should have medical consult prior to using osmotics. Glycerin should not be used in diabetic patients. Glycerin and isosorbide are unpalatable. In the nauseated patient, intravenous mannitol should be considered.

damage to the optic nerve. Therefore, if there is little or no drop in IOP within 3 hours after initiating medical treatment, plans should be made for intervention without further delay. If a laser is not available, prompt surgical iridectomy is indicated.

There are some historical but insightful comments to be considered. In the days before the availability of laser iridotomy, in discussing intensive medical therapy for acute angle-closure glaucoma, Chandler and Grant wrote:

> Since there are occasional cases that do not respond to the customary intensive treatment, some rethinking and re-evaluation of this treatment may be in order. The intensive use of miotics has been carried over, almost by habit, from times before the advent of aqueous suppressants and hypertonic osmotic agents. Yet it is known that in some eyes the application of strong miotics can shallow the anterior chamber and precipitate or aggravate angle-closure glaucoma. There is a conceptual case and some supporting evidence for starting out with less intensive miotic treatment, depending on aqueous suppressants and possibly osmotic agents to reduce the IOP sufficiently for the pupil to respond, aiming in this way to minimize contraction of the ciliary muscle that may favor unwanted forward movement of the lens. It seems to us that this less habitual but more reasoned approach to treatment of acute angle-closure glaucoma merits even more extensive clinical evaluation.

Surgical (Laser) Versus Medical Management

Two decades ago, there was considerable debate about whether patients after resolution of an event of acute angle-closure glaucoma in response to medical therapy could be managed with chronic miotics rather than surgical peripheral iridectomy. The advent of laser iridotomy (see Chapter 55) has made this a moot point. The ability to cure angle-closure glaucoma by a closed-eye outpatient procedure truly represents a major advance in treatment of acute angle-closure glaucoma.

To be clear, laser iridotomy should always be performed in cases of angle-closure glaucoma. However, there are rare cases in which laser treatment, whether argon or YAG, is not successful, and surgical iridectomy is required. Before the development of laser techniques, one would have performed a surgical peripheral iridectomy in the aftermath of angle-closure glaucoma instead of prescribing chronic medical therapy. The reader should understand the reasoning for this because it remains relevant today. Chandler wrote:

> In our hypothetical case in which the angle is still extremely narrow and capable of closing, one cannot predict what the subsequent course will be under miotic treatment. Since the success rate of a surgical peripheral iridectomy is very high after an attack of acute angle-closure glaucoma has been brought under control with medical treatment, as in this case, we believe it is best to operate on nearly all such

patients. Otherwise, without operation, the patient may suffer the second attack during a severe general illness or after injury, and then the condition may not be correctly diagnosed and treated until irreparable damage has been done. If the patient should happen to have general surgery somewhere else and be given atropine or scopolamine without appreciation of the danger, this may precipitate acute angle closure, and, in the presence of other postoperative pain and distress, the acute glaucoma may go unrecognized, even for several days. It appears that the risk of surgical peripheral iridectomy is less than the risk involved in going without operation. Far more eyes have been lost from a second or third attack of acute angle-closure glaucoma than from prompt operation after medical control of the initial attack. There may, of course, be general medical contraindication to operation, such as great age or serious illness, but this is unusual.

The same reasoning would thus apply to intervention by laser iridotomy. However, the risk of laser intervention is significantly lower than the risk of surgical iridectomy, so the point illustrated above holds even truer. The standard of care dictates that all cases of angle-closure glaucoma should now be treated by iridotomy.

Effect of Iris Atrophy

There is one rare circumstance in which iridotomy may be unnecessary after a violent attack of acute glaucoma. Commonly, the pupil remains somewhat dilated and fixed, or dilated in one meridian after an acute attack. This does not ordinarily prevent further attacks. However, if the dilation is sufficiently wide overall, or wide in one meridian to provide an easy communication from posterior to anterior chamber and thereby prevent relative pupillary block, then this can occasionally permit the angle to widen to the extent it would have in response to iridotomy.

Whether dilation of the pupil has been sufficient to widen the angle to a point where aqueous flows around the lens equator freely and the angle remains open can only be determined by gonioscopy. If there are permanent peripheral anterior synechiae in part of the circumference but the rest of the angle has widened, then there may be residual glaucoma due to the synechiae, but because of the large or displaced diameter of the pupil, this patient may never again have an acute attack.

In one definitive case of spontaneous cure of angle-closure glaucoma from atrophy of the iris and dilation of the pupil, the pupillary border was seen to have become retracted so far peripherally that it was actually lifted free of the lens in one quadrant, and there was a space sufficient for a view of ciliary processes. This case is the exception. As a rule, the definitive treatment for angle-closure glaucoma, in order to prevent a subsequent recurrent attack, is iridotomy.

EFFECTS OF MYDRIASIS

Inclusion of weak miotic therapy has become standard in medical treatment of acute angle-closure glaucoma, not only because of its potential "vector" efficacy (see Chapter 22), but because it makes laser iridotomy technically easier by thinning and stretching the iris and exposing the far peripheral iris tissue.

Several decades ago, there was interest in using mydriatic rather than miotic therapy to treat acute angle closure. At the time, there were not uncommon miotic therapy failures. These would sometimes respond to the opposite approach—mydriatic therapy. This approach is effective if the pupil dilates large enough to clear the equator of the lens.

The advent of potent topical aqueous suppressant therapy (combined with weak miotic therapy) has made such cases rare, but the reader should still keep in mind the potential efficacy of mydriatic therapy in unusual refractory cases of acute angle closure. Chandler and Grant have written on this subject extensively:

> Having considered spontaneous mydriasis as a possible mechanism by which angle closure may become relieved, let us consider the possibilities of mydriasis as a treatment for acute angle-closure glaucoma. We have accumulated several cases in which, instead of a miotic, mydriatic treatment was used investigationally, with a prompt fall in IOP in most cases. For a case of recent onset it might be that mydriasis would be better treatment than miotic treatment. If the pupil dilates quickly and fully, this completely relieves pupillary block and the angle opens as much as it does after iridectomy. Furthermore, there may be some effect similar to that obtained in the mydriatic-cycloplegic treatment of malignant glaucoma. When mydriatic-cycloplegic treatment is used to relieve pupillary block and acute angle-closure glaucoma, we are not certain how much benefit to attribute to dilation of the pupil and how much to the pulling back of the lens by tightening of the zonules. In certain instances, angle closure has been relieved by a cycloplegic, such as atropine, and in other instances by phenylephrine, which primarily affects the pupil and not the ciliary body and zonule tension. In some cases better results have been obtained when both were applied.
>
> Mydriasis as a treatment for acute angle-closure glaucoma is the exact opposite of the conventional treatment for this disorder, and we cannot advocate it as a routine treatment. For the present it would be best to confine mydriatic treatment, if used at all, to cases known to be recent in onset. For instance, in a case of acute angle-closure glaucoma in one eye, if prophylactic miotic treatment is given to the fellow eye, and this paradoxically sends the eye into an acute attack of angle-closure glaucoma, then counter treatment by mydriasis may be effective and may reduce the IOP rapidly. Mydriatic might also be justified in the treatment of acute angle-closure glaucoma in the first eye, if it is known definitely that the attack is of recent origin, ie, a matter of hours; however, in attacks of longer duration, such as several hours or a day or more, for the present it is better to employ miotic treatment.
>
> Mydriatic treatment may have a special place in angle-closure glaucoma that has been provoked by miotic treatment. For instance, if in an eye with open-angle glaucoma but a very narrow angle the use of strong miotics has provoked acute angle-closure glaucoma superimposed on the open-angle glaucoma, the treatment would be to use mydriatics, tropicamide or cyclopentolate, along with aqueous humor suppressants to relieve the attack in preparation for iridectomy.
>
> A paradoxical and potentially hazardous aspect of mydriatic administration is that sometimes the mydriatic will precipitate an attack of angle-closure in a predisposed eye. It is likely to do this when mydriasis is incomplete. If, for instance, the pupil is semidilated, this may only slightly reduce the resistance to flow through the pupil and may relax the iris sufficiently to let the pressure in the posterior chamber push the iris forward and close the angle. The hazardous state of mydriasis probably varies with different eyes, but in general is about 4 to 7 mm. This is exemplified by the mydriatic provocative test for acute angle-closure glaucoma. If the pupil dilates widely and fully the mydriasis test is usually negative, but later when the pupil is slowly becoming smaller, the patient may have acute closure.
>
> In general, older people do not get as wide of dilation with mydriatics as younger people, so mydriatic treatment in acute angle-closure glaucoma would not be advisable for a patient aged 70 or 80. Also, heavily pigmented dark-brown eyes do not dilate as rapidly and fully as blue eyes. Such patients would be expected to respond poorly to mydriatic treatment.
>
> A possible rationale to miotic treatment is that if good miosis is achieved, there is some reason to think that this may break peripheral anterior synechiae that have recently formed, whereas mydriasis would have no such effect. Mydriasis would just allow the iris to drop back if it were not already adherent to the angle wall.
>
> Another rationale for miotic therapy is that this prepares the eye for laser iridotomy by stretching and thinning the iris. Also, for the rarely performed surgical iridectomies, preoperative miotics allow easier repositing of the iris.

TIMING OF IRIDOTOMY

When should laser iridotomy be done? If the angle has opened completely under medical treatment, there is nothing to be lost by waiting, save the risk of another attack. Often, however, it is impossible to tell by gonioscopy immediately after the attack whether or not the angle is open completely, or nearly so. In any case, it is best to proceed at once with laser iridotomy.

If some degree of closure is still present after the IOP has been brought to normal, as occurs in many cases, this may be due to adhesions that are newly formed, weak, and easily separable. These new synechiae may quickly lead to permanent synechial closure. Iridotomy opens all portions of the angle capable of opening and may actually release recently formed peripheral anterior synechiae.

Hence, prompt laser iridotomy is indicated after the IOP has been brought to normal. In addition to bypassing pupillary block, iridotomy may serve to break new posterior synechiae, as brisk aqueous flow is restored to the anterior chamber and the anterior chamber deepens.

A delay in intervention "until the eye quiets down completely" or until recovery of vision can be evaluated may allow synechial closure to become firmly established. Even when one suspects that the entire angle may be closed by synechiae, laser iridotomy should be performed.

Following iridotomy, gonioscopy should be repeated to determine the extent of synechiae formation. Pigment and other debris may be liberated as a result of the iridotomy procedure. Thus, there may be a temporary elevation of IOP from an open-angle mechanism. If the IOP is at an elevated but acceptable level following laser, it is advisable to temporize for several weeks before deciding on the need for fistulizing surgery. In addition, the chances of success with a fistulizing operation are greater if the surgery is performed when the eye is quiet.

METHOD OF LASER IRIDOTOMY

Various lasers or combinations of lasers can be used to create the iridotomy. An Abraham contact lens is used to focus the energy into the desired area, usually into an iris crypt. There is some opinion that the iridotomy is best placed superiorly under the lid. Many clinicians[5] have reported problems with monocular diplopia or ghost images using this placement. They point out that the tear meniscus along the border of the superior lid may have a prismatic effect of introducing light through the superior opening. Thus, many advocate temporal placement of the iridotomy.

A yttrium-aluminum-garnet (YAG) laser works by photodisruption. In photo-disruption, no thermal energy is released. Rather, the energy is packaged in the form of intense light. As a benefit, YAG laser does not require a pigmented iris for absorption and effect. On the other hand, because there is no thermal component to the energy released by YAG, there is no corresponding coagulation of treated tissue. Specifically, irides treated by YAG may bleed at the site of application. This can occasionally create hyphema and reduced vision while the hyphema resolves, and may possibly induce IOP elevation. In addition, blood may obscure the area where the iridotomy is being created, inhibiting completion of the procedure.

When the iris bleeds, pressure against the eye for a few minutes with the focusing contact lens will usually stem the bleeding. Because of the presence of blood at the initial site, attempts at continuing YAG laser iridotomy at this site will sometimes need to be abandoned. The initial opening may not yet be full thickness and thus may not be effective at relieving angle closure. Treatment may be resumed after blood trickles away from the site or after a small clot over the site retracts, leaving the area visible again for continued treatment. One may also simply move to a different site for treatment.

An argon or diode laser, on the other hand, works by a thermal effect on the iris. Tissue is obliterated by heat in creating an opening. At the same time, coagulation takes place, and there is typically little or no bleeding from the site. However, a pigmented iris is required for absorption of energy. The challenge with argon or diode is that it does not work well in lightly colored irides. Such lightly pigmented eyes should instead be approached with YAG laser to achieve an iridotomy opening.

Eyes with pigmented and thick irides may be approached with both lasers sequentially. The iridotomy site is first treated with argon or diode. One sees thinning in the treated area and coagulation, but the deeper layers of the iris stroma, which are less pigmented, may not perforate. In that case, the patient may be moved to the YAG laser, and the deeper layer of iris can be easily perforated, resulting in a patent iridotomy. Some models of slit-lamp laser now available combine both thermal and YAG functionality into one unit, permitting easy switching between operational modes.

CHAMBER DEEPENING

Surgical anterior chamber deepening was a technique developed to ascertain the amount of peripheral anterior synechiae present following surgical peripheral iridectomy. This was developed before the use of indentation gonioscopy[6] and before laser iridotomy. The technique is presented here in part for historical perspective. It is also useful information because there may be exceptional situations in which argon laser gonioplasty either cannot technically be performed (shallow anterior chamber with high peripheral anterior synechiae) or laser iridotomy may not be effective because of a poor view. In addition, there may be rare occasions when a YAG laser or an argon laser is not available. Chamber deepening is then an alternate approach for dealing with a closed angle.

Older descriptions of chamber-deepening techniques refer to using sterile aqueous solutions through a paracentesis to create space in the anterior chamber. Currently, it is more advantageous to use dense surgical ophthalmic viscoelastic. Chamber deepening can also be combined with synechialysis—mechanical peripheral iris manipulation using an iris spatula through the paracentesis tract. The purpose is to break down synechiae and mechanically open the angle. This is usually accomplished in the operating room with gonioscopic visualization of the chamber angle during the procedure.[7-9]

Historical Perspective: Surgical Iridectomy or Filtering Procedure— Basis for Choice of Operation

Before the advent of laser iridotomy, in cases of angle closure, the surgeon would have to choose between surgical peripheral iridectomy and a filtration procedure. At the present time, there may be occasions where there is corneal clouding or a very thick inflamed iris, precluding successful iridotomy with either the argon or YAG laser. It may also be that there is no laser available. The surgeon may then be faced with deciding between these 2 surgical options. What are the factors to be considered? Chandler and Grant have written:

> Since its introduction by von Graefe, peripheral iridectomy has been the most widely used operation for acute angle-closure glaucoma. It is still the best operation in most cases. The principal alternative is a filtration operation. One must choose between them according to the condition of the angle. In eyes that have extensive closure after one or more acute attacks, there is no doubt that a filtration operation is necessary, but in the majority of cases, after IOP has been controlled medically and if there is no extensive synechial closure, iridectomy should be chosen.

How can one determine in an individual case whether to choose surgical iridectomy or a filtering operation? If it is a first attack and has a known duration of 36 hours or less, and failing laser iridotomy, surgical iridectomy is the operation of choice. An osmotic agent such as oral glycerol, IV mannitol, or urea may be required to bring the IOP under control. Experience has shown, in a case of such short duration, enough of the angle opens so that iridectomy will be sufficient. However, if the attack has been longer than 36 hours, even as long as several days, one should not automatically decide on a filtration operation. In certain eyes, the angle may still be capable of opening sufficiently, and a surgical iridectomy will suffice.

The level of IOP obtained with medical treatment is a poor guide and cannot be relied upon. Even if medical measures bring the IOP to subnormal levels, this does not automatically ensure that the angle has opened. The combined effect of CAIs, timolol, and hypertonic agents can present a misleading impression. They may lower IOP despite persistent synechiae.

The choice of whether iridectomy or a filtering operation should be performed is decided principally on the basis of gonioscopic findings, aided in some cases by gonioscopy during surgery.

If the cornea is sufficiently clear, it is usually possible to make a decision by preoperative gonioscopy. If most of the angle has opened in response to medical maneuvers, iridectomy is the appropriate choice. However, in some eyes, it is difficult to see definitely whether the angle has remained closed or almost closed. It is often impossible to determine by ordinary gonioscopy whether it is simple appositional contact or synechial closure. The situation may become more evident by repeating gonioscopy after deepening the anterior chamber with viscoelastic.

Forbes et al[6] have reported that using a Zeiss 4-mirror gonioscopy lens (Carl Zeiss Meditec AG, Berlin, Germany) at the slit-lamp microscope and purposely indenting the cornea helps in demonstrating whether synechiae are present.[6] This technique is known as *indentation gonioscopy*. It should always be attempted preoperatively, although corneal edema often limits visualization. With indentation, areas that are not involved by synechiae can be well-demonstrated. However, areas that are seen as still being closed can represent either true synechiae or areas of insufficient indentation. While the indented configuration of the iris in the suspected area can often help in understanding the anatomic situation, it must be remembered that, especially when performed at a time when the IOP is elevated, insufficient distortion may be generated by this technique to overcome appositional closure and allow a view of the angle.

Definitive results can be obtained by Koeppe gonioscopy after the anterior chamber is deepened with viscoelastic. One such use of gonioscopy during surgery was described by Shaffer in 1957.[10] Shaffer's technique consisted of performing a peripheral iridectomy, refilling the anterior chamber with saline solution, pulling up the suture, and tying one knot. He then placed a sterile Koeppe lens on the eye and examined the angle to see how much closure remained in order to decide whether to convert the iridectomy to a filtration procedure.

The choice between simple surgical iridectomy or a filtering procedure is made according to the extent of synechial closure that is found. If the angle is closed in one-quarter or less of the circumference, then a simple iridectomy is the appropriate choice. If the synechial closure involves one-third to one-half of the circumference of the angle, then information from previous tonography, if it has been conducted, may help with the decision. Poor facility of outflow would indicate a need for a filtering procedure. In borderline cases or when in doubt, it is generally advisable to first try iridectomy. This should not be performed at the 12 o'clock position, but at the half past 10 o'clock or half past 1 o'clock position. Subsequently, if the residual glaucoma cannot be controlled, an adequate untouched portion of the superior limbus is left available to provide a location where a filtering operation can be performed.

As the basis for deciding on a choice of operation, gonioscopy after surgical deepening of the anterior chamber with viscoelastic is a simple, safe procedure. Its practical value cannot be overemphasized. Deepening the anterior chamber in this way may actually separate recently formed, weak adhesions of iris to TM. After deepening the chamber with viscoelastic and re-applying gonioscopy, one sometimes sees little tabs of tissue on the TM that represent broken synechiae.

The following case, presented in part for historical interest, and in part for the circumstance where a laser is not available or may not be successful, illustrates the potential therapeutic benefit of chamber deepening. In this case, preoperative gonioscopy showed exactly the upper half of the angle closed, but after chamber deepening, almost the entire angle was found to be open, suggesting that the procedure of chamber deepening had broken the weak peripheral anterior synechiae.

Case 23-3

A 76-year-old woman had trace nuclear sclerosis in both eyes, more in the left. Corrected vision in the right eye was 6/6. Corrected vision in the left eye was 6/12. One month previously, she had experienced an attack of pain and blurred vision in the left eye with nausea and vomiting. The symptoms subsided. Eighteen hours prior to her presentation, the symptoms recurred, including pain, nausea, vomiting, and blurring of vision. These symptoms persisted. Vision in the left eye was counting fingers at 6 feet; the cornea was edematous. The pupil was in mid-dilation. The fundus could not be seen. IOP was 76. The angle appeared to be entirely closed. Six hours after the start of intensive treatment with 4% pilocarpine, acetazolamide, and glycerin, the IOP decreased to 17. Gonioscopy revealed that exactly the lower half of the angle appeared open. Peripheral iridectomy would be the operation of choice with half the angle open. Nevertheless, a chamber-deepening procedure was carried out to see if some recently formed peripheral anterior synechiae could be torn off. When that was accomplished, it was found that only about one clock-hour of the angle remained closed. It appeared that the chamber-deepening procedure had in fact broken nearly all the peripheral synechiae in the upper half of the angle and, therefore, served as a therapeutic procedure. Peripheral iridectomy was performed, and 2 months later, IOP was 15 without treatment.

Older and stronger peripheral anterior synechiae are not affected by deepening the anterior chamber. This procedure, if performed early in the course, demonstrates how much of the angle can be made to open and how much of the angle can be expected to remain functional. Clinical and experimental findings indicate that angles opened by this gentle procedure can be expected to function well. In extreme instances, almost the entire angle may appear closed by ordinary gonioscopy, but re-examination after deepening the anterior chamber may establish that most or all of the angle is capable of opening.

The choice of operation, peripheral iridectomy or filtering surgery, is greatly aided and usually decided by definitive gonioscopy. Still, there are other factors to be weighed in making the decision. These factors include the facility of outflow, the condition of the optic disc and field, and the age of the patient.

Angle-closure glaucoma commonly affects one eye before the other. The condition of the fellow eye with its angle still open can provide a guide as to what to expect from synechial closure of half of the circumference. If the contralateral eye with its angle open and in an unmedicated state has a low IOP and good facility of outflow, one can expect that synechial closure of half the circumference in the involved eye will not raise the IOP excessively, and peripheral iridectomy should suffice. If, instead, the contralateral eye with its angle open has an IOP at the upper limit of normal, the treatment of the eye with the angle closed by synechiae half its

---

ANTERIOR CHAMBER DEEPENING WITH MECHANICAL BREAKING OF PERIPHERAL ANTERIOR SYNECHIAE WITH AN IRIS SPATULA (GONIOSYNECHIALYSIS)

David L. Epstein, MD, MMM

Sometimes, postsurgical peripheral anterior synechaie (PAS) associated with a flat anterior chamber may extend far forward anterior to Schwalbe's line and be quite firm and not amenable to argon laser gonioplasty. Failure of laser gonioplasty may be due to the continued shallowness of the anterior chamber or to other technical problems, such as a lack of good corneal clarity. This clinical situation is the one exception to the rule that if the PAS does not separate easily with the argon laser gonioplasty technique, further treatment of that particular PAS is not warranted. In these situations, some have reported good success with surgical deepening of the anterior chamber using a viscoelastic, which itself might help break the PAS. Additionally, one may introduce a fine iris spatula into the anterior chamber through a paracentesis tract to mechanically directly break the synechiae by a posterior ballottement motion on the peripheral iris.[1-3] Ideally, this should be accomplished under gonioscopic control. Some have described performing this procedure without gonioscopy, especially in pseudophakic or aphakic eyes. There would be some risk of possible crystalline lens injury if gonioscopic control is not used in the phakic patient.

Such a method deserves further evaluation, especially in cases in which it is not possible to perform argon laser gonioplasty. Unfortunately, in some reports, this technique was combined with other methods of pressure lowering including cyclodestruction. Thus, it is not certain whether the synechialysis or the adjunctive therapy was responsible for the beneficial effects that have been reported.

Also, many such anterior PAS may be bridging over the TM, which is therefore functionally still open but not visualized in the tunnel under the anteriorly located synechiae. Despite the improved angle appearance, the residual postoperative glaucoma in these complicated eyes might be attributable to acute open-angle mechanisms, such as retained viscoelastic, inflammation, or the use of topical steroids. If these open-angle mechanisms are involved and if the IOP is not too high, tincture of time and medical therapy might prove effective, and the glaucoma might resolve.

REFERENCES
1. Forbes M. Gonioscopy with corneal indentation. *Arch Ophthalmol.* 1966;76:488-492.
2. Shaffer RN. Operating room gonioscopy in angle-closure glaucoma surgery. *Trans Am Ophthalmol Soc.* 1957;55:59-66.
3. Chandler PA, Simmons RJ. Anterior chamber deepening for gonioscopy at time of surgery. *Arch Ophthalmol.* 1965;74:177-190.

---

circumference will not be sufficiently treated by iridectomy alone. Postoperatively, the additional use of antiglaucoma medications will probably be required, especially if there has been damage to the optic disc.

The more evidence of damage to the disc and field, the more one would favor a primary filtering operation. In such a case, lower IOP would be required postoperatively to prevent progression of nerve damage and field loss. In a borderline case, limited life expectancy from age or disease would favor simple iridectomy.

PROGNOSIS FOR RECOVERY OF VISION

In acute angle-closure glaucoma, the degree of recovery of vision after control of IOP varies considerably. It is, therefore, difficult to make an absolutely accurate prediction about recovery of vision in any individual case. In general, the better the visual acuity at the height of the attack, the better will be the vision ultimately obtained.

One must take into consideration the condition of the cornea in prognosticating. If the cornea is clear, yet vision is low, most of the visual loss is due to damage to the optic nerve. The prognosis for recovery of vision is more guarded. If the cornea is cloudy with stromal and epithelial edema, then the condition of the cornea itself may be sufficient to cause marked reduction of vision. There may be little damage to the optic nerve. In such cases, when the cornea eventually clears, there may be a remarkable recovery of vision. Many weeks must elapse after resolution of an acute attack before one can be sure that no further recovery of vision is likely.

MANAGEMENT OF THE FELLOW EYE

In cases of acute angle-closure glaucoma, the fellow eye almost always has a narrow angle capable of closure. In a previous era, some such fellow eyes have been observed for many years with or without prophylactic miotic treatment and have remained without significant sequelae. However, the incidence of involvement of the fellow eye with angle closure is extremely high. Sometimes, an acute attack develops in the fellow eye while the patient is being treated for angle closure in the first eye.

Because it is usually not possible to predict if and when the fellow eye may suffer an attack of angle closure, it is strongly recommended that a prophylactic laser iridotomy be performed. Even before the advent of the laser procedure, prophylactic surgical peripheral iridectomy was similarly recommended.

In unusual situations, such as high degrees of anisometropia, one would not proceed if the fellow eye is noted to have a wide open angle. The burden is on the ophthalmologist to be certain that the angle of the fellow eye is not occludable. The use of systemic aqueous humor suppressants affecting vectors in the fellow eye may falsely lead one to conclude that the angle is not closeable. (This has been discussed in Chapter 22.) In the interval before iridotomy on the fellow eye, this eye may be left without treatment. Nevertheless, iridotomy should be planned and performed.

Chandler and Grant have written:

> The risk of a properly performed surgical prophylactic peripheral iridectomy seems much less than the risk of future attacks without operation. Many instances have been observed in which prophylactic operation was not done, and

the patient later had an acute attack of angle-closure glaucoma, but diagnosis and treatment were delayed, or improper treatment was carried out, and the eye was eventually lost. Prophylactic peripheral iridectomy in the fellow eye has been an important measure for the prevention of blindness in patients having proved angle-closure glaucoma in one eye.

The following case illustrates the unpredictable length of time that can pass before an attack of angle closure occurs in the fellow eye when there has been no prophylactic iridotomy.

Case 23-4

A woman, age 67, gave a history of acute glaucoma in the left eye 4 or 5 years previously. An operation had been performed, but the eye became blind. She was under treatment with 2% pilocarpine for her unaffected right eye. Corrected vision of the right eye was 6/5. The field was full. There was a little saucerization of the disc, but no pathologic excavation. IOP was 15. On gonioscopy, the angle was excessively narrow especially above and below, but the impression was that it was probably open throughout.

In view of the history of acute angle-closure glaucoma in the left eye, and the excessively narrow angle in the right, peripheral iridectomy was advised for the right eye, but this was not accomplished. The patient was next seen 13 years later with an attack of acute angle-closure in the right eye. IOP was 88. She was admitted to the hospital and given intensive treatment with miotics, acetazolamide, and glycerin. IOP fell to 30. A peripheral iridectomy was performed. Since that time, IOP has ranged from 17 to 30, but has mostly been under 20 on medical treatment of 2% pilocarpine 4 times a day, epinephrine twice a day, and acetazolamide 125 mg twice a day.

If she had undergone prophylactic iridectomy at the time of her initial presentation, this patient would have been spared an attack of glaucoma in her right eye and presumably would have required no medical treatment thereafter.

With limited and special exceptions, we therefore favor routinely performing laser iridotomy on all fellow eyes in patients who have experienced acute angle-closure glaucoma in one eye.

The rare exceptions to this rule are as follows:

- In few patients, the fellow eye may have a wide open angle. In that case, prophylactic peripheral iridotomy may be deferred. However, one must be cautious about dismissing the angle as being safely open. There are cases where the angle in the fellow eye is described as being open, yet it did subsequently close. Angle width varies from time to time, and one should not conclude that the angle of a fellow eye is safely open on the basis of a single gonioscopy. In particular, one may get a false impression if the patient is taking a systemic CAI for treatment of the angle-closure eye. Profound suppression of aqueous production may cause the angle in the fellow eye to appear wider than it will become when off such treatment (see Chapter 22).

- The most reliable finding of a safe, wide angle in the fellow eye is made in those unusual patients who have one hyperopic eye with a narrow angle, subject to angle closure, and the other myopic eye with the typical wide angle associated with myopia. There are occasional patients in whom the glaucomatous eye has a significantly smaller cornea and shallower anterior chamber than the fellow eye. In this exceptional case, one may feel secure in judging the angle of the fellow eye to be normal and safe without prophylactic iridotomy.

- If there is little refractive error in either eye, and if the fellow eye definitely has an angle of average width, one should consider the possibility that the shallowing of the anterior chamber and the angle closure in the affected eye may have been caused by a partial subluxation or dislocation of the crystalline lens in that eye. If this is indeed proven, then the normal fellow eye does not require prophylactic iridotomy.

REFERENCES

1. Anderson DR. Corneal indentation to relieve acute angle-closure glaucoma. *Am J Ophthalmol.* 1979;88:1091-1093.
2. Ritch R. Argon laser treatment for medically unresponsive attacks of angle-closure glaucoma. *Am J Ophthalmol.* 1982;94:197-204.
3. Wand M. Argon laser gonioplasty for synechial angle closure. *Arch Ophthalmol.* 1992;110:363-367.
4. Weiss HS, Shingleton BJ, Goode SM, Bellows AR, Richter CU. Argon laser gonioplasty in the treatment of angle-closure glaucoma. *Am J Ophthalmol.* 1992;114:14-18.
5. Spaeth GL, Idowu O, Seligsohn A, et al. The effects of iridotomy size and position on symptoms following laser peripheral iridotomy. *J Glaucoma.* 2005;14:364-367.
6. Forbes M. Indentation gonioscopy and efficacy of iridectomy in angle-closure glaucoma. *Trans Am Ophthalmol Soc.* 1974;74:488-515.
7. Campbell DG, Vela A. Modern goniosynechialysis for the treatment of synechial angle-closure glaucoma. *Ophthalmology.* 1984;91: 1052-1060.
8. Shingleton BJ, Chang MA, Bellows AR, et al. Surgical goniosynechialysis for angle-closure glaucoma. *Ophthalmology.* 1990;97:551-556.
9. Tanihara H, Nishiwaki K, Nagata M. Surgical results and complications of goniosynechialysis. *Graefes Arch Clin Exp Ophthalmol.* 1992;230:309-313.
10. Shaffer RN. Primary glaucomas. Gonioscopy, ophthalmoscopy, and perimetry. *Trans Am Acad Ophthalmol Otolaryngol.* 1960;62:112-127.

Subacute (and Chronic) Angle-Closure Glaucoma

George Ulrich, MD, FACS and David L. Epstein, MD, MMM

The principles underlying the pathogenesis, diagnosis, and treatment of subacute and chronic angle-closure glaucoma have been explained in the preceding 2 chapters. Certain important features will be highlighted in this chapter.

The incidence of subacute and chronic angle-closure glaucoma is probably considerably greater than the incidence of the acute type. However, just as in acute angle-closure glaucoma, the sole cause of the rise in intraocular pressure (IOP) is closure of the angle. When the angle is entirely open, the outflow is normal, and there is no glaucoma. The subacute type differs from the acute type in that the course may consist of less intense, intermittent attacks, usually over a long time. Symptoms are usually mild or may be absent entirely until the disease is far advanced.

As discussed in Chapter 22, the term *subacute* implies mini-attacks of angle closure, with or without symptoms, where the whole circumference of the angle is not simultaneously involved. The term *chronic*, however, is used to describe many different clinical situations: to connote the residua and continuation of subacute episodes when peripheral anterior synechiae commonly form over time; to connote residual synechial angle closure after laser iridotomy; or, perhaps most commonly, to connote a totally silent progressive condition of angle closure, either appositional or synechial, that may mimic primary open-angle glaucoma (POAG). The latter entity is critically important for the clinician to diagnose and understand and is discussed elsewhere.

The term *chronic* is thus quite imprecise. It is better to use specific descriptive terms such as *silent (appositional or synechial) angle closure, residual angle closure after iridotomy,* or *recurrent episodes of subacute angle closure leading to formation of synechiae.*

DIAGNOSIS

As a rule, there is more variation in the width of different portions of the angle in the subacute form than in the acute form. In the subacute form, some portions of the angle are excessively narrow while other portions may be considerably wider. The angle does not close in the whole circumference as is usually the case in the acute form. In both acute and subacute angle-closure, the anterior chamber is characteristically shallow, and the iris is convex. Angle closure with a relatively flat iris plane and less axial shallowing (plateau iris; see Chapter 26) presents more frequently as subacute angle closure than acute angle closure.

In the differential diagnosis of subacute angle closure with irregular narrowing of the angle, one should also consider cysts of the iris or ciliary body that may cause irregular closure of the angle. This condition is discussed in Chapter 34. Irregular synechial closure should also make one consider uveitis and, if unilateral, essential iris atrophy.

In rare cases, both open-angle and subacute or chronic angle-closure glaucoma occur in the same eye.

Intraocular Pressure Elevations in Subacute Closure

In subacute angle-closure glaucoma, the rise in IOP is proportional to the extent of closure at a given time. In some cases, during an episode of partial closure, there may be a considerable acute rise in IOP, giving symptoms of blurred vision, discomfort, or seeing colored haloes. In other cases in which the closure is less extensive or develops more

Kahook MY, Schuman JS, eds.
Chandler and Grant's Glaucoma, Fifth Edition (pp 269-270).
© 2013 SLACK Incorporated.

gradually (chronic silent angle closure), the patient remains asymptomatic. If symptomatic episodes do occur, they tend to recur much more frequently than do the dramatic attacks typical of acute angle closure. In subacute intermittent angle-closure glaucoma, episodes of elevated IOP causing symptoms may occur every week or 2, or even daily, whereas in severe acute angle-closure glaucoma, episodes giving rise to symptoms usually occur at intervals of several weeks, months, or even years. Violent acute irreversible episodes do not ordinarily occur in the subacute type.

Chronic Silent Angle Closure and Chronic Angle Closure From Subacute Closure Events

Cases of chronic silent angle-closure glaucoma are encountered that are truly asymptomatic and that mimic chronic open-angle glaucoma, a misdiagnosis for which patients are often mistakenly treated. Among referral patients, cases of undetected chronic silent angle closure are commonly found. Because this condition can be potentially cured by laser iridotomy, it is important to make this diagnosis correctly by employing the overall concepts already outlined. If there is a strong suspicion of this diagnosis in a patient with elevated IOP, laser iridotomy should be performed. In many such cases of chronic silent angle closure, the closure is more appositional rather than synechial; therefore, it is potentially reversible by iridotomy.

In addition to chronic silent angle-closure glaucoma, one also continues to encounter the term *chronic* applied to the residua, recurrence, and continual progression of subacute angle closure. The term *chronic*, in general, is confusing because it is defined often by past symptoms, and

it sometimes obscures the understanding of the entity of chronic silent angle-closure glaucoma that mimics POAG. Regardless, the treatment is the same: laser iridotomy. This is followed by a reassessment of the amount of peripheral anterior synechia formation. Further treatment and follow-up might include laser gonioplasty as described for acute angle-closure glaucoma.

Once the diagnosis of subacute or chronic angle-closure glaucoma is established, treatment should be laser iridotomy in nearly all cases.

However, in the early stages of this condition, when there is little or no synechial closure, the situation in the angle is often not recognized. Medical therapy for IOP elevation is applied indiscriminately and generically as though one is dealing with POAG. Moreover, the initial IOP response to medical therapy is normally satisfactory even without iridotomy.

This creates a dangerous long-term situation. In the short-term, by applying medical therapy, mostly with topical medications used in open-angle glaucoma, such as prostaglandin analogs, beta-blockers, or alpha-2 agonists, IOP may be brought to normal. Ironically, if medical therapy is to be applied, the patient might be better served with pilocarpine in order to alter iris apposition to the angle. However, in most cases in which medical treatment including pilocarpine is continued, sooner or later more synechial closure of the angle occurs.

The baseline IOP gradually rises, and additional medications are required to bring IOP temporarily to normal levels. This response to additional treatment also may give a false sense of security while synechial closure of the angle relentlessly progresses. Finally, after extensive synechial closure has occurred, IOP may remain at relatively high levels and may not be lowered by medical means.

Angle-Closure Glaucoma

Evaluation and Treatment After Iridotomy

Mina B. Pantcheva, MD; Malik Y. Kahook, MD; and David L. Epstein, MD, MMM

ROUTINE FOR EVALUATION OF PATIENT AFTER LASER IRIDOTOMY

The steps of handling patients' eyes before and immediately after laser iridotomy are detailed in Chapter 55. In brief, eyes are pretreated with 1% to 2% pilocarpine to stretch and thin the iris and to aid in peripheral placement of the iridotomy; they are also given alpha-adrenergic agonist to blunt a potential intraocular pressure (IOP) spike posttreatment by decreasing aqueous humor formation and to lessen the chance of iris bleeding with the yttrium-aluminum-garnet (YAG) laser by a vasoconstrictive action (see Chapter 12). Patients are then postoperatively treated with mild anti-inflammatory agents, such as weak steroids or nonsteroidal anti-inflammatory agents 4 times a day for 5 days and appropriate antiglaucoma therapy. The following section deals with the conceptual steps in the subsequent post-laser management.

Management begins with an evaluation before the laser as to the likely final diagnosis (ie, the likelihood of a combined open-angle and angle-closure mechanism) and thus the likelihood of a laser-induced IOP spike in the short term and residual open-angle glaucoma in the long term (see Chapter 22). This tentative understanding also aids in planning the needed frequency of patient visits after the laser procedure (Table 25-1).

The patient is seen the day after the iridotomy and every several days if the IOP is substantially elevated (in which case gonioscopy should be performed). Anti-inflammatory therapy can be extended if needed. Then, the patient is seen 7 to 10 days later when routine follow-up gonioscopy is performed. This visit is a convenient time to perform a prophylactic laser iridotomy on the fellow eye, assuming

there are no residua in the first eye. The patient is routinely asked if the first eye is back to baseline before performing a prophylactic iridotomy on the fellow eye (this is modified if there are urgent reasons to proceed more quickly with laser iridotomy in the second eye).

Gonioscopy identifies the need for argon laser gonioplasty that might be planned a few weeks and also allows correlation of the amount of synechiae with the measured IOP. IOP may be elevated for a few weeks after laser (and also surgical) iridotomy by an open-angle mechanism due to pigment or debris and the use of corticosteroids. Therefore, short-term antiglaucoma therapy (usually aqueous humor suppressants) is used only to protect against acute optic nerve damage, and an observed slightly high IOP, if safe for the optic nerve in the short-term, might be tolerated for a few weeks to evaluate, at a subsequent visit, the true steady-state. On the other hand, if more vigorous antiglaucoma therapy is initiated and the IOP later decreases into a range below the target, the need for continuation of such strong therapy should later be re-evaluated.

The patency of the iridotomy is assessed. At any visit during the 4- to 6-week post-laser period, late closure of the iridotomy may occur. This is much more common after argon laser iridotomy, but is still occasionally observed after YAG iridotomy. (If patent at the 6-week visit, it is rare for any laser iridotomy to close subsequently, except in patients with uveitis or neovascularization.) However, even if obviously patent, an iridotomy may be sequestered in the sense that there are adhesions between the posterior iris surface and the crystalline lens so that there is not free communication between the posterior and the anterior chamber. The iridotomy may be too central (especially if pre-laser pilocarpine was not used or the pupil was semidilated and fixed from the acute angle-closure attack) and, therefore, may not

Kahook MY, Schuman JS, eds.
Chandler and Grant's Glaucoma, Fifth Edition (pp 271-276).
© 2013 SLACK Incorporated.

TABLE 25-1. POSTOPERATIVE MANAGEMENT OF LASER IRIDOTOMY	
Immediate postoperative (1 to 2 hours)	Check patency of iridotomy; intraocular pressure (at all visits); start topical steroids (qid for 5 days).
Day 1	Check patency of iridotomy.
Day 7 to 10	Assess location and function of iridotomy; gonioscopy to assess angle status, laser iridogonioplasty if significant portions of angle synechially closed; iridotomy for fellow eye if indicated (some clinicians prefer to do iridotomy of fellow eye at same sitting as first eye).
Week 4 to 6	Assess iridotomy for patency, touch-up iridotomy if necessary, dilated exam; baseline disc photos and visual fields if indicated.
Every 3 to 12 months	25% of patients with acute angle closure develop an intraocular pressure rise after angle closure; (uniocular mydriatic provocative test); therefore, long-term follow-up is essential.

clear the equator of the crystalline lens. The iridotomy very rarely might be too small in size (less than 50 μm) or filled with iris stromal strands or some potentially plugging iris material on the posterior border. Many of these complications were more commonly encountered after argon laser iridotomy than YAG laser iridotomy, but are still sometimes observed.

Therefore, in addition to observing the apparent direct patency of the iridotomy, the functional status needs to be assessed separately by observing the contour of the iris. Has relative pupillary block been alleviated? If so, and there is resulting free communication between the posterior and anterior chambers through the iridotomy, the iris contour configuration should no longer be convex forward (an effect of increased fluid pressure in the posterior chamber). Sometimes, the crystalline lens convexity itself will hold the central iris forward from direct pressure, but the contour of the peripheral iris needs to be assessed by gonioscopy. Similarly, the peripheral chamber depth on slit-lamp examination (Van Herick's rule[1]) should have also deepened, reflecting the induced loss of iris convexity. If these findings are not observed, then the clinician needs to entertain the possibility that there is not a functionally patent iridotomy or that the patient has some other form of angle-closure glaucoma, such as plateau iris, or some entity with direct peripheral pressure on the peripheral posterior iris surface (eg, ciliary body cysts or detachment).

If pupillary block has not been alleviated, then the angle may still appear closed by gonioscopy. Thus, apparent synechiae may not be true synechiae but merely continued appositional closure. Therefore, repeat indentation gonioscopy after iridotomy because, if there is a patent iridotomy, then fluid pressure cannot be holding the peripheral iris in appositional closure over the trabecular meshwork (TM). Thus, with a patent iridotomy, indentation should not change the apparent amount of angle closure, in which case it would have to represent peripheral anterior synechiae formation. If indentation does open the angle, then either

the iridotomy is not patent or there is some secondary cause of the closure.

This refers to opening of the angle and not a possible indentation effect on the iris. Mirrored lenses, unfortunately, despite their advantages, have their greatest weakness in this post-laser iridotomy assessment of peripheral iris contour. Although there is free communication between anterior and posterior chambers, sudden indentation displacement of the anterior chamber contents with the Zeiss-style indentation lenses does seemingly cause a temporary posterior indentation of the iris in many, but not all, patients (the volume displaced by the indentation from the anterior chamber cannot pass quickly enough through the iridotomy into the posterior chamber, and thus posterior iris movement is commonly produced). This induced posterior movement of the iris makes it easier to see into the angle, but should not thereby change the functional status of the angle if there is a patent iridotomy. Such persisting posterior movement of the iris after iridotomy has led to much confusion for the glaucoma student. In an eye with a patent iridotomy and no other cause for angle closure except primary pupillary block, appositional closure of the angle cannot exist by definition. If it looked that way with this indirect approach, it was because the mirrored gonioscopy lens did not present a true view of the angle (commonly because there is a large crystalline lens holding the central half, but not the peripheral portion, of the iris forward). It is crucial to distinguish between central iris convexity, due directly to the position of the crystalline lens, and peripheral iris convexity, due to increased fluid pressure in the posterior chamber, because at this post-laser visit one must be sure that relative pupillary block is no longer present (Figure 25-1). If the examiner is uncertain, Koeppe gonioscopy should be performed, as it readily allows such discrimination.

If pupillary block has been eliminated, but the angle remains either closed or very narrow and therefore occludable, and this is not due to a misinterpretation from an indirect mirrored view or a large crystalline lens, then other diagnoses

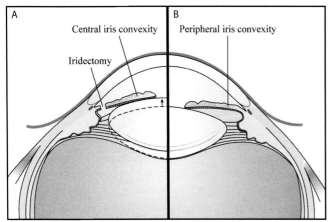

Figure 25-1. Iris convexity may be (A) secondary to forward location of the crystalline lens or (B) due to relative pupillary block. Iris convexity extends more peripherally in the latter case.

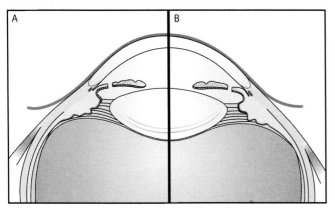

Figure 25-3. (A) Dilation in the presence of a peripheral iridotomy does not produce angle closure when due to relative pupillary block. (B) Because plateau iris configuration is not caused by relative pupillary block but rather by direct crowding of the iris into the angle, dilation does cause angle closure.

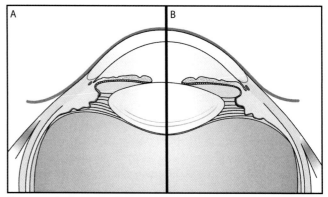

Figure 25-2. The iris configuration in pupillary block (A) demonstrates a gradual slope to the angle versus (B) that in plateau iris syndrome.

should be entertained at this post-laser visit. The possibility of peripheral anterior synechiae, or secondary direct mechanical closure from the ciliary body (see Chapter 28) producing continuing appositional closure, or a plateau iris should be considered (Figures 25-2 and 25-3). A mydriatic (using a sympathomimetic not a cycloplegic drug) provocative test to one eye can be performed, either at the 1-week visit or more often at a visit several weeks later, to rule out plateau iris.

Plateau iris[2-4] may be suspected pre-laser, or only post-laser when the access to the angle remains narrow. Most cases of possible plateau iris (plateau iris configuration) turn out after laser iridotomy not to have the true condition. However, there are also cases in which it was not suspected ahead of time, but proven to be a true plateau iris syndrome only after laser iridotomy.

At this post-laser visit (eg, 1 month after the second eye has had a laser iridotomy and all is quiet with patent iridotomies and the eyes are back to baseline), a mydriatic provocative test should be performed in one eye only (using the fellow eye as a control and avoiding precipitating a repeat of bilateral angle closure in a patient who had every expectation of being cured). A sympathomimetic drug, such as 2.5% or 5% phenylephrine, is administered to one eye once or twice to try to achieve wide dilatation, after which both the IOP and gonioscopy are reassessed. This should be a routine test administered to all post-laser iridotomy patients.

Sympathomimetic drugs should not elevate IOP, but rather can cause either no change or some transitory IOP lowering from a presumed decreased inflow effect. These agents rarely can cause elevation of IOP from liberation of pigment particles[5] into the anterior chamber. This can be assessed by repeating slit-lamp examination after dilation. An elevation of IOP of several millimeters of mercury or more compared with the control fellow eye needs to be explained, especially because, in plateau iris syndrome, the amount of functional angle closure increases progressively with wider dilation and resulting iris crowding of the angle. But, regardless of the IOP change after mydriatic challenge, the patient should be re-gonioscoped, and this should be documented in the chart for future reference.

Obviously, if the IOP increases during this mydriatic provocative test, gonioscopy should provide confirmation of angle closure as the responsible mechanism (otherwise, eg, suspect pigment liberation or other open-angle mechanisms). Also, the angle may look ominously closed after mydriatic treatment, even though the IOP did not increase, and this might indicate that, with wider mydriasis in the future, the angle might close in a plateau mechanism (not likely except when dilated in the ophthalmologist's office. There would be little risk of spontaneous closure, although long-term observations of such eyes over decades have not yet been made). Alternatively, it might indicate that the angle is functionally open beyond a peripheral iris roll, though it looks closed or close-to-closed with the mirrored gonioscopy lens. The latter appearance might be important to document in the chart for future reference when, for example, the patient might be dilated with a cycloplegic drug that could elevate the IOP in an open-angle mechanism[6,7] due to interference with ciliary muscle tone—the opposite effect of pilocarpine. In such a case, the IOP increase at this subsequent visit might be misinterpreted as angle closure due to plateau iris, and the patient would be mislabeled. Such a phenomenon is not rare, and it is surprising how many patients with prior angle closure were, at least in the previous era, both erroneously maintained on chronic pilocarpine therapy and told that their pupils should never be dilated, based on cycloplegic drug-induced IOP elevation due to a true open-angle mechanism that was never correlated with gonioscopy.

Performing gonioscopy on narrow-angled patients after pupillary dilation takes much experience because of the common presence of a peripheral iris roll. One learns to interpret correctly the open angle beyond this iris roll, but only if one routinely performs gonioscopy in all patients after pupillary dilatation (not just those with elevated IOP).

A cycloplegic (anticholinergic) drug, presumably by interfering with ciliary muscle tone to the outflow pathway, can cause an IOP increase with a maintained open angle in as many as one-third of patients with primary open-angle glaucoma (POAG).[6,7] This is supposedly uncommon in normal patients, and thus it would be unexpected in pure forms of angle-closure glaucoma.

When the pupil is dilated at this postoperative visit, a dilated slit-lamp examination should be performed, documenting the presence and extent of crystalline lens changes (there is a risk of lens changes long-term after laser iridotomy, but also occult exfoliation should be looked for[8]), the appearance of the optic nerve including stereo disc photos (due to the risk of residual open-angle glaucoma), and indirect ophthalmoscopy performed with examination of the retinal periphery as in any other patient with glaucoma (see Chapter 5).

For practical purposes, unilateral plateau iris has not been observed, and therefore if IOP does not increase or true angle closure is not observed with this unilateral mydriatic provocative test, at subsequent visits, it is safe to dilate both pupils with the physician's choice of mydriatic and/or cycloplegic.

If during the post-laser iridotomy visits it is suspected that there is direct mechanical pressure on the posterior iris surface acting to close the angle, cycloplegic drugs can and should be used to help diagnose this. Tightening the zonules and interfering with ciliary muscle contraction could cause posterior movement of the crystalline lens and potentially also some alteration in ciliary body position. Use of cycloplegic drugs for certain forms of secondary angle-closure glaucoma is described in Chapters 28 and 29.

Laser iridotomy establishes communication between the posterior and anterior chambers by creating a hole in the iris, but it does not change the position of the crystalline lens. Only the peripheral chamber depth can change after iridotomy. This has been confirmed by photogrammetric and biometric measurements.[9-11] The recording of both peripheral and axial anterior chamber depth measured in terms of corneal thicknesses is important, especially in case of subsequent shallowing of the anterior chamber. In malignant glaucoma syndromes, there is axial anterior chamber (as well as peripheral) shallowing (see Chapter 29). Although malignant glaucoma has not yet been unequivocally observed after laser iridotomy (there are only rare case reports[12]), it was not rare after surgical peripheral iridectomy. Eyes with previous angle closure may in the ensuing years experience some new occurrence, perhaps involving the posterior segment, unrelated to the past angle-closure event, and it may be very important to know that the axial depth has subsequently changed.

After laser iridotomy, residual open-angle glaucoma, possibly increasing nuclear sclerosis with the passage of time, etc, is still an issue in such eyes (see Chapter 22), and the patient should be checked 6 months later and then at yearly intervals and subsequently, assuming all is well, every 2 years.

RESIDUAL OPEN-ANGLE GLAUCOMA AFTER LASER IRIDOTOMY

There is a higher incidence of open-angle glaucoma in eyes that have had laser iridotomy than what would be predicted from the prevalence of POAG in the same aged population. Possible explanations include that the 2 diseases are linked genetically and that certain forms of open-angle glaucoma, such as exfoliation, commonly are associated with narrow angles.[8] Chronic iris touch from appositional closure may perhaps cause residual open-angle glaucoma, the original diagnosis of angle closure may be in error, and laser iridotomy might cause TM dysfunction presumably as a result of released pigment, debris, and inflammation, which all must leave the eye via the outflow pathways.[13]

Regardless, it behooves the clinician to establish the correct diagnosis as accurately as possible ahead of time (see Chapter 22) and both inform the patient and plan one's short-term and long-term follow-up accordingly. In a patient with exfoliation open-angle glaucoma and a narrow but functionally open angle, one should anticipate a potentially large IOP spike after laser iridotomy, which also would do nothing to improve the current IOP control (although potentially prevent future worsening). Inform the patient fully about this ahead of time. There are cases in which this scenario was not anticipated, resulting in loss of central visual acuity from the IOP spike, leading to medicolegal discussions.

LONG-TERM FOLLOW-UP AFTER IRIDOTOMY

The initial measurements of IOP after iridotomy are by no means a guide as to what the future is going to hold. If much of the angle is closed by synechiae, one should not be misled if the IOP at that time happens still to be low without treatment because, sooner or later, IOP can be expected to increase. This may not occur for some time. If there are synechiae, gonioplasty with the argon laser should be performed. Inform the patient that if the IOP increases to a level consistent with the extent of synechial closure, he or she may find that medical antiglaucoma therapy, additional laser therapy gonioplasty, or filtration surgery may be needed.

In addition, after laser iridotomy, IOP may be moderately elevated by an ill-defined open-angle mechanism for several weeks to months after the procedure. This may relate to the increased pigmentation of the TM, or perhaps to obstructing iris or inflammatory debris. Therefore, depending on disc and field status, one would like to delay if possible a decision concerning possible filtration surgery even in a patient with residual synechiae, until a month or so after the iridotomy.

TREATMENT OF RESIDUAL (CHRONIC) SYNECHIAL ANGLE-CLOSURE GLAUCOMA

Gonioscopy should always be performed at the first follow-up visit after laser iridotomy. As described, IOP can be elevated at this or subsequent visits by an open-angle mechanism, perhaps relating to pigment, debris, or inflammation in the TM, or can be lowered (giving a false sense of security) by hyposecretion, especially after a substantial acute attack. The clinician needs to ascertain the extent of residual peripheral anterior synechiae in the angle, no matter what the level of IOP.

In treating this residual synechial angle-closure glaucoma, one chooses medical therapy alone if there are minimal peripheral anterior synechiae and gonioplasty with supplemental medical antiglaucoma therapy if the synechiae are extensive. If this strategy fails because of the presence of extensive residual peripheral anterior synechiae, filtration surgery will be required.

MEDICAL THERAPY

Aqueous humor suppressant therapy is most commonly used in the short and intermediate term, but long-term, one is free to use any and all antiglaucoma therapy, including miotics and epinephrine (in the absence of previous malignant glaucoma or plateau iris).

ARGON LASER GONIOPLASTY (IRIDOPLASTY)

If 6 or more hours of the angle have synechiae, consideration should be given to performing gonioplasty[14-18] to break these synechiae, if possible. The overall clinical impression is that in perhaps 50% of patients with synechiae of less than 1-year duration, this procedure can restore normal or near-normal outflow function to the affected portion of the angle. Most likely, the more recent the synechia formation, the better the chances for a beneficial effect. On the other hand, the eye should be free from inflammation and fully recovered from the iridotomy procedure, and, therefore, the gonioplasty can usually be delayed for a few weeks after iridotomy.

In doing this laser gonioplasty technique, use of the angle mirror of a gonioscopy lens is preferred to directly place the argon laser burns (eg, 200 μm, 0.2 to 0.5 seconds, 300 mW) on the far peripheral iris as close to the angle as possible. Some synechiae will readily separate, yielding an apparent open angle to view (that still has only an approximate 50% chance of being functionally open). Other peripheral anterior synechiae do not readily separate with placement of the peripheral iris laser burn, and we recommend not persisting in treating such sites (because, even if it is anatomically possible to open the angle, the chance for functional recovery seems much less likely) and moving on to other sites. Because this procedure can induce inflammation in the eye and can liberate pigment debris, all of which might elevate the IOP by an open-angle mechanism, this procedure should be performed in 2 divided sessions, perhaps weeks apart. Pretreating the eye with 1% or 2% pilocarpine makes the procedure much easier to perform by stretching the peripheral iris.

Depending on other clinical factors such as the presumed filterability of the open angle (see Chapters 3 and 7) as well as the disc and field status, gonioplasty could also be performed for lesser amounts of residual peripheral anterior synechiae (eg, 3 to 6 hours of the angle). Probably for 3 or fewer hours of synechiae, except in unusual situations (the need for a very low IOP because of the vulnerability of the optic nerve), this procedure need not be performed.

Although not all clinicians would agree that this procedure is effective (and many would argue that, regardless, chronic iris touch to the TM in a narrow-angled eye can cause trabecular dysfunction even if the synechiae are anatomically separated), gonioplasty should be attempted before consideration of filtration surgery for uncontrolled residual synechial angle-closure glaucoma. Especially after certain secondary forms of angle closure, some have argued that surgical goniosynechialysis[19-21] should be attempted to break such peripheral anterior synechiae. In certain secondary forms of angle closure, the peripheral iris adjacent to the angle may not be accessible to the argon laser through the mirrored lens, and therefore this procedure may be used (see Chapter 23). However, in cases of primary angle-closure glaucoma, access of the peripheral iris to the argon laser is usually technically possible, and therefore surgical chamber deepening has only rare indication. Peripheral anterior synechiae that are difficult to separate with an argon laser burn probably indicate a portion of the angle with little if any chance for functional recovery.

After argon laser gonioplasty, patients are treated with topical steroids, probably a little more intensively than after iridotomy, for 4 to 5 days.

FILTRATION SURGERY

The techniques of filtration surgery in patients with residual (chronic) synechial angle-closure glaucoma are similar to those in other patients with glaucoma and are detailed in Chapter 59. There are, however, a few special considerations. Because the anatomy of the usual hyperopic eye is crowded anteriorly, special attention is made to carry the conjunctival and scleral flap incisions far enough anteriorly to avoid entering the eye and placing the fistula too far posteriorly, over the ciliary body. A good rule is that one is never far enough anteriorly, and extra time is taken at the limbus to move the dissection of tissue as far anterior as possible. Because shallowing of the anterior chamber intra- and postoperatively may be involved in the development of malignant glaucoma (see Chapter 29), there is special attention to the chamber intraoperatively in such hyperopic eyes to prevent anterior chamber shallowing. The glaucoma fistula might be designed to be tighter rather than looser (with potential future use of laser suture lysis) to try to avoid postoperative anterior chamber shallowing. The possibility of malignant glaucoma developing in the early postoperative period must always be on the surgeon's mind when performing filtration surgery on eyes with residual synechial angle closure.

REFERENCES

1. Van Herick W, Shaffer RN, Schwartz A. Estimation of width of angle of anterior chamber. Incidence and significance of the narrow angle. *Am J Ophthalmol.* 1969;68:626-629.
2. Tornquist R. Angle-closure glaucoma in an eye with a plateau type of iris. *Acta Ophthalmol.* 1958;36:419-423.
3. Wand M, Grant WM, Simmons RJ, et al. Plateau iris syndrome. *Trans Am Acad Ophthalmol Otolaryngol.* 1977;83:122-130.
4. Pavlin CJ, Ritch R, Foster FS. Ultrasound biomicroscopy in plateau iris syndrome. *Am J Ophthalmol.* 1992;113:390-395.
5. Epstein DL, Boger WP, Grant WM. Phenylephrine provocative testing in the pigmentary dispersion syndrome. *Am J Ophthalmol.* 1978;85:43-50.
6. Harris LS. Cycloplegic provocative testing. *Arch Ophthalmol.* 1969;81:544-547.
7. Harris LS. Cycloplegic provocative testing and topical administration of steroids. *Arch Ophthalmol.* 1971;86:12-14.
8. Gross FJ, Tingey D, Epstein DL. Increased prevalence of occludable angles and angle-closure glaucoma in patients with pseudoexfoliation. *Am J Ophthalmol.* 1993;117:333-336.
9. Lee DA, Brubaker RF, Ilstrup DM. Anterior chamber dimensions in patients with narrow angles and angle-closure glaucoma. *Arch Ophthalmol.* 1984;102:46-50.
10. Jin JC, Anderson DR. The effect of iridotomy on iris contour. *Am J Ophthalmol.* 1990;110:260-263.
11. Schrems W, Hofmann G, Krieglstein GK. Zur Biometrie der Augen-vorderkammer bei der Nd:YAG-Laseriridektomie. *Klin Monatsbl Augenheilkd.* 1990;196:128-131.
12. Cashwell LF, Martin TJ. Malignant glaucoma after laser iridotomy. *Ophthalmology.* 1992;99:651-659.
13. Robin AL, Pollack IP, Quigley HA, D'Anna S, Addicks EM. Histologic studies of angle structures after laser iridotomy in primates. *Arch Ophthalmol.* 1982;100:1665-1670.
14. Ritch R. Argon laser treatment for medically unresponsive attacks of angle-closure glaucoma. *Am J Ophthalmol.* 1982;94:197-204.
15. Wand M. Argon laser gonioplasty for synechial angle closure. *Arch Ophthalmol.* 1992;110:363-367.
16. Weiss HS, Shingleton BJ, Goode SM, Bellows AR, Richter CU. Argon laser gonioplasty in the treatment of angle-closure glaucoma. *Am J Ophthalmol.* 1992;114:14-18.
17. Lim AS, Tan A, Chew P, et al. Laser iridoplasty in the treatment of severe acute angle closure glaucoma. *Int Ophthalmol.* 1993;17:33-36.
18. Sassani JW, Ritch R, McCormick S, et al. Histopathology of argon laser peripheral iridoplasty. *Ophthalmic Surg.* 1993;24:740-745.
19. Campbell DG, Vela A. Modern goniosynechialysis for the treatment of synechial angle-closure glaucoma. *Ophthalmology.* 1984;91:1052-1060.
20. Shingleton BJ, Chang MA, Bellows AR, et al. Surgical goniosynechialysis for angle-closure glaucoma. *Ophthalmology.* 1990;97:551-556.
21. Tanihara H, Nishiwaki K, Nagata M. Surgical results and complications of goniosynechialysis. *Graefes Arch Clin Exp Ophthalmol.* 1992;230:309-313.

Plateau Iris

Joel S. Schuman, MD, FACS; Malik Y. Kahook, MD; and David L. Epstein, MD, MMM

PLATEAU IRIS CONFIGURATION AND PLATEAU IRIS SYNDROME

Clinical Features

In a minority of eyes that develop primary angle-closure glaucoma, the anterior chamber does not appear as shallow as we are accustomed to associate with angle-closure glaucoma, and the front surface of the iris lacks the overall convex curvature that usually involves the whole iris from pupil to angle. In angle-closure glaucoma associated with the so-called plateau iris or flat iris plane, the surface of the iris extending from the pupil toward the angle may appear nearly flat centrally; it may be convex only in the far periphery, where it conforms to the curvature of the angle wall and closes the angle. The profile of such an iris, if it could be seen in cross-section, can be conceived as resembling a plateau, as pointed out by Tornquist in 1958.[1]

It is now recognized that the major anatomic factor that results in plateau iris is the presence of anteriorly positioned ciliary processes that push forward on the iris root and crowd the angle.[2] Additionally, the iris often appears to be inserted more anteriorly along the face of the ciliary body, closer to the sclera spur, further crowding the angle.

In most cases in which angle closure is associated with plateau iris, the angle closure can be eliminated as successfully by iridectomy as in the more common cases in which the whole iris is convex. This indicates that relative pupillary block and accumulation of aqueous humor in the posterior chamber must be a significant factor contributing to the convexity of the iris in both the common and the plateau iris cases, though, with plateau iris, the convexity is usually limited to the periphery, and widening of the angle is not as striking after iridectomy as in eyes in which the whole iris is convex. However, there are cases of plateau iris that are not

apparent initially, because the additional presence of significant pupillary block may result in diffuse iris convexity, and the plateau iris only becomes evident after an iridectomy results in flattening of the iris contour.

Additionally, there may be a distinct phacomorphic component whereby the crystalline lens pushes the iris forward and crowds the angle, a factor that can be alleviated with cataract extraction. While the plateau configuration and the apposition of the ciliary processes against the peripheral iris may not resolve with cataract extraction, the anterior chamber does appear to deepen, and the angles may open.[4,5] In such cases, lens removal creates more space in the posterior chamber, and one can picture the entire iris plateau being able to rotate to some degree posteriorly, allowing the peripheral iris to move away from the trabecular meshwork.

Uncommonly, despite the creation of a patent iridectomy and elimination of any component of relative pupillary block, the angle of an eye with plateau iris remains occludable, and, rarely, it can be caused to close by dilating the pupil (see Chapter 25), and an attack of angle-closure glaucoma may result. Even more rarely, angle-closure glaucoma can occur spontaneously, without artificially dilating the pupil.

We have preferred to distinguish the preoperative condition of the iris from the postiridectomy recurrence of angle-closure glaucoma simply by calling the preoperative condition *plateau iris configuration* and the rare postoperative recurrence of glaucoma the *plateau iris syndrome*, as was done in a study of these conditions reported by Wand and colleagues.[6] The rarity of glaucoma due to plateau iris syndrome was also indicated in that report; only 8 cases could be identified among a large number of glaucoma patients in the Glaucoma Service of the Massachusetts Eye and Ear Infirmary and the referral practices of 2 of its members. It should be noted that, at present, the term *plateau iris syndrome* is often used in reference to a persistently closed or occludable angle, despite a patent iridectomy, regardless of

Kahook MY, Schuman JS, eds.
Chandler and Grant's Glaucoma, Fifth Edition (pp 277-280).
© 2013 SLACK Incorporated.

any intraocular pressure (IOP) elevation or glaucoma after dilation.

If following iridectomy, the IOP is found to increase with dilation, then plateau iris syndrome should be considered; however, the diagnosis needs to be established by performing gonioscopy and noting appositional angle closure. Other causes of IOP increase, spontaneously or from application of mydriatics, after iridectomy for angle-closure glaucoma include the following:

- Failure of the iridectomy to make a hole through all layers of the iris
- Residual peripheral anterior synechiae (see Chapter 24)
- Presence of multiple cysts of the ciliary body (see Chapter 34)
- Anterior lens subluxation or intumescence ("phacomorphic" glaucoma), which mechanically narrows the angle
- Presence of open-angle glaucoma (see Chapter 25)
- Malignant glaucoma

Slit-lamp biomicroscopy and gonioscopy can establish these diagnoses. Only if there is conspicuous axial shallowing of the anterior chamber associated with the postoperative increase of IOP and closure of the angle does one need to consider a diagnosis of malignant glaucoma (see Chapter 29). However, this distinction is important because the topical treatment of plateau iris syndrome and the treatment of malignant glaucoma are totally different. Plateau iris syndrome may be precipitated by cycloplegics and relieved by pilocarpine, whereas malignant glaucoma may be precipitated or aggravated by miotics and relieved or benefited by cycloplegics.

The conspicuous axial shallowing of the anterior chamber in malignant glaucoma (see Chapter 29) is the principal feature that should distinguish this condition from plateau iris syndrome. However, there is an important point in a rare case in which there is some uncertainty due to shallowness of the anterior chamber at the time of recurrent glaucoma after angle-closure glaucoma previously associated with plateau iris. The point we believe to be significant is the relationship of ciliary processes to lens equator, as viewed (when possible) through the iris coloboma (or the widely dilated pupil) with the aid of Koeppe lens gonioscopy. According to our observations so far, in malignant glaucoma, the lens equator tends to extend behind and peripheral to the tips of the ciliary processes, so that the lens equator is in a position to push ciliary processes and iris forward (see Chapter 28), whereas, in the plateau iris syndrome, we have not seen the lens extend peripherally beyond the tips of the ciliary processes.

DIAGNOSIS

Plateau iris may be suspected before laser iridectomy based upon the iris profile on gonioscopy and from the disparity of the axial/peripheral chamber depths on slit-lamp examination. The typical finding seen on indentation gonioscopy has been termed the *double-hump sign*, with a central elevation representing the portion of the iris supported by the lens, a mid-peripheral iris depression near the lens periphery, and a peripheral roll of iris that is supported by the iris processes (which can create loci of peripheral iris elevation). The most peripheral iris surface then steeply angulates posteriorly toward its insertion.[3]

To help confirm the clinical suspicion of plateau iris, ultrasound biomicroscopy can be performed (Figure 26-1). The typical features to look for are occludable angles (particularly in the dark), ciliary processes that push up against the iris root while closing the ciliary sulcus, and a relatively flat iris profile. The iris may be seen inserting anteriorly with respect to the face of the ciliary body.

Although a true plateau iris syndrome is rare, after laser iridectomy, the pupils should be dilated in each patient to rule out this condition (see Chapter 25) before reassuring the patient about his or her cure from the procedure. Each patient should have sequential unilateral mydriatic provocative tests (eg, 4 to 6 weeks postlaser). Measurement of IOP and gonioscopy should be performed before and after dilation. As discussed in Chapter 25, an additional benefit of this routine is to gain experience with the interpretation of gonioscopy in the presence of a dilated pupil because, often in narrow-angle eyes, a peripheral iris roll may partially obscure the viewing of a functionally open angle when the pupil is dilated.

CLINICAL COURSE

In patients who have a true plateau iris syndrome, the risk for the future could involve symptomatic attacks usually of subacute angle closure or, more commonly, asymptomatic progressive chronic angle closure with peripheral anterior synechia formation. Undiagnosed plateau iris can cause *creeping angle closure*—a term that is not favored because it indicates no mechanism and constitutes more than one entity—after iridectomy.

In the mechanism of true plateau iris syndrome, the angle becomes progressively crowded and occluded by the iris with increasing pupillary dilatation. Such full-blown attacks of angle-closure glaucoma from maximum mydriasis are, therefore, more common after pharmacological pupillary dilation in the ophthalmologist's office than spontaneously (where subacute attacks are more common). The potential for such an iatrogenic event makes it imperative that the results of routine unilateral mydriatic provocative testing be systematically studied in each patient after laser iridectomy, and the patient then appropriately classified at that time (not subsequently after an acute event).

Some have distinguished between cases where there is a high plateau that appears to occlude the entire angle and cases where the plateau is not as high, occluding only the posterior angle. Whereas in the former condition, termed *complete plateau iris syndrome*, there is IOP elevation with

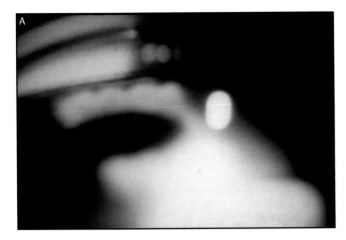
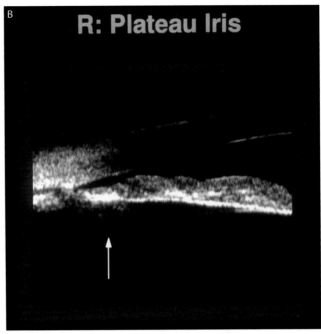

Figure 26-1. (A) Gonioscopy reveals a flat iris plane with a steep approach to the angle. (B) Ultrasound biomicroscopy reveals forward position of the anterior ciliary processes (arrow), pushing the iris into the angle.

mydriasis and a risk of acute angle closure, in the more common latter condition, termed *incomplete plateau iris*, there is a tendency toward chronic synechial closure.

TREATMENT AND FOLLOW-UP

In a patient with a newly diagnosed plateau iris syndrome, one initial strategy is to prevent significant spontaneous mydriasis by using a weak miotic sometimes just once a day at bedtime (for patient acceptance). The follow-up of plateau iris patients includes not only the history of possible episodes of subacute angle closure and the measurement of IOP, but careful gonioscopy with indentation looking for new peripheral anterior synechiae formation. Serial tonography may be useful in documenting functional outflow changes that correlate with the angle appearance. Even with miotic therapy, the angle usually continues to appear narrow, so it is sometimes difficult to discriminate whether there is progressive appositional closure in such patients. The IOP status is helpful, but one must be cautious with the interpretation in patients on aqueous humor suppressants that can mask a slowly progressive chronic angle closure (see Chapters 22 and 24). Therefore, the absence of new peripheral anterior synechiae formation on indentation gonioscopy (see Chapter 7) is a critical evaluation that the clinician needs to make to allow continuation of the existing therapy.

If weak miotic therapy is either undesirable (due to side effects) or unsuccessful in preventing progressive functional angle closure in plateau iris syndrome patients, patients should have argon laser gonioplasty[7-12] to contract the peripheral iris, and thus pull it away from the angle. The technique is similar to that used to break peripheral anterior synechiae and is described in Chapters 25 and 51. To avoid the potential side effects of miotic therapy, some may wish to proceed with gonioplasty at the first sight of a persistently occludable angle after laser iridotomy. In brief, the mirrored gonioscopy lens is used to place the argon laser burns (300 mW, 200 to 500 μm, 0.2 to 0.5 seconds) as far to the periphery of the iris as possible. In a few cases in which this has been used, there has been remarkable success, preventing the need for filtration surgery, which is the last resort after laser and full medical antiglaucoma therapy have been exhausted. Some glaucoma clinicians have reported anecdotally that the argon laser gonioplasty procedure may need to be repeated after a few years, but we have not yet observed this. In addition to gonioplasty, it should be kept in mind that cataract extraction (as mentioned above) has the potential to cure an occludable angle.

It is an intriguing question as to why this condition occurs. As mentioned, reports suggest, based on ultrasound findings, that the ciliary body is farther forward in this condition and holds the peripheral iris base close to the angle.[2,3] We have previously supposed that the iris base simply inserts farther forward onto the ciliary body band, as an anatomical variant. Other factors to consider are the thickness of the iris and its ability to lose volume upon dilation.[13] If such ability is impaired, one can see how a crowded angle may be more likely to become occluded in the maximally dilated state despite a patent iridectomy. While understanding that the exact pathophysiology does not currently alter clinical management, our continually expanding knowledge of the mechanisms of angle closure may allow us to tailor future therapies toward specific causes.

REFERENCES

1. Tornquist R. Angle-closure glaucoma in an eye with a plateau type of iris. *Acta Ophthamol.* 1958;36:419-423.

2. Ritch R. Plateau iris is caused by abnormally positioned ciliary processes. *J Glaucoma.* 1992;1:23-26.

3. Pavlin CJ, Ritch R, Foster FS. Ultrasound biomicroscopy in plateau iris syndrome. *Am J Ophthalmol.* 1992;113:390-395.

4. Tran HV, Liebmann JM, Ritch R. Iridociliary apposition in plateau iris syndrome persists after cataract extraction. *Am J Ophthalmol.* 2003;135:40-43.

5. Nonaka A, Kondo T, Kikuchi M, et al. Cataract surgery for residual angle closure after peripheral laser iridotomy. *Ophthalmology.* 2005;112:974-979.

6. Wand M, Grant WM, Simmons RJ, et al. Plateau iris syndrome. *Trans Am Acad Ophthalmol Otolaryngol.* 1977;83:OP-122-OP-130.

7. Ritch R. Argon laser treatment for medically unresponsive attacks of angle-closure glaucoma. *Am J Ophthalmol.* 1982;94:197-204.

8. Wand M. Argon laser gonioplasty for synechial angle closure. *Arch Ophthalmol.* 1992;110:363-367.

9. Weiss HS, Shingleton BJ, Goode SM, Bellows AR, Richter CU. Argon laser gonioplasty in the treatment of angle-closure glaucoma. *Am J Ophthalmol.* 1992;114:14-18.

10. Lim AS, Tan A, Chew P, et al. Laser iridoplasty in the treatment of severe acute angle closure glaucoma. *Int Ophthalmol.* 1993; 17:33-36.

11. Sassani JW, Ritch R, McCormick S, et al. Histopathology of argon laser peripheral iridoplasty. *Ophthalmic Surg.* 1993;24: 740-745.

12. Ritch R, Tham C, Lam D. Argon laser peripheral iridoplasty (ALPI): an update. *Surv Ophthalmol.* 2007;52:279-288.

13. Quigley HA. The iris is a sponge: a cause of angle closure. *Ophthalmology.* 2010;117:1-2.

27

The Use of Special Tests in Narrow-Angled Eyes

Joel S. Schuman, MD, FACS and David L. Epstein, MD, MMM

The advent of laser iridectomy with its favorable risk/benefit considerations has resulted in a clinical situation in which additional special tests are only rarely performed in eyes with potentially occludable angles. However, a firm understanding of the principles involved in evaluating these eyes is useful (see Chapter 22). These special tests are detailed both because of historical importance and also because they reinforce the understanding of these principles that are critical to appropriately treating such eyes. The beginning resident or student is urged to read and understand the conceptual basis for such tests.

GONIOSCOPY AND TONOGRAPHY

Reliable diagnosis of angle closure can only be made by gonioscopy, but tonography may be extremely helpful. In the early stages, if the patient is examined during an interval of normal intraocular pressure (IOP), one finds the angle open throughout, but at least a portion of the angle is very narrow. Under these conditions, tonography indicates a normal facility of outflow. During an interval of moderately elevated IOP, one finds that a portion of the angle appears closed, and tonography shows a proportionate decrease in facility of outflow. The significance of the tonographic measurements is that the change in facility of outflow is dependent on whether the angle is open or closed and is independent of current IOP. If open-angle glaucoma were present with the angle open and the IOP in a normal phase, the tonographic measurement would show persistently subnormal facility of aqueous outflow (and the implication would be that the IOP was normal due to a diurnal phase of decreased aqueous humor formation).

Sometimes, the situation is complicated at the initial examination because the patient may have started to take miotic treatment prescribed elsewhere. If there are no synechiae, the findings under the influence of miotic treatment may be the same as during a spontaneous remission: the IOP normal, angle open throughout, and facility of outflow normal. In such a case, to establish the diagnosis, all treatment is discontinued in the hope that IOP will increase considerably. Then, gonioscopy is repeated during the period of elevated IOP. If, with the IOP elevated, the angle is still entirely open, the diagnosis must be open-angle glaucoma, despite the narrow angle. If, on the other hand, one finds an extent of angle closure consistent with the elevation of IOP (see Chapters 7 and 22), the diagnosis is angle-closure glaucoma.

If, on discontinuation of treatment, IOP increases only moderately, such as to the high 20s, there is much more difficulty in making a diagnosis than cases in which the IOP goes to 40 or 50 mm Hg. Very little closure is necessary to cause an increase of IOP to the high 20s, and every gonioscopist realizes how difficult it may be to distinguish whether a small portion of the angle is closed or almost closed. During a period without treatment, with IOP at the general level of mid to high 20s, tonography may be helpful, although often not decisive. In this IOP range in angle-closure glaucoma, one finds a C value only 20% or 30% below normal. A considerably poorer C value, with the IOP in this range, suggests the presence of open-angle glaucoma. In such equivocal cases, the darkroom test, the bright-light test with or without thymoxamine, or possibly the mydriasis test may be helpful.

DARKROOM PRONE TESTS

The darkroom test is performed by having the patient remain in the dark, awake, for an hour, preferably face down.[1,2] This can be accomplished by having the patient

Kahook MY, Schuman JS, eds.
Chandler and Grant's Glaucoma, Fifth Edition (pp 281-284).

GONIOLENS CHARACTERISTICS
R. Rand Allingham, MD

Every ophthalmologist should be familiar with specific qualities of available goniolenses. This is particularly true in cases in which the functional status of the filtering angle is involved. Goniolenses with a small diameter (eg, Zeiss or Sussman) indent the central cornea and artifactually widen the angle. This is a useful quality that can be exploited to examine a narrow angle for peripheral anterior synechiae or to break an acute attack of angle-closure glaucoma. However, this same quality can lead the clinician to misjudge the true configuration of the filtering angle, leading to a false sense of security that the angle is not occludable when, in fact, it is. To view the angle without inducing artifactual changes, a goniolens with a wide diameter that bridges but does not indent the central cornea is necessary (eg, a Goldmann or Koeppe lens). An added benefit to these wider-diameter goniolenses is the superior view of the angle structures that is obtained with them. Therefore, the clinician must become familiar with the use of indenting and nonindenting goniolenses.

sitting in a chair with his or her head resting on his or her arms on an adjacent table, taking care not to press on the eyes. Immediately at the end of this period, the IOP is measured. In a negative test, IOP in both eyes is almost exactly the same as before the test and the same in both eyes. One may ordinarily think of a positive darkroom test as a situation in which IOP in one or both eyes increases considerably, to a level of 40 or 50 or more, but instances of such considerable increases after 1 hour in the dark are uncommon. It is much more common to find an increase of only 5 to 10 mm Hg. Because in a negative darkroom test, in patients who have no glaucoma of any sort, the IOP is usually exactly the same as before the test, an increase of only a few millimeters of mercury may be significant. If in the darkroom test there is a significant difference in the increase in IOP in the 2 eyes, even though the increase is moderate, this should be interpreted as a positive darkroom test.

However, a positive darkroom test based only on IOP change can occur in cases of open-angle glaucoma when a diurnal IOP increase happens to coincide with the test. Unless the increase of IOP is large and associated with a gonioscopically closed angle, other types of tests may be required to be sure.

If the darkroom test is completely negative, does this rule out angle-closure glaucoma in a given case? A negative darkroom test does not rule out angle-closure glaucoma.[3] If the angle is thought to be dangerously narrow and the darkroom test is negative, in the past (before the advent of laser iridectomy), we recommended that the patient have an IOP check twice a year indefinitely and repeat the darkroom test once or twice a year, for one cannot predict if and when such angles may close. Some patients were evaluated for 12 or more years, remaining normal and asymptomatic. Yet,

in other cases, the tests became positive in a few years or less, as in the following example.

Case 27-1

In this patient, the angles were extremely narrow, but IOP was normal and the darkroom test negative. IOP was checked regularly twice a year; it remained around 17 mm Hg, and the patient was asymptomatic. Finally, at a visit 6.5 years after the initial visit, IOP was right 22 mm Hg and left 27 mm Hg. The patient was still asymptomatic. A darkroom test was done, and IOP increased to 28 mm Hg in the right eye and 45 mm Hg in the left. A peripheral iridectomy was done on both eyes.

David Hill, MD conducted a survey of patients who underwent periodic darkroom tests in the Glaucoma Service of the Massachusetts Eye and Ear Infirmary purely because of extremely narrow angles. This survey indicated that, after a negative darkroom test, a patient was unlikely to develop acute angle closure within the next 6 months.

However, shortcomings of the darkroom test include the following:

- It is often negative even though the eye may be subject to spontaneous subacute angle-closure attacks.[3]

- It is difficult to perform gonioscopy as part of the test without causing some miosis with the light that is necessary for gonioscopy, and this may cause the angle to open even though it may have been closed previously in the dark. (We have performed gonioscopy in the dark with an infrared converter to get around this difficulty, but have found it difficult to evaluate the angle with the monochromatic, 2-dimensional image obtained.)

- An increase in IOP in the dark occurs in some open-angle glaucomatous eyes, sometimes as a coincidental part of spontaneous diurnal fluctuation, and this may cause error of interpretation unless the gonioscopy is done carefully and critically.

The evidence can be considerably strengthened by combining tonography with the darkroom test, because, with an increase in IOP, a concomitant decrease in facility of aqueous outflow is characteristic of angle closure, whereas an increase in IOP without change in facility of outflow (subnormal to begin with) is characteristic of the spontaneous diurnal fluctuation of open-angle glaucoma.

BRIGHT-LIGHT TEST

As an addendum to the darkroom test, when the darkroom test is positive, the bright-light test can be of great value in helping to determine more surely whether a positive result is truly due to angle closure. This has not been appreciated. The bright-light test should be used routinely in conjunction with positive darkroom tests as a confirmatory test. It potentially turns one of the weaknesses of the ordinary darkroom test into an advantage. One of the weaknesses already pointed out was that, if gonioscopy is done immediately after the darkroom test, the light may promptly cause the pupil to constrict and the angle to open. This often produces the dilemma that the pressure may have had a respectable increase in the dark, but when one then looks at the angle it is narrowly open, and we do not know whether it truly was closed in the dark or whether this was one of those coincidental diurnal IOP variations of open-angle glaucoma.

To differentiate a genuinely positive (angle closure) darkroom test from a spurious coincidental increase of IOP that is not due to closure of the angle, but is due simply to the diurnal IOP variation that occurs in some patients with open-angle glaucoma, apply the bright-light test immediately after the darkroom test. This is done as follows.

At the end of the darkroom test, after the IOP has been measured and the angle has been inspected in as dim illumination as possible, to see if the angle appears to have closed, the illumination is then greatly increased, to cause the pupils to constrict. This can be done by turning on bright ceiling lights while observing the angle through the goniolens. When the light is bright enough to make the angle clearly open in the entire circumference, one knows that if the IOP was elevated due to closure of the angle during the darkroom test, it should rapidly, within 5 to 15 minutes, drop back to its original level when the angle is reopened by bright light. However, if the IOP was elevated during the darkroom test due to coincidental diurnal IOP fluctuation, rather than by closure of the angle, we can expect no such rapid drop back to the original level. The time course of diurnal IOP fluctuations is much slower than the time course of the fall of IOP when a closed angle is reopened.

The bright-light test should be a routine procedure after apparently positive darkroom tests. Of course, in cases in which bright light does not open the angle, this test is of no value. Under such circumstances, one might have recourse to the bright-light and thymoxamine test.

BRIGHT-LIGHT AND THYMOXAMINE TEST

The bright-light and thymoxamine test[4,5] is the opposite of the darkroom test. The patient is placed under bright illumination to induce and maintain miosis, to favor opening of the angle. Accommodation is purposely avoided either by using diffuse illumination or by using a light source very close to the eye. (Perhaps application of plus lenses would be a worthwhile refinement.) The aim is to induce the pupillary sphincter to constrict, but to avoid constriction of the ciliary muscle, so that there will be no complicating alteration of the lens or the trabecular meshwork by the ciliary muscle.

The opening of the angle can be aided considerably by applying 0.5% thymoxamine hydrochloride eye drops in combination with exposure to bright light.[4] Thymoxamine is an alpha-adrenergic blocking agent that temporarily causes the radial muscle fibers of the iris to relax and allows the pupillary sphincter muscle to act unopposed in constricting the pupil and pulling the iris away from the angle wall. Thymoxamine does not appreciably affect the ciliary muscle, and if the angle is already open, it does not influence IOP or facility of aqueous outflow.[5] (In this respect, light and thymoxamine are unlike pilocarpine or cholinergic miotics, which are not well suited for use in testing for angle closure because they cause contraction of both the pupil and the ciliary muscle. By both mechanisms, pilocarpine and cholinergic miotics can influence IOP and aqueous outflow so that they do not serve to distinguish clearly between angle-closure and open-angle glaucoma. They can normalize IOP and outflow not only in angle closure, but also in open-angle glaucoma.) Thymoxamine should be administered to only one eye, and the other eye should be used as a control for diurnal variation.

One precaution to observe in the use of the bright-light test with or without thymoxamine is to avoid subjecting the eye to drying under the influence of local anesthesia and its attendant reduction in blink rate. The only shortcoming of the bright-light test and thymoxamine is that, in some eyes, the miosis induced is not enough to open the angle and lower the IOP; however, where it is positive, this test gives clear uncomplicated evidence.

When should one perform the darkroom test and when the bright-light and thymoxamine test? In patients with narrow angles but normal IOP, the question is whether this narrow, but presumably still functionally open, angle is capable of spontaneous closure. Such a patient should have a darkroom test to answer this question. However, in patients with narrow angles but elevated IOP, there is a separate question: Is the IOP elevation that is already present due to partial angle closure? For this question, the thymoxamine bright-light test should be performed first. This test, by inducing miosis, can reverse appositional (but not synechial) angle closure and lower IOP. It is a separate question (question one above) whether in this latter condition further angle is capable of closure in a darkroom test. Because the IOP is already elevated possibly due to an open-angle component, the potential for diurnal fluctuation due to open-angle glaucoma (and a spurious increase of IOP in the dark) must be kept in mind. This is further reason why a unilateral IOP lowering due to thymoxamine may be more definitive and why the latter test should be performed initially in such patients.

MYDRIATIC PROVOCATIVE TEST

The mydriasis test, which we have never favored (see Chapter 22), is performed by applying a short-acting mydriatic, such as eucatropine, homatropine, cyclopentolate, or phenylephrine, with measurement of IOP and inspection of the angle when the pupil has dilated, to determine if the angle has become closed. In many cases, the test may have been considered negative at the stage of widest mydriasis, and the patient had been dismissed to go home, with or without application of a counteracting drop of pilocarpine. After a few hours, the angle unexpectedly closed and an acute attack developed. This has had unfortunate consequences for patients who did not understand what was happening or who did not promptly obtain treatment for their condition.

The mydriasis test has many disadvantages. It is less natural and physiologic than the darkroom or bright-light test. It is often negative in eyes that are subject to actual spontaneous episodes of subacute angle closure, yet it can cause closure of narrow angles that might never close spontaneously. It is otherwise treacherous in that it may belatedly induce an angle-closure attack and, for greatest safety, would require surveillance of the patient for many hours. In certain cases of open-angle glaucoma,[6,7] cycloplegic mydriatics can cause an increase of IOP by impairment of facility of aqueous outflow without closure of the angle, necessitating careful, critical gonioscopy to minimize the chances of misinterpretation of an IOP increase with this test. If adrenergic mydriatics are used, it must be remembered that they have potentially confusing side effects, reducing aqueous formation in some eyes and, in rare instances, causing an increase of IOP in open-angle glaucomatous eyes without causing the angle to close, possibly from pigment particle liberation[8] (see Chapter 21).

Therefore, we rarely perform the mydriatic test to diagnose angle-closure glaucoma. However, as discussed in Chapter 25, we routinely perform a phenylephrine provocative test after laser iridectomy to rule out a plateau iris syndrome and establish baseline parameters for future evaluation.

Mapstone[9] proposed that phenylephrine combined with pilocarpine might be useful as a provocative test for angle closure, but long-term observation has not substantiated this theory.[10]

REFERENCES

1. Hyams SW, Friedman Z, Neumann E. Elevated intraocular pressure in the prone position. A new provocative test for angle-closure glaucoma. *Am J Ophthalmol.* 1968;66:661-672.
2. Friedman Z, Neumann E. Comparison of prone-position, darkroom, and mydriatic tests for angle-closure glaucoma before and after peripheral iridectomy. *Am J Ophthalmol.* 1972;74:24-27.
3. Wilensky JT, Kaufman PL, Frohlichstein D, et al. Follow-up of angle-closure glaucoma suspects. *Am J Ophthalmol.* 1993;115:338-346.
4. Wand M, Grant WM. The thymoxamine test: a test to differentiate angle-closure glaucoma from open-angle glaucoma with narrow angles. *Arch Ophthalmol.* 1978;96:1009-1011.
5. Wand M, Grant WM. Thymoxamine hydrochloride: effects on the facility of outflow and intraocular pressure. *Invest Ophthalmol.* 1976;15:400-403.
6. Harris LS, Galin MA. Cycloplegic provocative testing. *Arch Ophthalmol.* 1969;81:544-547.
7. Harris LS, Galin MA, Mittag TW. Cycloplegic provocative testing and topical administration of steroids. *Arch Ophthalmol.* 1971;86:12-14.
8. Epstein DL, Boger WP, Grant WM. Phenylephrine provocative testing in the pigmentary dispersion syndrome. *Am J Ophthalmol.* 1978;85:43-50.
9. Mapstone R. Outflow changes in positive provocative tests. *Br J Ophthalmol.* 1977;61:634-636.
10. Wishart PK. Can the pilocarpine phenylephrine provocative test be used to detect covert angle closure? *Br J Ophthalmol.* 1991;75:615-618.

SECONDARY ANGLE-CLOSURE GLAUCOMAS

28

Principles of
Secondary Angle-Closure Glaucomas

David L. Epstein, MD, MMM

In Chapter 22, the mechanisms underlying the primary angle-closure glaucomas were discussed. The fundamental concept was that of pupillary block, wherein fluid pressure in the posterior chamber from the normal secretion of aqueous humor ballooned the peripheral iris forward over the trabecular meshwork and thus closed the angle (see Figure 22-2). Peripheral iridectomy, by equalizing the pressure in the posterior and anterior chambers, eliminated this fluid pressure vector from the posterior chamber acting on the iris. The key concept in such a pupillary block mechanism is that of posterior chamber aqueous humor acting as the force, resulting in the angle closure. In contrast, in plateau iris syndrome, in addition to a relative pupillary block mechanism, the ciliary process causes direct crowding of the iris itself into the angle and is another mechanism for angle closure (see Figure 26-1).

In some secondary angle-closure glaucomas, such as that due to the iridocorneal endothelial (ICE) syndrome (see Chapter 32) or neovascular glaucoma (see Chapter 31), there are other abnormal local iris and angle factors acting to close the angle directly.

In other secondary angle-closure glaucomas, there is some additional force acting to close the angle. Conceptually, this additional force might act by itself to directly force the iris into the angle or by acting to move the crystalline lens forward, causing pupillary block (wherein the resulting increased fluid pressure from aqueous humor in the posterior chamber acts to force the peripheral iris over the angle). This may be termed a *secondary pupillary block*. The possibility for either or both of these 2 mechanisms in the secondary angle-closure glaucomas needs to be constantly kept in mind, for it is not rare for some patients in this category to respond favorably to laser iridectomy (even though primary pupillary block is not the initiating mechanism causing the disease).

Examples of the first mechanism include cysts of the ciliary body (see Chapter 34) or tumors, such as melanoma, that mechanically may push the iris into the angle (see Chapter 41); forward rotations of the ciliary body from choroidal detachment, hemorrhage, or scleral buckling that may then push the iris forward (see Chapter 33); and possible cases of ciliary body swelling, as seen in certain inflammatory syndromes and possibly after panretinal photocoagulation and in cases of transient myopia due to idiosyncratic systemic drug reaction (see Chapter 36). (In these cases, local accumulation of suprachoroidal fluid and forward rotation of the ciliary body may be an alternative explanation to that of ciliary body swelling and may also explain certain cases of so-called loose lens syndrome; see Chapter 29.) In all of these conditions, pathological processes affecting the ciliary body itself result in direct pressure of the ciliary processes on the iris to close the angle.

In other conditions, pathology involving vitreous volume, such as malignant glaucoma (see Chapter 29) and angle-closure glaucoma after vitreous hemorrhage, central retinal vein occlusion (see Chapter 35), and possibly panretinal photocoagulation, and certain volume-occupying massive forms of acute macular degeneration may result in pressure from the vitreous that shifts the entire lens-iris diaphragm forward (axial shallowing). Grant has observed that, in eyes with malignant glaucoma, the crystalline lens equator tends to extend behind and peripheral to the tips of the ciliary processes so that the lens equator is in a position to push the ciliary processes and the iris forward over the angle in response to this pressure from the vitreous. Likely, this relationship of the crystalline lens equator to the tips of the ciliary processes is an anatomical pre-condition in such eyes that have a narrowed middle segment that is accentuated by increasing lens size with increasing age. An expanded vitreous volume, as is

- 287 -

Kahook MY, Schuman JS, eds.
Chandler and Grant's Glaucoma, Fifth Edition (pp 287-288).
© 2013 SLACK Incorporated.

believed to occur acutely in the various malignant glaucoma syndromes, thus results in a secondary angle-closure glaucoma. However, whether angle closure in all such cases finally results from the ciliary processes themselves, in response to this posterior pressure, pushing the iris into the angle, or whether in some cases the forward shift of the lens-iris diaphragm from the increased fluid pressure in the expanded vitreous itself directly pushes the iris into the angle is not certain. Likely, in such eyes with expanded vitreous volume and a forward shift in the lens-iris diaphragm, there is some distortion of the anatomy of the posterior chamber and the zonules (the posterior zonules normally merge into the anterior hyaloid[1]).

In some cases in which vitreous pressure is hypothesized to be involved, the initiating event may be an increase in retinal volume (eg, after central retinal vein occlusion, acute exudative detachment of the macula,[2] or after panretinal photocoagulation) that conceptually acts on a noncompressible vitreous to shift the lens-iris diaphragm forward. Alternatively, these conditions may themselves result in fluid movement into the vitreous cavity, which itself is expanded in volume as presumably occurs in syndromes involving massive vitreous hemorrhage. In either case, vitreous volume acts as a mass to shallow the anterior chamber. The question as to why in some cases a shift in the lens-iris diaphragm occurs as a result of these diseases, and in other cases does not, will be discussed in Chapter 29, but it is believed to be a result of differences in constitutive "vitreous humor permeability" to fluid flow and transfer.

Thus, these secondary angle-closure glaucomas that involve pressure from behind the iris may result from mechanical forces from the ciliary body or the vitreous. As mentioned, the forward shift of the crystalline lens represents a separate additional mechanism—that of secondary pupillary block. A third possible mechanism, at least theoretically, is for the edge of the crystalline lens equator to itself directly push the iris into the angle. This might occur with a gross mismatch of the size of the crystalline lens to that of the middle segment of the eye, as might be conceived to occur in certain congenital conditions, nanophthalmos, or perhaps with cataract formation in certain phacomorphic glaucomas. We must all remember this possibility, especially as we face new entities of secondary angle-closure glaucoma, but our suspicion is that such a postulated direct crystalline lens force acting on the iris itself (without an intervening effect of the crystalline lens on ciliary processes as proposed for malignant glaucoma) and independent of pupillary block rarely if ever occurs because the equator of the crystalline lens likely does not extend far enough peripherally to close the angle. In fact, most cases of phacomorphic glaucoma (see Chapter 47) are not due to this mechanism, but rather pupillary block[3] from the enlarged crystalline lens. Thus, it is usually fluid pressure in the posterior chamber that exerts the force on the posterior iris surface to close the angle (ie, pupillary block).

All these secondary mechanisms should be kept in mind as we now discuss the various specific entities that constitute the secondary angle-closure glaucomas in the subsequent chapters. These mechanisms provide a unifying construct that explains how pressure from behind can cause the angle-closure glaucoma. However, these are usually complicated cases, and we still have much to learn about the actual mechanisms involved. New syndromes or subgroups are inevitable as we increase our understanding. These concepts likely oversimplify what is occurring in individual cases, but these constructs do allow a framework in which to initially classify these conditions to eventually increase our understanding. In the short term, this will enable effective patient management. Some of these cases only behave as if the above were the mechanisms, but if these concepts result in appropriate treatment, then this is worthwhile.

It is important to remember that these conditions of pressure from behind can cause a secondary pupillary block mechanism due to the forward movement of the crystalline lens. A diagnosis of pupillary block needs to be initially entertained as at least one contributing factor and the potential benefit of laser iridectomy contemplated. In fact, certain conditions, such as malignant glaucoma, require the presence of a patent peripheral iridectomy for both diagnosis and therapy.

REFERENCES

1. Streeten BW, Pulaski JP. Posterior zonules and lens extraction. *Arch Ophthalmol.* 1978;96(1):132-138.
2. Wood WJ, Smith TR. Senile disciform macular degeneration complicated by massive hemorrhagic retinal detachment and angle closure glaucoma. *Retina.* 1983;3(4):296-303.
3. Tomey KF, al-Rajhi AA. Neodymium:YAG laser iridotomy in the initial management of phacomorphic glaucoma. *Ophthalmology.* 1992;99(5):660-665.

29

The Malignant Glaucoma Syndromes

Ian P. Conner, MD, PhD; Joel S. Schuman, MD, FACS; and David L. Epstein, MD, MMM

The condition of malignant glaucoma,[1,2] sometimes called *ciliary block glaucoma*[3,4] or *aqueous misdirection syndrome*, either equivalently or only for certain clinical subtypes, is a dramatic form of secondary angle-closure glaucoma that is sustained despite the presence of a patent peripheral iridectomy. The signature of the condition is that of axial shallowing of the anterior chamber (ie, the crystalline lens has moved forward) (Table 29-1). Classically, malignant glaucoma is a postoperative condition after glaucoma filtration surgery, cataract or combined cataract/filtration surgery, or surgical peripheral iridectomy (Figure 29-1). It has not unequivocally been observed after laser iridotomy (although there have been a few reports[5-7]), in contrast to its noted occurrence after surgical iridectomy, and any explanation of possible pathogenesis must explain this difference.

Some have described forms of malignant glaucoma as a preoperative entity.[8] Although we still have an incomplete understanding of this complicated disorder and we should not be too quick to dismiss new observations, most of these latter observations probably can be explained by other phenomena, such as the normal forward movement of the crystalline lens under the influence of cholinergic drugs,[9] primary choroidal detachment syndromes resulting in loosening of zonular tension and forward lens movement that accompanies the forward rotation of the ciliary body, undiagnosed crystalline lens subluxation, and certain poorly understood loose lens syndromes. The malignant glaucoma syndromes may share common features (eg, limited vitreous fluid permeability) with other conditions, such as angle-closure glaucoma secondary to central retinal vein occlusion (see Chapter 35) or massive subretinal exudation.[10] However, these latter conditions frequently resolve (although there may be sequelae from the angle-closure episode). In contrast, malignant glaucoma is a sustained progressive process that characteristically results in blindness if not appropriately treated.[11] It is incorrect, therefore, to lump all flat chambers into a category of *malignant glaucoma*.

The latter term should only be used to describe a postoperative condition of axial shallowing of the anterior chamber where other causes, such as choroidal detachment and hemorrhage, have been ruled out.

It is because of this characteristic progression to blindness that malignant glaucoma truly deserves to be called malignant. (It is not appropriate to use the term *malignant* in front of patients because of the known connotation with cancer; alternative terms may be used. However, the term *malignant glaucoma* is well established in the literature, and among clinicians, it seems appropriate to continue to use this and especially to avoid implications of diverse unproven mechanisms implied with use of alternative terminology.)

There is a rich heritage of thought concerning malignant (ciliary block) glaucoma. We owe a great debt to Shaffer,[2-4] Chandler,[1,11-14] Grant,[13,14] and Simmons[14-16] for the evolution of our concepts.

DIFFERENTIAL DIAGNOSIS

It is important to state that not all postoperative angle-closure glaucoma is malignant glaucoma, nor are all postoperative flat chambers associated with elevated IOP (Table 29-2). The diagnosis of malignant glaucoma requires at a minimum axial shallowing of the anterior chamber, elevated intraocular pressure (IOP), the presence of a patent iridectomy or iridotomy, and the absence of suprachoroidal fluid or blood. There may, however, be supraciliary effusions present in malignant glaucoma.

When presented with postoperative angle-closure glaucoma, even with axial shallowing, the first diagnosis to be eliminated is pupillary block. A patent iridectomy or iridotomy (that is not sequestered posteriorly) that allows free communication between posterior and anterior chambers needs to be present. The surgical iridectomy or laser iridotomy must not be too central. If in doubt, the first step is to place another peripheral laser iridotomy. Again, it must be remembered that

Kahook MY, Schuman JS, eds.
Chandler and Grant's Glaucoma, Fifth Edition (pp 289-304).
© 2013 SLACK Incorporated.

TABLE 29-1. FEATURES OF MALIGNANT GLAUCOMA	
Feature	**Comment**
Postoperative condition	Malignant glaucoma only occurs in the postoperative setting, usually after fistulizing operations with or without cataract surgery, cataract surgery alone, or (historically) after surgical iridectomy.
Patient predisposition	Patients at greatest risk are those with a small, hyperopic eye, particularly those with a history of chronic angle-closure glaucoma with peripheral anterior synechiae.
Flat anterior chamber	Progressive axial shallowing of the anterior chamber is essential to the diagnosis.
Elevated IOP	IOP is higher than expected; with functioning filtering bleb, IOP may be in the teens; however, IOP usually rises progressively.
Additional requirements	Patients should have a patent peripheral iridectomy or iridotomy and a dilated exam and/or ultrasound (B scan) to rule out choroidal effusion or hemorrhage.

TABLE 29-2. DIFFERENTIAL DIAGNOSIS OF MALIGNANT GLAUCOMA	
Disorder	**Comment**
Suprachoroidal hemorrhage	Axial shallowing is often present; severe, acute pain; choroidal elevation on fundus exam or ultrasound; high IOP acutely but usually subsides within 12 to 24 hours.
Choroidal effusion	Usually, patients are hypotonous; peripheral anterior chamber shallowing is common; axial shallowing is usually less prominent but may progress as choroidal effusions enlarge; pain is unusual; choroidal elevation is usually visible by fundus exam or ultrasound.
Secondary postoperative angle closure following vitreoretinal surgery	Axial depth may be reduced in patients status postscleral buckling surgery, but usually only moderate in degree and not progressive; choroidal effusion may also be present in these patients.

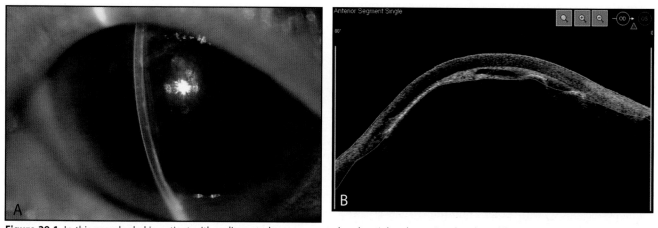

Figure 29-1. In this pseudophakic patient with malignant glaucoma, central and peripheral anterior chamber obliteration is readily noted. (A) Slit-beam photography shows near cornea-intraocular lens touch. (B) Visante anterior segment OCT shows obliteration of the anterior chamber with anterior rotation of the ciliary body and iris.

axial shallowing of the anterior chamber, perhaps initiated by a transient wound leak, can bring the crystalline lens to the pupil and thus lead to pupillary block. (But, as discussed in Chapter 22, pupillary block by itself does not cause axial shallowing of the anterior chamber, only peripheral shallowing.)

In malignant glaucoma, the IOP is elevated. However, in the presence of functioning fistulization, the IOP may not be very high (eg, only in the low teens). In contrast, when there is simply overfiltration and secondary choroidal detachment (see Chapter 60) after filtration surgery, the shallow or flat anterior chamber is associated with a very low IOP, in the low single digits, usually not in the low teens. Thus, although malignant glaucoma is commonly thought of as a flat chamber with high IOP, this concept should be modified in the presence of a functioning filtration bleb. In fact, a good rule is that a flat or shallow anterior chamber associated with IOP in the teens after fistulizing surgery is malignant glaucoma (or suprachoroidal hemorrhage) until proven otherwise.

Bleeding into the suprachoroidal space, which is not uncommon after fistulizing surgery (especially when antifibrotic therapy initially produces postoperative hypotony), actively occupies volume in the suprachoroidal space and thus acts as a mass that can rotate the ciliary body forward, release zonular tension, and result in forward crystalline lens movement. Delayed postoperative suprachoroidal hemorrhage can thus mimic malignant glaucoma. This condition can be diagnosed by indirect ophthalmoscopy, ultrasound, or at the time of interventional surgery where a posterior sclerotomy is performed prior to vitreous surgery. (Such suprachoroidal bleeding usually occurs in a setting of postoperative hypotony accompanied by secondary choroidal effusions, acting to prevent clotting of suprachoroidal blood.) Delayed suprachoroidal hemorrhage is a distinct entity, and the term *malignant glaucoma* should not be used to describe it.

In contrast, the usual postoperative serous choroidal detachment associated with hypotony and overfiltration after fistulizing surgery is a secondary event, which often does not act as a mass to shallow the anterior chamber. One might oversimply view this as a secondary response to fill the space in a soft eye. However, there are certain other conditions where a serous choroidal detachment can act as a mass to shallow the anterior chamber, appearing similar to the occurrence of suprachoroidal hemorrhage. Examples of such primary choroidal effusions include nanophthalmos (see Chapter 30), conditions of increased orbital venous pressure such as dural shunt and Sturge-Weber syndrome (see Chapter 46), and active uveal effusion syndromes including the one associated with human immunodeficiency virus (HIV) infection.[17,18] Each of these conditions can cause a secondary angle-closure glaucoma that is distinct from malignant glaucoma and need to be first ruled out for a diagnosis of malignant glaucoma to be established.

There are other flat chamber conditions associated with a localized anterior choroidal detachment that appears to be a primary phenomenon. These anterior uveal effusion syndromes have been characterized using ultrasound biomicroscopy and anterior segment optical coherence tomography.[19] Presumably, there is some inflammatory component to these conditions as they seem to respond to corticosteroids and cycloplegics. In the past, these conditions were probably described under categories of *ciliary body swelling*[20-22] or *loose lens syndromes*. The literature has reported numerous cases that appeared to be a result of an idiosyncratic systemic drug reaction (see Chapter 36). We obviously have much more to learn about these conditions and other related loose lens conditions, but these nonoperative conditions are not malignant glaucoma and do not involve a primary abnormality in the hyaloid, which we believe to be the underlying and unifying mechanism involved in malignant glaucoma.[23-26]

Malignant glaucoma is traditionally associated with smaller, hyperopic eyes. As will be discussed, we believe that this may relate to the small middle segment of such eyes and its relationship to the anterior hyaloid. Certainly, in such eyes that undergo intraocular surgery, the clinician should be on guard for postoperative malignant glaucoma. (It can even be argued that all such eyes should have a surgical peripheral iridectomy at the time of surgery, even if simple cataract surgery alone is performed. There is a strong clinical sense that, in many cases, pupillary block may occur first, followed by malignant glaucoma, and thus this simple surgical iridectomy procedure might lessen the occurrence. Alternatively, perioperative laser iridotomy could also be performed.) However, there are also other eyes that are not hyperopic that seem to develop a malignant glaucoma syndrome postoperatively. Some have used the term *aqueous misdirection* or other names to describe this occurrence, but clinically the condition behaves as malignant glaucoma, and discrimination in terminology potentially adds to confusion regarding management. As we will describe in this chapter, it is proposed that a similar pathogenic mechanism is involved in malignant glaucoma, whether the eye is hyperopic or not.

UNIFYING CONCEPTS IN PATHOGENESIS

There is evidently much more that we need to learn about this condition that will lead to a clearer understanding of the events involved. One does not wish to oversimplify what is a complex process in eyes with complicated disease and the potential for multiple mechanisms of pathology. Yet, there is a need for some template for our understanding; otherwise, worsening confusion about what to do for the patient can result. For example, lumping suprachoroidal hemorrhage or effusion into a malignant glaucoma category because of lack of clarity about the latter can interfere with appropriate clinical treatment.

What do we know about malignant glaucoma clinically and experimentally? We know that disruption of the anterior hyaloid with the yttrium-aluminum-garnet (YAG) laser by itself can cure phakic, aphakic, and pseudophakic forms of the disease.[25-31] We know from Chandler's observations[11,12] that puncture of the anterior hyaloid through an anterior approach can cure the condition both in phakic and aphakic eyes. We know that puncture of the hyaloid from a posterior sclerotomy approach,[14,15] as will be described, can cure the condition in phakic malignant glaucoma, if one is far enough anterior. If one goes too far posterior (presumably posterior to the anterior hyaloid) in performing surgical vitrectomy, the condition of malignant glaucoma can recur.[32] Also, although classically the posterior sclerotomy surgical operation was intended to aspirate a posterior pocket of aqueous humor "locked" in the vitreous, the procedure still worked even when liquid vitreous could not be aspirated[32] (presumably by the puncture itself disrupting the peripheral anterior hyaloid).

We know that mydriatic-cycloplegic therapy[13] can reverse malignant glaucoma in about 50% of affected phakic eyes, but there is risk of recurrence when the therapy is discontinued. Conversely, the use of miotics in postoperative eyes can precipitate the onset of malignant glaucoma.

We know that malignant glaucoma was not rare after surgical iridectomy, but is very rare[5-7] after laser iridotomy.

There is also a strong clinical sense that wound leak, even if transient, or overfiltration[33] may predispose an eye to malignant glaucoma, and such events seem to be a common theme in nonhyperopic eyes that develop this condition.

What do we know experimentally?[23,34] At least in enucleated human eyes, we know that if we direct the normal rate of aqueous humor flow (2 to 3 microliters/minute) entirely into the vitreous, malignant glaucoma does not result.[23,24] In fact, in such circumstances, the anterior hyaloid and vitreous offer insignificant resistance to forward fluid flow. Thus, it would seem that aqueous humor secreted into the posterior chamber normally has free access into (and out of) the vitreous cavity.[35] On the other hand, if one limits the amount of available hyaloid for fluid transfer,[34] then there is substantial resistance to forward fluid movement from the vitreous, and vitreous volume continues to expand if aqueous humor continues to be directed into the vitreous cavity, and the anterior chamber then shallows. Further, when the anterior chamber is initially decompressed (then re-established), this process is accentuated.[23]

Although the above is true experimentally for the normal aged (enucleated) human eye, in certain nonprimate species such as the enucleated calf eye, the hyaloid normally demonstrates much more resistance to fluid flow.[23] Thus, there are differences among species in hyaloid permeability and likely also among individuals. The hyperopic human vitreous may be more viscous and restrictive than that in the myopic eye.

Putting this all together, we propose that the anterior hyaloid, either because of inherent permeability or the amount of available hyaloid surface area for fluid transfer, is involved in the pathogenesis of the malignant glaucoma syndromes. Thus, a maintained increase in total vitreous volume (rather than the presence of sequestered pockets of aqueous humor

in the vitreous) is responsible for the axial flattening of the anterior chamber. Expanded vitreous volume can obliterate available peripheral anterior hyaloid for fluid transfer by movement of the hyaloid into apposition with the posterior ciliary body. In this "silent zone" just behind the posterior chamber (and in continuity with it), there is likely great variation in the amount of space between the hyaloid and ciliary body under baseline conditions.[36] In the hyperopic eye with a crowded middle segment, the peripheral anterior hyaloid in its normal position is probably quite close to the posterior ciliary body.

Decompression of the anterior chamber as happens with surgical procedures (but not laser iridotomy) might produce movement of the peripheral anterior hyaloid further forward into apposition with the ciliary body. In fact, if one accepts the concept of possible zonular distortion from anterior chamber decompression, one can hypothesize that, with this forward movement, the anterior hyaloid (which is continuous with the posterior zonules[37]) could be placed into direct apposition with portions of the secreting ciliary processes, even in phakic eyes. Thus, aqueous humor might move directly into the vitreous cavity. This is a hypothesis (and there are other possibilities for the cause of the initial expansion of vitreous volume that is then maintained in an expanded condition from the resulting obliteration of hyaloid surface area), because this process cannot be directly visualized in the phakic eye. On the other hand, this has been directly observed to have occurred in certain aphakic eyes where the hyaloid coated the surface of the ciliary processes.[2] Presumably, this can also develop in pseudophakic eyes[26] with any type of zonular disruption.

The decompression of the anterior chamber that occurs with surgical peripheral iridectomy does not occur with laser iridotomy and results in the movement forward (and peripheral) of the anterior hyaloid, contributing to the above events wherein the anterior hyaloid permeability/surface area is limited. An important clinical corollary of this would seem to be the imperative to minimize this decompression-related shallowing of the anterior chamber both intra- and postoperatively. For example, especially in hyperopic eyes at greater risk, using viscoelastic in the anterior chamber to prevent shallowing intraoperatively might be useful. Using a tighter rather than looser scleral flap with judicious use of suture lysis (one suture at a time) might minimize the chance of postoperative anterior chamber shallowing due to overfiltration that could then lead to a malignant glaucoma process.[33] We believe this approach is beneficial and, in fact, is what we would recommend as a general strategy.

This concept would explain the observed efficacy[25-31] of the YAG hyaloidotomy procedure in phakic, aphakic, and pseudophakic eyes and the above clinical experience with surgical techniques that have indicated the need for anterior enough positioning[32] to disrupt the anterior hyaloid. Surgical decompression during predisposing operations could be the initiating event that brings the hyaloid to the ciliary body, which leads to the sustaining effect of expanded vitreous volume that shallows the anterior chamber. Mydriatic-cycloplegic therapy might be effective, as originally intended, to tighten the lens-zonular diaphragm[13] to resist this force from behind, but also because cycloplegic drugs act to dilate the ciliary body ring[38] and thus potentially could move the ciliary body outward away from the peripheral anterior hyaloid. Conversely, cholinergic miotics might narrow the ciliary body ring and move the ciliary body closer to the hyaloid.

One also could conceptualize that if it is possible to restore the normal anatomy and the small space normally present between the peripheral hyaloid and the ciliary body in the "silent zone,"[36] then without other reinitiating events, such as repeat decompression of the anterior chamber, the vicious circle could be broken. There has been a strong clinical impression that, with the surgical technique for malignant glaucoma, an essential component was, in fact, to re-establish the normal anatomy and even expand the anterior chamber at the end of the operation and "push" things backward behind the iris.[32]

Understanding this construct allows one to appropriately diagnose and treat affected patients. For example, an attempt should always be made, at least in the pseudophakic eye, to disrupt the hyaloid (and intervening tissue, such as residual lens capsule) with the YAG laser to allow a channel for free communication between the posterior segment and anterior chamber before proceeding to surgical vitrectomy,[26] although some practitioners may choose to treat initially with vitrectomy. Nonetheless, the critical role of the anterior hyaloid in the pathogenesis seems clear from both clinical and experimental data.

What is missing in this (and any other) construct is an understanding of the initiating event in this whole process; that is, how is vitreous volume initially expanded?

Decompression of the anterior chamber surgically and the resulting movement of the peripheral hyaloid into apposition with the ciliary body would explain the different incidence of malignant glaucoma between surgical iridectomy and laser iridotomy, and there are some experimental data that are consistent with this.[23] With zonular distortion that might result from this anterior chamber decompression, it is possible that the peripheral hyaloid might come directly into apposition with the ciliary processes, and aqueous humor could conceivably be directly secreted into the vitreous across the apposed hyaloid. Still, this does not seem quite enough to fully explain the true initiating event.

Perhaps with the sudden onset of pupillary block, which may precede other events, aqueous humor is suddenly forced into the vitreous. That is, some nonsteady state event occurs. We do know clinically that, in the classically described surgical procedure for malignant glaucoma, one can inject balanced salt solution over the peripheral iridectomy too vigorously, and vitreous volume can suddenly expand and be maintained with a recurrence of malignant glaucoma. Alternatively, we

also know that there is a constant movement of fluid derived from aqueous humor posteriorly through the retina, presumably under the influence of the retinal pigment epithelium pump.[39-44] It is possible that, with the onset of pupillary block and high IOP, this posterior pump is impaired, and vitreous volume suddenly expands.[45] There is a report of one human eye enucleated shortly after an attack of untreated angle-closure glaucoma, which purportedly did show an expanded vitreous volume (and obliteration of the space between the peripheral hyaloid and ciliary body).[46]

Understanding the initiating event is nevertheless still a missing piece of the puzzle that, if elucidated, might provide important new insights. Yet, there still is good understanding based on both clinical experience and laboratory experimentation on which to successfully treat most patients with this condition, unlike in a former era when malignant glaucoma syndromes were truly blinding.[11] Most likely, the initiating event involves some nonsteady state phenomenon or anatomical distortion that results in a maintained increase in vitreous volume, which then requires disruption of the anterior hyaloid to re-establish the normal steady state. From a clinical point of view, the (peripheral) anterior hyaloid needs to be disrupted and thus eliminated as a fluid barrier.[47]

If there are sequestered spaces in the vitreous due to inflammation, etc, the hyaloid potentially needs to be disrupted in multiple locations to permit free communication between the vitreous cavity and the anterior chamber, as is normally the situation.[48]

CLINICAL OCCURRENCE AND THE EXAMINATION OF THE PATIENT

The usual clinical situation is that of a postoperative patient following fistulizing, combined cataract/fistulizing, or cataract surgery. Malignant glaucoma can occur any time during the usual postoperative period of a day to weeks, or even occasionally months. Most commonly, there is an indication of the condition on the first postoperative day.

Important times when the possibility of malignant glaucoma should be kept in mind are following suture lysis[33] at the filtration site (where shallowing of the anterior chamber associated with a sudden increase in outflow can subsequently lead to malignant glaucoma). Another time to keep in mind is when routine postoperative cycloplegics are stopped. In this situation, the cycloplegics may have prevented the occurrence of the condition by their therapeutic effects of tightening the lens-zonular diaphragm and dilating the ciliary body ring, and cessation can allow the syndrome to develop.

One begins by carefully examining the filtration bleb or cataract wound. As discussed above, shallowing of the anterior chamber due either to overfiltration or a wound leak (that may have been transient) might initiate the subsequent development of a malignant glaucoma process. More importantly, a shallow chamber from overfiltration or a wound leak needs to be differentiated from malignant glaucoma. In the former situation, the IOP is low, whereas in malignant glaucoma it is generally high, although again it must be emphasized that with a functioning filtration bleb, the IOP might appear within the normal range (eg, only in the low teens). In simple overfiltration with a shallow anterior chamber, the IOP should be in the low single digits, not in the low teens. Stated another way, following filtration surgery with an IOP in the low teens, the anterior chamber should not be shallow. Special attention to possible artifacts needs to be considered when measuring the IOP in the presence of a flat chamber.[49]

In a susceptible hyperopic eye, a postoperative shallow anterior chamber due to overfiltration should be more vigorously treated than that in a myopic eye. Such eyes need to be followed very carefully for development of a malignant glaucoma process.

What is the axial depth of the anterior chamber (as well as peripheral depth)? Has there in fact been axial shallowing? What is the contour of the iris (is there a convex forward peripheral ballooning of the iris suggestive of pupillary block)? Is the iridectomy or iridotomy patent? Is it far enough peripheral (ie, beyond the lens equator)? Could the iridectomy or iridotomy be sequestered posteriorly? Has swelling of the crystalline lens occurred (that might be simulating axial anterior chamber shallowing and malignant glaucoma)?

Gonioscopy should be performed to confirm suspected closure of the angle, to assess the contour of the iris and the patency of the iridectomy or iridotomy, as well as to look for retro-iridal abnormalities. In cases with choroidal effusions, the ciliary processes may be rotated forward, pressing against the base of the iris. Choroidal detachments or hemorrhage, if anterior, can sometimes be seen well through the mirrored Goldmann-type examination lens. In malignant glaucoma, quite commonly, the tips of the ciliary processes are observed to overlap anteriorly the edge of the crystalline lens equator. Presumably, this is a manifestation of the inherently crowded middle segment of the eye.

Indirect ophthalmoscopy should be performed, looking for possible choroidal detachment or hemorrhage as alternative diagnoses. In addition, possible conditions of acute central retinal vein occlusion (see Chapter 35), massive submacular[10] or vitreous hemorrhage, etc, which could cause a secondary angle-closure glaucoma with shallowing of the axial anterior chamber depth that may mimic malignant glaucoma (but possibly also share some common mechanisms wherein vitreous volume in only certain such patients does not decrease to accommodate the new mass of the lesion), should be evaluated.

Ultrasound[19,31] may aid in the determination of possible choroidal entities such as effusion or hemorrhage, which might simulate malignant glaucoma. As might be surmised from the above discussion of underlying mechanisms, ultrasound-detected abnormalities in the vitreous are not expected

(there is an increase in total vitreous volume with perhaps the usual normal areas of less dense lacunae occasionally, but no mystical pockets of trapped aqueous humor). In fact, except in the case of vitreous hemorrhage producing a pseudomalignant glaucoma syndrome, no vitreous pathology has been consistently observed in malignant glaucoma.

MANAGEMENT OF MALIGNANT GLAUCOMA

The approach to the management of patients with a flat anterior chamber postoperatively is methodical (Table 29-3). Any bleb or wound leak needs to be first addressed. Likely, if malignant glaucoma has developed as a subsequent process, the accompanying inflammation of the eye has resulted in a stoppage of such leakage, but not always. In fact, a continued wound leak, once malignant glaucoma has occurred, may confuse the clinical picture because the IOP may not be very high. If there is any suspicion of a wound leak or overfiltration, this should be treated first while the patient is in the office. If there is no bleb, a large soft contact lens that bridges well over the surgical site can be placed on the eye, and commonly if there is a wound leak, some deepening of the anterior chamber may be observed in 30 minutes. A pressure dressing could also be used in place of a large soft contact lens for a presumed wound leak, but is less predictable (see Chapter 60).

The use of a pressure dressing is both diagnostic and therapeutic—it often seems that once an anterior chamber deepens and presumably normal anatomy is restored, the eye may tend to "take over," and further resolution occurs. Obviously for this to occur, the wound leak will have to stop and/or overfiltration will have to decrease. The latter may have already begun spontaneously, but the anterior chamber is still shallow presumably because there is a new steady-state with the choroidal detachment, although originally only a secondary occurrence, now persisting until IOP can be more dramatically elevated by the pressure dressing (which suddenly can limit the outflow from the eye).

Next, the adequacy of the surgical iridectomy or laser iridotomy needs to be assessed. The iridectomy may be too central (which only became a problem when the initial overfiltration perhaps brought the crystalline lens forward) or sequestered posteriorly. Is the peripheral iris ballooned forward as if there were pupillary block? If in doubt whether pupillary block exists, another laser iridotomy should be performed, usually at a site remote from the surgical site. (Sometimes, at the surgical site, zonules may be partially dehisced, allowing vitreous to displace anteriorly and prevent free communication for aqueous humor secreted into the posterior chamber to come forward into the anterior chamber.) Peripheral iridectomy is performed at the time of filtration surgery to prevent pupillary block and also, perhaps even more importantly, to prevent the iris from rolling into the fistula site and thus

Medical Therapy	Comment
Rule out choroidal hemorrhage or effusion	Fundus exam and/or ultrasound
Rule out overfiltration or wound leak	Seidel test; oversized contact lens, pressure patch, or Simmons shell in hypotonus eyes
Rule out pupillary block	Laser iridotomy if functional iridectomy not present
Cycloplegics: cyclopentolate or tropicamide 1% qid	Short-term cycloplegics are more potent than those that are longer acting and are therefore preferred for initial management
Mydriatics: phenylephrine 2.5% to 5% qid Aqueous suppressants: timolol 0.5% or equivalent bid, brimonidine 0.2% tid, acetazolamide 250 mg po q6h (or dorzolamide 2% tid)	Question patient for contraindications for phenylephrine, beta-blocker, carbonic anhydrase inhibitor, or osmotic therapy and monitor for systemic side effects
Osmotics: glycerin, isosorbide, or mannitol 1 to 1.5 gm/kg q12 h for no more than 24 hours without medical consult	Osmotics should be considered optional therapy, but there may be a rational basis for their use (see text)
Chronic medical therapy (after acute medical treatment success): atropine 1% bid or scopolamine 0.25% bid	Patients may require permanent treatment with long-acting cycloplegics to prevent recurrence of malignant glaucoma; tapering medication should be done slowly and under close observation
Hyaloidotomy with Nd:YAG laser in aphakic or pseudophakic patients	Should be performed concomitantly with medical therapy in patients who have had cataract surgery
Surgical vitrectomy	It is essential that the retinal surgeon disrupt the hyaloid face and confirm that the normal anterior chamber depth has been restored at the end of surgery

TABLE 29-3. MANAGEMENT OF MALIGNANT GLAUCOMA

occluding it. If there is any doubt that the original surgical iridectomy might not be accomplishing these goals, then a laser iridotomy at the surgical site would be indicated.

Except in this circumstance, it is usually best to place a laser iridotomy at a site remote from the fistula wound to rule out the complicated situation described previously in the posterior chamber that may have been surgically induced (eg, broken zonules or inflammatory lacunae). The laser iridotomy should also be placed so that a YAG hyaloidotomy could be subsequently performed through it, because, often, there is overlying corneal edema and a hazy optical view overlying the original surgical iridectomy site. In the case of a superior wound, which may be extensive, one can still place the laser iridotomy superiorly, but perhaps away from the original iridectomy and also away from any location where there may have been an adjacent wound leak. It is technically easier in these usually "hot" eyes to perform the laser iridotomy prior to cycloplegic therapy, if this has not already been instituted, while the pupil is still somewhat miotic.

The next step classically (but now after laser iridotomy) would be the use of mydriatic-cycloplegic therapy[13] in phakic and pseudophakic patients with intact zonules for 5 days

prior to surgical vitrectomy. Presently, with the possibility of true cure with a successful YAG hyaloidotomy, and considering the danger of recurrence of malignant glaucoma once cycloplegics are stopped, it is not certain in straightforward cases whether the next step should be mydriatic-cycloplegic therapy or YAG hyaloidotomy. Two points are worth making here: often, these are complicated cases, and it is not known what the exact diagnosis is at the beginning, and if the IOP is controlled medically (see below) and there is no cornea lens touch, then it is not an emergency for YAG hyaloidotomy to be performed. In fact, there is a point for quieting the eye first with topical steroids, which might make the procedure easier to perform technically (certainly after corneal edema is reversed with lowering the IOP and there is quieting of the eye). Also, there might be less chance for a recondensation of the hyaloid[25] in a quieter eye. On the other hand, the longer the angle is closed, especially in a "hot" eye, the greater the risk of permanent peripheral anterior synechiae. Nevertheless, a reasonable tactic is to lower the IOP medically with aqueous suppressants (beta-blockers, brimonidine, and possibly carbonic anhydrase inhibitors) while simultaneously initiating mydriatic-cycloplegic drug therapy. Also, osmotics[50] should

THE HISTORY OF
MYDRIATIC-CYCLOPLEGIC THERAPY
David L. Epstein, MD, MMM

The origin in thought and history of mydriatic-cycloplegic therapy[1] for malignant glaucoma is of interest. Grant and Chandler in a dialogue about a specific patient with malignant glaucoma reasoned that if the lens-zonular diaphragm could be tightened by this therapy, it could resist the pressure from behind. In their first 8 subsequent cases, such mydriatic-cycloplegic therapy worked successfully in all 8. However, in their next 6 cases after this publication, this therapy did not work at all, and those trained by Chandler recall with much poignancy conversations with him and Dr. Grant where they with humility and humor wondered what would have happened if the latter 6 cases (where the treatment was unsuccessful) had been the initial patients chosen! They wondered how many other procedures for other glaucoma conditions that ultimately would prove to be effective might have been abandoned too prematurely. In the subsequent years, mydriatic-cycloplegic therapy has, in general, demonstrated a 50% success rate for the treatment of malignant glaucoma.

REFERENCE

1. Chandler PA, Grant WM. Mydriatic-cycloplegic treatment in malignant glaucoma. *Arch Ophthalmol.* 1962;62:353-359.

be considered to lower the IOP and also to temporarily dehydrate and thus decrease vitreous volume. The only caution should be that, if one does too many maneuvers simultaneously, it may be difficult to define exactly what is beneficial. Furthermore, the osmotic effect on vitreous volume may be only temporary. Theoretically, using the above construct of malignant glaucoma, decreasing aqueous humor formation with the aqueous suppressants alone might act to decrease vitreous volume by decreasing new fluid flow into the vitreous humor cavity.[35]

Mydriatic-Cycloplegic Therapy

It must be remembered that mydriatic-cycloplegic therapy is intended for phakic and pseudophakic, but not aphakic, eyes (where there are no zonules to tighten). In phakic eyes, mydriatic-cycloplegic therapy has a 50% success rate. Curiously, in the past, there were occasional aphakic cases and patients with anterior chamber intraocular lenses after intracapsular cataract surgery where this therapy appeared to be successful. Because cycloplegic therapy may move the ciliary body ring outward[38] away from the hyaloid, there may still be a role even in the absence of an intact zonule/lens diaphragm. Even in aphakic eyes, the vitreous may coat the whole posterior surface of the iris and ciliary body, thereby resulting in a limited hyaloid surface area for fluid transfer into the anterior chamber,[24,26] which might respond beneficially to dilation of the pupil (thus increasing the amount of hyaloid surface area in the pupil). In other words, it may be the mydriatic rather than the cycloplegic effect that is beneficial in aphakic eyes. In previous eras, there was much effort in distinguishing aphakic forms of this condition

from phakic, as obviously there are gross anatomic differences between such eyes. Yet, the above unifying concepts of malignant glaucoma relating to the anterior hyaloid seem applicable in all cases and, importantly, lead to effective therapeutic remedy in phakic, aphakic, and pseudophakic forms of this condition.

The use of a sympathomimetic mydriatic in addition to a cycloplegic drug has demonstrated empirical efficacy and perhaps can be explained by the above pupil effects in certain cases, perhaps also even in some phakic eyes, but more classically its effectiveness was felt to be due to the contraction of the iris dilator muscle and thus the tightening of the iris tone, which might then resist pressure from behind. In addition, the sympathomimetic drugs were believed, to a minor extent, to also contract the sympathetically innervated radial fibers of the ciliary muscle[51] and thus help tighten the zonules between the ciliary muscle and crystalline lens.

Originally, very high strengths of phenylephrine (10%) and atropine (up to 4%) with frequent (4 times a day) instillation were used and are still advocated by some. The clinician needs to be cautious about the occurrence of systemic side effects[52-54] with this, or even with a reduced, regimen. More commonly now, 1% cyclopentolate (or tropicamide) and 2.5% phenylephrine are instilled and the effects observed, especially on the axial anterior chamber depth. It must be remembered that the shorter-acting cycloplegics, such as cyclopentolate or tropicamide, actually produce a greater short-term effect than the longer-acting cycloplegics, such as atropine or scopolamine. The latter agents are more useful in maintaining cycloplegia and mydriasis once initiated. A regimen of 1% tropine and 2.5% phenylephrine twice a day (with monitoring for systemic side effects) may be initiated for the first 5 days of therapy, and, if successful, the phenylephrine can be discontinued and the 1% atropine maintained once a day.

There is substantial risk of recurrence of the malignant glaucoma process once the cycloplegics are stopped. Therefore, even with initial success of mydriatic-cycloplegic therapy, the performance of YAG hyaloidotomy as an elective procedure should be contemplated. In cases in which YAG hyaloidotomy is unsuccessful but cycloplegic therapy is successful, most clinicians have historically felt that continuance of the medical cycloplegic treatment indefinitely was indicated rather than performance of the surgical procedure. Such cases are becoming very rare as we have better established the role for YAG laser treatments and the need to establish communication from the posterior segment to the anterior chamber by removing intervening barriers (in pseudophakic eyes) in addition to the anterior hyaloid.

Yttrium-Aluminum-Garnet Hyaloidotomy

The goal of this procedure[25,26] is to disrupt the peripheral anterior hyaloid without injuring the crystalline lens (in the phakic patient), ciliary body, or zonules. A clear view and sharp focusing is required. Depending on circumstances, this procedure may be performed without any laser contact lens or with an iridotomy or gonioscopic lens.

The usual beginning laser energy is between 4 and 6 millijoules. Obviously, one needs to obtain optical breakdown at the level of the hyaloid, and with murky media or oblique angles of access, higher energy levels are sometimes required. With plasma formation[55] at the site of laser focus, energy moves anteriorly; therefore, it is common to focus posterior to the anterior hyaloid. Sometimes, in truth, one cannot visualize the hyaloid that readily, but one places the focus through the iridectomy or iridotomy behind the zonules but in front of the ciliary body with the intent of having anteriorly moving energy disrupt the hyaloid.

As indicated previously, in an inflamed eye with corneal edema, one may resort, after placing a new laser iridotomy, to using medical mydriatic-cycloplegic and antiglaucoma (aqueous suppressant) therapy for 12 hours or so. The goal of the new iridotomy is to eliminate any residual pupillary block component and permit another access site for a hyaloidotomy.

Clear media and sharp focusing are optimal requirements. Simpler aiming beam mechanisms on the YAG laser are an advantage because often there is some distortion due to the quality of the media. In choosing where to place the preliminary new iridotomy, these factors affecting the potential subsequent hyaloidotomy should be considered.

One attempts to obliterate the hyaloid within the circumference of the overlying (small) iridotomy, although sometimes one shot is all that is required. A single burst should be used for the first shot until one is certain one is in the retro-iridal space, but then a multiple burst mode can be chosen. If one uses the above retrofocusing strategy, one might then choose to come slightly forward with the second laser application. Sometimes, with suboptimal media clarity, one needs to proceed slowly and "feel one's way" forward in this retro-iridal space. But each shot should be precisely focused and orderly, and it is important to avoid a "machine-gunner" approach. That extra-wide shot potentially could injure the crystalline lens, if present, or the ciliary body and zonules.

It is usual to notice a slight deepening of the anterior chamber immediately after this YAG procedure, which increases somewhat over the next hour. Commonly, dramatic deepening of the anterior chamber is not noticed until 12 to 24 hours after the YAG hyaloidotomy. The explanation for this is not certain but possibly might relate to the relatively small size of the hyaloid opening in relation to the expanded vitreous volume. If no deepening is observed at all, then either one has not in fact obliterated the limiting anterior hyaloid membrane, or somehow, perhaps due to sequestered spaces of hyaloid secondary to inflammation, there is still not free communication from the posterior segment into the anterior chamber (through the iridectomy or iridotomy). In a pseudophakic eye, one needs to be certain that lens capsule, retained cortical material, inflammatory debris, or the intraocular lens is not blocking this path.[26] In

a phakic malignant glaucoma condition, these should not be factors, and one should choose to repeat this (including a new iridotomy) in another peripheral location or to perform a central hyaloidotomy,[27] carefully using the principle of retrofocusing (to avoid crystalline lens injury).

Many of these cases are complicated with somewhat hazy views and inexact focusing, but one of us (DLE) has had the opportunity in several, mostly pseudophakic, cases to proceed step by step, placing optical breakdown from the YAG in different discreet locations with the following clinical observations: in pseudophakic eyes, not only the peripheral hyaloid but also all intervening tissue (such as lens capsule and residual cortical lens material) must be perforated to allow full access of the flow pathway from vitreous space to the anterior chamber through the iridectomy or iridotomy. Also, a central hyaloidotomy may not be sufficient because the central space so created may not communicate sufficiently with the anterior chamber because of the intervening lens capsule and intraocular lens. For example, in one patient, after a central anterior hyaloidotomy that was ineffective, a subsequent posterior capsulotomy was also unsuccessful until the posterior capsule underlying a positioning hole in the intraocular lens was subsequently removed with the YAG. Then, the anterior chamber suddenly deepened! In another case, a peripheral and central hyaloidotomy and a central posterior capsulotomy were all unsuccessful until the posterior capsule in front of the original peripheral anterior hyaloidotomy was removed. There must be a free path for fluid to move from the posterior segment (vitreous cavity) to the anterior chamber. In general, this is easier to achieve through the peripheral rather than central hyaloid face.

Complicating this further has been the occurrence of inflammatory recondensations of the hyaloid. We have directly observed this in aphakic eyes[25] where the YAG procedure was initially successful, but then a recurrence of the malignant glaucoma occurred associated with an observed reformation of the anterior hyaloid. Especially in "hot" eyes that have malignant glaucoma, there is the potential for some restricted spaces in the vitreous cavity and in the "silent zone" of the peripheral middle segment of the eye, where ciliary body and hyaloid are in close proximity. We have suspected that this phenomenon may underlie some failures of the YAG procedure.

One must proceed more cautiously and deliberately in a phakic eye because of the risk and consequences of crystalline lens or zonular injury. Yet, there seem to be fewer problems with obstructing postsurgical intervening tissue, and, in fact, central hyaloidotomy has been reported to be effective by itself.[27] Nevertheless, one of us (DLE) would recommend a peripheral approach through a peripheral laser iridotomy with careful retrofocusing in the retro-iridal space, being attentive to remain anterior of the ciliary body and slowly moving forward while attempting also to avoid the zonules (as well as the edge of the crystalline lens). The clinician must be sensitive to the sudden partial deepening of the anterior chamber (which will evolve further to full deepening without need for additional laser applications) as a sign to cease additional laser applications.

Vitrectomy

For patients in whom YAG hyaloidotomy and medical therapy have failed, mechanical vitrectomy can almost always cure this condition. Pseudophakic eyes with malignant glaucoma are referred usually to the retina surgeon for vitrectomy, which is usually curative if care is taken to remove the peripheral anterior hyaloid as a result of the procedure. In fact, the most critical portion of the operation is removal of the anterior hyaloid barrier rather than the removal of the vitreous body itself. However, removal of vitreous may allow restoration of the normal anatomy more quickly by allowing anterior and mid-eye structures to move posteriorly into their more normal anatomic position. Such mechanical vitrectomy is the proper province of the vitreoretinal surgeon, but it must be remembered that the original *Chandler operation* was performed by anterior segment glaucoma surgeons. Such surgery is still curative, but should be undertaken only in exceptional circumstances, as the ready availability of mechanical vitrectomy and improved techniques in this arena have redefined the standard of care, decreasing the likelihood of retinal complications including retinal tears and detachments.[56]

A description of the Chandler operation was elegantly made by Simmons[57] and is included here for historical perspective. As detailed in the box "The Chandler Operation," steps 1 and 2 describe a standard approach for drainage of suprachoroidal fluid and are a critical tool in the glaucoma surgeon's armamentarium. Step 3, describing vitreous surgery, has been supplanted by modern mechanical vitrectomy. The interested reader is referred to prior editions of this text for the accompanying illustrations of this technique.

TREATMENT OF THE FELLOW EYE

If malignant glaucoma occurs in one eye, there is great risk of the fellow eye developing the condition postoperatively. Prophylactic laser iridotomy should almost always be performed in cases where there is evidence of chronic angle-closure or an occludable angle exists. If the fellow eye is at all hyperopic, it may be wise to perform the prophylactic laser iridotomy. Chandler and Grant had a strong clinical sense that eyes with functional angle closure, especially with peripheral anterior synechiae, were at greatest risk for the subsequent development of malignant glaucoma, and, as mentioned, there also is a sense that pupillary block may precede the occurrence of malignant glaucoma in many cases. Thus, it would seem wise to eliminate any pupillary block ahead of time in any eye that might be predisposed to malignant glaucoma.

As mentioned, at the time of intraocular surgery on such fellow eyes, steps should be taken to minimize intraoperative and postoperative anterior chamber shallowing.

OTHER ENTITIES RESEMBLING MALIGNANT GLAUCOMA

Principles

There are some nonoperative conditions that may, at first, behave similarly to malignant glaucoma in that they are characterized by high IOP and a flat (axial) anterior chamber depth. However, one should take care not to classify these entities as malignant glaucoma because it confuses the clinical management, as well as obscures understanding. The mechanisms involved in these other entities are likely each different and probably distinct from true malignant glaucoma at least with respect to the primary mechanism (which in malignant glaucoma involves some abnormality in the anterior hyaloid). And yet, secondarily, these processes might share some similar mechanisms.

Prior to discussing some of these entities such as loose lens or ciliary body swelling, the principles may be easiest to understand in the context of the unusual secondary angle-closure glaucoma that may occur following acute central retinal vein occlusion (see Chapter 35). In this condition, there is axial shallowing of the anterior chamber that is believed to be due to either an increase in retinal volume or vitreous fluid volume subsequent to the central retinal vein occlusion. Unlike true (postoperative) malignant glaucoma, this condition will spontaneously resolve.

The question for one of us (DLE) has always been not why this condition occurs, but why it occurs so uncommonly. The usual increase in retinal or vitreous volume that occurs in this condition should act as a mass in all patients to move the crystalline lens forward. However, it seems that, in most patients, this posterior volume mass does not transmit such a force through the vitreous to the crystalline lens. Rather, the vitreous gives up part of its own volume to accommodate this temporary increase in posterior segment volume. Fluid must move out of the vitreous in most such patients, and as discussed, experimental data suggest that normal vitreous, in fact, offers little resistance to such fluid flow. A minority of patients develop this secondary angle-closure syndrome. Perhaps, it occurs in those who are hyperopic or have restrictive hyaloid permeability or available surface area. The vitreous does not give up volume, and, therefore, the increase in posterior segment volume subsequent to the central retinal vein occlusion does act as a mass to shallow the anterior chamber axially. If this construct is correct, YAG hyaloidotomy should act in such cases to reverse the flat chamber, but unlike true malignant glaucoma, this process will spontaneously resolve with the decrease in posterior (retinal) volume that is part of the natural history of the vein occlusion.

Thus, in some cases with this other entity of secondary angle-closure glaucoma, some other process that occupies posterior segment volume may secondarily involve hyaloid factors in producing a shallow anterior chamber both

The Chandler Operation

Ian P. Conner, MD, PhD; Joel S. Schuman, MD, FACS; and David L. Epstein, MD, MMM

Step 1, Corneal Paracentesis

A beveled paracentesis incision is made peripherally in the cornea with a Wheeler knife or similar instrument to provide easy access to the anterior chamber for later injection of fluid and air. If the bevel follows a path through the cornea about 1.5 to 2 mm in length from the anterior to posterior surface of the cornea, a suture is not required at the end of the procedure to close it, because the wound will be self-sealing. This incision should be tested with a slender cannula or needle to be sure it provides easy entry.

Step 2, Exploration for Suprachoroidal Fluid

Radial sclerotomies are performed in both lower quadrants with a No. 15 Bard-Parker blade (Katena Eye Instruments, Denville, NJ; or a No. 57 Beaver blade [Beaver, Waltham, MA]). The sclerotomies should be about 3-mm long and centered at a measured distance of 3.5 mm from the limbus. If a choroidal separation or suprachoroidal hemorrhage is present, suprachoroidal fluid or blood will be found, but no fluid is found in malignant glaucoma. If the fluid is found, it should be allowed to drain. Whether or not fluid or blood escapes spontaneously from the sclerotomy openings, a smooth spatula such as a standard cyclodialysis spatula should be passed circumferentially from the lips of the sclerotomy in the suprachoroidal space parallel to the limbus in both directions, because, on occasion, fluid or blood can be present between choroid and sclera, which does not flow freely from the sclerotomy until this maneuver has been performed.

If suprachoroidal fluid is found and is drained, the anterior chamber should then be re-formed with saline solution through the preplaced corneal paracentesis wound, and the surgical procedure can be terminated, because a diagnosis of choroidal separation or suprachoroidal hemorrhage, instead of malignant glaucoma, will have been established with certainty. The sclerotomy procedure provides both diagnosis and treatment.

However, if no fluid is found and the anterior chamber remains shallow or flat, despite a patent iridectomy or iridotomy and posterior sclerotomies, the diagnosis of malignant glaucoma is established with certainty, and it can now be treated definitively by surgery on the vitreous body.

Step 3, Vitreous Surgery for Malignant Glaucoma

The rationale for surgery on the vitreous body is based on the working hypothesis that aqueous humor is somehow diverted and entrapped in or behind the vitreous body, pressing lens, ciliary processes, and iris forward. The surgery is intended to establish an opening through the anterior hyaloid membrane and vitreous body for aqueous humor to escape forward to the posterior and anterior chambers.

A ring of surface diathermy is placed around the scleral wound using a strong radiofrequency diathermy current with a conical electrode and sufficient power to produce brown discoloration of the sclera, and one must be sure that the ciliary body is touched with the diathermy. This diathermy is used to prevent bleeding from the ciliary body when it is later pierced. When this has been done, bleeding has not been a problem. A Wheeler knife is plunged in a quick motion through the ciliary body 3.5 mm from the limbus into the vitreous cavity with the point of the knife aimed toward the optic nerve to avoid injuring the lens. The wound in the ciliary body is slightly enlarged anteriorly and posteriorly to a total length of about 3 mm, with its center 3.5 mm behind the external limbus.

A sharp 18-gauge intravenous needle is then introduced, but first a hemostat is clamped on its shaft a measured distance of 12 mm from its point in order to prevent it from penetrating excessively deep into the globe. The needle is then passed through the scleral-uveal wound into the vitreous cavity toward the optic nerve. After it has been inserted to the measured depth of 12 mm, its tip is moved back and forth in an arc of about 4 mm, intending to cause slight separation of vitreous membranes in its path. (If the eye is extremely hyperopic, more than 8 D, the eye is shorter axially, and the needle should not be passed to a depth of more than 10 mm, because of the risk of injuring the retina in such a short eye.) Then, a glass hypodermic syringe, such as a 5-mL Luer-lock syringe (Becton, Dickinson and Co, Franklin Lakes, NJ), is attached to the needle. This is done by the assistant, because the surgeon must carefully observe and control the position of the needle within the eye using both hands. When the syringe is attached to the needle, the surgeon continues to maintain the position of the needle with one hand, and with the other hand aspirates 1 to 1.5 mL. The fluid thus obtained may be watery or may consist of vitreous of varying consistency. Before the needle is withdrawn from the vitreous cavity, approximately 0.25 mL of what has been aspirated is injected back into the eye in order to clear the tip of the needle of vitreous strands that may have been engaged within its lumen. The needle is then carefully drawn from the eye exactly along its path of entry. The eye at this point is expected to be markedly hypotonic, with folds in the cornea and sclera. The shape of the globe is now partially restored by injecting less than 1 mL of saline solution into the anterior chamber through the previously placed beveled corneal incision. It is important in this step that the amount of fluid injected is limited, so that the eye is not filled completely. If so much saline solution is injected that it fills the globe, it behaves in some cases as though it flows back into and behind the remaining vitreous humor and recreates the original malignant glaucoma. If this happens, a second operation must be done. Instead, after the shape of the globe is only partially restored with a limited amount of saline solution, a larger air bubble is injected into the anterior chamber to fill it completely and force the iris and lens posteriorly. The air bubble should be large enough to deepen the chamber artificially to a greater depth than is usually encountered in a normal myopic eye. This will be a much greater depth than is naturally found in eyes predisposed to primary angle-closure glaucoma or malignant glaucoma. Even after injection of the large air bubble, the eye should still be hypotonic. It is important not to fill the eye completely to normal shape or IOP. If there is measurable pressure within the eye, too much saline solution has been injected. A sterile Schiotz tonometer or palpation with a muscle hook can be used to be sure.

The scleral wounds are each closed with a single interrupted suture and then the conjunctival wounds are closed.

Postoperative Care

Atropine is instilled at the end of the operation and is continued for several weeks or until the eye is quiet. We have had no instances of recurrence of malignant glaucoma when cycloplegics were discontinued after a successful vitreous aspiration procedure. In 3 additional cases, miotics were later used, without a recurrence of malignant glaucoma. If shallowing of the anterior chamber should occur in some case in the future, we would immediately resume the use of cycloplegics.

(continued)

(continued)

RELIABILITY AND COMPLICATIONS

This procedure for malignant glaucoma has been used extensively by us and by some of our colleagues since it was first performed by Dr. Paul A. Chandler in 1965. The procedure has proved safe and effective when used precisely as described. We have learned, however, that careful attention to detail is essential. In a number of instances, colleagues have discussed with us complications or failures that have occurred in their hands. In each instance, when the exact methods they used in performing the procedure were reviewed, it was found that the procedure had been altered in one way or another, departing from the recommended protocol that we have outlined. For example, a colleague reported hemorrhage into the suprachoroidal space and vitreous cavity at the time the procedure was carried out, but review of the procedure revealed that diathermy had not been applied as prescribed around the wound of entry prior to piercing the ciliary body. In another instance, colleagues reported ineffectiveness of the procedure in their hands, but when the technique that they had employed was analyzed, it was found that in the last steps of the procedure, they had been inserting a much smaller air bubble than recommended, too small to deepen the anterior chamber effectively. When the same surgeons instilled a large quantity of air into the anterior chamber, as recommended to force the lens, iris, and anterior vitreous body posteriorly, the procedure became effective in their hands.

Another deviation that can cause failure and that has done so in a number of cases that we have learned of is making the incision in the sclera too far posteriorly (eg, centered 5 or 6 mm behind the limbus instead of the 3 to 5 mm recommended). We think that the specified anterior placement of the wound for vitreous puncture is probably essential, because it is calculated to be anterior to the normal vitreous base, so that the anterior hyaloid membrane is punctured as the knife and the needle are introduced into the vitreous cavity. The site of this wound would be measured carefully. We think it should not be less than 3.5 mm posteriorly to the limbus for fear of injuring the lens.

Another error is not to use a sharp needle for the procedure. We are aware of surgeons who mistakenly used a blunt-tip vitreous aspirating needle and were unsuccessful.

Occasionally, the air bubble instilled in the anterior chamber slips partially or totally behind the iris at the time of surgery or in the first day or 2 after surgery. The chamber then appears flat, but, on careful inspection, one can see that the air bubble is behind the iris. This should not be interpreted as a recurrence of malignant glaucoma. The air bubble can usually be shifted into the anterior chamber by movement of the patient's head or eye with the pupil dilated. Even if this cannot be immediately accomplished, the air bubble gradually absorbs, and the anterior chamber reforms.

Small punctate retinal hemorrhages have been detected postoperatively in a few eyes when they have been examined by indirect ophthalmoscopy, but these have not caused any difficulty.

Postoperative choroidal detachment has occurred in about one-third of our cases, but the choroidal separation has been transient. It is important to distinguish it from a recurrence of malignant glaucoma. With choroidal separation, the anterior chamber may be shallow or flat, but the eye is soft, and choroidal elevation in the peripheral fundus is usually visible.

Despite careful adherence to the surgical protocol, we have had several cases in which malignant glaucoma was not relieved the first time the vitreous aspiration procedure was performed. In these cases, we have merely resumed medical therapy for 2 to 3 days and then performed the procedure again. After the second operation, all eyes have responded with relief of the malignant glaucoma.

In 3 cases, all relatively young individuals, very little fluid could be drawn into the syringe when we tried to aspirate from the vitreous cavity with the 18-gauge needle. We withdrew the needle and attempted to inject air into the anterior chamber even though it was flat, but very little air could be injected. We then resumed atropine therapy and the full medical regimen for malignant glaucoma, and to our surprise, in all 3 cases, the eye responded to the medical therapy, although it had been unresponsive prior to the surgical procedure. This suggests that the puncture of anterior hyaloid and vitreous body, even without aspiration of fluid, was enough in these cases to disrupt the malignant glaucoma mechanism. In one of these cases, we found some months later that, for treatment of glaucoma due to residual peripheral anterior synechiae, miotic therapy could be resumed without causing a recurrence of malignant glaucoma.

The use of a miotic after operation for angle-closure glaucoma may precipitate malignant glaucoma, but after malignant glaucoma has been relieved by vitreous puncture and aspiration, the situation is changed. The following case is an instance in which a miotic was used postoperatively without a return of the malignant glaucoma. We know of several similar cases, including one in which echothiophate iodide 0.25% was used twice daily for years without recurrence of the malignant glaucoma. Thus, it appears safe to use a miotic where indicated after vitreous puncture and aspiration for malignant glaucoma.

CASE 29-1

A 49-year-old woman's ophthalmologist found a closed angle in both eyes and did a peripheral iridectomy on the left eye. The anterior chamber in that eye remained shallow or flat despite atropine, acetazolamide, and mannitol. When seen here, IOP was 60 mm Hg in the right eye and 30 mm Hg in the left eye. In the right eye, there was no light perception; the disc was cupped and atrophic. The left showed deep saucerization of the disc throughout; the anterior chamber was 1/2 corneal thickness deep in the center, flat elsewhere.

Vitreous puncture and aspiration were done. The chamber formed but remained somewhat shallow. Two weeks later, gonioscopy showed some peripheral anterior synechiae, but it was thought that the residual glaucoma could probably be controlled medically. IOP was 20 mm Hg. One week later, IOP was 27 mm Hg. She was given epinephrine, and 5 months later a report from her ophthalmologist stated that IOP had varied between 15 and 19 mm Hg, vision 6/7.5. One month later, IOP was found to be 34 mm Hg; she was then given pilocarpine. IOP with epinephrine and pilocarpine since then has been 18 to 20 mm Hg, and there has been no return of the malignant glaucoma.

axially and peripherally. Similarly, in conditions where there is an increased volume in the suprachoroidal space, either from hemorrhage, tumor, or primary effusion, there may occur, depending on inherent permeability factors of the hyaloid and such vitreous volume considerations, flattening of the anterior chamber. Also occurring in this situation is forward rotation of the ciliary body with loss of zonular tension and the potential loosening of the crystalline lens position. But even if these conditions require the maintenance of normal vitreous volume to transmit the force from behind, this is not the same clinical condition as postoperative malignant glaucoma, which arises from different causes and can only be cured through therapy directed at the hyaloid. In these other entities, which involve increased posterior segment volume, the disease can often be cured by draining the suprachoroidal blood or fluid (or perhaps in the latter case by treating the initiating inflammation) without the need or even indication for hyaloid therapy. Thus, these conditions are not only different in regard to primary events, but also as to required therapy, and, therefore, the term *malignant glaucoma* is not appropriate for these other entities.

Also, consider the following: there are cases of primary or secondary retinal detachment where the retina is completely detached and comes into close approximation with the posterior crystalline lens capsule, yet the observed anterior chamber depth axially is not shallow. How could this happen? Somehow, the vitreous "gave up its volume" to the detached retina without acting as a mass to move the crystalline lens forward. Such eyes, which have such a voluminous retinal detachment, are commonly myopic with vitreous that, unlike the hyperopic vitreous seen in malignant glaucoma, is quite freely permeable to fluid. One might (with some license) simplify this concept and suppose that in such cases the vitreous had its watery fluid easily "squeezed out" in response to this force from behind and, therefore, did not act as a force to move the crystalline lens forward.

There are many diseases that involve an increase in posterior segment volume as a primary process that may or may not shallow the anterior chamber depending on the inherent vitreous hyaloid permeability of the individual involved, but these diseases are distinct from primary malignant glaucoma.

Purported Loose Crystalline Lens Syndromes

There are a variety of clinical cases that are characterized by a forward crystalline lens position and the absence of pupillary block. These are usually but not always nonoperative eyes and, in this way and others, distinct from malignant glaucoma. Also, in these cases, there is no evidence for choroidal hemorrhage, central retinal vein occlusion, malignant melanoma, etc, that would occupy posterior segment volume. In the absence of any other apparent primary cause, they have often been called *loose lens syndrome*.

These cases are typically unilateral, and there is commonly no choroidal effusion visible on indirect ophthalmoscopy; otherwise, they would have been classified with the known primary uveal effusion syndromes that are usually but not always felt to be inflammatory. One such syndrome involves

the occurrence of primary uveal effusion and secondary angle closure with HIV infection.[17,18]

Ultrasound biomicroscopy techniques have indicated that some patients with presumed loose lens syndrome actually have unsuspected small anterior choroidal detachments. Such syndromes of far anterior choroidal detachment are probably not new and share features with what Phelps described as cases of ciliary body swelling.[20-22] In the latter entity, which was historically difficult to define because of the uncertainty of what a swollen ciliary body[58] or process actually looked like when viewed gonioscopically, inflammation was felt to be involved, and the eyes were commonly injected. Scleritis can cause such an inflammatory choroidal detachment syndrome.[59-62] These conditions usually resolved (probably this was not a single homogeneous entity) with use of topical steroids and cycloplegics. However, some cases of anterior choroidal detachment may not show obvious ocular inflammation, but may still respond to the use of cycloplegics and (often systemic) steroids.

The literature has reported numerous cases of unsuspected anterior choroidal detachment, only visible with ultrasound biomicroscopy techniques, which were due to an idiosyncratic systemic drug reaction (see Chapter 36). In general, the condition often resolves simply with cessation of such systemic therapy and fails to respond to cycloplegic therapy. Thus, a localized anterior choroidal (ciliary body) detachment may represent a common final mechanism from multiple causes for such an apparent syndrome.

In these conditions, the forward rotation of the ciliary body results in loosening of zonular tension and allows forward movement of the crystalline lens with attendant acute myopia.

However, it is doubtful that such localized anterior choroidal detachments can explain all such cases of apparent loose crystalline lens. Likely, there is more than one entity in this "basket," and we may learn further from some of our patients if we can understand these conditions better.

One of us (DLE) observed such a case, following blunt trauma to the eye, which demonstrated an apparent unilateral forward subluxation of the crystalline lens (without any horizontal or vertical component). The axial chamber depth shallowed further under the influence of cholinergic drugs (miotics), but did not deepen with cycloplegic therapy. No zonular dehiscence was visible with maximal pupillary dilatation, but the crystalline lens behaved as if it were loose in the anterior-posterior direction. Some have suggested that there are similar cases with spontaneous weak zonules due to exfoliation.[63,64]

There are also some cases that may be caused by swelling of the crystalline lens and slowly evolving cataract formation. In such cases, the axial depth of the anterior chamber is somewhat shallow and asymmetrical to the fellow eye, and the normal response (in some eyes) of cholinergic therapy to cause forward crystalline lens movement[9] may then simulate a loose lens.

In evaluating all such phenomena, it is important to contemplate and carry further the above concepts and discussion of the vitreous sometimes acting as a force to move the crystalline lens forward. We have discussed why sometimes with a new mass in the posterior segment (eg, retina or choroid), the vitreous may give up volume or not, and in the latter case act as a force to move the crystalline lens forward. But here we need also discuss why, in some patients with accommodation and release of zonular tension, does the crystalline lens not only change its curvature but move anteriorly. An exact understanding of this is not available, but it seems clear that in some patients with accommodation there is anterior crystalline lens movement and in others none. It would seem that the turgor of the vitreous might be an important factor contributing to this difference. In fact, it has been proposed that the normal mechanism of accommodation involves a narrowing of the ciliary body ring with resultant pressure on the vitreous, which transmits this pressure to the crystalline lens posterior surface, with the potential, at least in some patients, for anterior lens movement.[38] Such a construct could also explain the clinical observation that cholinergic miotics can precipitate the onset of malignant glaucoma by moving the ciliary body inward to apposition with the hyaloid.

Regardless, it would seem plausible that with loss of zonular tension from trauma as in the above case, or from forward rotation of the ciliary body with occult anterior choroidal detachment syndromes, or with other entities that can cause an apparent loose lens syndrome that we do not yet understand, loss of zonular tension is not enough in itself to explain forward movement of the crystalline lens. Rather, the position of the crystalline lens is also determined by the support (force) from the vitreous. Obviously, vitreous turgor may differ in different patients and might sensibly be expected to be greater in hyperopic eyes (thus with the potential for more anterior crystalline lens movement). However, such a mechanism is not equivalent to malignant glaucoma, although factors of vitreous turgor might be important in both conditions.

In these loose lens syndromes, the mechanism of angle-closure glaucoma is usually due to pupillary block, which can be effectively treated with laser iridectomy. Of course, the axial depth remains shallow and of concern to the clinician, especially if there is any possibility of crystalline lens-cornea touch. Very rarely (if ever), the crystalline lens might be so large (for the middle and anterior segments of the eye) that conceivably the edge of the crystalline lens might itself push the iris into the angle and cause a secondary angle closure by this mechanism (see Chapter 28).

Of course, if there is some dehiscence of zonules, vitreous can come forward into the posterior chamber and cause angle-closure glaucoma due to a pupillary block-type mechanism (aqueous humor normally secreted into the posterior chamber does not have free circumferential access to the iridectomy or iridotomy because of the vitreous coming forward through the broken zonules). It is in such cases that more than one iridectomy or iridotomy may be required to alleviate pupillary block, and the possibility of such a condition is another reason why the general first rule described above for dealing with flat chamber cases is to place a new iridectomy or iridotomy. Theoretically, if there is extensive zonular dehiscence, vitreous may move forward through enough of the posterior chamber circumference so that aqueous humor is being secreted into or behind the vitreous, and a malignant glaucoma-like condition (in a nonoperated eye) might be produced. One of us (DLE) has not seen this clinical situation, although it remains a theoretical possibility. For practical purposes, such cases of subluxed lenses usually involve mechanisms of pupillary block that respond to peripheral iridectomy or iridotomy (usually just one, but sometimes 2 in order to place one away from the area of zonular dehiscence).

This discussion should not imply that most cases of loose crystalline lens syndrome are in fact due to zonular dehiscence. There are likely a variety of causes that we have not fully categorized but we need to understand better. Commonly, there is some cataract formation in these cases, but, even if not, the condition seems to be cured by removal of the lens. It is noteworthy that the feeling among clinicians who have seen such cases is that such patients do well with cataract surgery with a posterior chamber lens. Obviously, if there were an underlying anterior choroidal detachment, this might not be expected, at least in these subgroups. This clinical observation raises the possibility that the abnormality might well have been in the crystalline lens itself (and the possibility therefore, for example, of having misinterpreted the findings of an evolving cataract with a normal response to miotics in terms of crystalline lens position or of some subclinical zonular weakness that the posterior chamber intraocular lens subsequently is not subject to). On the other hand, there might be other explanations for this observed benefit from cataract surgery.

These entities may constitute complicated clinical situations with more than one mechanism involved in individual cases. Regardless, in terms of malignant glaucoma, the following differentiating points, which are generally believed to be true, should be kept in mind: in true malignant glaucoma, cataract surgery, including the use of intracapsular surgery, was curative only when there was accompanying vitreous loss (and the hyaloid face was broken).[11] In contrast, in loose crystalline lens syndromes that ultimately seem to come to cataract surgery, the latter is most often curative by itself without the occurrence of vitreous loss. This suggests that malignant glaucoma and loose lens syndromes may share an abnormality in crystalline lens position (or size) but not in hyaloid permeability.

MALIGNANT GLAUCOMA IN APHAKIA

With the virtual disappearance of planned intracapsular cataract surgery, cases of aphakic malignant glaucoma with or without an anterior chamber lens are now rarely seen.

The one exception is when such eyes rendered previously aphakic must now undergo fistulizing surgery. Therefore, the clinician should still be aware of this entity. Also, the understanding and treatment of aphakic malignant glaucoma was an important milestone[25] in the development of the unifying concepts of this disease entity, which are explained above, but are now detailed further.

We explain this condition of aphakic malignant glaucoma as follows: in pure aphakic pupillary block, there is an aqueous humor-filled posterior chamber, at least in a portion of the circumference. Therefore, a laser iridotomy, by establishing communication with this aqueous humor space behind the iris, equalizes pressure in the posterior and anterior chamber and allows free communication of aqueous humor from ciliary body to anterior chamber. However, in aphakic malignant glaucoma, there is total obliteration of the posterior chamber aqueous space by vitreous humor and its hyaloid membrane, which is apposed to the posterior iris surface. Aqueous humor moves directly from the ciliary body into the vitreous humor and, in order to pass into the anterior chamber, must cross a limited surface area of anterior hyaloid, which may be thickened or abnormally impermeable. When a laser iridotomy is performed, there is no free communication of aqueous humor from posterior to anterior chamber, because vitreous is present behind the iridotomy. To establish free communication and equalize pressure in the posterior and anterior segments, the limiting membrane of the vitreous, the anterior hyaloid, must be disrupted.

In the past, this involved a deep surgical incision of the hyaloid or an anterior vitrectomy, but the neodymium (Nd):YAG laser has also been used to disrupt the hyaloid either in the pupillary area or through the iridotomy to cure this condition.[25] The observed dramatic cure with the YAG laser underscored the importance of the hyaloid in this condition. Often, the hyaloid appears thickened in this condition, but a limited hyaloid surface area for fluid flow may also be involved as indicated by our experimental studies.[23,24]

We observed this condition most commonly after anterior chamber intraocular lens implants with intracapsular surgery and wondered whether a slightly larger implant may have pushed the iris posteriorly toward the vitreous and favored the occurrence of this condition. However, it must be remembered that aphakic malignant glaucoma was a well-known entity prior to the advent of intraocular lenses.

In evaluating a patient with an aphakic (or pseudophakic) flat chamber postoperatively, one wants initially to rule out wound leak and choroidal detachment. IOP is usually low in such conditions, except with suprachoroidal hemorrhage or rare forms of choroidal effusion. However, a transient wound leak can lead to pupillary block by allowing vitreous to move forward and iridectomies to become adherent to the wound. This is less of a problem with fine, permanent sutures such as 10-0 nylon, which can be placed deeply, but can be quite common with sutures such as silk or various absorbable sutures that are placed too deep. Especially with silk sutures, a transient shallow chamber can occur several weeks after surgery when deep sutures develop a small amount of surrounding tissue necrosis.

The wound should be inspected, a Seidel test performed, and any suspected deep suture removed (especially if it is several weeks postoperative). If a wound leak is detected, a pressure patch with local tamponade over the limbus (as with use of the glaucoma shell or a soft contact lens or Simmons' shell) should be applied. Aqueous humor suppressant therapy can be used to reduce aqueous flow through the fistula. However, obvious wound leaks should be surgically repaired, the secondary choroidal detachment drained, and the anterior chamber reformed surgically.

Most often in such cases, no wound leak is apparent, and the IOP is at least moderately elevated. In these cases, laser iridotomy should then be performed to rule out pupillary block. If there is already a patent surgical iridectomy, then it is unlikely that pupillary block is the mechanism, but it is best to perform one additional iridotomy with the laser. This is to ensure that there is not an aqueous humor-filled posterior chamber space in at least one segment. If laser iridotomy fails to deepen the anterior chamber, then the YAG laser should be used to disrupt the anterior hyaloid through the iridotomy (or through the pupil if the hyaloid is easily visualized next to the pupillary margin). In many cases, this has proven dramatically successful in normalizing the anterior chamber depth, but in one observed case the effect was temporary, and surgical vitrectomy was required.[25]

References

1. Chandler PA. Malignant glaucoma. *Am J Ophthalmol.* 1951;34:993-1000.
2. Shaffer RN. The role of vitreous detachment in aphakic and malignant glaucoma. *Trans Am Acad Ophthalmol Otolaryngol.* 1954;58:217-231.
3. Weiss DI, Shaffer RN. Ciliary block (malignant) glaucoma. *Trans Am Acad Ophthalmol Otolaryngol.* 1972;76:450-461.
4. Shaffer RN, Hoskins HD. Ciliary block (malignant) glaucoma. *Trans Am Acad Ophthalmol Otolaryngol.* 1978,85:215-221.
5. Brooks AM, Harper CA, Gillies WE. Occurrence of malignant glaucoma after laser iridotomy. *Br J Ophthalmol.* 1989;73:617-620.
6. Cashwell LF, Martin TJ. Malignant glaucoma after laser iridotomy. *Ophthalmology.* 1992;99:651-659.
7. Aminlari A, Sassani JW. Simultaneous bilateral malignant glaucoma—following laser iridotomy. *Graefes Arch Clin Exp Ophthalmol.* 1993;231:12-14.
8. Levene R. A new concept of malignant glaucoma. *Arch Ophthalmol.* 1972;87:497-506.
9. Hitchings RA, Powell DJ. Pilocarpine and narrow-angle glaucoma. *Trans Ophthalmol Soc UK.* 1981;101:214-217.
10. Wood WJ, Smith TR. Senile disciform macular degeneration complicated by massive hemorrhagic retinal detachment and angle closure glaucoma. *Retina.* 1983;3:296-303.
11. Chandler PA. Progress in the treatment of glaucoma in my lifetime. *Surv Ophthalmol.* 1977;21:412-429.
12. Chandler PA. A new operation for malignant glaucoma: a preliminary report. *Trans Am Ophthalmol Soc.* 1964;62:408-424.
13. Chandler PA, Grant WM. Mydriatic-cycloplegic treatment in malignant glaucoma. *Arch Ophthalmol.* 1962;62:353-359.
14. Chandler PA, Simmons RJ, Grant WM. Malignant glaucoma, medical and surgical treatment. *Am J Ophthalmol.* 1968;66:495-502.

15. Simmons RJ. Malignant glaucoma. *Br J Ophthalmol.* 1972;56:263-272.

16. Simmons RJ. Laser shrinkage of ciliary processes: a treatment for malignant (ciliary block) glaucoma. *Ophthalmology.* 1980;87:1155-1159.

17. Nash RW, Lindquist TD. Bilateral angle-closure glaucoma associated with uveal effusion: presenting sign of HIV infection. *Surv Ophthalmol.* 1992;36:255-258.

18. Joshi N, Constable PH, Margolis TP, Hoyt CS, Leonard TJ. Bilateral angle closure glaucoma and accelerated cataract formation in a patient with AIDS. *Br J Ophthalmol.* 1994;78:656-657.

19. Troope GE, Pavlin CJ, Bau A, Baumal CR, Foster FS. Malignant glaucoma. Clinical and ultrasound biomicroscopic features. *Ophthalmology.* 1994;101:1030-1035.

20. Phelps CD. Angle-closure glaucoma secondary to ciliary body swelling. *Arch Ophthalmol.* 1974;92:297-290.

21. Saari KM. Acute glaucoma in hemorrhagic fever with renal syndrome (nephropathia epidemica). *Am J Ophthalmol.* 1976;81:455-461.

22. Letocha CE. Angle-closure secondary to ciliary body swelling. *Ann Ophthalmol.* 1977;9:597-598.

23. Epstein DL, Hashimoto JM, Anderson PJ, et al. Experimental perfusions through the vitreous and anterior chambers: possible relationship to malignant glaucoma. *Am J Ophthalmol.* 1979;88:1078-1086.

24. Epstein DL. Malignant glaucoma. In: Jakobiec F, Sigelman J, eds. *Advanced Techniques in Ocular Surgery.* Philadelphia, PA: WB Saunders Co; 1984:158-168.

25. Epstein DL, Steinert RF, Puliafito CA. Neodymium-YAG laser therapy to the anterior hyaloid in aphakic malignant glaucoma. *Am J Ophthalmol.* 1984;98:137-143.

26. Epstein DL. Pseudophakic malignant glaucoma—is it really pseudomalignant? *Am J Ophthalmol.* 1987;103:231-233.

27. Brown RH, Lynch MG, Tearse JE, et al. Neodymium-YAG vitreous surgery for phakic and pseudophakic malignant glaucoma. *Arch Ophthalmol.* 1986;104:1464-1466.

28. Luntz MH, Rosenblatt M. Malignant glaucoma. *Surv Ophthalmol.* 1987;32:73-93.

29. Melamed S, Ashkenazi I, Blumenthal M. Nd-YAG laser hyaloidotomy for malignant glaucoma following one-piece 7 mm intraocular lens implantation. *Br J Ophthalmol.* 1991;75:501-503.

30. Halkias A, Magauran DM, Joyce M. Ciliary block (malignant) glaucoma after cataract extraction with lens implant treated with YAG laser capsulotomy and anterior hyaloidotomy. *Br J Ophthalmol.* 1992;76:569-570.

31. Tello C, Chi T, Shepps G, Liebmann J, Ritch R. Ultrasound biomicroscopy in pseudophakic malignant glaucoma. *Ophthalmology.* 1993;100:1330-1334.

32. Simmons RJ. Malignant glaucoma. In: Chandler PA, Grant WM, eds. *Glaucoma.* Philadelphia, PA: Lea & Febiger; 1979.

33. DiSclafani M, Liebmann JM, Ritch R. Malignant glaucoma following argon laser release of scleral flap sutures after trabeculectomy. *Am J Ophthalmol.* 1989;108:597-598.

34. Grant WM. Experimental aqueous perfusions in enucleated human eyes. *Arch Ophthalmol.* 1963;69:783.

35. Bleeker GM. Variation in the depth of the anterior chamber and intraocular pressure. *Am J Ophthalmol.* 1963;55:964.

36. Jaffe NS. *The vitreous in clinical ophthalmology.* St Louis, MO: CV Mosby Co; 1969.

37. Streeten BW, Pulaski JP. Posterior zonules and lens extraction. *Arch Ophthalmol.* 1978;96:132-138.

38. Coleman DJ. Unified model for accommodative mechanism. *Am J Ophthalmol.* 1970;69:1063-1079.

39. VanHeuven WAJ, Lam KW, Ray GS. Source of subretinal fluid on the basis of ascorbate analyses. *Arch Ophthalmol.* 1982;100:976-978.

40. Pederson JE, Toris CB. Experimental retinal detachment. IX. Aqueous, vitreous, and subretinal protein concentrations. *Arch Ophthalmol.* 1985;103:835-836.

41. Tsuboi S, Pederson JE. Permeability of the isolated dog retinal pigment epithelium to carboxyfluorescein. *Invest Ophthalmol Vis Sci.* 1986;27:1767-1770.

42. Tsuboi S, Pederson JE. Volume flow across the isolated retinal pigment epithelium of cynomolgus monkey eyes. *Invest Ophthalmol Vis Sci.* 1988;29:1652-1655.

43. Marmor MF. Control of subretinal fluid: experimental and clinical studies. *Eye.* 1990;4:340-344.

44. Kawano S, Marmor MF. Metabolic influences on the absorption of serous subretinal fluid. *Invest Ophthalmol Vis Sci.* 1988;29:1255-1257.

45. Robbins RM, Galin MA. Vitreous response in glaucoma. *Am J Ophthalmol.* 1973;76:921-925.

46. Christensen L, Irvine AR. Pathogenesis of primary shallow chamber angle closure glaucoma. *Arch Ophthalmol.* 1966;75:490-495.

47. Quigley HA, Friedman DS, Congdon NG. Possible mechanisms of primary angle-closure and malignant glaucoma. *J Glaucoma.* 2003;12(2):167-180.

48. Massicotte EC, Schuman JS. A malignant glaucoma-like syndrome following pars plana vitrectomy. *Ophthalmology.* 1999;106(7):1375-1379.

49. Wright MM, Grajewski AL. Measurement of intraocular pressure with a flat anterior chamber. *Ophthalmology.* 1991;98:1854-1857.

50. Weiss DI, Shaffer RN, Harrington DO. Treatment of malignant glaucoma with intravenous mannitol infusion. *Arch Ophthalmol.* 1963;69:154-158.

51. Garner LF, Brown B, Baker R, et al. The effect of phenylephrine hydrochloride on the resting point of accommodation. *Invest Ophthalmol Vis Sci.* 1983;24:393-395.

52. Borromeo-McGrail V, Bordiuk JM, Keitel H. Systemic hypertension following ocular administration of 10 per cent phenylephrine in the neonate. *Pediatrics.* 1973;51:1032-1036.

53. Meyer SM, Fraunfelder FT. Phenylephrine hydrochloride. *Ophthalmology.* 1980;87:1177-1180.

54. Fraunfelder FT, Meyer SM. Systemic reactions to ophthalmic drug preparations. *Med Toxicol Adverse Drug Exp.* 1987;2:287-293.

55. Steinert RF, Puliafito CA, Kittrell C. Plasma shielding by Q-switched and mode-locked Nd-YAG lasers. *Ophthalmology.* 1983;90:1003-1006.

56. Debrouwere V, Stalmans P, Van Calster J, Spileers W, Zeyen T, Stalmans I. Outcomes of different management options for malignant glaucoma: a retrospective study. *Graefes Arch Clin Exp Ophthalmol.* 2012;250(1):131-141.

57. Simmons RJ. Malignant glaucoma. In: Epstein EL, ed. *Chandler and Grant's Glaucoma.* 3rd ed. Philadelphia, PA: Lea & Febiger; 1986.

58. Frayer WC, Laties AM. Some consequences of ciliary process swelling in the rabbit and in the human. *Trans Am Ophthalmol Soc.* 1977;74:107-121.

59. Oksala A, Koponen J. Choroidal detachment associated with scleritis—a case report with echograms. *Ultrasound Med Biol.* 1974;1:293-295.

60. Feldon SE, Sigelman J, Albert DM, Smith TR. Clinical manifestations of brawny scleritis. *Am J Ophthalmol.* 1978;85:781-787.

61. Benson WE. Posterior scleritis. *Surv Ophthalmol.* 1988;32:297-316.

62. Mangouritsas G, Ulbig M. Secondary angle-block glaucoma in posterior scleritis. *Klin Monatsbl Augenheilkd.* 1991;199:40-44.

63. Von Der Lippe I, Kuchle M, Naumann GO. Pseudoexfoliation syndrome as a risk factor for acute ciliary block angle closure glaucoma. *Acta Ophthalmol.* 1993;71:277-279.

64. Schlotzer-Schrehardt U, Naumann GO. A histopathologic study of zonular instability in pseudoexfoliation syndrome. *Am J Ophthalmol.* 1994;118:730-743.

Nanophthalmos
Diagnosis and Treatment

Zvia Burgansky-Eliash, MD and Richard J. Simmons, MD

Nanophthalmos is a relatively rare bilateral condition characterized by small ocular volume, typically associated with marked hyperopia and shallow anterior chamber.[1] The axial length is between 14 and 20.5 mm.[2,3] Exceptionally, nanophthalmic eyes may be emmetropic or myopic. The globe has a small equatorial diameter and a small corneal diameter, but the size of the lens is normal. The disproportion between lens and ocular volume contributes to iris convexity and anterior chamber shallowing. In nanophthalmos, the lens may occupy 10% to 30% of the volume of the globe, compared with approximately 4% in normal adult eyes.

In many cases, visual acuity is reduced due to macular hypoplasia presented with lack of foveal light reflex, lack of a normal foveal pit on ocular coherence tomography, and abnormal or absent foveal avascular zones on fluorescein angiography.[4] Retinal pigmentary dystrophy can accompany nanophthalmos as well.[5-7] A case of retinitis pigmentosa and optic nerve drusen associated with nanophthalmos was described.[8]

INHERITANCE

In some cases, nanophthalmos is inherited; in other cases, it is a sporadic occurrence. If inherited, transmission may be either autosomal recessive or autosomal dominant.[7,9,10] In one autosomal dominant nanophthalmos family, the abnormality was located on NNO1 locus on chromosome 11.[11] Often, the inheritance is unknown, but the patients have relatives who are blind from angle-closure glaucoma.[1,12] There is a controversy regarding female predominance.[1,13,14] Although nanophthalmos is usually not associated with systemic abnormalities, there are reports on cases with coexisting cryptorchidism,[15] Hallermann-Streiff syndrome,[16] and oculo-dento-digital syndrome.[17]

GLAUCOMA CHARACTERISTICS

Nanophthalmos is complicated by angle-closure glaucoma in many cases, which usually develops between 20 and 50 years of age.[2] In younger patients, the most characteristic findings are hyperopic eyes with small corneas and bulging forward of the lens and iris into a shallow anterior chamber. As the lens enlarges with age, there is an increase in relative pupillary block, and the anterior chamber becomes shallow, with progressive narrowing of the angle. This is the most common cause of angle-closure glaucoma in nanophthalmic eyes, which eventually leads to peripheral anterior synechia (PAS) formation.

Angle closure can also develop secondary to spontaneous choroidal thickening and effusions.[18] These choroidal changes may cause a forward rotation of the ciliary body that pushes the peripheral iris forward, allows the lens to move forward, and increases relative pupillary block. Severe uveal effusion and exudative retinal detachment is a frequent complication of anterior segment surgery. Choroidal effusion and exudative retinal detachment was reported also after laser peripheral iridotomy.[19,20]

HISTOPATHOLOGY

The sclera in eyes with nanophthalmos is both thicker and disorganized compared to normal sclera.[16,21-23] The collagen fibrils bundles are larger, less ordered, and more interwoven than normal.[21] High levels of fibronectin found in these cases affect the packing of collagen fibers and leads to

Kahook MY, Schuman JS, eds.
Chandler and Grant's Glaucoma, Fifth Edition (pp 305-307).
© 2013 SLACK Incorporated.

thickening of the sclera and occlusion of the vortex veins.[16] The thickened sclera reducing its permeability to protein[24] together with the constriction of vortex veins both contribute to uveal effusion in the nanophthalmic eye.

TREATMENT

In general, medication and laser therapy offer a safe and often sufficient option for treatment of nanophthalmic angle-closure glaucoma.[10,25]

Medical Treatment

Intraocular pressure (IOP) elevation is managed by aqueous suppressants: beta-blockers, alpha adrenergic agonists, and carbonic anhydrase inhibitors. Miotics may make the pupillary block worse by relaxing the lens zonules in these patients.[10]

Laser Iridectomy

It is recommended to perform a preventive peripheral iridectomy (PI) when angles are still open but so slit-like that angle closure is threatened. When glaucoma develops, laser iridotomy is beneficial to eliminate the pupillary block component in the early stage of glaucoma before the occurrence of PAS.[3,10]

Argon Laser Peripheral Iridoplasty

If angle remains narrow or becomes worse progressively with time, laser iridoplasty is the next step, providing widening of the angle in up to 91.6% of patients.[10,13] The widening effect of iridoplasty may gradually disappear. Therefore, a patient should have a slit-lamp examination and gonioscopy every 3 months. Iridoplasty is used repeatedly, attempting to open as much of the angle as possible.

Trabeculectomy

Filtration surgery alone is not advised as it is associated with high risk of permanent loss of vision caused by disastrous complications after the surgery.[10,26] Sudden decompression of the globe during surgery triggers the rapid progression of massive uveal effusion, which may lead to secondary retinal detachment, intraocular hemorrhage, and loss of vision (Figure 30-1). Therefore, glaucoma filtration surgery is considered as the last choice in the treatment of angle-closure glaucoma.[10,13] Prophylactic sclerectomy, anterior sclerotomy, or vortex vein decompression are needed to reduce disastrous complications.

During trabeculectomy, an effort is made to avoid intraoperative and postoperative hypotony to minimize the chance for choroidal effusions and exudative retinal detachments. This is achieved by filling the anterior chamber with viscoelastic agent prior to performing the sclerostomy,

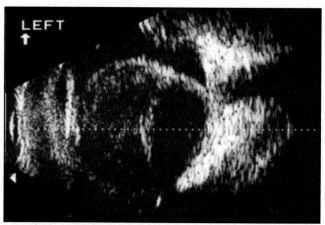

Figure 30-1. Ultrasound scan demonstrating severe choroidal effusion and hemorrhage after filtration surgery.

preplacing of trabeculectomy flap sutures so that they may be closed immediately, and tight suture closure.

When the glaucoma is such that trabeculectomy can be deferred, preoperative prophylactic sclerectomy is performed, preferably 4 to 6 weeks before the trabeculectomy to allow full recovery. In these cases, 2 inferior posterior sclerectomies are done, sparing the superior conjunctiva.

If the glaucoma is so severe that immediate surgery is necessary, anterior V-shaped sclerotomies can be done at the time of the trabeculectomy before the eye is opened. In a study of 20 patients who had trabeculectomy with mitomycin-C application and inferior sclerotomy, the cumulative probability of success was 85% at 1 year and 47% at 5 years after surgery. Complications were common and include uveal effusion in 50%, cataract formation in 35%, and late choroidal detachment in 25%.[3] In another small report, 2 patients underwent a similar procedure successfully.[25]

Sclerectomy and Sclerotomy

Several methods have been proposed to open areas in the sclera that allow drainage of existing uveal effusion and as a prophylactic measure before or at the beginning of filtration surgery.

Brockhurst[27] recommends including vortex vein decompression with lamellar scleral resection and posterior sclerotomies. In his description, 80% of subjects had a reattachment of the retina after this procedure. However, intraoperative bleeding may occur during scleral dissection around the vortex vein.[3]

The technique for posterior sclerectomies described by Gass[28] includes lamellar scleral resection and sclerotomy. Gass advocates the removal of a two-thirds thickness rectangle (5 mm × 7 mm) of sclera with the additional removal of a 1-mm full-thickness piece of sclera from the scleral bed.

The use of absorbable gelatin film to cover the sclerectomized area was tried successfully in one case of partial-thickness sclerectomy with a central sclerostomy. The gelatin film may prevent regeneration of scleral tissue and recurrence of the exudative retinal detachment.[20]

Jin and Anderson[13] described a V-shaped full-thickness sclerotomy anteriorly over the pars plana, leaving it unsutured to provide ongoing drainage postoperatively. The authors of this chapter recommend a similar technique with excising the flap completely at the base in high-risk cases, because the unsutured flaps may reseal within 7 days. The full thickness V-shaped scleral flaps (4 mm × 4 mm) are made in the inferior nasal and temporal quadrants (the point of the V should be 5 mm from the limbus directed toward the limbus). There is a risk related to large areas of uvea unprotected by sclera; however, anterior site is better protected than posterior area by thicker uveal layer and firm vitreous base.[3] Moreover, these eyes face certain blindness unless surgery is successful. Simple linear sclerotomies similar to that made for drainage of choroidal effusions are inadequate in true nanophthalmos.

PROGNOSIS

Although angle-closure glaucoma secondary to nanophthalmos can be treated with various techniques, the prognosis remains guarded.

REFERENCES

1. Brockhurst RJ. Nanophthalmos with uveal effusion. A new clinical entity. *Arch Ophthalmol.* 1975;93(12):1989-1999.
2. Ritch R, Chang BM, Liebmann JM. Angle closure in younger patients. *Ophthalmology.* 2003;110(10):1880-1889.
3. Yalvac IS, Satana B, Ozkan G, Eksioglu U, Duman S. Management of glaucoma in patients with nanophthalmos. *Eye (Lond).* 2008;22(6):838-843.
4. Walsh MK, Goldberg MF. Abnormal foveal avascular zone in nanophthalmos. *Am J Ophthalmol.* 2007;143(6):1067-1068.
5. Mandal AK, Das T, Gothwal VK. Angle closure glaucoma in nanophthalmos and pigmentary retinal dystrophy: a rare syndrome. *Indian J Ophthalmol.* 2001;49(4):271-272.
6. Ghose S, Sachdev MS, Kumar H. Bilateral nanophthalmos, pigmentary retinal dystrophy, and angle closure glaucoma—a new syndrome? *Br J Ophthalmol.* 1985;69(8):624-628.
7. MacKay CJ, Shek MS, Carr RE, Yanuzzi LA, Gouras P. Retinal degeneration with nanophthalmos, cystic macular degeneration, and angle closure glaucoma. A new recessive syndrome. *Arch Ophthalmol.* 1987;105(3):366-371.
8. Buys YM, Pavlin CJ. Retinitis pigmentosa, nanophthalmos, and optic disc drusen: a case report. *Ophthalmology.* 1999;106(3):619-622.
9. Neelakantan A, Venkataramakrishnan P, Rao BS, et al. Familial nanophthalmos: management and complications. *Indian J Ophthalmol.* 1994;42(3):139-143.
10. Singh OS, Simmons RJ, Brockhurst RJ, Trempe CL. Nanophthalmos: a perspective on identification and therapy. *Ophthalmology.* 1982;89(9):1006-1012.
11. Othman MI, Sullivan SA, Skuta GL, et al. Autosomal dominant nanophthalmos (NNO1) with high hyperopia and angle-closure glaucoma maps to chromosome 11. *Am J Hum Genet.* 1998;63(5):1411-1418.
12. Kimbrough RL, Trempe CS, Brockhurst RJ, Simmons RJ. Angle-closure glaucoma in nanophthalmos. *Am J Ophthalmol.* 1979;88(3 pt 2):572-579.
13. Jin JC, Anderson DR. Laser and unsutured sclerotomy in nanophthalmos. *Am J Ophthalmol.* 1990;109(5):575-580.
14. Calhoun FP Jr. The management of glaucoma in nanophthalmos. *Trans Am Ophthalmol Soc.* 1975;73:97-122.
15. Barad RF, Nelson LB, Cowchock FS, Spaeth GL. Nanophthalmos associated with cryptorchidism. *Ann Ophthalmol.* 1985;17(5):284-286, 288.
16. Yue BY, Kurosawa A, Duvall J, Goldberg MF, Tso MO, Sugar J. Nanophthalmic sclera. Fibronectin studies. *Ophthalmology.* 1988;95(1):56-60.
17. Widder RA, Engels B, Severin M, Brunner R, Krieglstein GK. A case of angle-closure glaucoma, cataract, nanophthalmos and spherophakia in oculo-dento-digital syndrome. *Graefes Arch Clin Exp Ophthalmol.* 2003;241(2):161-163.
18. Wu W, Dawson DG, Sugar A, et al. Cataract surgery in patients with nanophthalmos: results and complications. *J Cataract Refract Surg.* 2004;30(3):584-590.
19. Thapa SS, Paudyal G. Choroidal effusion following laser peripheral iridotomy for the treatment of angle closure glaucoma in a patient with nanophthalmos. *Nepal Med Coll J.* 2005;7(1):81-82.
20. Krohn J, Seland JH. Exudative retinal detachment in nanophthalmos. *Acta Ophthalmologica Scandinavica.* 1998;76(4):499-502.
21. Trelstad RL, Silbermann NN, Brockhurst RJ. Nanophthalmic sclera. Ultrastructural, histochemical, and biochemical observations. *Arch Ophthalmol.* 1982;100(12):1935-1938.
22. Stewart DH 3rd, Streeten BW, Brockhurst RJ, Anderson DR, Hirose T, Gass DM. Abnormal scleral collagen in nanophthalmos. An ultrastructural study. *Arch Ophthalmol.* 1991;109(7):1017-1025.
23. Shiono T, Shoji A, Mutoh T, Tamai M. Abnormal sclerocytes in nanophthalmos. *Graefes Arch Clin Exp Ophthalmol.* 1992;230(4):348-351.
24. Jackson TL, Hussain A, Morley AM, et al. Scleral hydraulic conductivity and macromolecular diffusion in patients with uveal effusion syndrome. *Invest Ophthalmol Vis Sci.* 2008;49(11):5033-5040.
25. Kocak I, Altintas AG, Yalvac IS, Nurozler A, Kasim R, Duman S. Treatment of glaucoma in young nanophthalmic patients. *Int Ophthalmol.* 1996;20(1-3):107-111.
26. Huang S, Yu M, Qiu C, Ye T. The management of secondary glaucoma in nanophthalmic patients. *Yan ke xue bao bian ji bu.* 2002;18(3):156-159.
27. Brockhurst RJ. Vortex vein decompression for nanophthalmic uveal effusion. *Arch Ophthalmol.* 1980;98(11):1987-1990.
28. Gass JD. Uveal effusion syndrome. A new hypothesis concerning pathogenesis and technique of surgical treatment. *Retina.* 1983;3(3):159-163.

Ruthanne B. Simmons, MD, now deceased, was an original author on this chapter.

31

Neovascular Glaucoma

Jeffrey R. SooHoo, MD; David K. Dueker, MD; and Malik Y. Kahook, MD

Neovascular glaucoma (NVG) is a potentially devastating secondary glaucoma that results from the growth of a fibrovascular membrane over the trabecular meshwork (TM) in the anterior chamber angle.

Predisposing Conditions

The changes in the anterior segment that lead to NVG arise in response to a predisposing condition elsewhere—most commonly to a disturbance of the retinal circulation resulting in ischemia. The 3 most common predisposing conditions are diabetic retinopathy, occlusion of the central retinal vein (ischemic type), and ocular ischemic syndrome. Other forms of retinal vascular disease (eg, Eales' disease and sickle cell retinopathy), intraocular neoplasm, chronic retinal detachment, and severe intraocular infection or inflammation are among numerous other disorders that have also been associated with NVG. Thus, a patient presenting with this disorder requires a rather broad-based diagnostic work-up to determine the underlying cause.[1,2] Conversely, any patient with a clinical condition known to predispose an eye to NVG deserves careful monitoring to detect the process in its earliest stages.

The conditions that predispose to NVG show large differences in their tendency to produce the disease. The incidence of NVG after central retinal vein occlusion (CRVO; of the ischemic type) is probably best known because both CRVO and NVG usually have clear signs and symptoms, and, when they occur in association, the time interval is short.[3-11] Classically known as *90-day glaucoma*, a high percentage of eyes that develop NVG after ischemic CRVO do so within the first 3 to 4 months after the CRVO. The overall risk of NVG after ischemic CRVO is 45%, with approximately 40% occurring in the first 7 months, after which NVG is rare.[3]

Fluorescein angiography has been advocated as a way to distinguish the 2 forms of CRVO.[7-10] The ischemic form of CRVO shows large areas of retinal capillary nonperfusion, a sign of severe retinal ischemia. When the capillaries are not filled, the retina remains dark (nonfluorescent), except for the major vascular branches. Because the risk of subsequent NVG resides almost entirely with the ischemic type of CRVO, identifying the type of occlusion is very helpful in guiding further management. However, a single angiogram showing well-perfused retinal capillary beds does not insure against all risk of NVG, because a percentage (approximately 15%) of nonischemic CRVOs later convert to the ischemic form.[5]

Furthermore, definitive angiograms may be unobtainable because of media opacities, widespread retinal hemorrhage, or failure to include peripheral capillary beds. Hayreh recommends a careful assessment of visual function (Table 31-1) as an aid in accurately separating ischemic from nonischemic CRVOs.[11]

The incidence of NVG in eyes with diabetic retinopathy is not as well-defined as in CRVO. In unselected populations of diabetics, the incidence of NVG is low. However, in the presence of proliferative retinopathy, the incidence is similar to that found with CRVO and may actually be higher.[12,13]

Among patients with one of the predisposing diseases, we do not yet know how to predict precisely which individual will develop neovascularization of the anterior segment. And if neovascularization of the iris or the angle develops, we do not yet know what factors determine which eyes will progress to NVG. Finally, in different patients with differing predisposing causes, the progression to full-blown NVG may take weeks, months, or years.

Against this background of multiple different causes and widely varying time course, the only sure method of detecting the earliest signs of anterior segment neovascularization is appropriate vigilance based on knowledge of the potential causes and knowledge of the early clinical signs of anterior segment neovascularization. The reward for this vigilance is the opportunity to intervene at a

Kahook MY, Schuman JS, eds.
Chandler and Grant's Glaucoma, Fifth Edition (pp 309-317).
© 2013 SLACK Incorporated.

TABLE 31-1. TESTS OF VISUAL FUNCTION THAT HELP DIFFERENTIATE ISCHEMIC FROM NONISCHEMIC CENTRAL RETINAL VEIN OCCLUSION[a]	
Visual acuity	Visual acuity 20/200 is seen in 60% of nonischemic and less than 2% of ischemic CRVO.
Perimetry	Goldmann VF with V4e target is normal in approximately 80% of nonischemic but less than 20% of ischemic CRVO.
RAPD	RAPD 0.70 log units in approximately 90% of ischemic and is normal in nonischemic CRVO (if no other optic nerve abnormality).
ERG	Scotopic b wave is reduced in 80% to 90% of ischemic and is usually normal in nonischemic CRVO.
[a]Data were derived from Hayreh et al.[11]	
CRVO: central retinal vein occlusion; ERG: electroretinogram; RAPD: relative afferent pupillary defect.	

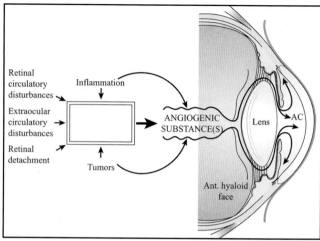

Figure 31-1. Retinal ischemia seems to be the common factor in all or most cases of anterior segment neovascularization. The pathogenic sequence leading to NVG may be modeled as depicted here. A variety of disorders may cause ischemia of the retina. The ischemic retina, in turn, produces angiogenic factor(s) that diffuse forward, causing new vessel growth on the iris and angle. Forward diffusion may be impeded by the vitreous or lens, explaining why there may be a burst of angiogenic activity after vitrectomy, lensectomy, or capsulotomy. Tumors and inflammation may stimulate angiogenesis directly through elaboration of angiogenic factors or indirectly by causing retinal ischemia.

relatively harmless stage of the process, slowing or even arresting it with appropriate therapy. Most often, the intervention takes the form of retinal ablation, though, in certain cases, other forms of therapy are also useful with particular interest in recent years on the promise of anti-angiogenic factors. The rationale for retinal ablation and antiangiogenic therapy derives from clinical observation and theoretical models of the disease (Figure 31-1).

NATURAL CLINIC HISTORY OF NEOVASCULAR GLAUCOMA

Although the pathologic conditions predisposing to NVG are numerous and varied, the sequence of anterior segment change is sufficiently uniform to suggest that the various causes of NVG act through a common pathway, though with variable intensities. When a patient has a disorder with known potential to cause NVG, the first sign that new vessel growth in the anterior segment is beginning is a leakage of intravenously injected fluorescein dye from vessels at the pupillary margin. This leakage of dye may be conspicuous even when the iris appears completely normal on careful slit-lamp examination at high magnification. This abnormal permeability to fluorescein reflects an alteration of the pre-existing vasculature—an opening of the tight junctions normally found between endothelial cells in iris vessels, which is probably a necessary prelude to neovascular proliferation. When vascular proliferation occurs, it is observable by

clinical slit-lamp biomicroscopy without fluorescein, though one cannot appreciate by regular slit-lamp examination as much abnormality as is revealed by fluorescein angiography.

Vascular proliferation is usually first evident at the pupil. Careful attention to the pupillary margin is therefore of great clinical importance for early detection of neovascularization. When an abnormality in vessels of the pupillary margin is suspected, gonioscopy should be done to search for vessels in the chamber angle. In a small proportion of patients (especially those with dark irides), there may be significant vascular proliferation in the angle before any change at the pupil is recognized by slit-lamp examination. Therefore, any patient at risk of developing NVG in a useful eye should have not only a careful and repeated high-magnification slit-lamp examination of the iris (with an undilated pupil), but also a periodic inspection of the anterior chamber angle by gonioscopy.

When proliferating vessels are limited to the iris surface, they do not seem to cause clinically significant disturbance in the anterior chamber, even though they show an abnormal permeability to fluorescein during angiography. But when vessels proliferate in the angle, they cause a progressive decrease of outflow facility and eventually severe glaucoma. New vessels growing in the chamber angle develop from the base of the iris as individual trunks that cross the ciliary body and scleral spur in a direct path to the filtration area of the corneoscleral TM. On the meshwork, the individual vessels branch into a complex pattern of fine vessels that eventually involve the entire circumference, intertwining with branches from other trunk vessels.[14] This fibrovascular tissue may severely compromise aqueous outflow, with

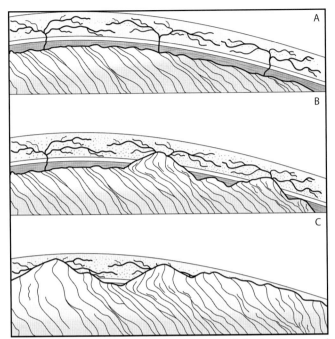

Figure 31-2. Stages of anterior segment neovascularization. New vessel proliferation begins at the pupillary margin and occurs subsequently in the anterior chamber angle. (A) New angle vessels begin as trunks growing up from the iris base, crossing the ciliary body band and scleral spur to reach the TM where they branch and grow circumferentially, often connecting with branches from adjacent trunks. (B) Intermediate: Contractile processes along the vessels lead to synechiae formation. (C) Late: The final stage is total angle closure.

TABLE 31-2. CAROTID ARTERY DISEASE: UNDERAPPRECIATED CAUSE FOR NEOVASCULAR GLAUCOMA UNIQUE FEATURES
1. IOP may be normal, with poor outflow facility masked by decreased aqueous production.
2. Correction of carotid occlusion may lead to marked elevation of IOP.
3. PRP may be less effective.[23]
IOP: intraocular pressure; PRP: panretinal photocoagulation.

resultant glaucoma, even while the angle remains open.[15] Next, a contractile process begins along one or more of the major vessels that run from the iris base to the TM, producing localized anterior synechiae that tend to spread and ultimately to join, causing complete closure of the angle (Figure 31-2).

The rate at which peripheral synechiae spread to involve, eventually, the whole circumference is remarkably variable. In some eyes, once the formation of synechiae is started, the angle may become fully closed within a week. In other eyes, the process is much slower, for reasons unknown. The onset of high pressure is often acute and painful, whether or not the angle has been closed by neovascular tissue or synechiae, and frequently the patient comes for attention as an emergency with a red eye, edematous cornea, and rubeosis of the iris.

DIAGNOSIS

A patient with acute NVG occasionally presents a challenge in diagnosis because the cornea may be so hazy that it obscures a view of details in the anterior chamber. Under such circumstances, the differential diagnosis includes acute angle-closure glaucoma or acute glaucoma secondary to an inflammatory disease. A careful history is frequently helpful in diagnosing the underlying problem. For instance,

most patients developing glaucoma after CRVO recall a painless blurring or loss of vision in the affected eye weeks or months prior to developing pain. Likewise, a diabetic patient with retinal vasculopathy sufficient to cause NVG is almost sure to be aware that he or she has diabetes. Also, a diabetic patient frequently, but not always, has a history of reduced vision before development of glaucoma. Careful examination of the patient's other eye can also provide valuable information, particularly regarding the appearance of the chamber angle, the intraocular pressure (IOP), and the condition of the retina. For example, most patients with acute primary angle closure have a predisposition to the same problem in the opposite eye (especially if the refractive error of both eyes is similar). Therefore, gonioscopy of the opposite eye will usually show a narrow angle. An elevated IOP in the opposite eye, coupled with a normal gonioscopic appearance, will suggest open-angle glaucoma, a common finding in the eye opposite one with NVG after a CRVO. When diabetic retinopathy is the underlying cause for NVG in one eye, the opposite retina will almost always show some evidence of retinopathy as well.

Carotid artery disease may produce NVG (Table 31-2). These patients may demonstrate only peripheral retinal hemorrhages and a relatively low IOP despite advanced angle closure. If carotid artery disease is treated surgically, the IOP may markedly increase due to improved ocular perfusion.

Even a severely edematous cornea in the involved eye can usually be cleared enough with topical glycerin to allow some of the superficial new vessels on the iris and angle to be seen. Occasionally, an acute iritis will cause a rubeotic appearance because the major vessels, and even the capillaries, may dilate markedly, becoming much more visible and imparting a red hue to the iris. But these inflamed vessels, though dilated and tortuous, are still within the iris stroma and still in a predominantly radial pattern consistent with normal iris vasculature. One must differentiate this finding from the rubeosis associated with a true vasoproliferative response that derives from the growth of irregular networks of newly formed vessels on the iris surface. Frequently, a contractile element associated with these new surface vessels causes an ectropion of the posterior iris pigment epithelium; this finding can be a useful clinical clue to the diagnosis.

TABLE 31-3. CONDITIONS ASSOCIATED WITH NEOVASCULAR GLAUCOMA

Diabetic retinopathy (common)
Retinal disorders
Vascular occlusive disorders
Central retinal vein occlusion (common)
Central retinal artery occlusion
Branch retinal artery or vein occlusion
Retinal detachment (chronic)
Retinopathy of prematurity
Coat's disease
Sickle cell retinopathy
Syphilitic retinopathy
Retinoschisis
Radiation-induced retinopathy
Ocular tumors
Ocular melanoma
Retinoblastoma
Reticulum cell sarcoma
Metastatic tumors
Uveitis (chronic)
Vascular disorders (associated with ocular ischemia)
Carotid artery occlusive disease (common)
Carotid cavernous fistula
Temporal (giant cell) arteritis
Pulseless disease
Postsurgical
Strabismus surgery (interruption of anterior ciliary vessels)
Vitrectomy (with associated diabetic retinopathy)
Cataract surgery (with associated diabetic retinopathy)

Having determined that the case is a true NVG, the clinician will then want to ensure that the underlying cause has been correctly identified. This is important because the underlying pathologic condition may require specific treatment (eg, diabetes, systemic hypertension, carotid artery occlusion, or retinal detachment; Table 31-3). Diagnostic ultrasound is uniquely helpful in revealing occult malignancy or retinal detachment presenting as NVG and should be considered for all cases in which the cause of anterior neovascularization is unclear or the fundus cannot be seen.

The management of NVG is guided by the underlying cause. Enucleation was, in the past, a common outcome for a painful and sightless eye. Enucleation may still be the proper approach for cases in which NVG has been caused by a posterior neoplasm or a devastating inflammation or infection. However, most cases do not fall into this category, and treatment to preserve remaining vision and maintain a comfortable eye is increasingly effective.

PROPHYLAXIS

Before any discussion of treatment, however, prevention of NVG is now possible in a large proportion of eyes that would have been destined for this disease in the past. Preventive treatment is based on careful assessment of the setting in which anterior segment neovascularization develops and recognition of the progressive stages leading to fully manifest glaucoma. With continuing improvements in early detection and prophylaxis, the need to treat the disease in full-blown form may eventually become uncommon.

The keystone for prevention of NVG at this time is retinal ablation in which, by means of photocoagulation or cryotherapy, a portion of the retinal tissue is destroyed. Reducing the mass of viable retina with photocoagulation therapy seems to inhibit and even reverse new vessel proliferation in the anterior segment. Several authors have reported regression of new vessels on the surface of the iris after panretinal photocoagulation (PRP),[16-22] and a large retrospective study demonstrated a significantly lower incidence of neovascularization of the iris and angle in the eyes of diabetic patients treated by panretinal photocoagulation.[23]

These findings are in agreement with the observation that anterior segment neovascularization characteristically occurs in close association with retinal hypoxia. This is compatible with the hypothesis put forth by Michaelson[24] that ischemic retinal tissue calls forth new vessel growth by releasing a diffusible angiogenic substance. Forward diffusion of such an angiogenic factor could initiate neovascularization in the anterior segment as well[25] (see Figure 31-2). A factor with angiogenic properties has been found in solid tumors,[26] and there is indication that retinal tissue also harbors an angiogenic substance.[27] Vascular endothelial growth factor (VEGF) has been measured in the ocular fluids of eyes with ischemic retinas, suggesting it may mediate the neovascular response.[28] Although characterization of chemical mediators of angiogenesis, as well as means to block their effect, have become available in recent years, large-scale destruction of retinal tissue by photocoagulation continues to play an important role in reducing the vasoproliferative stimulus in both the posterior and the anterior segment. Furthermore, the retinal ablation need not be accomplished solely by photocoagulation. If media opacities preclude photocoagulation, widespread retinal cryoablation is an alternative approach that is also effective in reducing anterior segment vasoproliferation.[29,30]

Although panretinal treatment of the retina is the primary laser-based preventive treatment for NVG, a second means of prophylaxis using direct laser coagulation of the new vessels growing in the chamber angle, an approach

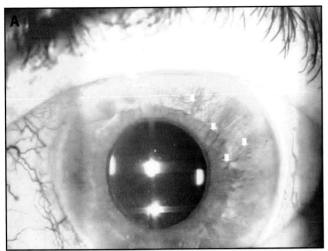 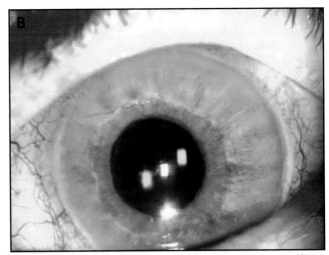

Figures 31-3. (A) Before and (B) after bevacizumab injections. (Reprinted with permission from Kahook MY, Schuman JS, Noecker RJ. Intravitreal bevacizumab in a patient with NVG. *Ophthalmic Surg Lasers Imaging.* 2006;37[2]:144-146.)

developed by Simmons et al[31,32] has also been used. This method, *goniophotocoagulation*, requires meticulous application of small laser burns to the trunks of new vessels as they cross the ciliary band and scleral spur between the iris base and the TM. Successful occlusion of these vessels at the level of the ciliary band or scleral spur causes blanching of the fine vascular network that arborizes on the TM. Thus, goniophotocoagulation interrupts a critical tissue response to the angiogenic stimulus, while retinal photocoagulation appears to reduce the stimulus itself.

When solid indications for PRP exist (eg, in diabetes according to Diabetic Retinopathy Study guidelines),[33,34] timely use of retinal ablation may decrease the angiogenic stimulus and prevent significant vasoproliferation in the anterior segment. When a diabetic eye presents with new vessels already actively growing on the iris and/or chamber angle, possibly with early synechia formation, rapid initiation of retinal ablation may successfully reduce the proliferative stimulus, leading to regression of the new vessels and preservation of an open angle. In some cases, however, the progression to angle closure is so rapid that it occurs before the eye has time to respond to retinal treatment. In such cases, goniophotocoagulation may provide a direct, though transient, interruption in the anatomic chain of events in the anterior segment, providing time for retinal treatment to achieve a reduction in the driving stimulus. In recent years, the development of antivascular endothelial growth factor (anti-VEGF) compounds has provided an alternative, remarkably effective means for inducing rapid regression of new vessels in the anterior segment.

It is well-established that PRP is an effective and long-lasting treatment for reducing/preventing anterior neovascularization in proliferative diabetic retinopathy. However, Michaelson's hypothetical concept of a diffusible angiogenic substance (Factor X) produced by ischemic retina now has confirmation, with the presumed role of Factor X well-filled

by VEGF. Direct attack on this stimulus is now available in the form of anti-VEGF antibodies (eg, bevacizumab [Avastin]). Initial trials of intravitreal injections of anti-VEGF agents showed dramatic reduction in anterior segment neovascularization, and subsequent larger series and controlled trials have confirmed these initial impressions.[35] In addition, because of widespread use of anti-VEGF agents for other ocular diseases, the safety profile and dosing for intravitreal use are well-established.

A single intravitreal dose of anti-VEGF antibody can have a dramatic effect on reversing anterior segment neovascularization (Figure 31-3) and seems, as well, to offer reduction in IOP, inflammation, and pain in some patients. Furthermore, administration is straightforward and does not require the clarity of media needed for PRP. In an acute presentation of NVG, intravitreal VEGF can be given along with initial medical treatment for pressure reduction and inflammation. Iris fluorescein angiography has demonstrated that leakage from iris neovascularization decreases as soon as the first day after injection with intracameral bevacizumab.[36] Use of anti-VEGF agents can quickly lead to lower pressures and clearing of the cornea and thus allow supplemental PRP, if indicated. The regression of iris and angle neovascularization induced by anti-VEGF therapy may be temporary and can be addressed by repeat treatment with anti-VEGF therapy, PRP, or surgery.[37] If the anterior chamber angle remains open in substantial areas, the glaucoma may be controlled medically. If the neovascular process has already closed most of the anterior chamber angle, adequate pressure control may still require surgery. But the rapid coordinated use of these treatments will have produced, in many instances, an eye with much greater chance of surgical success and reduced risk of complications.

Because various forms of prophylaxis are available, it is prudent to identify eyes at risk for, or in early stages of, anterior segment neovascularization to allow intervention before the more advanced stages of NVG have a chance to develop. Because the onset of NVG after CRVO can be very rapid, these cases have been subject to careful study. First of all, it is established that the ischemic form of CRVO carries the risk for developing CRVO, so early identification by fluorescein angiography and tests of visual function is important. Because NVG can be such a devastating disease, there have been reports advocating PRP for all cases of ischemic CRVO.[20,38,39] Others have advocated following the high-risk ischemic CRVO patients carefully to monitor for early signs of anterior segment neovascularization[38,40] and, when found, administering PRP. Hayreh has pointed out evidence suggesting that the value of PRP for preventing NVG after ischemic CRVO may have been over-estimated and prefers to monitor such patients closely and to use treatment other than PRP to avoid compromising peripheral visual field.[41]

The Central Retinal Vein Occlusion Study (CRVOS)[5] was a randomized NIH-sponsored multicenter trial of early panretinal photocoagulation for ischemic CRVO. In the CVOS, eyes with an ischemic CRVO were randomly assigned either to early PRP or to PRP only in the event that anterior segment neovascularization developed. Per study protocol,[5] after initial intervention, "panretinal photocoagulation is mandated after appropriate photographic documentation for any eye that develops 2 clock hoursof INV (iris neovascularization) or any angle neovascularization (ANV) at any time during the study."

The CVOS concluded that PRP is effective treatment for neovascularization of the anterior segment caused by ischemic CRVO.[42] However, there was no benefit from PRP performed prior to the development of iris or angle neovascularization when frequent follow-up examinations were being performed.[5] It was recommended that all eyes with CRVO should be evaluated with retinal angiography to identify occlusions of the ischemic type. Where this is not possible due to media opacity or nonavailability, eyes with CRVO should be managed as if they were of the ischemic type. In cases where follow-up examinations are problematic, prophylactic PRP was recommended. The identification of early neovascularization of the pupillary border was felt to be particularly important in patients after recent CRVO to assess the need for initial or additional PRP. This study is in agreement with the general impression that PRP is an effective treatment for the prevention of NVG after ischemic CRVO, an opinion that is widely held but not universal.[41,43]

In diabetes, the main risk for neovascularization of the anterior segment occurs with proliferative diabetic retinopathy. These cases should receive panretinal photocoagulation as treatment for their retinopathy[33,34] and consequently gain the additional benefits of reducing their risk for iris and angle neovascularization. However, even eyes treated with adequate PRP may, in fact, still harbor significant areas of ischemic retina and, therefore, have a persisting risk for neovascularization of the anterior segment. Thus, eyes with

proliferative diabetic retinopathy deserve careful monitoring of the iris and angle, even after a standard course of PRP, so that further retinal ablation can be done if new vessels develop or progress in the anterior segment.

There are other events that may initiate or aggravate new vessel growth in a previously quiet diabetic eye. One is surgical intervention. The anterior hyaloid and lens represent a barrier to forward movement of angiogenic substances from the retina (see Figure 31-2). Removal of this barrier by vitrectomy/lensectomy or intracapsular cataract extraction may lead to rapid progression of anterior segment neovascularization in a predisposed eye.[44-47] Cataract surgery that preserves the posterior capsule appears to preserve this useful barrier, but that benefit may be lost if posterior capsulotomy is required later.[48]

Diabetics may also develop tractional retinal detachments. Because chronic retinal detachment is an important cause of NVG, this introduces another risk factor for NVG that requires increased monitoring of the anterior segment. Finally, diabetics may develop retinal ischemia on the basis of ocular or extraocular circulatory compromise that does not present as classic retinopathy but that can lead to NVG.

MEDICAL TREATMENT

Careful monitoring of at-risk eyes and vigorous use of prophylactic intervention has reduced but not eliminated the need to treat more advanced stages of NVG. Medical therapy of NVG is based on aqueous suppressants—carbonic anhydrase inhibitors, beta-adrenergic blockers, and alpha-2 agonists. The outflow system of these eyes is usually not responsive to miotics, and because they may aggravate inflammation, they should be avoided. Use of prostaglandin analogs is advised on a cautious trial basis because their ability to improve uveoscleral flow is likely to be reduced in the presence of extensive angle closure, and they hold some risk for increasing inflammation. Antiglaucoma medication is often supplemented with anti-inflammatory treatment, corticosteroids, and cycloplegics. If the angle is fully closed by synechiae, such combined aqueous suppressant/anti-inflammatory therapy may bring comfort and some reduction in pressure, but it will seldom provide a normal pressure. On the other hand, if the angle is wholly or partly open, and particularly if the vessels can be made to regress using retinal ablation and/or administration of anti-VEGF therapy, medical therapy alone may then provide adequate long-term glaucoma control.

SURGICAL TREATMENT

Surgical therapy for intractable NVG has been considered a major clinical challenge. Fortunately, the situation has evolved in recent years to the point that these cases can now be approached with increasing confidence, though they remain demanding and retain a higher failure rate than most other forms of glaucoma. A recurring theme for NVG has been the positive benefit of retinal ablation, now often supplemented by anti-VEGF therapy. Retinal ablation can be considered most effective when used in appropriate circumstances to prevent NVG altogether. When used at a somewhat later stage, with new vessels proliferating on the iris and angle, retinal ablation (again, now often in conjunction with anti-VEGF therapy) remains extremely useful for its potential to regress the neovascular process and salvage remaining outflow function. Even when the angle is completely closed by irreversible fibrous contraction, retinal ablation and anti-VEGF therapy are extremely effective as a means to quiet inflammation, reduce new vessel growth, and prepare the eye for glaucoma surgery. The full preparation of an NVG eye for surgery thus includes aqueous suppressants to reduce pressure, corticosteroids and cycloplegics to reduce inflammation, and PRP and/or anti-VEGF antibodies to reduce the vasoproliferative stimulus.[49]

While not yet conclusive, data continue to emerge that support the use of anti-VEGF agents as adjuncts to glaucoma filtration surgery. In addition to the previously mentioned effects these agents have on neovasculature, it has been suggested that antibodies such as bevacizumab may modulate wound healing and improve the efficacy of drainage procedures.[50-52] A rabbit model has demonstrated a possible synergistic effect when 5-FU and bevacizumab are used in combination to modulate wound healing after filtration surgery.[53]

The exact agent, dose, route of administration, and timing of administration are all currently under investigation; at present, there is no clear consensus regarding the optimal use of these therapies. In the setting of trabeculectomy, bevacizumab has been used preoperatively, intraoperatively, postoperatively, and for treatment of failing filtering blebs or during bleb revision. These studies have looked at intracameral, intravitreal, and subconjunctival administration.[50,51,54-56] Use of topical ranibizumab after trabeculectomy with MMC has also been proposed.[57]

The selection of a surgical procedure for NVG has evolved over time, with emphasis shifting toward conventional drainage procedures rather than ablation of the ciliary body (by cryo or, more recently, laser) as initial treatment. Hayreh[58] and Netland[59] have provided thorough reviews of the pros and cons of the available surgical therapies.

Trabeculectomy remains an option favored by some, with its success rate improved by the introduction of antimetabolites. However, even with antimetabolite use, initial success is not as high as, and failure over time is more common than, other glaucomas. As mentioned above, adjunctive use of anti-VEGF compounds may increase filtration surgery success in NVG, but, at this time, there is insufficient long-term evidence to draw this conclusion. The cases most likely to do well with trabeculectomy are those with less active inflammation and neovascularization. In more severe cases, many surgeons will favor a tube-shunt implant.

In fact, the development of tube-shunts was largely driven by the need to find alternate effective ways to manage difficult glaucomas such as NVG surgically.[60-62] Scarred conjunctiva, active inflammation, vigorous new vessel growth, and prior failure of trabeculectomy are all reasons to consider tube-shunt surgery in NVG. There is little evidence to select one model shunt over another, just as there is no clear and consistent basis for choosing between trabeculectomy or drainage implant—the selection is based primarily on individual surgical judgment and consideration of multiple variables. As Netland[59] notes: "Because of lack of direct comparative evidence in the literature, the choice between trabeculectomy and drainage implants is surgeon preference at this time."

In eyes with little visual potential, cilioablation, most often performed now by trans-scleral diode laser, remains an effective initial option. Cilioablation can also be used as an effective supplement to a drainage implant to improve pressure control. Hayreh has pointed out the relative safety of graduated doses of cyclophotocoagulation to avoid hypotony and phthisis. He notes that this can provide safe, effective pressure control even in eyes without a drainage implant. He advocates this approach particularly for eyes with ischemic CRVO, which, he notes, may resolve spontaneously without PRP, a treatment he prefers to avoid in such cases because of its adverse impact on peripheral vision.

Unfortunately, despite concerted effort, some eyes with NVG still end up without sight and with significant pain. In such cases, it is reasonable to try retrobulbar alcohol nerve block. In some intractable cases, removal of the eye by evisceration or enucleation will be required.

CONCLUSION

Understanding the fundamental pathophysiology of NVG has increased the opportunities to prevent its development and reverse the process in the early, less difficult, stages. Certainly, the greatest advance in NVG therapy recently has been the development and use of anti-VEGF compounds to reverse new vessel growth in the anterior segment. This exciting new capability, along with judicious use of retinal ablation, modern glaucoma surgery and medicine, and heightened ability to identify a high-risk eye, produces an improved outlook for successful management, even of full-blown NVG. Nevertheless, NVG remains a difficult, and all too often devastating, form of glaucoma, challenging us to still further improve our methods of treatment and to continue to search for more effective therapies for the underlying disorders that cause this secondary glaucoma.

REFERENCES

1. Wand M. Neovascular glaucoma. In: Albert DM, Jakobiec FA, eds. *Principles and Practice of Ophthalmology. Clinical Practice.* Philadelphia, PA: WB Saunders Co; 1994:1485-1510.

2. Gartner S, Henkind P. Neovascularization of the iris (rubeosis iridis). *Surv Ophthalmol.* 1978;22:291.

3. Hayreh SS, Rojas P, Podhajsky P, Montague P, Woolson RF. Ocular neovascularization with retinal vascular occlusion—III. Incidence of ocular neovascularization with retinal vein occlusion. *Ophthalmology.* 1983;90:488-506.

4. Hayreh SS. Classification of central retinal vein occlusion. *Ophthalmology.* 1983;90:458-474.

5. Central Vein Occlusion Study Group, The Central Vein Occlusion Study, Baseline and Early Natural History Report. *Arch Ophthalmol.* 1993;111:1087-1095.

6. Hayreh SS. Retinal vein occlusion. Current ophthalmology. *Indian J Ophthalmol.* 1994;42:3, 109-132.

7. Laatikainen L, Kohner EM. Fluorescein angiography and its prognostic significance in central retinal vein occlusion. *Br J Ophthalmol.* 1976;60:411-418.

8. Laatikainen L, Blach RK. Behaviour of the iris vasculature in central retinal vein occlusion: a fluorescein angiographic study of the vascular response of the retina and the iris. *Br J Ophthalmol.* 1977;61:272-277.

9. Sinclair SH, Gragoudas ES. Prognosis for rubeosis iridis following central retinal vein occlusion. *Br J Ophthalmol.* 1979;63:735-743.

10. Magargal LE, Brown GC, Augsburger JJ, Parrish RK 2nd. Neovascular glaucoma following central retinal vein obstruction. *Ophthalmology.* 1981;88:1095-1101.

11. Hayreh SS, Klugman MR, Beri M, et al. Differentiation of ischemic from nonischemic central retinal vein occlusion during the early acute phase. *Graefes Arch Clin Exp Ophthalmol.* 1990;228:201-217.

12. Ohrt V. The frequency of rubeosis iridis in diabetic patients. *Acta Ophthalmol.* 1971;49:301-307.

13. Madsen PH. Rubeosis of the iris and haemorrhagic glaucoma in patients with proliferative diabetic retinopathy. *Br J Ophthalmol.* 1971;55:368-371.

14. Jocson VL. Microvascular injection studies in rubeosis iridis and neovascular glaucoma. *Am J Ophthalmol.* 1977;483:508-517.

15. Grant WM. Management of neovascular glaucoma. In: Leopold IH, ed. *Symposium on Ocular Therapy.* Vol 7. St Louis, MO: CV Mosby; 1974.

16. Krill AC, Archer D, Newell FW. Photocoagulation in complications secondary to branch vein occlusion. *Arch Ophthalmol.* 1971;85:48-60.

17. Callahan MA. Letter: photocoagulation and rubeosis iridis. *Am J Ophthalmol.* 1974;78:873-874.

18. Little HL, Rosenthal AR, Dellaporta A, Jacobson DR. The effect of pan-retinal photo-coagulation on rubeosis iridis. *Am J Ophthalmol.* 1976;81:804-809.

19. Laatikainen L. Preliminary report on effect of retinal panphotocoagula-tion on rubeosis iridis and neovascular glaucoma. *Br J Ophthalmol.* 1977;61:278-284.

20. Laatikainen L, Kohner EM, Khoury D, Blach RK. Panretinal photocoagulation in central retinal vein occlusion. A randomized controlled clinical study. *Br J Ophthalmol.* 1977;61:741-753.

21. Murphy RP, Egbert PR. Regression of iris neovascularization following panretinal photocoagulation. *Arch Ophthalmol.* 1979;97:700-702.

22. Tasman W, Magargal LE, Augsburger JJ. Rubeosis iridis and angle neovascularization. *Ophthalmology.* 1980;87:400-402.

23. Wand M, Dueker DK, Aiello LM, Grant WM. Effects of panretinal photocoagulation on rubeosis iridis, angle neovascularization and neovascular glaucoma. *Am J Ophthalmol.* 1978;86:332-339.

24. Michaelson IC. The mode of development of the vascular system of the retina with some observations of its significance in certain retinal diseases. *Trans Ophthalmol Soc UK.* 1948;68:137.

25. Ashton N. Retinal vascularization in health and disease. *Am J Ophthalmol.* 1957;44:7-17.

26. Folkman J. The vascularization of tumors. *Sci Am.* 1976:234-259.

27. Glaser BM, D'Amore PA, Michels RG, et al. The demonstration of angiogenic activity from ocular tissues. Preliminary report. *Ophthalmology.* 1980;87:440-446.

28. Aiello L, Avery RL, Arrigg PG, et al. Vascular endothelial growth factor in ocular fluid of patients with diabetic retinopathy and other retinal disorders. *N Engl J Med.* 1994;331:1480-1487.

29. Hilton G. Panretinal cryotherapy of diabetic rubeosis. *Arch Ophthalmol.* 1979;97:776.

30. May DR, Bergstrom TJ, Parmet AJ, Schwartz JG. Treatment of neovascular glaucoma with transcleral panretinal cryotherapy. *Ophthalmology.* 1980;87:1106-1111.

31. Simmons RJ, Dueker DK, Kimbrough RL, Aiello LM. Goniophotocoagulation for neovascul glaucoma. *Trans Am Acad Ophthalmol Otolaryngol.* 1977;83:80-89.

32. Simmons RJ, Depperman SR, Dueker DK. The role of goniophotocoagulation in neovascularization of the anterior chamber angle. *Ophthalmology.* 1980;87:79-82.

33. Preliminary report on effects of photocoagulation therapy. The Diabetic Retinopathy Study Research Group. *Am J Ophthalmol.* 1976;81:383-396.

34. Four risk factors for severe visual loss in diabetic retinopathy. Diabetic Retinopathy Study Research Group. *Arch Ophthalmol.* 1979;97:654-655.

35. Horsley MB, Kahook MY. Anti-VEGF therapy for glaucoma. *Curr Opin Ophthalmol.* 2010;21:112-117.

36. Grisanti S, Biester S, Peters S, Tatar O, Ziemssen F, Bartz-Schmidt KU. Intracameral bevacizumab for iris rubeosis. *Am J Ophthalmol.* 2006;142(1):158-160.

37. Gheith ME, Siam GA, de Barros DS, Garg SJ, Moster MR. Role of intravitreal bevacizumab in neovascular glaucoma. *J Ocul Pharmacol Ther.* 2007;23(5):487-491.

38. May DR, Klein ML, Peyman GA, Raichand M. Xenon arc panretinal photocoagulation for central retinal vein occlusion: a randomized prospective study. *Br J Ophthalmol.* 1979;63:725-734.

39. Laatkainen L, Kohner EM, Khoury D, et al. Panretinal photocoagulation in central vein occlusion: a randomized controlled clinical study. *Br J Ophthalmol.* 1977;61:741-753.

40. Magargal LE, Brown GC, Augsburger JJ, et al. Efficacy of panretinal photocoagulation in preventing neovascular glaucoma following ischemic central retinal vein obstruction. *Ophthalmology.* 1982;89:780-784.

41. Hayreh SS, Klugman MR, Podhajsky P, et al. Argon laser panretinal photocoagulation in ischemic central retinal vein occlusion. *Graefes Arch Ophthalmol.* 1990;228:281-296.

42. The Central Vein Occlusion Study Group. A randomized clinical trial of early panretinal photocoagulation for ischemic central vein occlusion. *Ophthalmology.* 1995;102:1434-1444.

43. Hayreh SS, Klugman MR, Podhajsky P, et al. Argon laser panretinal photocoagulation in ischemic central retinal vein occlusion. *Graefes Arch Clin Ophthalmol.* 1990;228:281-296.

44. Aiello LM, Wand M, Liang G. Neovascular glaucoma and vitreous hemorrhage following cataract surgery in patients with diabetes mellitus. *Ophthalmology.* 1983;90:814-820.

45. Blankenship G. The lens influence on diabetic vitrectomy results; report of a prospective randomized study. *Arch Ophthalmol.* 1980;98:2196-2198.

46. Aaberg TM. Pars plana vitrectomy for diabetic traction retinal detachment. *Ophthalmology.* 1981;88:639-642.

47. Rice TA, Michels RG, Maguire MG, Rice EF. The effect of lensectomy on the incidence of iris neovascularization and neovascular glaucoma after vitrectomy for diabetic retinopathy. *Am J Ophthalmol.* 1983;95:1-11.

48. Weinreb RN, Wasserstrom JP, Parker W. Neovascular glaucoma following neodymium: YAG laser posterior capsulotomy. *Arch Ophthalmol.* 1986;104:730-731.

49. Allen RC, Bellows AR, Hutchinson BT, et al. Filtration surgery in the treatment of neovascular glaucoma. *Ophthalmology.* 1982;89:1181.

50. Cornish KS, Ramamurthi S, Saidkasimova S, Ramaesh K. Intravitreal bevacizumab and augmented trabeculectomy for neovascular glaucoma in young diabetic patients. *Eye (Lond).* 2009;23(4):979-981.

51. Grewal DS, Jain R, Kumar H, Grewal SP. Evaluation of subconjunctival bevacizumab as an adjunct to trabeculectomy a pilot study. *Ophthalmology.* 2008;115(12):2141-2145.

52. Kapetansky FM, Krasnow MA. Suconjunctival injection(s) of bevacizumab for failing filtering blebs. *Invest Ophthalmol Vis Sci.* 2007;E-Abstract 837.

53. How A, Chua JL, Charlton A, et al. Combined treatment with bevacizumab and 5-fluorouracil attenuates the postoperative scarring response after experimental glaucoma filtration surgery. *Invest Ophthalmol Vis Sci.* 2010;51(2):928-932.

54. Kahook MY, Schuman JS, Noecker RJ. Intravitreal bevacizumab in a patient with neovascular glaucoma. *Ophthalmic Surg Lasers Imaging.* 2006;37(2):144-146.

55. Kahook MY, Schuman JS, Noecker RJ. Needle bleb revision of encapsulated filtering bleb with bevacizumab. *Ophthalmic Surg Lasers Imaging.* 2006;37(2):148-150.

56. Choi JY, Choi J, Kim YD. Subconjunctival bevacizumab as an adjunct to trabeculectomy in eyes with refractory glaucoma: a case series. *Korean J Ophthalmol.* 2010;24(1):47-52.

57. Bochmann F, Kaufmann C, Becht CN, et al. ISRCTN12125882—influence of topical anti-VEGF (Ranibizumab) on the outcome of filtration surgery for glaucoma—study protocol. *BMC Ophthalmol.* 2011;11:1.

58. Hayreh SS. Neovascular glaucoma. *Prog Retin Eye Res.* 2007;26:470-485.

59. Netland PA. The Ahmed glaucoma valve in neovascular glaucoma (an AOS thesis). *Trans Am Ophthalmol Soc.* 2009;107:325-342.

60. Molteno ACB, Von Rooyen MMB, Bartholomew RS. Implants for draining neovascular glaucoma. *Br J Ophthalmol.* 1977;61:120-125.

61. Krupin R, Kaufman P, Mandell A, et al. Filtering valve implant surgery for eyes with neovascular glaucoma. *Am J Ophthalmol.* 1980;89:338-343.

62. Schocket SS, Lakhanpal V, Richards RD. Anterior chamber tube shunt to an encircling band in the treatment of neovascular glaucoma. *Ophthalmology.* 1982;89:1188-1194.

Iridocorneal Endothelial Syndromes

Sarwat Salim, MD, FACS and M. Bruce Shields, MD

Iridocorneal endothelial (ICE) syndrome represents a spectrum of disease, comprising 3 clinical variations: Chandler's syndrome, progressive iris atrophy, and Cogan-Reese syndrome. These 3 variants, initially described separately and with distinct clinical manifestations, have been shown by histopathological and ultrastructural studies to be linked by a fundamental defect of the corneal endothelium. The spectrum is an acquired, unilateral disorder, which typically occurs in early to middle adulthood and predominantly affects women. Clinically, anterior segment changes are most notable, affecting the cornea, anterior chamber angle, and iris. The progressive nature of this disease is associated with a high incidence of visual loss, either from corneal decompensation or refractory glaucoma, frequently requiring surgical intervention with variable success rates.

HISTORY AND TERMINOLOGY

There were several isolated case reports in the late 19th century of patients with extreme iris atrophy and associated glaucoma, but it was the paper by Harms in 1903[1] that led to our current understanding of the condition that has been called *essential iris atrophy* or *progressive essential iris atrophy*. In 1956, Chandler[2] reported cases that were similar but differed by having less severe iris atrophy and more frequent corneal edema, which often occurred with intraocular pressures (IOPs) that were normal or only slightly elevated. In all of his cases, Chandler noted an abnormality of the corneal endothelium that he described as having a fine, hammered silver appearance. The condition became known as *Chandler's syndrome*.

Given the similar clinical features and associated secondary angle-closure glaucoma in patients with either essential iris atrophy or Chandler's syndrome, Chandler and Grant[3] concluded, in the first edition of their textbook, that the 2 conditions are likely variations of a spectrum of disease.

In 1969, Cogan and Reese[4] described 2 patients with pigmented nodules of the iris. Malignant melanoma was suspected, and the eyes were enucleated, but the nodules were found to be benign, composed of tissue resembling that of the iris stroma.

Subsequent studies revealed that these nodules may occur on the surface of the iris in association with the other changes seen with essential iris atrophy and Chandler's syndrome, and this condition became known as the *Cogan-Reese syndrome*.

Continued study of these 3 conditions revealed the common denominator of a characteristic abnormality of the corneal endothelium, which may lead to corneal edema, progressive closure of the anterior chamber angle with associated glaucoma, and the spectrum of iris abnormalities. Scheie and Yanoff[5] described a fourth condition with flat nevi on the surface of the iris that they called the *iris nevus syndrome*, and lumped it with the Cogan-Reese syndrome as a single entity. However, the iris lesions in the 2 conditions are distinctly different, and the iris nevus syndrome has not been shown to have the corneal endothelial abnormality, as with the other 3 conditions.

Eagle and associates[6] suggested the term *ICE syndrome*, and this has now become the most commonly used term for the spectrum of disease, which includes essential iris atrophy, Chandler's syndrome, and the Cogan-Reese syndrome. Because atrophy of the iris is neither an essential nor fundamental aspect of these disorders, the term *progressive iris atrophy* may be preferable for the first of these 3 clinical variations. In any case, Chandler and Grant were correct in believing that these conditions do represent a broad spectrum of ocular disease.

CLINICAL FEATURES

The ICE syndrome is typically a unilateral disorder that usually manifests in early to middle adulthood with a predilection for women, although bilateral involvement and

Kahook MY, Schuman JS, eds.
Chandler and Grant's Glaucoma, Fifth Edition (pp 319-326).
© 2013 SLACK Incorporated.

its occurrence in a child have been reported.[7-10] In some cases, subclinical abnormalities of the corneal endothelium may be seen in the asymptomatic fellow eye.[11-13] Kupfer and colleagues[13] also demonstrated decreased aqueous outflow facility without IOP elevation in the contralateral eye of 4 out of 6 patients with the ICE syndrome. Familial cases are rare, and there is no consistent association with systemic diseases, although an isolated case was recently described with progressive iris atrophy and sensorineural deafness.[14] The report[14] suggested re-evaluation of the neural crest hypothesis (discussed in the Differential Diagnosis section of this chapter) as an etiological association for these findings with abnormal proliferation and degeneration of undifferentiated neural crest-derived cells in the cornea, iris, and superior cervical ganglion, with the latter causing microcirculation dysregulation of the internal ear.

In a study of 37 consecutive cases of the ICE syndrome, approximately half were Chandler's syndrome, while the other 2 clinical variations each accounted for about one-fourth of all cases.[15] Chandler's syndrome was characterized by more severe corneal edema, even though the glaucoma tended to be less severe than in the other 2 variations. However, another study[16] reported a higher incidence of elevated IOP in Chandler's syndrome and reported similar response to treatment among different variants.

ICE syndrome has been described in different ethnic groups, although the prevalence of the 3 clinical variations may vary among ethnicities. For example, Cogan-Reese syndrome has been reported to be the most common form of ICE syndrome in a Thai population, with other characteristics of the spectrum being similar to the White population, including age of onset and gender predilection.[17] This article also described a clinically discernible translucent membrane by slit-lamp examination on the dark irides.

A common presenting manifestation is the recognition of an abnormal shape or position of the pupil, which the patient may describe as a localized or diffused dark spot on the iris. Other patients may present with a chief complaint of reduced vision that is typically worse in the morning, due to the corneal edema that develops while the lids are closed during sleep, and which improves during the day as the cornea dehydrates with exposure to air. Corneal permeability and hydration control have been investigated in ICE syndrome in a few in vivo studies.[18,19] Reduced corneal swelling secondary to decreased endothelial permeability and slower de-swelling responses have been demonstrated in eyes with ICE syndrome. Some patients may also present with pain, which is usually due to the corneal edema. Patients with more advanced disease may have persistent reduction in vision due to severe corneal edema or glaucomatous optic atrophy. Kocaoglan and colleagues[20] reported cystoid macular edema (CME) in a patient with Chandler's syndrome and proposed increased levels of prostaglandin-like inflammatory mediators inducing CME, possibly secondary to a viral infection. The role of viral etiology in the

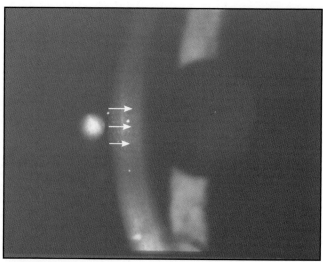

Figure 32-1. Slit-lamp view showing fine, hammered silver appearance of corneal endothelial abnormality (arrows) in ICE syndrome. (This article was published in *Am J Ophthalmol*, 85, Shields MB, Campbell DG, Simmons RJ, The essential iris atrophies, 749-759, Copyright Elsevier 1978.)

pathogenesis of ICE syndrome will be discussed in detail in Theories of Mechanism section of this chapter.

Clinical examination of a patient with ICE syndrome typically reveals abnormalities of the cornea, anterior chamber angle, and iris.

The corneal abnormality, which is a common feature throughout the ICE syndrome, is seen by slit-lamp examination as a fine hammered silver appearance of the posterior cornea, similar to that of Fuchs' dystrophy, but less coarse (Figure 32-1). The cornea may be otherwise clear with no associated symptoms, or there may be corneal edema with variable degrees of reduced vision and pain, as noted above. In some cases, islands of the endothelial abnormality may be seen in the fellow eye, which is otherwise unaffected by the disease process.

Specular microscopy of the corneal endothelial cells reveals a characteristic, diffuse abnormality with variable degrees of pleomorphism in size and shape and loss of hexagonal margins. These abnormal cells also show dark-light reversal, with cell boundaries appearing bright and cell surfaces dark[21] (Figure 32-2). These cells have been called *ICE cells*, and the tissue they form has been termed *ICE tissue*.[22] In some cases, the cells cover the entire posterior cornea (total ICE), while in other eyes they are scattered throughout the cornea (disseminated ICE) or occur in areas that are sharply demarcated from endothelial cells that are normal, abnormally large (subtotal ICE minus), or abnormally small (subtotal ICE plus). In some cases, the focal area of abnormal cells may spread over time to eventually cover the entire cornea, although one case has been reported in which the abnormal cells disappeared almost entirely over a 10-year observation period.[23]

The typical anterior chamber angle abnormality, which is also common to all variations of ICE syndrome, is seen

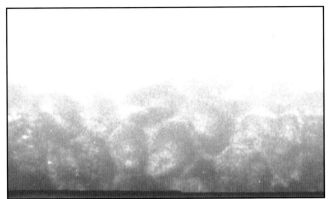

Figure 32-2. Specular microscopic appearance of corneal endothelial cells in ICE syndrome showing pleomorphism in size and shape, dark areas within the cells, and loss of clear hexagonal margins. (Reprinted with permission from Shields MB. *Textbook of Glaucoma*. 3rd ed. Baltimore, MD: Williams and Wilkins; 1992:261.)

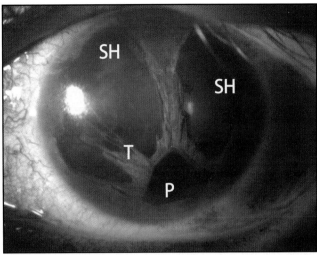

Figure 32-3. Progressive iris atrophy, a variation of the ICE syndrome, with pupillary distortion (P), thinning of the iris (T), and stretch holes (SH).

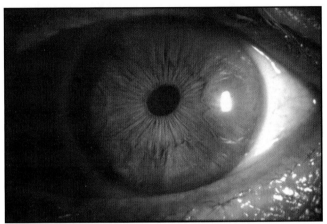

Figure 32-4. Chandler's syndrome, a variation of the ICE syndrome, with slight pupillary distortion and thinning of iris stroma at the vertical poles.

by gonioscopy as peripheral anterior synechiae that extend to or beyond Schwalbe's line. These iridotrabecular adhesions are broad based and typically progress around the circumference of the angle, eventually leading to IOP elevation. Glaucoma occurs in approximately half of all patients with ICE syndrome. Most studies indicate that glaucoma is more severe and difficult to control in patients with progressive iris atrophy and Cogan-Reese variations, as opposed to those with Chandler's syndrome.[15,17,24] However, Laganowski and colleagues[16] reported both a higher prevalence of glaucoma in eyes with Chandler's syndrome and similar response to treatment among different variants. The latter authors also correlated the occurrence of glaucoma with the specular microscopic appearance and found a greater prevalence of glaucoma when abnormal endothelial cells involved the entire posterior surface of the cornea (total ICE). In general, glaucoma is believed to be related to the angle closure in most cases of ICE syndrome but it does not correlate precisely with the degree of synechial closure. It may be observed in eyes with entirely open

angles due to the presence of a transparent Descemet's-like basement membrane over the trabecular meshwork (TM) that is secreted by the ICE cells, obstructing aqueous outflow.[25]

The iris abnormalities constitute the primary basis for distinguishing the clinical variations within the ICE syndrome. Progressive iris atrophy is characterized by marked atrophy of the iris, associated with variable degrees of corectopia and ectropion uvea (Figure 32-3). The latter 2 features are usually directed toward the quadrant with the most prominent area of peripheral anterior synechia. The hallmark of progressive iris atrophy is hole formation of the iris, which occurs in 2 forms: stretch holes and melting holes.[26] With stretch holes, the iris is markedly thinned in the quadrant away from the direction of pupillary distortion, and the holes develop within the stretched area. Melting holes develop without associated corectopia or iris thinning, and fluorescein angiographic studies suggest that these holes are associated with iris ischemia.[26]

In Chandler's syndrome, there is typically minimal corectopia and mild atrophy of the iris stroma (Figure 32-4). In some cases, there may be no detectable change in the iris.

Intermediate variations may also occur in which the degree of corectopia and stromal iris atrophy is more extensive than that of typical Chandler's syndrome, but the characteristic hole formation of progressive iris atrophy is lacking.

Eyes with the Cogan-Reese syndrome may have any degree of iris atrophy, but are distinguished by the presence of pigmented, pedunculated nodules on the surface of the iris (Figure 32-5). The iris stroma surrounding the nodules is typically flat, with loss of the normal iris architecture. In some cases, other features of ICE syndrome may be present for many years before the nodules appear.

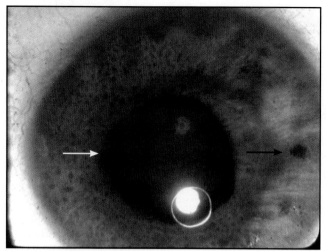

Figure 32-5. Cogan-Reese syndrome, a variation of the ICE syndrome, showing ectropion uvea (white arrow) and numerous dark nodules (black arrow) on area of flattened iris stroma.

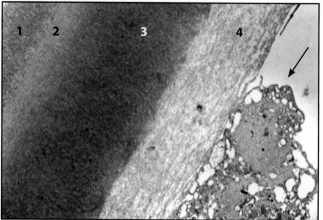

Figure 32-6. Transmission electron microscopic view of inner corneal surface in ICE syndrome showing part of an abnormal cell (arrow) on a 4-layered membrane, composed of the anterior nonbanded (1) and posterior banded (2) portions of Descemet's membrane with abnormal compact collagenous (3) and loose collagenous (4) layers (x6,875). (This article was published in *Ophthalmology*, 86, Shields MB, McCracken JS, Klintworth GK, et al, Corneal edema in essential iris atrophy, 1533-1550, Copyright Elsevier 1979.)

HISTOPATHOLOGIC FEATURES

Numerous ultrastructural and immunohistochemical studies have enhanced our understanding of the abnormal endothelial cells in ICE syndrome.[27-35] These cells display marked alterations in size, shape, and density. Abnormal intercellular junctions are noted, consistent with loss of contact inhibition and migratory features that these cells exhibit. Both metabolically active and necrotic cells have been demonstrated. Examination of the endothelial apical surfaces revealed presence of filopodial cytoplasmic projections and cytoplasmic actin filaments, indicative of cellular mitosis and migration.[28] Kramer and colleagues[29] demonstrated increased expression of cytokeratins in corneal endothelium, although another immunohistochemical study revealed no evidence of epithelial characteristics.[30] Hirst and colleagues,[33] in addition to demonstrating epithelial-like characteristics of ICE cells, also reported cross-reactivity with vimentin, suggesting that these cells retain some endothelial features as well. The abnormal ICE cells have been shown to secrete a basement membrane with multilayered collagenous tissue posterior to Descemet's membrane[27,28] (Figure 32-6). Description of this cellular membrane differs among studies and may be related to the extent or stage of the disease at the time of examination. Compared to the 2 layers of normal Descemet's membrane, additional layers are seen in eyes with ICE syndrome. In addition to a striated prenatal layer and a normal early postnatal layer, there is a thicker, nonstriated third layer that is formed postnatally and is composed of a variety of collagenous and noncollagenous material.[27,31] This pattern of membrane deposition supports an acquired etiology of this spectrum of disease. Occasional lymphocytes have been seen on or within the abnormal cellular layer.[28,30]

Histologic studies of the anterior chamber angle reveal a cellular membrane, consisting of a single layer of endothelial cells and a Descemet's-like membrane, extending down from the peripheral cornea. The membrane may cover an open anterior chamber angle that could explain those cases of glaucoma with open angles. Far more typically, however, the membrane is associated with synechial closure of tshe chamber angle.

Histopathology of the iris in all variations of ICE syndrome includes a cellular membrane on portions of the anterior surface of the iris, which is similar to and continuous with that seen over the anterior chamber angle. The membrane is most often found in the quadrant toward which the pupil is distorted. Eagle and colleagues[6] reported the presence of this membrane deep to peripheral anterior synechiae, indicating that the endothelialization is the primary defect and occurs prior to synechiae formation. In progressive iris atrophy, there is marked iris atrophy and hole formation in the opposite quadrant. The histopathology is the same in Chandler's syndrome with the exception of less extensive iris atrophy and no hole formation. In the Cogan-Reese syndrome, the nodular lesions have an ultrastructure similar to that of the underlying stroma of the iris. The presence of these nodules on the endothelialized portion of the iris, attenuation of the cellular membrane under the nodules, and openings within the membrane and continuity with the underlying stroma suggest that the proliferating endothelium encircles and pinches off portions of the stroma to create the nodules.[36,37]

THEORIES OF MECHANISM

The precise etiology of ICE syndrome is unknown. The infrequency of familial cases and the histologic evidence that corneal alterations begin in postnatal life argues in favor of an acquired disorder, rather than an inherited or congenital condition. The possibility of an inflammatory etiology was first postulated by Harms.[1] Eagle and colleagues[6] reported mild chronic iridocyclitis in 10 of 16 eyes with Cogan-Reese syndrome. The observation of lymphocytes on or in the corneal endothelial layer suggests the presence of chronic inflammation and has led to the theory of a viral etiology.[28] Serologic studies[38] in 13 patients with ICE syndrome suggested, but did not prove, a role for the Epstein-Barr virus. More compelling evidence from primer pair and polymerase chain reaction methods revealed herpes simplex viral DNA in 16 of 25 corneal specimens of ICE patients with localization within the endothelium.[39] This finding was absent in normal corneas and in corneas from patients with 3 other chronic corneal diseases. In addition, samples from positive ICE syndrome specimens yielded negative results for herpes simplex virus (HSV) after the endothelial layer was removed, indicating that HSV resided in the abnormal endothelium and may play a vital role in pathogenesis of ICE syndrome.

Although the initial event in the pathogenesis of the ICE syndrome is not established, the corneal endothelial abnormality is most likely the fundamental alteration that leads to the other clinicopathologic features. According to the theory of Campbell and associates,[40] the abnormality of the corneal endothelium in the ICE syndrome causes the corneal edema in some cases and leads in other cases to the proliferation of the cellular membrane across the anterior chamber angle and onto the iris surface. Contraction of the cellular portion of this membrane causes the formation of peripheral anterior synechiae, corectopia, and ectropion uvea. Stretching of the iris in the direction away from the corectopia is believed to contribute to the atrophy and hole formation, although additional factors, such as ischemia, may also be involved. The cellular membrane is also felt to be responsible for the development of the nodular lesions of the iris in the Cogan-Reese syndrome, possibly by encircling and pinching off portions of the iris stroma.[41]

The mechanism of glaucoma in ICE syndrome, as previously noted, is also believed to be related to the cellular membrane. In some cases, the membrane may cover the TM, which is still visible gonioscopically, thereby obstructing aqueous outflow. In most cases, however, the IOP does not begin to rise until contraction of the membrane has led to some degree of synechial closure of the anterior chamber angle.

DIFFERENTIAL DIAGNOSIS

There are several other disorders of the cornea and iris, many of which have associated glaucoma, that could be confused with various forms of the ICE syndrome. It may be helpful to consider them in 3 categories as those with disorders of the corneal endothelium, iris dissolution, and iris nodules. The 2 main differential diagnoses for corneal endothelial disorders are posterior polymorphous dystrophy (PPMD) and Fuchs' endothelial dystrophy.[42,43] PPMD is a bilateral disorder with autosomal dominant inheritance. Clinically, blisters and vesicles with scalloped edges are seen on the posterior cornea. A small percentage of patients may exhibit an irregular pupil, iris changes, and alterations in the anterior chamber angle that might resemble the ICE syndrome, but careful analysis of specular microscopy findings helps differentiate the 2 entities.[43] On gonioscopy, a high insertion of iris, as seen in congenital glaucoma, may be seen. Glaucoma is infrequent in PPMD and is reported to occur in approximately 15% of the cases with or without iridocorneal adhesions. Ultrastructural studies of the posterior cornea in PPMD revealed an incomplete Descemet's membrane covered by multiple layers of collagen and abnormal endothelial cells, whereas a fully developed membrane was seen in ICE syndrome.[44] These findings suggest that PPMD abnormality started during gestation while the defect in ICE syndrome is acquired after birth. The corneal endothelial changes of Fuchs' endothelial dystrophy more closely resemble those of the ICE syndrome, but these patients have none of the anterior chamber angle or iris features of the latter condition.

Conditions with iris dissolution that could be confused with ICE syndrome include the Axenfeld-Rieger (A-R) syndrome, which has striking clinical and histopathologic similarities to ICE syndrome, but differs by the bilateral and congenital nature of the condition. The clinical findings in A-R syndrome are usually stationary, although some progression may be seen over time. The mechanism of both ICE and A-R syndromes involves an abnormal membrane, but of different origin.[45] In the A-R syndrome, the iris and angle alterations are due to retention and contraction of a primordial endothelial layer, whereas changes in ICE syndrome are secondary to migration and subsequent contraction of abnormal corneal endothelial cells. Because A-R syndrome is thought to be secondary to a developmental arrest of tissues derived from neural crest cells, other systemic abnormalities involving tissues derived from the same progenitor cells are seen, most commonly involving the teeth and facial bones. As previously noted, a possible neural crest etiology has also been suggested for ICE syndrome,[14] but there is little support for this theory. The iris abnormalities of aniridia and iridoschisis might also lead to confusion with ICE syndrome. Aniridia is a bilateral disease affecting both the anterior and posterior segments of the eye and is predominantly inherited as an autosomal dominant disorder. Some forms of aniridia are associated with systemic findings. Iridoschisis is characterized by separation of superficial layers of the iris. This condition is seen mostly in the elderly and is infrequently associated with glaucoma.

Nodular lesions of the iris that could be confused with the Cogan-Reese syndrome include melanomas of the iris, recalling that the first 2 reported cases were enucleated because of this confusion. Melanosis of the iris is characterized by verrucous-like elevations that could also be confused with the iris nodules of the Cogan-Reese syndrome. In addition, differentiation must be made from the Lisch nodules of neurofibromatosis, as well as inflammatory nodules, as seen with granulomatous uveitic conditions such as sarcoidosis.

MANAGEMENT

Patients with ICE syndrome may require treatment for corneal edema, glaucoma, or both.

Mild cases of corneal edema are often managed conservatively with the bandage soft contact lenses and/or hypertonic saline solutions. Warm air, as with a hair dryer, in the morning may also be helpful in accelerating corneal deturgescence. In some cases, reduction of IOP, even in the absence of glaucoma, may be helpful in clearing the edema, although even an extremely low IOP may not reverse corneal edema in advanced cases. Furthermore, corneal edema may develop as a postoperative complication of glaucoma-filtering surgery in eyes with ICE syndrome. Therefore, filtering surgery is not recommended as a specific treatment for the corneal edema.

In more advanced cases of corneal edema, surgical intervention is often required with either penetrating or endothelial keratoplasty. Most studies have reported favorable results with penetrating keratoplasty (PK), particularly in eyes with Chandler's syndrome. Buxton and Lash[46] reported 1 failure among 5 cases after a mean follow-up of almost 3 years. Crawford and colleagues[47] reported no graft failure in their series, with 44% of the eyes achieving a final visual acuity of 20/40 or better with a mean follow-up of 43 months. Chang and colleagues[48] reported a success rate of 83% (10/12 eyes) with a mean follow-up of 30 months. Alvim and colleagues[49] reported clear grafts in 12 of 14 eyes with an average follow-up of 58 months, although 43% required repeat PK. On the other hand, DeBroff and Thoft[50] reported a very high rate of graft failure in patients with progressive iris atrophy undergoing PK. Persistent low-grade to moderate inflammation was seen in all 6 eyes, with 5 eyes ultimately leading to graft failure (83.3%). Most of these studies indicate that the limiting factor in maintaining graft survival is adequate glaucoma control.

Endothelial keratoplasty (EK), which selectively replaces diseased endothelium, has been gaining popularity, and results with this technique have been reported in eyes with ICE syndrome.[51-53] EK offers numerous advantages over PK including rapid visual rehabilitation, less astigmatism, avoidance of suture-related complications, and better corneal structural integrity. Two variants of EK—Descemet's stripping with endothelial keratoplasty (DSEK) and deep lamellar endothelial keratoplasty (DLEK)—have been performed in patients with ICE syndrome. Price and colleagues[52] reported resolution of corneal edema with visual acuity better than 20/30 and mean refractive cylinder of 1.2 D at 14 months in 3 eyes that underwent DSEK. Huang and colleagues[53] reported success after DLEK in 7 eyes at 20 months follow-up

with postoperative visual acuity ranging from 20/30 to 20/60 and mean corneal astigmatism of 2 D. In this study, it was also noted that eyes with ICE syndrome present numerous intraoperative challenges due to the extensive peripheral anterior synechiae and shallow anterior chamber and suggest the superiority of DLEK over DSEK in these patients. The recessed edge created at the recipient bed with DLEK improved tucking and adhesion of the donor graft with less manipulation and requirement for air tamponade when compared with DSEK.

Glaucoma management in patients with ICE syndrome is extremely challenging. It may be controlled medically in the early stages, especially with drugs that reduce aqueous production, such as beta-blockers, alpha-2 agonists, and carbonic anhydrase inhibitors. Miotics are usually ineffective, and the role of hypotensive lipids has not been fully explored in these eyes. When the IOP can no longer be controlled medically, surgical intervention is indicated.

Laser trabeculoplasty is usually not effective in these cases due to the structural alterations in the angle recess. Even in eyes where the angle appears to be open, the translucent membrane in stretched areas adjacent to the treated TM will obstruct aqueous outflow. In addition, laser-induced inflammation may cause reactivation of the pathogenic virus.[17]

The potential benefit of a goniotomy-like procedure with incision of a glassy membrane was speculated for a patient with ICE syndrome, who presented with glaucoma without peripheral anterior synechiae.[25] However, the subsequent growth of abnormal ICE cells in the anterior chamber angle may limit the long-term benefit of this approach. Goniotomy was performed in a child with ICE syndrome, but failed after 18 months due to endothelialization of the drainage angle and recurrence of peripheral anterior synechiae, eventually requiring trabeculectomy.[10]

Trabeculectomy is the most commonly performed surgery for glaucoma in patients with ICE syndrome. One report[26] described a success rate of 69% in 33 cases after glaucoma filtration surgery, which included trephination procedures. Laganowski and colleagues[16] reported a success rate of 60% at 1 year after trabeculectomy, which declined significantly following subsequent procedures. In contrast, Kidd and colleagues[54] reported higher success rates for repeated trabeculectomies in ICE syndrome and found these rates to be similar to those of initial surgery in patients with primary open-angle glaucoma. The success rates of glaucoma filtration surgery may be slightly better with the use of antifibrosis agents. Doe and colleagues[55] reported a survival rate of 73% at 1 year following trabeculectomy with antifibrotics, although this fell to 29% at 5 years. In one report of 9 eyes with the ICE syndrome, 8 of which had prior unsuccessful trabeculectomies, filtration surgery with postoperative subconjunctival injections of 5-fluorouracil controlled the IOP in only 4 eyes.[56] Lanzl and colleagues[57] reported IOP of 21 mm Hgor less without medications in 8 of 10 eyes with ICE syndrome with a mean follow-up of 15 months after trabeculectomy with mitomycin C. In general, a higher failure rate after trabeculectomy is attributed to a younger patient population with excessive scarring. Endothelialization with accumulation of an abnormal basement membrane in the ostium of a filtering bleb has also been reported to result in late failures.[58]

Aqueous drainage implants have shown favorable outcomes in a small series, but additional surgeries were required for revisions and tube positioning.[59] The study recommended a few modifications to avoid risk of occlusion or anterior migration of the tube from continued contraction of the abnormal endothelial membrane: longer distal tubes, curved course of the tube to the anterior chamber and placement of the tube in the pars plana in pseudophakic eyes.[59]

As with other forms of glaucoma, when the IOP cannot be controlled with the more conventional therapies, cyclodestructive procedures, especially trans-scleral cyclophotocoagulation, may be beneficial.

FUTURE CONSIDERATIONS

The ultimate treatment for all forms of glaucoma is to identify the initial events and treat these before they lead to obstruction of aqueous outflow, elevation of IOP, and glaucomatous damage. The ICE syndrome provides an example of how this concept of early glaucoma intervention may someday be invoked. For example, if the viral etiology is confirmed, this might provide a means of early diagnosis through the patient's past medical history and possibly through identification of a viral antibody or other evidence of previous viral infection. Specular microscopy, or some other screening technique, could then be used in this high-risk population to detect those patients with an abnormal corneal endothelium, ideally before it leads to alterations in the anterior chamber angle. Recently, a role for in vivo confocal microscopy has been suggested in early detection of ICE syndrome.[60-64] This technology offers numerous advantages over specular microscopy, such as high resolution, superior image contrast, ability to provide information in the presence of an opaque cornea, and the ability to image all cellular layers of the cornea. Confocal microscopy has also demonstrated alterations in the stromal structure of the cornea, with prominent corneal nerves, in addition to the typical morphologic changes of the corneal endothelium of the affected eyes.[60,64] These findings are consistent with the etiology of herpetic infection in ICE syndrome, because this virus is known to have a high affinity for nerve fibers. In addition, this technology may allow early diagnosis and intervention to prevent the proliferation of the abnormal endothelium over the anterior chamber angle and iris. Fulcher and associates,[65] for example, described an immunotoxin that inhibits the proliferation of human corneal endothelium in tissue culture. Alternatively, Alvarado and associates have suggested that topical and systemic antiviral agents may one day prove to be an effective treatment.[39] While there is still much work to be done before the concept of early glaucoma intervention

can be applied to the treatment of ICE syndrome, we have seen considerable advances in our understanding of this condition since it was first recognized as a spectrum of disease by Chandler and Grant more than 45 years ago.

REFERENCES

1. Harms C. Einseitige spontane Liickenbildung der Iris durch Atrophie ohne mechanische Zerrung. *Klin Monatsbl Augenheilkd.* 1903;41:522-528.
2. Chandler PA. Atrophy of the stroma of the iris. Endothelial dystrophy, corneal edema, and glaucoma. *Am J Ophthalmol.* 1956;41:607-615.
3. Chandler PA, Grant WM. *Lectures on Glaucoma.* Philadelphia, PA: Lea and Febiger; 1965:276.
4. Cogan DG, Reese AB. A syndrome of iris nodules, ectopic Descemet's membrane, and unilateral glaucoma. *Doc Ophthalmol.* 1969;26:424-432.
5. Scheie HG, Yanoff M. Iris nevus (Cogan-Reese) syndrome. A cause of unilateral glaucoma. *Arch Ophthalmol.* 1975;93:963-970.
6. Eagle RC Jr, Font RL, Yanoff M, et al. Proliferative endotheliopathy with iris abnormalities. The iridocorneal endothelial syndrome. *Arch Ophthalmol.* 1979;97:2104-2111.
7. Huna R, Barak A, Melamed S. Bilateral iridocorneal endothelial syndrome presented as Cogan-Reese and Chandler's syndrome. *J Glaucoma.* 1996;5:60-62.
8. Des Marchais B, Simmons RB, Simmons RJ, et al. Bilateral Chandler syndrome. *J Glaucoma.* 1999;8(4):276-277.
9. Gupta V, Kumar R, Gupta R, et al. Bilateral iridocorneal endothelial syndrome in a young girl with Down's syndrome. *Indian J Ophthalmol.* 2009;57:61-63.
10. Salim S, Shields MB, Walton D. Iridocorneal endothelial syndrome in a child. *J Pediatr Ophthalmol Strabismus.* 2006;43(5):308-310.
11. Eagle RC, Shields JA. Iridocorneal endothelial syndrome with contralateral guttate endothelial dystrophy—a light and electron microscopic study. *Ophthalmology.* 1987;94:862-870.
12. Lucas-Glass TC, Baratz KH, Nelson LR, et al. The contralateral corneal endothelium in the iridocorneal endothelial syndrome. *Arch Ophthalmol.* 1997;115:40-43.
13. Kupfer C, Kaiser-Kupfer MI, Datiles M, et al. The contralateral eye in the iridocorneal endothelial (ICE) syndrome. *Ophthalmology.* 1983;90:1343-1350.
14. Hu R, Gu Y, Li X. Coexistence of unilateral iridocorneal endothelial syndrome and sensorineural deafness. *Can J Ophthalmol.* 2007;42:626-627.
15. Wilson MC, Shields MB. A comparison of the clinical variations of the iridocorneal endothelial syndrome. *Arch Ophthalmol.* 1989;107:1465-1468.
16. Laganowski HC, Kerr Muir MG, Hitchings RA. Glaucoma and the iridocorneal syndrome. *Arch Ophthalmol.* 1992;110:346-350.
17. Teekhasaenee C, Ritch R. Iridocorneal endothelial syndrome in Thai patients. *Arch Ophthalmol.* 2000;118:187-192.
18. Bourne WM, Brubaker RF. Decreased corneal endothelial permeability in the iridocorneal endothelial syndrome. *Ophthalmology.* 1982;89:591-595.
19. Ohguro N, Matsuda M, Fukuda M, et al. Gas stress test for assessment of corneal endothelial function. *Jpn J Ophthalmol.* 2000;44:325-333.
20. Kocaoglan H, Unlu N, Kanpolat A, et al. Macular edema and iridocorneal endothelial syndrome. *Cornea.* 2005;24:221-223.
21. Hirst LW, Quigley HA, Stark WJ, et al. Specular microscopy of iridocorneal endothelia syndrome. *Am J Ophthalmol.* 1980;89:11-21.
22. Sherrard ES, Frangoulis MA, Kerr MG, et al. The posterior surface of the cornea in the iridocorneal endothelial syndrome: a specular microscopical study. *Trans Ophthalmol Soc UK.* 1985;104:766-774.

23. Bourne WM, Brubaker RF. Progression and regression of partial corneal involvement in the iridocorneal endothelial syndrome. *Am J Ophthalmol.* 1992;114:171-181.

24. Shields MB. Progressive essential iris atrophy, Chandler's syndrome, and the iris nevus (Cogan-Reese) syndrome: a spectrum of disease. *Surv Ophthalmol.* 1979;24:3-20.

25. Weber, PA, Gibb G. Iridocorneal endothelial syndrome: glaucoma without peripheral anterior synechiae. *Glaucoma.* 1984;6:128-130.

26. Shields MB, Campbell DG, Simmons RJ. The essential ins atrophies. *Am J Ophthalmol.* 1978;85:749-759.

27. Shields MB, McCracken JS, Klintworth GK, et al. Corneal edema in essential iris atrophy. *Ophthalmology.* 1979;86:1533-1548.

28. Alvarado JA, Murphy CG, Maglio M, et al. Pathogenesis of Chandler's syndrome, essential iris atrophy and the Cogan-Reese syndrome. I. Alterations of the corneal endothelium. *Invest Ophthalmol Vis Sci.* 1986;27:853-872.

29. Kramer TR, Grossniklaus HE, Vigneswaran N, et al. Cytokeratin expression in corneal endothelium in the iridocorneal endothelial syndrome. *Invest Ophthalmol Vis Sci.* 1992;33:3581-3585.

30. Rodrigues MM, Stulting RD, Waring GO III. Clinical, electron microscopic, and immunohistochemical study of the corneal endothelium and Descemet's membrane in the iridocorneal endothelial syndrome. *Am J Ophthalmol.* 1986;101:16-27.

31. Alvarado JA, Murphy CG, Juster RP, et al. Pathogenesis of Chandler's syndrome, essential iris atrophy and the Cogan-Reese syndrome. II. Estimated age of disease onset. *Invest Ophthalmol Vis Sci.* 1986;27:873-882.

32. Richarson TM. Corneal decompensation in Chandler's syndrome—a scanning and transmission electron microscopic study. *Arch Ophthalmol.* 1979;97:2112-2119.

33. Hirst LW, Bancroft J, Yamauchi K, et al. Immunohistochemical pathology of the corneal endothelium in iridocorneal endothelial syndrome. *Invest Ophthalmol Vis Sci.* 1995;36:820-827.

34. Levy SG, McCartney ACE, Baghai MH. Pathology of the iridocorneal endothelial syndrome—the ICE cell. *Invest Ophthalmol Vis Sci.* 1995;36:2592-2601.

35. Levy SG, Kirkness CM, Moss J, et al. The histopathology of the iridocorneal endothelial syndrome. *Cornea.* 1996;15:46-53.

36. Shields MB, Campbell DG, Simmons RJ, et al. Iris nodules in essential iris atrophy. *Arch Ophthalmol.* 1976;94:406-410.

37. Eagle RC, Font RL, Yanoff M, et al. The iris nevus (Cogan-Reese) syndrome: light and electron microscopic observations. *Br J Ophthalmol.* 1980;64:446-452.

38. Tsai CS, Ritch R, Straus SE, et al. Antibodies to Epstein-Barr virus in iridocorneal endothelial syndrome. *Arch Ophthalmol.* 1990;108:1572-1576.

39. Alvarado J, Underwood J, Green R, et al. Detection of herpes simplex viral DNA in the iridocorneal endothelia syndrome. *Arch Ophthalmol.* 1994;112:1601-1609.

40. Campbell DG, Shields MB, Smith TR. The corneal endothelium and the spectrum of essential iris atrophy. *Am J Ophthalmol.* 1978;86:317-324.

41. Campbell DG. Formation of iris nodules in primary proliferative endothelial degeneration. *Invest Ophthalmol Vis Sci.* 1979;(suppl):142.

42. Hirst LW. Congenital anterior segment epithelialisation (case). *Aust J Ophthalmol.* 1983;11:209-213.

43. Krachmer JH. Posterior polymorphous corneal dystrophy: a disease characterized by epithelial-like endothelial cells which influence management and prognosis. *Trans Am Ophthalmol Soc.* 1985;83:413-475.

44. Salim S, Shields MB. Pretrabecular mechanisms of intraocular pressure elevation. In: Tombran-Tink J, Barnstable CJ, Shields MB, eds. *Mechanisms of the Glaucomas.* New York, NY: Humana Press; 2008:83-97.

45. Shields MB. Axenfeld-Rieger and iridocorneal endothelial syndromes: 2 spectra of disease with striking similarities and differences. *J Glaucoma.* 2001;5:536-538.

46. Buxton JN, Lash RS. Results of penetrating keratoplasty in the iridocorneal endothelial syndrome. *Am J Ophthalmol.* 1984;98: 297-301.

47. Crawford GJ, Stulting Rd, Cavanagh HD, et al. Penetrating keratoplasty in the management of iridocorneal endothelial syndrome. *Cornea.* 1989;8:34-40.

48. Chang PC, Soong HK, Couto MF, et al. Prognosis for penetrating keratoplasty in iridocorneal endothelial syndrome. *Refract Corneal Surg.* 1993;9:129-132.

49. Alvim PDT, Cohen EJ, Rapuano CJ, et al. Penetrating keratoplasty in iridocorneal endothelial syndrome. *Cornea.* 2001;20:134-140.

50. DeBroff BM, Thoft RA. Surgical results of penetrating keratoplasty in essential iris atrophy. *J Cataract Refract Surg.* 1994;10:428-432.

51. Bahar I, Kaiserman I, Buys Y, et al. Descemet's stripping with endothelial keratoplasty in iridocorneal endothelial syndrome. *Ophthalmic Surg Lasers.* 2008;39:54-56.

52. Price MO, Price FW. Descemet stripping with endothelial keratoplasty for treatment of iridocorneal endothelial syndrome. *Cornea.* 2007;26:493-497.

53. Huang T, Wang Y, Ji J, et al. Deep lamellar endothelial keratoplasty for iridocorneal endothelial syndrome in phakic eyes. *Arch Ophthalmol.* 2009;127:33-36.

54. Kidd M, Hetherington J, Magee S. Surgical results in iridocorneal endothelial syndrome. *Arch Ophthalmol.* 1988;106:199-201.

55. Doe EA, Budenz DL, Gedde SJ, et al. Long-term surgical outcomes of patients with glaucoma secondary to the iridocorneal endothelial syndrome. *Ophthalmology.* 2001;108:1789-1795.

56. Wright MM, Grajewski AL, Chstal SM, et al. 5-fluorouracil after trabeculectomy and the iridocorneal endothelial syndrome. *Ophthalmology.* 1991;98:314-316.

57. Lanzl IM, Wilson RP, Dudley D, et al. Outcome of trabeculectomy with mitomycin c in the iridocorneal endothelial syndrome. *Ophthalmology.* 2000;107:295-297.

58. Yanoff M, Scheie H, Allman M. Endothelialization of filtering bleb in iris nevus syndrome. *Arch Ophthalmol.* 1976;94:1933-1936.

59. Kim DK, Aslanides IM, Schmidt CM, et al. Long-term outcome of aqueous shunt surgery in ten patients with iridocorneal endothelial syndrome. *Ophthalmology.* 1999;106:1030-1034.

60. Grupcheva CN, McGhee CNJ, Dean S, et al. In vivo confocal microscopic characteristics of iridocorneal endothelial syndrome. *Clin Exp Ophthalmol.* 2004;32:275-283.

61. Sheppard JD, Lattanzio FA, Williams PB, et al. Confocal microscopy used as the definitive, early diagnostic method in Chandler syndrome. *Cornea.* 2005;24:227-229.

62. Mocan MC, Bozkurt B, Orhan M, et al. Chandler syndrome manifesting as ectropion uvea following laser in situ keratomileusis. *J Cataract Refract Surg.* 2008;34:871-873.

63. Pezzi PP, Marenco M, Cosimi P, et al. Progression of essential iris atrophy studied with confocal microscopy and ultrastructural biomicroscopy: a 5 year report. *Cornea.* 2009;28:99-102.

64. Le QH, Sun XH, Xu JJ. In-vivo confocal microscopy of iridocorneal syndrome. *Int Ophthalmol.* 2009;29:11-18.

65. Fulcher S, Lui G, Houston LL, et al. Use of immunotoxin to inhibit proliferating human corneal endothelium. *Invest Ophthalmol Vis Sci.* 1988;29:755-759.

33

Glaucoma After Vitreoretinal Procedures

Ron A. Adelman, MD, MPH, MBA, FACS and Martin Wand, MD

Vitreoretinal surgery is the third most common ocular surgery following cataract surgery and laser vision correction with more than 200,000 procedures performed each year in the United States.[1] There is a complex relationship between intraocular pressure (IOP) and vitreoretinal procedures.[1-10] Ocular hypertension may present after vitrectomy, scleral buckle, and/or intravitreal injections.[1,2] Although transient or persistent ocular hypertension following vitreoretinal procedures is not infrequent, vitrectomy may be helpful in the treatment of a select group of glaucoma patients, such as those with aqueous misdirection. Of interest is that reversible loss of light perception after vitreoretinal surgery does occur in some patients.[9] In postvitrectomy patients with high IOP and no light perception, decreasing the IOP may be associated with return of light perception.[9]

Glaucoma after vitreoretinal surgery requires special attention to its etiology, pathophysiology, diagnosis, treatment, and prevention. Direct communication between the retina surgeon and glaucoma specialist will result in early diagnosis and appropriate management based on the likely etiology. It is important to distinguish between early (first week) and late (second week and later) ocular hypertension following vitreoretinal procedures. In the early postoperative period, ocular hypertension is usually due to viscoelastics, expanding gas bubble, pupillary block, angle closure, inflammation, hemorrhage, choroidal edema, silicone oil, or steroid response.[1] Late glaucoma may be a result of angle closure, neovascularization of the angle, emulsified silicone oil, or new open-angle glaucoma. As a rule, the more complicated the vitreoretinal surgery, the higher the risk of development of ocular hypertension.

Soon after a retina operation, the eye is often congested, painful, and with poor vision; the patient may be uncomfortable, somnolent, and at times nauseated, particularly if the surgery is performed under general anesthesia. Thus, the signs and symptoms of a secondary glaucoma in the early postoperative period can be confused with the expected side effects of vitrectomy or scleral buckle surgery. An awareness of this complication and its different presentations will facilitate recognition as well as allow for timely treatment and, in some instances, prevention of the complication.

ANGLE-CLOSURE GLAUCOMA

The reported incidence of clinically detectable angle narrowing after scleral buckle procedures ranges from 11.9% at 1 month[11] to 29% at 2 months after surgery[12]; the incidence reaches 50% in eyes examined within 1 week after surgery.[13] The reported incidence of actual angle-closure glaucoma ranges from 1% to 4%.[11,14-16] The etiology of the angle shallowing is probably multifactorial (Table 33-1). Experimentally, occlusion of vortex veins in monkey eyes results in uveal tract congestion, forward movement of the iris-lens diaphragm, shallowing or closure of the anterior chamber angle, and, in some eyes, elevated IOP.[17] Grant has shown that fluid injected into the choroid of human eyebank eyes results in choroidal detachment and angle closure.[18] Clinically, a choroidal detachment is frequently, but not always, detectable after retinal detachment surgery.[16] Ultrasound biomicroscopic studies have shown that choroidal effusion is present in eyes after scleral buckling procedures even when there are no signs of anterior chamber

Kahook MY, Schuman JS, eds.
Chandler and Grant's Glaucoma, Fifth Edition (pp 327-335).
© 2013 SLACK Incorporated.

TABLE 33-1. RISK FACTORS FOR ANGLE-CLOSURE GLAUCOMA AFTER SCLERAL BUCKLING SURGERY
Pre-existing narrow angles (hyperopic patient)
Older age
Encircling band
High scleral buckle
Scleral buckle anterior to equator
Episcleral implants (versus intrascleral implant)

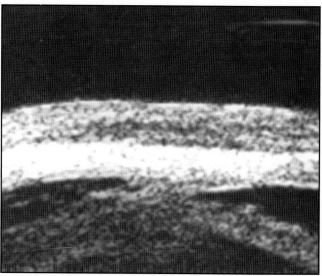

Figure 33-1. Ultrasound biomicroscopy of an eye one week after a 360-degree encircling band procedure for a rhegmatogenous retinal detachment. Postoperatively, the IOP was normal, the anterior chamber was deep, and no choroidal detachment was noted. Choroidal effusion (left side of picture) was present 360 degrees with detachment of the ciliary body except for its attachment to the scleral spur. There is anterior rotation of the ciliary processes, narrowing of the peripheral angle, anterior displacement of the lens, and relative pupillary block as shown by the anterior bowing of the iris. (Reprinted with permission from Charles J. Pavlin, MD.)

shallowing or clinical findings of choroidal detachment (Figure 33-1). This confirms the impression of retinal surgeons that virtually all eyes undergoing retinal surgery have some degree of choroidal effusion. Angle narrowing and angle closure are just at one end of the spectrum of choroidal effusion after retinal detachment.

Other clinical situations where there is inflammation and/or swelling of the uveal tract have also been shown to result in shallowing of the anterior chamber axially, anterior rotation of the ciliary body, and shallowing or closure of the anterior chamber angle. A similar pathophysiologic process may be implicated in the following conditions, all of which have been associated with angle-closure glaucoma: panretinal photocoagulation,[19,20] uveal[21] and orbital pseudotumor,[22] uveal effusion,[23] central retinal vein occlusion,[24,25] choroidal hemorrhage,[26] and idiopathic ciliary body swelling.[27] The ciliary body is firmly attached to the scleral spur. With uveal swelling from these diverse causes, including postscleral buckling, there is an anterior rotation of the ciliary body with anterior movement of the lens-iris diaphragm (Figure 33-1). In phakic or pseudophakic eyes, there may be enough forward movement to produce pupillary block with resultant angle-closure glaucoma.

However, angle closure may also occur in the absence of pupillary block. In such cases, anterior rotation of the ciliary body may be limited to pushing the peripheral iris against the trabecular meshwork. The result is similar to the plateau iris syndrome (ie, there is a relatively deep central anterior chamber depth, flat iris plane, and peripheral angle closure).[28] This is attested to by the finding that angle-closure glaucoma has been noted in aphakic as well as phakic eyes and in eyes with patent iridectomies.[11,16] The incidence and extent of angle shallowing and closure has been related to myriad conditions including a preexisting narrow angle,[11,15] high myopia,[15] older age of patient,[15] use of an encircling band versus a scleral implant without an encircling band,[13] large buckle elements, intravitreal injection of gas, placement of the encircling band anterior to the equator,[11] episcleral implants versus intrascleral implants,[16] choroidal detachment extending to the ciliary body,[11] and the extent of the surgical procedure.[15] In most cases, the shallowing of the angle resolves with time as the choroidal effusion is absorbed.[11-13,15]

Prevention and Treatment

The critical point in the treatment of this problem is an awareness of the potential for angle closure after retinal detachment surgery. Frequently, there is no more discomfort or pain than from the normal sequelae of retinal surgery. Findings are minimal, and a hazy cornea with a mid-dilated pupil is often the only clue that glaucoma may be present.[16] Ocular rigidity is decreased to one-quarter normal after a scleral buckle,[29] and Schiotz tonometry gives a falsely low IOP.[12] Thus, an IOP measurement by applanation or Tono-Pen (Reichert Technologies, Depew, NY) and slit-lamp examination should be done preferably within the first 24 hours after surgery. If the cornea is not clear enough for gonioscopy, and the IOP is elevated, angle closure must be presumed to be present. With the advent of anterior segment optical coherence tomography (OCT), the diagnosis of angle closure in such cases may be easier.

Treatment of angle-closure glaucoma after scleral buckling surgery progresses from medical management through surgical intervention (Table 33-2). Maximal dilation and cycloplegia with atropine and phenylephrine should be aggressively continued, along with topical steroids, which may decrease ocular and choroidal congestion and effusion. Miotics should be avoided; beta-blockers, carbonic anhydrase inhibitors, and alpha-adrenergics should be used as tolerated. Regardless of the medical therapy, a laser iridotomy is indicated. With mild corneal haziness, a

TABLE 33-2. TREATMENT OF ANGLE-CLOSURE GLAUCOMA AFTER SCLERAL BUCKLING SURGERY	
Treatment	Comments

Medical
    Cycloplegics
    Beta-blockers
    Apraclonidine
    Carbonic anhydrase inhibitors
    Osmotics
	Continue cycloplegics (pilocarpine may further shallow anterior chamber, worsen angle closure, and cause pain)
	If more than 7 to 10 days since surgery, consider topical steroids as the source of elevated IOP

Laser iridotomy	Topical glycerin may help clear cornea
Laser gonioplasty	May help open angle enough to delay or prevent operative intervention

Surgical intervention
    Choroidal tap
    Consider loosening excessively tight scleral buckle
    Trabeculectomy with antimetabolites, seton implantation, or cyclophotocoagulation in late stages
	Surgical intervention is a last resort; choroidal effusions generally clear with time

neodymium:yttrium-aluminum-garnet (Nd:YAG) laser may often be successful in iris penetration where the argon laser might fail.[30] If the cornea is very hazy, clarity can frequently be achieved with topical glycerin. When the cornea is too hazy to allow even Nd:YAG laser iridotomy, argon laser peripheral iridoplasty might be helpful, as this has been reported to be successful in primary angle-closure glaucoma under such circumstances.[31] As a last resort, angle closure from pupillary block may require a surgical iridectomy, but the advent of the different lasers has virtually eliminated the need for such intervention.

When a patent laser iridotomy does not resolve the angle closure, then choroidal detachment with anterior rotation of the ciliary body is commonly the cause of the angle closure. With the availability of argon laser gonioplasty,[32] the angle can often be opened enough to lower the IOP, keeping in mind that once past the acute crisis, the choroidal effusion and secondary angle closure will resolve with time. However, there can be so much choroidal effusion that the only solution is to drain the choroidal fluid, the traditional technique of treating this type of glaucoma.[14] Surgical anterior chamber deepening and mechanical breaking of peripheral anterior synechiae can be performed at the time of this surgery, if persistent angle closure is present (see Chapter 23).

Case 33-1

A 69-year-old man with a rhegmatogenous retinal detachment underwent a successful scleral buckle operation with a 200-degree scleral implant and a 360-degree encircling band. The course of his postoperative hospital stay was not well-documented, but at his 1-week postoperative visit, the visual acuity was counting fingers, the IOP was 40 mm Hg, and the eye was congested. Various antiglaucoma medications were instituted without success. At 7 weeks after the retina surgery, the visual acuity was 20/100, and the IOP was 57 mm Hg, the cornea clear, the anterior chamber deep, and the iris was flat with a 6-mm pupil. No pupillary block was evident, but the angle was closed 360 degrees (Figure 33-2). Argon laser gonioplasty was performed 360 degrees with immediate opening of the angle, and the IOP decreased to 31 mm Hg. The next day, the IOP was 21 mm Hg, and the angle remained open (Figure 33-3). Subsequently, his IOPs have remained under control on a topical beta-blocker only.

This case illustrates several important points. Angle closure after retinal detachment surgery is easily overlooked if not specifically sought for and may persist long after the acute postoperative inflammatory period. It can occur in the absence of pupillary block, making the diagnosis more elusive. With the availability of laser iridotomy and laser gonioplasty, many, if not most, cases of angle closure, even of several weeks duration, can now be resolved without further surgical intervention.

OPEN-ANGLE GLAUCOMA

Postoperative open-angle glaucoma requires special consideration because it frequently is a reflection of the preoperative status of the eye. The prevalence of open-angle glaucoma in eyes that develop retinal detachment is reported to be 4 to 12 times higher than that in the general population.[33] The reason is unknown, but the commonality of high myopia[34] and the use of miotics in open-angle glaucoma resulting in retinal detachment[35] have been cited as possible explanations. A higher incidence of both open-angle glaucoma and retinal detachment in diabetics may be another factor. Because the IOP is often lower in

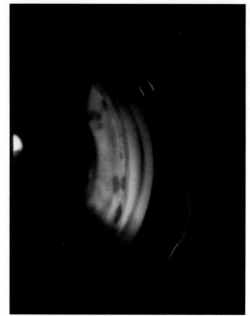

Figure 33-2. Persistent angle closure glaucoma 7 weeks after a sclera buckling procedure. Goniophotograph shows peripheral appositional angle closure without a papillary block component. (Reprinted with permission from Martin Wand, MD.)

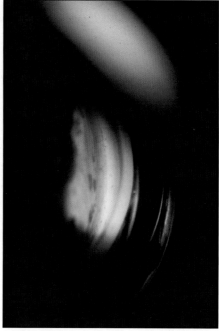

Figure 33-3. Same eye as in Figure 33-2. Goniophotograph showing open angle after argon laser gonioplasty. (Reprinted with permission from Martin Wand, MD.)

eyes with retinal detachment due to decreased aqueous formation or increased outflow through the retinal break and uvea, successful reattachment usually but not always results in a return to at least the predetachment level of IOP. Additionally, debris, inflammation, blood breakdown products, and steroid response contribute to the decreased facility of outflow postoperatively.[36] All things considered, re-emergence of preexisting open-angle glaucoma should be looked for carefully after retinal detachment surgery and appropriately treated.

Chang[1] has reported that vitrectomy increases the risk of unilateral open-angle glaucoma in the operated eye. Following vitrectomy, up to 15% to 20% of eyes may develop open-angle glaucoma. Given the fact that there are more than 200,000 vitrectomies per year in the United States, up to 30,000 new cases of glaucoma following vitrectomy may develop each year. The open-angle glaucoma may present months or years after vitrectomy. In a large series, the average time from vitrectomy to open-angle glaucoma in phakic eyes and pseudophakic eyes was 46 and 18 months, respectively. The presence of a crystalline lens may have a protective effect. The etiology of delayed-onset open-angle glaucoma following vitrectomy may be due to inflammation and debris that reduce aqueous outflow, increased susceptibility of the optic nerve to damage, or alteration in the biochemical environment of the eye. Chang[1] postulated that the high level of oxygen in the vitreous cavity after vitrectomy results in oxidative stress of the trabecular meshwork.

Postoperative open-angle glaucoma may also be associated with Schwartz's syndrome[37] in which the preoperative IOP elevation is caused by obstruction of the trabecular meshwork by photoreceptor outer segments from a retinal tear or dialysis[38] and is improved by retinal surgery. If the retinal break is sealed and the retina reattached, the source of trabecular meshwork obstruction (photoreceptor outer segments) is eliminated, and the secondary open-angle glaucoma usually resolves. In this unique situation, persistent postoperative open-angle glaucoma should lead one to suspect an undetected persistent retinal detachment.

NEOVASCULAR GLAUCOMA

Chronic retinal detachment with its resultant retinal hypoxia has long been recognized as a cause of neovascular glaucoma (NVG).[39] Occasionally, the surgery for retinal detachment has been implicated in neovascularization of the iris, presumably due to anterior segment ischemia from damage to the anterior ciliary vessels.[40,41] Recently, vitrectomy in diabetic eyes has been associated with a high incidence of NVG if the eye is already aphakic or has concurrent lensectomy.[42] Aphakia may have resulted in the elimination of a diffusion barrier for the passage of some angiogenic substance from the posterior to the anterior segment.[43] Subsequently, although the presence of the lens does seem to provide a relative protective barrier, of greater importance in the development of NVG is the presence of an angiogenic stimulus.[44,45]

In both diabetic and nondiabetic eyes[46] where there is posterior segment hypoxia from a persistent retinal detachment, aphakia is only of secondary importance. The highest incidence of NVG after vitrectomy for complications of diabetic retinopathy is in eyes with a persistent retinal detachment and aphakia (92%); the lowest incidence is in phakic eyes with an attached retina (0%), and intermediate incidence in phakic eyes with a detached retina (40%)[45] (see Chapter 31).

In eyes already predisposed toward the development of NVG, such as eyes with diabetic retinopathy, previous central retinal vein occlusion, or carotid obstructive disease, retinal detachment surgery, with or without vitrectomy, further stimulates the inflammatory and angiogenic responses.[47,48] One must be alert to the potential development of NVG postretinal detachment surgery, and one should specifically look for neovascularization of the iris on slit-lamp examination. If neovascularization of the iris is detected, a dilated fundus examination with scleral depression must be performed. When a retinal detachment is found, a successful re-attachment will usually resolve the anterior segment neovascularization.[49] Occasionally, neovascularization of the iris and NVG may appear after successful retinal detachment surgery. If this occurs in eyes with preexisting diabetic retinopathy or previous central retinal vein occlusion, intravitreal antivascular endothelial growth factor injections and/or panretinal photocoagulation either must be performed, if not already done, or, if done, it must be augmented. Indirect laser ophthalmoscopy and photocoagulation can be useful in treating the peripheral retina in this situation. With the extra inflammatory and angiogenic stimuli from the surgery, supplemental panretinal photocoagulation often needs to be performed. We and others have noted resolution of neovascularization of the iris and NVG after supplemental panretinal photocoagulation in such cases.[40,44] In recent years, development of antivascular endothelial growth factor has improved the outcome of patients with rubeosis. Intravitreal bevacizumab (Avastin) and ranibizumab (Lucentis) quickly improve recent-onset neovascularization of the iris. However, the duration of the therapeutic effect of these medications is about 1 month. Thus, multiple intravitreal injections may become necessary.[7]

GLAUCOMA AFTER INTRAVITREAL GAS

The use of various intraocular gases in vitreoretinal surgery has become increasingly popular over the past decades.[50] Because of their surface tension, all gases exert a tamponading effect on the retinal breaks. However, air has the disadvantage of being absorbed (in 2 to 7 days[51]) before firm choroidal-retinal adhesions can develop. Fluorinated hydrocarbon gases have an advantage over air because they are expansile and have a longer intraocular duration, attributed to their high molecular weight, low diffusion coefficient, and low water solubility. The most commonly used gases are sulfa hexafluoride (SF6) and perfluoropropane

(C3F8). SF6 remains in the eye for about 2 weeks; C3F8, with a higher molecular weight than SF6, remains in the eye for about 2 months.[50,51] When injected into the vitreous cavity, the volume of these gases expands because of diffusion of nitrogen, oxygen, and carbon dioxide from ocular tissue. Pure SF6 expands to 2 to 2.5 times its original volume within 24 to 36 hours, and pure C3F8 expands to 3 to 4 times its original volume within the first 3 days.[50,51] With both gases, the maximum expansion occurs within the first 6 hours. When the gas gets diluted to a 40% concentration, further expansion occurs slowly and is balanced by vitreous loss.[52,53] The nonexpansile concentration for SF6 is 18% and for C3F8 is 14%.

With an expansile intravitreal gas bubble, anterior displacement of the lens can occur, despite proper positioning of the patient's head in a prone position, resulting in pupillary block. This can occur even after the period of maximum expansion, and one must be aware of this possibility for the duration of the intravitreal gas. Because the gas bubble is compressible, high-displacement tonometers, such as the Schiotz tonometer, result in significant under-evaluation of the true IOP.[54] With 1 mL of intraocular gas, there is a 7- to 8-mm Hg under-evaluation when the IOP is in the 30- to 40-mm Hg range.[50] Even with low-displacement applanation tonometers, there can be a significant under-evaluation of the true IOP. The Tono-Pen was found to under-estimate true IOP (as measured in eye bank eyes with an intraocular manometer) by 15% and the pneumotonometer by 21%.[55] Therefore, not only is it imperative that only a low-displacement tonometer, such as the Goldmann applanation tonometer (Haag-Streit, Koeniz, Switzerland) or Tono-Pen, be used, but to realize that there could still be up to a 20% under-estimation in eyes with intraocular gas.

More common than pupillary block is the glaucoma resulting directly from the expansile gas. The highest incidence and the highest IOP are during the rapid expansile phase when egress of liquid vitreous and aqueous cannot keep pace with the increasing gas volume. In an early study, 45% of 101 patients who had SF6 during surgery developed IOPs greater than 30 mm Hg within the first postoperative day; in 33 patients, the elevated IOPs persisted beyond the second postoperative day. More alarmingly, 11 of the 101 patients developed central retinal artery occlusion, 10 of whom had elevated IOPs; none of these eyes achieved functional vision.[56] Eyes that developed postoperative anterior chamber fibrinous exudates appear more likely to develop elevated IOPs, and diabetic eyes are more likely to develop these exudates.[56] Thus, eyes likely to have retinal vascular diseases, such as with diabetes, hypertension, sickle cell trait, or chronic open-angle glaucoma, may be at even greater risk for vascular occlusion associated with an elevated IOP.[57]

Patients with intraocular gas who subsequently have surgery under general anesthesia with nitrous oxide will have a significant increase in IOP during anesthesia. Wolf and colleagues[58] found that SF6 gas volume in an eye increased

INTRAOCULAR GAS AND ALTITUDE
Martin Wand, MD and
Ron A. Adelman, MD, MPH, MBA, FACS

With the use of intraocular gas, another unusual complication should be considered. With any decrease in atmospheric pressure, there is a corresponding decrease in the absolute IOP, which results in expansion of the intraocular gas. Because there is a delay between the decrease in the atmospheric pressure and the decrease in the absolute IOP, there is a net increase in the IOP.[1] Experimental studies in monkeys show that with only 0.25 mL of intraocular gas, simulated decompression as experienced in commercial airline cabins (300 feet per minute to a cabin altitude of 8000 feet above sea level) resulted in IOPs greater than 40 mm Hg.[2] Transient central retinal artery occlusion was noted in these eyes. In a 79-year-old man who had undergone recent intraocular fluid-gas exchange, IOP was measured with a Tono-Pen and the intraocular gas bubble observed with an indirect ophthalmoscope during a low-altitude airplane trip.[3] In an unpressurized small plane, the gas fill went from 65% at sea level to 85% at 3000 feet; the IOP went from 16 mm Hg to 49 mm Hg. Although it might be safe to fly for short periods at low altitudes, commercial air flights pose more serious potential problems.[4] Current jets fly at up to 42,000 feet (as high as 60,000 feet for the Concorde), and cabin pressurization varies greatly from a high of 1000 feet in a Concorde to a low of 8000 feet in a B737; the average pressurization was 5670 feet as measured on 204 commercial flights in different types of airplanes.[5] Standard pressure differential for the commercial airline industry is 8:6:1. These pressurization levels clearly put an eye with intraocular gases at great risk. In addition, should sudden depressurization occur on a commercial airplane, the ocular consequences would be disastrous. Thus, it is essential to warn patients to avoid flying at cabin pressures less than 2000 feet (706 mm Hg)[2] or preferably not at all until all the intraocular gas is absorbed.

In addition, rapid ascent or descent when traveling in automobiles or in high-rise elevators should be avoided. Although experimental studies suggest that up to 0.6 mL of gas can be safe in a flight,[1] clinically, up to 1 mL of gas may be tolerated.

REFERENCES
1. Lincoff H, Weinberger D, Reppucci V, et al. Air travel with intraocular gas: I. The mechanisms for compensation. *Arch Ophthalmol.* 1989;107:902-906.
2. Dieckert JP, O'Connor PS, Schacklett DE, et al. Air travel and intraocular gas. *Ophthalmology.* 1986;93:642-645.
3. Kokame GT, Ing MR. Intraocular gas and low altitude air flight. *Retina.* 1994;14:356-358.
4. Mills MD, Devenyi RG, Lam WC, et al. An assessment of intraocular pressure rise in patients with gas-filled eyes during simulated air flight. *Ophthalmology.* 2001;108:40-44.
5. Contrell JJ. Altitude exposures during aircraft flight: flying higher. *Chest.* 1988;92:81-84.

who had C3F8 in their eyes from vitreoretinal surgery 10 to 30 days earlier experienced loss of vision from central retinal artery occlusion after general anesthesia with nitrous oxide. Thus nitrous oxide anesthesia should be contraindicated in all patients who still have expansile gas in their eyes.

Prevention and Treatment

Titrating the concentration and volume of these intraocular gases is the recognized approach to their safe use.[57] Recent studies using 20% SF6 showed only 6% of eyes had an IOP greater than 30 mm Hg on one postoperative occasion,[60] and only 9% had an IOP greater than 30 mm Hg when a 14% concentration of C3F8 was used.[61] Regardless of the amount and concentration of gas used, close monitoring of the IOP postoperatively and attention to proper positioning of the patient's head are imperative. An unusual condition is that encountered with changes of IOP with altitude in eyes with intraocular gas[62-65] (see the box "Intraocular Gas and Altitude"). Carbonic anhydrase inhibitors, beta-blockers, and alpha-adrenergic agonists may be employed to control the IOP, but if the IOP is extremely high, or in eyes susceptible to central retinal artery occlusion, aliquots of intraocular gas are sequentially removed until normotension is achieved.

GLAUCOMA AFTER INTRAOCULAR SILICONE OIL

Silicone oil is a vitreous substitute and is used for retinal tamponade, was introduced in 1962. Initially, serious associated complications and pending progress in modern vitreoretinal surgery and bioengineering limited its use.[66] Subsequently, the use of silicone oil in complex vitrectomies has enjoyed a resurgence.[67] Like air, silicone oil is lighter than aqueous or vitreous, and, because of its buoyancy, it can compress the superior angle of an eye in the upright position. In aphakic eyes, it can occlude the pupil and cause pupillary block. A 5% incidence of angle closure and a 29% incidence of angle compromise in 93 patients 3 years after intravitreal silicone use have been reported.[68]

Open-angle glaucoma is a more common complication after the use of silicone oil. A definite correlation exists between the appearance of the oil in the anterior chamber and elevated IOP,[69] as well as a significant decrease in the IOP with subsequent removal of the oil from the anterior chamber.[70] Silicone oil was thought to be more likely to enter the anterior chamber in aphakic rather than phakic or pseudophakic eyes. With time, foamy silicone bubbles may appear in the anterior chamber of phakic eyes as well[71,72] (Figure 33-4). Silicone-laden microphages have been detected within the trabecular meshwork, which otherwise appears normal,[68] and emulsified oil in the anterior chamber may not be detectable except on gonioscopy.[69] Thus, obstruction of the outflow by silicone oil appears to be at least a

300% with nitrous oxide ventilation compared with a 50% increase with air ventilation and 35% increase with oxygen ventilation. Fu[5] reported 4 out of 5 patients with intraocular gas and subsequent nitrous oxide anesthesia had final visual acuity of 20/200 or worse and significant optic atrophy. Hart and associates[59] also reported that 3 patients

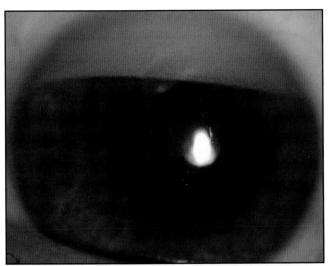

Figure 33-4. Silicone oil emulsification. Slit-lamp photo shows emulsified silicone oil in the superior part of the anterior chamber (inverted hypopyon).

contributory cause of the elevated IOP. After intravitreal silicone oil, the incidence of ocular hypertension has been reported to be 56% (increase > 10 mm Hg) in the immediate postoperative period.[73] It decreases to 48% (> 25 mm Hg or increase > 10 mm Hg) 16 months postoperatively[74] and to 12% (> 22 mm Hg) 3 years postoperatively.[68] However, there are probably other contributory causes to the elevated IOP in these cases because oil in the anterior chamber is not always related to elevated IOPs, and elevated IOPs have been reported in eyes with no oil in the anterior chamber.[74] Peripheral anterior synechiae, inflammatory cells, and debris have been implicated,[73] and preoperative elevated IOP is a major risk factor (90% chance) in the development of glaucoma after intravitreal silicone oil.[74]

Prevention and Treatment

To avoid angle closure from pupillary block, because silicone oil is buoyant within the eye, a prophylactic inferior peripheral iridotomy at the time of the vitrectomy in aphakic eyes and a selected group of pseudophakic eyes has been recommended.[75] With an inferior peripheral iridotomy, should silicone oil get into the anterior chamber, positioning the patient in the prone position will allow the silicone oil an avenue of egress from the anterior chamber to the vitreous cavity through the pupil and ingress of aqueous through the iridectomy. In a recent study[74] affirming the protective value of an inferior iridectomy, all 21 eyes requiring glaucoma surgery after intravitreal silicone oil either had a scleral buckle and/or lacked an intraoperative peripheral iridectomy. Once pupillary block is detected, an inferior peripheral iridectomy should be performed either with the laser or by surgery depending on the clarity of the cornea. Fibrinous closure of a peripheral iridectomy can occur, in which case reopening

it with the Nd:YAG laser may be successful.[70] In addition, silicone oil should be removed when the retina is completely and firmly attached and adequate chorioretinal adhesion has sealed the breaks, keeping in mind that there is a significant incidence of re-detachment of the retina associated with this procedure.[71]

With secondary open-angle glaucoma, preventive measures include avoidance of superior iridectomies or superior iris trauma at the time of vitrectomy, avoidance of overfilling the eye with silicone oil, instillation of air into the anterior chamber in aphakic eyes at the time of surgery and removal of silicone oil from the anterior chamber as soon as possible when this is noted postoperatively.[70] Unfortunately, even an inferior peripheral iridectomy does not always prevent the movement of silicone oil into the anterior chamber angle.[69] Once glaucoma is noted, conservative measures include vigorous mydriasis-cycloplegia, topical steroids to decrease inflammation, and topical beta-blockers and carbonic anhydrase inhibitors as tolerated. With concurrent removal of silicone oil, the majority (60%)[70,74] of cases[76] of such a glaucoma can be controlled.

GLAUCOMA SURGERY AFTER VITREORETINAL DETACHMENT SURGERY

In all cases of glaucoma secondary to vitreoretinal detachment surgery, if conservative therapy does not control the IOP, surgical intervention must be undertaken to save vision. Filtration surgery with 5-fluorouracil (5-FU),[77] Molteno (Molteno Ophthalmic Ltd, Dunedin New Zealand) or other implants, Schocket procedures, and Nd:YAG laser trans-scleral cyclophotocoagulation have been reported to be successful,[74] but the number of cases reported has been small. If filtration surgery is contemplated, because of conjunctival scarring from the vitreoretinal surgery, antifibrotics will increase the likelihood of successful filtration. After a retina operation, to augment the chances of successful filtration, retina surgeons should be encouraged to close the peritomy tightly with multiple sutures and eschew the tendency to use only 2 tack sutures at the 3 o'clock and 9 o'clock positions. With the latter closure, the superior conjunctival flap often does not attach to the limbus, and a superior pocket is formed, sometimes extending 3- to 4-mm posterior to the limbus. Therefore, before the glaucoma surgeon starts to dissect the posterior conjunctiva for a limbus-based flap, determine the status of the conjunctiva at the limbus because it may indicate the need for a fornix-based conjunctival flap. Based on personal experience, the success rate of trabeculectomy with intraoperative mitomycin-C is not different from the success rate of other high-risk glaucoma eyes, and good pressure control without antiglaucoma medications is in the 80% success range.

Ocular Hypertension After Intravitreal Injections

In recent years, intravitreal injections have become the most common retina procedure. Intravitreal medications such as ranibizumab (Lucentis), bevacizumab (Avastin), and triamcinolone acetate (Kenalog) are injected into the vitreous cavity. Both transient and persistent ocular hypertension may occur after intravitreal injection of these medications. Several studies[78-81] have investigated the short-term IOP changes after intravitreal injections. These studies have shown that intravitreal injection of these medications led to an expected short-term and transient elevation of IOP immediately after injection. IOP usually returned to a lower level (below 25 mm Hg) within 30 to 60 minutes without using therapy for IOP control. Hollands et al[78] noted that phakic patients might have a slightly higher IOP compared to pseudophakic patients shortly after intravitreal injections. It should be noted that eyes with a history of glaucoma may take longer to return to the baseline IOP.[79] About one-third of patients who receive intravitreal triamcinolone develop a delayed-onset ocular hypertension.[82] Ocular hypertension may develop weeks or months after intravitreal steroid. Recently, we and others reported persistent ocular hypertension in patients who received intravitreal injections of ranibizumab and/or bevacizumab.[2,81-84] Persistent ocular hypertension usually occurs following multiple injections, although it might happen after only one injection. These patients may require IOP-lowering therapy.[2]

References

1. Chang S. LXII Edward Jackson lecture: open angle glaucoma after vitrectomy. *Am J Ophthalmol.* 2006;141(6):1033-1043.
2. Adelman RA, Zheng Q, Mayer H. Persistent ocular hypertension following intravitreal bevacizumab and ranibizumab injections. *J Ocul Pharmacol Ther.* 2010;26(1):105-110.
3. Sato EA, Shinoda K, Inoue M, Ohtake Y, Kimura I. Reduced choroidal blood flow can induce visual field defect in open angle glaucoma patients without intraocular pressure elevation following encircling scleral buckling. *Retina.* 2008;28(3):493-497.
4. Pavlidis M, Scharioth G, Ortueta DD, Baatz H. Iridolenticular block in heavy silicone oil tamponade. *Retina.* 2010;30(3):516-520.
5. Fu AD, McDonald HR, Eliott D, et al. Complications of general anesthesia using nitrous oxide in eyes with preexisting gas bubbles. *Retina.* 2002;22(5):569-574.
6. Luk FO, Kwok AK, Lai TY, Lam DS. Presence of crystalline lens as a protective factor for the late development of open angle glaucoma after vitrectomy. *Retina.* 2009;29(2):218-224.
7. Yazdani S, Hendi K, Pakravan M, Mahdavi M, Yaseri M. Intravitreal bevacizumab for neovascular glaucoma: a randomized controlled trial. *J Glaucoma.* 2009;18(8):632-637.
8. Bakri SJ, McCannel CA, Edwards AO, Moshfeghi DM. Persistent ocular hypertension following intravitreal ranibizumab. *Graefes Arch Clin Exp Ophthalmol.* 2009;246(7):955-958.
9. Kangas TA, Bennet SR, Flynn HW, et al. Reversible loss of light perception after vitreoretinal surgery. *Am J Ophthalmol.* 1995;120(6):751-756.
10. Chang S. Intraocular gases. In: Ryan S, ed. *Retina.* 4th ed. Philadelphia, PA: Elsevier Mosby; 2006:2165-2179.
11. Sebestyen JG, Schepens CL, Rosenthal ML. Retinal detachment and glaucoma. I. Tonometric and gonioscopic study of 160 cases. *Arch Ophthalmol.* 1962;67:736-745.
12. Fiore JV, Newton JC. Anterior segment changes following the scleral buckling procedure. *Arch Ophthalmol.* 1970;84:284-287.
13. Hartley RE, Marsh RJ. Anterior chamber depth changes after retinal detachment. *Br J Ophthalmol.* 1973;57:546-550.
14. Smith TR. Acute glaucoma developing after scleral buckling procedure. *Am J Ophthalmol.* 1967;63:1807-1808.
15. Kreiger AE, Hodgkinson BJ, Frederick AR, et al. The results of retinal detachment surgery. *Arch Ophthalmol.* 1971;86:385-394.
16. Perez RN, Phelps CD, Burton TC. Angle closure glaucoma following scleral buckling operations. *Trans Am Academy Ophthalmol Otolaryngol.* 1976;81:247-252.
17. Hayreh SS, Baines JAB. Occlusion of the vortex veins. An experimental study. *Br J Ophthalmol.* 1973;57:217-238.
18. Grant WM. Experimental aqueous perfusion in enucleated human eyes. *Arch Ophthalmol.* 1963;69:783-801.
19. Mensher JH. Anterior chamber depth alteration after retinal photocoagulation. *Arch Ophthalmol.* 1977;95:113-116.
20. Liang JC, Huamonte FU. Reduction of immediate complications after panretinal photocoagulation. *Retina.* 1984;4:166-170.
21. Gass JD. Retinal detachment and narrow angle glaucoma. *Am J Ophthalmol.* 1967;63:94-103.
22. Kurtz S, Moisseier J, Gutman I, et al. Orbital pseudotumor presenting as acute glaucoma with choroidal and retinal detachment. *Ophthalmology.* 1993;2:61-62.
23. McDonald PR, de la Paz V, Sarin LK. Non-rhegmatogenous retinal separation with choroidal detachment (uveal effusion). *Am J Ophthalmol.* 1965;59:820-827.
24. Grant WM. Shallowing of the anterior chamber following occlusion of the central retinal vein. *Am J Ophthalmol.* 1973;75:384-389.
25. Bloome MA. Transient angle closure glaucoma in central retinal vein occlusion. *Ann Ophthalmol.* 1977;9:44-48.
26. Holland PM, Smith TR. Broad scleral buckle in the management of retinal detachments with giant tears. *Am J Ophthalmol.* 1977;83:518-525.
27. Phelps CD. Angle closure glaucoma secondary to ciliary body swelling. *Arch Ophthalmol.* 1974;92:287-290.
28. Pavlin CJ, Ritch R, Foster FS. Ultrasound biomicroscopy in plateau iris syndrome. *Am J Ophthalmol.* 1992;113:390-395.
29. Pemberton JW. Schiotz-applanation disparity following retinal detachment surgery. *Arch Ophthalmol.* 1969;81:534-537.
30. Wand M. Diagnosis and management of angle closure glaucoma. *Focal Points VI.* 1994;10:1-12.
31. Ritch R. Argon laser treatment for medically unresponsive attacks of angle closure glaucoma. *Am J Ophthalmol.* 1982;94:197-204.
32. Wand M. Argon laser gonioplasty for synechial angle closure. *Arch Ophthalmol.* 1992;110:363-367.
33. Phelps CD, Burton TC. Glaucoma and retinal detachment. *Arch Ophthalmol.* 1977;95:418-422.
34. Podos SM, Becker B, Morton WR. High myopia and primary open angle glaucoma. *Am J Ophthalmol.* 1966;62:1039-1043.
35. Ackerman AL. Retinal detachments and miotic therapy. In: Pruett RL, Regan CDJ, eds. *Retinal Congress.* New York, NY: Appleton-Century-Crofts Inc; 1972:533-539.
36. Minckler D. Glaucoma after vitrectomy—role of intravitreal gas and silicone oil. *J Glaucoma.* 1994;3:165-167.
37. Schwartz A. Chronic open angle glaucoma secondary to rhegmatogenous retinal detachment. *Am J Ophthalmol.* 1973;75:205-211.
38. Matsuo N, Takabatake M, Ueno H, et al. Photoreceptor outer segments in the aqueous humor in rhegmatogenous retinal detachment. *Am J Ophthalmol.* 1986;101:673-679.

39. Schulze RR. Rubeosis iritis. *Am J Ophthalmol.* 1967;63:487-495.
40. Wand M. Neovascular glaucoma. In: Albert DM, Jakobiec FA, eds. *Principles and Practice of Ophthalmology.* Philadelphia, PA: WB Saunders Co; 1994:1485-1510.
41. Tanaka S, Ideta H, Yonemoto J, et al. Neovascularization of the iris in rhegmatogenous retinal detachment. *Am J Ophthalmol.* 1991;112:632-634.
42. Rice TA, Michaels RG, Maguire MG, et al. The effects of lensectomy on the incidence of iris neovascularization and neovascular glaucoma after vitrectomy in diabetic eyes. *Am J Ophthalmol.* 1983;95:1-11.
43. Thompson JT, Glaser BM. Role of lensectomy and posterior capsule in movement of tracers from vitreous to aqueous. *Arch Ophthalmol.* 1985;103:420-421.
44. Kokame GT, Flynn HW, Blankenship GW. Posterior chamber intraocular lens implantation during diabetic pars plana vitrectomy. *Ophthalmology.* 1989;96:603-610.
45. Wand M, Madigan JC, Gaudio AR, et al. Neovascular glaucoma following pars plana vitrectomy for complications of diabetic retinopathy. *Ophthalmic Surg.* 1990;21:113-118.
46. Camaratta MR, Chang S, Sparrow J. Iris neovascularization in proliferative vitreoretinopathy. *Ophthalmology.* 1992;99:898-905.
47. Azzolini C, Brancato R, Camesasca FI, et al. Influence of silicone oil on iris microangiopathy in diabetic vitrectomized eyes. *Ophthalmology.* 1993;100:1152-1159.
48. Oldenoerp J, Spitznas M. Factors influencing the results of vitreous surgery in diabetic retinopathy: I. Iris rubeosis and/or active neovascularization at the fundus. *Graefes Arch Clin Exp Ophthalmol.* 1989;227:1-8.
49. Scuder JJ, Blumenkranz MS, Blankenship GW. Regression of diabetic rubeosis iridis following successful surgical reattachment of the retina by vitrectomy. *Retina.* 1982;2:193-196.
50. Hilton GF, Grizzard WS. Pneumatic retinopexy. A 2-step outpatient operation without conjunctival incision. *Ophthalmology.* 1986;93:626-641.
51. Norton EWD. Intraocular gas in the management of selected retinal detachments. *Trans Am Academy Ophthalmol Otolaryngol.* 1973;77:85-88.
52. Peyman GA, Vygantas CM, Bennett TO, et al. Octafluorocyclobutane in vitreous and aqueous humor replacement. *Arch Ophthalmol.* 1975;93:514-517.
53. Killey FP, Edelhauser HF, Aaberg TM. Intraocular sulfur hexafluoride and octofluorocyclobutane. *Arch Ophthalmol.* 1978;96:511-515.
54. Aronowitz JD, Brubaker RF. Effect of intraocular gas on intraocular pressure. *Arch Ophthalmol.* 1976;94:1191-1196.
55. Lim JI, Blair NP, Higginbotham EJ, et al. Assessment of intraocular pressure in vitrectomized gas-containing eyes: A clinical and manometric comparison of the Tono-Pen to the pneumotonometer. *Arch Ophthalmol.* 1990;108:684-688.
56. Abrams GW, Swanson DE, Sabates W. The results of sulfur hexafluoride gas in vitreous surgery. *Am J Ophthalmol.* 1982;94:165-171.
57. Sabates WI, Abrams GW, Swanson DE, et al. The use of intraocular gases. The results of sulfur hexafluoride gas in retinal detachment surgery. *Ophthalmology.* 1981;88:447-454.
58. Wolf G, Capuano C, Hartung J. Effect of nitrous oxide on gas bubble volume in the anterior chamber. *Arch Ophthalmol.* 1985;103:418-419.
59. Hart RH, Vote BJ, Borthwick JH, McGeorge AJ, Worsley DR. Loss of vision caused by expansion of intraocular perfluoropropane (C_3F_8) gas during nitrous oxide anesthesia. *Am J Ophthalmol.* 2002;134:761-763.
60. Vitrectomy with silicone oil or sulfur hexafluoride gas in eyes with severe proliferative vitreoretinopathy: results of a randomized clinical trial. Silicone Study Report 1. *Arch Ophthalmol.* 1992;110:770-779.
61. Vitrectomy with silicone oil or perfluoropropane gas in eyes with severe proliferative vitreopathy: results of a randomized clinical trial. Silicone Study Report 2. *Arch Ophthalmol.* 1992;110:780-792.
62. Lincoff H, Weinberger D, Reppucci V, et al. Air travel with intraocular gas: I. The mechanisms for compensation. *Arch Ophthalmol.* 1989;107:902-906.
63. Dieckert JP, O'Connor PS, Schacklett DE, et al. Air travel and intraocular gas. *Ophthalmology.* 1986;93:642-645.
64. Kokame GT, Ing MR. Intraocular gas and low altitude air flight. *Retina.* 1994;14:356-358.
65. Contrell JJ. Altitude exposures during aircraft flight: flying higher. *Chest.* 1988;92:81-84.
66. Cox MS, Trese MT, Murphy PL. Silicone oil for advanced proliferative vitreoretinopathy. *Ophthalmology.* 1986;93:646-649.
67. McCuen BW, Landers MB, Machemer R. The use of silicone oil following failed vitrectomy for retinal detachment with advanced proliferative vitreoretinopathy. *Ophthalmology.* 1985;92:1029-1034.
68. Leaver PK, Gray RMB, Garner A. Silicone oil injection in the treatment of massive periretinal retraction. II: late complications in 93 eyes. *Br J Ophthalmol.* 1979;63:361-367.
69. Valone J, McCarthy M. Emulsified anterior chamber silicone oil and glaucoma. *Ophthalmology.* 1994;101:1908-1912.
70. Gao R, Neubauer L, Tang S, et al. Silicone oil in the anterior chamber. *Graefe's Arch Clin Exp Ophthalmology.* 1989;227:106-109.
71. Pearson RV, McLeod D, Gregor ZJ. Removal of silicone oil following diabetic vitrectomy. *Br J Ophthalmol.* 1993;77:204-207.
72. Chan C, Okun E. The question of ocular tolerance to intravitreal liquid silicone. A long-term analysis. *Ophthalmology.* 1986;93:651-660.
73. de Corral LR, Cohen SB, Peyman GA. Effect of intravitreal silicone oil on intraocular pressure. *Ophthalmic Surg.* 1987;8:446-449.
74. Nguyen QH, Lloyd MA, Heuer DK, et al. Incidence and management of glaucoma after intravitreal silicone oil injection for complicated retinal detachments. *Ophthalmology.* 1992;99:1520-1526.
75. Ando F. Intraocular hypertension resulting from pupillary block by silicone oil. *Am J Ophthalmol.* 1985;99:87-88.
76. Moisseier J, Barah A, Manaim J, et al. Removal of silicone oil in the management of glaucoma in eyes with emulsified silicone. *Retina.* 1993;13:290-295.
77. Ophir A, Ticho U. Trabeculectomy with 5-fluorouracil subsequent to circular buckling operation and cataract extraction. *Ann Ophthalmol.* 1992;24:386-390.
78. Hollands H, Wong J, Bruen R, Campbell RJ, Sharma S, Gale J. Short-term intraocular pressure changes after intravitreal injection of bevacizumab. *Can J Ophthalmol.* 2007;42:807-811.
79. Kim JE, Mantravadi AV, Hur EY, Covert DJ. Short-term intraocular pressure changes immediately after intravitreal injections of antivascular endothelial growth factor agents. *Am J Ophthalmol.* 2008;146:930-934.
80. Mojica G, Hariprasad SM, Jager RD, Mieler WF. Short-term intraocular pressure trends following intravitreal injections of ranibizumab (Lucentis) for the treatment of wet age-related macular degeneration. *Br J Ophthalmol.* 2008;92:584.
81. Bakri SJ, Pulido JS, McCannel CA, Hodge DO, Diehl N, Hillemeier J. Immediate intraocular pressure changes following intravitreal injections of triamcinolone, pegaptanib, and bevacizumab. *Eye.* 2009;23:181-185.
82. Baath J, Ells AL, Crichton A, Kherani A, Williams RG. Safety profile of intravitreal triamcinolone acetonide. *J Ocul Pharmacol.* 2007;23(3):304-310.
83. Kahook MY, Kimura AE, Wong LJ, Ammar DA, Maycotte MA, Mandava N. Sustained elevation in intraocular pressure associated with intravitreal bevacizumab injections. *Ophthalmic Surg Lasers Imaging.* 2009;40(3):293-295.
84. Good TJ, Kimura AE, Mandava N, Kahook MY. Sustained elevation of intraocular pressure after intravitreal injections of anti-VEGF agents. *Br J Ophthalmol.* 2011;95:1111-1114.

Angle-Closure Glaucoma Due to Multiple Cysts of the Iris and Ciliary Body

Ian P. Conner, MD, PhD; Joel S. Schuman, MD, FACS; and David L. Epstein, MD, MMM

Intra-epithelial cysts[1] (Figure 34-1) of the iris and ciliary body, if multiple, may gradually push the peripheral iris forward so as to close the angle and cause elevated intraocular pressure (IOP). Angle-closure glaucoma caused by cysts of the iris and ciliary body is rare compared with angle-closure glaucoma from other causes.

The onset of the glaucoma is sometimes rapid with the typical picture of acute angle-closure glaucoma. The diagnosis may be suspected by finding on gonioscopic examination a considerable difference in the width of the chamber angle in various parts of the circumference. In some areas, the angle may appear closed but in other areas, the angle may be wide, with a broad ciliary body band visible. Such marked variation in angle width is unknown in primary acute angle-closure glaucoma and should alert the astute clinician as to the possibility of posterior iris pathology, either in the form of pigment epithelium cysts or tumor. There is often also a characteristic irregularly spaced bumpy contour to the peripheral iris. Occasional patients have been observed with 1 or 2 such areas in the total angle circumference. Presumably, occasional cysts may not be as rare as once thought. From a practical point of view, the presence of only a few such areas does not substantially affect aqueous outflow.

It is important to recognize this entity, especially from the standpoint of prognosis. In primary angle-closure glaucoma, laser iridotomy, if performed in a timely fashion, usually affects a cure of the glaucoma. If the angle closure is caused by cysts of the iris and ciliary body, the prognosis must be more guarded.

The true state of affairs may not be recognized until after there is an iridectomy or iridotomy. After surgical iridectomy (eg, in cataract or filtration surgery), one or more cysts of the ciliary processes may be seen in the iris opening.

Even through typically small laser iridotomies, cysts may occasionally be seen through the iris opening by gonioscopy. Also, either with the miotic pupil or, more commonly, after dilation, an iris cyst can be seen presenting at or behind the pupillary border. These iris cysts are dark brown and may be mistaken for a melanoma. In the area of an iris cyst, the iris is usually lifted off the lens sufficiently so that, on gonioscopic examination, one can look under the iris on either side of the cyst and sometimes see smaller cysts of the ciliary processes. These cysts of the ciliary processes may be heavily pigmented like iris cysts, or they may be perfectly clear.

Iris cysts can be punctured with an argon or neodymium:yttrium-aluminum-garnet (Nd:YAG) laser using a mirrored gonioscopy lens if they extend into or beyond the pupillary border and apparently show little tendency to recur. Puncture of an iris cyst results in considerable widening of the angle in the region of the cyst if peripheral anterior synechiae have not already formed. Ciliary body cysts likely could be similarly easily treated with the laser, if visualized. (Occasionally, one may see 2 or 3 ciliary body cysts on either side of an iris cyst.)

In one eye that we observed after intracapsular cataract extraction, we could easily see behind the iris during gonioscopy and could view a continuous row of cysts of the ciliary processes in the entire circumference. In cases in which cysts of the ciliary body appear to be present in the whole circumference, the angle may remain extremely narrow after iridectomy or iridotomy and may close again, causing another acute increase in IOP. In most cases, the glaucoma can be controlled medically after iridotomy but, in exceptional cases, a filtering operation may be necessary. Ciliary body cysts in particular may continue to grow and cause further closure of the angle, requiring a filtering operation.

Kahook MY, Schuman JS, eds.
Chandler and Grant's Glaucoma, Fifth Edition (pp 337-339).
© 2013 SLACK Incorporated.

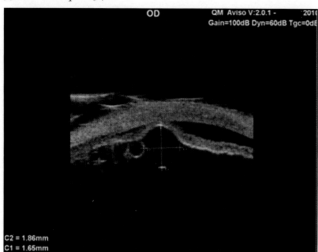

OD   QM Aviso V:2.0.1 -   2011
                      Gain=100dB Dyn=60dB Tgc=0dE

C2 = 1.86mm
C1 = 1.65mm

Figure 34-1. Cysts of the iris and ciliary body may be visible only as an irregular iris surface contour gonioscopically, but are visualized by ultrasound biomicroscopy.

In some cases of multiple cysts of the iris and ciliary body, a heavy deposition of pigment is present in the trabecular meshwork, similar to that seen in pigmentary glaucoma. This pigment can cause a permanent obstruction to outflow and a form of open-angle glaucoma.

Iris and ciliary body cysts have occurred within families.[2] This suggests that cysts of the iris and ciliary body may be genetically determined, and all members of the immediate family should be examined. In one member of such a family, marked fluctuations in the size of these cysts were documented (by author DLE) that may have been related to the woman's menstrual cycle.

In addition to causing or potentiating angle-closure glaucoma, peripheral iris cysts can also create the appearance of the plateau iris syndrome.[3] Similar to true plateau iris configuration, the peripheral iris may not appreciably change its appearance in response to peripheral iridotomy in these cases and may require further treatment, including laser treatment of iris cysts or laser gonioplasty.[4]

Finally, isolated cases of iris cyst formation and growth have been reported as a consequence of treatment with the prostaglandin analog class of topical medications.[5] Although angle closure secondary to this specific pattern of iris cyst growth has not yet been reported, it remains a possibility of which the clinician should have some awareness.

The following case reports are instances of angle-closure glaucoma caused by cysts of the iris or ciliary body or both.

Case 34-1

A 55-year-old man had a history of an attack of acute glaucoma in the left eye. He was treated with miotics and acetazolamide. When first seen 3 weeks after the attack, IOP was OD 17 and OS 20. The right disc was normal; the left showed no pathologic cupping but seemed a little paler than

the right. Gonioscopy was as follows: in the right eye, nasally, the angle was moderately wide with a fairly broad ciliary band, but below and temporally the angle was extremely narrow in 2 clock-hours of the circumference and the iris was much more convex in this region. Above and temporally, there were another 2 clock-hours of excessively narrow angle, very striking and suggestive of iris and ciliary body cysts. The trabecular meshwork showed heavy pigmentation. In the left eye, approximately two-thirds of the angle was open but irregularly and excessively narrow, likely closed in another 1 to 2 clock-hours of the circumference.

A surgical peripheral iridectomy was performed on the left eye (this was before the era of laser iridotomy). Two days later, the pupil was widely dilated in the right eye. One could then see a large cyst behind the iris below and temporally. The cyst lifted the iris off the lens in this region, and one could see for a short distance on either side a continuous row of cysts of the ciliary processes. An operation was performed to collapse the iris cyst by inserting a Haab needle through the peripheral cornea across the anterior chamber and by incising the cyst where it was exposed behind the edge of the pupil. When the left pupil was widely dilated, a large iris cyst could be seen presenting between the iris and the lens from about 3 o'clock to 5 o'clock. This cyst was similarly incised with a needle. Over the next 8 years, the right eye required no medication but the left required 4% pilocarpine and epinephrine to maintain IOPs less than 20 mm Hg. Vision then was OD 20/30 and OS 20/60. The right lens was clear; the left had a little nuclear sclerosis.

In this case, as in other similar cases, there seems to be no tendency for iris cysts to reform after they have been incised. Twenty years after these cysts were incised, there was still no sign of them reforming.

Case 34-2

A 35-year-old man had been told he had a suspicion of glaucoma. He was asymptomatic and using 1% pilocarpine 3 times daily. The discs were normal, fields full. On gonioscopy, the picture was striking. In exactly the nasal half of the angle in both eyes, the iris plane was flat; the angle was wide with scleral spur visible and even a little ciliary band. In the temporal half, the iris contour was very convex, a marked contrast to the flat iris plane on the nasal side, and the angle was excessively narrow, portions possibly closed. IOP in both eyes was in the mid-20s. He was seen later when off treatment. The gonioscopic picture was unchanged and the IOP was still in the mid-20s in both eyes. The pupils were then widely dilated to about 8 mm. In both eyes, there were 2 iris cysts temporally touching each other. In the left eye in the upper temporal quadrant, the iris cyst projected a little beyond the 8-mm pupil. Elsewhere, the cysts just reached the border of the 8-mm pupil. These iris cysts were treated with the argon laser. The temporal angle widened, and no iris cysts were now visible, even when the pupil was widely dilated.

This latter case re-emphasizes the important point that most hyperopic narrow-angled eyes are symmetrically narrow around the circumference of the angle (except for the superior angle, which is narrowest in most eyes, including emmetropic eyes). If there is great disparity between the nasal and temporal halves of the angle in terms of narrowness, then the attentive clinician should suspect iris or ciliary body cysts, or other ciliary body pathology, including tumors such as melanoma (see Chapters 7 and 41).

REFERENCES

1. Shields JA. Primary cysts of the iris. *Trans Am Ophthalmol Soc.* 1981;79:771-809.
2. Vela A, Rieser JC, Campbell DG. The heredity and treatment of angle-closure glaucoma secondary to iris and ciliary body cysts. *Ophthalmology.* 1984;91:332-337.
3. Shukla S, Damji KF, Harasymowycz P, et al. Clinical features distinguishing angle closure from pseudoplateau versus plateau iris. *Br J Ophthalmol.* 2008;92(3):340-344.
4. Crowston JG, Medeiros FA, Mosaed S, Weinreb RN. Argon laser iridoplasty in the treatment of plateau-like iris configuration as result of numerous ciliary body cysts. *Am J Ophthalmol.* 2005;139(2):381-383.
5. Lai IC, Kuo MT, Teng LM. Iris pigment epithelial cyst induced by topical administration of latanoprost. *Br J Ophthalmol.* 2003;87(3):366.

35

Angle-Closure Glaucoma Secondary to Occlusion of the Central Retinal Vein

Malik Y. Kahook, MD and David L. Epstein, MD, MMM

Occlusion of the central retinal vein is not ordinarily thought to affect the depth of the anterior chamber, but occasionally, within a few days after vein occlusion, the lens and iris move forward, producing conspicuous shallowing of the anterior chamber in the affected eye. This is especially appreciated when one compares the axial depth of the anterior chamber in the affected eye with that in the contralateral normal eye.[1-4] In some cases, there has been enough shallowing to cause the angle to close. In such cases, angle-closure glaucoma has usually been diagnosed within 2 or 3 weeks after vein occlusion. The shallowing is reversible, and the anterior chamber does return to its original depth within a few weeks. The problem of angle-closure glaucoma then disappears if no synechiae have formed, but subsequent neovascular glaucoma may develop.

In the past, before this entity was clearly distinguished from other forms of angle-closure glaucoma, most cases were treated with pilocarpine and aqueous humor suppressants, which sufficed to keep the angle open until the spontaneous deepening and resolution of the glaucoma took place. We encountered one case in which treatment with pilocarpine, a carbonic anhydrase inhibitor, and oral osmotics did not relieve unilateral angle-closure glaucoma secondary to occlusion of the central retinal vein. However, when the pilocarpine was discontinued and a cycloplegic (cyclopentolate) was administered, the anterior chamber deepened, and the angle opened. Bloome reported 2 cases in which there was a good response to a cycloplegic and acetazolamide.[3] Treatment with cycloplegic agents seems logical in this condition, and, although we still have much to learn, cycloplegics should be used as initial treatment instead of miotics.

We assume that an abnormal accumulation of blood or fluid in the posterior segment is responsible for pushing the vitreous and lens forward. This fluid is gradually reabsorbed, allowing the vitreous and lens to recede to their normal position. Angle closure appears to be caused by abnormal resistance to flow of aqueous humor through the pupil from the posterior chamber to anterior chamber due to the forward position of the lens, analogous to the mechanism in primary angle-closure glaucoma in which the lens is also forward, but on a permanent rather than a transient basis; that is, the mechanism for the closure of the angle in this entity seems to involve a secondary pupillary block mechanism. In some cases of this type, peripheral iridectomy has been done and has relieved the angle-closure glaucoma without altering the position of the crystalline lens.

Before the availability of laser iridectomy, we believed that, in this particular kind of angle-closure glaucoma, it was best to treat the condition medically rather than by iridectomy. We learned that in most cases, the underlying condition cleared in a few weeks, even if the angle was only minimally open in this interval. With the relative ease of laser iridectomy, we now recommend that it be performed if the eye is not totally blind to prevent chronic synechial glaucoma, unless medical (cycloplegic) therapy opened the angle so well that synechia formation would be unlikely. Gonioscopy of the fellow eye is important because it may be occludable.

The occurrence of shallowing of the anterior chamber and angle-closure glaucoma secondary to occlusion of the central retinal vein is not directly related to the risk of developing neovascular glaucoma later.[5] The proportion of eyes that have developed neovascular glaucoma has not been more or less than is expected after ordinary occlusion of the central retinal vein without axial shallowing.

This condition must always be considered in the differential diagnosis of unilateral angle closure. Other causes

Kahook MY, Schuman JS, eds.
Chandler and Grant's Glaucoma, Fifth Edition (pp 341-342).
© 2013 SLACK Incorporated.

of transient unilateral shallowing of the anterior chamber with or without angle-closure glaucoma include panretinal photocoagulation,[6,7] choroidal hemorrhage,[8] massive retinal detachment secondary to macular degeneration,[9] uveal effusion,[10] and massive vitreous hemorrhage.[11]

The capacity of the vitreous to normally give up fluid and reduce its volume to compensate for the expanded posterior segment volume from the central retinal vein occlusion, is believed to explain why this syndrome of angle-closure glaucoma is uncommon. Presumably, the condition occurs in patients with more turgid vitreous. A systematic analysis of the difference between affected and unaffected patients with central retinal vein occlusion would be of interest. However, we suspect that slight axial shallowing (without angle closure) occurring acutely after central retinal vein occlusion may be more common than realized.

REFERENCES

1. Hyams SW, Neumann E. Transient angle-closure glaucoma after retinal vein occlusion. *Br J Ophthalmol.* 1972;56:535-355.
2. Grant WM. Shallowing of the anterior chamber following occlusion of the central retinal vein. *Am J Ophthalmol.* 1973;75:384-389.
3. Bloome MA. Transient angle-closure glaucoma in central retinal vein occlusion. *Ann Ophthalmol.* 1977;9:44-48.
4. Mendelsohn AD, Jampol LM, Shoch D. Secondary angle-closure glaucoma after central retinal vein occlusion. *Am J Ophthalmol.* 1985;100:581-585.
5. Hayreh SS, Rojas P, Montague P, et al. Ocular neovascularization with retinal vascularization occlusion-III. Incidence of ocular neovascularization with retinal vein occlusion. *Ophthalmology.* 1983;90:488-506.
6. Boulton PE. A study of the mechanisms of transient myopia following extensive xenon arc photocoagulation. *Trans Ophthalmol Soc UK.* 1973;93:287-300.
7. Mensher JH. Anterior chamber depth alteration after retinal photocoagulation. *Arch Ophthalmol.* 1977;95:113-116.
8. Christensen L. Narrow angle glaucoma. *Trans Am Acad Ophthalmol Otolaryngol.* 1963;67:71-74.
9. Wood WJ, Smith TR. Senile disciform macular degeneration complicated by massive hemorrhagic retinal detachment and angle closure glaucoma. *Retina.* 1983;3:296-303.
10. McDonald PR, de la Paz V Jr, Sarin LK. Nonrhegmatogenous retinal separation: With choroidal detachment (uveal effusion). *Am J Ophthalmol.* 1965;59:820-827.
11. Doden W. Sekundarglaukom bei Periphlebitis retinae. *Ophthalmologica.* 1961;142:506-511.

36

Angle-Closure Glaucoma Secondary to Acute Myopia

Malik Y. Kahook, MD and David L. Epstein, MD, MMM

Angle-closure glaucoma secondary to acute myopia is a relatively rare condition that an ophthalmologist may see a handful of times during an entire career, but it is a distinct entity that can be puzzling diagnostically. Acute transient myopia due to an idiosyncratic reaction to systemic drugs that have no cholinergic or parasympathomimetic activity is well known, but in only the rarest instances has the episode been accompanied by shallowing of the anterior chamber.[1-11] More than 20 different drugs of several different kinds, but most commonly diuretics[12-14] and sulfa-type drugs,[2,4,7,10,15-17] have induced acute transitory myopia. Other drugs reported include tetracycline,[3] aspirin,[5] corticosteroids,[18] bromocriptine,[19] prochlorperazine,[20] and promethazine.[21] More recently, topiramate has been implicated in cases of angle-closure glaucoma associated with acute myopia and suprachoroidal effusions.[22]

Sometimes, there is no past history of drug exposure. Typically, however, the patient has taken some medication weeks or months previously, such as a diuretic or sulfonamide antibiotic, without notable visual side effects, but after discontinuing the medication for a while and then taking it again, an acute reaction develops. Characteristically, within a few hours or a few days after resuming the medication, the patient experiences blurring of vision for distant objects due to the development of several diopters of myopia. Visual acuity can be restored to normal with a suitable refraction but not by anticholinergics. There is no miosis and no evidence of cyclotonia.

Good evidence, including ultrasonographic measurements,[8,13] indicates that swelling of the crystalline lens is responsible, at least in part, for the myopia in most cases and that it is reversible.[4] However, others have attributed at least some of the myopia to the forward movement of the crystalline lens.[7,10,11] We have seen one patient in whom

accumulation of anterior choroidal fluid was implicated not only in the pathogenesis of secondary angle-closure glaucoma, but also in the induced myopia.[11] The choroidal effusion presumably caused forward rotation of the ciliary body, which led to forward movement of the entire crystalline lens due to loss of zonular tension and angle closure. The latter presumably occurred from direct mechanical pressure of the ciliary body on the iris because laser iridectomy was without effect. The forward position of the crystalline lens could explain about half of the myopic shift. A similar case of induced myopia and angle closure has been reported in which one eye had a pseudophakos, and therefore, presumably lens swelling was ruled out as a cause of the myopia, which was attributed to the forward shift in the intraocular lens position.[10] This condition has also been observed commonly in young women, often during the first few months of pregnancy.

When the suspect drug is discontinued, the myopia disappears spontaneously within a few days. In all cases, similar changes have occurred in both eyes, except for an instance of unilateral aphakia that in contrast to the aforementioned, there was no change in the refraction of the aphakic eye. Either crystalline lens swelling or forward positioning of the crystalline lens or both may be involved in the etiology of the induced myopia.

Only in rare cases does crystalline lens swelling and/or forward shift of the crystalline lens cause sufficient shallowing of the anterior chamber to induce bilateral angle-closure glaucoma from pupillary block, and it is usually subacute rather than acute. When the process resolves in a few days, the myopia disappears, the anterior chambers return to normal depth, and the angles reopen to their former width. The following case is another example.

Kahook MY, Schuman JS, eds.
Chandler and Grant's Glaucoma, Fifth Edition (pp 343-345).
© 2013 SLACK Incorporated.

ACUTE BILATERAL TRANSITORY MYOPIA ASSOCIATED WITH OPEN-ANGLE GLAUCOMA

Joel S. Schuman, MD, FACS

I have seen a patient with bilateral transitory myopia associated with open-angle, rather than angle-closure, glaucoma. At the initial presentation, the patient, a 36-year-old woman, reported blurred vision after awakening. She had a low-grade fever (100°F) and a flu-like syndrome of aches, pains, and malaise. She did not recall taking any unusual medications, only loratadine (antihistamine) and nonsteroidal anti-inflammatory drugs (NSAIDs). She had no hypertension or diabetes, and a blood glucose was normal.

On examination, visual acuity was 20/200 OU, refracting to 20/25 OU with -2.00 D in each eye. IOPs were 23 and 24 mm Hg, and her angle was open in each eye to ciliary body band. Her examination otherwise was completely unremarkable. She was given her prescription and sent home. When she returned 3 weeks later, visual acuity was 20/20 without correction, and IOPs were 15 mm Hg in each eye. Angles were again open, and her examination was unchanged except that her axial anterior chamber depth seemed slightly greater than on the previous visit.

Two months later, the patient presented again with the same constitutional and ophthalmologic complaints. Vision was again correctable to 20/25 with -2.00 D sphere, but this time her IOPs were 36 and 38 mm Hg, although her angles were still open to scleral spur. She denied taking any new medications, but during the examination recalled that she had taken quinine for leg cramps just before the previous episode, and again before the current episode. This was the 31st quinine tablet she had ever taken, though she had only 2 recognized episodes of blurred vision.

Ultrasound biomicroscopy (UBM) showed her angles to be open to ciliary body band, confirming the gonioscopy, but also revealed very anterior ciliochoroidal effusions bilaterally (Figure 36-1). On follow-up examination 2 weeks later, the IOPs had returned to the mid-teens, the patient was again emmetropic, and the UBM demonstrated that the angles were now significantly wider than previously. The effusions were gone (Figure 36-2). An A-scan ultrasound at the time of the myopia compared with one taken after its resolution showed deepening of the anterior chamber and thinning of the crystalline lens with the resolution of the episode.

Quinine has been associated with acute bilateral transitory myopia with angle-closure glaucoma in one case.[1] Our patient appears to have developed an acute sensitivity to the drug, having taken it with no known adverse effects on 29 previous occasions, but with marked systemic and ocular side effects during the last 2. The mechanism for the ciliochoroidal effusion and, indeed, of the open-angle glaucoma itself remains mysterious, but the former may be related to a change in vascular permeability causing the effusion. The increased volume of the supraciliochoroidal space may have accounted for the increase in IOP, as this patient's angle was clearly open throughout each episode. Alternately, the change in the ciliary muscle[2,3] induced by the effusion may have relaxed the tone in the trabecular meshwork and Schlemm's canal, resulting in a decrease in outflow facility, thus explaining the IOP rise.

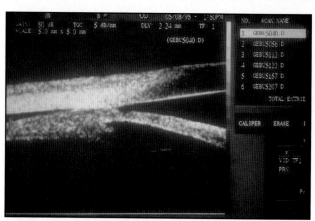

Figure 36-1. Ultrasound biomicroscopy during an episode of acute bilateral transitory myopia associated with open-angle glaucoma demonstrates anterior ciliochoroidal effusion with narrowing of the angle inlet, but the angle is open to ciliary body band.

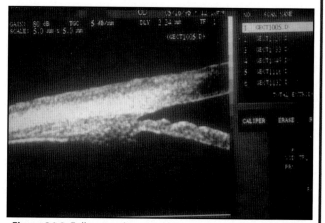

Figure 36-2. Follow-up ultrasound biomicroscopy after resolution of the episode (Figure 36-1) shows disappearance of supraciliochoroidal fluid and deepening of angle. Note change in angle configuration, although it was open both during and after the episode.

Whatever the mechanism, this rare condition of glaucoma associated with acute bilateral transitory myopia is no longer limited to angle closure alone.

REFERENCES

1. Segal A, Aisemberg A, Ducasse A. Quinine transitory myopia and angle-closure glaucoma. *Bull Soc Ophthalmol France.* 1983;83:247-249.
2. Grant WM. Experimental aqueous perfusion in enucleated human eyes. *Arch Ophthalmol.* 1963;69:783-801.
3. Rosenquist RC, Melamed S, Epstein DL. Anterior and posterior axial lens displacement and human aqueous outflow facility. *Invest Ophthalmol Vis Sci.* 1988;29:1159-1164.

CASE 36-1

A woman, aged mid-20s, accustomed to good vision without glasses, had rapid onset of blurring of vision in the course of several hours. The patient had a history of numerous allergies, but during the previous year she had taken a thiazide diuretic without adverse effects. She had stopped the diuretic 9 months before the present episode but had resumed taking it just before the onset of the blurring of vision, having taken 5 tablets during 2 or 3 days but none since. She had 4 diopters (D) of myopia in each eye, with vision correctable to normal by lenses. The anterior chambers were shallowed to 1.5 corneal thicknesses axially, and intraocular pressure (IOP) was 30 in each eye. The angles were extremely narrow and appeared closed in portions of the circumference. Pilocarpine and acetazolamide were started. The next day, IOP was 14 in each eye. The media were clear and the fundi normal, but myopia had increased to 7 D, and the anterior chambers were still very shallow. In 2 more days, the anterior chambers regained normal depth, the angles attained normal width, vision became normal without the need for glasses, and IOP was normal without further treatment.

The reversible myopia from lens swelling as an idiosyncratic reaction to drugs may be in some way allied to the changes in refraction that occasionally occur in diabetes mellitus. A bilateral transitory angle-closure glaucoma has been reported in one case in an insulin-treated diabetic patient during an episode of several diopters of myopia and marked shallowing of the anterior chambers.[23]

Also, acute bilateral transitory myopia with shallowing of the anterior chambers and angle-closure glaucoma has in 3 cases been reported in association with a febrile illness, but whether the mechanism differed from that in drug idiosyncrasy and diabetes mellitus is unproven.[24]

Treatment for this particular type of angle-closure glaucoma is discontinuance of any recently resumed systemic medication and temporary administration of aqueous humor suppressants. In the past, miotics have been used with good success, presumably due to considerations of net vectors. With lens swelling leading to pupillary block, such traditional medical therapy would make sense. However, in those cases where there may have also occurred a forward movement of the crystalline lens, it is possible that miotics may actually worsen the condition. Cycloplegics theoretically might be beneficial but in a recent case[11] there was no benefit, which we attribute to the maintained forwardly rotated position of the ciliary body that resulted from the supraciliary fluid accumulation.

Supraciliary effusion resulting from idiosyncratic drug reaction may be a more common mechanism in these cases that demonstrate secondary angle-closure glaucoma than is currently appreciated. Thus, there are 2 potential mechanisms for such secondary angle-closure glaucoma:

1. Pupillary block secondary to swelling of the crystalline lens or its induced forward position (as a result of loss of zonular tension accompanying suprachoroidal fluid accumulation)

2. Direct mechanical pressure (secondary to supraciliary effusion) of the forwardly rotated ciliary body on the iris forcing it into the angle

Laser iridectomy would alleviate the angle-closure glaucoma only if the first mechanism were involved. In our case, laser iridectomy was totally without effect, thus indicating that secondary pupillary block was not involved in the mechanism for the secondary angle-closure glaucoma.

Because sulfonamide drugs of the carbonic anhydrase inhibitor type are used for glaucoma therapy and influence fluid movement at the level of the ciliary body, it is theoretically possible that misdirection of flow into the suprachoroidal space might rarely occur from an idiosyncratic reaction.

REFERENCES

1. Grant WM, Schuman JS. *Toxicology of the Eye.* 4th ed. Springfield, IL: Charles C. Thomas; 1993.

2. Muirhead JF, Scheie HG. Transient myopia after acetazolamide. *Arch Ophthalmol.* 1960;63:315-318.

3. Edwards TS. Transient myopia due to tetracycline. *J Am Med Assoc.* 1963;186:69-70.

4. Maddalena MA. Transient myopia associated with acute glaucoma and retinal edema following vaginal administration of sulfanilamide. *Arch Ophthalmol.* 1968;80:186-188.

5. Sanford-Smith JH. Transient myopia after aspirin. *Br J Ophthalmol.* 1974;58:698-700.

6. Schroeder W, Schwarzer J. Transitorische Myopie mit Winkelblockglaukom. *Klin Monatsbl Augenheilkd.* 1978;172:762-766.

7. Bovino JA, Marcus DF. The mechanism of transient myopia induced by sulfonamide therapy. *Am J Ophthalmol.* 1982;94:99-102.

8. Hook SR, Holladay JT, Prager TC, et al. Transient myopia induced by sulfonamides. *Am J Ophthalmol.* 1986;101:495-496.

9. Ryan EH, Jampol LM. Drug-induced acute transient myopia with retinal folds. *Retina.* 1986;6:220-223.

10. Fan JT, Johnson DH, Burk RR. Transient myopia, angle closure glaucoma, and choroidal detachment after oral acetazolamide. *Am J Ophthalmol.* 1993;115:813-814.

11. Postel E, Assalian F, Epstein DL. Drug-induced transient myopia and angle closure associated with supraciliary choroidal effusion. *Am J Ophthalmol.* 1996;122(1):110-112.

12. Michaelson JJ. Transient myopia due to hygroton. *Am J Ophthalmol.* 1962;54:1146-1147.

13. Pallin O, Ericsson R. Ultrasound studies in a case of hygroton-induced myopia. *ACTA Ophthalmol.* 1965;43:692-696.

14. Beasley FJ. Transient myopia and retinal edema during hydrochlorothiazide (hydrodiuril) therapy. *Arch Ophthalmol.* 1961;65:212-213.

15. Granstrom KO. Transient myopia following the administration of sulphonamides. *ACTA Ophthalmol.* 1949;27:59-68.

16. Galin MA, Baras I, Zweifach P. Diamox-induced myopia. *Am J Ophthalmol.* 1957;35:478-484.

17. Beasley FJ. Transient myopia and retinal edema during ethoxzolamide (cardrase) therapy. *Arch Ophthalmol.* 1962;68:490-491.

18. Stern JJ. Transient myopia in a case of dermatitis treated with corticotropin. *Arch Ophthalmol.* 1956;54:762.

19. Manor RS, Dickerman Z, Llaron Z. Myopia during bromocriptine treatment. *Lancet.* 1981;1(8211):102.

20. Yasuna E. Acute myopia associated with promethazine (compazine) therapy. *Am J Ophthalmol.* 1962;54:783-796.

21. Bard L. Transient myopia associated with prochlorperazine (phenergan) therapy: report of a case. *Am J Ophthalmol.* 1964;58:682-686.

22. Fraunfelder FW, Fraunfelder FT, Keates EU. Topiramate-associated acute, bilateral, secondary angle-closure glaucoma. *Ophthalmology.* 2004;111(1):109-111.

23. Birnbaum F, Leu P. Akute Myopisierung mit intraokularer Drucksreigerung bei Entgleisung eines juvenilen Diabete mellitus. *Klin Monatsbl Augenheilkd.* 1975;167:613-615.

24. Saari KM. Acute glaucoma in hemorrhagic fever with renal syndrome (nephropathia epidemica). *Am J Ophthalmol.* 1976;31:455-461.

Glaucoma After
Penetrating Keratoplasty

Mina B. Pantcheva, MD; Joel S. Schuman, MD, FACS;
Malik Y. Kahook, MD; and David L. Epstein, MD, MMM

A common form of glaucoma that is difficult to manage is one that occurs after penetrating keratoplasty (PKP).[1-3] Most often, the mechanism involves peripheral anterior synechiae (PAS) formation and represents a form of chronic angle-closure glaucoma. However, the chronic use of topical steroids is responsible for some cases of secondary open-angle glaucoma. This latter diagnosis, which is often unrecognized because the time of onset may be late and the steroid dosage low, should always be suspected in these patients. Attempts should be made to reduce or discontinue the topical steroids. intraocular pressure (IOP) may be substantially lower only a few days after steroids are totally discontinued, thus indicating an extreme sensitivity to these agents. It is important to note that increases in IOP place the corneal transplant at risk for rejection (Figure 37-1). One of the main risk factors for developing glaucoma post-PKP is the indication for surgery. Keratoconus is reported to have 1% incidence of induced glaucoma, whereas the incidence rises to 29% to 44% in patients undergoing surgery for aphakic bullous keratopathy.[2,4]

The mechanism of angle-closure glaucoma is not well understood in these patients (Table 37-1). Pupillary block can occur, and for this reason, peripheral iridectomy should be routinely performed at the time of surgery. However, cases are encountered in which surgical iridectomy was performed, but, in the postoperative period, the iris and iridectomy were observed to be adherent to the cornea and thus was nonfunctional. A transient wound leak must always be suspected. Some have questioned whether the iris may be more reactive after keratoplasty and whether iris swelling may lead to PAS formation and angle closure, especially if the iris is in contact with an intraocular lens haptic.[5] Eyes with corneal disease often do demonstrate inflammatory ocular

disease and the iris may thus be more "sticky." Alternatively, one of us (DLE) has questioned whether choroidal detachment may occur intraoperatively from ocular hypotension, which may develop more commonly than suspected, leading to rolling forward of the ciliary body and iris into the angle. A choroidal detachment postoperatively from a transient wound leak would have the same effect. In addition, choroidal detachment may result in forward lens movement similar to that seen after retinal detachment surgery, which may add a pupillary block component to the angle closure. Lens swelling, if it occurs, may also cause pupillary block.

If acute angle-closure glaucoma is observed, laser iridectomy can alleviate the glaucoma. In the case of a choroidal detachment, surgical drainage may be required.

More commonly, acute postoperative glaucoma is not observed in these patients, but several weeks to months after keratoplasty, elevated IOP due to angle-closure glaucoma is first detected. In some of these cases, earlier elevations of IOP may simply have been missed, but in others, hyposecretion, perhaps due to a choroidal detachment, may have masked the angle closure and delayed IOP elevation. It is only later after the choroidal detachment resolves, and aqueous humor production returns to normal, that elevated IOP is observed.

Unfortunately, most of these cases are complicated, and the factors that have led to the chronic angle-closure glaucoma are unclear. With regard to prevention, a peripheral iridectomy should be performed at the time of surgery and the period of ocular hypotony minimized. Sodium hyaluronate can be used to maintain the anterior chamber. However, this agent can cause substantial IOP elevation postoperatively[6] and should be removed from the anterior chamber at the conclusion of the operation. The anterior chamber should be

Kahook MY, Schuman JS, eds.
Chandler and Grant's Glaucoma, Fifth Edition (pp 347-350).
© 2013 SLACK Incorporated.

| TABLE 37-1. GLAUCOMA AFTER PENETRATING KERATOPLASTY ||
Cause	Comment
Open-angle glaucoma • Angle compression • Postoperative inflammatory products (pigment, blood, viscoelastics) • Steroids • Pre-existing glaucoma	Angle compression may be reduced with meticulous wound closure and by using a donor graft that is larger than the recipient bed; viscoelastics should always be thoroughly removed at end of procedure; chronic use of topical steroids should be considered a cause of elevated intraocular pressure.
Closed-angle glaucoma • Progressive angle closure • Pupillary block	Iris sutures at pupillary margin to tighten iris plane can be used to reduce incidence of late angle closure. All patients should have a patent iridectomy.

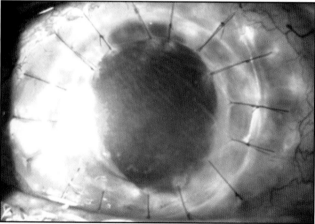

Figure 37-1. An eye with post-PKP glaucoma showing an edematous cornea and rejection of the donor tissue that coincided with high IOP.

well formed at the conclusion of surgery. Tightening the iris by direct suturing at the time of surgery may decrease the occurrence of angle closure.[7]

Experimental tight suturing close to the limbus in enucleated eyes can cause obstruction to outflow through an open-angle mechanism (not involving iris-trabecular apposition).[6,8,9] However, if this occurs in living eyes, it most likely is a short-lived phenomenon. Slightly oversized corneal grafts may decrease the occurrence of such a secondary open-angle glaucoma.[10-12] Laser trabeculoplasty may be effective for patients with open-angle glaucoma after penetrating keratoplasty.[13] Secondary pigmentary glaucoma after anterior segment surgery can also occur.[14]

In the last several years, many forms of endothelial keratoplasty have been developed. The techniques aim to replace the diseased corneal endothelium with donor corneal endothelium, Descemet's membrane, and a small amount of posterior stroma. The Descemet's stripping with endothelial keratoplasty (DSAEK) has several advantages over conventional PKP. The most impressive

is the rapid healing and early visual rehabilitation, but it also requires few, if any, corneal sutures. Another major advantage is that the structural integrity of the recipient eye is maintained throughout the surgery. However, it involves injecting air into the anterior chamber, which can lead to pupillary block glaucoma if the air bubble extends beyond the inferior pupillary border when the patient is upright.[15,16] PAS can be formed if pupillary block occurs. PAS may also be formed if air enters the posterior chamber during the procedure and remains behind the iris while the patient remains supine. Lee and colleagues[15] described a patient with pupillary block glaucoma and 6 patients with air in the posterior chamber leading to iridocorneal adhesions and increased IOP. The true incidence of glaucoma after DSAEK is not clearly known. It has been reported to be from zero to 18%.[17] Recently, Vajaranant and colleagues[18] reported a relatively high incidence of IOP elevation after DSAEK in 35% of patients with no prior glaucoma, 45% of patients with prior glaucoma, and 43% of patients with prior glaucoma with preexisting glaucoma surgery, but no adverse visual outcomes related to IOP elevation in any group.

Patients who have had prior large iridectomy are at increased risk of air passage through the iridectomy into the posterior chamber. Superior iridotomies and iridectomies can be particularly challenging in the setting of unicameral eye, as air escapes from the anterior chamber into the vitreous cavity.

The major long-term clinical glaucoma problem after PKP and DSAEK is chronic synechial angle closure. Medical therapy (Table 37-2) of this form of glaucoma is challenging because drugs that facilitate outflow, such as pilocarpine, are limited due to PAS formation. However, a trial of miotics is warranted because, in some cases, the PAS may be bridging over an otherwise functional trabecular meshwork to the cornea. Aqueous suppressants are useful. For surgical therapy, if PAS formation is recent, then, as discussed elsewhere, lysing

TABLE 37-2. MANAGEMENT OF GLAUCOMA AFTER PENETRATING KERATOPLASTY	
Treatment	**Comment**
Medical management • Beta-blockers • Adrenergic agonists • Miotics (direct and indirect acting) • Apraclonidine • Carbonic anhydrase inhibitors	Both direct- and indirect-acting miotics can be very effective after the early postoperative period if the angle is open; adrenergic agents may cause or worsen cystoid macular edema.
Laser therapy • Laser iridectomy • Laser trabeculoplasty • Laser gonioplasty	To prevent pupillary block, all patients should have a patent iridectomy; laser trabeculoplasty can be effective in patients with open angles. Laser gonioplasty should be reserved for patients with peripheral anterior synechaie of recent onset (less than 1 to 2 months).
Surgical therapy • Trabeculectomy with antimetabolites • Seton implantation • Cyclodestructive procedure	Tight flap with cautious suture lysis recommended to avoid flat chamber and graft injury, setons can be effective but may cause increased graft rejection; laser cyclodestructive procedures are useful in patients with poor potential visual acuity.

of synechiae should be contemplated by use of argon laser gonioplasty or surgically.[19-21] In long-standing cases with good central acuity, filtration surgery should be attempted initially, but special attention to the problem of flat anterior chamber is required due to the vulnerability of the recently transplanted cornea. Immediate or delayed suprachoroidal hemorrhage as a complication of filtration surgery may be more common in these eyes. Ciliodestructive procedures are effective means of IOP control,[22-26] but there is risk of macular edema in eyes with good acuity and risk of cataract formation in phakic eyes. Such treatment, however, is often the only effective means for pressure control. The use of glaucoma drainage devices can be effective but are accompanied by a high incidence of corneal graft rejection.[27,28]

REFERENCES

1. Karesh JW, Nirankari VS. Factors associated with glaucoma after penetrating keratoplasty. *Am J Ophthalmol*. 1983;96:160-164.
2. Foulks GN. Glaucoma associated with penetrating keratoplasty. *Ophthalmology*. 1987;94:871-874.
3. Simmons RB, Stern RA, Teekhasaenee C, et al. Elevated intraocular pressure following penetrating keratoplasty. *Trans Am Ophthalmol Soc*. 1989;87:79-91.
4. Kirkness CM, Ficker LA. Risk factors for the development of post-keratoplasty glaucoma. *Cornea*. 1992;11:427-432.
5. Chu MW, Font RL, Koch DD. Visual results and complications following posterior iris-fixated posterior chamber lenses at penetrating keratoplasty. *Ophthalmic Surg*. 1992;23:608-613.
6. Berson FG, Patterson MM, Epstein DL. Obstruction of aqueous outflow by sodium hyaluronate in enucleated human eyes. *Am J Ophthalmol*. 1983;95:668-672.
7. Cohen EJ, Kenyon KR, Dohlman CH. Iridoplasty for prevention of postkeratoplasty angle closure and glaucoma. *Ophthalmic Surg*. 1982;13:994-996.
8. Campbell DG, Grant WM. Unpublished data cited in Berson FG, Patterson MM, Epstein DL: Obstruction of aqueous outflow by sodium hyaluronate in enucleated human eyes. *Am J Ophthalmol*. 1983;95:668-672.
9. Zimmerman TJ, Krupin T, Grodski W, et al. The effect of suture depth on outflow facility in penetrating keratoplasty. *Arch Ophthalmol*. 1978;96:505-506.
10. Zimmerman T, Olson R, Waltman S, et al. Transplant size and elevated intraocular pressure postkeratoplasty. *Arch Ophthalmol*. 1978;96:2231-2233.
11. Bourne WM, Davison JA, O'Fallon WM. The effects of oversize donor buttons on postoperative intraocular pressure and corneal curvature in aphakic penetrating keratoplasty. *Ophthalmology*. 1982;89:242-246.
12. Heidemann DG, Sugar A, Meyer RF, et al. Oversized donor grafts in penetrating keratoplasty. A randomized trial. *Arch Ophthalmol*. 1985;103:1807-1811.
13. Van Meter WS, Allen RC, Waring GO, et al. Laser trabeculoplasty for glaucoma in aphakic and pseudophakic eyes after penetrating keratoplasty. *Arch Ophthalmol*. 1988;106:185-858.
14. Insler MS, Zatzkis SM. Pigment dispersion syndrome in pseudo-phakic corneal transplants. *Am J Ophthalmol*. 1986;102:762-765.
15. Lee JS, Desai NR, Schmidt GW, et al. Secondary angle closure caused by air migrating behind the pupil in Descemet stripping endothelial keratoplasty. *Cornea*. 2009;28:652-656.
16. Suh LH, Yoo SH, Deobhakta A, et al. Complications of Descemet's stripping with automated endothelial keratoplasty: survey of 118 eyes at one institute. *Ophthalmology*. 2008;115:1517-1524.
17. Bannit MR, Chopra V. Descemet's stripping with automated endothelial keratoplasty and glaucoma. *Curr Opin Ophthalmol*. 2010;21:144-149.

18. Vajaranant TS, Price MO, Price FW, et al. Visual acuity and intraocular pressure after Descemet's stripping endothelial keratoplasty in eyes with and without preexisting glaucoma. *Ophthalmology.* 2009;116:1644-1650.

19. Campbell DG, Vela A. Modern goniosynechialysis for the treatment of synechial angle-closure glaucoma. *Ophthalmology.* 1984;91:1052-1060.

20. Shingleton BJ, Chang MA, Bellows AR, et al. Surgical goniosynechialysis for angle-closure glaucoma. *Ophthalmology.* 1990;97:551-556.

21. Tanihara H, Nishiwaki K, Nagata M. Surgical results and complications of goniosynechialysis. *Graefes Arch Clin Exp Ophthalmol.* 1992;230:309-313.

22. West CE, Wood TO, Kaufman HE. Cyclocryotherapy for glaucoma pre or postpenetrating keratoplasty. *Am J Ophthalmol.* 1973;76:485-489.

23. Thoft RA, Gordon JM, Dohlman CH. Glaucoma following keratoplasty. *Trans Am Acad Ophthalmol Otolaryngol.* 1974;78:352-364.

24. Binder PS, Abel R Jr, Kaufman HE. Cyclocryotherapy for glaucoma after penetrating keratoplasty. *Am J Ophthalmol.* 1975;79:489-492.

25. Cohen EJ, Schwartz LW, Luskind RD, et al. Neodymium: YAG laser transscleral cyclophotocoagulation for glaucoma after penetrating keratoplasty. *Ophthalmic Surg.* 1989;20:713-716.

26. Wheatcroft S, Singh A, Casey T, et al. Treatment of glaucoma following penetrating keratoplasty with transscleral YAG cyclophotocoagulation. *Int Ophthalmol.* 1992;16:397-400.

27. McDonnell PJ, Robin JB, Schanzlin DJ, et al. Molteno implant for control of glaucoma in eyes after penetrating keratoplasty. *Ophthalmology.* 1988;95:364-369.

28. Sherwood MB, Smith MF, Driebe WT Jr, et al. Drainage tube implants in the treatment of glaucoma following penetrating keratoplasty. *Ophthalmic Surg.* 1993;24:185-189.

COMBINED MECHANISMS

38

Combined Open-Angle and Angle-Closure Glaucoma

Joel S. Schuman, MD, FACS and David L. Epstein, MD, MMM

The obstruction to aqueous outflow in primary open-angle glaucoma (POAG) is due mainly to abnormalities within or just beyond the trabecular meshwork, whereas in angle-closure glaucoma, the cause of obstruction to aqueous outflow is contact between the periphery of the iris and the corneoscleral trabecular meshwork, preventing access of aqueous humor to the normal aqueous outflow system. There is no reason why both conditions could not occur in the same eye. Because each has an independent basis, a certain number of coincidences of this sort can be expected. On the other hand, there are more cases of residual open-angle glaucoma after laser iridectomy than would be expected by chance.

There is also a hypothetical possibility that repeated episodes of angle closure could cause permanent damage to the corneoscleral trabecular meshwork even without formation of peripheral anterior synechiae (PAS) and that they could in this way induce a form of permanent open-angle glaucoma that would persist between episodes of angle closure and after angle-closure attacks were terminated by iridectomy. This has been mentioned previously (open-angle glaucoma due to chronic iris touch). As yet, however, we lack clear evidence for this mechanism.

Occasionally, patients present evidence of having both open-angle and angle-closure glaucomas. In some of these patients, one may be certain that only 2, 3, or 4 clock-hours of the angle are closed, but one may find an IOP of 40 mm Hg, and tonography may indicate an impairment of facility of outflow consistent with the intraocular pressure (IOP), but disproportionately more than the extent of angle closure. When the findings are this clear and definitive, the diagnosis is easy. One has to conclude that there is not enough angle closure to account for this amount of glaucoma.

In many other cases, it is much more difficult to establish whether one is dealing with pure angle-closure glaucoma or a combination of angle-closure with open-angle glaucoma. Difficulty in establishing a definite diagnosis of combined open-angle and angle-closure glaucoma, or distinguishing between open-angle and angle-closure glaucoma, is greatest when a question of chronic appositional angle closure is involved. The other varieties of angle closure seldom present a problem in this regard. For instance, in acute angle-closure glaucoma, when all the typical symptoms and signs are present, we are seldom confronted with glaucoma out of proportion to the extent of closure during an attack or out of proportion to any residual peripheral anterior synechiae after iridectomy is done. Also, in chronic synechial angle-closure glaucoma in which a considerable portion of the angle has gradually become closed by synechiae, it is uncommon to find glaucoma out of proportion to the extent of angle closure or residual glaucoma after iridectomy out of proportion to the extent of synechiae.

The greatest problem is encountered in eyes in which the angle is so narrow in a portion of the circumference that we think, but cannot be sure, that some of it is actually closed, while at the same time measurements of IOP and facility of outflow suggest that the glaucoma is more severe than would be expected from the conceivable extent of angle closure. When closure of only a portion of the circumference is in question, it may be very difficult to prove whether angle closure is actually taking place. If laser iridectomy is done in these cases, and the angle becomes widened so that we can rule out future episodes of angle closure, we may find that IOP and facility of outflow are not improved and that the open-angle glaucoma that is present requires continuing treatment. However, peripheral iridectomy in such cases

Kahook MY, Schuman JS, eds.
Chandler and Grant's Glaucoma, Fifth Edition (pp 353-355).
© 2013 SLACK Incorporated.

confers the real benefit of eliminating concern about future attacks of angle-closure glaucoma. The benefit/risk ratio of laser iridectomy is such that it is often used to eliminate any angle-closure component. However, it is important to realize that surgical iridectomy was also previously so used. The following case illustrates this situation.

CASE 38-1

A man, age 47 years with hypermetropia of 5 diopters (D), a history of hypermetropia in many relatives, and acute glaucoma in his hypermetropic grandfather, was referred to us because of extremely narrow angles in both eyes. Optic nerve heads and fields were normal.

We found applanation IOPs 26 to 30 mm Hg on different occasions and tonographic C value of 0.11 in both eyes. The anterior chambers were not excessively shallow axially (equivalent to 4 or 5 corneal thicknesses) but the irides were convex peripherally, and the angles appeared to be closed in one-third to one-half the circumference, very narrow in the remainder. Trial of 2% and later 4% pilocarpine in one eye did not improve the facility of outflow, but under this treatment, IOP was 20 mm Hg; the angle remained so narrow that it was impossible to say whether the angle in the superior quadrant opened; in the rest of the circumference, the angle was definitely open but extremely narrow.

The tonographic measurements indicated more obstruction to aqueous outflow than would be explained by closure of a small fraction of the angle, so we concluded that the glaucoma was mainly of the open-angle variety, but because of the extreme narrowness of the angle and probably closure of a portion, peripheral iridectomy was performed on each eye as a protective measure.

Several months after the iridectomies, when the eyes were entirely healed and quiet, examination without treatment showed applanation IOPs of 25 mm Hg and tonographic C values of 0.12 in both eyes, all essentially the same as before the operation. The angles were only slightly less narrow than before iridectomy, but now discernibly open superiorly and definitely open in the rest of the circumference. A view obtained through the surgical colobomas suggested that the persistent narrowness of the angles might be attributable to the position of the ciliary processes that were in contact with the back of the iris and appeared possibly to be holding the periphery of the iris forward. (Certainly, the persistent narrowness of these angles could not be due to accumulation of aqueous in the posterior chamber after iridectomy.)

We concluded that, as suspected preoperatively, the glaucoma in this patient was principally open-angle glaucoma, but that the peripheral iridectomies had been worthwhile. Although the iridectomies caused only slight widening of the angles in this case, that amount appeared critical. Furthermore, by eliminating all hindrance to the flow of aqueous from the posterior to anterior chamber, the iridectomies made safe and feasible the future use of all types of

miotics and epinephrine-like drugs that eventually may be needed for control of the open-angle glaucoma during the patient's expected 30 or 40 remaining years of life.

As a principle of treatment, when the angle is extremely narrow, and especially when it is certain that a portion of the angle can close when the eye is without treatment, but there is conclusive evidence of open-angle glaucoma with the facility of outflow persistently subnormal when the angle is open, either spontaneously or under miotics, there is justification for performing laser iridectomy to eliminate the pupillary block angle-closure element and to permit use of all types of medication for the open-angle glaucoma. In eyes having open-angle glaucoma with a very narrow angle that have developed acute angle-closure glaucoma, the status of the previously open-angle glaucoma is unchanged after iridectomy. The iridectomy is intended purely to prevent or relieve angle-closure glaucoma.

Eyes that have been under intensive treatment for open-angle glaucoma and have angles that are only moderately narrow, with full width of trabecular meshwork visible gonioscopically and not therefore threateningly narrow, and never having closed spontaneously, merit assessment by modified darkroom testing. In such testing, the patient is scanned with a ultrasound biomicroscopy under lightroom and darkroom conditions, and the relative state of the angle is assessed. A similar test can be done in a darkened examination room using slit-lamp gonioscopy. Should the angle close under dark conditions, the patient should undergo laser peripheral iridectomy.

Many of these issues have been discussed in previous chapters, especially in terms of the indication for laser iridectomy and the categories of residual open-angle glaucoma after iridectomy. The physiological principles of correlating the extent of angle closure with the IOP elevation have been discussed in other chapters. In addition to these considerations of open-angle glaucoma in eyes with angle closure, the reverse category of a superimposed angle-closure component to a basic open-angle glaucoma process needs to be considered and has been discussed in another chapter. In particular, the occurrence of a subsequent additional angle-closure component to an open-angle glaucoma due to pseudoexfoliation[1] needs to be kept in mind as it is not rare.

Patients with presumed POAG need periodic repeated gonioscopy and should always have gonioscopy when the IOP is elevated at a follow-up visit. In addition to identifying a superimposed angle-closure component, other causes such as occult inflammatory precipitates or new blood vessels need to be ruled out. When a patient with POAG seems to demonstrate some functional angle closure (usually 4 clock-hours or more) but there is no PAS formation on indentation gonioscopy, and thus there is some uncertainty whether there is truly a functional appositional angle-closure component or whether the angle is narrow but still functionally open, the benefit/risk considerations are such that after fully informing the patient about these considerations as well as one's diagnostic uncertainty (and what the clinician would do if it were his or her eye), it is usually wisest to proceed with laser iridectomy. This is because the risk of not treating a possible angle-closure glaucoma component is greater than the risk of the procedure.

Nevertheless, the clinician and the patient need to be fully prepared for an IOP spike that may be substantial if, for example, the glaucoma is entirely due to an open-angle pseudoexfoliation mechanism rather than some functional angle-closure component. In this situation, pigment and other iris debris from the iridectomy and inflammation may provide further short-term and possibly long-term insult to trabecular meshwork function. Regardless, the iridectomy may be indicated for prophylactic purposes, but the patient and clinician need to know ahead of time that the iridectomy will not improve the IOP in the short-term and may cause a substantial acute IOP spike.

Finally, chronic silent angle closure may masquerade as open-angle glaucoma, given the absence of symptoms.

The usual aqueous suppressant therapy for such presumed open-angle glaucoma, by decreasing the vectors acting on the posterior iris surface, may somewhat deepen the angle perpetuating the misdiagnosis. Such an action needs to be evaluated in any patient suspected of having combined mechanism glaucoma.

REFERENCE

1. Gross FJ, Tingey D, Epstein DL. Increased prevalence of occludable angles and angle-closure glaucoma in patients with pseudoexfoliation. *Am J Ophthalmol.* 1993;117:333-336.

Glaucoma in the Pseudophakic and Aphakic Eye

Ian P. Conner, MD, PhD; Joel S. Schuman, MD, FACS; and David L. Epstein, MD, MMM

A major revolution has occurred in the techniques of cataract surgery in the past 30 years, with a transition from intracapsular to extracapsular surgery (including phaco-emulsification) with smaller and smaller incisions. Many of the former, seemingly unique aspects of glaucoma in aphakia now in hindsight, clearly relate to the larger wounds and the removal of the mechanical support structure of the crystalline lens that occurred in intracapsular cataract surgery. Although intracapsular cataract surgery is rarely performed today, there are still aphakic eyes that face glaucoma surgery where some of the former issues still have relevance.

The major issue in pseudophakic and aphakic eyes is the guarded prognosis for filtration surgery because of previous cataract surgery with conjunctival manipulation. Even clear corneal cataract surgery increases the risk of filtration surgery failure. The use of antimetabolites has improved the surgical prognosis for such eyes and is discussed in Chapter 59. If the conjunctiva is mobile, then filtration surgery with antimetabolites can and should be performed as in phakic eyes. Sometimes, if there is scarring of the conjunctiva only at the limbus, the scleral flap dissection can be used to carry the surgical site anterior to the limbus underneath this external scarring, or a fornix-based conjunctival flap technique can be used. Subconjunctival fibrosis from previous cataract surgery is not simply a technical barrier to an adequate surgical procedure, but is also a sign indicating the likelihood of exuberant postfiltration wound healing with a higher risk of bleb failure (the conjunctiva always remembers). In cases in which the conjunctiva is severely scarred, one may consider using a glaucoma drainage device, which may be placed more posteriorly away from the scar tissue. In the past, trabeculectomy was occasionally performed in the inferior quadrants in cases of significant superior scarring, but this is rarely performed today due to concern for serious postoperative complications, including endophthalmitis.[1] With careful technique, tube shunt surgery can be used successfully in inferior quadrant locations. In addition, cyclodestructive procedures (see Chapter 56) are other surgical options in these challenging cases (Table 39-1).

THE POSTOPERATIVE EYE THAT IS APHAKIC

With intracapsular surgery, a large wound was employed. Wound closure was frequently inadequate in these patients, and there was significant potential for wound leaks to occur that would allow the vitreous to displace anteriorly, potentially initiating pupillary block or malignant glaucoma-type conditions (see Chapter 29). There were many descriptive terms used to explain a postoperative flat anterior chamber, but it often was not fully appreciated how often a wound leak, albeit transient, may have precipitated the condition. In addition, alpha-chymotrypsin was instilled into the eye to disrupt the zonules and allow intracapsular delivery of the crystalline lens, but the zonular fragments[2-4] could obstruct the trabecular meshwork (TM) and produce a temporary but substantial postoperative glaucoma with intraocular pressure (IOP) commonly above 50 mm Hg.[5] It is amazing, in retrospect, how late the understanding of this postoperative enzyme glaucoma was achieved, and especially the potential for acute posterior pole vascular events (eg, acute ischemic optic neuropathy) or wound leaks as a result of this severe IOP elevation. In the intracapsular surgery era, it was common practice to delay postoperative IOP measurement for several days because of concerns about infection.

Kahook MY, Schuman JS, eds.
Chandler and Grant's Glaucoma, Fifth Edition (pp 357-366).
© 2013 SLACK Incorporated.

TABLE 39-1. SURGICAL MANAGEMENT FOR GLAUCOMA IN PSEUDOPHAKIA (APHAKIA)		
Trabeculectomy With Antimetabolites	Seton (Tube Shunt)	Laser Cyclophotocoagulation
Mobile conjunctiva	Scarred conjunctiva	Scarred conjunctiva
Good visual potential (20/100 or better) or only eye	Visual potential fair to good (20/200 or better)	Fair to poor visual potential (20/200 or worse)
Little or no ocular inflammation or active neovascularization	Active ocular inflammation or neovascularization	Not a candidate for more invasive procedure

In retrospect, it seems obvious that the corneal edema commonly observed and the usual postoperative pain that the patient experienced was likely due to high levels of IOP.

When anterior chamber lens implant techniques were added to intracapsular surgery, the acute postoperative open-angle glaucoma was exaggerated by the use of viscoelastic material that was placed into the anterior chamber. Viscoelastic was not removed because of the danger of vitreous loss in these aphakic eyes. As we now know, thorough irrigation of viscoelastic from the anterior chamber may reduce the incidence and severity of postoperative acute IOP elevation, although in some cases the material is already present in the outflow pathway and can be difficult, if not impossible, to completely wash out.[6]

Intracapsular cataract surgery is now rarely if ever performed (except perhaps for partially dislocated crystalline lenses or in the Third World). The following description is included for those rare occasions, but also for general orientation, historical importance, and context.

Open-Angle Glaucoma Due to Immediate Postoperative Reaction After Intracapsular Cataract Extraction

In the immediate postoperative period after cataract extraction, the IOP should be measured routinely. It is not uncommon for there to be substantial IOP elevation.[5] The cornea may be deceptively clear or show only trace edema, despite high IOP. The anterior chamber maintains normal aphakic depth throughout, and the angle remains open.

Although IOP will return to normal usually in several days, these higher levels of pressure should be treated to prevent acute damage. Instances of optic atrophy have been observed from this temporary glaucoma. Aqueous suppressants are effective in lowering IOP in this condition,[5] but osmotic therapy may also be required. The glaucoma has sometimes been blamed on postoperative iritis, but with little evidence. When alpha-chymotrypsin was introduced as an aid to intracapsular extraction, the incidence of acute, transitory, postoperative secondary open-angle glaucoma increased. In a careful study of a large series of cases, Kirsch[7] found the incidence of transitory postoperative glaucoma to

be much higher in eyes in which the enzyme was used than in a control series without the enzyme.

We have the clinical impression that the greater the volume of enzyme solution used, the greater the incidence of glaucoma and the higher the IOP.

The tendency for cataract surgeons to use a large number of interrupted sutures in closing the wound resulted in an increased number of cases of elevated IOP in the immediate postoperative period. In some cases, the IOP reached quite high levels—50 to 70 mm Hg. IOP usually returned to normal within a few days. Formerly, when fewer sutures were used, these considerable elevations of IOP were less common. Perhaps a small wound leak commonly behaved as a safety valve, whereas numerous tight sutures prevented this inadvertent accessory aqueous outflow.

Clinical and experimental investigations by D. G. Campbell (personal communication, 1977). have shown that, in patients who had intracapsular cataract extraction with alpha-chymotrypsin and multiple sutures, the IOP was usually at its maximum on the day of the operation and gradually fell thereafter. Campbell found that this might be explained by a mechanism that he demonstrated in enucleated normal human eyes. In these eyes, when the facility of aqueous outflow was measured by perfusion before and after limbal sutures were inserted and were tied tightly as in cataract operations, the aqueous outflow was significantly obstructed.[8] This pathologic obstruction was shown to be related to compression of limbal tissues and to gross distortion of the aqueous outflow system by the sutures. The distortion of the tissues and the obstruction to outflow were readily reversible by loosening the sutures. These effects have been confirmed by others.[6,9] Kirsch and colleagues[10] performed gonioscopy immediately after cataract surgery and described seeing a ridge formed inside the eye; however, this was unrelated to sutures and appears to be different from Campbell's suture-induced effect.

In patients, the postoperative glaucoma that may be attributable to this mechanism generally subsided in a few days, presumably because the sutures spontaneously loosened and the distortion of the tissues became less.

Another factor that can cause impairment of outflow facility and a postoperative elevation of IOP is the use of viscoelastics, such as sodium hyaluronate, during cataract

GLAUCOMA SURGERY IN PSEUDOPHAKIA AND
APHAKIA: A HISTORICAL PERSPECTIVE

R. Rand Allingham, MD

Glaucoma surgery is frequently required in pseudophakic and, less common today, aphakic patients. There are many options available to the surgeon, and the question often arises as to how to decide which procedure to undertake. The major surgical choices include trabeculectomy with antimetabolites, glaucoma drainage device implantation (ie, tube-shunt surgery), or laser cyclophotocoagulation. The primary determinants I use in selecting 1 procedure are the overall status of the patient, visual status, and ocular condition.

STATUS OF THE PATIENT

For patients with frail health, or who for whatever reason are unable to tolerate an incisional procedure but require IOP reduction, I use laser cyclophotocoagulation (see Chapter 56).

VISUAL STATUS

In my experience, filters and glaucoma drainage device implantation are less likely to cause postoperative vision loss than cyclodestructive procedures, which are often associated with this complication. If actual or potential visual acuity is better than 20/200 and the visual field is functional, I feel that a fistulizing procedure is indicated. If the visual acuity is worse than 20/200, I do laser cyclophotocoagulation. An exception is the patient with only 1 functional eye. In these patients, if vision is ambulatory, I favor performing a fistulizing procedure before considering cyclodestruction.

CONDITION OF THE EYE

Where a fistulizing procedure is contemplated and the anterior chamber is deep with mobile conjunctiva in a superior quadrant (usually the case in patients who have had a phacoemulsification procedure), I will perform a trabeculectomy with mitomycin C (see Chapter 59). If the conjunctiva is scarred and immobile, then I will implant a glaucoma drainage device (see Chapter 62).

If the anterior chamber is shallow and there is insufficient room to insert a tube, I favor performing a trabeculectomy with antimetabolites. If the patient has had a complete vitrectomy (including meticulous amputation of the vitreous base), then the tube of the glaucoma drainage device can be inserted through the pars plana, which can minimize corneal injury.

If vitreous is present in the anterior chamber, which is a particular problem in aphakic patients, a limited (but thorough) anterior vitrectomy must be performed prior to a trabeculectomy or glaucoma drainage device implantation in order to prevent occlusion of the sclerotomy or tube, respectively.

For trabeculectomies in these patients, I use mitomycin C 0.3 mg/mL for 3 to 5 minutes. Additionally, adjunctive 5-fluorouracil (3 to 7 injections) can be used postoperatively if there are signs of bleb failure. If an implant is required, I prefer either valved glaucoma drainage devices (eg, Ahmed [New World Medical, Rancho Cucamonga, CA]) or nonvalved glaucoma drainage devices with the use of a stent or ligature, in order to prevent postoperative hypotony in these patients, who are at relatively higher risk for suprachoroidal hemorrhage (due to previous intraocular surgery).

surgery.[6] Experimentally, a severe obstruction to outflow in enucleated human eyes occurs, and this is additive to the effects of limbal suture compression.[6] Curiously, in simulated surgical maneuvers with hyaluronate, it proved difficult to alleviate the impairment of outflow by irrigation of the anterior chamber. Clinically, severe postoperative glaucoma, presumably due to sodium hyaluronate, has been observed, sometimes persisting for several days.

Especially in patients with preexisting glaucoma and optic nerve damage, acute postoperative IOP elevations can be dangerous and, at times, difficult to treat.

THE POSTOPERATIVE PSEUDOPHAKIC EYE

With a historical background concerning intracapsular cataract surgery, one should not be surprised to learn that postoperative open-angle glaucoma also occurs after modern extracapsular cataract surgery, including phacoemulsification (Table 39-2). In extracapsular surgery, such severe IOP elevation is much less common, likely owing to several factors: omission of alpha-chymotrypsin, the smaller size wound, and the more efficient removal of ophthalmic viscoelastic material with irrigating/aspirating devices. However, substantial residual cortical material can impair outflow facility (lens-particle glaucoma) acutely (see Chapter 47). It is for this reason that IOP also must be carefully monitored after yttrium-aluminum-garnet (YAG) capsulotomy, especially in patients with known glaucoma and/or decreased outflow facility.

Although postoperative glaucoma after extracapsular surgery may not be as severe or sustained as that after intracapsular surgery, it still requires attention, especially in patients with glaucomatous optic nerve cupping and field loss. Similar to that described above, IOP may be substantially elevated after extracapsular cataract extraction for the first several hours after surgery, although it is not routinely measured in this time period.

The mechanism for open-angle glaucoma after extracapsular surgery most likely involves retained viscoelastic in the eye despite intraoperative irrigation, crystalline lens fragments that may have entered the outflow pathway intraoperatively, and wound compression and inflammation. Postoperative hyphema, although uncommon in phacoemulsification, can also contribute to the IOP elevation because the red blood cells are cleared through the trabecular outflow pathway[11] and can temporarily obstruct it.

Especially in patients with susceptible optic nerves, the postoperative IOP must be carefully monitored with judicious use of preventative antiglaucoma therapy. In patients with such susceptible nerves and borderline IOP control, consideration should be given to performing a combined cataract extraction/filtration procedure (see Chapter 61) not only to establish better long-term IOP control, but also to blunt this potentially damaging early postoperative IOP spike.

TABLE 39-2. INTRAOCULAR PRESSURE ELEVATION FOLLOWING CATARACT SURGERY	
Cause	**Comment**
Early IOP elevation (first 24 to 48 hours) Inflammatory debris (cells, pigment, or blood) Lens products Viscoelastic Zonular fragments (intracapsular cataract extraction with alpha chymotrypsin) Suprachoroidal hemorrhage Pupillary block	Lens products, blood, and viscoelastics should always be completely removed from the anterior chamber at the end of the procedure, especially in patients with preexisting IOP elevation. Postoperative hypotony, vitrectomized patients, and high myopia increase risk of intra- and postoperative suprachoroidal hemorrhage.
Midterm IOP elevation (2 to 30 days) Pupillary block (intraocular lens or vitreous) Malignant glaucoma Steroid-induced	Pupillary block is uncommon after extracapsular cataract extraction with posterior chamber Intraocular lens but can occur (all eyes with an anterior chamber Intraocular lens require an iridectomy); axial shallowing that occurs with an elevated IOP is malignant glaucoma until proven otherwise. Topical steroids are a common and overlooked cause of postoperative elevated IOP.
Late onset Open-angle glaucoma Synechial angle closure Pupillary block glaucoma (intraocular lens or vitreous)	Whether late-onset open-angle glaucoma is secondary to surgery or is a manifestation of a preexisting process is often not known; however, treatment is the same.

The choice of added antiglaucoma therapy depends on the patient's existing regimen. Beta-blockers and/or alpha-agonists are commonly given at the end of surgery (if there is no contraindication), and some clinicians routinely employ a single administration of (often intravenous) carbonic anhydrase inhibitors. Except for the very small risk of blood dyscrasia in patients without a known systemic contraindication, such one-time use of carbonic anhydrase therapy is usually well tolerated. Miotics should be used sparingly because of the usual postoperative inflammatory reaction, and epinephrine-like compounds, used in the past, may cause cystoid macular edema as well as unwanted vascular effects in the acute postoperative eye.

It is important to measure the IOP, especially in patients at an increased risk, perhaps even several hours after surgery, but certainly no later than the next day.

DIFFERENTIAL DIAGNOSIS OF ACUTE POSTOPERATIVE GLAUCOMA IN THE PSEUDOPHAKIC EYE

The key question is whether the mechanism of the postoperative glaucoma involves an open-angle or an angle-closure basis. This can usually be determined from the slit-lamp examination, evaluating the anterior chamber depth and configuration of the iris. The clinician should not hesitate to gently perform gonioscopy on the eye and examine the angle. It is fundamental to know whether one is dealing with angle-closure or open-angle process. In fact, one of the great lessons learned from the previous era of intracapsular cataract surgery and anterior chamber intraocular lenses was how common it was for the clinician to miss a treatable form of angle closure (due to pupillary block) on the basis of the slit-lamp examination alone.[12] Not uncommonly, such unsuspected pupillary block had a delayed onset. Unanticipated pupillary block has also been reported with use of posterior chamber intraocular lenses.[13]

If one is dealing with an open-angle postoperative glaucoma in the pseudophakic eye, then medical antiglaucoma therapy is used as above. The most common mechanism relates to retained viscoelastic material if the IOP is severely elevated and sustained. Such a viscoelastic-induced secondary open-angle glaucoma is usually self-limited over 4 to 5 days (although the now discontinued viscoelastic Orculon [4% polyacrylamide] could potentially cause elevated IOP to persist indefinitely[14,15]). Newer, more cohesive viscoelastics can also lead to longer term spikes in IOP commonly related to inadequate intraoperative removal of these materials. Rarely, it may be necessary to take the patient back to the operating room and repeat irrigation of the anterior chamber. Anterior chamber washout could also be employed for a postoperative hyphema that is judged to be responsible for the IOP elevation. Of course, if a combined cataract/filtering surgery was performed, then suture lysis could be performed in the face of high postoperative IOP. However, in an additional 4 or 5 days, the temporary added obstruction to outflow from the viscoelastic material will have spontaneously cleared (by the normal action of the TM), and therefore, one does not want to have produced overfiltration by creating too loose a flap through which the much less viscous aqueous humor is leaving the eye.

Sometimes, if a paracentesis was performed at the time of surgery, the site can be gently manipulated at the slit-lamp postoperatively to temporarily lower the IOP, although one should avoid substantially shallowing the anterior chamber, as this could produce other problems such as peripheral anterior synechiae (PAS). In the best-case scenario, a glob of cohesive viscoelastic material can occasionally be observed to exit the anterior chamber through the paracentesis with this maneuver. Otherwise, postoperative manipulation of the paracentesis site is commonly effective only in lowering the IOP for a few hours, so if the ocular hypertension recurs, then probably other choices for IOP lowering should be employed. (Experimentally, such viscoelastic-induced secondary open-angle glaucoma can be cured by placing hyaluronidase into the anterior chamber.[6] Unfortunately, such an orphan drug of very pure hyaluronidase for human use has not yet been developed.)

As a general rule, intraocular retention of a dispersive viscoelastic (eg, Viscoat [Alcon, Fort Worth, TX]) is more likely to result in a temporary, self-limited rise in IOP postoperatively, while retention of a more cohesive viscoelastic (eg, Healon) is more likely to require anterior chamber washout maneuvers in order to normalize IOP. Of course, meticulous removal of all viscoelastic material at the end of the extracapsular or phacoemulsification procedure is the best technique for avoiding this issue entirely.

If the angle is closed, then the most likely diagnosis in the postoperative period is pupillary block. This has been discussed in Chapters 22 and 23, but the typical findings are a normal axial depth but shallow peripheral depth with a ballooning forward, or convex appearance, of the iris. Residual cortical material that has fluffed up behind the iris or capsular fragments may produce postoperative pupillary block. Inflammatory adhesions postoperatively may do likewise. The treatment is to either dilate the pupil or place a laser iridotomy.

It is routine now not to place a surgical peripheral iridectomy at the time of cataract surgery. However, one of us (DLE) still believes that glaucomatous eyes, even with routine primary open-angle glaucoma, are higher risk sick eyes and advocates the routine placement of a surgical peripheral iridectomy at the time of cataract surgery. The concept of possible bad things hypothesized to happen when one touches the iris during the surgery has achieved unsubstantiated popularity. On the occasion that one sees these postoperative eyes with preexisting open-angle glaucoma, which now have developed a superimposed angle closure with the severe complications that can ensue, one wishes that all such eyes had received routine surgical peripheral iridectomy at the time of cataract surgery. Overall, one of us (DLE) truly believes that the benefit of surgical peripheral iridectomy outweighs the risk (mainly of transient postoperative hyphema) to justify its routine use in all glaucoma eyes. Especially when eyes have been on previous miotic therapy, there is both the potential for more substantial postoperative inflammation that can lead to pupillary block (most clinicians will perform an iridectomy if a patient has a history of previous uveitis), and there is also greater potential for there to be residual cortical material (due to submaximal pupillary dilation) that also could lead to pupillary block. All patients who have an anterior chamber intraocular lens require an iridectomy or iridotomy.

Angle-closure glaucoma postoperatively that persists despite a patent laser iridotomy is not pupillary block and must be further investigated to determine the true cause and optimal subsequent course of treatment. In brief, the differential diagnosis involves choroidal hemorrhage or effusion, and secondarily, the diagnosis is malignant glaucoma until proven otherwise. A careful slit-lamp examination along with a skilled B-scan should be sufficient to determine the nature of the postoperative angle closure without pupillary block.

Primary Open-Angle Glaucoma and the Pseudophakic Eye

In the past, some clinicians felt that (intracapsular) cataract surgery could improve long-term IOP control.[16,17] There was considerable controversy about this, and interestingly there have been swings of opinion.

The following is what we judge to represent current clinical information about the effect of extracapsular cataract surgery alone on the course of open-angle glaucoma, but this is being continuously evaluated. In the immediate postoperative period,[18,19] there can be instances of acute worsening of the open-angle glaucoma (Table 39-2) from a few days to weeks that should lead to consideration of combined cataract and fistulizing surgery being performed. Beginning several months after cataract surgery (when routine corticosteroids have been stopped), there is the strong clinical impression of some beneficial effect on IOP control in some patients,[20,21] but unfortunately not all. Because this effect of cataract surgery on IOP is not predictable ahead of time, cataract surgery alone should not generally be employed as a strategy for patients with borderline IOP control, and yet some patients do seem to benefit. Classically, it has been felt that at this intermediate time period, the possible beneficial effect was due to hyposecretion of aqueous humor in the continuing postoperative period. However, this mechanism has not been adequately confirmed. Another hypothesis involves a stress response as part of usual postoperative inflammation that may clear debris from the outflow pathway, as has been proposed to occur following the "inflammation" that accompanies laser trabeculoplasty.[22,23] In fact, such an occurrence might explain the generally poorer response of pseudophakic and aphakic eyes to laser trabeculoplasty in that they have already participated in such a TM inflammatory response.

Historically, it has been felt that in the long term (after a year) the open-angle glaucoma returns to baseline with no residual beneficial effect. In fact, the long-term beneficial effect that was reported by some in the intracapsular era was likely due to continued occult filtration that was probably initiated because of a wound that was not tightly sutured. However, the final word may not have been spoken in this regard, especially in light of numerous more recent publications demonstrating modest sustained IOP lowering after phacoemulsification.[21] Unfortunately, more work is needed to better understand the mechanism, magnitude, and duration of this effect. Given the common coexistence of cataract and glaucoma, it nonetheless seems clear that cataract extraction at least plays a role in the management of IOP in glaucoma patients.

Patients with open-angle glaucoma who are pseudophakic can be treated with the usual antiglaucoma medications, with the exception that epinephrine-like compounds should be avoided in both the pseudophakic as well as aphakic eye in order to avoid the potentiation of cystoid macular edema. Fortunately, these agents are uncommonly used today. Miotics can play an important role in pseudophakic eyes but require proper attention to the retina because of the slightly increased risk of retinal detachment in these eyes. Indeed, miotics are usually well tolerated visually by the pseudophakic patient, and weak concentrations of strong miotics, such as echothiophate iodide (Phospholine Iodide) are often remarkably effective. Both echothiophate and pilocarpine gel also offer the advantage of infrequent dosing and are usually very patient-friendly.

Eyes with pseudoexfoliation have a tendency toward earlier cataract formation,[24] and the clinician should be alert to possible previously undiagnosed pseudoexfoliation in pseudophakic eyes, especially because pseudoexfoliation eyes also have some tendency for rapid worsening of glaucoma control. (Removing the cataract does not by itself improve the exfoliation glaucoma; the crystalline lens capsule is just one source for the abnormal exfoliation material.) In the pseudophakic eye with an absent anterior lens capsule, the light-gray amorphous exfoliation material may still be seen on the pupillary border, the posterior surface of the iris, the ciliary processes, the zonules, and the anterior capsular remnants.

When considering cataract surgery in the pre-phacoemulsification era on a patient with currently well-controlled POAG, it was prudent to save some of the superior conjunctiva (eg, in the superonasal quadrant) for possible future filtration surgery and, therefore, to perform the cataract surgery more temporally. With the dominance of phacoemulsification and the clear cornea approach, this is much less of a concern.

Glaucoma Due to Peripheral Anterior Synechiae in Pseudophakic Eyes

Gonioscopy should be routinely performed on all eyes with open-angle glaucoma several months after cataract surgery (if not sooner in response to acute problems) to establish a new baseline. An unpleasant surprise is sometimes experienced when one views the presence of new PAS and thus loss of some of the angle circumference for outflow in a situation where the trabecular outflow process was already abnormal due to POAG with a previous open angle. Such PAS formation may result from an undetected transient wound leak or pupillary block, or may be a result of inflammation. Sometimes, residual lens cortex will fluff up postoperatively in one area and mechanically force the iris into the angle (without pupillary block) and result in synechiae formation. An anteriorly displaced intraocular lens haptic may do the same.[25] After a combined cataract/filter operation where there is overfiltration and a transient shallow chamber, there may also be resulting formation of PAS. This is much more common after (combined) cataract surgery than after filtration surgery alone, presumably because of the greater amount of usual postoperative inflammation that seals the iris to the apposed TM.

If extensive formation of PAS is observed, then consideration should be given to laser iridogonioplasty. Recently formed PAS can sometimes be pulled from the angle using this technique. Unfortunately, such PAS are often tightly cemented in the angle and not able to be broken.

Sometimes, PAS formation may seem extensive but the IOP, and especially the response to outflow drugs, such as miotics, is normal. In such cases of normal or supranormal outflow, one wants to be certain that one is not dealing with a rare inadvertent cyclodialysis cleft that was produced at the time of surgery (although if the IOP is controlled and not hypotonous, antiglaucoma therapy should just be continued; cyclodialysis was at one time a very useful surgical procedure for glaucoma but was unfortunately unpredictable). More likely now, with controlled clear-corneal incisions, one must be certain that the low IOP following initiation of miotic therapy is not due to a retinal detachment. However, it is also possible that the angle synechiae are actually bridging the TM to the peripheral cornea at

Schwalbe's line and that there is functional underlying TM. With shallow anterior chambers due to overfiltration (and usually quiet eyes), it is not rare for such bridging synechiae to occur.

Nevertheless, it is a cause for great concern when a patient with open-angle glaucoma, especially one with marginal control, now develops a superimposed chronic angle-closure component. Unobserved, transient pupillary block[12,13] in the postoperative period may have been the cause of occult PAS.

APHAKIC PUPILLARY BLOCK

Aphakic pupillary block is rarely seen now except in previously aphakic eyes undergoing subsequent additional surgery. Chandler and Grant offer a classic description of the clinical findings, which should be treated with a laser iridotomy:

Among the signs of pupillary block in aphakia, one occasionally observes iris bombé, but what one usually finds is overall shallowing of the anterior chamber or complete flatness, with IOP elevated. If the anterior chamber is shallow or flat in an aphakic eye and the IOP is elevated, even if only slightly, one must consider this to be positive evidence of pupillary block. If the anterior chamber is shallow or flat in association with separation of the ciliary body or choroid, IOP is almost invariably very low. (We have seen only 1 or 2 cases with choroidal separation and flat anterior chamber in which IOP was moderately elevated, among the hundreds of cases in which IOP was very low.) Less commonly, instead of uniform shallowing or absence of the anterior chamber, one finds unevenness in its depth. The anterior chamber may be normally deep in one area, shallow in another. Unevenness of depth of the anterior chamber is more common after extracapsular extraction, because there is generally more postoperative reaction than after intracapsular extraction. If there has been an unusual degree of postoperative inflammation, an unevenness in depth of the anterior chamber may sometimes be seen even after intracapsular extraction. The reason for the unevenness in depth of the anterior chamber is that there is an inflammatory membrane on the posterior surface of the iris in the area of deep anterior chamber, which prevents the iris from bowing forward. In the area where the iris bows forward, there is no inflammatory membrane behind it. The unevenness in depth of the anterior chamber is particularly common in pupillary block in children after discission or lens extraction. We know of no cause other than pupillary block for such unevenness in depth of the anterior chamber in aphakic eyes with elevated IOP.

After a round-pupil intracapsular extraction with a peripheral opening or openings in the iris, these openings may become closed by adhesion to the wound, by filling with blood or fibrin, or by adhesion to the hyaloid, after which pupillary block may develop. In such cases, the hyaloid membrane may herniate further and further through the round pupil until it eventually reaches the cornea (and rarely causes edema). The anterior chamber itself may remain at normal or almost-normal depth for a period, but the hyaloid eventually reaches the cornea. If the block is not relieved, the anterior chamber finally becomes shallow, at least in the periphery, and the angle closes.

OPEN-ANGLE GLAUCOMA DUE TO VITREOUS HUMOR FILLING THE ANTERIOR CHAMBER

In certain aphakic eyes, glaucoma is apparently due to vitreous humor completely filling the anterior chamber and blocking the corneoscleral meshwork itself.[26-28] Evidence for this mechanism has been both clinical and experimental. In the laboratory, vitreous humor introduced to fill the anterior chamber of an enucleated normal human eye clearly obstructs aqueous outflow, and this obstruction is quickly eliminated by addition of hyaluronidase.[29] The clinical situation may develop within a few weeks after cataract operation, but may be delayed for several months. It may be initiated, at least in some cases, by an extensive posterior vitreous separation, so that the remaining vitreous body tends to move forward. One sees in such cases that the angle is open. On slit-lamp and gonioscopic examination, the vitreous appears to fill the entire anterior chamber.

IOP is sometimes lowered by miotic treatment, but in other cases it is made higher. Mydriatic treatment is usually more effective. If the pupil is kept dilated, in most cases, the IOP gradually falls and vitreous eventually withdraws from the angle of the anterior chamber. This form of glaucoma appears to be self-limited and usually does not require surgical treatment. Aqueous humor suppressants are used during the period of elevated IOP. If this does not suffice, peripheral iridectomy and evacuation of vitreous from the anterior chamber should cure the condition.

In making a diagnosis, it is easy to be certain by gonioscopy that the angle is open. With slit-lamp examination, one must determine if the vitreous humor extends into the angle. However, clinically, it is almost impossible to be certain that it reaches the TM, and the diagnosis must be partially presumptive.

In 1963, Dr. Grant[26] collected 4 cases of this condition, but since then, we have only suspected it in 1 or 2 additional cases.[26] It must be an extremely rare condition.

EPITHELIALIZATION OF THE ANTERIOR CHAMBER

Diagnosis

After cataract extraction, the eye occasionally remains injected and irritable with photophobia and discomfort. One commonly sees cells in the aqueous. If there is little or no response to local steroid and cycloplegic treatment following cataract extraction, then this should lead to a suspicion of epithelial downgrowth. (Also, entities such as *Propionibacterium acnes* endophthalmitis[30-32] need to be considered.) One may see a delicate membrane on the back of the cornea advancing from the limbal area of the wound, through which it has invaded the anterior chamber (Figure 39-1). Characteristically, the advancing edge appears slightly thickened. This membrane sometimes extends onto the iris or in aphakic eyes onto the hyaloid membrane. If it extends onto the hyaloid membrane, there are often smooth-edged holes or oval windows in the membrane. These are very suggestive that the membrane is epithelial because one does not expect to see the same type of hole in an ordinary inflammatory membrane.

Because of the sheer number of procedures performed, epithelial membranes most frequently occur after cataract extraction but have also been seen after perforating injuries in which the crystalline lens has been damaged or lost, in children as well as in adults. The most significant risk factor for epithelial downgrowth is instability of the cataract wound in the postoperative period, especially when involving iris incarceration.

In epithelialization of the anterior chamber, if there is an open fistula in the wound at the site of epithelial downgrowth, the IOP may be low. When there is a fistula through the wound and the eye is soft, any evidence of a membrane on the back of the cornea or on the iris, however slight, nearly always indicates epithelialization.

If there is no fistula, IOP may be normal or elevated. When eyes are lost as a result of epithelialization of the anterior chamber, in the majority of cases, it is because the eyes become blind and painful from glaucoma. It appears that the mechanism of this severe glaucoma is usually pupillary block by the epithelial membrane, leading to closure of the angle and high IOP. However, in some cases of glaucoma, an epithelial membrane has been described in the angle, presumably blocking the escape of aqueous humor from the angle.[33] With the use of more extensive anterior segment reconstructive procedures to treat this condition, this latter mechanism for secondary glaucoma is being observed more commonly.

Gonioscopically, if one can see ciliary processes through an iridotomy or iridectomy, the processes commonly may be seen to be enveloped by a delicate, gray cocoon of epithelium, which is diagnostically helpful.

When the other signs and symptoms suggestive of epithelialization of the anterior chamber are present, even if no membrane is seen on cornea, iris, or hyaloid, it is appropriate to aspirate aqueous humor from the anterior chamber and examine the cellular material thus obtained. This may reveal epithelial cells and thus establish the diagnosis.[34,35] Argon laser application to the involved iris produces a characteristic whitening. A biopsy through a small limbal incision may also establish the diagnosis.[36,37]

After cataract extraction or penetrating injury, an implantation, serous, or pearl cyst in the anterior chamber that gradually increases in size is almost always an epithelial cyst. Manipulation of the cyst with laser treatment or

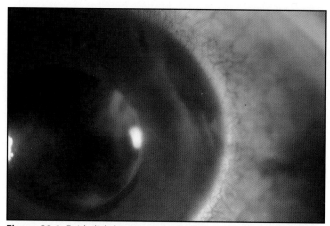

Figure 39-1. Epithelial downgrowth after cataract surgery. This patient had an unstable corneal incision with iris tissue incarcerated in the wound at her first postoperative visit. The downgrowth progressed over several months until she presented to the tertiary care eye clinic.

incomplete surgical removal can produce rapidly progressive frank epithelialization of the anterior chamber[38] and secondary glaucoma. It is best in these cases to completely remove the cyst.

Treatment

Epithelial membranes in the anterior chamber have been treated with radiation,[39] beta irradiation,[40] cryotherapy,[41-43] curettage of the membrane from the back of the cornea and application of 70% alcohol,[44-50] photocoagulation,[51] corneal transplant,[52] intraocular application of 5-fluorouracil,[53] and en bloc resection.[54] A few eyes have been saved by one or another of these forms of treatment.[55,56] Although radical procedures were once commonly favored, these are less enthusiastically embraced at the time of this writing, especially when widespread involvement of anterior chamber structures is present. Instead, attention has been focused on the control of IOP to maximize the longevity of the affected eye. However, filtration procedures typically fail, presumably due to involvement of the epithelialization process and the accompanying inflammation. In one reported case, antimetabolites used for the glaucoma filtration surgery did not alter the relentless progression of epithelialization.[57] Sometimes, cyclodestructive laser procedures are temporarily effective in controlling the secondary glaucoma. Most practitioners would now advocate attempting a glaucoma drainage device procedure if cyclodestruction is not a satisfactory option.[58,59]

After an epithelial membrane has produced pupillary block, transient relief may be obtained by incising the membrane or by iridotomy or iridectomy, but no permanent relief has been obtained in this manner in any case of which we are aware, and there seems to be a strong tendency to form PAS.[33]

Epithelial implantation cysts have been treated by block dissection of the iris, a portion of ciliary body band, and the cyst itself.[56,60]

Prevention

If a fistula is seen in the wound shortly after cataract extraction, then this calls for prompt reformation of the anterior chamber and suturing of the wound, which is usually effective in preventing this devastating complication. A fistula found a longer time after cataract extraction is a more serious matter and may lead to epithelialization. Such fistulas should be widely excised and the wound tightly closed with multiple sutures, but severe complications including glaucoma may still ensue.[61]

Concerning eyes that have had a filtration operation for glaucoma and have subsequently had cataract extraction, a leak or rupture of a filtration bleb has different implications in an aphakic eye than in one that is phakic. In the phakic eye, on occasion, a thin bleb will rupture or leak so that the anterior chamber becomes shallow or flat. This is often a very manageable, not emergent matter. In most cases, one protects the eye from infection with topical antibiotics, the leak gradually closes, and the anterior chamber resumes normal depth. If the leak is slow in healing, a bridging soft contact lens may be applied to promote healing, or if the anterior chamber remains flat, a blowout patch may be applied over the leaky bleb to reform the anterior chamber. Regardless, in the phakic eye with a leaking bleb, one need not fear epithelialization of the anterior chamber.

If the eye is aphakic, however, a shallow or flat anterior chamber from a leaking bleb is a far more serious matter. We have seen a few cases in which there was rapid epithelialization of the anterior chamber, and the eyes were lost. We, therefore, feel that if a leak develops in a bleb in an aphakic eye sufficient to produce a shallow or flat anterior chamber, surgical repair should be implemented immediately. In a pseudophakic eye after phacoemulsification or extracapsular cataract surgery, there likely is not as great a risk as in the aphakic eye, but there is still cause for concern.

It is not yet known why epithelialization of the anterior chamber rarely develops when an intact crystalline lens is present, but as a rule it develops only when the lens has been removed or has been grossly injured.

We clearly need better understanding of the pathogenesis[62,63] of this condition. Our current treatments are vastly inadequate and most commonly ineffective. Pharmacological approaches, such as those involving immunotoxins,[64] and new concepts currently being tested in preclinical studies are desperately needed.

REFERENCES

1. Wolner B, Liebmann JM, Sassani JW, et al. Late bleb-related endophthalmitis after trabeculectomy with adjunctive 5-fluorouracil. *Ophthalmology.* 1991;98:1053-1060.

2. Chee P, Hamasaki DI. The basis for chymotrypsin-induced glaucoma. *Arch Ophthalmol.* 1971;85:103-106.

3. Anderson DR. Experimental alpha-chymotrypsin glaucoma studied by scanning electron microscopy. *Am J Ophthalmol.* 1971;71:470-476.

4. Worthen DM. Scanning electron microscopy after alpha-chymotrypsin perfusion in man. *Am J Ophthalmol.* 1972;73:637-642.

5. Packer AJ, Fraioli AJ, Epstein DL. The effects of timolol and acetazolamide on transient intraocular pressure elevation following cataract extraction with alpha-chymotrypsin. *Ophthalmology.* 1981;88:239-243.

6. Berson FG, Patterson MM, Epstein DL. Obstruction of aqueous outflow by sodium hyaluronate in enucleated human eyes. *Am J Ophthalmol.* 1983;95:668-672.

7. Kirsch RE. Glaucoma following cataract extraction associated with use of alpha-chymotrypsin. *Arch Ophthalmol.* 1964;72:612-620.

8. Campbell DG, Grant WM. Obstruction of aqueous outflow by sodium hyaluronate in enucleated human eyes. *Am J Ophthalmol.* 1983;95:668-672.

9. Zimmerman TJ, Krupin T, Gordski W, et al. The effect of suture depth on outflow facility in penetrating keratoplasty. *Arch Ophthalmol.* 1978;96:505-506.

10. Kirsch RE, Levine O, Singer JA. Further studies on the ridge at the internal edge of the cataract incision. *Trans Am Acad Ophthalmol Otolaryngol.* 1977;83:OP-224-OP-231.

11. Campbell DG, Simmons RJ, Grant WM. Ghost cells as a cause of glaucoma. *Am J Ophthalmol.* 1976;81:441.

12. Van Buskirk EM. Pupillary block after intraocular lens implantation. *Am J Ophthalmol.* 1983;95:55-59.

13. Samples JR, Bellows AR, Rosenquist RC, et al. Pupillary block with posterior chamber intraocular lenses. *Arch Ophthalmol.* 1987;105:335-337.

14. Siegel MJ, Spiro HJ, Miller JA, et al. Secondary glaucoma and uveitis associated with Orculon [letter]. *Arch Ophthalmol.* 1991;109:1496-1497.

15. Kaufman PL, Lütjen-Drecoll E, Hubbard WC, et al. Obstruction of aqueous humor outflow by cross-linked polyacrylamide microgels in bovine, monkey, and human eyes. *Ophthalmology.* 1994;101:1672-1679.

16. Bigger JF, Becker B. Cataracts and primary open-angle glaucoma: the effect of uncomplicated cataract extraction on glaucoma control. *Trans Am Acad Ophthalmol Otolaryngol.* 1971;75:260.

17. Randolph ME, Maumenee AE, Iliff CE. Cataract extraction in glaucomatous eyes. *Am J Ophthalmol.* 1971;71:328-330.

18. Savage JA, Thomas JV, Belcher CD 3rd, Simmons RJ. Extracapsular cataract extraction and posterior chamber intraocular lens implantation in glaucomatous eyes. *Ophthalmology.* 1985;92:1506-1516.

19. Krupin T, Feitl ME, Bishop KI. Postoperative intraocular pressure rise in open-angle glaucoma patients after cataract or combined cataract-filtration surgery. *Ophthalmology.* 1989;96:579-584.

20. McGuigan LJ, et al. Extracapsular cataract extraction and posterior chamber lens implantation in eyes with preexisting glaucoma. *Arch Ophthalmol.* 1986;104:1301-1308.

21. Shrivastava A, Singh K. The effect of cataract extraction on intraocular pressure. *Curr Opin Ophthalmol.* 2010;21(2):118-122.

22. Melamed S, Epstein DL. Alterations of aqueous humor outflow following argon laser trabeculoplasty in monkeys. *Br J Ophthalmol.* 1987;71:776-781.

23. Puska P. Lens opacity in unilateral exfoliation syndrome with or without glaucoma. *Acta Ophthalmol.* 1994;72:290-296.

24. Wang N, Chintala SK, Fini ME, Schuman JS. Ultrasound activates the TM ELAM-1/IL-1/NF-kappaB response: a potential mechanism for intraocular pressure reduction after phacoemulsification. *Invest Ophthalmol Vis Sci.* 2003;44(5):1977-1981.

25. Evans RB. Peripheral anterior synechia overlying the haptics of posterior chamber lenses. Occurrence and natural history. *Ophthalmology.* 1990;97:415-423.

26. Grant WM. Open-angle glaucoma associated with vitreous filling the anterior chamber. *Trans Am Ophthalmol Soc.* 1963;61:196-218.

27. Iuglio N, Tieri O. Glaucoma ad angolo aperto da vitreo in camera anteriore. *Arch Ophthalmol.* 1964;68:481-484.

28. Schneider J. The treatment of aphakic pupillary block. *Eye Ear Nose Throat Mon.* 1969;48(2):89-95.

29. Grant WM. Experimental aqueous perfusion in enucleated human eyes. *Arch Ophthalmol.* 1963;69:783.

30. Roussel TJ, Olson ER, Rice T, Meisler D, Hall G, Miller D. Chronic postoperative endophthalmitis associated with Actinomyces species. *Arch Ophthalmol.* 1991;109:60-62.

31. Whitcup SM, Belfort R Jr, de Smet MD, Palestine AG, Nussenblatt RB, Chan CC. Immunohistochemistry of the inflammatory response in *Propionibacterium acnes* endophthalmitis. *Arch Ophthalmol.* 1991;109:978-979.

32. Owens SL, Lam S, Tessler HH, et al. Preliminary study of a new intraocular method in the diagnosis and treatment of *Propionibacterium acnes* endophthalmitis following cataract extraction. *Ophthalmic Surg.* 1993;24:268-272.

33. Bernardino VV, Kim JC, Smith TR. Epithelialization of the anterior chamber after cataract extraction. *Arch Ophthalmol.* 1969:742-750.

34. Verrey F. Cytologic de l'humeur aqueuse et invasion epitheliale de la chambre anterieure. *Ophthalmologics.* 1967;154:310-311.

35. Verrey F. Invasion epitheliale de la chambre anterieure: confirmation anatomique par l'examen cytologique de l'humeur aqueuse. *Ophthalmoligica.* 1967;153:467-473.

36. Calhoun FP. An aid to the clinical diagnosis of epithelial downgrowth into the anterior chamber following cataract extraction. *Am J Ophthalmol.* 1966;61:1055-1059.

37. Soong HK, Meyer RF, Wolter JR. Fistula excision and peripheral grafts in the treatment of persistent limbal wound leaks. *Ophthalmology.* 1988;95:31-36.

38. Orlin SE, et al. Epithelial downgrowth following the removal of iris inclusion cysts. *Ophthalmic Surg.* 1991;22:330-335.

39. Gallardo E. Epithelial membrane in anterior chamber after cataract surgery: case report and comments on X-ray treatment. *Am J Ophthalmol.* 1955;39:868-870.

40. Zarzycka M, Kornacki B. The use of beta-rays in cases of anterior chamber epithelial ingrowth after bulbus surgery. *Klin Oczna.* 1971;41:401-406.

41. Maumenee AE, Paton D, Morse P, et al. Review of 40 histologically proven cases of epithelial downgrowth following cataract extraction and suggested surgical management. *Am J Ophthalmol.* 1970;69:598-603.

42. Dixon WS, Speakman JS. Epithelial downgrowth following cataract surgery. Cryotherapy for an intraocular foreign body. *Arch Ophthalmol.* 1970;84:303-305.

43. Brown SI. Treatment of advance epithelial downgrowth. *Trans Am Acad Ophthalmol Otolaryngol.* 1973;77:OP-618-OP-622.

44. Long JC. Three cases of epithelial invasion of anterior chamber treated surgically. *Arch Ophthalmol.* 1957;58:396-400.

45. Maumenee AE. Treatment of epithelial downgrowth and intraocular fistula following cataract extraction. *Trans Am Ophthalmol Soc.* 1964;62:153-166.

46. Nakamura Y, Nakamura S. Two cases of epithelial downgrowth cured by a surgical technique. *Folia Ophthalmol Jpn.* 1968;19:881-885.

47. Witmer R. Therapie der Epithelinvasion der Vorderkammer nach Staro-peration. *Ophthalmologica.* 1970;161:286-291.

48. Fock V. A case of epithelialization of the anterior chamber treated operatively according to Maumenee's method. *Acta Ophthalmol.* 1971;49:11-15.

49. Harbin TS, Maumenee AE. Epithelial downgrowth after surgery for epithelial cyst. *Am J Ophthalmol.* 1974;78:1-4.

50. Laflamme MY. L'invasion epitheliale de la chambre anterieure: a propos de 8 cas opérés selon la technique de Maumenee. *Can J Ophthalmol.* 1976;11:17-20.

51. Okun E, Mandell A. Photocoagulation as a treatment of epithelial implantation cysts following cataract surgery. *Trans Am Ophthalmol Soc.* 1974;74:170-183.

52. Sullivan GL. Epithelialization of the anterior chamber following cataract extraction: a new approach to treatment. *Trans Am Ophthalmol Soc.* 1958;56:606-654.

53. Shaikh AA, Damji KF, Mintsioulis G, Gupta SK, Kertes PJ. Bilateral epithelial downgrowth managed in one eye with intraocular 5-fluorouracil. *Arch Ophthalmol.* 2002;120(10):1396-1398.

54. Friedman AH. Radical anterior segment surgery for epithelial invasion of the anterior chamber: report of 3 cases. *Trans Sect Ophthalmol Am Acad Ophthalmol Otolaryngol.* 1977;83(2):216-223.

55. Schaeffer AR, Nalbandian RM, Brigham DW, et al. Epithelial down-growth following wound dehiscence after extracapsular cataract extraction and posterior chamber lens implantation: surgical management. *J Cataract Refract Surg.* 1989;15:437-441.

56. Sugar HS. Further experience with posterior lamellar resection of the cornea for epithelial implantation cysts. *Am J Ophthalmol.* 1967;64:291-299.

57. Loane ME, Weinreb RN. Glaucoma secondary to epithelial downgrowth and 5-fluorouracil. *Ophthalmic Surg.* 1990;21:704-706.

58. Rubin B, et al. Histopathologic study of the Molteno glaucoma implant in 3 patients. *Am J Ophthalmol.* 1990;110:371-379.

59. Costa VP, Katz LJ, Cohen EJ, et al. Glaucoma associated with epithelial downgrowth controlled with Molteno tube shunts. *Ophthalmic Surg.* 1992;23:797-800.

60. Sugar HS. Deep lamellar resection of intra- and extraocular epithelial implantation cyst. *Am J Ophthalmol.* 1973;76:451-454.

61. Anseth A, Dohlman CH, Albert DM. Epithelial downgrowth—fistula repair and keratoplasty. *Refract Corneal Surg.* 1991;7:23-27.

62. Rodrigues MM, Krachmer JH, Sun TT. Clinical, electron microscopic, and monoclonal antibody studies of intraocular epithelial downgrowth. *Trans Am Ophthalmol Soc.* 1986;84:146-169.

63. Weiner MJ, Trentacoste J, Pon DM, et al. Epithelial downgrowth: a 30-year clinicopathological review. *Br J Ophthalmol.* 1989;73:6-11.

64. Fulcher S, Foulks GN, Wilkerson M, Cobo LM, Houston LL, Hatchell D. Suppression of human corneal epithelial proliferation with breast carcinoma immunotoxin. *Cornea.* 1993;12:391-396.

40

Characteristically Unilateral Glaucomas
Differential Diagnosis

Joel S. Schuman, MD, FACS; Malik Y. Kahook, MD; and David L. Epstein, MD, MMM

Certain kinds of glaucomas are typically unilateral, whereas other kinds regularly affect both eyes. This chapter is intended to provide a synopsis for the differential diagnosis of certain unilateral glaucomas, most of which are described individually in greater detail elsewhere in this book.

In this chapter, we will provide an outline of unilateral glaucomas that belong to the following general categories:

- Unilateral angle-closure glaucomas
- Unilateral peripheral synechial glaucomas
- Unilateral secondary open-angle glaucomas

For this synopsis, unilateral angle-closure glaucomas are defined as those glaucomas in which there is axial shallowing of the anterior chamber and ballooning forward of the periphery of the iris to close the angle. Peripheral synechial glaucomas are defined for this discussion as those glaucomas in which there is no axial shallowing or pupillary block to explain the development of peripheral synechiae, but peripheral anterior synechiae are present. The term *secondary open-angle glaucomas* is self-explanatory.

UNILATERAL ANGLE-CLOSURE GLAUCOMAS

In primary acute angle-closure glaucoma, a closed angle and elevated IOP in only one eye are very common. In the subacute and chronic forms of primary angle closure, unilateral glaucoma is less common. When one finds angle closure and elevated IOP in one eye, in most cases, the angle in the fellow eye is narrow and predisposed to closure. Occasionally, the angle in the fellow eye appears of good width, and one might conclude that it would not close, but

this is generally an erroneous conclusion, particularly if the iris is convex. In several cases, despite knowledge of spontaneous closure of the angle in the first eye, at our initial gonioscopic examination, we estimated that the angle in the fellow eye was of safe width and have been chagrined to find that it subsequently closed. One may be misled in a single gonioscopic examination by a transient deepening of the anterior chamber and widening of the angle due to the action of agents, such as aqueous humor suppressants or hypertonic agents, given systemically for treatment of the contralateral glaucomatous eye.

The cases that one can tell with some assurance that the angle in the fellow eye will not close are those in which there is considerable anatomical asymmetry, such as when one eye is hypermetropic and the other is myopic, or when the cornea is smaller in the affected eye than in the fellow uninvolved eye, and the configuration of the anterior segment is quite different in the 2 eyes.

True unilateral angle-closure glaucoma can be produced by the following:

- Dislocation of the lens
- Hypermature swollen lens
- Intraocular tumor
- Central retinal vein occlusion
- Panretinal photocoagulation
- Choroidal hemorrhage
- Massive vitreous hemorrhage
- Scleral buckling surgery
- Orbital venous congestion
- Retrobulbar tumor

Kahook MY, Schuman JS, eds.
Chandler and Grant's Glaucoma, Fifth Edition (pp 367-368).
© 2013 SLACK Incorporated.

- Iris bombé from inflammation
- Iris bombé from epithelialization
- Pupillary block or malignant glaucoma in aphakia or pseudophakia
- Persistent primary hyperplastic vitreous in childhood

UNILATERAL PERIPHERAL SYNECHIAL GLAUCOMAS

With the anterior chamber not significantly shallowed, unilateral glaucoma due to peripheral anterior synechiae occurs in the following conditions:

- Neovascular glaucoma
- Progressive essential iris atrophy, Chandler's syndrome, and Cogan-Reese syndrome
- Uveitis
- Keratic precipitates on the trabecular meshwork
- Cysts of the iris or ciliary processes
- Malignant tumor of the ciliary body
- After trauma
- After intraocular surgery with postoperative flat chamber

UNILATERAL SECONDARY OPEN-ANGLE GLAUCOMAS

In cases in which there is unilateral glaucoma with a clearly open angle and no peripheral anterior synechiae, the diagnosis is aided by special signs in the aqueous humor, on the back of the cornea, at the pupillary margin, and in the angle. These distinguish the following types:

- Pseudoexfoliation and open-angle glaucoma
- Glaucoma from contusion of the eye
- Hemolytic or ghost-cell glaucoma
- Lens-induced (phacolytic) glaucoma
- Extraocular venous congestion and open-angle glaucoma
- Corticosteroid glaucoma
- Herpes simplex keratitis, uveitis, and glaucoma
- Herpes zoster keratitis, uveitis, and glaucoma
- Chorioretinitis and glaucoma
- Glaucomatocyclitic crisis
- Heterochromic cyclitis
- Detached retina and glaucoma (Schwartz's syndrome)
- Malignant melanoma

Glaucoma Secondary to Intraocular Tumors

Sumit P. Shah, MD and Jay S. Duker, MD

The association between unilaterally elevated intraocular pressure (IOP) and intraocular tumor has been appreciated for many years.[1] Because intraocular neoplasms are far from common, this occurrence is rarely encountered in general ophthalmologic practice. However, when present, it is critically important to recognize. The presence of intraocular cancer represents one of the few situations in ophthalmology in which delay in diagnosis and/or inappropriate surgical intervention (eg, filtering surgery) can not only threaten vision but life as well.

In determining the proper treatment for elevated IOP in an eye with a tumor, the histopathologic cell type and therefore the risk of tumor growth and/or metastasis greatly impacts the treatment decisions. In such cases, definitive histologic diagnosis may be required. Contrary to widespread thought, the mere presence of elevated IOP associated with an intraocular neoplasm does not necessarily indicate that the underlying tumor is malignant.

In a study published 100 years ago, elevated IOP was documented in more than 50% of eyes enucleated with intraocular tumors.[1] Because of increased familiarity with intraocular tumors, modern improvements in diagnostic techniques, including indirect ophthalmoscopy and ultrasonography, as well as earlier therapeutic interventions, at the present time, only 5% of eyes harboring intraocular tumors will have elevated IOP at the time of diagnosis.[2] In the setting of melanoma of the uveal tract (iris, ciliary body, and choroid), location of the tumor is key in determining the risk of IOP elevation. Elevated IOP is much more common with ciliary body melanomas (17%) than with iris melanomas (7%) or choroidal melanoma (2%).[2] With anterior, pigmented tumors, tumor invasion of the angle followed by pigment dispersion are the most common causes of elevated IOP. For posterior tumors, iris neovascularization with secondary angle closure is the usual cause.

INSIGHTS INTO MECHANISMS OF ELEVATED INTRAOCULAR PRESSURE

Nine well-recognized mechanisms (Table 41-1) by which an intraocular tumor can abnormally elevate IOP[2,3] include the following:

- Direct tumor invasion and/or seeding of the angle structures

- Pigmentary dispersion mechanically obstructing the outflow apparatus

- Melanophagic, in which macrophages with ingested melanin mechanically obstruct the outflow apparatus (melanophagic or melanomalytic)

- Hemolytic as a result of bleeding from neovascular vessels, inherent tumor vessels, tumor necrosis, or invasion of the tumor into normal vessels

- Uveitic from secondary inflammatory cells mechanically obstructing the outflow apparatus

- Iris neovascularization with secondary angle closure (neovascular glaucoma)

- Angle closure from choroidal detachment with anterior displacement of the lens/iris diaphragm

- Angle closure from massive suprachoroidal hemorrhage with anterior displacement of the lens-iris diaphragm

- Angle closure from anterior displacement of the lens-iris diaphragm due to mass effect by extremely large posterior tumors or ring melanomas

As in any case of elevated IOP, gonioscopy is the critical diagnostic procedure to determine the mechanism. Whenever a diagnosis of unilateral glaucoma secondary to

Kahook MY, Schuman JS, eds.
Chandler and Grant's Glaucoma, Fifth Edition (pp 369-375).
© 2013 SLACK Incorporated.

TABLE 41-1. MECHANISMS OF ELEVATED INTRAOCULAR PRESSURE

Tumor invasion of the angle structures
Pigmentary dispersion
Melanophagic or melanomalytic
Hemolytic
Uveitic
Neovascular
Angle closure due to: <ul><li>Choroidal detachment</li><li>Massive suprachoroidal hemorrhage</li><li>Mass effect by extremely large posterior tumors or ring melanoma</li></ul>

one of these mechanisms is made, the clinician must rule out the presence of an intraocular neoplasm with further appropriate studies. In the setting of acutely elevated IOP, clinicians must not forget to fully evaluate the mechanism of elevated IOP after the acute episode is resolved.

Ancillary testing helps greatly in determining the location, size, site of origin, and growth characteristics of intraocular masses. Depending on the clinical situation, dilated examination with indirect ophthalmoscopy, B-scan ultrasonography, ultrasound biomicroscopy (UBM), transillumination, computed tomography (CT) scanning, magnetic resonance imaging (MRI) scanning, diagnostic paracentesis, fine-needle aspiration biopsy, incisional biopsy, and excisional biopsy may all be considered.[4,5]

STEPS IN MANAGEMENT

Previously Undiagnosed and Untreated Intraocular Tumor

The first critical step in managing patients with glaucoma secondary to an intraocular tumor is to recognize the presence of the tumor. Depending on location of the tumor, cell type, size, and growth characteristics, this may be either an exercise in the obvious or an arduous undertaking punctuated by multiple follow-up examinations and ancillary tests. In the setting of grossly elevated IOP, immediate medical management is usually indicated to forestall rapid optic disc damage or a retinal vascular obstruction. Further management of the glaucoma, however, will be intimately intertwined with the future management of the underlying tumor.

Based on patient history, clinical characteristics of the tumor, and the results of ancillary testing, a systemic search for either a primary malignancy or secondary metastases from the intraocular primary lesion may be indicated. If this search yields evidence of systemic malignancy and/or

metastases, then the systemic prognosis will impact further future interventions with respect to the glaucoma.

Eyes that may harbor malignant tumors should not undergo partial resection of the tumor through a full-thickness scleral incision as this may predispose to local seeding through the incision site (extrascleral extension). If biopsy is necessary, several options exist:

- Complete excision for diagnosis and therapy, preferably through a trap-door lamellar scleral incision or, if anterior, a limbal or clear-corneal incision

- Incisional biopsy with frozen section histopathologic evaluation followed by immediate enucleation if the tumor proves to be malignant

- Fine-needle aspiration biopsy through the clear cornea or trans-pars plana

In eyes with elevated IOP on the basis of pigment dispersion or melanophagic glaucoma, complete excision of the tumor can result in clearing of the pigment and/or macrophages from the trabecular meshwork with accompanying normalization of the IOP.[6,7] Alternatively, radiation therapy of the underlying tumor has been noted to yield similar results in selected cases.

As a general rule, treatment of the tumor should supersede treatment of the glaucoma. When enucleation is indicated to manage the tumor, glaucoma therapy is no longer a concern. In eyes that retain useful vision, however, medical management of the elevated IOP becomes the mainstay. Eyes with benign tumors such as nevi and adenomas have no contraindication to filtering surgery. Eyes that may harbor actively growing malignant tumors, especially melanomas, should not undergo filtering surgery as this may lead to orbital and eventually systemic dissemination of tumor cells. Alternatively, in eyes with unresponsive glaucoma secondary to a malignant tumor, enucleation may be the only therapeutic option, even if therapy of the primary tumor does not require it.

Treated Intraocular Tumors

Radiation therapy (Figure 41-1) has become the mainstay of treatment for uveal melanomas as it can salvage the eye and preserve vision while maintaining a survival rate comparable to enucleation.[8] But, this paradigm shift has made the possibility of secondary mixed mechanism glaucoma more likely as a long-term sequelae. Surgical intervention for glaucoma, whether laser cyclophotocoagulation or incisional, should be avoided if at all possible in the setting of a previous intraocular malignancy.

Exceptions may exist. For instance, under certain circumstances, a choroidal melanoma successfully treated with radiation therapy but complicated by secondary angle closure from neovascular glaucoma could be considered for filtering surgery depending on the potential visual outcome, timing of the treatment, and location of the tumor.

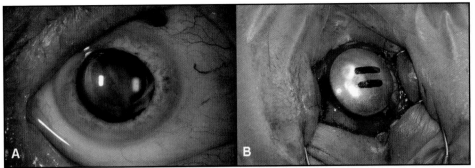

Figure 41-1. (A) Iridociliary melanoma with pigment dispersion anteriorly and extraocular extension treated with plaque radiotherapy (B) to the entire anterior segment and ciliary body. (Reprinted with permission from Drs. Carol and Jerry Shields.)

Likewise, there is a single case report in the literature of a patient who developed intractable vitreous hemorrhage and secondary hemorrhagic glaucoma arising 7 years after plaque brachytherapy for a choroidal melanoma. The patient continued to rebleed with secondary glaucoma despite undergoing 3 pars plana vitrectomies and a trabeculectomy with mitomycin C. Endoresection of the irradiated choroidal melanoma was done to treat the refractory vitreous hemorrhage and glaucoma. The patient maintained 20/200 vision at 1 year with no reported local recurrence or metastasis.[9]

If indicated, ciliary body destructive procedures can be safely and effectively performed in eyes with intraocular tumors; however, ciliary body destructive procedures do lead to a breakdown in the blood-aqueous barrier. It is not currently known whether this breakdown might predispose to cellular elements (eg, viable tumor cells), gaining access to the systemic circulation. No definite data implying an increased risk of metastases with ciliary destructive procedures exist, but common sense and caution should be used in such circumstances.

Ultimately, in these refractory secondary glaucoma cases involving radiation-treated intraocular malignant tumors, therapeutic intervention should be tailored on a case-by-case basis. The patient and ophthalmologist must carefully review the risks and benefits of the various treatment options before embarking upon a management plan.

The Role of Vascular Endothelial Growth Factor

Recent immunohistochemical evidence suggests ocular melanoma angiogenesis may be vascular endothelial growth factor (VEGF) dependent.[10] Bevacizumab is a recombinant humanized anti-VEGF IgG1 monoclonal antibody that has been approved as an antiangiogenic agent for the treatment of metastatic colorectal cancer. In addition, it has been shown to be effective in reducing anterior and posterior segment neovascularization of varying etiologies.

Although, with limited experience, it has not shown any evidence for efficacy as a primary treatment for uveal melanoma. There may be an adjunctive role of bevacizumab in addition to brachytherapy in ocular melanomas associated with neovascular glaucoma (Figure 41-2).[11,12] Furthermore, radiation therapy is known to cause retinal and choroidal ischemia manifested as neovascularization of the iris, neovascular glaucoma, and exudative retinal detachment (Figure 41-3). These late complications may also be amenable to anti-VEGF therapy.[12]

LOCATION: IRIS

Tumor Type: Primary

In most instances, iris tumors are easily detected at the slit-lamp. Differentiation between benign and malignant lesions may not be quite as straightforward. If definite differentiation is required by the clinical circumstances, an invasive procedure like anterior chamber paracentesis, fine-needle aspiration biopsy, or excisional biopsy will be required.

Benign iris melanocytic lesions (iris nevi) rarely cause elevated IOP. When they do, pigment dispersion is the most likely mechanism. Iris nevi are usually solitary while malignant iris melanocytic lesions are classified as either solitary or diffuse melanomas. Diffuse iris nevus has been reported to cause elevated IOP.[13] Iris nevi tend to be stable over time and can safely be observed.

Melanocytoma is a type of nevus that most commonly occurs in the posterior segment of the eye. Rarely, they occur as solitary iris lesions that are dark brown or jet black in color. Melanocytomas have a strong tendency to undergo necrosis leading to pigment dispersion and secondarily elevated IOP.[2]

An iris pigment epithelial adenoma is a rare, benign tumor arising from the posterior pigment epithelial layer. They are typically dark-brown or black in color and may elevate IOP via pigment dispersion. Complete surgical excision is often possible if the tumor involves less than half the iris.

In any patient with unilateral glaucoma and acquired heterochromia, diffuse melanoma of the iris must be considered. These tumors, like their solitary counterparts (see

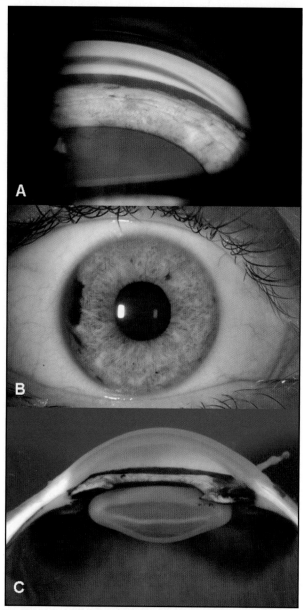

Figure 41-2. (A, B) Ring melanoma causing elevated IOP secondary to significant involvement of the trabecular meshwork seen on histologic specimen (C) after enucleation. (Reprinted with permission from Drs. Carol and Jerry Shields.)

Figure 41-2), may cause elevated IOP by direct invasion of the angle structures, pigment dispersion, or rarely, spontaneous bleeding leading to hemorrhage-associated glaucoma. Diffuse iris melanomas are apt to be confused with congenital melanocytosis, hemosiderosis, siderosis bulbi, or one of the irido-corneal endothelial syndromes.[14]

Because iris tumors are rarely life-threatening, they are typically treated by observation alone, assisted by periodic photographic documentation. Any associated increased IOP should be controlled medically. Surgery should be considered only if the glaucoma is uncontrolled medically with progressive field loss and/or unequivocal tumor growth

is documented. Location of the tumor (eg, involvement of the angle structures) alone is not an indication for surgical excision or enucleation. In a definite iris melanoma that cannot reliably be removed completely by surgical excision (ie, greater than half the iris involved), enucleation should be considered.

Tumor Type: Metastasis

Metastases to the iris are rare. However, when they occur, elevated IOP is often a prominent finding. About two-thirds of iris metastases will show elevated IOP usually due to direct invasion of the trabecular meshwork by tumor cells.[2] Lung and breast carcinoma are the most common primary sites, while cutaneous melanoma and kidney tumors may metastasize to the iris as well. Occasionally, a definite primary site is never located.

Metastatic iris carcinomas may present as either a solitary or a diffuse process. Tumor cells freely floating in the anterior chamber can mimic uveitis, and layered cells may accumulate inferiorly in the angle forming a pseudohypopyon. Uveitis, iris melanoma, intraocular lymphoma, and endogenous endophthalmitis are all in the differential diagnosis.

In the presence of a known primary cancer, metastatic iris carcinoma may not be a difficult diagnosis to make. Anterior chamber paracentesis or even fine-needle aspiration biopsy can be used through the clear cornea to obtain cells for histologic diagnosis.

Beyond medical therapy, further interventions to control elevated IOP may be dependent on both the local control of the tumor as well as the systemic treatment of the primary tumor. Systemic chemotherapy can shrink intraocular metastases, and local radiation therapy is highly effective for many cell types as well.

LOCATION: CILIARY BODY

Tumor Type: Primary

In contradistinction to iris masses, ciliary body masses are rarely visible with routine ophthalmologic examination techniques, including gonioscopy. Because of this fact, delay in diagnosis and/or extended treatment for a secondary manifestation of the tumor, such as uveitis or elevated IOP, is quite common. Clinicians should be versed in the varied clinical presentations for ciliary body tumors as well as current techniques available to image such lesions like transillumination and UBM.

Like their iris counterparts, benign ciliary body tumors such as nevi, melanocytomas, and pigment epithelial adenomas can lead to elevated IOP due to pigment dispersion and/or melanophagic mechanisms. Because of their location, it is virtually impossible to rule out the diagnosis of ciliary body melanoma without histopathologic examination of the lesions.

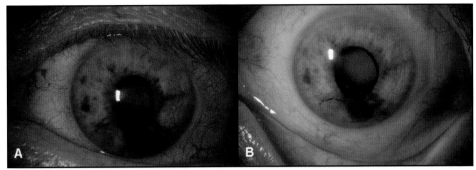

Figure 41-3. (A) Neovascularization of the iris secondary to iris melanoma. (B) There was complete regression of the neovascularization after treatment with combination plaque brachytherapy and intravitreal bevacizumab. (Reprinted with permission from Drs. Carol and Jerry Shields.)

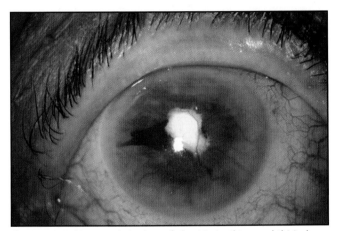

Figure 41-4. Neovascularization of the iris in this prephthisical eye as a late sequelae to plaque brachytherapy for choroidal melanoma. (Reprinted with permission from Drs. Carol and Jerry Shields.)

Ciliary body melanomas will result in elevated IOP in about 17% of cases.[2] Along with the mechanisms mentioned above, invasion into the angle by the growing tumor can occur as well (Figure 41-4). Diagnostic procedures that are helpful in the setting of ciliary body tumors include transillumination and UBM. UBM allows very high-resolution, 2-dimensional imaging of the angle structures, iris, ciliary body region, and the pars plana. B-scan ultrasonography can be useful as well, but small, anterior tumors may not be imaged well with this technique. CT and MRI can also add useful information in certain cases.

Medulloepithelioma (diktyoma) is an exceedingly rare, embryonal tumor that presents in infants or young children. Secondary glaucoma from a variety of mechanisms including angle closure, iris neovascularization, angle seeding, and hyphema have all been observed.[15] The treatment of choice for most medulloepitheliomas is enucleation despite their frequently benign cytology. Typically, the tumors cannot be completely excised locally, and end-stage glaucoma results in a blind, painful globe.

Ciliary body lesions may be amenable to surgical resection. In general, if greater than 4 clock-hours are affected, complete surgical excision is difficult and ocular morbidity

is high. Alternatively, radiation therapy can be used for growing tumors in this location.

Tumor Type: Metastasis

Isolated metastases to the ciliary body are quite rare. When they occur, however, they are notoriously difficult to diagnose due to their protean presentation and lack of direct visibility using standard ophthalmic examination procedures. Seeding of the anterior segment may cause a uveitic syndrome and/or pseudohypopyon if the cells are loosely cohesive. Alternatively, a solid metastasis may mimic a melanoma in growth characteristics.

B-scan ultrasonography and/or UBM can detect isolated ciliary body metastases reliably. Treatment will depend on cell type, location of the primary tumor, systemic prognosis, and visual prognosis.

LOCATION: CHOROID

Tumor Type: Melanocytic

While the choroid is the most common location for melanocytic tumors of the uveal tract, elevated IOP rarely results from neoplasms in this location. The incidence of secondary glaucoma from choroidal melanomas has been reported to be only 2%.[2] The incidence of secondary elevated IOP from benign choroidal melanocytic lesions (choroidal nevi) is vanishingly small.

In most instances, the diagnosis of secondary glaucoma from a choroidal melanoma is not subtle. The typical mechanism is secondary angle closure from anterior segment neovascularization. Rarely, a necrotic tumor can produce a form of hemorrhagic glaucoma or inflammatory glaucoma. The ring melanoma, a rare variant consisting of a multilobular, anterior tumor, can produce secondary angle closure as well (see Figure 41-4). This variant is apt to be confused with multiple choroidal detachments. In most instances of secondary angle closure, the posterior segment tumor is large and a secondary retinal detachment may also be present. B-scan ultrasonography, CT scanning, and MRI can be helpful when the media are opaque.

Enucleation is the treatment of choice for larger melanomas with secondary glaucoma, although, rarely, other modalities like radiation therapy or resection may be employed in highly selective cases. Alternatively, if advanced age, metastatic disease, or poor systemic health is present, observation may be suggested.

Tumor Type: Metastases

Like their melanocytic counterparts, the choroid is the most common site in the uveal tract for a hematogenously spread metastatic tumor to develop.[2] Similarly, the risk of elevated IOP in this location is quite small. Only large tumors that are accompanied by choroidal detachments, significant necrosis, or secondary retinal detachments typically produce glaucoma.[16,17]

Breast and lung are by far the most common primary locations for metastases to the uveal tract. It is not uncommon for lung metastases to appear prior to detection of the primary mass. This is quite rare for breast carcinoma, however.

Management will be dependent on the systemic status of the patient, size, number and location of the choroidal metastases, cell type, and status of the fellow eye. Enucleation, radiation therapy (episcleral plaque or external beam), and observation are all possibilities. Medical management and/or ciliary body destruction procedures to manage the underlying elevated IOP may be indicated if eye-preserving therapies are to be attempted.

LOCATION: RETINA

Primary retinal tumors of adults are rare and secondary glaucoma does not usually develop. Rare cases of retinal capillary hemangioma and retinal astrocytoma in association with retinal detachment may lead to secondary iris neovascularization.

Retinoblastoma is the most common intraocular malignancy of children. Secondary glaucoma can ensue due to a variety of mechanisms including iris neovascularization (about 20% of cases), tumor necrosis, and angle closure.[18] Heterochromia may result and may be a prominent presenting sign of retinoblastoma. Therapy of the secondary glaucoma is rarely an issue; however, affected eyes usually have far advanced tumors that typically require enucleation for treatment. In general, filtering operations should not be considered in these eyes due to the risk of extraocular spread.

LOCATION: OPTIC NERVE

Optic nerve tumors rarely result in secondarily elevated IOP. There is a single case report of a necrotic optic nerve

TABLE 41-2. COMMON MISDIAGNOSES: ANTERIOR TUMORS

Iritis
Granulomatous iris nodule (sarcoid, syphilis, tuberculosis)
Fuchs' heterochromic iridocyclitis
Iris nevus syndromes
Pigmentary dispersion syndrome
Endogenous endophthalmitis
Unilateral angle-closure glaucoma without occludable contralateral angle

melanocytoma resulting in a vascular obstruction and subsequent neovascular glaucoma.[19]

MISDIAGNOSES

Common misdiagnoses for anterior tumors are listed in Table 41-2.

CONCLUSION

With current advances in ophthalmic evaluation and earlier detection, only 5% of patients harboring intraocular tumors will have elevated IOP.[2] Despite this relatively small percentage, making the correct diagnosis in these patients represents one of the few times in ophthalmology that not only impacts vision, but life as well. Elevated IOP in the setting of intraocular tumors occurs as a result of 9 potential mechanisms. As a general rule, treatment of the tumor should precede treatment of the glaucoma with medical management being the mainstay when possible. Surgical intervention for glaucoma, whether laser cyclophotocoagulation or incisional, should be avoided if at all possible in the setting of a previous intraocular malignancy, but exceptions may exist. In the end, the patient and ophthalmologist must carefully review the risks and benefits of the various treatment options before embarking upon a management plan.

ACKNOWLEDGMENTS

The authors would like to thank Drs. Carol and Jerry Shields for their contributions and insight in preparing this book chapter.

REFERENCES

1. Marshall CD. On tension in cases of intra-ocular tumour. *Trans Ophthalmol Soc UK*. 1896;16:155-170.
2. Shields CL, Shields JA, Shields MB, Augsburger JJ. Prevalence and mechanisms of secondary intraocular pressure elevation in eyes with intraocular tumors. *Ophthalmology*. 1987;94(7):839-846.

3. Ozment R. Ocular tumors and glaucoma. In: Albert DM, Jakobiec FA, eds. *Principles and Practice of Ophthalmology*. Philadelphia, PA: WB Saunders Co; 1994.

4. Shields JA, Shields CL. *Intraocular Tumors. A Text and Atlas.* Philadelphia, PA: WB Saunders Co; 1992.

5. Shields JA, Shields CL, Shields MB. *Glaucomas associated with intraocular tumors*. In: Ritch R, Shields MB, Krupin T, eds. *The Glaucomas*. St. Louis, MO: CV Mosby; 1990:1111-1124.

6. Shields JA, Annesley WH Jr, Spaeth GL. Necrotic melanocytoma of iris with secondary glaucoma. *Am J Ophthalmol.* 1977;84(6): 826-829.

7. Shields JA, Augsburger JJ, Sanborn GE, Klein RM. Adenoma of the iris-pigment epithelium. *Ophthalmology.* 1983;90(6):735-739.

8. Diener-West M, Earle JD, Fine SL, et al. The COMS randomized trial of iodine 125 brachytherapy for choroidal melanoma, III: initial mortality findings. COMS Report No. 18. *Arch Ophthalmol.* 2001;119(7):969-982.

9. Ferreyra HA, Goldbaum MH, Weinreb RN. Endoresection of irradiated choroidal melanoma as a treatment for intractable vitreous hemorrhage and secondary blood-induced glaucoma. *Semin Ophthalmol.* 2008;23(2):135-138.

10. Lee ES, Baratz KH, Pulido JS, Salomao DR. Expression of vascular endothelial growth factor in iris melanoma. *Arch Ophthalmol.* 2006;124(9):1349-1350.

11. Bianciotto C, Shields CL, Kang B, Shields JA. Treatment of iris melanoma and secondary neovascular glaucoma using bevacizumab and plaque radiotherapy. *Arch Ophthalmol.* 2008;126(4):578-579.

12. Vasquez LM, Somani S, Altomare F, Simpson ER. Intracameral bevacizumab in the treatment of neovascular glaucoma and exudative retinal detachment after brachytherapy in choroidal melanoma. *Can J Ophthalmol.* 2009;44(1):106-107.

13. Nik NA, Hidayat A, Zimmerman LE, Fine BS. Diffuse iris nevus manifested by unilateral open angle glaucoma. *Arch Ophthalmol.* 1981;99(1):125-127.

14. Brown D, Boniuk M, Font RL. Diffuse malignant melanoma of iris with metastases. *Surv Ophthalmol.* 1990;34(5):357-364.

15. Broughton WL, Zimmerman LE. A clinicopathologic study of 56 cases of intraocular medulloepitheliomas. *Am J Ophthalmol.* 1978;85(3):407-418.

16. Bloch RS, Gartner S. The incidence of ocular metastatic carcinoma. *Arch Ophthalmol.* 1971;85(6):673-675.

17. Khawly JA, Shields MB. Metastatic carcinoma manifesting as angle-closure glaucoma. *Am J Ophthalmol.* 1994;118(1):116-117.

18. Shields JA, Augsburger JJ. Current approaches to the diagnosis and management of retinoblastoma. *Surv Ophthalmol.* 1981;25(6):347-372.

19. Croxatto JO, Ebner R, Crovetto L, Morales AG. Angle closure glaucoma as initial manifestation of melanocytoma of the optic disc. *Ophthalmology.* 1983;90(7):830-834.

SECONDARY OPEN-ANGLE GLAUCOMA

Glaucoma Due to Intraocular Inflammation

Zvia Burgansky-Eliash, MD; Guy Aharon Weiss, MD; and R. Rand Allingham, MD

Ocular inflammation may result in elevated intraocular pressure (IOP) and glaucoma. The inflammatory process can be an isolated idiopathic finding or a manifestation of systemic inflammation or infection. Therefore, diagnosing glaucoma secondary to inflammatory disease deserves careful evaluation and investigation. Furthermore, treatment of uveitic glaucoma is frequently challenging to the ophthalmologist despite the numerous available therapies.

GENERAL CONSIDERATIONS

A diagnosis of glaucoma subsequent to intraocular inflammation is self-evident in cases in which glaucoma develops in conjunction with diagnosed uveitis. However, in many instances, clinical symptoms may be mild; the aqueous humor may be deceptively clear with only trace flare and a rare circulating white cell. Occasionally, the signs and symptoms of glaucoma develop rapidly over a period of a few days, and the first evidence of inflammation may appear only after several days. Indications of an inflammatory process, such as accumulation of inflammatory cells on the trabecular meshwork (TM), posterior synechiae, or inflammatory foci in the fundus, may be present. Clues that might prompt one to consider intraocular inflammation as a possible etiology are unilateral open-angle glaucoma and open-angle glaucoma of rapid onset. These features are atypical for primary open-angle glaucoma (POAG). Common causes of uniocular glaucoma, such as exfoliation, trauma, and pigmentary dispersion syndrome, can be eliminated after careful examination. Exclusion of these differential diagnoses should suggest inflammatory glaucoma as a possibility. It is important to make the correct diagnosis promptly because, in many respects, the management of glaucoma due to intraocular inflammation is different from that of other types of glaucoma.

Mechanism of Glaucoma

In association with various types of uveitis, the IOP may be normal, below, or well above normal. Inflammation tends to increase aqueous outflow resistance while reducing aqueous humor inflow. Because these forces act in opposite directions, IOP varies considerably; the IOP is low in most acute forms of uveitis while a tendency for elevated IOP is more common in the chronic forms of uveitis. Acute uveitis that tends to present with acute IOP elevation includes herpetic anterior uveitis[1] and the Posner-Schlossman syndrome[2] as well as less common entities, such as sarcoid uveitis, toxoplasmic retinochoroiditis, listeria endophthalmitis, cytomegalovirus infection, and syphilis.[3]

In active inflammatory processes, if the character or intensity of the inflammation changes, IOP can change dramatically. If the formation of aqueous humor returns to a normal rate, then while the resistance to outflow remains high, the IOP will rise. The reverse is also true; if an eye has elevated IOP because of high resistance to aqueous outflow, change in intraocular inflammation may reduce aqueous formation and decrease IOP. Therefore, a careful monitoring of IOP in patients with uveitis is crucial.

Ocular inflammation is associated with production of prostaglandins, which affects the eye in various mechanisms.[4] These effects may be mediated through alteration of aqueous humor production, uveoscleral outflow, or aqueous outflow resistance via the TM.

Aqueous Production

The decrease in IOP associated with intraocular inflammation can be completely reversible. The IOP may return promptly to normal level after the inflammation has subsided in some cases or very slowly in others. In some cases,

Kahook MY, Schuman JS, eds.
Chandler and Grant's Glaucoma, Fifth Edition (pp 379-412).
© 2013 SLACK Incorporated.

a permanent decrease in aqueous formation appears to be induced by structural damage to the ciliary processes mediated by chronic intraocular inflammation. When this occurs, the ciliary processes, if visible, may appear atrophic. Occasionally, a distinct cyclitic membrane may be seen overlying the ciliary processes.

Outflow Resistance

Intraocular inflammation can affect aqueous outflow resistance through various mechanisms.

In most cases, the angle appears normal and the cause of elevated outflow resistance cannot be detected by gonioscopy. The TM may be obstructed by inflammatory cells or debris.[5] Experimentally, serum proteins have been shown to increase aqueous outflow resistance.[6] Swelling of phagocytic cells lining the lamellae within the TM or adjacent to Schlemm's canal may also contribute to elevated IOP.[7]

In certain types of uveitis, focal accumulations of inflammatory cells resembling keratic precipitates (KPs) may be visible on the inner surface of the TM by gonioscopy. These trabecular precipitates can completely resolve as inflammation subsides, leaving few, if any, persistent changes in the angle.

Frequently, inflammatory changes in the TM are not reversible. The most conspicuous form of irreversible obstruction to aqueous outflow is caused by peripheral anterior synechiae (PAS), which form when the iris adheres to the TM. PAS are produced as a result of organization of inflammatory exudates in the angle or from secondary pupillary block. Permanent obstruction can also be caused by endothelial or fibrovascular membranes that may line the inner surface of the TM. Other alterations of the TM that may affect the permeability of the angle structures may only produce a dirty appearance of the TM gonioscopically. Occasionally, the TM does not have this appearance, but is blank, white, and lacking its normal, finely granular surface texture.

Pupillary block due to inflammatory membrane at the pupillary margin readily seals the iris to the lens, which causes considerable elevation of IOP. The iris is bowed forward in a characteristic fashion, iris bombé (Figure 42-1), by elevated posterior chamber pressure, which closes the angle. Laser iridectomy should be performed to relieve the angle closure. If extensive synechial closure of the angle is found after iris bombé is relieved by iridectomy, a filtering operation may be necessary. If synechiae are of recent onset and inflammation is well controlled, iridoplasty or synechiolysis can, on occasion, restore aqueous outflow.

In some cases, ocular inflammation might induce uveal effusion or massive serous retinal detachment that can cause acute closure of the anterior chamber angle by uveal effusion with forward rotation of the ciliary body.

In acute inflammation, the blood vessels of the anterior segment may be conspicuously dilated, but no demonstration has shown that this in itself has an influence on the facility of aqueous outflow. Occasionally, dilated iris vessels can be confused with those seen in neovascular glaucoma. However, blood vessels found in association with inflammation have a normal radial pattern and do not bridge the scleral spur or arborize over the TM as do those seen in neovascularization of the anterior segment (see Chapter 31). Neovascular glaucoma might complicate ocular inflammation as well, especially when severe ischemia of the posterior segment exists.

Corticosteroid treatment, commonly used to control inflammation, may adversely increase IOP (see Chapter 44). When evaluating the effect of steroids on IOP in patients with uveitis, possible separate actions on aqueous humor secretion and outflow must be considered. Steroids may suppress inflammation in the ciliary body so that aqueous humor formation returns to a more normal rate. If outflow facility is impaired by inflammation, the improvement in aqueous humor formation may produce an increase in IOP that is not secondary to steroid-induced outflow obstruction. If there is actual inflammation in the TM, steroids may, in fact, improve outflow facility, but the resulting IOP represents the balance between aqueous humor inflow and outflow effects. Steroid-induced IOP elevations typically occur after 7 to 10 days but may occur much sooner. Where this is a concern, topical steroid treatment should be tapered, or less potent steroid formulations can be substituted (eg, fluorometholone 0.12%). If possible, taper steroid therapy gradually to avoid rebound inflammation that may occur after rapid discontinuation.

Terminology

Ocular inflammation can affect any ocular tissue—the most common site is the uvea, causing uveitis. Uveitis was classified by the International Uveitis Study Group[8] (IUSG) according to location, clinical course, and laterality. The anatomical categories include the following 4 groups:

1. Anterior uveitis where inflammation involves the iris (formally known as iritis) and ciliary body (formally known as iridocyclitis)

2. Intermediate uveitis where inflammation is centered primarily in the vitreous, pars plana, or anterior retina

3. Posterior uveitis affecting the choroid (choroiditis) or extending to the retina (chorioretinitis)

4. Panuveitis when 2 or more segments of the uvea are involved[8]

The clinical course is classified as acute, recurrent, or chronic if inflammation persists for more than 2 to 3 months. The chronic type is more prone to complications, including glaucoma.

In this chapter, we will discuss different disease entities as well as idiopathic forms of uveitis. Unfortunately, many cases remain undiagnosed despite extensive diagnostic evaluation.

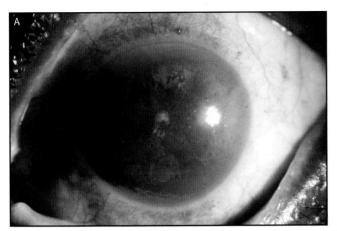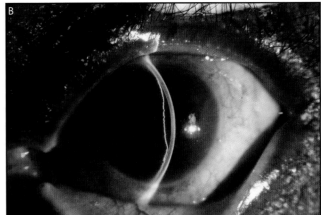

Figure 42-1. (A) Iris bombé and angle-closure glaucoma caused by posterior synechiae from chronic uveitis. (B) Ultrasound biomicroscopic image of a patient with iris bombé and secondary angle closure. (Reprinted with permission from Joel S. Schuman, MD, FACS.)

Treatment

Medical Control of Inflammation

The treatment of ocular inflammation depends on the specific disease causing it. Most inflammatory processes are treated with topical, periocular, or systemic corticosteroids. Other therapeutic measures are topical or systemic non-steroidal anti-inflammatory drugs (NSAIDs), cycloplegic agents to prevent synechiae formation, systemic immunosuppressive therapy, and biological agents.

Immunosuppressive Therapy Corticosteroids have a wide range of adverse effects associated with their long-term use, such as hypertension, osteoporosis, hyperglycemia, and growth retardation in children; therefore, the use of corticosteroid-sparing agents is considered. These agents are also used when severe inflammation is threatening vision or in cases in which an associated systemic disorder exists.[9,10] Corticosteroid-sparing agents include antimetabolites (mycophenolate mofetil, methotrexate [MTX], and azathioprine), T cell calcineurin inhibitors (cyclosporine and tacrolimus), and alkylating agents (cyclophosphamide and chlorambucil).

Immunosuppressive agents have been proven effective in several uveitic conditions.[11,12] Nevertheless, the use of these therapeutic agents requires careful clinical and laboratory monitoring due to potential side effects. The antimetabolite medications were proven efficient in controlling a variety of uveitic conditions.[13-15] The T cell calcineurin inhibitors have also been used successfully in uveitis.[16,17] The alkylating agents are the least commonly used immunomodulatory agents for uveitis due to their serious side effects. Alkylating agents are reserved for cases with severe, bilateral refractory uveitis with a potential for visual recovery.[18,19]

Biologic Agents Biologic agents are a group of medications that target cytokines and other soluble inflammatory mediators. Three groups of biologic medications have been used for ophthalmic indications:

1. Tumor necrosis factor (TNF)-α antagonists (infliximab, adalimumab, and etanercept)

2. Interleukin (IL)-2 receptor antagonist (daclizumab)

3. IL-1 receptor antagonist (anakinra)

Infliximab was reported effective in the treatment of refractory uveitis like sarcoidosis, Behçet's disease, pars planitis, Crohn's disease, juvenile idiopathic arthritis, and human leukocyte antigen (HLA)-B27-associated acute anterior uveitis.[20] It was used successfully alone as well as in combination with immunosuppressive therapy. Nevertheless, serious effects were reported with this treatment, including development of antinuclear antibodies, congestive heart failure, pulmonary emboli, vitreous hemorrhage, reactivation of latent tuberculosis, unmasking of demyelinating disease, and possible development of lymphoma. Therefore, the exact application of this treatment for ocular diseases requires further investigation.[20] Adalimumab showed good response in 81% to 88% of pediatric uveitis patients.[21,22] Good efficacy was also reported in a small series of patients with Behçet's disease.[23,24] Reported side effects are mainly at the site of injection, herpes simplex virus (HSV), keratitis and elevation of liver enzymes. Etanercept is probably the least effective TNF-α antagonist in the treatment of uveitis.[25] Daclizumab has shown efficacy in the treatment of several uveitic disorders like sarcoidosis, Vogt-Koyanagi-Harada syndrome, idiopathic intermediate uveitis, anterior uveitis, idiopathic panuveitis, and multifocal choroiditis.[26] No serious side effects were reported with this treatment.[27] Anakinra has only limited but encouraging experience in treating ocular diseases.[28]

Medical Control of Glaucoma

If IOP elevation secondary to uveitis requires treatment, aqueous suppressants, including topical beta-blockers, α2-adrenergic agonists, and systemic or topical carbonic anhydrase inhibitors (CAIs), are often effective.[29,30] Frequent monitoring of IOP is needed in these patients because the lowering effect of most ocular hypotensive agents is highly variable in uveitis. The responses range from no response at all to profound reductions of IOP (70% to 80%) on relatively small amounts of ocular hypotensive medication, especially topical CAIs.[31]

Prostaglandin analogs are used with caution in cases of uveitic glaucoma. Although prostaglandins are mediators of inflammatory process in the eye, the antiglaucoma prostaglandin analogs have a very low dose and altered compounds and do not show breakdown of the blood-aqueous barrier in healthy subjects.[32] However, there are rare reports of anterior uveitis associated with latanoprost therapy in subjects with no history of uveitis[33] or in patients with prior inflammation or surgery.[34] Moreover, these agents are prone to induce cystoid macular edema in uveitis patients[35-38] and reactivation of herpetic keratouveitis[39,40]; therefore, caution should be used in these cases.

Miotic treatment is generally contraindicated in the presence of anterior uveitis. Miotics can cause pain, intensify anterior segment inflammation, and increase formation of posterior synechiae, which can produce complete pupillary block.

If the optic nerve head is entirely normal, as is usual in acute anterior uveitis, treatment of moderate elevation of IOP may not be indicated. In these cases, once inflammation is controlled, the IOP will probably return to safe levels long before optic nerve damage occurs. Typically, a normal optic nerve can tolerate an IOP in the mid-30s for many weeks without damage. Only if there are frequent recurrences, or if inflammation becomes chronic, significant optic nerve damage is likely. In eyes with corneal endothelial disease, a moderate elevation of IOP may cause corneal edema, which calls for more vigorous efforts to lower the IOP.

Surgical Management of Glaucoma

Medical treatment may not adequately control glaucoma in cases associated with ocular inflammation. Surgical treatment must be directed at the mechanism responsible for outflow obstruction.

Laser Therapy   In cases in which pupillary block exists (eg, iris bombé), an iridectomy is indicated. Laser iridectomy is possible in these cases. In the presence of active inflammation, a tendency for small iridectomy to close exists. Additional sessions may be needed, or, in some cases, a surgical iridectomy may be required.

Argon laser trabeculoplasty (ALT) is not only ineffective in cases in which glaucoma is secondary to an inflammatory process, but it may produce acute flare-up of uveitis and significant increase in IOP; therefore, it is not recommended for patients with uveitis-related glaucoma.[41]

Trans-scleral diode laser cyclophotocoagulation (TDLC) can be used in cases in which advanced optic nerve damage exists and visual potential is limited (see Chapter 56).[42]

Cycloablative procedures often increase intraocular inflammation or cause unpredictable severe hypotony with visual loss and phthisis due to further damage of an already sick ciliary body. In a report on 16 patients, the success rate was 75%, but 19% of eyes developed hypotony that was higher than in any diagnostic category other than uveitis.[43] Contradicting results were recently reported[44] in 18 uveitic glaucoma eyes with a 1-year success rate of 72%, but no case of phthisis, hypotony, or marked activation of the underlying inflammatory. In this study, however, the repeated treatment rate was higher than in others (63.6%).[44]

Incisional Surgery   Filtering surgery is prone to failure in patients who have uveitis (see Chapter 59). It is crucial to minimize ocular inflammation preoperatively by topical or systemic steroids before the operation. Unfortunately, glaucoma is, at times, an immediate threat to vision and it is not possible to completely control inflammation prior to surgery.

In general, the use of adjuvant antimetabolites, such as 5-fluorouracil (5-FU) and mitomycin C (MMC), is important and improves surgical results.[31] A qualified success rate (IOP of 21 mm Hg or higher with or without topical medications) of 78% at 1 year and 62% at 2 years was reported in 44 eyes with MMC (primarily) or 5-FU trabeculectomy.[45] Interestingly, the use of the less potent 5-FU in 50 eyes resulted in a similar, if not better, effect with a qualified success rate of 82% at 1 and 2 years after surgery and 67% at 5 years.[46] This rate of success is influenced largely by risk factors for surgical failure, such as prior incisional surgery, Black patients, idiopathic uveitis, and the degree of inflammation control before surgery. Therefore, in a cohort with minimal risk factors and long preoperative control of inflammation, even trabeculectomy without antimetabolites resulted in a comparatively good qualified success rate—78% in 5 years.[47] Cataract formation after filtration and antimetabolites was noted in more than half of the phakic patients. After cataract surgery, 25% required repeat glaucoma surgery due to failure of the filtering bleb and loss of IOP control.[45]

Small pilot reports on the use of nonpenetrating deep sclerectomy demonstrate 1-year qualified success of 90%[48] to 100%[49] with a low rate of surgical complications.

For chronic childhood uveitis, goniotomy was suggested as a good first-line surgical option with a qualified success rate of 75% after 1 year and minimal complications.[50]

Glaucoma drainage devices (GDDs) are preferred in many high-risk cases for trabeculectomy failure, especially when significant postoperative inflammation is likely.[51] The long-term qualified success rate of Molteno implants (Molteno Ophthalmic Ltd, Dunedin, New Zealand) in 40 eyes with uveitic glaucoma was 87% at 5 years and 93% at 10 years.[52] The reported 2-year success rate with a Baerveldt glaucoma drainage device (Abbott Medical Optics Inc., Chicago, IL) was 91.7% in 24 uveitic eyes.[53] Two studies[54,55] with the Ahmed glaucoma drainage device (New World Medical, Rancho Cucamonga, CA) report a 1-year success rate of 94%,

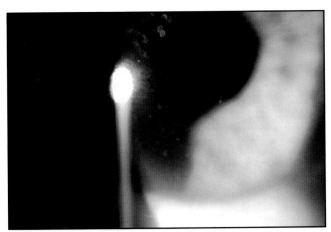

Figure 42-2. Acute anterior uveitis. Note KPs. (Reprinted with permission from Haggay Avizemer, MD.)

although this rate drops to 60% at 2 years.[55] The most common complication was valve occlusion, which is probably related to the inflammatory process.

ANTERIOR UVEITIS

Most inflammatory-associated IOP elevations and glaucoma are caused by anterior uveitis.

Acute Anterior Uveitis

Acute anterior uveitis (AAU) is typically associated with anterior segment hyperemia, cells and flare in the anterior chamber, and KPs (Figure 42-2). Usually, IOP remains normal or low despite common increases in outflow resistance because the rate of aqueous humor formation is typically lowered to a degree that is compensatory or even disproportionately greater.

In AAU, the angle is typically open gonioscopically. The treatment of the inflammation is the same whether glaucoma is present or not, relying principally upon topical administration of cycloplegic agents and corticosteroids (except in herpetic epithelial keratopathy). If inflammation has caused an increase in outflow resistance, topical steroids may improve aqueous outflow over the short term. In cases where a cause for the uveitis is discovered, a specific treatment is required.

Recurrent and Chronic Anterior Uveitis

The majority of cases of recurrent or chronic anterior uveitis are idiopathic. The uveitic glaucoma subtypes related to specific disease entities represent a small proportion of all cases of recurrent anterior uveitis and will be discussed individually later in this chapter. In idiopathic chronic anterior uveitis, the signs of inflammation, particularly cells, flare, and KPs, come and go, or persist over a long period, responding incompletely to treatment. Glaucoma becomes a serious

problem in some of these cases because of significantly elevated IOP and a chronic course.

In cases in which anterior segment inflammation has been prolonged, IOP may remain normal for a long time because of a low rate of aqueous production, but when the inflammation subsides, the rate of aqueous formation may return to normal. The IOP may then rise considerably if outflow facility remains reduced secondary to changes in the TM. In some instances, control of inflammation may result in an IOP that is uncontrollable by any medical means. Under these circumstances, one may be forced to choose between reducing anti-inflammatory treatment and permitting mild inflammation, or proceeding with invasive high-risk glaucoma surgery.

IDIOPATHIC INFLAMMATORY CONDITIONS

Posner-Schlossman Syndrome

Posner-Schlossman syndrome (PSS), also termed glaucomatocyclitic crisis, was first described by Posner and Schlossman[2] in 1948 as a rare self-limiting unilateral condition characterized by recurring acute attacks of mild anterior uveitis with an IOP elevation. In between attacks, the IOP is normal with open angles. Although originally considered a benign syndrome, it was shown that there is an association between PSS and concomitant POAG.[56] Moreover, a quarter of PSS patients' eyes might develop glaucoma due to repeated attacks. Patients with disease duration of a decade or more have a 2.8 times higher risk of developing glaucomatous optic nerve and visual field damage in comparison to patients with shorter disease duration.[57]

The syndrome appears between the third and sixth decades of life, with a mean age at onset of 35 years.[57] Diagnosing PSS can be challenging at presentation of the first attack, with only mild inflammation that may go undetected, or the elevated IOP might be confused with acute angle-closure glaucoma. There are no specific diagnostic laboratory tests, and the diagnosis is based on clinical findings.

Onset of symptoms is usually acute. Patients present with slight ocular discomfort, blurred vision, or appearance of colored haloes around lights secondary to corneal edema. Examination reveals a highly elevated IOP, usually between 40 and 70 mm Hg. The eye is generally quiet with little or no hyperemia. The cornea may have mild to moderate epithelial edema with a few fine KPs. KPs may not be noted for 2 or 3 days after the onset of symptoms and tend to vary in number and position from day to day. In some cases, there is focal segmental ischemia of the iris during the attack.[56] Gonioscopy reveals a normal-appearing angle, open throughout, with no abnormal pigmentation.

Occasionally, one may find a few tiny inflammatory precipitates on the TM. Characteristically, no posterior or anterior synechiae are formed. If tonography is performed, it demonstrates a highly elevated resistance to aqueous outflow in the affected eye but a normal value in the unaffected eye.

The etiology of this PSS is unknown. Herpes simplex virus may play a role in this syndrome, as viral DNA was found in aqueous humor samples of PSS patients during acute attacks.[58] Cytomegalovirus (CMV) was demonstrated in half of the patients in aqueous analysis.[59] Immunogenetic factors might also play a role in PSS. An association with the major HLA-Bw54 was found in 41% of Japanese patients.[60]

During the acute attack, the optic nerve head undergoes morphologic as well as hemodynamic changes. These changes are usually transient and mostly do not cause permanent damage.[61]

A selective reduction in the S-cone component of an electroretinogram b-wave was demonstrated during acute PSS attacks. This finding may reflect the relative susceptibility to damage of the S-cone pathway, in comparison to the L- and M-cone systems, as a result of elevated IOP.[62]

The IOP elevation might be due to trabeculitis, with histological evidence of mononuclear cells in the meshwork, blocking the aqueous outflow.[63] In addition to a decrease in the outflow facility, increased levels of aqueous prostaglandin, mainly prostaglandin E, might also explain the elevated IOP, through excessive aqueous production.[64] The correlation of PSS to chronic open-angle glaucoma may have a role in the elevated IOP mechanism.[56]

An attack of glaucomatocyclitic crisis generally subsides within 1 to 3 weeks, with or without treatment. Medical treatment is indicated to prevent pressure-related optic nerve damage and to reduce inflammation. The condition usually responds to topical corticosteroids and aqueous-suppressant ocular hypotensive drugs: beta-blockers, α_2-adrenergic agonists, and CAIs. The use of 1% apraclonidine lowered IOP during attacks by half, regardless of the initial level of IOP, and had a more significant hypotensive effect in PSS in comparison to POAG.[65] It is unclear whether cycloplegics are beneficial.

Surgery should be restricted to cases with severe and disabling symptoms or progressive glaucomatotic optic neuropathy with visual field loss.[61] Filtering surgery with antimetabolites might be used to control elevated IOP, although reports concerning efficacy are controversial.[57]

The risk of developing chronic glaucoma in some cases dictates funduscopic follow-up and visual field monitoring in all subjects. Glaucomatocyclitic crises are prone to recur at intervals of a few months to a year or 2 over 15 to 25 years. Eventually, episodes appear to stop; this condition is almost never seen after age 60. Repeated episodes usually occur in the same eye but rarely occur in one eye and then the other.

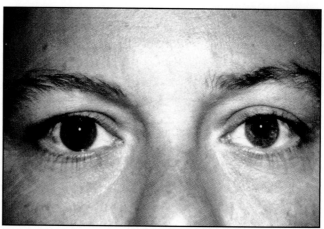

Figure 42-3. Patient with Fuchs' heterochromic iridocyclitis. Iris stromal atrophy of the left eye is responsible for the heterochromia. (Reprinted with permission from Glenn J. Jaffe, MD.)

Fuchs' Heterochromic Iridocyclitis

Fuchs' heterochromic iridocyclitis (FHI) is a chronic low-grade anterior uveitis, associated with iris stromal atrophy, cataract formation, and glaucoma. It accounts for 2% to 3% of all cases of uveitis[66] and continues to be underdiagnosed (Figure 42-3). Because of the diverse number of abnormalities that may be present, this may be one of the more difficult uveitides to diagnose. FHI occurs mainly in the third and fourth decades of life and affects men and women equally.[66] FHI typically affects only one eye; however, in up to 15.6% of cases, it affects both eyes.[67]

Patients are usually asymptomatic. When symptomatic, the most common presenting symptoms are floaters[68] and visual deterioration.[67,69] The eye is typically white and quiet. The prominent signs reported are typical KP in all cases, cataract in nearly 80% of cases, and heterochromia in 70% to 80% of patients.[67-69] Characteristically, the KPs are fine and colorless; some are round, but the most typical are filamentary or star-shaped, scattered over the posterior surface of the cornea (Figure 42-4). The KPs are best seen by retroillumination. There may be trace flare in the aqueous humor with an occasional white cell. A cataract in the affected eye is the rule, initially presenting as a posterior subcapsular cataract. The iris is infiltrated with plasma cells with accompanying degeneration and atrophy.[70] Clinically, atrophy of the iris affects the pupil collarette (transforming it to a hyaline border) and produces hypochromia of the iris stroma with abnormal transillumination of the posterior pigment layer.[71] Fluorescein may leak from vessels at the pupil, but these are not new vessels. In 50% of patients, there is only discrete iris heterochromia,[68] which may delay diagnosis. The iris heterochromia depends on the level of stromal atrophy, iris color, and pigment amount in the iris pigmented epithelium; it may not be recognized in darkly pigmented irides.[66] Some patients develop iris nodules mainly on the pupillary margin and less frequently on the iris stroma.[72] In some cases,

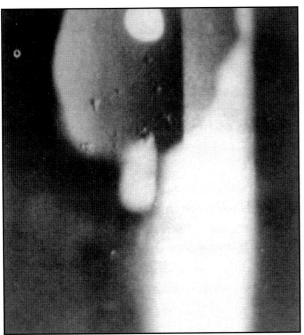

Figure 42-4. Typical filamentary star-shaped KPs seen in Fuchs' heterochromic iridocyclitis.

congenital Horner's syndrome has been reported.[73] Vitreous opacities are frequent.[74] Chorioretinal scars similar to those seen in toxoplasmosis have been described in Fuchs' FHI, but the association of these 2 diseases is unclear.[75]

Gonioscopy characteristically reveals a few fine new blood vessels on the surface of the ciliary band, scleral spur, and on the corneoscleral meshwork. These blood vessels appear to be different from those associated with neovascular glaucoma because they do not proliferate or produce synechial closure of the angle. Abnormal vessels in the angle may also be seen in cases of heterochromia without glaucoma.[76] These abnormal blood vessels may lead to hyphema. Most affected eyes do not develop synechia.[66] The angle typically remains open, and the TM may be covered by an inflammatory membrane that is demonstrable only histologically.[77] In some cases, Schlemm's canal appears to be collapsed.[78]

One of the most serious complications is glaucoma.[68] Fourteen percent to 27% of patients develop glaucoma and nearly 10% of FHI patients require filtration surgery.[67,69,79,80] After diagnosis, there is a 0.5% risk per year to develop glaucoma, decreasing substantially after 15 years of follow-up.[80] Typically, glaucoma is of the open-angle variety, but a number of mechanisms have been observed, including secondary synechial angle closure, neovascular glaucoma, lens-induced, and glaucoma secondary to recurrent hyphemas.[80] Cataract surgery might also precipitate glaucoma.[80]

The pathogenesis of FHI is unknown; however, many reports suggest an infectious origin. Intraocular antibody production against rubella virus was demonstrated, with evidence of the rubella genome in the aqueous humor of

FHI patients.[81] Another potential causative agent is herpes simplex.[82] Its DNA was found in the aqueous humor of FHI patients.[82] In another report, the serology of toxoplasma was found positive in one-third of patients.[68] An infectious origin of the disease might explain the low efficacy of corticosteroid therapy in treating this disease.[83] Another theory suggests there is an immunological impairment in FHI. Various reports discovered depressed suppressor-T-cell activity,[84] cellular immunity to corneal antigens (demonstrated in most patients),[85] autoantibodies against corneal epithelium present in nearly 90% of cases,[86] and nonspecific immune complexes found in the iris vessel walls.[87]

Active treatment is not required in 75% of patients,[69] though all should be screened routinely for glaucoma.[67] Symptomatic exacerbations are treated with a short course of corticosteroids.[66] More than 40% of patients required cataract surgery.[67,69]

In most cases of heterochromic iridocyclitis, once glaucoma develops, it appears to be permanent. Unfortunately, control of the associated inflammation has little influence on the IOP, and it is questionable whether it is even worthwhile, especially because there is little tendency to form synechiae. The inflammation usually continues for many years, but even if the inflammation eventually clears, the glaucoma invariably remains. Medical antiglaucoma treatment may be effective initially. As time passes, the glaucoma responds poorly to medical treatment. In one series, 73% of glaucoma patients did not respond successfully to maximal medical treatment.[79] Glaucoma filtration surgery is generally well tolerated and causes little or no increase in the inflammation. Trabeculectomy had a 72% rate of successful IOP control for more than 2 years of follow-up.[79] Adjunctive antimetabolites appear to improve the glaucoma surgical success rate.[79,80,88]

In general, the visual prognosis of FHI is good,[66] with glaucoma, posterior capsule opacification, and vitreous opacity causing most of the visual impairment following cataract surgery.[69]

Keratic Precipitates on the Trabecular Meshwork (Grant's Syndrome)

Chandler and Grant were the first to describe a relatively rare cause of idiopathic secondary glaucoma consisting of inflammatory precipitates on the TM[89] subsequently given the eponym *Grant's syndrome*. Although it is uncommon, it is important to diagnose this disorder correctly because treatment with topical steroids in most cases is effective.[90]

Typically, onset of the syndrome is acute,[90] the IOP is elevated in both eyes, and the eyes are white and quiet, with few (if any) inflammatory precipitates on the cornea endothelium. There may be a few cells in the aqueous, but, in most cases, no cells are seen.

Gonioscopy is crucial to differentiate this condition from POAG. Gonioscopy reveals inflammatory precipitates projecting from the surface of the corneoscleral meshwork. These are generally colorless or tapioca-colored and tend to be broader and flatter than KPs seen on the cornea endothelium and may be confluent. In rare instances, the KPs in the angle are large and striking in appearance. In all other cases, the KPs have been small and inconspicuous and therefore easily overlooked. It is not unusual that after careful examination of the entire angle, only a few KP may be identified; however, with repeated examinations, more KP may be observed. Irregularity in the level of the attachment of the iris root might also be noted. KP in the angle tend to organize and thus cause irregularities in the width of the angle. In POAG, although the angle may be narrower above or below, there are never any abrupt changes in the width of the angle. Such abrupt changes are almost certainly the result of organization of KPs in the angle or trauma. The only other conditions in which such abrupt changes in the width of the angle are seen include old interstitial keratitis, multiple cysts of the iris and ciliary body, essential atrophy of the iris, and Chandler's syndrome.

Ultrasound biomicroscopy may demonstrate the pathology and supplement gonioscopy. Sonographic findings may include inflammatory precipitates overlying the TM and PAS, without abnormalities of the TM or ciliary body.[90]

The level of IOP elevation may not be proportional to the number of inflammatory precipitates observed in the angle. In some cases, many KPs are visible in the angle, but the IOP is normal or only slightly elevated and vice versa. High IOP despite few KPs suggests that inflammatory debris must be present within the TM, which is blocking the outflow pathways but cannot be seen gonioscopically.

In early cases of glaucoma associated with inflammatory precipitates on the TM, the disc is normal and the field is full, but in long-standing cases, cupping of the disc with field loss is found. If the true condition is not recognized and the patient is treated mistakenly as POAG, there is usually a poor response. Moreover, the exudates in the angle may gradually organize to bring about synechial closure of the angle and permanent glaucoma.

The cause of this disorder is unknown. Some patients who initially present with this disorder will develop other inflammatory conditions, such as sarcoidosis, ankylosing spondylitis, rheumatoid arthritis, or chronic uveitis.[5]

Medical treatment consists of topical corticosteroids and aqueous-suppressant ocular hypotensive drugs, as required. Topical corticosteroids are given at first every hour during the day, and then are gradually tapered. Trabecular precipitates typically clear over a 1- to 2-week period and, in the absence of advanced peripheral synechial closure, the IOP returns to normal levels.

In the majority of cases, when the topical corticosteroids are reduced below a certain level or are discontinued, the precipitates in the angle tend to recur and IOP again becomes elevated. In such cases, the maintenance dose of topical steroids in preventing recurrence is determined by trial and error. Once the KPs have cleared after treatment, the IOP returns to normal, but if there are many recurrences, eventually, the patient may have a permanent open-angle glaucoma. Individuals with this condition should be monitored indefinitely because of a significant risk of recurrence, which is usually asymptomatic.

If there is extensive synechial closure of the angle when the diagnosis is first established, eliminating the precipitates in the open portions of the angle may improve the condition, but there may be severe residual glaucoma because of the secondary angle closure. In such cases, a glaucoma filtering operation may be necessary.

Sarcoidosis

Sarcoidosis is a multisystem disorder of unknown etiology, characterized by the formation of noncaseating granulomas and a remissions and exacerbations pattern. Sarcoidosis usually presents with bilateral hilar adenopathy, pulmonary infiltrates, and cutaneous and ocular involvement. Incidence of sarcoidosis varies between different geographical areas and ethnic groups. It is more prevalent in Black patients compared to White patients. Sarcoidosis affects mainly young adults between 20 and 40 years of age.[91]

Ocular involvement exists in up to 80% of the sarcoidosis patients.[91] Sarcoid uveitis can affect individuals at any age; the mean age is around 40 years.[92] It has a higher prevalence in postmenopausal women.[93] Ocular disease may present with acute or chronic granulomatous or nongranulomatous eye disease. A report of 60 patients described 81% of cases as granulomatous, while only 15% had nongranulomatous uveitis. In that cohort, the majority of patients (91%) suffered from a chronic disease, 7% had recurrent flares, and only one patient had a monophasic acute uveitis.[92] Young patients commonly suffer from an acute disease, whereas in older patients, the chronic disease is more common.[93]

There is a wide spectrum of ocular inflammation in sarcoidosis; the most common manifestation is sole anterior or intermediate uveitis.[92] Ninety percent of sarcoid uveitis cases are bilateral.[93] Sarcoid uveitis may clinically include some distinctive features. KPs may appear in a form of mutton-fat KP or small granulomatous KP. Sarcoid nodules may appear on the iris (Koeppe or Busacca nodules), the TM, or ciliary body and create tent-shaped PAS or posterior synechiae (Figure 42-5). In the vitreous, opacities with snowballs or strings of pearls appear. Posterior manifestations include multiple chorioretinal peripheral lesions, segmental periphlebitis, candle-wax-like drippings, retinal macroaneurysm, optic disc nodules or granulomas, and solitary choroidal nodule. Other ocular manifestations include Sicca syndrome and orbital and lacrimal gland involvement. Causes of vision loss include cataract,

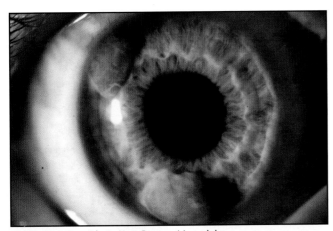

Figure 42-5. Sarcoidosis. Note Bussaca iris nodules.

glaucoma, macular edema, vitreous hemorrhage, and retinal detachment.[94]

Glaucoma was found in approximately 10% of patients with sarcoid uveitis.[95] The most prominent glaucoma mechanism is aqueous outflow obstruction due to granulomatous infiltration of the angle.[96] Sarcoidosis inflammatory precipitates in the angle are sometimes the only sign of inflammation in a subacute uveitis and may result in IOP elevation.[5] Histologically, there are inflammatory mononuclear cells infiltrates around the inner and outer walls of Schlemm's canal and granulomatous and fibrotic tissue obstructing its lumen.[97] A chronic course of the uveitis may induce the development of secondary angle-closure glaucoma due to PAS formation.[93] Neovascularization of the iris and angle causing neovascular glaucoma may also develop in these patients.[98]

The etiology of sarcoidosis is unclear and multifactorial. The immunological response might be triggered by an environmental antigen exposure in genetically predisposed individuals. Several different microorganisms, including mycobacteria, human herpes virus type 8,[99] *Propionibacterium acnes*, and *Propionibacterium granulosum*,[100] were isolated from sarcoid tissues, suggesting an infectious origin.[101] First-degree and second-degree relatives of sarcoidosis patients have an increased risk of developing sarcoidosis supporting a genetic theory.[102] A linkage was found to chromosomes 5 and 6 in sarcoidosis patients[103] as well as association to HLA-DRB1.[104]

The diagnosis of ocular sarcoidosis is made according to clinical ocular signs and ancillary investigations. In 2006, the International Workshop on Ocular Sarcoidosis[91] (IWOS) published a combined criteria based on a combination of clinical, laboratory, and histologic findings. Laboratory studies include serum angiotensin-converting enzyme (ACE), lysozyme, serum and urinary calcium, chest radiography, computed tomography scan, bronchoscopy with bronchoalveolar lavage, and gallium scan.[91] Measuring the levels of

ACE and performing whole-body gallium scan are good in diagnosing patients with clinically suspicious ocular sarcoidosis with normal chest radiographs.[105] Gallium uptake in the eye was found in one-fifth of the cases, while uptake in the lacrimal glands was found in two-thirds of cases.[105] The definitive test is biopsy, showing typical noncaseating granulomas.[91]

Effective treatment consists primarily of long-term use of corticosteroids.[93] Half of the patients with uveitis require treatment with oral corticosteroids, and another 11% required additional immunosuppressive therapy.[106] Severe systemic disease, refractory cases, or sight-threatening conditions require immunosuppressive (mainly MTX) or biological treatments.[91,101] TNF has been found to be a contributing factor in the formation of sarcoid granulomas. Infliximab, a TNF-α antagonist, has been used for refractory sarcoidosis and produced successful results, while etanercept, another TNF-α antagonist, failed to show improvement and may even precipitate the disease.[107]

Glaucoma associated with uveitis resolved with treatment of uveitis in nearly 90% of cases.[105] Glaucoma may respond well to topical corticosteroids early in the disease course, but later it may become increasingly difficult to control, especially when PAS are extensive. There is evidence showing controlled ocular inflammation following a surgical excision of iris nodules in patients with refractory granulomatous uveitis.[108] In some cases, despite extensive PAS, IOP may remain well-controlled. In this situation, topical corticosteroid treatment may cause an IOP elevation by increasing aqueous humor formation or in conjunction with a true steroid response.

Anterior uveitis is related to a better visual outcome, in comparison to multifocal choroiditis or panuveitis.[94] After 6 months, half of patients had improvement in visual acuity,[92] and after a decade, more than half of patients retained normal visual acuity.[106] Nevertheless, despite the mild nature of the uveitis, 15% of patients suffer from poor visual outcome.[93] Glaucoma is one of the risk factors for unfavorable visual prognosis.[92]

AUTOIMMUNE DISORDERS

Juvenile Idiopathic Arthritis

Juvenile idiopathic arthritis (JIA), also known as juvenile rheumatic arthritis, is the most common disorder associated with uveitis in children and usually presents as anterior uveitis. This disorder accounts for approximately 70% of all cases of juvenile arthritis.[109,110] The following are the 3 major forms:

1. Systemic-onset JIA is associated with fever, generalized lymphadenopathy, hepatosplenomegaly, pericarditis, or rash and accounts for 20% of cases

2. Polyarticular-onset JIA affects 5 or more joints within the first 3 months

3. Pauciarticular-onset JIA affects 4 or fewer joints within the first 3 months

Uveitis occurs rarely in systemic-onset JIA, in about 10% to 15% of those children with polyarticular-onset JIA, but in more than 75% of those with pauciarticular-onset JIA.[109,110] Overall, 8% to 20% of JIA pediatric patients suffer from uveitis.[111-113] This incidence also varies geographically, being highest in Scandinavia, followed by the United States, then Asia, and lowest in India.[113] In more than 60% of cases, arthritis precedes uveitis, while in about 25% they appear simultaneously, and in up to 13%, uveitis precedes arthritis.[112,114] Children who developed uveitis prior to or along with arthritis suffered from a more chronic ocular disease and high rate of complications.[112] JIA patients who develop uveitis are significantly younger at presentation than those without uveitis.[111] The average age of uveitis diagnosis is 4.5 years.[114] Female gender was not found as a risk factor for the development of uveitis among JIA patients.[111,113] Uveitis is more frequent in antinuclear antibody (ANA)-positive patients.[113]

Uveitis is bilateral in more than two-thirds of the cases.[109,110] Patients with uveitis are usually asymptomatic even when inflammation is marked; this might delay diagnosis and increases the rate of complications.[114] The uveitis is typically nongranulomatous in nature. KPs are small and frequently confined to the inferior cornea. When inflammation is marked, there may be cells in the anterior vitreous. Nearly 70% have chronic anterior uveitis, 16% acute anterior, 12% recurrent anterior, and only 3.5% panuveitis.[115] JIA is associated with a high rate of complications in adulthood like cataract, glaucoma, posterior synechiae, band keratopathy, papilledema, macular edema, and hypotonia[111-114] (Figure 42-6).

Secondary glaucoma is a major cause of vision loss in JIA and carries a poor prognosis. The rate of secondary glaucoma ranges between 5% and 33%.[113] Glaucoma is usually caused by pupillary block, although direct infiltration of outflow facility with inflammatory process was observed as well.[116]

Treatment mainly includes the use of topical cycloplegic agents and corticosteroids. Systemic corticosteroids, immunomodulating agents (like MTX and cyclosporine), and biological agents (like TNF-α antagonists) are needed in severe cases or to help reduce the use of topical corticosteroids.[111,114]

Aqueous suppressants are useful in managing glaucoma. However, systemic CAIs (as well as MTX) should be used with caution in these patients because it might interact with the NSAIDs used to treat the arthritis. Unfortunately, 9% to 30% require surgical intervention for IOP control.[114,115] Goniotomy was proved an effective and safe first-line surgery, although most patients

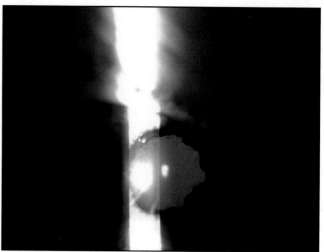

Figure 42-6. Juvenile idiopathic arthritis. Patient with a long history of anterior uveitis. Note posterior synechiae. (Reprinted with permission from Vicktoria Vishnevskia-Dai, MD.)

require antiglaucoma therapy after the surgery.[50] Nonpenetrating deep sclerectomy with the placement of collagen glaucoma drainage device was tried successfully in one report.[117] Overall, JIA-associated glaucoma outcomes with trabeculectomy are disappointing, and primary drainage device implantation is preferred by many with good long-term IOP control, even better than in other types of refractory glaucoma.[118] Trans-scleral diode cyclophotocoagulation (TD-CPC) was proved to be unsatisfactory as a primary surgical treatment.[119]

Patients with JIA need routine ophthalmic evaluation, even while their arthritis is inactive, because of the silent asymptomatic nature of the eye disease.[112,114] Parents should be educated to be aware of first signs and symptoms.[112] Secondary glaucoma is a diagnostic and therapeutic challenge, but if treated with an aggressive approach, early in the course of the disease, most patients will have a good visual prognosis. Good visual acuity was found in nearly 90% of cases, despite uveitic complications.[113,115]

Human Leukocyte Antigen-B27-Associated Uveitis

Approximately 50% of patients with acute anterior uveitis (AAU) have human leukocyte antigen (HLA)-B27 haplotype,[120,121] either when uveitis is the only disorder or when it is a part of a systemic immunological disease. The incidence of AAU in patients with HLA-B27 is between 33% and 88% depending on the population studied.[122,123]

Fifty percent to 77% of the patients with HLA-B27-associated AAU have a systemic inflammatory disorder (ie, seronegative spondyloarthropathies [SSA]).[123,124] SSA is a group of inflammatory conditions that involve the spine, sacroiliac, and shoulder joints. The disease entities are described separately in the following sections. This group has a strong genetic association to the HLA-B27 haplotype. Patients with SSA had an earlier onset of uveitis and more uveitis attacks compared to AAU patients without associated systemic disease.[124] Thirty-three percent of SSA patients develop uveitis, most commonly unilateral AAU, which is typically self-limited. This prevalence is higher in HLA-B27-positive patients and varied according to the specific SSA type. At the onset of AAU, the prevalence of HLA-B27-associated systemic disease is higher in males, but after the onset of uveitis, the risk of developing a HLA-B27-associated systemic disease has no gender discrepancy.[125]

HLA-B27-positive patients, either with or without systemic disease, have a more severe anterior chamber inflammation with hypopyon formation, higher frequency of uveitis attacks, and more complications than HLA-B27-negative patients.[126] Ocular complications include secondary glaucoma, cataract, pupillary synechiae, vitritis, cystoid macular edema, and optic disc edema.[126]

During acute inflammation, pressure is usually lowered due to ciliary body underproduction of aqueous. However, secondary glaucoma may develop due to synechial angle and pupillary closure.[120] Extensive persistent pupillary synechiae were found in one-fifth of HLA-B27-associated AAU.[126] In this study, secondary glaucoma developed in 2% of HLA-B27-associated AAU patients with no systemic disease and in 6% of patients with systemic disease. Another study[125] reported a higher rate of secondary glaucoma (11%) among 80 HLA-B27-positive uveitis patients.

The exact mechanism of HLA-B27-associated uveitis is not known. There is antigenic similarities between gram-negative bacteria, including *Helicobacter pylori* and HLA-B27.[123] HLA-B27-associated uveitis was associated with high levels of serum prolactin.[127]

The treatment of HLA-B27-positive uveitis requires more aggressive treatment than in HLA-B27-negative patients.[126] The use of periocular and systemic corticosteroid therapy is often effective.[128] Immunomodulatory therapy, such as MTX, is effective in patients resistant to conventional steroid treatment[128,129]; it may reduce recurrence of uveitic attacks when initiated within 3 years of the disease onset.[129] TNF-α antagonists, such as infliximab and etanercept, were found to be highly efficient in these cases.[128] Secondary pupillary block glaucoma is treated with peripheral iridectomy. Intracameral tissue plasminogen activator (tPA) was reported to be successful in dissolving the fibrinous membranes and in breaking the synechiae in a patient with posterior synechiae.[130]

Recurrence of severe AAU attacks occurs frequently among HLA-B27-positive patients, usually in the same eye.[122] Despite that, visual prognosis is fairly good.[121]

Ankylosing Spondylitis

Ankylosing spondylitis (AS) is the most frequent subtype of SSA. It mainly affects the spine and sacroiliac joints. The mean age at onset is 26 years. According to different reports,

14% to 33% of AS patients develop uveitis.[131,132] AS uveitis is typically a unilateral AAU. Recurrences are common, often involving the contralateral eye. Presence of AAU in AS patients is in correlation with higher disease activity and poor functional ability. Of patients with AS uveitis, HLA-B27 haplotype was detected in 36%.[133] On the other hand, among patients with HLA-B27-associated uveitis, AS was found in more than 40%, more in males than in females.[124,133]

Reactive Arthritis

Reactive arthritis, formerly termed *Reiter's syndrome*, is a multiorgan disease characterized by arthritis, conjunctivitis, and mucocutaneous lesions.[134] Reactive arthritis is precipitated by Gram-negative intestinal or genitourinary tract flora bacteria.[135] Most patients can report on a history of infection, most frequently urethritis.[134] Patients are commonly young adult males; 85% are HLA-B27-positive.[134] The risk of reactive arthritis development in HLA-B27 carriers is more than 27 times higher than the mean incidence in the general population.[136] Most patients have a positive family history.[134]

Ocular manifestations were reported in 58% of 113 reactive arthritis patients[137]; the most common manifestation is conjunctivitis with papillary reaction and mucopurulent discharge. Anterior uveitis developed in 7.8% of 254 patients and can be recurrent and chronic. Other possible manifestations are pars planitis scleritis and episclertitis.[134,137] Secondary glaucoma occurs in up to 2% of reactive arthritis patients.[136,137]

Systemic therapy with corticosteroids is typically required for intraocular inflammation control, with additional immunosuppressive therapy, mainly MTX.[134]

Inflammatory Bowel Disease-Associated Arthritis

Inflammatory bowel diseases (IBDs) include Crohn's disease and ulcerative colitis and may have extra-intestinal manifestations, mainly arthritis and ocular inflammation.

Anterior uveitis is the most common ocular manifestation in IBD. Bilateral relapsing uveitis has been reported to be synchronous with bowel relapse.[138] HLA-B27 is significantly more common in IBD patients who develop uveitis than in those who do not.[139] Secondary glaucoma may develop as a result of posterior synechiae causing pupillary block, or neovascular glaucoma due to retinal vasculitis.[138]

Treatment with topical corticosteroids, sometimes combined with systemic corticosteroids, controls the ocular inflammation.[138] Glaucoma is treated according to manifestation with peripheral iridectomy,[135] panretinal photocoagulation, or surgically.[138]

Psoriatic Arthritis

Psoriatic arthritis is a chronic inflammatory arthropathy. The prevalence of uveitis in psoriatic arthritis patients ranges between 18% and 25%[132,140] and is associated with the rate of HLA-B27.[140] Predicting factors for development of uveitis in psoriatic arthritis patients include extensive axial involvement and the HLA-DR13 antigen.[140]

The uveitis is solely anterior in almost 80% of patients, with indigos onset in two-thirds of the cases. Nearly 40% of uveitis cases are bilateral.[140] Psoriasis-associated uveitis presents at an older age and has a more prolonged course compared to idiopathic or HLA-B27-associated AAU.[141]

Oral corticosteroids are required in many cases. Many patients also require additional immunosuppressive therapy[140] and oral NSAIDs.[141]

Synovitis-Acne-Pustulosis-Hyperostosis-Ostitis Syndrome

Synovitis-acne-pustulosis-hyperostosis-ostitis (SAPHO) syndrome is considered another member of the SSA family. Clinical manifestations may include skeletal changes, mainly in the chest wall and skull, arthritis, and dermatologic involvement.[142] Cases have frequent association with sacroiliitis.[143] SAPHO syndrome was also described in association with IBD and Behçet's disease (BD).[143] Ocular complications of the syndrome include recurrent uveitis, which may induce severe secondary bilateral glaucoma.[143]

Behçet's Disease

BD, also named *Adamantiades-Behçet disease*, is a multi-organ immune-mediated vasculitis of unknown origin. The disorder is characterized by recurrent oral and/or urogenital ulcerations, skin lesions, intraocular involvement, central nervous system manifestations, arthritis, and gastrointestinal lesions.[144,145] It is rare in the United States, occurring more commonly in the Middle and Far East. At the onset of the symptoms, most patients are younger than 40 years old.[146]

Sixty percent to 80% of BD patients develop an ocular disease.[145] Most patients experience recurrent bilateral anterior uveitis, frequently with hypopyon that resolves spontaneously with little or no evidence of inflammation between attacks.[144,147] The minority of patients suffer from chronic posterior uveitis with retinal vaso-occlusive disease causing visual loss[146] (Figure 42-7). Men tend to suffer from a more severe disease with worse visual prognosis and a higher incidence of panuveitis.[144] BD might be complicated with retinal and optic atrophy, vitreous hemorrhage, neovascular glaucoma, and retinal detachment.[147]

Glaucoma was diagnosed in about 11% of eyes, either open-angle glaucoma secondary to inflammation or corticosteroid treatment (44%), angle-closure glaucoma with PAS and pupillary block (44%), or neovascular glaucoma (12%).[146]

Although the pathogenesis of the disease was not fully discovered, genetic factors play an important role. The disease has been associated with HLA-B5 and HLA-B51 alleles in populations of various ethnicities.[148] The ocular inflammation is associated with both innate immune response

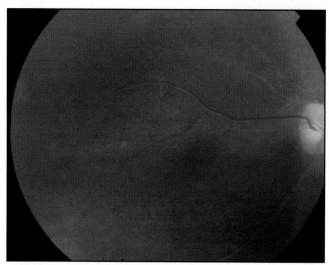

Figure 42-7. Behçet's disease: chronic posterior uveitis with retinal vaso-occlusive disease. (Reprinted with permission from Asaf Bar, MD and Susan Lightman, MD.)

(neutrophils, NK cells) and adaptive immune response (T cells).[145] Selenium-binding protein was found to be an auto-antigen in BD-associated uveitis.[149]

Treatment includes a high-dose intravenous corticosteroid, which is effective initially. Eventually, most patients require treatment with cytotoxic agents like cyclosporine, FK506, antimetabolites, or biologic drugs.[147] Biological drugs like infliximab, adalimumab, and interferon-alpha have been proven beneficial and safe in controlling BD-associated uveitis.[145]

Antiglaucoma medication is effective in some cases; laser iridotomy is recommended for angle-closure and pupillary block. However, nearly one-third of the patients required trabeculectomy, glaucoma drainage device implantation, or diode-laser cyclodestruction.[146,150] A one-year follow-up after primary trabeculectomy with MMC demonstrated a success rate of more than 80%.[151] If ocular surgery is required, complete preoperative control of inflammation is essential.[152] Using interferon-alpha, prior, during, and after vitrectomy and trabeculectomy was tried effectively.[153]

Throughout the 1990s, following the use of immunosuppressive regimens, the clinical outcome of BD has improved significantly.[154] Nevertheless, an international case series of 1465 patients with ocular disease published[144] in 2007 found that, despite modern therapy, one-quarter of the patients were legally blind.

Vogt-Koyanagi-Harada Syndrome

Vogt-Koyanagi-Harada syndrome (VKH) is a chronic systemic autoimmune disease characterized by alopecia, vitiligo, poliosis, dysacousia, and meningeal irritation. In a study of 101 patients, two-thirds of patients were female, and the mean age was 34 years, although it may present in a wide range of ages (8 to 75 years).[155] VKH is more prevalent

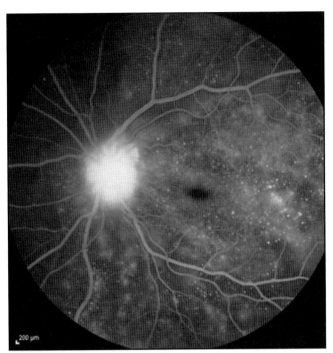

Figure 42-8. Vogt-Koyanagi-Harada syndrome. Fluorescein angiography demonstrating typical, multifocal, "starry sky" pattern of retinal pigment epithelium leakage. (Reprinted with permission from Asaf Bar, MD and Susan Lightman, MD.)

in Asian, Middle Eastern, Indian American, and Hispanic populations.[156]

Ocular involvement is characterized by granulomatous uveitis and exudative retinal detachment (Figure 42-8).[157] Half of the eyes develop at least one complication, such as cataract, glaucoma, choroidal neovascularization (CNV), and subretinal fibrosis.[155,156] Complicated cases are associated with longer disease duration and a higher number of intraocular inflammatory episodes.[155]

Glaucoma is a common complication in VKH, occurring in 27% to 33% of patients. In a study of 16 patients with VKH glaucoma, 56% had open-angle, and 44% closed-angle glaucoma.[158] Angle-closure glaucoma is often secondary to uveal effusion with forward displacement of the lens-iris diaphragm, which may be acute and cause extensive PAS formation.[159,160] Ultrasound biomicroscopy (UBM) demonstrates swelling of the ciliary body and supraciliary space with anterior rotation of the ciliary body.[161] Similar findings were described with anterior segment optical coherence tomography (AS-OCT).[162]

The autoimmune process responsible for the disease is directed against melanocytes-associated antigen.[156] There is a genetic contribution as well; several HLA-DQB1 alleles were associated with VKH.[163] On histopathologic examination, there is a nonnecrotizing diffuse granulomatous panuveitis and formation of Dalen-Fuchs' nodules. Choriocapillaris are spared initially but are involved later.[164]

VKH treatment includes initial high-dose intravenous corticosteroid therapy followed by prolonged oral corticosteroid treatment.[164] Other immunosuppressive therapy, such as cyclosporine or cytotoxic agents, may be required.[156,164] In a report on adjunctive oral MTX in refractory pediatric cases, MTX was shown to be safe and effective in controlling inflammation.

Nearly one-third of glaucoma cases can be controlled medically with systemic corticosteroids,[165] cycloplegics, and aqueous suppressants. Two-thirds require surgical treatment by iridectomy, trabeculectomy, or glaucoma drainage device implantation.[158] In cases where there are multiple complications, such as severe cataracts and secondary glaucoma, a one-stage procedure including pars plana lensectomy-vitrectomy and peripheral anterior synechiolysis is optional. Following the procedure, IOP control was achieved with timolol only in all 6 operated eyes.[166]

Pediatric cases present with an aggressive course,[166] although their visual prognosis is usually favorable.[167] Overall, nearly 60% of patients retained 20/30 vision or better.[164] Prognostic factors associated with a worse visual prognosis include multiple complications, older age at onset, worse acuity at presentation, delayed treatment, recurrence of inflammation, and use of intravenous corticosteroids.[155,167]

Sympathetic Ophthalmia

Fortunately rare but potentially devastating, sympathetic ophthalmia (SO) occurs weeks to months after trauma or ocular surgery, mainly pars plana vitrectomy and cyclodestructive procedures,[168] and causes a bilateral nonnecrotizing, granulomatous uveitis.[168] More than 70% of patients are male,[168,169] with an average patient age of 30 to 46 years in different reports.[168,169]

Most patients present with reduced vision, redness, and photophobia.[168,170] More than one-quarter of SO patients have a visual acuity (VA) of 20/200 or worse at presentation, with further vision loss to 20/200 or worse at a rate of 10% per person-year.[171] In more than half of patients, only fundus lesions are evident, mainly exudative retinal detachment, yellowish-white mid-peripheral lesions (Dalen-Fuchs' nodules), papilledema, vasculitis, peripapillary choroidal neovascularization, and choroidal scarring.[172] The pathology is similar to that seen in VKH syndrome, although chorioretinal scarring is less severe here. Recurrence, mainly in the anterior segment, occurs in 30% of eyes, even years after the resolution of the initial episode.[169,172]

Secondary glaucoma developed in more than 40% of cases in one study.[173] The glaucoma mechanism is unclear, though plasma cell infiltration of the iris and ciliary body was found in many SO biopsy samples.[173]

SO is caused by bilateral autoimmune hypersensitivity reaction against exposed ocular antigens, possibly found on choroidal melanocytes, in the injured eye.[168] Photoreceptor mitochondrial oxidative stress mediated by iNOS and TNF-α was found in SO, which might lead to photoreceptor apoptosis and subsequent decreased visual outcome.[174] HLA-DR15 has been associated with SO.[175]

Treatment includes oral or high-dose intravenous corticosteroid, sub-Tenon dexamethasone, intravitreal corticosteroid treatments, or immunomodulator therapy.[168,170,171] Intravitreal fluocinolone slow-release device was found to be an effective and safe alternative to multiple intravitreal triamcinolone injections in chronic SO.[176] Although enucleation of the injured exciting eye before the disease develops in the contralateral sympathizing eye is the only known prevention of SO, this remains a controversial procedure and is not justified in most cases.[172,177] The glaucoma is difficult to treat, requiring frequent adjustments of corticosteroid therapy and possible glaucoma surgery.[172]

Despite the high ocular complication rate in the sympathizing eye, 50% of patients regain a VA better than 20/40 after a decade.[169,177] Prompt and aggressive therapy is key in obtaining a good visual prognosis. Poor visual prognosis is associated with complications such as glaucoma, chorioretinal macular scars, and exudative retinal detachment.[171,177]

Systemic Lupus Erythematosus

Systemic lupus erythematosus (SLE) is an autoimmune disorder involving multiple organs. It is more prevalent in females. The prevalence of SLE in patients with uveitis varies in the literature from 0.1% to 4.8%.[178-180]

Ocular involvement in SLE patients is fairly common, consisting of mostly dry eye syndrome, and is found in 31% of patients. Steroid-related complications like bilateral subcapsular cataract and glaucoma are also prevalent, up to 21% and 2.9%, respectively.[181,182] Nearly all parts of the eye and visual pathways might be involved by inflammation or thrombus.[182] Possible sight-threatening manifestations include uveitis, optic neuritis, ischemic optic neuropathy, scleritis, episcleritis, and retinopathy.[182] Retinopathy can manifest as drusen, retinal pigment epithelium atrophy, vascular changes, macular chorioretinitis scar, or branch retinal vein occlusion.[181]

Several mechanisms were described as causing glaucoma: bilateral uveal effusions,[183] posterior scleritis causing angle-closure glaucoma,[184] as well as open-angle glaucoma.[185] In patients with antiphospholipid antibodies, retinal vascular occlusive disease may result in neovascular glaucoma.[182]

Anterior uveitis, as well as episcleritis and dry eyes, are commonly treated topically, whereas scleritis and severe retinopathy require systemic therapy ranging from NSAIDs to corticosteroids and other immunosuppressive agents.[182] Vaso-occlusive disease is treated with anticoagulation and laser photocoagulation.[182]

Treatment of glaucoma requires antiglaucoma medications in addition to inflammation control. In refractory cases, sclerectomies and choroidal drainage were reported as effective.[183] Glaucoma secondary to scleritis was treated with corticosteroids and antiglaucoma therapy, with a good response.[184]

Multiple Sclerosis

Multiple sclerosis (MS) is a chronic autoimmune disease with inflammatory demyelinization of the central nervous system.[186] Fifteen percent to 40% of MS patients develop uveitis, although more than half of them are asymptomatic.[187] The uveitis preceded the onset of MS in 25% to 56% of cases.[188,189]

The most common form of uveitis is pars planitis. The next most common form is granulomatous anterior uveitis, characterized by development of extensive posterior synechiae and large mutton fat KPs.[187] The uveitis is bilateral in almost all cases.[188] Complications of uveitis include cataracts, symptomatic vitritis, occlusive peripheral retinal vasculitis with neovascularization, macular edema, and epiretinal macular membrane.[187] Glaucoma was found in 15% of patients with MS uveitis.[187]

Uveitis treatment includes systemic corticosteroids and immunosuppressive treatment.[187,189] Glaucoma is treated with aqueous suppressants and trabeculectomy with antimetabolites as needed. In a study[187] describing 5 operated eyes, 60% achieved normal IOP with surgery alone, whereas the rest needed additional antiglaucoma medication for IOP control.

Visual prognosis is fairly good in treated patients.[188] More than 80% of patients had the same or better VA during follow-up.[189]

INFECTIOUS DISEASES

Viral Infections

Herpes Virus Family

The herpes virus family includes 8 human herpes viruses—herpes simplex virus type 1 (HSV-1), type 2 (HSV-2), varicella zoster virus (VZV), cytomegalovirus (CMV) Epstein-Barr virus (EBV), human herpes virus type 6 (HHV6), type 7 (HHV7), and type 8 (HHV8). Several of these DNA viruses may cause ocular manifestations, including keratitis, uveitis, and secondary glaucoma.[190]

Herpes Simplex Virus Ocular involvement in HSV infection may include conjunctivitis, keratitis, and uveitis. HSV keratouveitis is often accompanied by IOP elevation and secondary glaucoma.[191] HSV uveitis might present without keratitis. In these cases, the uveitis is more severe than uveitis with previous corneal involvement and results in a worse glaucoma.[192]

In different reports, 28% to 54% of patients with ocular HSV developed increased IOP, mostly with corneal disciform or stromal disease[193-195] (Figure 42-9). Increased IOP is usually related to obstruction of the TM by trabeculitis or

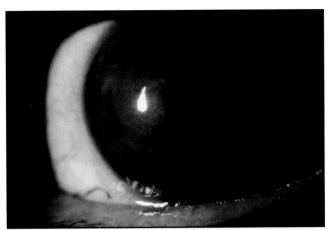

Figure 42-9. Herpes simplex stromal keratitis. Note corneal disciform keratitis. (Reprinted with permission from Haggay Avizemer, MD.)

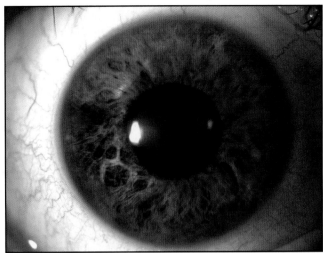

Figure 42-10. Herpes zoster keratouveitis. Note large areas of iris atrophy from iridocyclitis. (Reprinted with permission from Vicktoria Vishnevskia-Dai, MD.)

inflammatory debris.[196] HSV-1 was found to have the ability to enter and produce infection of the TM, through a receptor named herpes virus entry mediator (HVEM).[197] A rabbit model of herpetic uveitis showed biphasic elevation of IOP. The primary uveitis is caused by the active HSV infection of uveal tissue during the first few days, whereas the secondary uveitis derives from immunological mechanisms.[198] A devastating condition consisting of anterior segment ischemia secondary to chronic keratouveitis has been reported.[199] In these cases, severe secondary angle-closure glaucoma developed due to extensive corneoscleral and intraocular inflammation that was unresponsive to maximal medical therapy.

HSV type 1 is the dominant causative agent of herpetic uveitis, although there are reports of keratouveitis caused by HSV type 2.[200,201] Diagnosis of HSV keratouveitis can be confirmed by polymerase chain reaction (PCR) from the aqueous humor.[193]

Treatment of herpetic uveitis is complex and involves close monitoring and balance between antiviral and anti-inflammatory therapy. Treatment includes inhibiting activation of the virus with antiviral therapy in conjunction with topical corticosteroids in tapered doses and aqueous suppressants.[191] Long-term prophylaxis with oral antiviral medications is effective in preventing recurrences.[193,202] Periocular and systemic corticosteroids are required more frequently in HSV patients in comparison to VZV patients.[194] Filtration surgery is rarely required.[191,193]

Herpes Zoster Herpes zoster ophthalmicus involves the ophthalmic division of the fifth cranial nerve. The infection usually manifests with typical cutaneous vesicular eruptions, yet ocular involvement may present without zoster dermatitis (zoster sine herpete).[203] Fifty percent to 70% of herpes zoster ophthalmicus patients develop some form of ocular involvement like keratitis, uveitis, secondary glaucoma, scleritis, and ocular nerve palsy.[204] Two-thirds of patients have a single episode of uveitis, while one-third have a chronic relapsing course of uveitis.[204] Ocular involvement typically

occurs 1 to 2 weeks after the appearance of the skin lesions. In these cases, the ipsilateral eye demonstrates anterior chamber cells and flare, often with associated KPs. The KPs tend to become dark with pigment. Usually, there is inconspicuous localized irregularity of the corneal epithelium at the onset of ocular involvement, but later, deep keratitis may develop, and the zoster virus can cause dendritic ulcers resembling those of herpes simplex. The stroma of the iris in the affected eye may develop one or more gray atrophic patches that transilluminate (Figure 42-10). This presumably results from virus-induced arteritis that causes ischemic necrosis of the iris stroma and posterior pigmented epithelium. Fluorescein iris angiography demonstrates areas of abnormal leakage of iris blood vessels.

More than half of the patients with keratouveitis develop elevated IOP.[194,204] The IOP may rise to 30 to 50 mm Hg, with the angle remaining open. Obstruction to aqueous outflow causes glaucoma and it is generally reversible. Formation of PAS is uncommon but may appear.

The uveitis is caused by infiltration of VZV-reactive T cells.[205] VZV uveitis is confirmed by PCR demonstrating VZV-DNA in the aqueous humor. Immunohistological test can detect VZV antigen in the iris.[206]

Early treatment with antiviral therapy lowers the risk of serious inflammatory complications.[207] In addition to antiviral therapy, corticosteroids are used for inflammation and aqueous suppressants are used for reduction of IOP. Cycloplegic medications may be useful to relieve ciliary pain and, if significant inflammation exists, to prevent formation of posterior synechiae. Treatment for uveitis and secondary glaucoma is usually necessary for several months, but it may be required indefinitely. If the IOP remains high despite maximal medical treatment, a filtering operation may be required.

Cytomegalovirus CMV can cause unilateral anterior uveitis in immunocompetent patients, mainly in a chronic form, but also recurrent granulomatous uveitis was described.[208-210] CMV was also reported as the cause of anterior uveitis in an acquired immune deficiency syndrome (AIDS) patient with CMV retinitis, characterized by acute inflammatory cell infiltration with cytomegalic cells.[211]

Increased IOP and glaucoma were reported secondary to keratouveitis with a median IOP of 30 mm Hg.[208,209,212] Some of the glaucoma patients have iris atrophy and hypopigmentation of the anterior chamber angle compared to the fellow eye.[208,212]

Diagnosis of CMV uveitis is confirmed by PCR detection of CMV-DNA and anti-CMV antibodies in the aqueous humor.[208] There is a correlation between the inflammatory activity and the number of virus copies in the aqueous humor.[210]

Treatment includes topical corticosteroids, antiglaucoma medications, and usually additional oral valganciclovir with good control of the inflammation and IOP.[208,212] Systemic ganciclovir was also reported as effective,[213] as well as intravitreal ganciclovir injection as a loading dose with or without the following oral valganciclovir.[214] Relapsing cases require maintenance with valganciclovir. In one report,[209] 1 of 5 patients needed glaucoma surgery despite medical treatment.

Epstein-Barr Virus EBV uveitis is characterized by bilateral severe acute anterior uveitis with fibrinous exudates or granulomatous anterior uveitis in the chronic stage. In the posterior segment, there is little vitreous inflammation, disc edema with hyperemia, and early depigmentation of the fundus.

Patients with uveitis have elevated antibody titers to EBV compared to normal controls, suggesting that uveitis might be correlated with EBV reactivation.[215] The existence of EBV-DNA can be detected in ocular fluids by PCR analysis.[216]

EBV uveitis usually responds well to steroid treatment but has common recurrence; nevertheless, final visual acuity is usually good.[217]

Acute Retinal Necrosis Acute retinal necrosis (ARN) syndrome, also known as Kirisawa's uveitis, is characterized by severe diffuse uveitis, retinal vasculitis, and retinal necrosis,[218,219] usually bilaterally[219] (Figure 42-11). It is caused by the herpes virus family, including HSV type 1, VZV,[218] CMV, EBV,[219] and less frequently HSV-2.[220] It usually affects immunocompetent patients[219] but can also affect immunocompromised individuals.[221]

Glaucoma is not common.[222] It can appear as both open-angle glaucoma in association with mild anterior chamber inflammation or as angle closure due to iris bombé. In several cases, despite secondary angle closure, the IOP can be normal or low due to damage to the ciliary body and reduced aqueous production.

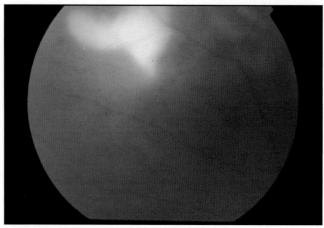

Figure 42-11. Acute retinal necrosis. Note the gray area of retinal necrosis. (Reprinted with permission from Asaf Bar, MD and Susan Lightman, MD.)

Diagnosis is confirmed by PCR detection of viral DNA in intraocular specimens.[218]

The treatment of ARN includes intravenous acyclovir, corticosteroids, and aspirin. Intravenous acyclovir is followed by oral acyclovir for 14 weeks for the prevention of contralateral involvement.[219]

Acquired Immune Deficiency Syndrome

AIDS is a disorder caused by the human immunodeficiency virus (HIV) and characterized by severe immunocompromisation. Patients are subject to opportunistic infections, many of which involve the eye, most commonly CMV retinitis.[223] Other possible infections are herpes simplex and zoster, syphilis, toxoplasma gondii, tuberculosis (TB), pneumocystis carinii, histoplasma capsulatum, candida, and others.[224,225]

Anterior uveitis is a very common sign of AIDS, affecting more than half of patients and responsible for one-third of cases with decreased visual acuity.[226,227] Mild anterior uveitis is often the result of a herpes simplex and zoster infection, unlike severe inflammation evident in toxoplasmosis retinochoroiditis and syphilis chorioretinitis.[228] Several antiretroviral medications, such as cidofovir, rifabutin, nevirapine, and indinavir, are also a frequent cause of anterior uveitis.[223]

The most commonly described glaucoma affecting AIDS patients has been acute bilateral angle closure secondary to anterior uveal effusion with secondary anterior rotation of the ciliary body.[229,230] Clinically, mild central shallowing with prominent peripheral shallowing are evident.[229] Diagnosis can be confirmed with ultrasound, demonstrating the ciliochoroidal effusion.[229,230] The glaucoma is treated with cycloplegic agents to retract the iris lens diaphragm, corticosteroids, and aqueous suppressants.[229] Miotics exacerbate this form of angle closure and are, therefore, contraindicated. Drainage of suprachoroidal fluid may be required.

Immune recovery uveitis (IRU) is a condition where intraocular inflammation caused by a response to a latent infectious antigen (mainly CMV but also toxoplasma or TB) appears within weeks from the start of highly active antiretroviral therapy (HAART).[223,228] It always affects only a previously infected eye. Complications include retinal neovascularization or posterior synechiae and iris bombé causing acute angle-closure glaucoma. Treatment includes topical and periocular steroids and peripheral iridectomy for the treatment of glaucoma.[231]

Congenital Rubella Syndrome

Rubella infection within the first trimester of pregnancy in nonimmunized pregnant women is associated with a high incidence of ophthalmic, auditory, and cardiac anomalies, as well as psychomotor and mental retardation, endocrine disorders, hematologic disorders, and a wide variety of other manifestations.[232] The age-adjusted prevalence of the syndrome was 73.2 per million in Omani patients younger than 20 years of age, with an incidence of 0.6 per 1000 live births.[233]

The ocular complications of congenital rubella are bilateral in nearly 90% of cases.[234] Possible complications are cataract, micro-ophthalmia, pigmentary retinopathy, and glaucoma.[232-234] Congenital glaucoma was found in 6.25% to 29% of patients with congenital rubella syndrome.[232,233,235,236] Glaucoma is significantly correlated with micro-ophthalmia and cataract,[232] contradicting previous impressions suggesting no correlation between cataract and glaucoma.[237]

The glaucoma can present in different forms depending on the mechanism. Infantile type can develop secondary to micro-ophthalmic eyes causing angle closure, angle anomalies, or anterior uveitis. Usually, the anterior chamber shows little evidence of active inflammation. However, in some cases, there are KP signaling an inflammatory component to the glaucoma with open angle on gonioscopy.[238] Aphakic glaucoma typically has a late onset, months to years following cataract surgery.[232,236]

The glaucoma seen in congenital rubella patients is frequently severe and difficult to manage. Glaucoma may present with acute exacerbations of IOP elevation that initially respond to medical treatment of aqueous humor suppressants and topical steroids. These acute exacerbations may be followed by long periods of good IOP control. In most of these patients, control of glaucoma proves increasingly difficult and ultimately requires surgical intervention. The main surgical procedure is goniotomy, and usually patients require repeat glaucoma surgeries.[232]

Visual prognosis, despite medical and surgical progress, is poor. In one study, 8 of 15 children were blinded by glaucoma.[239] Prevention is the main goal. Vaccination significantly reduced the prevalence of this syndrome in the past 4 decades.[240]

Human T-Lymphotropic Virus Type I Uveitis

The human T-lymphotropic virus type I (HTLV-1) is a prevalent infection in some parts of the world, mostly in Japan, Africa, the Caribbean Islands, and South America, where more than 1% of the general population is infected.[241,242] This human RNA retrovirus has been associated with several conditions, including neurological conditions such as HTLV-1-associated myelopathy/tropical spastic paraparesis (HAM/TSP)[243]; hematological disorders such as adult T cell leukemia/lymphoma (ATLL)[244]; endocrine diseases such as Graves' disease[243]; and infective dermatitis.[242]

The rate of reported ocular involvement in patients infected by HTLV-1 varies. In Japan, a high proportion (4% to 17.1%) of cases of uveitis are related to HTLV-1 uveitis (HU).[241] Among asymptomatic HTLV-1 carriers in Brazil, the incidence of HU is under 2%.[245] Females are affected twice as often as males.

Ocular manifestations include uveitis, retinal degeneration, neuro-ophthalmic disorders, and keratoconjunctivitis sicca.[246] Nearly 80% of patients with HU have intermediate uveitis, presenting with floaters and vision that is foggy and blurry.[243] A relapsing course appears in half of the patients; the interval varies between 2 weeks and a decade.[243,246] In approximately 60% of cases, the disease is unilateral.[246] Nearly 45% of patients develop complications like cataract and persistent vitreous opacity. Secondary glaucoma develops in 14% to 16% of patients with HU.[243,247]

The uveitis is probably caused by virus-infected T cells that produce inflammatory cytokines, such as IL 2, 6, and 8, TNF-α, and interferon gamma. HTLV-1 carriers with uveitis show antibodies against HTLV-I in the aqueous humor.[248]

Most cases of uveitis reach complete resolution within a month or 2 of treatment with topical or systemic corticosteroids. Yet, up to half of patients suffer from recurrence.[246] Recent reports, contradicting the earlier impression, suggest that the disease is associated with poor visual prognosis due to severe ocular complications.[246]

West Nile Virus

The West Nile virus is frequent worldwide and is usually asymptomatic or causes a self-limiting febrile illness with malaise, myalgia, nausea, vomiting, headache, rash, lymphadenopathy, and rare neurological complications.[249,250]

The majority of patients with ocular involvement experience floaters or decreased vision.[250,251] Ocular findings include anterior uveitis, vitritis, multifocal chorioretinitis, retinal vasculitis, optic neuritis, choroidal neovascularization, and VI nerve palsy.[250,251] The anterior uveitis is nongranulomatous and might cause an IOP elevation.[250] Ocular involvement is usually self-limiting, and treatment is targeted against specific manifestation, with most patients regaining their VA.[249]

Dengue Fever

Dengue fever (DF) is endemic worldwide and may cause headache, myalgia, thrombocytopenia, purpuric rash, and hypotension in severe cases.[249] Ocular manifestations were present in 7.1% of 1686 of DF patients.[252]

Onset of visual symptoms coincided with the nadir of serum thrombocytopenia.[253]

Ophthalmologic manifestations include subconjunctival hemorrhage, dengue maculopathy with macular edema, hemorrhages and cotton wool spots, retinal vasculitis, exudative retinal detachment, and anterior uveitis.[249,253] The uveitis, observed in 7.7% of patients with ocular involvement, is mostly solely anterior and might appear a few months after the acute stage of the disease.[252,254] Secondary glaucoma due to synechiae is not uncommon and can present bilaterally.[252,255,256]

Treatment includes topical, periocular, systemic steroids and immune globulins with variable success.[252,254] Antiglaucoma treatment is administrated if needed.[252] The prognosis of postdengue uveitis is good.[252,253]

Chikungunya Fever

Chikungunya virus is prevalent in Africa and Asia, causing a disease characterized by acute fever, crippling arthralgia, rash, and myalgia.

Ocular manifestations include acute granulomatous and nongranulomatous anterior uveitis, dendritic lesions, retinitis, nodular episcleritis, and optic neuritis.[257,258] Posterior synechiae are not common.[249,258,259] IOP elevation with open angles was found in 33% of the patients in a small study.[259] Chikungunya fever is a benign and self-limiting disease. The uveitis is also transient and resolved with topical corticosteroids and topical antiglaucoma treatment with preservation of good vision.[249,257-259]

Hemorrhagic Fever With Renal Syndrome

Hemorrhagic fever with renal syndrome (HFRS) is caused by several Hantavirus subtypes, including Puumala, Seoul, Hantaan, and Dobrava viruses, according to the geographical location. The disease is characterized by fever, nausea, headache, abdominal pain, proteinuria, oliguria, hematuria, and uremia.[260,261] Nearly half of 29 patients studied with acute-phase HFRS suffered from ocular involvement.[262]

Ocular HFRS includes eyelid edema, chemosis, anterior uveitis, retinal edema, anisocoria, and transient myopia (due to a forward movement of the ocular anterior diaphragm and thickening of the lens).[261,262] Acute anterior uveitis was present in 13.5% of patients.[263]

There are reports of acute angle-closure glaucoma in HFRS patients that can be bilateral.[262] Some cases are due to anterior uveitis with posterior synechiae. In some patients, angle-closure glaucoma appears with retinal edema

or corneal edema.[260,264,265] In these cases, vascular abnormality causes edema and hemorrhage in the ciliary body with anterolateral rotation and anterior movement of the lens.[260,261] However, in most cases, shallowing of the anterior chamber and narrowing of the anterior chamber angle does not cause acute angle-closure attack but a decrease in IOP.[262,263,266] Ultrasound scanning demonstrated narrowing of the anterior chamber in nearly 95% of eyes and thickening of the lens in more than 85% during the acute phase of the disease.[263]

The acute glaucoma resolved rapidly with topical cycloplegic and corticosteroid treatment.[260,261] Acetazolamide should not be used because of the risk of metabolic acidosis.[265]

Mumps

A rare complication of mumps is unilateral painless interstitial keratitis and uveitis.[267] Mumps infection can rarely also cause transient secondary glaucoma with little or no sign of anterior uveitis except for redness of the eye.[268] There is also a report[268] on 2 cases of anterior uveitis following combined vaccination for measles, mumps, and rubella.[269] Short treatment with topical corticosteroids and oral acetazolamide normalized the IOP.

Adenovirus

Adenovirus type 10 was reported as the cause of bilateral keratoconjunctivouveitis following pharyngitis, with transient elevated IOP.[270]

Bacterial Infections

Tuberculosis

The prevalence of ocular involvement in TB patients varies from 0.5% to 1.4%.[271] Ocular TB usually involves the anterior segment of the eye with keratitis, anterior uveitis, and conjunctival granulomas, but can also present with intermediate uveitis, panuveitis, scleritis, choroidal granulomas, subretinal abscesses, or optic neuritis.[271] Only a very few cases present with mutton fat KPs or anterior chamber granulomas.[272] Glaucoma might develop in chronic cases due to posterior synechiae and pupillary block.[273] Glaucoma also was described in an acute panuveitis case.[274]

Diagnosis of TB uveitis is based on a purified protein derivative (PPD) skin test, the detection of mycobacterium TB, or its DNA in ocular fluids or tissues, with staining, culture, histopathological analysis, or interferon gamma assay. Positive ocular response to anti-TB therapy supports the diagnosis.[275]

Anterior uveitis is treated with topical corticosteroids and cycloplegics,[276] combined with anti-TB therapy. This controls inflammation and IOP and reduces the recurrence of uveitis episodes.[277-279] Laser iridectomy is safe and effective for therapeutic and prophylactic purposes in chronic TB uveitis with glaucoma.[280]

The use of Bacille-Calmette-Guérin (BCG) intravesical injection[276] or vaccine[281] has been reported to cause anterior uveitis, probably due to autoimmune reaction. This is caused by similarity between proteins of BCG, mycobacterium TB, and retinal antigens.[276,281]

Hansen's Disease

Multibacillary Hansen's disease (HD), or leprosy, is a chronic granulomatous condition that involves the eye and ocular adnexa, the skin, and peripheral nerves.[282] HD remains a significant cause of preventable blindness in developing nations worldwide.[283] Ocular leprosy is rarely seen in developed countries, yet immigration from endemic areas has increased the incidence of HD. Leprosy uveitis is a common finding in HD and a major cause of blindness in patients with ocular disease.[284] The overall blindness rate in Nigerian HD patients was 8.7%, nearly 10-fold the local population rate.[285]

Sight-threatening complications include corneal anesthesia, lagophthalmos causing exposure keratopathy, uveitis, scleritis, and chorioretinal lesions.[285-287] Uveitis may occur acutely (plastic iridocyclitis) or may be chronic. The iris may have ciliary or nodular lepromata (nodules).[288] Low-grade anterior uveitis is common and requires periodic examinations for detection.[284]

Glaucoma was diagnosed in 10% of 193 American HD-treated patients. Uveitis, causing open-angle glaucoma or chronic angle-closure glaucoma, was the cause of glaucoma in most patients.[289] Other studies report on lower rates of secondary glaucoma.[286,287] In 15% of 72 patients with early HD, the IOP was lower than 7 mm Hg, and 60% of these patients exhibit postural changes in IOP.[290] This may result from early ocular autonomic neuropathy causing reduction in aqueous humor production or increase in uveoscleral outflow.[290] Untreated chronic plastic iridocyclitis also significantly lowers IOP.[291]

Diagnosis is made by biopsies of iris and aqueous humor. In addition to skin biopsies, these biopsies demonstrate the causative acid-fast bacilli, *Mycobacterium leprae*.[292]

Combined treatment with dapsone, corticosteroids, and rifampin achieved resolution of the uveitis.[288] Unfortunately, even patients who have completed their multidrug HD treatment suffer from poor ocular outcome. It is important to check patients routinely for IOP elevation and low-grade uveitis to prevent the ocular damage before it becomes irreversible.[284,285,289]

Cat Scratch Disease

Cat scratch disease, caused by *Bartonella henselae*, is a common and self-limiting infection characterized by fever and lymphadenopathy.[293]

Ocular involvement includes Parinaud's oculoglandular conjunctivitis, panuveitis, neuroretinitis with papillitis, macular edema, multiple foci of retinal vasculitis, and diffuse choroidal thickening. KPs are typically large and nonpigmented.[293] There are 2 reports of glaucoma: one case of neovascular glaucoma due to central retinal artery and vein occlusion[294] and one case of glaucoma secondary to uveitis.[295] Uveitis can precede the appearance of typical neuroretinitis by a long period and a high level of suspicion is needed.[296] Interestingly, the frequency of HLA-B27 in patients with positive *B. henselae* uveitis is higher than in the general population.[297]

Diagnosis is confirmed with serological tests.[296] Immunodetection and molecular detection of the organism can be done from the aqueous humor and vitreous as well.[298] Treatment by fluoroquinolone or macrolide combined with uveitis treatment with topical corticosteroids and cycloplegic agents resulted in complete resolution.[293,296,299]

Brucellosis

Brucellosis, caused by the gram-negative bacteria *Brucella melitensis*, has been eradicated successfully from many countries; yet, endemic regions still exist in developing countries.[300] Brucellosis symptoms include fever, arthralgia, hepatomegaly, splenomegaly, anorexia, and weight loss.[301]

Ocular brucellosis presents in up to one-fifth of brucellosis patients in accordance to their geographical location.[302] The most common ocular manifestation is uveitis (in 83%), mainly anterior uveitis, followed by choroiditis and panuveitis. Papilledema and retinal hemorrhages were found in less than 10% of patients.[302] Patients may suffer from recurrent attacks of uveitis that is resistant to corticosteroid therapy.[300]

The diagnosis of brucellosis is based on clinical criteria, positive agglutination titers, and blood cultures.[301,302] Intraocular serological tests may be helpful in the diagnosis of ocular brucellosis.[303] Treatment includes 2 months of systemic antibiotics, such as tetracycline and streptomycin, and topical or systemic corticosteroids.[302]

Meningococcemia

Endophthalmitis and anterior uveitis are rare complications of meningococcemia.[304,305] The anterior chamber typically has fibrinous exudate and multiple posterior synechiae.[304,305] Glaucoma may develop secondary to outflow obstruction by inflammation. In addition to antibiotic therapy, topical steroids and cycloplegic agents lead to resolution of ocular inflammation.[304,305]

Listeria Monocytogenes

Listeria monocytogenes-induced endophthalmitis (LMIE) is a rare condition; there are about 30 reported cases worldwide.[306,307] LMIE may present with uveitis, iris pigment epithelial detachment, and iris tissue changes. The release of iris pigment produces a dark hypopyon and highly elevated IOP.[306,308] UBM scan can demonstrate iris pigment epithelial detachment.[308] Microbiological cultures and PCR analysis of aqueous humor sampling confirm the diagnosis.[306-308] Treatment included anterior chamber lavage and intravitreal, systemic, and topical antibiotics.[306] Pars plana vitrectomy might be necessary.[307] Treatment leads to a significant improvement in inflammation, IOP control, and recovery of visual acuity.[306-308]

Whipple Disease

Whipple disease is a rare systemic infectious disorder that involves the gastrointestinal system and may present with weight loss, diarrhea, abdominal pain, and arthralgia. In the eye, acute posterior uveitis, leading to the development of uveitis-induced neovascular glaucoma as well as superficial punctate keratitis, was reported.[309,310] Diagnosis is confirmed by PCR analysis of small bowel biopsy, immunohistochemistry, or electron microscopy, detecting the causative bacteria, *Tropheryma whippelii.*[309]

Spirochetal Infections

Syphilis

Syphilis is one of the leading types of uveitis associated with secondary glaucoma.[41] Glaucoma is associated most commonly with congenital syphilis but also in the acquired form of the disease (Figure 42-12).

Interstitial keratitis occurs in about 15% of cases of congenital syphilis. The onset of symptoms is usually in the first 2 decades of life and consists of lacrimation and photophobia and is usually bilateral. Vascularization of the deep layers of the cornea, corneal infiltrates, and anterior uveitis is typically present. Glaucoma can develop in congenital syphilis during attacks of acute interstitial keratitis or soon after the inflammation has subsided. With the advent of early diagnosis and treatment of syphilis, patients with acute interstitial keratitis and secondary glaucoma are rare today.

The common sequelae of interstitial keratitis include ghost vessels in the deeper layers of the cornea, PAS, irregular pigmentation of the open portions of the anterior chamber angle, and chorioretinal atrophy.[311] Late secondary glaucoma in these patients can present with deep-chamber or angle-closure type in about equal frequency.[311] In patients with the deep-chamber type of glaucoma, there are no signs of active inflammation. In the angle, there are varying amounts of old synechiae combined with portions of dirty appearance open angle. The IOP in most cases is higher than one would anticipate from the extent of visible synechiae. Glaucoma may be present in one or both eyes. Commonly, there is glaucomatous damage in the optic discs and visual fields at the time of diagnosis. The pathology of this condition is probably endothelialization of open portions of the angle and formation of an impermeable membrane.[311] Additionally, there have been reports of iridoschisis and glaucoma in patients with luetic interstitial keratitis.[312,313] In patients with angle-closure

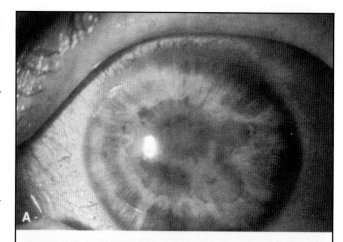
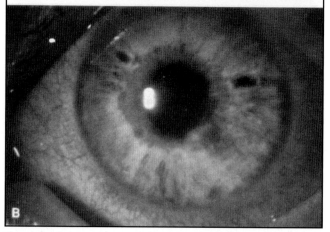

Figure 42-12. Acute anterior uveitis with iris bombé in a patient with secondary syphilis. (A) On presentation, the patient had intense anterior chamber reaction, iris bombé, and high IOP. (B) Marked improvement in patient 3 days after medical treatment for secondary syphilis and laser iridectomies for iris bombé. (Reprinted with permission from Glenn J. Jaffe, MD.)

late secondary glaucoma, the eyes characteristically have small anterior segments, possibly as a consequence of the childhood disease. The portions of the angle that are open are subject to reversible closure by forward movement of the iris, as in primary angle-closure glaucoma. The onset of angle-closure glaucoma is occasionally acute, but more often is subacute.

Young adult cases with acquired syphilis may present with active anterior uveitis and secondary glaucoma. Raised IOP during the acute phase of inflammation was reported in 14% to 18% of patients with syphilis uveitis.[3,314] Glaucoma can also develop due to posterior synechiae in patients with chronic inflammation.[314]

Diagnosis includes dark field examination of aqueous humor detecting *Treponema pallidum* and is confirmed by immunofluorescence.[315] Modalities such as enzyme immunoassays and PCR are useful in detecting intraocular *Treponema pallidum.*[316] CSF analysis is needed in syphilitic uveitis patients to exclude associated neurosyphilis.[316] Syphilis uveitis patients should be tested for HIV as HIV and syphilis have similar risk factors, and uveitis is a common manifestation of syphilis in HIV-positive patients.[316]

Treatment of all stages of uveitis includes systemic penicillin (parenteral penicillin G) or oral tetracycline in cases of penicillin allergy.[315,316] Treatment of congenital syphilitic keratitis usually includes topical corticosteroids and cycloplegics. A report describes a successful treatment of a pediatric case with a combination of immunosuppressive therapy (oral cyclosporine) and oral low-dose corticosteroids, with no recurrences of uveitis.[317]

In most cases of the deep-chamber type of glaucoma, there is a poor response to medical treatment, and a filtering operation is required. The results of filtering operations appear to be as good as in POAG. In patients with late secondary angle-closure glaucoma, if the closure is mostly appositional and reversible, peripheral iridectomy is curative. With extensive synechial closure, a filtering operation is indicated. In cases of acute inflammatory IOP elevation that is associated with active acquired uveitis, antiglaucoma medications and topical corticosteroids are highly effective.[314]

Lyme Disease

Lyme borreliosis is a worldwide multisystem disease, caused by the spirochete *Borrelia burgdorferi*.[318,319] Lyme disease presents with dermatological and neurological symptoms, and the latter are often associated with ocular involvement.[318]

Conjunctivitis, episcleritis, and uveitis are the most frequent manifestations during the early stage. Uveitis and neuro-ophthalmic disorders with neuroretinitis and involvement of multiple cranial nerves occur during the second stage. The most common ocular manifestations that appear during the late stage of the disease include keratitis, chronic intraocular inflammation, and orbital myositis.[320] In this phase, all patients with uveitis had posterior segment involvement with retinal vasculitis in most cases.[321]

The diagnosis of borreliosis is based on serology or DNA detection, depending on the stage of the disease.[322] PCR analysis can detect *Borrelia burgdorferi* DNA in the cerebral spinal fluid, urine, or vitreous tap.[320] Treatment includes a course of oral antibiotics combined with topical corticosteroids for the anterior uveitis.[319] Management of ocular manifestations might require intravenous therapy.[320] Early diagnosis and treatment are keys to achieving good response.[319]

Leptospirosis

Leptospirosis is a spirochetal disease that can result in systemic infection and ocular involvement. Ocular signs may appear in the acute systemic bacteremic phase; however, uveitis appears in the second immune phase of the disease and might be overlooked due to a long asymptomatic period between the systemic and ocular disease.[323] Inflammatory ocular manifestations include acute nongranulomatous panuveitis, hypopyon, vasculitis, membranous vitreous

opacities, and optic disc edema.[323] Complications include cataract and glaucoma.[324,325]

Aqueous humor studies of patients with leptospiral uveitis detected neutrophil infiltration, high levels of cytokines, and leptospiral lipopolysaccharide. The latter finding suggests an endotoxin as the causative factor for this condition.[326]

Treatment of leptospiral uveitis includes topical, periocular, or systemic corticosteroids, according to the severity and anatomical location of inflammatory process. Typically, treatment results in complete resolution and good visual prognosis, even with severe inflammation.[323] The glaucoma responds well to antiglaucoma therapy.[324,325]

Fungal Infections

Coccidioidomycosis

Coccidioidomycosis is a fungal systemic disease that can cause severe and/or chronic multiorgan involvement, including pulmonary, cutaneous, meningeal, and skeletal infections.[327,328] The causative fungus, *Coccidioides immitis*, is prevalent in South and Central America and western and southwestern United States.[327,329]

The infection might involve extraorbital or ocular tissue.[327] The ocular disease may present as a chronic granulomatous anterior uveitis, asymptomatic focal chorioretinitis, or fulminate granulomatous panuveitis.[327,330] Intraocular involvement might be unilateral or bilateral and usually presents together with evident systemic involvement.[329] Eye examination reveals granulomatous uveitis, multiple iris nodules, or possible large vascularized anterior chamber mass.[327,328] The anterior segment involvement is probably due to hypersensitivity response.[330] In very rare instances, this infection has resulted in secondary glaucoma due to anterior segment inflammation and exudates.[331,332]

The diagnosis is confirmed by systemic evaluation, serologic tests, and skin biopsy, revealing *Coccidioides immitis* spherules.[328] Anterior chamber centesis and iris biopsy demonstrate granulomatous or fibrinopurulent inflammatory exudates with fungal spherules.[329]

Treatment includes local and systemic amphotericin B and oral fluconazole. Fluconazole is an effective and safe agent, with less severe adverse effects.[328-330] A high index of suspicion is needed in patients from endemic areas with granulomatous uveitis and iris mass, resistant to corticosteroid treatment.[329]

Histoplasmosis

Histoplasmosis is a systemically disseminated fungal disorder that can cause asymptomatic multifocal choroiditis. There are reports of endogenous endophthalmitis in immunocompromised patients[333,334] that may cause total angle closure and severe glaucoma due to budding yeast and inflammatory infiltrates in the anterior chamber angle. Treatment includes intravenous amphotericin B and oral voricanozole, causing

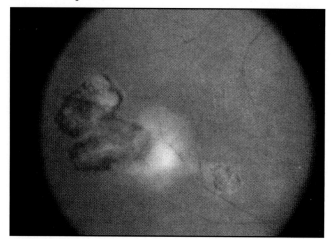

Figure 42-13. Toxoplasmosis: an active retinal lesion adjacent to an old chorioretinal scar. (Reprinted with permission from Glenn J. Jaffe, MD.)

inactivation of chorioretinal lesions. However, in immunocompromised patients, eradication of *H. capsulatum* from the anterior segment is difficult.[333] In one of the reported cases, despite medical antiglaucoma treatment, laser iridotomy, and cyclophotocoagulations, only moderate control of IOP was achieved and loss of vision occurred.[333]

Parasitic Infections

Toxoplasmosis

Toxoplasmosis, caused by *Toxoplasma gondii*, is a common cause of vitritis and necrotizing retinitis (Figure 42-13).[335] Toxoplasmosis is the most common cause of posterior uveitis in immunocompetent subjects worldwide[336] and is a prominent cause for uveitis in general.[121] Among immunocompromised patients with uveitis, 26% had toxoplasmosis.[337] The level of intraocular inflammation varies geographically, with a greater severity among patients in Brazil compared to patients in Europe and North and South America.[338]

Toxoplasmosis can be either congenital or acquired postnatally. Nearly one-quarter of reported ocular toxoplasmosis is acquired, nearly 15% is congenital, and more than 60% is of unknown origin.[339] The ocular lesions might present at birth or appear later in life. The average age at diagnosis of congenital cases is 9 years and of acquired ocular toxoplasmosis is 22 years.[336,339] Nearly 90% of patients had unilateral involvement.[340]

Congenital toxoplasmosis results in birth defects varying from blindness and severe mental retardation to insignificant retinochoroidal lesions of minimal consequence.[236] The ocular presentation of young children is mainly micro-ophthalmia and strabismus but also reduced visual acuity, nystagmus, and leukocoria.[341] In adults, typical symptoms are reduced visual acuity, floaters, photophobia, pain, and redness.[341]

Toxoplasmic retinochoroiditis typically affects the posterior pole. Active lesions present as grey-white focus of retinal necrosis with adjacent inflammation and hemorrhage. Scarring occurs from the periphery toward the center, with variable pigmentary hyperplasia.[341] Although posterior segment involvement is most common, anterior uveitis is frequent, presenting with cells and flare, mutton fat KPs, fibrin, iris nodules, and posterior synechiae.[341]

Forty percent of the patients with active toxoplasmosis retinochoroiditis have an elevated IOP. The elevated IOP is usually transitory and corresponds with the episode of uveitis.[342] Elevated IOP is associated with more severe inflammation in the anterior chamber and macular involvement.[338] Retinal nerve fiber layer atrophy associated with a retinal lesion might mimic glaucomatous damage.[343]

Autoimmunity may play a role in ocular toxoplasmosis. IL-5 and IL-12 were found to be markers for ocular toxoplasmosis, and IL-17 was found to be a marker for disease severity.[344]

Interferon gamma is associated with resistance to toxoplasmosis; homozygocity for the A allele in its gene (+874T/A) might increase susceptibility to ocular toxoplasmosis.[345] Genotypes associated with a low production of IL-10, an anti-inflammatory cytokine, may be correlated with the incidence of toxoplasmic retinochoroiditis.[346]

The diagnosis is based on clinical criteria. The detection of *T. gondii* DNA using PCR and anti-*T. gondii* antibodies in patients' tears and aqueous humor may confirm the diagnosis.[341]

Toxoplasmosis treatment includes oral, topical, or sub-Tenon corticosteroids[342] combined with specific antiprotozoal therapy, including primarily pyrimethamine and sulfadiazine, although other drug combinations are available.[341] Most patients with elevated IOP are treated temporarily with antiglaucoma therapy. Only a few (3.3%) require chronic therapy or glaucoma surgery.[342] The prognosis is fairly good, as long as the central macula is spared.[341] Eighty percent of patients suffer from recurrence; the interval between recurrences shortens over time.[340]

Toxocariasis

Toxocariasis is a parasitic systemic infectious disease that may affect the eye, respiratory tract, and liver. Other findings include fever, leukocytosis, and eosinophilia. The parasitic causative agent is *Toxocara canis*, an intestinal nematode usually found in dogs.[347] It primarily affects animals and less frequently humans. As opposed to toxoplasmosis, toxocariasis is always an acquired disease.[348] It mainly affects younger patients with an average age of 16.5 years.[349] Distribution is worldwide.[347,349]

Ocular findings include posterior uveitis, vitreal infiltrates mimicking endophthalmitis in severe cases, epiretinal membranes, and subretinal granulomas.[347] Toxocara uveitis is unilateral in more than 90% of cases.[349] Because this disorder commonly presents as a uniocular painless white retinal mass in a child's eye, it can be confused with retinoblastoma. Although posterior segment pathology is most common, anterior uveitis may occur,[350] which may cause posterior synechiae and angle-closure glaucoma.[351]

Diagnosis is confirmed by sera antibody detection with enzyme-linked immunosorbent assay testing (ELISA).[352] Unclear cases can be diagnosed with ELISA testing of vitreous fluid.[347] Treatment includes a combination of an antihelmintic, such as albendazole, and oral corticosteroids to control the inflammation.[348,352] Pars plana vitrectomy may be needed when vitreoretinal complications are evident.[347] Reactivation might occur even years after the initial episode has resolved.[352] Early diagnosis and treatment of ocular toxocariasis is crucial to preserve visual acuity.[347,352]

Onchocerciasis

This microfilarial disease occurs in individuals infected by *Onchocerca volvulus*. Larvae of the nematode are transmitted to humans by the bite of the black fly genus *Simulium*. Onchocerciasis is prevalent throughout much of the Third World. It is complicated by a high incidence of uveitis.[353] It is a significant cause of blindness in countries where it is widespread, especially in Africa. Systemic findings include skin microfilaria, onchocercal subcutaneous nodules, and eosinophilia.[354]

Ocular manifestations included punctate keratitis (41%), visible microfilaria in the anterior chamber (39%), chorioretinitis (7.2%), and anterior uveitis (6.0%). Other ophthalmic manifestations, such as lid nodules, corneal leucomas, and conjunctival injection, were evident in more than half of the population with onchocerciasis.[354]

Reports of association between onchocerciasis and glaucoma have been contradicting. A cross-sectional case-control study in Ghana found a higher prevalence of onchocerciasis in operated glaucoma patients than in cataract patients (10.6% and 2.6%, respectively).[355] In patients with glaucoma and onchocerciasis, microfilaria infiltration was found around Schlemm's canal, efferent veins, and vessels in Tenon's capsule.[356] In a report[357] on onchocercal infection from Nigeria, IOP was reduced in spite of PAS formation, probably due to a low-grade inflammation. Another report[354] from Brazil also did not find an association between onchocerciasis and glaucoma.

Community-based treatment with ivermectin (microfilaricide) reduces the incidence of ocular manifestations of the disease, including anterior uveitis.[358]

Malaria

Malaria infection might have ocular manifestations including acute bilateral panuveitis or anterior uveitis with secondary glaucoma, multiple superficial retinal hemorrhages with or without perivasculitis, and subconjunctival hemorrhages. Histopathology demonstrated plasmodium vivax-infected erythrocytes, schizonts, and gametocytes within the blood vessels of the choroid and retina.[359] Antimalaria and local therapies were used successfully to control IOP and improve visual acuity.[359] A high index of suspicion is needed in patients residing in or travelling to endemic areas.

Schistosomiasis

Schistosomiasis, caused by the parasite *Schistosoma mansoni*, is endemic in many areas of the world, mainly Africa, South America, and Asia, causing diarrhea, fever, cough, and rash.[360,361] The parasite's eggs may penetrate into the eye and form a granuloma and inflammation.[361] This process might involve the retina and choroid or present as keratouveitis with mutton-fat KPs, large inflammatory cells, and flare.[360] There is a report of secondary glaucoma due to keratouveitis, where inflammatory material as well as parasite eggs blocked outflow channels and caused an increase in IOP.[360] Treatment of ocular schistosomiasis includes combined antiparasitic therapy and corticosteroids; antiglaucoma therapy is given as needed.[360]

Acanthamoeba Keratitis

Acanthamoeba keratitis is associated primarily with the use of homemade saline or tap water solutions for contact lenses.[362,363]

Acanthamoeba keratitis may cause inflammatory complications, including anterior scleritis and anterior uveitis. It is also associated with cataract and iris atrophy.[362,364] Secondary glaucoma is not uncommon and is often severe.[365,366] Glaucoma is caused by chronic inflammation of the TM and posterior synechiae.[365,367] *Acanthamoeba* organisms were not present in the angle structures.[365] Diagnosis of *Acanthamoeba* keratitis is confirmed by positive confocal microscopy or culture.[365]

Treatment includes topical antibiotics, chlorhexidine hydrochloride, oral ketoconazole, and varying amounts of topical steroids.[363,366,367] Refractory cases are treated with penetrating keratoplasty,[362,366] and even enucleation.[367] Antiglaucoma drugs are given to treat the secondary glaucoma, but it frequently requires trabeculectomy and glaucoma drainage device implantation.[363-365,367] Secondary glaucoma is a poor prognostic sign in patients with *Acanthamoeba* keratitis and is a major cause of severe vision loss.[365,367]

OTHER CAUSES OF INFLAMMATORY GLAUCOMA

Pars Planitis

Pars planitis is a chronic inflammatory disorder primarily involving the vitreous, pars plana, or anterior retina. It is frequently associated with cystoid macular edema.[368] Other manifestations are retinal vascular sheathing, snowballs, snowbanks, cataract, and retinal detachment.[369]

Secondary glaucoma occurs in less than 10% of patients.[369,370] The anterior chamber angle is mainly open, but scattered PAS also have been observed, with inflammatory precipitates on the TM.

Histopathological examination shows the intravitreal snowbank made of fibroglial tissue with scattered mononuclear inflammatory cells.[371]

Medical treatment includes topical, periocular, and systemic corticosteroids combined with aqueous-suppressant antiglaucoma medications.[369] Peripheral cryotherapy has been used with some success to treat the snowbanking.[370] Chronic steroid use is frequently required with this disorder. Corticosteroid-sparing treatment with NSAIDs or antimetabolites may be required to avoid steroid-related IOP elevation.

Scleritis and Episcleritis

Scleritis is a disorder characterized by severe pain in association with variable anterior or posterior segment inflammation. A number of diseases are associated with the development of scleritis, and the most common associated condition is rheumatoid arthritis. Other disorders associated with scleritis include herpes zoster ophthalmicus, IgA nephropathy, *Acanthamoeba* keratitis, toxoplasmosis, systemic lupus erythematosus, rheumatic fever, and other systemic immune-mediated conditions.[372]

Anterior scleritis can be divided into diffuse, nodular, or necrotizing types. Diffuse and nodular scleritis are characterized by pain with variable degrees of erythema (Figure 42-14). Clinically, these forms are more benign. Necrotizing scleritis is associated with rheumatoid arthritis. It presents with severe inflammation and, if untreated, may result in irreversible destruction of ocular tissues. This form of scleritis accounts for approximately 10% of scleritis cases and has a higher risk of glaucoma than other forms of anterior scleritis. Posterior scleritis mainly appears in elderly women and tends to recur.[373] Posterior segment imaging with ultrasound, computerized tomography (CT), and magnetic resonance imaging (MRI) are helpful in confirming the diagnosis.[373,374]

Secondary glaucoma is more common in anterior than in posterior scleritis. It has been reported to develop in 11% or more of cases of anterior scleritis but to be rare in association with posterior scleritis.[375] The mechanism of glaucoma in anterior scleritis is usually damage to the TM by uveitis, PAS formation, or elevated episcleral venous pressure.[376,377] Glaucoma in posterior scleritis is usually secondary to ciliochoroidal effusion and detachment causing angle closure.[372,378-382] Resolution of this process was achieved by antiglaucoma therapy—topical and oral corticosteroids.[373,378,379]

Episcleritis is typically a benign, self-limited syndrome consisting of mild to moderate pain and episcleral injection and edema; it is often recurrent. Of 100 patients with episcleritis, one-third had bilateral involvement.[383] Permanent damage to ocular structures is rare. Complications are not common and may include secondary glaucoma, uveitis, and

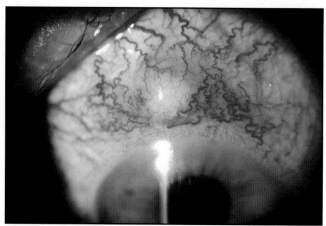

Figure 42-14. Anterior nodular scleritis. (Reprinted with permission from Haggay Avizemer, MD.)

corneal involvement. Episcleritis is usually managed with topical anti-inflammatory drugs, systemic NSAIDs, or corticosteroids.[383]

Retinal Detachment, Uveitis, and Glaucoma (Schwartz-Matsuo Syndrome)

In the majority of cases of retinal detachment, IOP is normal or subnormal. In a small percentage of patients with retinal detachment or dialysis, the IOP may become elevated to a moderate or high level in association with a mild anterior chamber reaction. The first mention of this form of anterior segment inflammation and glaucoma was by Shaffer in 1963.[384] Schwartz[385,386] presented 11 cases of severe anterior inflammation with glaucoma in which he found retinal detachment. Approximately half of the cases were secondary to ocular trauma with resultant peripheral retinal dialysis. In 1986, Matsuo and colleagues[387] reported on 7 patients with the syndrome.

The syndrome is characterized by cellular reaction in the anterior chamber, tobacco dust pigmentation in the anterior vitreous,[388] elevated IOP with open angle, and rhegmatogenous retinal detachment. The IOP elevations often occur in the evening and may present with a fairly rapid onset.[385,386] Typically, the retinal detachment is caused by an anterior dialysis at the ora serrata or a break in the nonpigmented epithelium of the ciliary body.[387]

The anterior chamber reaction and the glaucoma in this condition are probably secondary to the release of photoreceptor outer segments through the retinal break into the aqueous humor, which then obstruct the TM, resulting in elevated IOP.[387] Aqueous humor sampling shows melanic pigment and degenerated photoreceptor outer segments rather than inflammatory cells, which confirm this diagnosis.[389]

Local treatment with steroids, cycloplegics, and aqueous suppressants may be of some benefit temporarily but typically these interventions fail to control the anterior chamber reaction or glaucoma. Retinal detachment repair must be performed as soon as possible.[390] The elevated IOP resolves, even within 48 hours, without specific treatment, following retinal reattachment.[388,389]

Epidemic Dropsy

Epidemic dropsy is a toxic multiorgan condition that might cause pitting pedal edema, skin erythema, diarrhea, hepatomegaly, and cardiac and renal failure.[391,392] It is the result of the ingestion of *Argemone mexicana* in contaminated edible mustard oil.[393] Ocular findings include retinal vasculitis with venous dilatation, tortuosity, and hemorrhages.[391,392]

Four percent to 11% develop bilateral glaucoma characterized by open-angle without anterior uveitis.[391,392] Visual field defects may appear in epidemic dropsy, more frequently in early stages of the disease.[393]

The TM appears normal on histopathologic and histochemical testing. Aqueous analysis, however, reveals elevated prostaglandin E2 levels, histamine activity, and total protein levels, suggesting hypersecretory as the etiology of IOP elevation.[394] The toxic damage is mainly caused by free radicals affecting cell membranes.[395]

Treatment is mostly symptomatic, along with administration of antioxidants, multivitamins, and aqueous-suppressant agents for the glaucoma.[395] The elevated IOP is transitory—after 3 months, only 0.43% of patients needed antiglaucoma medications, and none needed them after 5 months.[396] Therefore, weekly titration of antiglaucoma treatment is recommended.

Blau Syndrome

Blau syndrome (BS), also named *Jabs disease*, is a rare familial disease with an autosomal dominant inheritance, characterized by granulomatous polyarthritis, uveitis, and dermatitis.[397-400] The disease was first described by Blau in 1985,[399] the same year Jabs reported a similar family.[400] So far, BS has been diagnosed in 136 members of 28 families, and in 4 sporadic cases.[397]

Clinically, BS resembles early-onset sarcoidosis with a triad of arthritis-uveitis-dermatitis.[398,399] Several ocular complications have been reported in recent years like cataract formation and secondary glaucoma due to inflammatory process or posterior synechiae with pupillary block.[397,400]

BS results from mutations in the caspase recruitment domain-15 (CARD 15)/nucleotide oligomerization domain (Nod2) that activates the up-regulation of pro-inflammatory cytokine transcription.[397] This mutation probably plays a role in the autoinflammatory reactions to unknown microorganisms in BS.[397] BS is not associated with HLA-B27.[399]

Diagnosis is based on skin and joint biopsies, demonstrating noncaseating granulomatous infiltration with multinucleated giant cells.[397,401] Iridectomy specimen demonstrated nonspecific inflammation.[401] Genetic analysis of the CARD 15/Nod2 gene is a useful diagnostic tool.[401]

Treatment includes topical and systemic corticosteroids, or a combination of NSAIDs with systemic corticosteroids as needed.[397,401] This therapy helps control the disease fairly well and reduces the ocular inflammation.[397,401] Peripheral iridectomy might be needed to release iris bombé.[397]

REFERENCES

1. Womack LW, Liesegang TJ. Complications of herpes zoster ophthalmicus. *Arch Ophthalmol.* 1983;101:42-45.
2. Posner A, Schlossman A. Syndrome of unilateral recurrent attacks of glaucoma with cyclitic symptoms. *Arch Ophthal.* 1948;39:517-535.
3. Reddy S, Cubillan LD, Hovakimyan A, Cunningham ET Jr. Inflammatory ocular hypertension syndrome (IOHS) in patients with syphilitic uveitis. *Br J Ophthalmol.* 2007;91:1610-1612.
4. Chiang TS, Thomas RP. Consensual ocular hypertensive response to prostaglandin E 2. *Invest Ophthalmol.* 1972;11:845-849.
5. Roth M, Simmons RJ. Glaucoma associated with precipitates on the trabecular meshwork. *Ophthalmology.* 1979;86:1613-1619.
6. Epstein DL, Hashimoto JM, Grant WM. Serum obstruction of aqueous outflow in enucleated eyes. *Am J Ophthalmol.* 1978;86:101-105.
7. Freddo TF, Patterson MM, Scott DR, Epstein DL. Influence of mercurial sulfhydryl agents on aqueous outflow pathways in enucleated eyes. *Invest Ophthalmol Vis Sci.* 1984;25:278-285.
8. Bloch-Michel E, Nussenblatt RB. International Uveitis Study Group recommendations for the evaluation of intraocular inflammatory disease. *Am J Ophthalmol.* 1987;103:234-235.
9. Andrasch RH, Pirofsky B, Burns RP. Immunosuppressive therapy for severe chronic uveitis. *Arch Ophthalmol.* 1978;96:247-251.
10. Benezra D, Cohen E. Treatment and visual prognosis in Behcet's disease. *Br J Ophthalmol.* 1986;70:589-592.
11. Jabs DA, Akpek EK. Immunosuppression for posterior uveitis. *Retina.* 2005;25:1-18.
12. Jabs DA, Rosenbaum JT, Foster CS, et al. Guidelines for the use of immunosuppressive drugs in patients with ocular inflammatory disorders: recommendations of an expert panel. *Am J Ophthalmol.* 2000;130:492-513.
13. Doycheva D, Deuter C, Stuebiger N, Biester S, Zierhut M. Mycophenolate mofetil in the treatment of uveitis in children. *Br J Ophthalmol.* 2007;91:180-184.
14. Kim SJ, Yu HG. The use of low-dose azathioprine in patients with Vogt-Koyanagi-Harada disease. *Ocul Immunol Inflamm.* 2007;15:381-387.
15. Samson CM, Waheed N, Baltatzis S, Foster CS. Methotrexate therapy for chronic noninfectious uveitis: analysis of a case series of 160 patients. *Ophthalmology.* 2001;108:1134-1139.
16. Nussenblatt RB, Palestine AG, Chan CC, Stevens G Jr, Mellow SD, Green SB. Randomized, double-masked study of cyclosporine compared to prednisolone in the treatment of endogenous uveitis. *Am J Ophthalmol.* 1991;112:138-146.
17. Hogan AC, McAvoy CE, Dick AD, Lee RW. Long-term efficacy and tolerance of tacrolimus for the treatment of uveitis. *Ophthalmology.* 2007;114:1000-1006.
18. Goldstein DA, Fontanilla FA, Kaul S, Sahin O, Tessler HH. Long-term follow-up of patients treated with short-term high-dose chlorambucil for sight-threatening ocular inflammation. *Ophthalmology.* 2002;109:370-377.

19. Mudun BA, Ergen A, Ipcioglu SU, Burumcek EY, Durlu Y, Arslan MO. Short-term chlorambucil for refractory uveitis in Behcet's disease. *Ocul Immunol Inflamm.* 2001;9:219-229.

20. Suhler EB, Smith JR, Wertheim MS, et al. A prospective trial of infliximab therapy for refractory uveitis: preliminary safety and efficacy outcomes. *Arch Ophthalmol.* 2005;123:903-912.

21. Vazquez-Cobian LB, Flynn T, Lehman TJ. Adalimumab therapy for childhood uveitis. *J Pediatr.* 2006;149:572-575.

22. Biester S, Deuter C, Michels H, et al. Adalimumab in the therapy of uveitis in childhood. *Br J Ophthalmol.* 2007;91:319-324.

23. van Laar JA, Missotten T, van Daele PL, Jamnitski A, Baarsma GS, van Hagen PM. Adalimumab: a new modality for Behcet's disease? *Ann Rheum Dis.* 2007;66:565-566.

24. Mushtaq B, Saeed T, Situnayake RD, Murray PI. Adalimumab for sight-threatening uveitis in Behcet's disease. *Eye (Lond).* 2007;21:824-825.

25. Foeldvari I, Nielsen S, Kummerle-Deschner J, et al. Tumor necrosis factor-alpha blocker in treatment of juvenile idiopathic arthritis-associated uveitis refractory to second-line agents: results of a multinational survey. *J Rheumatol.* 2007;34:1146-1150.

26. Nussenblatt RB, Thompson DJ, Li Z, et al. Humanized antiinterleukin-2 (IL-2) receptor alpha therapy: long-term results in uveitis patients and preliminary safety and activity data for establishing parameters for subcutaneous administration. *J Autoimmun.* 2003;21:283-293.

27. Bumgardner GL, Hardie I, Johnson RW, et al. Results of 3-year phase III clinical trials with daclizumab prophylaxis for prevention of acute rejection after renal transplantation. *Transplantation.* 2001;72:839-845.

28. Teoh SC, Sharma S, Hogan A, Lee R, Ramanan AV, Dick AD. Tailoring biological treatment: anakinra treatment of posterior uveitis associated with the CINCA syndrome. *Br J Ophthalmol.* 2007;91:263-264.

29. Koskela T, Brubaker RF. Apraclonidine and timolol. Combined effects in previously untreated normal subjects. *Arch Ophthalmol.* 1991;109:804-806.

30. Gharagozloo NZ, Brubaker RF. Effect of apraclonidine in long-term timolol users. *Ophthalmology.* 1991;98:1543-1546.

31. Sung VC, Barton K. Management of inflammatory glaucomas. *Curr Opin Ophthalmol.* 2004;15:136-140.

32. Stjernschantz JW. From PGF(2alpha)-isopropyl ester to latanoprost: a review of the development of xalatan: the Proctor Lecture. *Invest Ophthalmol Vis Sci.* 2001;42:1134-1145.

33. Warwar RE, Bullock JD, Ballal D. Cystoid macular edema and anterior uveitis associated with latanoprost use. Experience and incidence in a retrospective review of 94 patients. *Ophthalmology.* 1998;105:263-268.

34. Fechtner RD, Khouri AS, Zimmerman TJ, et al. Anterior uveitis associated with latanoprost. *Am J Ophthalmol.* 1998;126:37-41.

35. Moroi SE, Gottfredsdottir MS, Schteingart MT, et al. Cystoid macular edema associated with latanoprost therapy in a case series of patients with glaucoma and ocular hypertension. *Ophthalmology.* 1999;106:1024-1029.

36. Wand M, Gaudio AR. Cystoid macular edema associated with ocular hypotensive lipids. *Am J Ophthalmol.* 2002;133:403-405.

37. Ayyala RS, Cruz DA, Margo CE, et al. Cystoid macular edema associated with latanoprost in aphakic and pseudophakic eyes. *Am J Ophthalmol.* 1998;126:602-604.

38. Rowe JA, Hattenhauer MG, Herman DC. Adverse side effects associated with latanoprost. *Am J Ophthalmol.* 1997;124:683-685.

39. Wand M, Gilbert CM, Liesegang TJ. Latanoprost and herpes simplex keratitis. *Am J Ophthalmol.* 1999;127:602-604.

40. Kroll DM, Schuman JS. Reactivation of herpes simplex virus keratitis after initiating bimatoprost treatment for glaucoma. *Am J Ophthalmol.* 2002;133:401-403.

41. Merayo-Lloves J, Power WJ, Rodriguez A, Pedroza-Seres M, Foster CS. Secondary glaucoma in patients with uveitis. *Ophthalmologica.* 1999;213:300-304.

42. Schuman JS, Puliafito CA, Allingham RR, et al. Contact transscleral continuous wave neodymium:YAG laser cyclophotocoagulation. *Ophthalmology.* 1990;97:571-580.

43. Murphy CC, Burnett CA, Spry PG, Broadway DC, Diamond JP. A two centre study of the dose-response relation for transscleral diode laser cyclophotocoagulation in refractory glaucoma. *Br J Ophthalmol.* 2003;87:1252-1257.

44. Schlote T, Derse M, Zierhut M. Transscleral diode laser cyclophotocoagulation for the treatment of refractory glaucoma secondary to inflammatory eye diseases. *Br J Ophthalmol.* 2000;84:999-1003.

45. Ceballos EM, Beck AD, Lynn MJ. Trabeculectomy with antiproliferative agents in uveitic glaucoma. *J Glaucoma.* 2002;11:189-196.

46. Towler HM, McCluskey P, Shaer B, Lightman S. Long-term follow-up of trabeculectomy with intraoperative 5-fluorouracil for uveitis-related glaucoma. *Ophthalmology.* 2000;107:1822-1828.

47. Stavrou P, Murray PI. Long-term follow-up of trabeculectomy without antimetabolites in patients with uveitis. *Am J Ophthalmol.* 1999;128:434-439.

48. Auer C, Mermoud A, Herbort CP. Deep sclerectomy for the management of uncontrolled uveitic glaucoma: preliminary data. *Klin Monbl Augenheilkd.* 2004;221:339-342.

49. Arruabarrena C, Munoz-Negrete FJ, Marquez C, Rebolleda G. Results of nonpenetrating deep sclerectomy in inflammatory glaucoma: one year follow up. *Arch Soc Esp Oftalmol.* 2007;82:483-487.

50. Freedman SF, Rodriguez-Rosa RE, Rojas MC, Enyedi LB. Goniotomy for glaucoma secondary to chronic childhood uveitis. *Am J Ophthalmol.* 2002;133:617-621.

51. Hill RA, Nguyen QH, Baerveldt G, et al. Trabeculectomy and Molteno implantation for glaucomas associated with uveitis. *Ophthalmology.* 1993;100:903-908.

52. Molteno AC, Sayawat N, Herbison P. Otago glaucoma surgery outcome study: long-term results of uveitis with secondary glaucoma drained by Molteno implants. *Ophthalmology.* 2001;108:605-613.

53. Ceballos EM, Parrish RK 2nd, Schiffman JC. Outcome of Baerveldt glaucoma drainage implants for the treatment of uveitic glaucoma. *Ophthalmology.* 2002;109:2256-2260.

54. Da Mata A, Burk SE, Netland PA, Baltatzis S, Christen W, Foster CS. Management of uveitic glaucoma with Ahmed glaucoma valve implantation. *Ophthalmology.* 1999;106:2168-2172.

55. Ozdal PC, Vianna RN, Deschenes J. Ahmed valve implantation in glaucoma secondary to chronic uveitis. *Eye (Lond).* 2006;20:178-183.

56. Raitta C, Vannas A. Glaucomatocyclitic crisis. *Arch Ophthalmol.* 1977;95:608-612.

57. Jap A, Sivakumar M, Chee SP. Is Posner Schlossman syndrome benign? *Ophthalmology.* 2001;108:913-918.

58. Yamamoto S, Pavan-Langston D, Tada R, et al. Possible role of herpes simplex virus in the origin of Posner-Schlossman syndrome. *Am J Ophthalmol.* 1995;119:796-798.

59. Chee SP, Jap A. Presumed Fuchs' heterochromic iridocyclitis and Posner-Schlossman syndrome: comparison of cytomegalovirus-positive and negative eyes. *Am J Ophthalmol.* 2008;146:883-889.

60. Hirose S, Ohno S, Matsuda H. HLA-Bw54 and glaucomatocyclitic crisis. *Arch Ophthalmol.* 1985;103:1837-1839.

61. Darchuk V, Sampaolesi J, Mato L, Nicoli C, Sampaolesi R. Optic nerve head behavior in Posner-Schlossman syndrome. *Int Ophthalmol.* 2001;23:373-379.

62. Maeda H, Nakamura M, Negi A. Selective reduction of the S-cone component of the electroretinogram in Posner-Schlossman syndrome. *Eye (Lond).* 2001;15:163-167.

63. Harstad HK, Ringvold A. Glaucomatocyclitic crises (Posner-Schlossman syndrome). A case report. *Acta Ophthalmol (Copenh).* 1986;64:146-151.

64. Nagataki S, Mishima S. Aqueous humor dynamics in glaucomato-cyclitic crisis. *Invest Ophthalmol.* 1976;15:365-370.

65. Hong C, Song KY. Effect of apraclonidine hydrochloride on the attack of Posner-Schlossman syndrome. *Korean J Ophthalmol.* 1993;7:28-33.

66. Bonfioli AA, Curi AL, Orefice F. Fuchs' heterochromic cyclitis. *Semin Ophthalmol.* 2005;20:143-146.

67. Fearnley IR, Rosenthal AR. Fuchs' heterochromic iridocyclitis revisited. *Acta Ophthalmol Scand.* 1995;73:166-170.

68. Norrsell K, Sjodell L. Fuchs' heterochromic uveitis: a longitudinal clinical study. *Acta Ophthalmol.* 2008;86:58-64.

69. Velilla S, Dios E, Herreras JM, Calonge M. Fuchs' heterochromic iridocyclitis: a review of 26 cases. *Ocul Immunol Inflamm.* 2001;9:169-175.

70. Wobmann P. [Fuchs' heterochromic cyclitis. Electron-microscopic study of nine iris biopsies (author's transl)]. *Albrecht Von Graefes Arch Klin Exp Ophthalmol.* 1976;199:167-178.

71. Saari M, Vuorre I, Nieminen H. Infra-red transillumination stereophotography of the iris in Fuchs' heterochromic cyclitis. *Br J Ophthalmol.* 1978;62:110-115.

72. Rothova A, La Hey E, Baarsma GS, Breebaart AC. Iris nodules in Fuchs' heterochromic uveitis. *Am J Ophthalmol.* 1994;118: 338-342.

73. Regenbogen LS, Naveh-Floman N. Glaucoma in Fuchs' heterochromic cyclitis associated with congenital Horner's syndrome. *Br J Ophthalmol.* 1987;71:844-849.

74. La Hey E, Baarsma GS, De Vries J, Kijlstra A. Clinical analysis of Fuchs' heterochromic cyclitis. *Doc Ophthalmol.* 1991;78:225-235.

75. Arffa RC, Schlaegel TF Jr. Chorioretinal scars in Fuchs' heterochromic iridocyclitis. *Arch Ophthalmol.* 1984;102:1153-1155.

76. Huber A. [Glaucoma in complicated heterochromia of Fuchs]. *Ophthalmologica.* 1961;141:122-135.

77. Perry HD, Yanoff M, Scheie HG. Rubeosis in Fuchs heterochromic iridocyclitis. *Arch Ophthalmol.* 1975;93:337-339.

78. Francois J. [New contribution on Fuchs' heterochromia]. *Bull Soc Belge Ophtalmol.* 1952;102:607-624.

79. La Hey E, de Vries J, Langerhorst CT, Baarsma GS, Kijlstra A. Treatment and prognosis of secondary glaucoma in Fuchs' heterochromic iridocyclitis. *Am J Ophthalmol.* 1993;116:327-340.

80. Jones NP. Glaucoma in Fuchs' heterochromic uveitis: aetiology, management and outcome. *Eye (Lond).* 1991;5(pt 6):662-667.

81. Quentin CD, Reiber H. Fuchs heterochromic cyclitis: rubella virus antibodies and genome in aqueous humor. *Am J Ophthalmol.* 2004;138:46-54.

82. Barequet IS, Li Q, Wang Y, O'Brien TP, Hooks JJ, Stark WJ. Herpes simplex virus DNA identification from aqueous fluid in Fuchs heterochromic iridocyclitis. *Am J Ophthalmol.* 2000;129:672-673.

83. Quentin CD, Reiber H. Fuchs heterochromic cyclitis: Rubella virus antibodies and genome in aqueous humor. *Am J Ophthalmol.* 2004;138:46-54.

84. O'Connor GR. Doyne lecture. Heterochromic iridocyclitis. *Trans Ophthalmol Soc U K.* 1985;104(pt 3):219-231.

85. van der Gaag R, Broersma L, Rothova A, Baarsma S, Kijlstra A. Immunity to a corneal antigen in Fuchs' heterochromic cyclitis patients. *Invest Ophthalmol Vis Sci.* 1989;30:443-448.

86. la Hey E, Baarsma GS, Rothova A, Broersma L, van der Gaag R, Kijlstra A. High incidence of corneal epithelium antibodies in Fuchs' heterochromic cyclitis. *Br J Ophthalmol.* 1988;72:921-925.

87. La Hey E, Mooy CM, Baarsma GS, de Vries J, de Jong PT, Kijlstra A. Immune deposits in iris biopsy specimens from patients with Fuchs' heterochromic iridocyclitis. *Am J Ophthalmol.* 1992;113:75-80.

88. Jones NP. Fuchs' heterochromic uveitis: an update. *Surv Ophthalmol.* 1993;37:253-272.

89. Chandler PA, Grant WM. *Lectures on Glaucoma.* Philadelphia, PA: Lea & Febiger; 1965:431.

90. Cohen RG, Wu HK, Schuman JS. Glaucoma with inflammatory precipitates on the trabecular meshwork: a report of Grant's syndrome with ultrasound biomicroscopy of precipitates. *J Glaucoma.* 1996;5:266-270.

91. Bonfioli AA, Orefice F. Sarcoidosis. *Semin Ophthalmol.* 2005;20: 177-182.

92. Dana MR, Merayo-Lloves J, Schaumberg DA, Foster CS. Prognosticators for visual outcome in sarcoid uveitis. *Ophthalmology.* 1996;103:1846-1853.

93. Uyama M. Uveitis in sarcoidosis. *Int Ophthalmol Clin.* 2002;42: 143-150.

94. Lobo A, Barton K, Minassian D, du Bois RM, Lightman S. Visual loss in sarcoid-related uveitis. *Clin Experiment Ophthalmol.* 2003;31:310-316.

95. Obenauf CD, Shaw HE, Sydnor CF, Klintworth GK. Sarcoidosis and its ophthalmic manifestations. *Am J Ophthalmol.* 1978;86:648-655.

96. Iwata K, Nanba K, Sobue K, Abe H. Ocular sarcoidosis: evaluation of intraocular findings. *Ann N Y Acad Sci.* 1976;278:445-454.

97. Hamanaka T, Takei A, Takemura T, Oritsu M. Pathological study of cases with secondary open-angle glaucoma due to sarcoidosis. *Am J Ophthalmol.* 2002;134:17-26.

98. Mayer J, Brouillette G, Corriveau LA. Sarcoidosis and rubeosis iridis [in French]. *Can J Ophthalmol.* 1983;18:197-198.

99. Di Alberti L, Piattelli A, Artese L, et al. Human herpesvirus 8 variants in sarcoid tissues. *Lancet.* 1997;350:1655-1661.

100. Eishi Y, Suga M, Ishige I, et al. Quantitative analysis of mycobacterial and propionibacterial DNA in lymph nodes of Japanese and European patients with sarcoidosis. *J Clin Microbiol.* 2002;40: 198-204.

101. Jones NP. Sarcoidosis. *Curr Opin Ophthalmol.* 2002;13:393-396.

102. Rybicki BA, Iannuzzi MC, Frederick MM, et al. Familial aggregation of sarcoidosis. A case-control etiologic study of sarcoidosis (ACCESS). *Am J Respir Crit Care Med.* 2001;164:2085-2091.

103. Gray-McGuire C, Sinha R, Iyengar S, et al. Genetic characterization and fine mapping of susceptibility loci for sarcoidosis in African Americans on chromosome 5. *Hum Genet.* 2006;120:420-430.

104. Margolis R, Lowder CY. Sarcoidosis. *Curr Opin Ophthalmol.* 2007;18:470-475.

105. Hegab SM, Al-Mutawa SA, Sheriff SM. Ocular sarcoidosis in Kuwait with a review of literature. *Int Ophthalmol.* 1997;21: 255-260.

106. Edelsten C, Pearson A, Joynes E, Stanford MR, Graham EM. The ocular and systemic prognosis of patients presenting with sarcoid uveitis. *Eye (Lond).* 1999;13(pt 6):748-753.

107. Baughman RP, Drent M, Kavuru M, et al. Infliximab therapy in patients with chronic sarcoidosis and pulmonary involvement. *Am J Respir Crit Care Med.* 2006;174:795-802.

108. Ocampo VV Jr, Foster CS, Baltatzis S. Surgical excision of iris nodules in the management of sarcoid uveitis. *Ophthalmology.* 2001;108:1296-1299.

109. Chylack LT Jr, Bienfang DC, Bellows AR, Stillman JS. Ocular manifestations of juvenile rheumatoid arthritis. *Am J Ophthalmol.* 1975;79:1026-1033.

110. Kanski JJ, Shun-Shin GA. Systemic uveitis syndromes in childhood: an analysis of 340 cases. *Ophthalmology.* 1984;91:1247-1252.

111. Reininga JK, Los LI, Wulffraat NM, Armbrust W. The evaluation of uveitis in juvenile idiopathic arthritis (JIA) patients: are current ophthalmologic screening guidelines adequate? *Clin Exp Rheumatol.* 2008;26:367-372.

112. Benezra D, Cohen E, Behar-Cohen F. Uveitis and juvenile idiopathic arthritis: a cohort study. *Clin Ophthalmol.* 2007;1: 513-518.

113. Carvounis PE, Herman DC, Cha S, Burke JP. Incidence and outcomes of uveitis in juvenile rheumatoid arthritis, a synthesis of the literature. *Graefes Arch Clin Exp Ophthalmol.* 2006;244: 281-290.

114. Marvillet I, Terrada C, Quartier P, Quoc EB, Bodaghi B, Prieur AM. Ocular threat in juvenile idiopathic arthritis. *Joint Bone Spine.* 2009;76:383-388.

115. Sabri K, Saurenmann RK, Silverman ED, Levin AV. Course, complications, and outcome of juvenile arthritis-related uveitis. *J AAPOS.* 2008;12:539-545.

116. Merriam JC, Chylack LT Jr, Albert DM. Early-onset pauciarticular juvenile rheumatoid arthritis. A histopathologic study. *Arch Ophthalmol.* 1983;101:1085-1092.

117. Price FW Jr, Ziemba SL. Placement of a collagen glaucoma drainage device to control intraocular pressure and chronic iritis secondary to juvenile rheumatoid arthritis. *Ophthalmic Surg Lasers.* 2002;33:233-236.

118. Valimaki J, Airaksinen PJ, Tuulonen A. Molteno implantation for secondary glaucoma in juvenile rheumatoid arthritis. *Arch Ophthalmol.* 1997;115:1253-1256.

119. Heinz C, Koch JM, Heiligenhaus A. Transscleral diode laser cyclophotocoagulation as primary surgical treatment for secondary glaucoma in juvenile idiopathic arthritis: high failure rate after short term follow up. *Br J Ophthalmol.* 2006;90:737-740.

120. Suhler EB, Martin TM, Rosenbaum JT. HLA-B27-associated uveitis: overview and current perspectives. *Curr Opin Ophthalmol.* 2003;14:378-383.

121. Jakob E, Reuland MS, Mackensen F, et al. Uveitis subtypes in a german interdisciplinary uveitis center—analysis of 1916 patients. *J Rheumatol.* 2009;36:127-136.

122. Chang JH, McCluskey PJ, Wakefield D. Acute anterior uveitis and HLA-B27. *Surv Ophthalmol.* 2005;50:364-388.

123. Otasevic L, Zlatanovic G, Stanojevic-Paovic A, et al. *Helicobacter pylori:* an underestimated factor in acute anterior uveitis and spondyloarthropathies? *Ophthalmologica.* 2007;221:6-13.

124. Chung YM, Liao HT, Lin KC, et al. Prevalence of spondyloarthritis in 504 Chinese patients with HLA-B27-associated acute anterior uveitis. *Scand J Rheumatol.* 2009;38:84-90.

125. Braakenburg AM, de Valk HW, de Boer J, Rothova A. Human leukocyte antigen-B27-associated uveitis: long-term follow-up and gender differences. *Am J Ophthalmol.* 2008;145:472-479.

126. Power WJ, Rodriguez A, Pedroza-Seres M, Foster CS. Outcomes in anterior uveitis associated with the HLA-B27 haplotype. *Ophthalmology.* 1998;105:1646-1651.

127. Proenca H, Ferreira C, Miranda M, Castanheira-Dinis A, Monteiro-Grillo M. Serum prolactin levels in HLA-B27-associated uveitis. *Eur J Ophthalmol.* 2008;18:929-933.

128. Ali A, Samson CM. Seronegative spondyloarthropathies and the eye. *Curr Opin Ophthalmol.* 2007;18:476-480.

129. Androudi S, Brazitikos P, Iaccheri B, et al. Outcomes of early and late immunomodulatory treatment in patients with HLA-B27-associated chronic uveitis. *Graefes Arch Clin Exp Ophthalmol.* 2003;241:1000-1005.

130. Skolnick CA, Fiscella RG, Tessler HH, Goldstein DA. Tissue plasminogen activator to treat impending pupillary block glaucoma in patients with acute fibrinous HLA-B27 positive iridocyclitis. *Am J Ophthalmol.* 2000;129:363-366.

131. Sampaio-Barros PD, Conde RA, Bonfiglioli R, Bertolo MB, Samara AM. Characterization and outcome of uveitis in 350 patients with spondyloarthropathies. *Rheumatol Int.* 2006;26:1143-1146.

132. Zeboulon N, Dougados M, Gossec L. Prevalence and characteristics of uveitis in the spondyloarthropathies: a systematic literature review. *Ann Rheum Dis.* 2008;67:955-959.

133. Niederer R, Danesh-Meyer H. Uveitis screening: HLAB27 antigen and ankylosing spondylitis in a New Zealand population. *N Z Med J.* 2006;119:U1886.

134. Kiss S, Letko E, Qamruddin S, Baltatzis S, Foster CS. Long-term progression, prognosis, and treatment of patients with recurrent ocular manifestations of Reiter's syndrome. *Ophthalmology.* 2003;110:1764-1769.

135. Singleton EM, Hutson SE. Anterior uveitis, inflammatory bowel disease, and ankylosing spondylitis in a HLA-B27-positive woman. *South Med J.* 2006;99:531-533.

136. Kovalev Iu N, Il'in, II. Ophthalmological aspects of Reiter's disease [in Russian]. *Vestn Oftalmol.* 1990;106:65-69.

137. Lee DA, Barker SM, Su WP, Allen GL, Liesegang TJ, Ilstrup DM. The clinical diagnosis of Reiter's syndrome. Ophthalmic and non-ophthalmic aspects. *Ophthalmology.* 1986;93:350-356.

138. Chaoui Z, Bernoussi A, Belmekki M, Berraho A. Uveitis and chronic intestinal inflammatory diseases: three case studies [in French]. *J Fr Ophthalmol.* 2005;28:854-856.

139. Turkcapar N, Toruner M, Soykan I, et al. The prevalence of extraintestinal manifestations and HLA association in patients with inflammatory bowel disease. *Rheumatol Int.* 2006;26:663-668.

140. Queiro R, Torre JC, Belzunegui J, et al. Clinical features and predictive factors in psoriatic arthritis-related uveitis. *Semin Arthritis Rheum.* 2002;31:264-270.

141. Durrani K, Foster CS. Psoriatic uveitis: a distinct clinical entity? *Am J Ophthalmol.* 2005;139:106-111.

142. Smith M, Buller A, Radford R, Laitt R, Leatherbarrow B. Ocular presentation of the SAPHO syndrome. *Br J Ophthalmol.* 2005;89:1069-1070.

143. Yabe H, Takano Y, Nomura E, et al. Two cases of SAPHO syndrome accompanied by classic features of Behcet's disease and review of the literature. *Clin Rheumatol.* 2008;27:133-135.

144. Kitaichi N, Miyazaki A, Iwata D, Ohno S, Stanford MR, Chams H. Ocular features of Behcet's disease: an international collaborative study. *Br J Ophthalmol.* 2007;91:1579-1582.

145. Deuter CM, Kotter I, Wallace GR, Murray PI, Stubiger N, Zierhut M. Behcet's disease: ocular effects and treatment. *Prog Retin Eye Res.* 2008;27:111-136.

146. Elgin U, Berker N, Batman A. Incidence of secondary glaucoma in behcet disease. *J Glaucoma.* 2004;13:441-444.

147. Nussenblatt RB. Uveitis in Behcet's disease. *Int Rev Immunol.* 1997;14:67-79.

148. de Menthon M, Lavalley MP, Maldini C, Guillevin L, Mahr A. HLA-B51/B5 and the risk of Behcet's disease: a systematic review and meta-analysis of case-control genetic association studies. *Arthritis Rheum.* 2009;61:1287-1296.

149. Okunuki Y, Usui Y, Takeuchi M, et al. Proteomic surveillance of autoimmunity in Behcet's disease with uveitis: selenium binding protein is a novel autoantigen in Behcet's disease. *Exp Eye Res.* 2007;84:823-831.

150. Elgin U, Berker N, Batman A, Soykan E. Nd:YAG laser iridotomy in the management of secondary glaucoma associated with Behcet's disease. *Eur J Ophthalmol.* 2007;17:191-195.

151. Elgin U, Berker N, Batman A, Soykan E. Trabeculectomy with mitomycin C in secondary glaucoma associated with Behcet disease. *J Glaucoma.* 2007;16:68-72.

152. Foster CS, Fong LP, Singh G. Cataract surgery and intraocular lens implantation in patients with uveitis. *Ophthalmology.* 1989;96:281-288.

153. Krause L, Hoffmann F, Zouboulis CC, Foerster MH. Vitrectomy and trabeculectomy combined with interferon alpha treatment in Adamantiades-Behcet's disease: a case report. *Graefes Arch Clin Exp Ophthalmol.* 2003;241:871-874.

154. Yoshida A, Kawashima H, Motoyama Y, et al. Comparison of patients with Behcet's disease in the 1980s and 1990s. *Ophthalmology.* 2004;111:810-815.

155. Read RW, Rechodouni A, Butani N, et al. Complications and prognostic factors in Vogt-Koyanagi-Harada disease. *Am J Ophthalmol.* 2001;131:599-606.

156. Read RW. Vogt-Koyanagi-Harada disease. *Ophthalmol Clin North Am.* 2002;15:333-341, vii.

157. Ohno S, Char DH, Kimura SJ, O'Connor GR. Vogt-Koyanagi-Harada syndrome. *Am J Ophthalmol.* 1977;83:735-740.

158. Forster DJ, Rao NA, Hill RA, Nguyen QH, Baerveldt G. Incidence and management of glaucoma in Vogt-Koyanagi-Harada syndrome. *Ophthalmology.* 1993;100:613-618.

159. Lugossy G. [Vogt-Koyanagi-Harada syndrome and cortisone]. *Bull Mem Soc Fr Ophtalmol.* 1976:44-46.

160. Perry HD, Font RL. Clinical and histopathologic observations in severe Vogt-Koyanagi-Harada syndrome. *Am J Ophthalmol.* 1977;83:242-254.

161. Kishi A, Nao-i N, Sawada A. Ultrasound biomicroscopic findings of acute angle-closure glaucoma in Vogt-Koyanagi-Harada syndrome. *Am J Ophthalmol.* 1996;122:735-737.

162. Yamamura K, Mori K, Hieda O, Kinoshita S. Anterior segment optical coherence tomography findings of acute angle-closure glaucoma in Vogt-Koyanagi-Harada disease. *Jpn J Ophthalmol.* 2008;52:231-232.

163. Min HY, Liu Y, Niu NF, Zhang MF, Zhu XL, Zhao JL. Polymorphism of HLA-DQB1 alleles in Chinese Han patients with Vogt-Koyanagi-Harada syndrome [in Chinese]. *Zhonghua Yan Ke Za Zhi.* 2007;43:355-360.

164. Moorthy RS, Inomata H, Rao NA. Vogt-Koyanagi-Harada syndrome. *Surv Ophthalmol.* 1995;39:265-292.

165. Shirato S, Hayashi K, Masuda K. Acute angle closure glaucoma as an initial sign of Haradas disease—report of 2 cases. *Jpn J Ophthalmol.* 1980;24:260-266.

166. Soheilian M, Aletaha M, Yazdani S, Dehghan MH, Peyman GA. Management of pediatric Vogt-Koyanagi-Harada (VKH)-associated panuveitis. *Ocul Immunol Inflamm.* 2006;14:91-98.

167. Abu El-Asrar AM, Al-Kharashi AS, Aldibhi H, Al-Fraykh H, Kangave D. Vogt-Koyanagi-Harada disease in children. *Eye (Lond).* 2008;22:1124-1131.

168. Castiblanco CP, Adelman RA. Sympathetic ophthalmia. *Graefes Arch Clin Exp Ophthalmol.* 2009;247:289-302.

169. Gupta V, Gupta A, Dogra MR. Posterior sympathetic ophthalmia: a single centre long-term study of 40 patients from North India. *Eye (Lond).* 2008;22:1459-1464.

170. Kuo YH, Juang CJ. Sympathetic ophthalmia associated with cyclitis: case report. *Changgeng Yi Xue Za Zhi.* 1999;22:328-333.

171. Galor A, Davis JL, Flynn HW Jr, et al. Sympathetic ophthalmia: incidence of ocular complications and vision loss in the sympathizing eye. *Am J Ophthalmol.* 2009;148:704-710, e702.

172. Makley TA Jr, Azar A. Sympathetic ophthalmia. A long-term follow-up. *Arch Ophthalmol.* 1978;96:257-262.

173. Lubin JR, Albert DM, Weinstein M. Sixty-five years of sympathetic ophthalmia. A clinicopathologic review of 105 cases (1913-1978). *Ophthalmology.* 1980;87:109-121.

174. Parikh JG, Saraswathy S, Rao NA. Photoreceptor oxidative damage in sympathetic ophthalmia. *Am J Ophthalmol.* 2008;146:866-875.

175. Du L, Kijlstra A, Yang P. Immune response genes in uveitis. *Ocul Immunol Inflamm.* 2009;17:249-256.

176. Jonas JB, Rensch F. Intravitreal steroid slow-release device replacing repeated intravitreal triamcinolone injections for sympathetic ophthalmia. *Eur J Ophthalmol.* 2008;18:834-836.

177. Chan CC, Roberge RG, Whitcup SM, Nussenblatt RB. 32 cases of sympathetic ophthalmia. A retrospective study at the National Eye Institute, Bethesda, Md., from 1982 to 1992. *Arch Ophthalmol.* 1995;113:597-600.

178. Jimenez-Alonso J, Martin-Armada M, Toribio M, Herranz-Marin MT, Rivera-Civico F, Perez-Alvarez F. Incidence of systemic lupus erythematosus among 255 patients with uveitis of unknown origin. *Ann Rheum Dis.* 2002;61:471.

179. Rodriguez A, Calonge M, Pedroza-Seres M, et al. Referral patterns of uveitis in a tertiary eye care center. *Arch Ophthalmol.* 1996;114:593-599.

180. Rosenbaum JT, Wernick R. The utility of routine screening of patients with uveitis for systemic lupus erythematosus or tuberculosis. A Bayesian analysis. *Arch Ophthalmol.* 1990;108:1291-1293.

181. Klejnberg T, Moraes Junior HV. [Ophthalmological alterations in outpatients with systemic lupus erythematosus]. *Arq Bras Oftalmol.* 2006;69:233-237.

182. Sivaraj RR, Durrani OM, Denniston AK, Murray PI, Gordon C. Ocular manifestations of systemic lupus erythematosus. *Rheumatology (Oxford).* 2007;46:1757-1762.

183. Wisotsky BJ, Magat-Gordon CB, Puklin JE. Angle-closure glaucoma as an initial presentation of systemic lupus erythematosus. *Ophthalmology.* 1998;105:1170-1172.

184. Wagemans MA, Bos PJ. Angle-closure glaucoma in a patient with systemic lupus erythematosus. *Doc Ophthalmol.* 1989;72:201-207.

185. Brock-Utne JG, Good CJ. Glaucoma and systemic lupus erythematosus. *Br Med J.* 1971;4:747.

186. Jankowska-Lech I, Terelak-Borys B, Grabska-Liberek I, Palasik W. Glaucoma neuropathy and neuropathy in multiple sclerosis—common elements of pathogenesis? [in Polish]. *Klin Oczna.* 2007;109:317-320.

187. Towler HM, Lightman S. Symptomatic intraocular inflammation in multiple sclerosis. *Clin Experiment Ophthalmol.* 2000;28:97-102.

188. Zein G, Berta A, Foster CS. Multiple sclerosis-associated uveitis. *Ocul Immunol Inflamm.* 2004;12:137-142.

189. Siskova A, Rihova E, Havrdova E. Uveitis and multiple sclerosis [in Czech]. *Cesk Slov Oftalmol.* 2005;61:235-244.

190. Sugita S, Shimizu N, Watanabe K, et al. Use of multiplex PCR and real-time PCR to detect human herpes virus genome in ocular fluids of patients with uveitis. *Br J Ophthalmol.* 2008;92:928-932.

191. Jones R 3rd, Pasquale LR, Pavan-Langston D. Herpes simplex virus: an important etiology for secondary glaucoma. *Int Ophthalmol Clin.* 2007;47:99-107.

192. Santos C. Herpes simplex uveitis. *Bol Asoc Med P R.* 2004;96:71-74, 77-83.

193. Sungur GK, Hazirolan D, Yalvac IS, Ozer PA, Aslan BS, Duman S. Incidence and prognosis of ocular hypertension secondary to viral uveitis. *Int Ophthalmol.* 2010;30(2):191-194.

194. Miserocchi E, Waheed NK, Dios E, et al. Visual outcome in herpes simplex virus and varicella zoster virus uveitis: a clinical evaluation and comparison. *Ophthalmology.* 2002;109:1532-1537.

195. Falcon MG, Williams HP. Herpes simplex kerato-uveitis and glaucoma. *Trans Ophthalmol Soc U K.* 1978;98:101-104.

196. Hogan MJ, Kimura SJ, Thygeson P. Pathology of herpes simplex kerato-iritis. *Trans Am Ophthalmol Soc.* 1963;61:75-99.

197. Tiwari V, Clement C, Scanlan PM, Kowlessur D, Yue BY, Shukla D. A role for herpesvirus entry mediator as the receptor for herpes simplex virus 1 entry into primary human trabecular meshwork cells. *J Virol.* 2005;79:13173-13179.

198. Oh JO. Effect of cyclophosphamide on primary herpes simplex uveitis in rabbits. *Invest Ophthalmol Vis Sci.* 1978;17:769-773.

199. Johns KJ, O'Day DM, Webb RA, Glick A. Anterior segment ischemia in chronic herpes simplex keratouveitis. *Curr Eye Res.* 1991;(10 suppl):117-124.

200. Inoda S, Wakakura M, Hirata J, Nakazato N, Toyo-Oka Y. Stromal keratitis and anterior uveitis due to herpes simplex virus-2 in a young child. *Jpn J Ophthalmol.* 2001;45:618-621.

201. Usui N, Kashiwase M, Minoda H, et al. Typing of herpes simplex virus in patients with uveitis. *Jpn J Ophthalmol.* 2001;45:112.

202. Gaynor BD, Margolis TP, Cunningham ET Jr. Advances in diagnosis and management of herpetic uveitis. *Int Ophthalmol Clin.* 2000;40:85-109.

203. Nakamura M, Tanabe M, Yamada Y, Azumi A. Zoster sine herpete with bilateral ocular involvement. *Am J Ophthalmol.* 2000;129:809-810.

204. Thean JH, Hall AJ, Stawell RJ. Uveitis in Herpes zoster ophthalmicus. *Clin Experiment Ophthalmol.* 2001;29:406-410.

205. Milikan JC, Kuijpers RW, Baarsma GS, Osterhaus AD, Verjans GM. Characterization of the varicella zoster virus (VZV)-specific intraocular T-cell response in patients with VZV-induced uveitis. *Exp Eye Res.* 2006;83:69-75.

206. Nakashizuka H, Yamazaki Y, Tokumaru M, Kimura T. Varicella-zoster viral antigen identified in iridocyclitis patient. *Jpn J Ophthalmol.* 2002;46:70-73.

207. Severson EA, Baratz KH, Hodge DO, Burke JP. Herpes zoster ophthalmicus in olmsted county, Minnesota: have systemic antivirals made a difference? *Arch Ophthalmol.* 2003;121:386-390.

208. van Boxtel LAA, van der Lelij A, van der Meer J, Los LI. Cytomegalovirus as a cause of anterior uveitis in immunocompetent patients. *Ophthalmology.* 2007;114:1358-1362.

209. de Schryver I, Rozenberg F, Cassoux N, et al. Diagnosis and treatment of cytomegalovirus iridocyclitis without retinal necrosis. *Br J Ophthalmol.* 2006;90:852-855.

210. Kawaguchi T, Sugita S, Shimizu N, Mochizuki M. Kinetics of aqueous flare, intraocular pressure and virus-DNA copies in a patient with cytomegalovirus iridocyclitis without retinitis. *Int Ophthalmol.* 2007;27:383-386.

211. Cheng L, Rao NA, Keefe KS, Avila CP Jr, Macdonald JC, Freeman WR. Cytomegalovirus iritis. *Ophthalmic Surg Lasers.* 1998;29:930-932.

212. Yamauchi Y, Suzuki J, Sakai J, Sakamoto S, Iwasaki T, Usui M. A case of hypertensive keratouveitis with endotheliitis associated with cytomegalovirus. *Ocul Immunol Inflamm.* 2007;15:399-401.

213. Mietz H, Aisenbrey S, Ulrich Bartz-Schmidt K, Bamborschke S, Krieglstein GK. Ganciclovir for the treatment of anterior uveitis. *Graefes Arch Clin Exp Ophthalmol.* 2000;238:905-909.

214. Hwang YS, Lin KK, Lee JS, et al. Intravitreal loading injection of ganciclovir with or without adjunctive oral valganciclovir for cytomegalovirus anterior uveitis. *Graefes Arch Clin Exp Ophthalmol.* 2009.

215. Touge C, Agawa H, Sairenji T, Inoue Y. High incidence of elevated antibody titers to Epstein-Barr virus in patients with uveitis. *Arch Virol.* 2006;151:895-903.

216. Yamamoto S, Sugita S, Sugamoto Y, Shimizu N, Morio T, Mochizuki M. Quantitative PCR for the detection of genomic DNA of Epstein-Barr virus in ocular fluids of patients with uveitis. *Jpn J Ophthalmol.* 2008;52:463-467.

217. Usui M, Sakai J. Three cases of EB virus-associated uveitis. *Int Ophthalmol.* 1990;14:371-376.

218. Usui Y, Goto H. Overview and diagnosis of acute retinal necrosis syndrome. *Semin Ophthalmol.* 2008;23:275-283.

219. Bonfioli AA, Eller AW. Acute retinal necrosis. *Semin Ophthalmol.* 2005;20:155-160.

220. Miserocchi E, Modorati G, Azzolini C, Foster CS, Brancato R. Herpes simplex virus type 2 acute retinal necrosis in an immunocompetent patient. *Eur J Ophthalmol.* 2003;13:99-102.

221. Fisher JP, Lewis ML, Blumenkranz M, et al. The acute retinal necrosis syndrome. Part 1: clinical manifestations. *Ophthalmology.* 1982;89:1309-1316.

222. Kalman A, Vogt M, Bernasconi E, Gloor B. Bilateral acute retinal artery necrosis—healing of the second affected eye [in German]. *Klin Monbl Augenheilkd.* 1994;204:235-240.

223. Biswas J, Sudharshan S. Anterior segment manifestations of human immunodeficiency virus/acquired immune deficiency syndrome. *Indian J Ophthalmol.* 2008;56:363-375.

224. Blumenkranz MS, Penneys NS. Acquired immunodeficiency syndrome and the eye. *Dermatol Clin.* 1992;10:777-783.

225. Rao NA. Acquired immunodeficiency syndrome and its ocular complications. *Indian J Ophthalmol.* 1994;42:51-63.

226. Cunningham ET Jr. Uveitis in HIV positive patients. *Br J Ophthalmol.* 2000;84:233-235.

227. Otiti-Sengeri J, Colebunders R, Kempen JH, Ronald A, Sande M, Katabira E. The prevalence and causes of visual loss among HIV-infected individuals with visual loss in Uganda. *J Acquir Immune Defic Syndr.* 2010;53(1):95-101.

228. Moraes HV Jr. Ocular manifestations of HIV/AIDS. *Curr Opin Ophthalmol.* 2002;13:397-403.

229. Nash RW, Lindquist TD. Bilateral angle-closure glaucoma associated with uveal effusion: presenting sign of HIV infection. *Surv Ophthalmol.* 1992;36:255-258.

230. Joshi N, Constable PH, Margolis TP, Hoyt CS, Leonard TJ. Bilateral angle closure glaucoma and accelerated cataract formation in a patient with AIDS. *Br J Ophthalmol.* 1994;78:656-657.

231. Robinson MR, Reed G, Csaky KG, Polis MA, Whitcup SM. Immune-recovery uveitis in patients with cytomegalovirus retinitis taking highly active antiretroviral therapy. *Am J Ophthalmol.* 2000;130:49-56.

232. Givens KT, Lee DA, Jones T, Ilstrup DM. Congenital rubella syndrome: ophthalmic manifestations and associated systemic disorders. *Br J Ophthalmol.* 1993;77:358-363.

233. Khandekar R, Al Awaidy S, Ganesh A, Bawikar S. An epidemiological and clinical study of ocular manifestations of congenital rubella syndrome in Omani children. *Arch Ophthalmol.* 2004;122:541-545.

234. Vijayalakshmi P, Kakkar G, Samprathi A, Banushree R. Ocular manifestations of congenital rubella syndrome in a developing country. *Indian J Ophthalmol.* 2002;50:307-311.

235. Lahbil D, Souldi L, Rais L, Lamari H, El Kettani A, Zaghloul K. [Manifestation of congenital rubella syndrome: clinical and epidemiologic aspects]. *Bull Soc Belge Ophtalmol.* 2007:13-20.

236. O'Neill JF. The ocular manifestations of congenital infection: a study of the early effect and long-term outcome of maternally transmitted rubella and toxoplasmosis. *Trans Am Ophthalmol Soc.* 1998;96:813-879.

237. Boniuk M. Glaucoma in the congenital rubella syndrome. *Int Ophthalmol Clin.* 1972;12:121-136.

238. Boger WP 3rd. Late ocular complications in congenital rubella syndrome. *Ophthalmology.* 1980;87:1244-1252.

239. Sundmacher R, Neumann-Haefelin D. Herpes simplex virus isolations from the aqueous humor of patients suffering from focal iritis, endotheliitis, and prolonged disciform keratitis with glaucoma (author's transl) [in German]. *Klin Monbl Augenheilkd.* 1979;175:488-501.

240. Armstrong NT. The ocular manifestations of congenital rubella syndrome. *Insight.* 1992;17:14-16.

241. Miyanaga M, Shimizu K, Kawaguchi T, Miyata K, Mochizuki M. A clinical survey of uveitis in HTLV-1 endemic region. *Ocul Immunol Inflamm.* 2009;17:335-341.

242. Proietti FA, Carneiro-Proietti AB, Catalan-Soares BC, Murphy EL. Global epidemiology of HTLV-I infection and associated diseases. *Oncogene.* 2005;24:6058-6068.

243. Takahashi T, Takase H, Urano T, et al. Clinical features of human T-lymphotropic virus type 1 uveitis: a long-term follow-up. *Ocul Immunol Inflamm.* 2000;8:235-241.

244. Ohshima K. Pathological features of diseases associated with human T-cell leukemia virus type I. *Cancer Sci.* 2007;98:772-778.

245. Pinheiro SR, Martins-Filho OA, Ribas JG, et al. Immunologic markers, uveitis, and keratoconjunctivitis sicca associated with human T-cell lymphotropic virus type 1. *Am J Ophthalmol.* 2006;142:811-815.

246. Buggage RR. Ocular manifestations of human T-cell lymphotropic virus type 1 infection. *Curr Opin Ophthalmol.* 2003;14:420-425.

247. Takahashi T, Ohtani S, Miyata K, Miyata N, Sirato S, Mochizuki M. A clinical evaluation of uveitis-associated secondary glaucoma [in Japanese]. *Nippon Ganka Gakkai Zasshi.* 2002;106:39-43.

248. Nakao K, Ohba N, Matsumoto M. Noninfectious anterior uveitis in patients infected with human T-lymphotropic virus type I. *Jpn J Ophthalmol.* 1989;33:472-481.

249. Khairallah M, Chee SP, Rathinam SR, Attia S, Nadella V. Novel infectious agents causing uveitis. *Int Ophthalmol.* 2010;30(5):465-483.

250. Kuchtey RW, Kosmorsky GS, Martin D, Lee MS. Uveitis associated with West Nile virus infection. *Arch Ophthalmol.* 2003;121:1648-1649.

251. Koevary SB. Ocular involvement in patients infected by the West Nile virus. *Optometry.* 2005;76:609-612.

252. Gupta A, Srinivasan R, Setia S, Soundravally R, Pandian DG. Uveitis following dengue fever. *Eye (Lond).* 2009;23:873-876.

253. Chan DP, Teoh SC, Tan CS, et al. Ophthalmic complications of dengue. *Emerg Infect Dis.* 2006;12:285-289.

254. Bacsal KE, Chee SP, Cheng CL, Flores JV. Dengue-associated maculopathy. *Arch Ophthalmol.* 2007;125:501-510.

255. Pierre Filho Pde T, Carvalho Filho JP, Pierre ET. Bilateral acute angle closure glaucoma in a patient with dengue fever: case report. *Arq Bras Oftalmol.* 2008;71:265-268.

256. Richardson S. Ocular symptoms and complications observed in Dengue. *Trans Am Ophthalmol Soc.* 1933;31:450-477.

257. Mahendradas P, Ranganna SK, Shetty R, et al. Ocular manifestations associated with chikungunya. *Ophthalmology.* 2008;115:287-291.

258. Lalitha P, Rathinam S, Banushree K, Maheshkumar S, Vijayakumar R, Sathe P. Ocular involvement associated with an epidemic outbreak of chikungunya virus infection. *Am J Ophthalmol.* 2007;144:552-556.

259. Mittal A, Mittal S, Bharathi JM, Ramakrishnan R, Sathe PS. Uveitis during outbreak of Chikungunya fever. *Ophthalmology.* 2007;114:1798.

260. Saari KM. Acute glaucoma in hemorrhagic fever with renal syndrome (nephropathia epidemica). *Am J Ophthalmol.* 1976;81:455-461.

261. Tedeschi-Reiner E, Mandic Z, Grgic D. [Ocular changes in hemorrhagic fever with renal syndrome]. *Acta Med Croatica.* 2003;57:415-419.

262. Parssinen O, Klemetti A, Rossi-Rautiainen E, Forslund T. Ophthalmic manifestations of epidemic nephropathy. *Acta Ophthalmol (Copenh).* 1993;71:114-118.

263. Kontkanen M, Puustjarvi T, Kauppi P, Lahdevirta J. Ocular characteristics in nephropathia epidemica or Puumala virus infection. *Acta Ophthalmol Scand.* 1996;74:621-625.

264. Saari KM, Luoto S. Ophthalmological findings in nephropathia epidemica in Lapland. *Acta Ophthalmol (Copenh).* 1984;62:235-243.

265. Saari M, Alanko H, Jarvi J, Vetoniemi-Korhonen SL, Rasanen O. Nephropathia epidemica. The Scandinavian form of hemorrhagic fever with renal syndrome. *JAMA.* 1977;238:874-877.

266. Kontkanen MI, Puustjarvi TJ, Lahdevirta JK. Intraocular pressure changes in nephropathia epidemica. A prospective study of 37 patients with acute systemic Puumala virus infection. *Ophthalmology.* 1995;102:1813-1817.

267. Onal S, Toker E. A rare ocular complication of mumps: keratouveitis. *Ocul Immunol Inflamm.* 2005;13:395-397.

268. Polland W, Thorburn W. Transient glaucoma as a manifestation of mumps. A case report. *Acta Ophthalmol (Copenh).* 1976;54:779-782.

269. Islam SM, El-Sheikh HF, Tabbara KF. Anterior uveitis following combined vaccination for measles, mumps and rubella (MMR): a report of two cases. *Acta Ophthalmol Scand.* 2000;78:590-592.

270. Hara J, Ishibashi T, Fujimoto F, Danjyo S, Minekawa Y, Maeda A. Adenovirus type 10 keratoconjunctivitis with increased intraocular pressure. *Am J Ophthalmol.* 1980;90:481-484.

271. Donahue HC. Ophthalmologic experience in a tuberculosis sanatorium. *Am J Ophthalmol.* 1967;64:742-748.

272. Rathinam SR, Cunningham ET Jr. Infectious causes of uveitis in the developing world. *Int Ophthalmol Clin.* 2000;40:137-152.

273. Militaru C. [Chronic tuberculous iridocyclitis]. *Oftalmologia.* 1997;41:40-43.

274. de Popa DP, Smochina S. Therapeutical difficulties in a patient with TB panuveitis and open angle glaucoma [in Romanian]. *Oftalmologia.* 2002;54:23-26.

275. Vasconcelos-Santos DV, Zierhut M, Rao NA. Strengths and weaknesses of diagnostic tools for tuberculous uveitis. *Ocul Immunol Inflamm.* 2009;17:351-355.

276. Garip A, Diedrichs-Mohring M, Thurau SR, Deeg CA, Wildner G. Uveitis in a patient treated with Bacille-Calmette-Guerin: possible antigenic mimicry of mycobacterial and retinal antigens. *Ophthalmology.* 2009;116:2457-2462 e2451-2452.

277. Hamade IH, Tabbara KF. Complications of presumed ocular tuberculosis. *Acta Ophthalmol.* 2009.

278. Bansal R, Gupta A, Gupta V, Dogra MR, Bambery P, Arora SK. Role of antitubercular therapy in uveitis with latent/manifest tuberculosis. *Am J Ophthalmol.* 2008;146:772-779.

279. Cimino L, Herbort CP, Aldigeri R, Salvarani C, Boiardi L. Tuberculous uveitis, a resurgent and underdiagnosed disease. *Int Ophthalmol.* 2009;29:67-74.

280. Ustinova EI, Baranov I, Kliavina AE. Laser iridectomy in tuberculous uveitis complicated by glaucoma and ophthalmic hypertension [in Russian]. *Oftalmol Zh.* 1990:14-18.

281. Spratt A, Key T, Vivian AJ. Chronic anterior uveitis following bacille Calmette-Guerin vaccination: molecular mimicry in action? *J Pediatr Ophthalmol Strabismus.* 2008;45:252-253.

282. Schwab IR. Ocular leprosy. *Infect Dis Clin North Am.* 1992;6:953-961.

283. Reddy SC, Raju BD, Achary NR. Survey of eye complications in leprosy in Prakasam district (Andhra Pradesh). *Lepr India.* 1981;53:231-237.

284. Espiritu CG, Gelber R, Ostler HB. Chronic anterior uveitis in leprosy: an insidious cause of blindness. *Br J Ophthalmol.* 1991;75:273-275.

285. Nwosu SN, Nwosu MC. Ocular findings in leprosy patients in Nigeria. *East Afr Med J.* 1994;71:441-444.

286. Parikh R, Thomas S, Muliyil J, Parikh S, Thomas R. Ocular manifestation in treated multibacillary Hansen's disease. *Ophthalmology.* 2009;116:2051-2057, e2051.

287. Hogeweg M, Faber WR. Progression of eye lesions in leprosy: ten-year follow-up study in The Netherlands. *Int J Lepr Other Mycobact Dis.* 1991;59:392-397.

288. Michelson JB, Roth AM, Waring GO 3rd. Lepromatous iridocyclitis diagnosed by anterior chamber paracentesis. *Am J Ophthalmol.* 1979;88:674-679.

289. Walton RC, Ball SF, Joffrion VC. Glaucoma in Hansen's disease. *Br J Ophthalmol.* 1991;75:270-272.

290. Hussein N, Courtright P, Ostler HB, Hetherington J, Gelber RH. Low intraocular pressure and postural changes in intraocular pressure in patients with Hansen's disease. *Am J Ophthalmol.* 1989;108:80-83.

291. Brandt F, Malla OK, Anten JG. Influence of untreated chronic plastic iridocyclitis on intraocular pressure in leprous patients. *Br J Ophthalmol.* 1981;65:240-242.

292. Messmer EM, Raizman MB, Foster CS. Lepromatous uveitis diagnosed by iris biopsy. *Graefes Arch Clin Exp Ophthalmol.* 1998;236:717-719.

293. Rehman S, Metcalfe TW, Barnham M. Anterior uveitis associated with cat scratch disease. *Br J Ophthalmol.* 1998;82:587-588.

294. Gray AV, Michels KS, Lauer AK, Samples JR. Bartonella henselae infection associated with neuroretinitis, central retinal artery and vein occlusion, neovascular glaucoma, and severe vision loss. *Am J Ophthalmol.* 2004;137:187-189.

295. Ziemssen F, Bartz-Schmidt KU, Gelisken F. Secondary unilateral glaucoma and neuroretinitis: atypical manifestation of cat-scratch disease. *Jpn J Ophthalmol.* 2006;50:177-179.

296. Martinez-Osorio H, Calonge M, Torres J, Gonzalez F. Cat-scratch disease (ocular bartonellosis) presenting as bilateral recurrent iridocyclitis. *Clin Infect Dis.* 2005;40:e43-45.

297. Kerkhoff FT, Rothova A. Bartonella henselae associated uveitis and HLA-B27. *Br J Ophthalmol.* 2000;84:1125-1129.

298. Drancourt M, Bodaghi B, Lepidi H, Le Hoang P, Raoult D. Intraocular detection of Bartonella henselae in a patient with HLA-B27 uveitis. *J Clin Microbiol.* 2004;42:1822-1825.

299. Soheilian M, Markomichelakis N, Foster CS. Intermediate uveitis and retinal vasculitis as manifestations of cat scratch disease. *Am J Ophthalmol.* 1996;122:582-584.

300. Tabbara KF, al-Kassimi H. Ocular brucellosis. *Br J Ophthalmol.* 1990;74:249-250.

301. Gedalia A, Watemberg N, Rothschild M. Childhood brucellosis in the Negev [in Hebrew]. *Harefuah.* 1990;119:313-315.

302. Sungur GK, Hazirolan D, Gurbuz Y, Unlu N, Duran S, Duman S. Ocular involvement in brucellosis. *Can J Ophthalmol.* 2009;44: 598-601.

303. Rolando I, Vilchez G, Olarte L, et al. Brucellar uveitis: intraocular fluids and biopsy studies. *Int J Infect Dis.* 2009;13:e206-211.

304. Gorrono-Echebarria MB, Guzman-Blazquez J, Teus-Guezala MA, Martin-Villa JM. Anterior uveitis and meningococcemia: a case report. *Ocul Immunol Inflamm.* 2006;14:193-194.

305. Mason W, Igdaloff S, Friedman R, Wright HT Jr. Meningococcal sepsis with endophthalmitis. *Am J Dis Child.* 1979;133:1151-1152.

306. Lohmann CP, Gabel VP, Heep M, Linde HJ, Reischl U. Listeria monocytogenes-induced endogenous endophthalmitis in an otherwise healthy individual: rapid PCR-diagnosis as the basis for effective treatment. *Eur J Ophthalmol.* 1999;9:53-57.

307. Berger E, Donat M, Guthoff RF, Podbielski A. Listeria endophthalmitis [in German]. *Ophthalmologe.* 2005;102:888-890.

308. Mendez-Hernandez C, Garcia-Feijoo J, Garcia-Sanchez J. Listeria monocytogenes-induced endogenous endophthalmitis: bioultrasonic findings. *Am J Ophthalmol.* 2004;137:579-581.

309. Nishimura JK, Cook BE Jr, Pach JM. Whipple disease presenting as posterior uveitis without prominent gastrointestinal symptoms. *Am J Ophthalmol.* 1998;126:130-132.

310. Leland TM, Chambers JK. Ocular findings in Whipple's disease. *South Med J.* 1978;71:335-338.

311. Grant WM. Late glaucoma after interstitial keratitis. *Am J Ophthalmol.* 1975;79:87-91.

312. Salvador F, Linares F, Merita I, Amen M. Unilateral iridoschisis associated with syphilitic interstitial keratitis and glaucoma. *Ann Ophthalmol.* 1993;25:328-329.

313. Foss AJ, Hykin PG, Benjamin L. Interstitial keratitis and iridoschisis in congenital syphilis. *J Clin Neuroophthalmol.* 1992;12:167-170.

314. Anshu A, Cheng CL, Chee SP. Syphilitic uveitis: an Asian perspective. *Br J Ophthalmol.* 2008;92:594-597.

315. Hong MC, Sheu SJ, Wu TT, Chuang CT. Ocular uveitis as the initial presentation of syphilis. *J Chin Med Assoc.* 2007;70:274-280.

316. Aldave AJ, King JA, Cunningham ET Jr. Ocular syphilis. *Curr Opin Ophthalmol.* 2001;12:433-441.

317. Orsoni JG, Zavota L, Manzotti F, Gonzales S. Syphilitic interstitial keratitis: treatment with immunosuppressive drug combination therapy. *Cornea.* 2004;23:530-532.

318. Boye T. [What kind of clinical, epidemiological, and biological data is essential for the diagnosis of Lyme borreliosis? Dermatological and ophtalmological courses of Lyme borreliosis]. *Med Mal Infect.* 2007;37(suppl 3):S175-S188.

319. Zaidman GW. The ocular manifestations of Lyme disease. *Int Ophthalmol Clin.* 1997;37:13-28.

320. Lesser RL. Ocular manifestations of Lyme disease. *Am J Med.* 1995;98:60S-62S.

321. Mikkila HO, Seppala IJ, Viljanen MK, Peltomaa MP, Karma A. The expanding clinical spectrum of ocular lyme borreliosis. *Ophthalmology.* 2000;107:581-587.

322. Ness T, Pleyer U, Neudorf U, Frosch M. [Infectious uveitis in infancy: borreliosis, tuberculosis, lues]. *Klin Monbl Augenheilkd.* 2007;224:488-493.

323. Rathinam SR. Ocular manifestations of leptospirosis. *J Postgrad Med.* 2005;51:189-194.

324. Rathinam SR, Rathnam S, Selvaraj S, Dean D, Nozik RA, Namperumalsamy P. Uveitis associated with an epidemic outbreak of leptospirosis. *Am J Ophthalmol.* 1997;124:71-79.

325. Rathinam SR, Namperumalsamy P, Cunningham ET Jr. Spontaneous cataract absorption in patients with leptospiral uveitis. *Br J Ophthalmol.* 2000;84:1135-1141.

326. Priya CG, Rathinam SR, Muthukkaruppan V. Evidence for endotoxin as a causative factor for leptospiral uveitis in humans. *Invest Ophthalmol Vis Sci.* 2008;49:5419-5424.

327. Hwang JM, Pian D. Iritis presumed as secondary to disseminated coccidioidomycosis. *Optometry.* 2006;77:547-553.

328. Cunningham ET Jr, Seiff SR, Berger TG, Lizotte PE, Howes EL Jr, Horton JC. Intraocular coccidioidomycosis diagnosed by skin biopsy. *Arch Ophthalmol.* 1998;116:674-677.

329. Moorthy RS, Rao NA, Sidikaro Y, Foos RY. Coccidioidomycosis iridocyclitis. *Ophthalmology.* 1994;101:1923-1928.

330. Rodenbiker HT, Ganley JP. Ocular coccidioidomycosis. *Surv Ophthalmol.* 1980;24:263-290.

331. Pettit TH, Learn RN, Foos RY. Intraocular coccidioidomycosis. *Arch Ophthalmol.* 1967;77:655-661.

332. Bell R, Font RL. Granulomatous anterior uveitis caused by Coccidioides immitis. *Am J Ophthalmol.* 1972;74:93-98.

333. Ala-Kauhaluoma M, Aho I, Ristola M, Karma A. Involvement of intraocular structures in disseminated histoplasmosis. *Acta Ophthalmol.* 2008.

334. Gonzales CA, Scott IU, Chaudhry NA, et al. Endogenous endophthalmitis caused by Histoplasma capsulatum var. capsulatum: a case report and literature review. *Ophthalmology.* 2000;107: 725-729.

335. Perkins ES. Ocular toxoplasmosis. *Br J Ophthalmol.* 1973;57:1-17.

336. Commodaro AG, Belfort RN, Rizzo LV, et al. Ocular toxoplasmosis: an update and review of the literature. *Mem Inst Oswaldo Cruz.* 2009;104:345-350.

337. Westeneng AC, Rothova A, de Boer JH, de Groot-Mijnes JD. Infectious uveitis in immunocompromised patients and the diagnostic value of polymerase chain reaction and Goldmann-Witmer coefficient in aqueous analysis. *Am J Ophthalmol.* 2007;144: 781-785.

338. Dodds EM, Holland GN, Stanford MR, et al. Intraocular inflammation associated with ocular toxoplasmosis: relationships at initial examination. *Am J Ophthalmol.* 2008;146:856-865, e852.

339. Delair E, Monnet D, Grabar S, Dupouy-Camet J, Yera H, Brezin AP. Respective roles of acquired and congenital infections in presumed ocular toxoplasmosis. *Am J Ophthalmol.* 2008;146:851-855.

340. Accorinti M, Bruscolini A, Pirraglia MP, Liverani M, Caggiano C. Toxoplasmic retinochoroiditis in an Italian referral center. *Eur J Ophthalmol.* 2009;19:824-830.

341. Bonfioli AA, Orefice F. Toxoplasmosis. *Semin Ophthalmol.* 2005;20:129-141.

342. Westfall AC, Lauer AK, Suhler EB, Rosenbaum JT. Toxoplasmosis retinochoroiditis and elevated intraocular pressure: a retrospective study. *J Glaucoma.* 2005;14:3-10.

343. Sheets CW, Grewal DS, Greenfield DS. Ocular toxoplasmosis presenting with focal retinal nerve fiber atrophy simulating glaucoma. *J Glaucoma.* 2009;18:129-131.

344. Garweg JG, Candolfi E. Immunopathology in ocular toxoplasmosis: facts and clues. *Mem Inst Oswaldo Cruz.* 2009;104:211-220.

345. Albuquerque MC, Aleixo AL, Benchimol EI, et al. The IFN-gamma +874T/A gene polymorphism is associated with retinochoroiditis toxoplasmosis susceptibility. *Mem Inst Oswaldo Cruz.* 2009;104:451-455.

346. Cordeiro CA, Moreira PR, Andrade MS, et al. Interleukin-10 gene polymorphism (-1082G/A) is associated with toxoplasmic retinochoroiditis. *Invest Ophthalmol Vis Sci.* 2008;49:1979-1982.

347. Goto H, Mochizuki M, Yamaki K, Kotake S, Usui M, Ohno S. Epidemiological survey of intraocular inflammation in Japan. *Jpn J Ophthalmol.* 2007;51:41-44.

348. Deuter CM, Garweg JG, Pleyer U, Schonherr U, Thurau S. Ocular toxoplasmosis and toxocariasis in childhood [in German]. *Klin Monbl Augenheilkd.* 2007;224:483-487.

349. Stewart JM, Cubillan LD, Cunningham ET Jr. Prevalence, clinical features, and causes of vision loss among patients with ocular toxocariasis. *Retina.* 2005;25:1005-1013.

350. Smith PH, Greer CH. Unusual presentation of ocular Toxocara infestation. *Br J Ophthalmol.* 1971;55:317-320.

351. Shields JA. Ocular toxocariasis. A review. *Surv Ophthalmol.* 1984;28:361-381.

352. Frazier M, Anderson ML, Sophocleous S. Treatment of ocular toxocariasis with albendazole: a case report. *Optometry.* 2009;80:175-180.

353. Newland HS, White AT, Greene BM, Murphy RP, Taylor HR. Ocular manifestations of onchocerciasis in a rain forest area of west Africa. *Br J Ophthalmol.* 1991;75:163-169.

354. Neto GH, Jaegger K, Marchon-Silva V, et al. Eye disease related to onchocerciasis: a clinical study in the Aratha-u, Yanomami Tribe, Roraima State, Brazil. *Acta Trop.* 2009;112:115-119.

355. Egbert PR, Jacobson DW, Fiadoyor S, Dadzie P, Ellingson KD. Onchocerciasis: a potential risk factor for glaucoma. *Br J Ophthalmol.* 2005;89:796-798.

356. Stilma JS. Onchocerciasis and glaucoma: ophthalmo-pathological aspects of the limbus and Tenon's capsule in 25 surgical patients from Ghana. *Doc Ophthalmol.* 1981;50:327-335.

357. Yang YF, Cousens S, Murdoch IE, Babalola OE, Abiose A, Jones B. Intraocular pressure and gonioscopic findings in rural communities mesoendemic and nonendemic for onchoceriasis, Kaduna State, Nigeria. *Eye (Lond).* 2001;15:756-759.

358. Somo RM, Ngosso A, Dinga JS, Enyong PA, Fobi G. A community-based trial of ivermectin for onchocerciasis control in the forest of southwestern Cameroon: clinical and parasitologic findings after three treatments. *Am J Trop Med Hyg.* 1993;48:9-13.

359. Kravchinina VV, Dushin NV, Beliaev VS, Barashkov VI, Gonchar PA, Frolov MA. [A case of relapsing iridocyclitis in tropical malaria]. *Vestn Oftalmol.* 1997;113:41-42.

360. Bialasiewicz AA, Hassenstein A, Schaudig U. [Subretinal granuloma, retinal vasculitis and keratouveitis with secondary open-angle glaucoma in schistosomiasis]. *Ophthalmologe.* 2001;98:972-975.

361. Creed TD. Unilateral optic atrophy presumed secondary to schistosomiasis of the optic nerve. *J Am Optom Assoc.* 1993;64:440-445.

362. Bacon AS, Frazer DG, Dart JK, Matheson M, Ficker LA, Wright P. A review of 72 consecutive cases of Acanthamoeba keratitis, 1984-1992. *Eye (Lond).* 1993;7(pt 6):719-725.

363. Doren GS, Cohen EJ, Higgins SE, et al. Management of contact lens associated Acanthamoeba keratitis. *CLAO J.* 1991;17:120-125.

364. Herz NL, Matoba AY, Wilhelmus KR. Rapidly progressive cataract and iris atrophy during treatment of Acanthamoeba keratitis. *Ophthalmology.* 2008;115:866-869.

365. Kelley PS, Dossey AP, Patel D, Whitson JT, Hogan RN, Cavanagh HD. Secondary glaucoma associated with advanced acanthamoeba keratitis. *Eye Contact Lens.* 2006;32:178-182.

366. Wright P, Warhurst D, Jones BR. Acanthamoeba keratitis successfully treated medically. *Br J Ophthalmol.* 1985;69:778-782.

367. Kosrirukvongs P, Wanachiwanawin D, Visvesvara GS. Treatment of acanthamoeba keratitis with chlorhexidine. *Ophthalmology.* 1999;106:798-802.

368. TugalTutkun I, Havrlikova K, Power WJ, Foster CS. Changing patterns in uveitis of childhood. *Ophthalmology.* 1996;103:375-383.

369. Ortega-Larrocea G, Arellanes-Garcia L. Pars planitis: epidemiology and clinical outcome in a large community hospital in Mexico City. *Int Ophthalmol.* 1995;19:117-120.

370. Henderly DE, Genstler AJ, Rao NA, Smith RE. Pars planitis. *Trans Ophthalmol Soc U K.* 1986;105(pt 2):227-232.

371. Pederson JE, Kenyon KR, Green WR, Maumenee AE. Pathology of pars planitis. *Am J Ophthalmol.* 1978;86:762-774.

372. Benson WE. Posterior scleritis. *Surv Ophthalmol.* 1988;32:297-316.

373. Mangouritsas G, Ulbig M. Secondary angle-block glaucoma in posterior scleritis [in German]. *Klin Monbl Augenheilkd.* 1991;199:40-44.

374. Erdol H, Kola M, Turk A. Optical coherence tomography findings in a child with posterior scleritis. *Eur J Ophthalmol.* 2008;18: 1007-1010.

375. Watson PG, Hayreh SS. Scleritis and episcleritis. *Br J Ophthalmol.* 1976;60:163-191.

376. Jorgensen JS, Guthoff R. The role of episcleral venous pressure in the development of secondary glaucomas [in German]. *Klin Monbl Augenheilkd.* 1988;193:471-475.

377. Wilhelmus KR, Grierson I, Watson PG. Histopathologic and clinical associations of scleritis and glaucoma. *Am J Ophthalmol.* 1981;91:697-705.

378. Nasser LS, Liendo da Costa VL, Taniguchi MP, Bolanho A, Petrilli AM. Angle-closure glaucoma secondary to nonspecific orbital inflammatory: case report [in Portuguese]. *Arq Bras Oftalmol.* 2007;70: 1029-1033.

379. Jain SS, Rao P, Kothari K, Bhatt D, Jain S. Posterior scleritis presenting as unilateral secondary angle-closure glaucoma. *Indian J Ophthalmol.* 2004;52:241-244.

380. Pavlin CJ, Easterbrook M, Harasiewicz K, Foster FS. An ultrasound biomicroscopic analysis of angle-closure glaucoma secondary to ciliochoroidal effusion in IgA nephropathy. *Am J Ophthalmol.* 1993;116:341-345.

381. Quinlan MP, Hitchings RA. Angle-closure glaucoma secondary to posterior scleritis. *Br J Ophthalmol.* 1978;62:330-335.

382. Fourman S. Angle-closure glaucoma complicating ciliochoroidal detachment. *Ophthalmology.* 1989;96:646-653.

383. Akpek EK, Uy HS, Christen W, Gurdal C, Foster CS. Severity of episcleritis and systemic disease association. *Ophthalmology.* 1999;106:729-731.

384. Shaffer R. Glaucoma in uveitis. In: Kimura SJ, Goodner EK, eds. *Ocular Pharmacology and Therapeutics and the Problems of Medical Management.* Philadelphia: Davis; 1963:viii, 267.

385. Schwartz A. Chronic open-angle glaucoma secondary to rhegmatogenous retinal detachment. *Am J Ophthalmol.* 1973;75: 205-211.

386. Schwartz A. Chronic open-angle glaucoma secondary to rhegmatogenous retinal detachment. *Trans Am Ophthalmol Soc.* 1972;70:178-189.

387. Matsuo N, Takabatake M, Ueno H, Nakayama T, Matsuo T. Photoreceptor outer segments in the aqueous humor in rhegmatogenous retinal detachment. *Am J Ophthalmol.* 1986;101: 673-679.

388. Callender D, Jay JL, Barrie T. Schwartz-Matsuo syndrome: Atypical presentation as acute open angle glaucoma. *Br J Ophthalmol.* 1997;81:609-610.

389. Gutierrez C, Merayo J, Cuevas J, Lazaro M, Rebolleda G, Munoz-Negrete FJ. Glaucoma related with photoreceptor outer segments in aqueous humor. Schwartz-Matsuo syndrome [in Spanish]. *Arch Soc Esp Oftalmol.* 2001;76:315-318.

390. Heatley G, Pro M, Harasymowycz P. Schwartz-Matsuo syndrome. *J Glaucoma.* 2006;15:562-564.

391. Rathore MK. Ophthalmological study of epidemic dropsy. *Br J Ophthalmol.* 1982;66:573-575.

392. Singh NP, Anuradha S, Dhanwal DK, et al. Epidemic dropsy—a clinical study of the Delhi outbreak. *J Assoc Physicians India.* 2000;48:877-880.

393. Singh K, Singh MJ, Das JC. Visual field defects in epidemic dropsy. *Clin Toxicol (Phila).* 2006;44:159-163.

394. Sachdev MS, Sood NN, Verma LK, Gupta SK, Jaffery NF. Pathogenesis of epidemic dropsy glaucoma. *Arch Ophthalmol.* 1988;106:1221-1223.

395. Thatte U, Dahanukar S. The Mexican poppy poisons the Indian mustard facts and figures. *J Assoc Physicians India.* 1999;47:332-335.

396. Malik KP, Dadeya S, Gupta VS, Sharan P, Guliani, Dhawan M. Pattern of intraocular pressure in epidemic dropsy in India. *Trop Doct.* 2004;34:161-162.

397. Punzi L, Furlan A, Podswiadek M, et al. Clinical and genetic aspects of Blau syndrome: a 25-year follow-up of one family and a literature review. *Autoimmun Rev.* 2009;8:228-232.

398. Becker ML, Rose CD. Blau syndrome and related genetic disorders causing childhood arthritis. *Curr Rheumatol Rep.* 2005;7:427-433.

399. Blau EB. Familial granulomatous arthritis, iritis, and rash. *J Pediatr.* 1985;107:689-693.

400. Jabs DA, Houk JL, Bias WB, Arnett FC. Familial granulomatous synovitis, uveitis, and cranial neuropathies. *Am J Med.* 1985;78:801-804.

401. Kurokawa T, Kikuchi T, Ohta K, Imai H, Yoshimura N. Ocular manifestations in Blau syndrome associated with a CARD15/Nod2 mutation. *Ophthalmology.* 2003;110:2040-2044.

43

Glaucoma Due to Trauma

Carla I. Bourne, MD and Bradford J. Shingleton, MD

Glaucoma due to trauma is a multifactorial disease. Intraocular pressure (IOP) may increase after blunt trauma, lacerating trauma, chemical exposure, electromagnetic radiation, or surgery. Elevated IOP may develop immediately after the injury or years later. The angle may be open or closed. The injured eye may demonstrate obvious signs of damage, or clinical signs of trauma may be largely unapparent. Eyes that are predisposed to glaucoma after ocular injury may actually have a low IOP initially rather than a high IOP. Low IOP may result from aqueous hyposecretion due to ciliary contusion and inflammation, increased uveoscleral/vortex outflow due to a cyclodialysis cleft, tears through trabecular meshwork (TM) into Schlemm's canal, or loss of integrity of the globe due to scleral or corneal perforation. Low IOP can often convert to high IOP as a result of treatment, normal healing processes, and the long-lasting effect of the injury itself on TM outflow. Elevated IOP has multiple causes, but they all tend to reflect a reduced facility of outflow of aqueous humor through the TM drainage channels (Table 43-1).[1]

Glaucoma causing injuries to the anterior segment most commonly follow blunt injury, and the United States Eye Injury Registry[2] reports that, at 6 months following the injury, the incidence of glaucoma was 3.39%. Factors highly predictive of developing glaucoma have been identified as poor initial visual acuity, advancing age, lens injury, angle recession, higher initial IOP, and hyphema.[2-4]

The impact from the blunt injury results in a sudden compressive deformation of the eye. The cornea and anterior sclera are displaced posteriorly, and there is a compensatory expansion of the globe in the equatorial direction.[5] Campbell[6] has graphically described 7 rings, or circles, of tissue anterior to the equator of the globe that suddenly expand with blunt impact. Because the internal fluids of the eye cannot compress, the forces are transmitted to the 7 rings of tissue. This often results in splitting or tearing of tissues that may manifest as radial sphincter tears, iridodialysis, angle recession, cyclodialysis, TM tears, zonule separation, or peripheral retinal dialysis. Damage in many of these areas may result in either early onset or delayed onset glaucoma.

EARLY-ONSET GLAUCOMA AFTER EYE INJURY

Contusion With Intraocular Inflammation

Blunt trauma commonly results in inflammation of the anterior segment visualized as flare and cells at the slit-lamp. Red blood cells and gross angle disruption are often not identified but IOP may still be elevated. The elevation of IOP in this setting is presumably due to reduced aqueous outflow as a result of inflammatory cells and debris obstructing TM outflow channels. Edema and direct damage to TM beams may not be identified on gonioscopy but may still contribute to a temporary rise in IOP. This situation tends to be self-limited and clears spontaneously or with the use of topical steroids.

Trabecular Meshwork Damage

Herschler[7] has shown that gonioscopy early after blunt injury may demonstrate trauma-related changes in the trabecular zone. A full-thickness tear in TM may occur, and a trabecular flap may be created at the point of rupture. This tends to arise just below the insertion of the trabecular sheets at Schwalbe's line. Inflammation is invariably associated with this type of injury. IOP may or may not be elevated depending on the amount of aqueous production. Indeed, IOP may actually be subnormal in the early peritraumatic period due to direct access of aqueous to Schlemm's canal, bypassing the TM. A small clot may be noted in the area of

Kahook MY, Schuman JS, eds.
Chandler and Grant's Glaucoma, Fifth Edition (pp 413-422).
© 2013 SLACK Incorporated.

TABLE 43-1. KEY POINTS: DIFFERENTIAL DIAGNOSIS OF ELEVATED INTRAOCULAR PRESSURE AFTER TRAUMA
Early-Onset Glaucoma
Contusion injury
Trabecular meshwork damage
Traumatic hyphema
Chemical injury
Late-Onset Glaucoma
Angle recession
Ghost-cell glaucoma
Lens-induced glaucoma
Peripheral anterior synechiae
Closure of cyclodialysis cleft
Epithelial downgrowth
Retained intraocular foreign body
Choroidal hemorrhage
Rhegmatogenous retinal detachment

the TM tear due to bleeding from Schlemm's canal. Healed TM tears are difficult to see, as gonioscopy is more commonly performed at a time remote from the injury. If IOP elevation develops at a later time, it is probably associated with more extensive angle recession.

Traumatic Hyphema

Significant bleeding in the anterior chamber associated with blunt ocular trauma increases the chance for elevation of IOP.[8] The high-impact compression and expansion secondary to blunt injury leads to rupture of iris stromal or ciliary body blood vessels. The IOP may be elevated due to all the factors noted under "Contusion With Intraocular Inflammation" and "Trabecular Meshwork Damage" as well as red blood cell obstruction of the outflow pathway.

Moderate IOP elevation up to 10 mm Hg above baseline may occur in as many as 30% of patients with traumatic hyphema.[9] Because the vast majority of these patients have healthy optic nerves, they can tolerate an elevation of IOP for a moderate period of time. The elevation tends to be self-limited and clears as the blood cells are normally processed through the aqueous drainage channels. A given patient's susceptibility to IOP elevation in the setting of trauma is highly variable. Read and Goldberg[9,10] found that IOP levels to 35 mm Hg or more that persist beyond 5 to 7 days may be associated with an increased risk of glaucomatous optic atrophy, particularly in the presence of sickle cell disease, but not restricted to that group. Higher pressures for a shorter period may be even more poorly tolerated.

One of the groups at highest risk for optic nerve damage in the setting of traumatic hyphema are those patients with sickle cell hemoglobinopathy.[10] These patients are susceptible to even marginal IOP elevation and are also predisposed to profound IOP spikes. The sensitivity of the optic nerve to marginal IOP elevation is presumably related to restricted blood flow to the optic nerve in the setting of the sickle cell disease. A high increase of IOP that may occur in these patients seems to be related to the restricted egress of rigid, sickled red blood cells through the TM outflow pathway. A vicious circle develops in that the sickle cells cannot clear from the anterior chamber, and there is a stagnation of cells. A relatively acidotic pH develops in the anterior chamber, leading to further sickling. The accumulating sickled red cells have no greater chance of clearing through the trabecular outflow pathway, and the cycle feeds on itself. Treatment has been proposed to increase the oxygen content of aqueous with the goal of reducing sickling and theoretically lowering IOP. Early positive results have been demonstrated in an animal study using intracameral hyperbaric oxygen[11] and another study using humidified oxygen delivered transcorneally in human eyes.[12] Our traditional means for treating glaucoma in this setting may actually contribute to an exacerbation of the sickling process. These are theoretical concerns without confirmation clinically, but these factors must be considered by any physician treating patients with sickle disease or sickle trait. Use of a carbonic anhydrase inhibitor (CAI) and the associated metabolic acidosis that results may increase sickling. Methazolamide theoretically causes less systemic acidosis than acetazolamide. If a systemic CAI is required in this situation, methazolamide may be the preferred choice. Epinephrine derivatives may exacerbate sickling due to their vasoconstrictive effect and subsequent hypoxia that develops in the anterior chamber. Miotics and prostaglandin agonists may increase inflammation. Topical aqueous suppressants are the treatment of choice, and the role of topical apraclonidine remains to be determined.

In patients with normal hemoglobin, the greatest concern for serious elevation of IOP is in those hyphema patients who suffer re-bleeding. The incidence of re-bleeding is highly variable depending on type of injury and patient population. It may be associated with clot lysis and clot retraction from damaged blood vessels. If re-bleeding occurs, it tends to occur in the first 2 to 5 days after the injury. Although the majority of patients who lose vision in the setting of traumatic hyphema do so secondary to macular problems rather than secondary to glaucoma, every effort should be made to minimize the risk for sudden elevation of IOP. Treatment is directed toward minimizing the rate of re-bleeding.

Several studies[13-18] prove the efficacy of oral aminocaproic acid and tranexamic acid in reducing the rate of re-bleeding; however, there is variability in the reports dealing with its side effects (eg, nausea, vomiting, or postural hypotension) and extension of duration of the clot. Some patients have a dramatic elevation of IOP on cessation of aminocaproic acid,[19] and for this reason, we rarely use this drug. In low-risk groups, the side effects of oral antifibrinolytic therapy may actually outweigh the risks of no treatment at all. The use of topical aminocaproic acid[20] is also being studied. One randomized study[21] showed a decreased risk of re-bleeding by approximately 67% in patients receiving topical aminocaproic acid. However, the continued need for a large-scale trial has left many questions unanswered, including its efficacy in sickle cell patients. Groups that appear to be at higher risk from re-bleeding are Black Americans, patients who present more than 24 hours after injury,[22] and patients taking anticoagulants. Antifibrinolytics are not the only oral medicines used to decrease rate of re-bleeding. A study in 1992 by Farber and colleagues[23] claimed efficacy for systemic prednisone at a dosage of 40 mg per day to reduce re-bleeding. This dosage was equivalent in effect to the reduction in re-bleeding obtained at the same institution several years earlier with aminocaproic acid. However, as with aminocaproic acid and tranexamic acid, there are no large trials demonstrating a definitive improvement in outcomes.[24,25] Current recommendations include discontinuation of salicylates and anticoagulant therapy to decrease the risk of rebleed.[25] Intracameral tissue plasminogen activator (tPA) has been suggested to speed clot resorption. However, use is limited to eyes with no active bleeding site and results are mixed in reducing rebleeding.[26-28]

Medical treatment for glaucoma in the setting of traumatic hyphema involves aqueous suppressants as the first line of defense (Table 43-2). Cycloplegic agents and topical steroids are often used to reduce the associated iritis and minimize outflow pathway edema. Activity limitation, shield protection, and elevation of the bed have traditionally been used during the first 5 to 7 days following injury.

Surgical treatment is indicated for those patients who do not respond satisfactorily to medical therapy. Traditional indications for surgery have included an IOP higher than 40 mm Hg for more than 48 hours, corneal blood staining in the setting of a large hyphema, or a stagnant, nonresorbing blood clot involving a significant amount of the angle circumference. The threshold for surgery is less in sickle cell patients with intervention recommended for IOP higher than 30 mm Hg at any time or more than 24 mm Hg for more than 24 hours (see Table 43-2). A host of surgical procedures have been described, including anterior chamber washout,[29] clot expression,[30] delivery of the clot with a cryoprobe,[31] automated hyphemectomy,[32] ultrasonic fragmentation or aspiration,[33] and peripheral iridectomy and/or trabeculectomy.[34,35] Washing out of the circulating red cells from the anterior chamber may be all that is required. If that does not lower IOP to an acceptable level, the washout can be repeated or additional techniques employed as noted in Table 43-2. Paracentesis and anterior chamber washout seems to be the simplest procedure,[29] and this may be coupled with a coaxial manual irrigation system. The entire clot does not need to be

TABLE 43-2. MANAGEMENT OF HYPHEMA ASSOCIATED WITH GLAUCOMA

First Line of Therapy: Medical Management
Aqueous suppressants
Topical steroids
Cycloplegic agents
Aqueous suppressants

Second Line of Therapy: Surgical Management
Anterior chamber washout
Expression of blood clot
Delivery of clot with cryoprobe
Ultrasonic emulsification of clot
Peripheral iridectomy
Trabeculectomy/glaucoma drainage device
Cyclophotocoagulation

removed as only the circulating red blood cells obstruct the outflow pathways. Subsequent release of aqueous and blood can be achieved via the paracentesis at the slit-lamp postoperatively, as needed.

Chemical Trauma

Alkaline agents have the capability of penetrating ocular tissues and may lead to glaucoma. This is uncommon with acid burns. A number of researchers have studied the nature of the IOP rise following alkali exposure.[36] A dicrotic pressure rise has been noted with an immediate IOP rise up to the level of 40 to 50 mm Hg within the first 10 minutes of the injury. The pressure tends to return to normal after a short time and then gradually rises to high levels at the end of the first hour or 2. It is believed that shrinkage of the outer collagen coats of the eye resulting in distortion of the TM[37] may cause the initial IOP spike. Prostaglandin release has been implicated as the major factor in the second hypertensive phase. Weeks to months later, the IOP may be elevated due to angle closure as a result of peripheral anterior synechia formation. In addition, if aqueous pH remains elevated higher than 11.5 for prolonged periods, ciliary body damage can lead to hypotony and phthisis bulbi, and decreased secretion of ascorbate can limit keratocyte collagen repair.[37] Studies[38,39] on rabbits have shown that rinsing with borate-buffered eyewash is significantly better at neutralizing pH compared to isotonic saline.

Because of the impressive corneal changes that may arise from a chemical injury, IOP elevation may be overlooked. It is critical to monitor IOP because Kuckelkorn has shown early development of glaucoma in 15.6% of chemically injured eyes and late-onset secondary glaucoma in 22.2% of such eyes.[40]

Treatment of the IOP elevation, if necessary, is focused on aqueous suppressant therapy, both topically and systemically. Miotics are generally avoided because of the intense inflammation that is associated with chemical burns. Topical steroids, if not contraindicated from a corneal basis, may reduce inflammation, and cycloplegic agents may maximize comfort and help to stabilize the blood-aqueous barrier. Brodovsky et al[41] and Ralph[42] demonstrated that in cases of severe burns, oral vitamin C and tetracycline, in addition to topical citrate, ascorbate, and tetracycline drops, decrease collagenolytic activity. However, no large, long-term randomized studies on humans have been documented. Anterior chamber paracentesis had been favored by some in the past but is less commonly used at this time. Trabeculectomy is largely unsuccessful due to extensive conjunctival scarring. Glaucoma drainage devices and cyclophotocoagulation procedures may have better IOP outcomes. Cyclophotocoagulation has been shown to have a reasonably low complication rate and may be a better option when the anterior chamber view and ocular surface are compromised.[43]

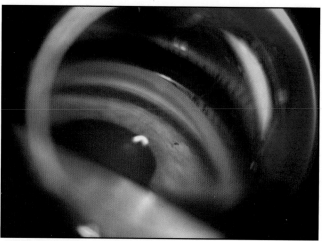

Figure 43-1. Angle recession in trauma. Angle recession must always be considered in the setting of asymmetrical IOP or unilateral glaucoma. Careful gonioscopy is critical. This figure demonstrates classic findings of a broadened ciliary body band with iris retrodisplacement, reduced ciliary processes, and an abnormally white scleral spur.

LATE-ONSET GLAUCOMA AFTER EYE INJURY

Angle Recession

A tear in the ciliary body results in angle recession. The typical tear occurs between the circular and longitudinal muscles in the ciliary body. There is a resulting posterior displacement of the iris root, which results in the clinical appearance of a broadening of the ciliary body band. Collins[44] was the first to give a pathologic description of angle recession in 1892. Wolff and Zimmerman[45] presented a classic correlation between traumatic glaucoma and angle recession in 1962.

Angle recession is remarkably common after blunt injury. The incidence of angle recession in the setting of traumatic hyphema has been reported from 50% to 100%.[22,46,47] The incidence of glaucoma with angle recession appears to be directly related to the extent of angle involvement. The risk of glaucoma appears to be greatest if 240 degrees or more of the angle are involved. The elevation in IOP after blunt trauma with angle recession may occur months or years after the initial injury. Blanton observed a bimodal pattern with glaucoma occurring within the first year or after 10 years of injury.[47]

The diagnosis of angle recession is made by careful gonioscopic examination (Figure 43-1). The ciliary body band tends to be broader in certain zones, and there may be baring of ciliary processes. The scleral spur may appear abnormally white. Differences between the eyes may be remarkably subtle. The most useful technique for documenting angle recession is to compare quadrants between the injured eye and the noninvolved eye of a given patient.

Traditionally, bilateral, simultaneous Koeppe gonioscopy (Ocular Instruments, Seattle, WA)[48] with 2 lenses has been an excellent way to detect these differences. Anterior segment optical coherence topography (OCT) and ultrasound biomicroscopy are newer techniques that permit objective and quantitative documentation of the angle configuration.[49,50]

The treatment of angle-recession glaucoma follows the pattern used for primary open-angle glaucoma. Inadequate control with topical and oral therapy may lead one to consider laser trabeculoplasty (LTP). LTP is rarely effective and may also be associated with a higher incidence of acute IOP elevation. Filtration surgery is often required. Trabeculectomy success is strongly dependent on the use of adjunctive antimetabolites, as most patients are young and predisposed to fibrosis.[51,52]

The mechanism for glaucoma in angle recession depends on the timing of the IOP elevation after injury. Early IOP increase is due to trabecular inflammation and the presence of circulating blood and inflammatory products. This often resolves within weeks to months, and the patient may enter a honeymoon period with normalization of IOP. The ophthalmologist must be aware that this period of normal IOP can be short-lived; eyes with significant angle recession deserve close follow-up at least every 6 months initially.

Late angle-recession glaucoma may be secondary to the formation of a glass-like membrane over the TM, thought to be an extension of Descemet's membrane. This explains the poor response to conventional medical and laser treatment in angle-recession glaucoma. Indeed, in such eyes treated with LTP, the surgeon may see a spreading, whitening of cracked glass-like appearance at the site of laser impact. In contrast, if instead of LTP the surgeon performs neodymium:yttrium-aluminum-garnet (Nd:YAG)

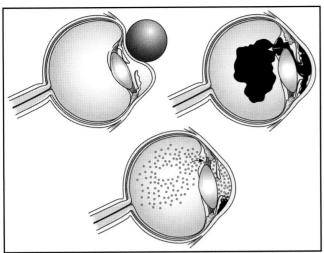

Figure 43-2. Ghost-cell glaucoma in trauma. The mechanism involved in the development of ghost-cell glaucoma is critical to diagnosis and management. This schematic demonstrates the effects of blunt injury, equatorial globe expansion, hyphema and vitreous hemorrhage, disruption of the anterior hyaloid face, passage of rigid khaki-colored ghost cells into the anterior chamber, and blockage of TM. If medical therapy of glaucoma fails, treatment must involve removal of the ghost cells via anterior chamber washout, usually combined with a pars plana vitrectomy.

TABLE 43-3. MANAGEMENT OF GHOST-CELL GLAUCOMA
Initial Medical Management
Aqueous suppressants
Topical steroids
Cycloplegic agents
Aqueous suppressants
Stepwise Surgical Management
Anterior chamber washout
Pars plana vitrectomy
Trabeculectomy/Schlemm's canal directed surgery/glaucoma drainage device
Cyclophotocoagulation

goniopuncture (YLT), a transient reduction in IOP is seen, supporting the suggestion that obstruction to outflow in angle-recession glaucoma is due to the presence of a glass-like membrane covering the TM. Unfortunately, such IOP reductions tend to be short-lived, as Melamed and colleagues[53-55] have shown in monkeys that the openings made by goniopuncture tend to be covered by Descemet's membrane over time. When goniopuncture was repeated in humans, more than 50% required further surgery within a year of YLT.[56]

Ghost-Cell Glaucoma

Ghost-cell glaucoma can occur when injury to the globe causes disruption of the anterior hyaloid face and is associated with blood accumulation in the vitreous (Figure 43-2); however, disruption of the hyaloid face is not a prerequisite for the development of ghost-cell glaucoma. Campbell and colleagues[57] have shown that 1 to 3 weeks after the injury, or rarely even sooner, a secondary elevation of IOP can occur. This occurs when red blood cells, usually in the vitreous but occasionally in long-standing hyphema, convert to less pliable, rigid, khaki-colored ghost cells that do not pass easily through the TM. The cells obstruct aqueous outflow with a resulting rise in IOP. The khaki ghost cells can often be identified at the slit-lamp and may occasionally layer in the inferior angle recess as tan hypopyon. Anterior chamber aspirates demonstrate cells with a characteristic shrunken appearance by phase contrast microscopy. Heinz bodies represent denatured hemoglobin present in the cytoplasm of some ghost cells.[58]

The treatment of ghost-cell glaucoma includes conventional medical therapy with surgery as necessary (Table 43-3). Anterior chamber washout may temporarily control IOP. If the reservoir of khaki ghost cells is large enough, there may be recurrent elevation of IOP despite anterior chamber washout. A pars plana vitrectomy may be necessary to ensure complete removal of all blood components trapped in the vitreous. Filtration surgery, glaucoma drainage devices, or cyclophotocoagulation are sometimes coupled with anterior chamber washout and pars plana vitrectomy.[59]

Lens-Induced Glaucoma

Lens-induced glaucoma is a varied group of secondary glaucomas that has the lens as a factor in the cause of IOP elevation. The 4 major categories include lens dislocation, lens swelling, phacolytic glaucoma, and lens particle glaucoma. Each type may develop with trauma to the globe (Table 43-4).[60,61]

Lens Dislocation or Subluxation

Dislocation or subluxation of the crystalline lens most commonly occurs with blunt trauma. Disruption of the zonules allows the lens to move anteriorly or posteriorly. Depending on the position of the lens and vitreous status, pupillary block may occur and may lead to angle closure with a precipitous increase in IOP. Creeping angle closure may develop in a more subacute or chronic form, leading to late-onset development of glaucoma. Rarely, complete dislocation of the lens may allow vitreous to come forward to fill the anterior chamber and lead to vitreous block glaucoma.

Treatment of lens-induced glaucoma depends on the type of glaucoma presenting. Careful examination is critical to determine the presence or absence of pupillary block. If pupillary block is present, a laser iridectomy or surgical iridectomy is indicated.[62] Lensectomy may be required for visual reasons and for recurrent episodes of pupillary block.

SECONDARY GLAUCOMA IN BLACK PATIENTS: A HISTORICAL PERSPECTIVE

Morton F. Goldberg, MD

Approximately 9% of North American Black individuals carry the gene for sickle cell hemoglobin.[1] When this mutation is inherited from only one parent, creating the heterozygous condition called sickle cell trait, this unique cell trait is considered nonpathologic because sickling of erythrocytes is uncommon. This valid principle does not apply to the anterior chamber where all sickle cell hemoglobinopathies can induce a specific type of secondary glaucoma.

Sickled erythrocytes are elongated and rigid (like miniaturized pencils) and unlike normal, pliable red blood cells are not easily pushed through the interstices of the TM into Schlemm's canal. The log-jam of sickled and nonsickled erythrocytes produces mechanical blockade of these outflow channels, creating mild to severe elevation of IOP. This sequence of events can occur even when the total amount of blood in the aqueous humor is small (eg, a 1- or 2-mm layered hyphema and occasionally even a dispersed microhyphema showing no gravitational settling). The elevation in IOP can occur when only a relatively small percentage of erythrocytes (eg, 5% to 15%) becomes sickled. These events also occur regardless of the etiology of the hemorrhage (eg, blunt trauma, perforating trauma, or postoperatively, for example, with passage of red cells from the vitreous to the aqueous humor after vitrectomy in an aphakic eye or after cataract surgery).

The physico-chemical environment of the aqueous humor is uniquely constituted (ie, in comparison with circulating whole blood). The aqueous has a low pO_2, low pH, high pCO_2, and a particularly high concentration of ascorbate (a reducing agent). These parameters, individually and in the aggregate, are capable of initiating and maintaining the sickled, rigid conformation of affected erythrocytes. Moreover, the presence of nonaerobically metabolizing erythrocytes and aerobically metabolizing leukocytes in the stagnant, sequestered aqueous humor contributes to further acidosis, hypoxia, and hypercarbia, thereby making a bad situation worse by contributing to a vicious cycle as follows: trabecular blockade, then sequestered blood in the anterior chamber, then sickling, then trabecular blockage (which, of course, can lead to elevated IOP).

Secondary glaucoma appears to be substantially more dangerous for the optic nerve in patients with a sickle cell hemoglobinopathy than in individuals with normal hemoglobin. Permanent, visually disabling infarctions of the optic nerve have occurred in several sickle cell hemoglobinopathy patients with only small amounts of intracameral blood and only mildly or transiently elevated IOPs

(eg, low 30s mm Hg). The mechanism is somewhat unclear, but may involve insufficient perfusion pressure within the small vessels of the optic nerve that are subjected to modest but sudden elevation of the IOP. Sluggish flow can lead to excessive oxygen extraction from the blood (inducing intravascular sickling), increased viscosity of the blood, and, in some cases, total cessation of flow, with infarction of dependent tissue.

Conventional treatment regimens for hyphema-induced secondary glaucoma are inherently conservative and are often ineffective in the sickle cell patient. Some components of the usual treatment program, such as frequently repeated doses of osmotic agents or acetazolamide, may be deleterious because they can exacerbate the sickling process in the anterior chamber and elsewhere. Therefore, serious consideration should be given to the following clinical guidelines:

- All Black patients (and possibly individuals with Mediterranean or Hispanic ancestry) should have a routine, quick solubility screening test for the presence of sickle cell hemoglobin (a formal hemoglobin electrophoresis is not necessary for initial clinical decision making)

- Patients who are known or discovered to be positive should have regular measurements of IOP made every 6 hours

- Whenever the measurements during any consecutive 24-hour period of time exceed 24 mm Hg (mnemonic: 24 for 24) or demonstrate spikes higher than 30 mm Hg, some of the blood should be removed from the anterior chamber to lower the burden of cells within the outflow pathways

If the hyphema is small, a simple paracentesis (which can be repeated if necessary) is usually sufficient; if the hyphema is large and blocks the pupil, a more extensive surgical washout is often indicated. Concomitant usage of the following regimen is sometimes effective: topical beta-blockers, atropine, and corticosteroids, plus oral epsilon-aminocaproic acid and/or corticosteroids.

These suggestions are based on clinical success in a limited number of patients. Optic nerve function cannot easily be assessed during the period of time when blood is in the anterior chamber. Because the optic nerve may be undergoing occult infarction during this time, a high index of suspicion accompanied by aggressive attempts to lower the IOP, as suggested here, may well be in the best interests of this physiologically vulnerable group of patients.

REFERENCE

1. Goldberg MF. The diagnosis and treatment of sickled erythrocytes in human hyphemas. *Trans Am Ophthalmol Soc.* 1978;76:481-501.

The technique of lensectomy will depend on the degree of subluxation. Surgical removal may involve a planned extracapsular or phacoemulsification approach, intracapsular extraction, or pars plana lensectomy with vitrectomy.[63,64]

Lens Swelling

Blunt or penetrating trauma may alter lens fibers or capsule sufficiently to result in lens swelling. The lens may hydrate and become a mature cataract with development of phacomorphic glaucoma. Pupillary block may occur or the lens may swell enough to directly close angle structures. Cataract surgery is required for visual rehabilitation and

correction of the glaucoma. Gonioscopy at the time of surgery is helpful because residual peripheral anterior synechiae may best be treated directly at that time with surgical goniosynechialysis.

Phacolytic Glaucoma

Phacolytic glaucoma is typically seen in the setting of a mature cataract. Open-angle glaucoma occurs as a result of leakage of high molecular weight proteins through an intact lens capsule.[61] Macrophages also are present in the anterior chamber. This entity is described in detail in another chapter.

TABLE 43-4. INSIGHTS INTO MECHANISMS OF LENS-INDUCED GLAUCOMA

Lens-Induced Glaucoma
Lens dislocation/subluxation— pupillary block with 2-degree angle closure, direct mechanical angle closure, or vitreous block glaucoma
Lens swelling—mass effect leading to direct mechanical angle closure or pupillary block glaucoma
Phacolytic—high molecular weight proteins obstructing trabecular meshwork with an open angle
Lens particle—lens and inflammatory material obstructing trabecular meshwork with an open angle

Lens Particle Glaucoma

Frank disruption of the lens due to penetrating trauma, and rarely blunt trauma, may lead to fragments of lens material in the anterior chamber. Most of the time, this will be obvious at the time of initial injury and will require surgical decision-making based on other associated findings. Most of these cases are associated with corneoscleral lacerations that require primary repair with a primary lensectomy at the time of surgery. A few case reports have described lens particle glaucoma secondary to posterior capsular rupture following blunt trauma. Here, also, primary lensectomy has been the main treatment.[65]

Peripheral Anterior Synechiae

Ocular injury often results in inflammation and blood in the anterior chamber. If these persist and there is pupillary block, iridocorneal apposition may occur. Peripheral anterior synechiae may then form. Hyphemas that persist for an extended period of time in the setting of significant inflammation are the most common cause of peripheral anterior synechia formation in the setting of blunt trauma. Stagnant clots may be an indication for anterior chamber washout.[66] Penetrating trauma commonly results in peripheral anterior synechia formation, particularly if the laceration crosses the limbus. Careful attention to an intraoperative sweep of the angle and avoiding iris apposition to the wound will minimize peripheral anterior synechia formation when corneoscleral lacerations are repaired. If peripheral anterior synechiae have not been firmly established, argon laser gonioplasty may be a means of reducing synechiae or surgical goniosynechialysis may be performed.[67,68] If synechial closure is restricted to one quadrant, no treatment may be required.

Late Closure of a Cyclodialysis Cleft

A separation of ciliary body from the scleral spur results in a cyclodialysis cleft. This may occur following blunt trauma or after surgical intervention. This can result in temporary or permanent hypotony. The presence of a small cyclodialysis cleft can be protective of the development of traumatic glaucoma. Sihota et al[4] and Goldmann[69] have postulated that a reduction in the normal flow of aqueous across the TM results in a reduced permeability of the meshwork to aqueous outflow. This may account for the marked, acute IOP elevation that can occur following closure of cyclodialysis clefts. The IOP increase tends to be severe and is associated with significant pain. Treatment involves the use of aqueous suppressants, oral or intravenous hyperosmotics, as well as alpha-agonists. Most cases can be managed medically through the short period of time that the IOP is elevated. Miotics are generally avoided because they can lead to reopening of the cleft and subsequent recurrence of hypotony. As with angle recession, anterior segment OCT and ultrasound biomicroscopy are invaluable for diagnosis.[49,50]

Epithelial Downgrowth

Lacerating trauma to the eye may lead to a fistula that develops from the external surface of the eye into the anterior chamber. This provides a conduit for epithelium to enter the anterior segment. This is an uncommon problem in the setting of microsurgical repair but must be searched for in eyes that develop glaucoma at a time remote from the initial lacerating injury. The characteristic slit-lamp appearance of a scalloped endothelial membrane is diagnostic for epithelial downgrowth (Figure 43-3). Argon laser applications to involved iris make a white spot. These 2 findings confirm the diagnosis, although histopathologic confirmation via iris biopsy may be required in certain cases. Treatment involves excision of all involved iris and explantation of the intraocular lens, if present. Cryotherapy is applied to the involved ciliary body and cornea. Visual prognosis is guarded in these cases. Glaucoma drainage device procedures may also be effective. Cases of success with injection of 5-fluorouracil and endocylophotocoagulation have been reported.[70,71]

Retained Intraocular Foreign Body

A rare and late manifestation of iron-containing foreign bodies is siderotic glaucoma. Luo and colleagues[72] found a 7.69% incidence of secondary glaucoma in patients with siderosis. The classic slit-lamp findings include iris heterochromia, mydriasis, and rust-like discoloration of the anterior subcapsular lens surface. However, iron-containing foreign bodies can cause secondary open angle without these pathognomonic findings.[73] Copper-containing foreign bodies result in chalcosis, but a definite link with glaucoma has not been shown.[74] If these findings are present, foreign bodies

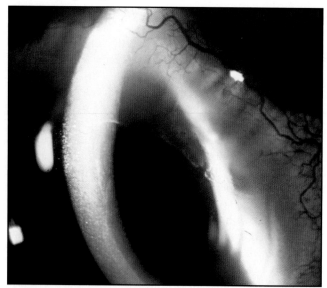

Figure 43-3. Epithelial downgrowth after trauma. This figure demonstrates the classic, scalloped advancing border of epithelial cells on the endothelium of a patient with epithelial downgrowth. At this stage, IOP is usually elevated, and patients are troubled by photophobia and eye pain. Argon laser applications (100 μm, 0.1 seconds, 300 mW) to areas of iris involved with epithelium will blanch white to aid diagnosis, but occasionally, incisional biopsy is required.

should be searched for carefully with a complete ophthalmoscopic examination including gonioscopy. Further studies may include plain radiographs, computed tomographic scanning, and ultrasound. Electroretinography may be helpful in advanced cases of siderosis.

Choroidal Hemorrhage

Contusion injury can result in rupture of choroidal blood vessels and vortex veins with resultant subchoroidal hemorrhage. Signs include pain, shallowing of the anterior chamber, and decrease of red reflex.[75] The lens-iris diaphragm may move anteriorly, blocking the TM, and, if long-term, can lead to synechia. Initial management includes pain control and medical management of IOP. Aqueous suppressants and alpha-agonists are the mainstay of medical therapy. Miotics should be avoided because they may shallow the anterior chamber. Cycloplegics are indicated to tighten zonules and deepen the anterior chamber. In addition, aggressive topical and oral steroids have been recommended to stabilize choroidal vessels.[75]

Surgical drainage is indicated when there is lens-corneal touch, uncontrolled IOP, or retina-to-retina apposition. It is advised to wait 3 to 10 days, if possible, to allow for liquefaction of the clot and sequestration of the blood into the suprachoroidal space. Even if the clot resorbs or is removed, visual prognosis is poor.[76]

IRIS RETRACTION SYNDROME
Joel S. Schuman, MD, FACS

An interesting phenomenon can occur in some cases of Schwartz's syndrome. Exceptional patients with the syndrome and posterior synechiae will develop an excessively deep anterior chamber, with dramatic iris concavity, when placed on aqueous suppressants, especially CAIs. The chamber will return to normal depth when the medications are discontinued and can be made extremely deep again with their reinstatement. Dramatic presentations can even have an initially elevated intraocular pressure with iris bombé, alternating with hypotony and an exceedingly deep anterior chamber once aqueous suppressants are started. The presumed mechanism for this occurrence, called *iris retraction syndrome*, by Campbell,[1] who described the entity requires the presence of both a retinal hole and 360-degree posterior synechiae and depends on a decrease in aqueous production and an increase in aqueous outflow by an unconventional route—through the retinal pigment epithelium. Aqueous humor moves freely through the vitreous cavity,[2] and the subretinal fluid of some eyes with retinal detachment has contained a high ascorbic acid level, suggesting the presence of aqueous humor in this space.[3]

CAIs can stimulate the retinal pigment epithelial pump and so are particularly likely to result in this uncommon circumstance, given the proper underlying conditions. This is essentially a situation of reverse pupillary block, with a lower pressure occurring in the posterior segment than the anterior, due to the 360-degree posterior synechiae, the decreased aqueous production, and the aqueous outflow via the retinal pigment epithelium through the retinal hole. Although a peripheral iridectomy will eliminate the anterior chamber deepening and is required given the pupillary block, a more definitive cure is repair of the retinal break.

REFERENCES
1. Campbell DG. Iris retraction associated with rhegmatogenous retinal detachment syndrome and hypotony: a new explanation. *Arch Ophthalmol.* 1984;102(10):1457-1463.
2. Epstein DL, Hashimoto JM, Anderson PJ, et al. Experimental perfusions through the vitreous and anterior chambers; possible relationship to malignant glaucoma. *Am J Ophthalmol.* 1979;88(6):1078-1086.
3. Van Heuven WAJ, Lam KW, Ray GS. Source of subretinal fluid on the basis of ascorbate analyses. *Arch Ophthalmol.* 1982;100(6):976-978.

Rhegmatogenous Retinal Detachment

Rhegmatogenous retinal detachment is most commonly associated with ocular hypotension due to a decrease in aqueous production.[77] However, 5% to 10% of the patients may develop elevated IOP (Schwartz's syndrome). The mechanism for increased IOP is most likely due to direct photoreceptor outer segment obstruction of aqueous outflow in the anterior segment.[78,79] Schwartz's syndrome can be difficult to diagnose and commonly occurs in the setting of a shallow, peripheral retinal detachment with the appearance of an anterior chamber inflammatory reaction. It is not unusual for Schwartz's syndrome to be misdiagnosed as inflammatory glaucoma, and it is the ophthalmologist who is alert to the possibility of rhegmatogenous retinal detachment as a cause of elevated IOP who will make the correct diagnosis. For this reason, consider this diagnosis in any case of uveitic glaucoma and dilate all such patients, with a full examination of the peripheral retina to rule out the possibility of Schwartz's syndrome.

It is of particular importance to establish the correct diagnosis of Schwartz's syndrome, as it is a curable entity, with a treatment different from that for inflammatory glaucoma. Repair of the retinal detachment most commonly results in a prompt and permanent return of IOP to normal, assuming there are no associated problems in the anterior segment that might exacerbate a tendency toward glaucoma.

CONCLUSION

Glaucoma due to trauma is complicated by its acute and chronic manifestations. After the acute situation has been rectified, it is important for patients to appreciate that elevated IOP may develop months to decades later. All patients with glaucoma should have a careful history and complete examination to search for signs of trauma as a possible cause. In addition, all patients with significant ocular trauma should be followed indefinitely on a regular basis to monitor for IOP elevation.

REFERENCES

1. Tingey DP, Shingleton BJ. Glaucoma associated with ocular trauma. In: Albert, DM, Miller JW, eds. *Principles and Practice of Ophthalmology.* 3rd ed. Philadelphia, PA: WB Saunders Co; 2008:2623-2631.
2. Girkin CA, McGwin G Jr, Long C, Morris R, Kuhn F. Glaucoma after ocular contusion: a cohort study of the United States Eye Injury Registry. *J Glaucoma.* 2005;14(6):470-473.
3. Ozer PA, Yalvac IS, Satana B, Eksioglu U, Duman S. Incidence and risk factors in secondary glaucomas after blunt and penetrating ocular trauma. *J Glaucoma.* 2007;16(8):685-690.
4. Sihota R, Kumar S, Gupta V, et al. Early predictors of traumatic glaucoma after closed globe injury trabecular pigmentation, widened angle recession, and higher baseline intraocular pressure. *Arch Ophthalmol.* 2008;126(7):921-926.
5. Thompson JT. Traumatic retinal tears and detachments. In: Shingleton BJ, Hersh PS, Kenyon KR, eds. *Eye Trauma.* St Louis, MO: Mosby Year Book; 1991:196-213.
6. Campbell DG. Traumatic glaucoma. In: Shingleton BJ, Hersh PS, Kenyon KR, eds. *Eye Trauma.* St Louis, MO: Mosby Year Book; 1991:117-125.
7. Herschler J. Trabecular damage due to blunt anterior segment injury and its relationship to traumatic glaucoma. *Trans Am Acad Ophthalmol Otolaryngol.* 1972;83:229-248.
8. Walton W, Von Hagen S, Grigorian R, Zarbin M. Management of traumatic hyphema. *Surv Ophthalmol.* 2002;47(4):297-334.
9. Read J, Goldberg MF. Comparison of medical treatment for traumatic hyphema. *Trans Am Acad Ophthalmol Otolaryngol.* 1974;78:799.
10. Goldberg MF. The diagnosis and treatment of sickled erythrocytes in human hyphemas. *Trans Am Ophthalmol Soc.* 1978;76:481-501.
11. Wallyn CR, Jampol LM, Goldberg MF, Zanetti CL. The use of hyperbaric oxygen therapy in the treatment of sickle cell hyphema. *Invest Ophthalmol Vis Sci.* 1985;26(8):1155-1158.
12. Benner JD. Transcorneal oxygen therapy for glaucoma associated with sickle cell hyphema. *Am J Ophthalmol.* 2000;130(4):514-515.
13. McGetrick JJ, Jampol LM, Goldberg MF, et al. Aminocaproic acid decreases secondary hemorrhage after traumatic hyphema. *Arch Ophthalmol.* 1983;101:1031.
14. Palmer DJ, Goldberg MF, Frenkel M, Fiscella R, Anderson RJ. A comparison of two dose regimens for epsilon-aminocaproic acid in the prevention and management of secondary traumatic hyphemas. *Ophthalmology.* 1986;93:102-108.
15. Deans R, Noël LP, Clarke WN. Oral administration of tranexamic acid in the management of traumatic hyphema in children. *Can J Ophthalmol.* 1992;27(4):181-183.
16. Clarke WN, Noël LP. Outpatient treatment of microscopic and rim hyphemas in children with tranexamic acid. *Can J Ophthalmol.* 1993;28(7):325-327.
17. Teboul BK, Jacob JL, Barsoum-Homsy M, et al. Clinical evaluation of aminocaproic acid for managing traumatic hyphema in children. *Ophthalmology.* 1995;102:1646-1653.
18. Albiani DA, Hodge WG, Pan YI, Urton TE, Clarke WN. Tranexamic acid in the treatment of pediatric traumatic hyphema. *Can J Ophthalmol.* 2008;43(4):428-431.
19. Dieste MC, Hersh PS, Kylstra JA, et al. Intraocular pressure increase associated with epsilon-aminocaproic acid therapy for traumatic hyphema. *Am J Ophthalmol.* 1988;106:383-390.
20. Crouch ER Jr, Williams PB, Gray MK, et al. Topical aminocaproic acid in the treatment of traumatic hyphema. *Arch Ophthalmol.* 1997;115:1106-1112.
21. Pieramici DJ, Goldberg MF, Melia M, et al. A phase III, multicenter, randomized, placebo-controlled clinical trial of topical aminocaproic acid (Caprogel) in the management of traumatic hyphema. *Ophthalmology.* 2003;110(11):2106-2112.
22. Volpe NJ, Larrison WI, Hersh PS, et al. Secondary hemorrhage in traumatic hyphema. *Am J Ophthalmol.* 1991;112:507-513.
23. Farber MD, Fiscella R, Goldberg MF. Aminocaproic acid versus prednisone for the treatment of traumatic hyphema. *Ophthalmology.* 1991;98:279-286.
24. Rahmani B, Jahadi HR. Comparison of tranexamic acid and prednisolone in the treatment of traumatic hyphema. A randomized clinical trial. *Ophthalmology.* 1999;106:375-379.
25. Recchia FM, Saluja RK, Hammel K, Jeffers JB. Outpatient management of traumatic microhyphema. *Ophthalmology.* 2002;109(8):1465-1470.
26. Howard GR, Vukich J, Fiscella RG, Farber MD, Goldberg MF. Intraocular tissue plasminogen activator in a rabbit model of traumatic hyphema. *Arch Ophthalmol.* 1991;109(2):272-274.
27. Laatikainen L, Mattila J. The use of tissue plasminogen activator in posttraumatic total hyphaema. *Graefes Arch Clin Exp Ophthalmol.* 1996;234:67-68.
28. WuDunn D. Intracameral urokinase for dissolution of fibrin or blood clots after glaucoma surgery. *Am J Ophthalmol.* 1997;124(5):693-695.
29. Belcher CD, Brown SVL, Simmons RJ. Anterior chamber washout for traumatic hyphema. *Ophthalmic Surg.* 1985;16:475-479.
30. Sears ML. Surgical management of black ball hyphema. *Trans Acad Ophthalmol Otolaryngol.* 1970;74:820-825.
31. Hill K. Cryoextraction of total hyphema. *Arch Ophthalmol.* 1968;80:368-370.
32. McCuen BW, Fang WE. The role of vitrectomy instrumentation in the treatment of severe traumatic hyphema. *Am J Ophthalmol.* 1979;71:930-934.
33. Kelman CD, Brooks DL. Ultrasonic emulsification and aspiration of traumatic hyphema. A preliminary report. *Am J Ophthalmol.* 1971;71:1289-1291.
34. Parrish RK, Bernardino V. Iridectomy in the surgical management of eight ball hyphema. *Arch Ophthalmol.* 1982;100:435-437.
35. Weiss JS, Parrish RK, Anderson DR. Surgical therapy of traumatic hyphema. *Ophthalmic Surg.* 1983;14:343-345.

36. Paterson CA, Pfister RR. Intraocular pressure changes after alkali burns. *Arch Ophthalmol.* 1974;91:211-218.

37. Wagoner M. Chemical injuries of the eye: current concepts in pathophysiology and therapy. *Surv Ophthalmol.* 1997;41(4):275-313.

38. Rihawi S, Frentz M, Schrage NF. Emergency treatment of eye burns: which rinsing solution should we choose? *Graefes Arch Clin Exp Ophthalmol.* 2006;244(7):845-854.

39. Rihawi S, Frentz M, Reim M, Schrage NF. Rinsing with isotonic saline solution for eye burns should be avoided. *Burns.* 2008;34(7):1027-1032.

40. Kuckelkorn R, Keller GK, Redbrake C. Glaucoma after extremely severe chemical and thermal eye burns. Surgical possibilities. *Ophthalmologe.* 2001;98(12):1149-1156.

41. Brodovsky SC, McCarty CA, Snibson G, et al. Management of alkali burns. An 11-year retrospective review. *Ophthalmology.* 2000;107:1829-1835.

42. Ralph RA. Tetracyclines and the treatment of corneal stromal ulceration: a review. *Cornea.* 2000;19(3):274-277.

43. Kuckelkorn R, Kottek A, Reim M. Intraocular complications after severe chemical burns—incidence and surgical treatment [in German]. *Klin Monatsbl Augenheilkd.* 1994;205:86-92.

44. Collins ET. On the pathologic examination of three eyes lost from concussion. *Trans Ophthalmol Soc UK.* 1992;12:180.

45. Wolff SM, Zimmerman LE. Chronic secondary glaucoma associated with retrodisplacement of iris root and deepening of the anterior chamber angle secondary to contusion. *Am J Ophthalmol.* 1962;84:547-563.

46. Canavan YM, Archer DB. Anterior segment consequences of blunt ocular injury. *Br J Ophthalmol.* 1982;66:549-555.

47. Blanton FM. Anterior chamber angle recession and secondary glaucoma. A study of the after effects of traumatic hyphema. *Arch Ophthalmol.* 1964;72:39-43.

48. Alper MG. Contusion angle deformity and glaucoma. Gonioscopic observation and clinical course. *Arch Ophthalmol.* 1963;69:455-467.

49. Friedman DS, He M. Anterior chamber angle assessment techniques. *Surv Ophthalmol.* 2008;53(3):250-273.

50. Wylegala E, Dobrowolski D, Nowińska A, Tarnawska D. Anterior segment optical coherence tomography in eye injuries. *Graefes Arch Clin Exp Ophthalmol.* 2009;247(4):451-455.

51. Mermoud A, Salmon F, Straker C, Murray AD. Post-traumatic angle recession glaucoma: a risk factor for bleb failure after trabeculectomy. *Br J Ophthalmol.* 1993;77:631-634.

52. Manners T, Salmon JF, Barron A, Willies C, Murray ADN. Trabeculectomy with mitomycin C in the treatment of posttraumatic angle recession glaucoma. *Br J Ophthalmol.* 2001;85:159-163.

53. Melamed S, Pei J, Puliafito CA, et al. Q-switched neodymium-YAG laser trabeculopuncture in monkeys. *Arch Ophthalmol.* 1985;103:129-133.

54. Epstein DL, Melamed S, Puliafito CA, et al. Neodymium-YAG laser trabeculopuncture in open-angle glaucoma. *Ophthalmology.* 1985;92:931-937.

55. Melamed S, Ashkenazi I, Gutman I, Blumenthal M. Nd:YAG laser trabeculopuncture in angle-recession glaucoma. *Ophthalmic Surg.* 1992;23(1):31-35.

56. Mermoud A, Salmon F, Straker C, Murray AD. Post-traumatic angle recession glaucoma: a risk factor for bleb failure after trabeculectomy. *Br J Ophthalmol.* 1993;77:631-634.

57. Campbell DG, Simmons RJ, Grant WM. Ghost cells as a cause of glaucoma. *Am J Ophthalmol.* 1973;97:2141.

58. Campbell DG. Ghost cell glaucoma following trauma. *Ophthalmology.* 1981;88:11511158.

59. Abu el-Asrar AM, al-Obeidan SA. Pars plana vitrectomy in the management of ghost cell glaucoma. *Int Ophthalmol.* 1995;19(2):121-124.

60. Irvine JA, Smith RF. Lens injuries. In: Shingleton BJ, Hersh PS, Kenyon KR, eds. *Eye Trauma.* St Louis, MO: Mosby Year Book; 1991:126-135.

61. Epstein DL. Diagnosis and management of lens-induced glaucoma. *Ophthalmology.* 1982;89:227-230.

62. Peng SX, Zhou WB. Traumatic lens dislocation-related glaucoma. *Zhonghua Yan Ke Za Zhi.* 1993;29(6):332-335.

63. Synder A, Latecka-Krajewska B, Omulecki W. Secondary glaucoma in patients with lens subluxation or luxation. *Klin Oczna.* 2000;102(6):409-412.

64. Lam DS, Chua JK, Kwok AK, Wong AK, Leung AT, Fan DS, Gopal L. Combined surgery for severe eye trauma with extensive iridodialysis, posterior lens dislocation, and intractable glaucoma. *J Cataract Refract Surg.* 1999;25(2):285-288.

65. Jain SS, Rao P, Nayak P, Kothari K. Posterior capsular dehiscence following blunt injury causing delayed onset lens particle glaucoma. *Indian J Ophthalmol.* 2004;52(4):325-327.

66. Deutsch TA, Feller DB. *Paton and Goldberg's Management of Ocular Injuries.* 2nd ed. Philadelphia, PA: WB Saunders; 1985.

67. Weiss HS, Shingleton BJ, Bellows AR, et al. Argon laser gonioplasty for the treatment of angle-closure glaucoma. *Am J Ophthalmol.* 1992;114:14-18.

68. Shingleton BJ, Chang MA, Bellows AR, et al. Surgical goniosynechialysis for angle-closure glaucoma. *Ophthalmology.* 1990;97:551-556.

69. Goldmann H. Clinical studies on the glaucoma problem. I. The role of Schlemm's canal after arrangement of new outflow channels [in Undetermined Language]. *Ophthalmologica.* 1953;125:16.

70. Lenhart PD, Randleman JB, Grossniklaus HE, Stulting RD. Confocal microscopic diagnosis of epithelial downgrowth. *Cornea.* 2008;27:1138-1141.

71. Jadav DS, Rylander NR, Vold SD, Fulcher SF, Rosa RH Jr. Endoscopic photocoagulation in the management of epithelial downgrowth. *Cornea.* 2008;27:601-604.

72. Luo Y, Lin X, Wang Z. Clinical analysis of ocular siderosis [in Chinese]. *Yan Ke Xue Bao.* 2007;23(4):231-237.

73. Shiar K, Ji XC, Sun XH. A clinical analysis of subclinical siderosis and secondary glaucoma [in Chinese]. *Zhonghua Yan Ke Za Zhi.* 1994;30(6):420-422.

74. Teichmann KD, Pülhorn G. Glaucoma in the presence of chalcosis [in German]. *Klin Monbl Augenheilkd.* 1978;173(3):295-298.

75. Pesin SR, Katz LJ, Augsburger JJ, Chien AM, Eagle RC Jr. Acute angle-closure glaucoma from spontaneous massive hemorrhagic retinal or choroidal detachment. An updated diagnostic and therapeutic approach. *Ophthalmology.* 1990;97(1):76-84.

76. Viestenz A, Küchle M. Blunt ocular trauma. Part II. Blunt posterior segment trauma [in German]. *Ophthalmologe.* 2005;102(1):89-99.

77. Cinner E. Intraocular pressure in retinal detachment. *Arch Ophthalmol.* 1966;84:101.

78. Matsuo N, Takabatake M, Ueno H, et al. Photoreceptor outer segment in the aqueous humor in rhegmatogenous retinal detachment. *Am J Ophthalmol.* 1986;101:673-679.

79. Mitry D, Constable I, Singh J. Photoreceptor outer segment glaucoma in rhegmatogenous retinal detachment. *Arch Ophthalmol.* 2009;127(8):1053-1054.

44

Corticosteroid Glaucoma

Mina B. Pantcheva, MD

Corticosteroid-induced elevation of intraocular pressure (IOP) may accompany the use of topical, periocular, intravitreal, oral, intravenous, or inhaled corticosteroid therapy. The potential for steroids to increase IOP and cause subsequent glaucomatous optic neuropathy mandates a regular monitoring of IOP in patients on steroids.

Use of corticosteroids in ophthalmic conditions started within 2 years of the preparation and clinical use of cortisol by Hench and colleagues[1] at the Mayo Clinic in 1949.[2] In 1950, McLean[3] reported elevated IOP associated with systemic administration of adrenocorticotrophic hormone (ACTH). A report by Francois[4] on pressure elevation caused by topical steroids appeared in 1954. Landmark studies by Armaly[5-8] and Becker et al[9-11] in 1963 led to a profusion of studies on the effect of corticosteroids on IOP in the years to follow.

The clinical resemblance of corticosteroid-induced glaucoma to primary open-angle glaucoma (POAG) led to the initial hope that corticosteroids could be used to create a model of POAG, allowing insights into its development and possible genetic nature.[5-12] In addition, the finding of high-responder patients, with a marked elevation of IOP after steroid provocative tests, was hoped to identify patients at risk for the later development of POAG. The similarities between corticosteroid-induced glaucoma and POAG are indeed striking: asymptomatic, quiet eyes with open angles and no distinguishing or specific findings on clinical examination. Unfortunately, the relationship between the 2 conditions may not be as close as was originally thought as these initial hopes were not realized in later studies.[13-15]

KEY CLINICAL POINTS

- How common is corticosteroid glaucoma? Although all patients may respond with some change in pressure after prolonged corticosteroid use, studies by Armaly[5-8] and Becker et al[9-11] indicate that 30% to 40% of the normal population may be intermediate responders, with a pressure increase of at least 6 mm Hg or attain pressure levels of 20 mm Hg or higher. A small group of high responders had elevations of 16+ mm Hg or achieved levels of 32+ mm Hg (Table 44-1).

- How soon after starting steroids can IOP increase? Although most prospective studies used topical corticosteroids for 3 to 6 weeks to assess pressure response, some elevation of pressure can be found in most patients as early as the first or second week.[5-9] Armaly noted a hypertensive effect at the end of the first week in normal patients, with a mean increase in pressure of 19%.[5] High responders had more rapid and higher increases in pressure, with a few patients developing an increase of 60% at the end of the first week of therapy.[5,6] Patients with POAG, most of whom were considered high responders, also show a faster rate of pressure increase than normal patients. One study found more than 50% of patients with POAG developed elevations of pressure 15 mm Hg higher than baseline by the end of the second week. (In some cases, elevation in IOP from the use of frequent, potent topical steroid preparations, such as hourly prednisolone acetate 1%, may occur within 3 to 5 days. Additionally, patients on chronic lower-dose steroids may not develop IOP elevation for months, which may make this diagnosis more problematic.)

  It is unknown whether patients with little elevation of pressure after a 6-week steroid provocative test would develop higher pressures with prolonged use.

- How long will the elevated pressure remain once corticosteroids are stopped? The IOP increase is usually short-lived. Both Armaly and Becker reported pressures to return to baseline values in a matter of days to weeks after stopping steroids in the majority of subjects; Armaly[5] found this to occur by 2 weeks in all subjects. The duration of corticosteroid use, or the height of the

Kahook MY, Schuman JS, eds.
Chandler and Grant's Glaucoma, Fifth Edition (pp 423-429).
© 2013 SLACK Incorporated.

TABLE 44-1. CORTICOSTEROID TESTING AND INTRAOCULAR PRESSURE			
Patient Group	Response		
	Low Armaly: <6 mm Hg Becker: IOP <20 mm Hg	Intermediate Armaly: 6 to 15 mm Hg Becker: IOP 20 to 31 mm Hg	High Armaly: 16+ mm Hg Becker: IOP 32+ mm Hg
Normals			
Armaly	66%	29%	5%
Becker	58%	36%	6%
Primary open-angle glaucoma			
Armaly	6%	48%	46%
Becker	0%	8%	92%

Adapted from Becker B, Mills DW. Corticosteroids and intraocular pressure. *Arch Ophthalmol.* 1963;70:500-507 and Armaly MF. Inheritance of dexamethasone hypertension and glaucoma. *Arch Ophthalmol.* 1967;77(6):747-751.

pressure, may not necessarily predict the time course for the decrease of pressure. Case reports include that of increased pressure discovered in a patient after 1 year of topical corticosteroid use in which the pressure returned to normal 19 days after discontinuing the medication, whereas a second patient with a pressure increase that occurred after 8 weeks of corticosteroid use required 5 weeks to decrease.[16] Pressure elevation accompanying several years of steroid use may not decrease, however, once steroids are discontinued.[17] In other situations, pressure may attain such a high level, or enough damage may have occurred, that laser trabeculoplasty or filtering surgery is required before the IOP would have a chance to diminish.

- Are certain patients more likely to develop the problem? Patients with POAG are particularly susceptible to the pressure-elevating effect of corticosteroids. Steroid provocative tests in this population indicate that 94% to 100% of these patients will develop IOP increases of at least 6 mm Hg or IOPs between 20 and 31 mm Hg.[6,7,9,11] At least half of these were actually considered high responders, with pressures elevating at least 16 mm Hg or to levels above 31 mm Hg. Studies[18] in patients with secondary open-angle glaucoma generally do not find such high response rates.

Although older patients are at an increased risk, the frequency of steroid responsiveness with age may occur in a bimodal distribution. A study by Lam and colleagues[19] showed that 71.2% of children receiving topical dexamethasone 0.1% 4 times a day responded with an IOP rise greater than 21 mm Hg. Among children under 6 years of age, the peak IOP was greater, the net increase in IOP was greater, and the time required to obtain the peak IOP was less. Those older than 6 years (up to age 10 studied) had a similar net increase in IOP, but did not

show a significant difference in peak IOP or the time required to reach a peak IOP. This potential should be kept in mind when prescribing steroids for uveitis, after strabismus surgery, or for other conditions in children, especially as lack of cooperation may make it difficult to measure the IOP in these patients. First-degree relatives of patients with POAG, diabetics, high myopes, and patients with rheumatoid arthritis or other connective tissue diseases have also been reported to be likely steroid-responders.[8,10,13,20-22]

- Can systemic or other forms of corticosteroids elevate IOP? All methods of corticosteroid use have the potential to elevate IOP. Systemic steroid use is less likely to cause elevations of IOP than topical application; a study[23] found a 10% incidence of ocular hypertension in renal transplant patients receiving systemic steroids after transplant, although pretreatment pressures were not obtained.

Endogenous corticosteroids may cause elevation of IOP in patients with Cushing's syndrome and other forms of hypersecretion.

Periocular injections of corticosteroids may elevate IOP. Long-acting preparations, such as triamcinolone acetonide, may be especially likely to cause increases, as reports indicate active steroid may be released for months.[24] Some patients may require the surgical removal of a repository steroid injection for IOP control. In consideration of this, such injections should be given in an easily retrievable spot, such as the inferior fornix.

Recently, the use of intravitreal corticosteroid injections or implants for macular edema, adjunctive therapy in the treatment of choroidal neovascularization, and noninfectious posterior segment uveitis has led to increased incidence of steroid-induced ocular hypertension.[25-29]

Dermal applications of corticosteroids have caused elevation of IOP, whether administered to the periocular region or at distant sites.[30] Inhaled corticosteroids may also cause an increase in pressure.[31]

- Steps in the management of corticosteroid-induced glaucoma. Recognition of the condition is the most important step in its management. Measurement of IOP on a regular basis in any patient placed on long-term topical corticosteroids is essential. Prevention is also key: use of nonsteroidal anti-inflammatory agents rather than steroids, use of steroid preparations less likely to elevate IOP when possible[32-34] (rimexolone [Vexol], fluorometholone [FML], medrysone [HMS]), and avoidance of using extremely long-acting steroid preparations for subconjunctival injections. Prevention of the unmonitored use of steroids by patients should be considered by writing nonrefillable prescriptions for only small quantities of corticosteroids, when possible.

Once the possibility of steroid glaucoma is seriously considered, stopping steroid treatment and observation of the eye for several weeks will usually result in spontaneous lowering of the IOP. If the IOP has reached a dangerous or worrisome level, the use of IOP-lowering agents or surgery may be required.[35] No specific treatment, such as an antisteroid eye drop, is available.

More perplexing is the situation of elevation of IOP in an eye that has been on steroid therapy for chronic iritis or uveitis (see Chapter 42). It is difficult to know if the inflammatory condition has worsened and caused elevation of the pressure or whether the patient has now become a steroid-responder. It is usually advisable to increase the steroid therapy for several days to attempt to suppress any increase in inflammation. If the IOP decreases with the increased steroid, inflammation, not a steroid response, was the explanation for the increased IOP. If, however, the IOP remains unchanged or elevates, then a steroid response in IOP, whether due to obstruction of aqueous outflow or increased aqueous inflow, is likely and the amount of steroid use must be decreased. This may entail using the drops less often, decreasing the strength of the drops, or switching to a preparation less likely to affect IOP. Addition of an IOP-lowering agent may also be considered if steroid use cannot be decreased.

CORTICOSTEROID PREPARATIONS

Corticosteroids are a family of compounds related in structure to the cholesterol molecule from which they are derived. They share structural similarities with the 2 other major classes of steroids: mineralocorticoids and sex steroids (Figure 44-1). Addition of an extra double bond in the ring structures or small modifications of side groups of the steroid base molecule may cause significant changes in both effect and potency; prednisolone, which has a second double bond in the A ring, has significantly greater anti-inflammatory activity and less fluid-retaining effects than cortisol (Table 44-2).[36,37] The creation of derivative compounds (ie, the addition of an acetate group) can also change the clinical effect of the base molecule by affecting its penetration into the eye, release characteristics, and degradation rate. Although these factors determine bioavailability, other factors, such as affinity of binding to the steroid receptor, are also involved in determining anti-inflammatory activity.[36] In topical therapy, experimental studies of inflammatory keratitis indicate that the acetate derivative (more lipophilic) is the most effective, followed by the alcohol and finally the steroid-phosphate compounds (relatively hydrophilic).[38]

Attempts to separate the IOP-elevating effect from the anti-inflammatory effect have been met with mixed results. While studies indicate that rimexolone (Vexol), fluorometholone (FML), and medrysone (HMS) are less likely to cause elevation of IOP,[32-34] they also appear less efficacious for intraocular inflammation than prednisolone or dexamethasone (Table 44-3).[36,38] The decreased tendency of fluorometholone to elevate IOP may be due to an increased degradation rate in the ocular tissues, resulting in a shorter duration of action or a smaller amount reaching the target tissue.[36]

The efficacy and duration of action of periocular injections of corticosteroids is dependent on both the steroid base and the derivative formulation. The solubility of the compound appears to play a major role in its duration of action. Poorly soluble compounds are considered long-acting, while water-soluble compounds are considered short-acting (Table 44-4).[24,36]

PATHOPHYSIOLOGY

The mechanism of corticosteroid-induced ocular hypertension is increased aqueous outflow resistance. Reports of histologic findings in the trabecular meshwork (TM) of eyes with corticosteroid glaucoma are variable. Some reports find no pathological change, whereas others have described the accumulation of excess basement membrane-like material.[23,39-44] The variable time course for both the development and resolution of the IOP increase makes it likely that several mechanisms may be involved. Clark and colleagues[45] showed that the actin stress fibers were reorganized into actin networks that resembled geodesic-dome-like polygonal lattices in human TM cells cultured in the presence of dexamethasone. Upon discontinuing dexamethasone, cross-linking of the actin networks was reversible. The effect was thought to be mediated via TM glucocorticoid receptors. In perfusion-cultured human eyes, the steroid treatment had similar microstructural changes and was associated with an increased outflow resistance.[46]

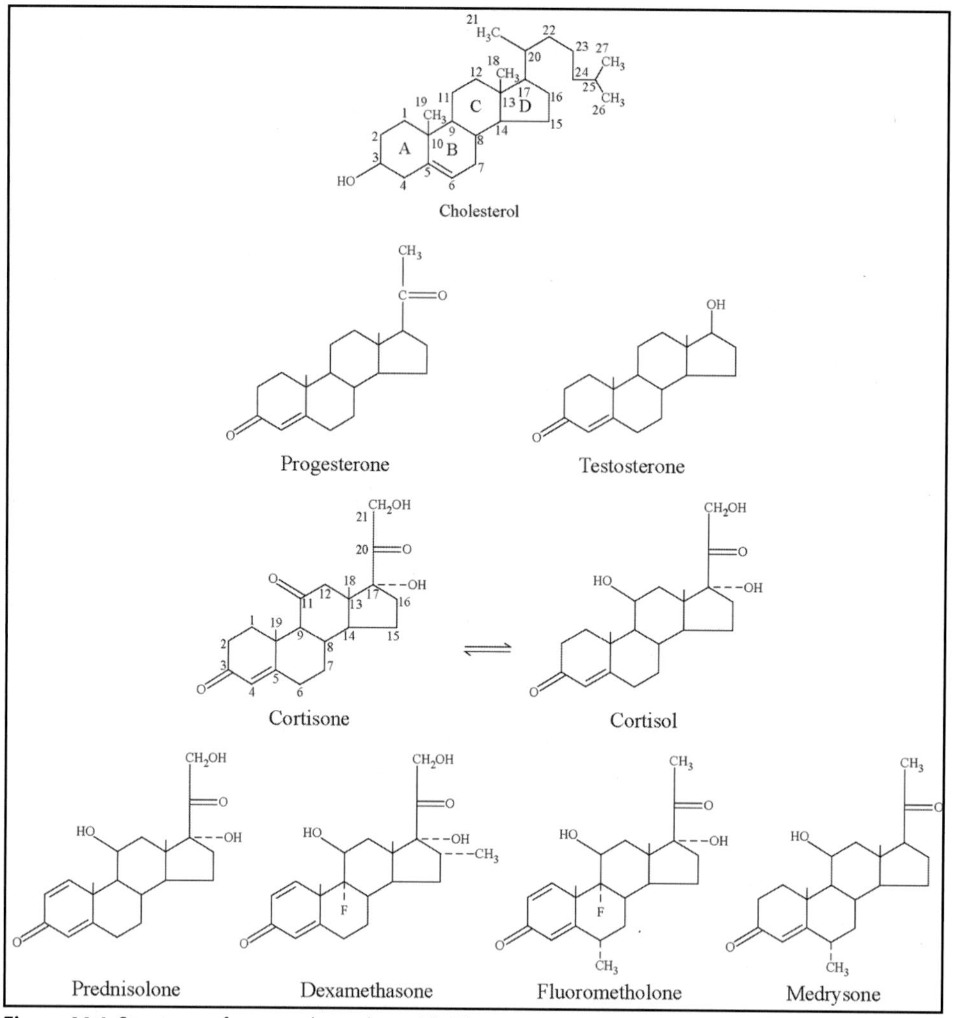

Figure 44-1. Structures of commonly used steroids. The parent molecule, cholesterol, has 4 rings and 27 carbon atoms. Progesterone and the corticosteroids keep the basic 4-ring structure and have 21 carbon atoms; testosterone has 19. Cortisone, initially termed *compound E*, has a keto group at position II, while cortisol, *compound F*, has a hydroxyl group in this position.

Wilson and colleagues[47] found an increased deposition of extracellular matrix material altering the ultrastructure of the juxtacanalicular region. The corticosteroid dexamethasone increases glycosaminoglycan, elastin, and fibronectin production in cultured TM[48]; the glycosaminoglycan deposition increases further with prolonged steroid exposure.[49,50] Immunohistochemical evaluation of the extracellular material in the TM in steroid-induced glaucoma showed that there is, in fact, an accumulation of type IV collagen and fibronectin in the TM.[51]

The decreased outflow facility may be caused by reduced degradation of substances in the TM. Levels of tissue plasminogen activator, stromelysin, and metalloproteases have been shown to decrease in TM cultures treated with dexamethasone.[50,52,53] Furthermore, dexamethasone treatment inhibits TM cell arachidonic acid metabolism and reduces the phagocytic properties of the cells.[52,54,55] Because these cells function to remove debris deposited in the meshwork, reduced functional activity may lead to reduced outflow facility.

RELATIONSHIP TO PRIMARY OPEN-ANGLE GLAUCOMA

The marked sensitivity to corticosteroids of high responder normal eyes and eyes with POAG led to initial thought that such patients had a similar genetic inheritance of a recessive gene for glaucoma.[8,10] Moreover, having a first-degree relative with POAG could make one susceptible to being a steroid-responder.[10,56] High responders were thought to be at risk for the later development of POAG. Subsequent work did not support this hypothesis; high responders did not develop POAG with the frequency predicted from such a model.[13,15] An explanation for the large

TABLE 44-2. RELATIVE POTENCY OF CORTICOSTEROIDS

Steroid Base	Relative Anti-Inflammatory Activity
Short acting (8 to 2 hr)	
Cortisone	0.8
Cortisol	1.0
Intermediate acting (12 to 36 hr)	
Prednisone	4
Prednisolone	4
Triamcinolone	5
Long acting (36 to 72 hr)	
Dexamethasone	25
Betamethasone	25

Adapted from Haynes RC, Murad F. Adrenocorticotropic hormone; adrenocortical steroids and their synthetic analogs; inhibitors of adrenocortical steroid biosynthesis. In: Gilman AG, Goodman LS, Rail TW, Murad F, eds. *The Pharmacological Basis of Therapeutics.* 7th ed. New York, NY: MacMillan Publishing Co; 1985.

TABLE 44-3. ANTI-INFLAMMATORY ACTIVITY OF TOPICAL CORTICOSTEROIDS IN EXPERIMENTAL KERATITIS

Steroid Compound	Anti-Inflammatory Activity (%)
Dexamethasone acetate 0.1%	55
Prednisolone acetate 1% (Pred Forte; Enconopred Plus)	51
Dexamethasone alcohol 0.1% (Maxidex)	40
Fluorometholone alcohol 0.25% (FML Forte)	35
0.1% (FML)	31
Prednisolone phosphate 1% (Inflamase Forte)	28
Dexamethasone phosphate 0.1% (Decadron Phosphate)	19
Medrysone (HMS)	Not tested

Adapted from Leibowitz HM. Management of inflammation in the cornea and conjunctiva. *Ophthalmology.* 1980;87(8):753-758.

TABLE 44-4. INJECTABLE CORTICOSTEROIDS

Short Acting
- Dexamethasone sodium phosphate (Decadron)
- Hydrocortisone sodium succinate (Solu-Cortef)
- Methylprednisolone sodium succinate (Solu-Medrol)
- Intermediate acting
- Triamcinolone diacetate (Aristocort)
- Methylprednisolone acetate (Depo-Medrol)

Long Acting
- Triamcinolone acetonide (Kenalog)
- Triamcinolone hexacetonide (Aristospan)

This article was published in *Am J Ophthalmol,* 82, Herschler J, Increased intraocular pressure induced by repository corticosteroids, 90-93, Copyright Elsevier 1976.

number of high responders among POAG patients may be the pre-existing condition of the TM.[5]

THE FUTURE

Diurnal Variations

Numerous studies[57-60] have examined the relationship between the diurnal variation in IOP, aqueous humor flow, and the diurnal pattern of endogenous cortisone secretion, yet the exact relationship remains unclear. Several studies[61-63] have found a 3- to 4-hour lag time between the administration of systemic corticosteroids and an elevation in IOP. Interestingly, this elevation of IOP lasts only a few hours. Understanding the mechanism of corticosteroids in elevating IOP and understanding their presumed role in the diurnal variations in aqueous humor flow will provide fundamental insights into the mechanisms controlling aqueous dynamics. Such an understanding may help with the design of new and more effective therapy for glaucoma.

Antisteroids

Outflow facility increases during pregnancy, and several studies have considered the elevated progesterone levels during this time to be responsible.[64,65] The effect of other steroids and their metabolites have been examined, finding that a metabolite of cortisol, 3α, 5β-tetrahydrocortisol, may lower IOP in patients with POAG.[66] An anabolic androgenic steroid, 17a-methyltestosterone, reversed the steroid-induced elevation of IOP in a series of monkeys.[67] This compound also possesses angiostatic activity and may represent a new class of therapeutic agents.[68] RU486 is a progesterone blocker and a corticosteroid blocker that has been shown to decrease IOP when administered topically or subconjunctivally in a rabbit model.[69,70] This agent has not been investigated in humans for this purpose to date. However, none of these studies have looked at the potential inflammatory effect that such blocking of normal steroid metabolism may cause.

Although steroids may play a key role in understanding fundamental aspects of aqueous inflow and outflow and antisteroid compounds hold promise for the future at the present time, corticosteroids must still be used with discretion and the awareness of their potential to elevate IOP.

REFERENCES

1. Hench PS, Kendall EC, Slocumb CH, et al. The effect of a hormone of the adrenal cortex (17-hydroxy-11-dehydrocorticosterone: compound E) and of pituitary adrenocorticotropic hormone on rheumatoid arthritis. *Proc Staff Meet Mayo Clin.* 1949;24(8):181-197.
2. Woods AC. Clinical and experimental observation on the use of ACTH and cortisone in ocular inflammatory disease. *Am J Ophthalmol.* 1950;33(9):1325-1349.
3. McLean JM. In discussion of Woods AC. Clinical and experimental observation on the use of ACTH and cortisone in ocular inflammatory disease. *Trans Am Ophthalmol Soc.* 1950;48:259-296.
4. Francois J. Cortisone et tension oculaire. *Ann Oculist.* 1954;187:805.
5. Armaly MF. Effect of corticosteroids on intraocular pressure and fluid dynamics. I. The effect of dexamethasone in the normal eye. *Arch Ophthalmol.* 1963;70:482-491.
6. Armaly MF. Effect of corticosteroids on intraocular pressure and fluid dynamics. II. The effect of dexamethasone in the glaucomatous eye. *Arch Ophthalmol.* 1963;70:492-499.
7. Armaly MF. Statistical attributes of the steroid hypertensive response in the clinically normal eye. *Invest Ophthalmol Vis Sci.* 1965;4:187-197.
8. Armaly MF. The heritable nature of dexamethasone-induced ocular hypertension. *Arch Ophthalmol.* 1966;75(1):32-35.
9. Becker B, Mills DW. Corticosteroids and intraocular pressure. *Arch Ophthalmol.* 1963;70:500-507.
10. Becker B, Hahn KA. Topical corticosteroids and heredity in primary open-angle glaucoma. *Am J Ophthalmol.* 1964;57:543-551.
11. Becker B. Intraocular pressure response to topical corticosteroids. *Invest Ophthalmol Vis Sci.* 1965;4:198.
12. Grant WM. Glaucoma from topical corticosteroids. *Arch Ophthalmol.* 1963;70:445-446.
13. Armaly MF. Inheritance of dexamethasone hypertension and glaucoma. *Arch Ophthalmol.* 1967;77(6):747-751.
14. Kitazawa Y, Horie T. The prognosis of corticosteroid-responsive individuals. *Arch Ophthalmol.* 1981;99(5):819-823.
15. Lewis JM, Priddy T, Judd J, et al. Intraocular pressure response to topical dexamethasone as a predictor for the development of primary open-angle glaucoma. *Am J Ophthalmol.* 1988;106(5):607-612.
16. Epstein DL, ed. *Chandler and Grant's Glaucoma.* 3rd ed. Philadelphia, PA: Lea & Febiger; 1986.
17. Espildora J, Vicuna P, Diaz E. Cortisone-induced glaucoma: a report on 44 affected eyes. *J Fr Ophthalmol.* 1981;4:503-508.
18. Becker B. The effect of topical corticosteroids in secondary glaucomas. *Arch Ophthalmol.* 1964;72:769-771.
19. Lam DSC, Fan DSP, Ng JSK, et al. Ocular hypertensive and antiinflammatory responses to different dosages of topical dexamethasone in children: a randomized trial. *Clin Exp Ophthalmol.* 2005;33(3):252-258.
20. Podos SM, Becker B, Morton WR. High myopia and primary open-angle glaucoma. *Am J Ophthalmol.* 1966;62(6):1038-1043.
21. Becker B. Diabetes mellitus and primary open-angle glaucoma. The XXVII Edward Jackson Memorial Lecture. *Am J Ophthalmol.* 1971;71:1-16.
22. Gaston H, Absolon MJ, Thurtle OA, et al. Steroid responsiveness in connective tissue diseases. *Br J Ophthalmol.* 1983;67(7):487-490.
23. Adhikary HP, Sells RA, Basu PK. Ocular complications of systemic steroids after renal transplantation and their association with HLA. *Br J Ophthalmol.* 1982;66(5):290-291.
24. Herschler J. Increased intraocular pressure induced by repository corticosteroids. *Am J Ophthalmol.* 1976;82(1):90-93.
25. Smithen LM, Ober MD, Maranan L, et al. Intravitreal triamcinolone acetonide and intraocular pressure. *Am J Ophthalmol.* 2004;138(5):740-743.
26. Singh IP, Ahmad SI, Yeh D, et al. Early rapid rise in intraocular pressure after intravitreal triamcinolone acetonide injection. *Am J Ophthalmol.* 2004;138(2):286-287.
27. Gillies MC, Simpson JM, Billson FA, et al. Safety of an intravitreal injection of triamcinolone: results from a randomized clinical trial. *Arch Ophthalmol.* 2004;122(3):336-340.
28. Jonas JB, Degenring RF, Kreissing I, et al. Intraocular pressure elevation after intravitreal triamcinolone acetonide injection. *Ophthalmology.* 2005;112(4):593-598.
29. Bollinger KE, Smith SD. Prevalence and management of elevated intraocular pressure after placement of an intravitreal sustained-release steroid implant. *Curr Opin Ophthalmol.* 2009;20(2):99-103.
30. Spaeth GL, Rodrigues MM, Weinreb S. Steroid-induced glaucoma: A. Persistent elevation of intraocular pressure. B. Histopathological aspects. *Tr Am Ophthalmol Soc.* 1977;75:353-381.
31. Bergmann J, Witmer MT, Slonim CB. The relationship of intranasal steroids to intraocular pressure. *Curr Allergy Asthma Rep.* 2009;9(4):311-315.
32. Cantrill HL, Palmberg PF, Zink II A, et al. Comparison of in vitro potency of corticosteroids with ability to raise intraocular pressure. *Am J Ophthalmol.* 1975;79(6):1012-1017.
33. Stewart RH, Kimbrough RL. Intraocular pressure response to topically administered fluorometholone. *Arch Ophthalmol.* 1979;97(11):2139-2140.
34. Kass M, Cheetham J, Duzman E, et al. The ocular hypertensive effect of 0.25% fluorometholone in corticosteroid responders. *Am J Ophthalmol.* 1986;102(2):159-163.
35. Spaeth GL, Monteiro de Barros DS, Fudemberg SJ. Visual loss caused by corticosteroid-induced glaucoma: how to avoid it. *Retina.* 2009;29(8):1057-1061.
36. Polansky JR, Weinreb RN. Anti-inflammatory agents. Steroids as anti-inflammatory agents. In: Sears ML, ed. *Handbook of Experimental Pharmacology.* Vol 69. Berlin: Heidelberg, Springer-Verlag; 1984.
37. Haynes RC, Murad F. Adrenocorticotropic hormone; adrenocortical steroids and their synthetic analogs; inhibitors of adrenocortical steroid biosynthesis. In: Gilman AG, Goodman LS, Rail TW, Murad F, eds. *The Pharmacological Basis of Therapeutics.* 7th ed. New York, NY: MacMillan Publishing Co; 1985:1466-1496.
38. Leibowitz HM. Management of inflammation in the cornea and conjunctiva. *Ophthalmology.* 1980;87(8):753-758.
39. Rohen JW, Linnér E, Witmer R. Electron microscopic studies on the trabecular meshwork in two cases of corticosteroid-glaucoma. *Exp Eye Res.* 1973;17(1):19-31.
40. Toriyama K. An electron microscopic study on the trabecular meshwork in corticosteroid-glaucoma. *Bull Jpn Ophthalmol.* 1979;30:1583.
41. Roll P, Benedikt O. Elektronenoptische Untersuchung des Trabekelwerkes bei einem Kortikosteroidglaukom. *Klin Mbl Augenheilk.* 1979;174(3):421-428.
42. Kayes J. Pore structure of the inner wall of Schlemm's canal. *Invest Ophthalmol.* 1967;6:381.
43. Kayes J, Becker B. The human trabecular meshwork in corticosteroid-induced glaucoma. *Trans Am Ophthalmol Soc.* 1969;67:339-354.
44. Sano T, Miyata Y. Autopsy findings in a case with steroid glaucoma. *Jpn J Clin Ophthalmol.* 1971;25:17.

45. Clark AF, Wilson K, McCartney MD, et al. Glucocorticoid-induced formation of cross-linked actin networks in cultured human trabecular meshwork cells. *Invest Ophthalmol Vis Sci.* 1994;35(1):281-294.

46. Clark AF, Brotchie D, Read AT, et al. Dexamethasone alters F-actin architecture and promotes cross-linked actin network formation in human trabecular meshwork tissue. *Cell Motil Cytoskeleton.* 2005;60(2):83-95.

47. Wilson K, McCartney MD, Miggans ST, Clark AF. Dexamethasone induced ultrastructural changes in cultured human trabecular meshwork cells. *Curr Eye Res.* 1993;12(9):783-793.

48. Yun AJ, Murphy CG, Polansky JR, Newsome DA, Alvarado JA. Proteins secreted by human trabecular cells. Glucocorticoid and other effects. *Invest Ophthalmol Vis Sci.* 1989;30(9):2012-2022.

49. Yue BY. The extracellular matrix and its modulation in the trabecular meshwork. *Surv Ophthalmol.* 1996;40(5):379-390.

50. Johnson DH, Bradley JM, Acott TS. The effect of dexamethasone on glycosaminoglycans of human trabecular meshwork in perfusion organ culture. *Invest Ophthalmol Vis Sci.* 1990;31(12):2568-2571.

51. Tawara A, Tou N, Kubota T, et al. Immunohistochemical evaluation of the extracellular matrix in trabecular meshwork in steroid induced glaucoma. *Graefes Arch Clin Exp Ophthalmol.* 2008;246(7):1021-1028.

52. Wordinger RJ, Clark AF. Effects of glucocorticoids on the trabecular meshwork: towards a better understanding of glaucoma. *Prog Retina Eye Res.* 1999;18(5):629-667.

53. Snyder RW, Stamer WD, Kramer TR, Seftor REB. Corticosteroid treatment and trabecular meshwork proteases in cell and organ culture supernatants. *Exp Eye Res.* 1993;57(4):461-468.

54. Weinreb RN, Polansky JR, Kramer SG, Baxter JD. Acute effects of dexamethasone on intraocular pressure in glaucoma. *Invest Ophthalmol Vis Sci.* 1985;26(2):170-175.

55. Shirato S, Bloom E, Polansky J, et al. Phagocytic properties of confluent human trabecular meshwork cells. *Invest Ophthalmol Vis Sci.* 1988;29:S125.

56. Davies TG. Tonographic survey of the close relatives of patients with chronic simple glaucoma. *Br J Ophthalmol.* 1968;52(1):32-39.

57. Linner E. Adrenocortical hormones and glaucoma. *Acta Ophthalmologics.* 1966;44(3):299-305.

58. Smith JL, Stempfel RS, Campell HS, Hudnell AB Jr, Richman DW. Diurnal variation of plasma 17-hydroxycorticoids and intraocular pressure in glaucoma. *Am J Ophthalmol.* 1962;54:411.

59. Maus TL, Young WF Jr, Brubaker RF. Aqueous flow in humans after adrenalectomy. *Invest Ophthalmol Vis Sci.* 1994;35(8):3325-3331.

60. Sheridan PT, Brubaker RF, Larsson LI, Rettig ES, Young WF Jr. The effect of oral dexamethasone on the circadian rhythm of aqueous humor flow in humans. *Invest Ophthalmol Vis Sci.* 1994;35(3):1150-1156.

61. Weitzman ED, Henkind P, Leitman M, et al. Correlative 24-hour relationships between intraocular pressure and plasma Cortisol in normal subjects and patients with glaucoma. *Br J Ophthalmol.* 1975;59(10):566-572.

62. Boyd TAS, McLeod LE, Hassard DTR, et al. Relation of diurnal variation of plasma corticoid levels and intraocular pressure in glaucoma. *Can Med Ass J.* 1962;86:772-775.

63. Weinreb RN, Polansky JR, Kramer SG, et al. Acute effects of dexamethasone on intraocular pressure in glaucoma. *Invest Ophthalmol Vis Sci.* 1985;26(2):170-175.

64. Becker B, Friedenwald JS. Clinical aqueous outflow. *Arch Ophthalmol.* 1953;50(5):557-571.

65. Ziai N, Ory SJ, Khan AR, et al. β-human chorionic gonadotropin, progesterone, and aqueous dynamics during pregnancy. *Arch Ophthalmol.* 1994;112(6):801-806.

66. Southren AL, Wandel T, Gordon GG, et al. Treatment of glaucoma with 3 alpha, 5 beta-tetrahydrocortisol: a new therapeutic modality. *J Ocular Pharmacol.* 1994;10(1):385-391.

67. Knepper PA, Collins JA, Frederick R. Effect of 17-alpha-methyl-testosterone on IOP and GAG profile of dexamethasone-induced ocular hypertension in primates. *Invest Ophthalmol Vis Sci.* 1991;32:871.

68. Clark AF, McNatt L, Knepper PA. Angiostatic steroids as a new class of IOP lowering compounds. *Invest Ophthalmol Vis Sci.* 1994;35(ARVO suppl):1483.

69. Tsukahara S, Sasaki T, Phillips CI, et al. Subconjunctival injection of RU486 lowers intraocular pressure in normal rabbits. *Br J Ophthalmol.* 1986;70(6):451-455.

70. Green K, Phillips CI, Gore SM, et al. Ocular fluid dynamics response to topical RU486, a steroid blocker. *Curr Eye Res.* 1985;4(5):605-612.

Douglas H. Johnson, MD, now deceased, was an original author on this chapter.

Hemolytic or Ghost-Cell Glaucoma

David L. Epstein, MD, MMM

CLINICAL FINDINGS

The term *hemolytic glaucoma* was introduced by Fenton and Zimmerman[1] to describe the clinical and histologic findings in a patient who had spontaneous hemorrhage into the vitreous humor and several weeks later had high intraocular pressure (IOP) and pain, leading to enucleation. Hemorrhagic debris and pigment-laden macrophages were found in sections of the anterior chamber angle. Fenton and Zimmerman[1] postulated that the glaucoma was caused by a mechanical blockage of aqueous outflow by broken-down red blood cells and macrophages, analogous to phacolytic glaucoma, which was conceived of as being due to obstruction by lens material and macrophages. Clinical and experimental investigations by Campbell and colleagues[2-5] have led us to believe that ghost cells, resulting from degeneration of red blood cells, are a particularly important factor in obstructing aqueous outflow and causing glaucoma as an occasional consequence of hemorrhage in the vitreous humor, and also in some cases of glaucoma associated with hemorrhage into the anterior chamber from blunt injury to the globe.

Retinal vascular disease or injury often produces hemorrhage into the vitreous humor, but the blood seldom passes the barrier of the anterior hyaloid membrane to reach the anterior chamber. However, a few such cases have been reported in phakic eyes.[6,7] Most commonly, the anterior hyaloid is not intact, often from accidental injury or surgery, particularly after cataract extraction or vitrectomy, and thereby the products of hemorrhage can enter the anterior chamber and produce severe open-angle glaucoma. Fresh hemorrhage into the vitreous humor appears red when viewed with the slit-lamp biomicroscope, but within 2 to 4 weeks, the color of the material in the vitreous changes to a light-tan or khaki color due to loss of the red-colored hemoglobin and degeneration of the red cells to ghosts. The red blood cells change from biconcave discs to spherical forms with Heinz bodies. Ghost-cell glaucoma tends to develop within 3 to 4 weeks after the occurrence of a hemorrhage into the vitreous humor in an eye with a defective anterior hyaloid membrane. Myriad small cells appear in the aqueous humor and the IOP rises into the range of 30 to 70 mm Hg, with the angle remaining open.

In many instances, the appearance of myriad cells in the aqueous humor associated with a severe open-angle glaucoma has been misinterpreted as an iritis or uveitis, in the belief that the cells were inflammatory cells. In such cases, topical or systemic treatment with corticosteroids has often been used, generally to no avail. In fact, corticosteroids may delay the reabsorption of the blood cells from the eye. (It is interesting to contemplate how corticosteroids might interfere with this blood reabsorption within the trabecular meshwork [TM] by interfering with normal trabecular cell actions. Similar cellular actions may be involved in steroid-induced open-angle glaucoma or even primary open-angle glaucoma [POAG].)

Ghost-cell glaucoma with such tan-colored cells in the anterior chamber may be misinterpreted as postsurgical endophthalmitis. In these cases, there are no inflammatory keratic precipitates. If, with the slit-lamp biomicroscope the color of the light-tan, old blood in the vitreous is compared with that of the fine cells circulating in the anterior chamber, they have the same hue, characteristic of ghost cells.

Aspiration of material from the anterior chamber in a series of cases of this sort and immediate examination of the fluid by phase-contrast microscopy without drying, staining, or filtering have shown great numbers of ghost cells with characteristic Heinz bodies. These cells have occasionally been called erythroclasts. Their identity has been confirmed by transmission and scanning electron microscopy both in the aqueous and vitreous humors. Variable amounts of amorphous debris accompany the ghost cells, but in at least 15 samples of aqueous humor from eyes with hemolytic glaucoma examined by Campbell and colleagues,[2] macrophages were remarkably scarce and there was no cellular evidence of inflammatory reaction.

Kahook MY, Schuman JS, eds.
Chandler and Grant's Glaucoma, Fifth Edition (pp 431-434).
© 2013 SLACK Incorporated.

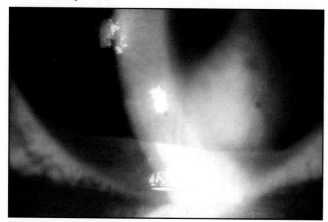

Figure 45-1. Tan hyphema, which may at times be mixed with red blood cells, are associated with glaucoma. The tan layer is composed of ghost cells, red blood cells that have lost their hemoglobin and elasticity. These cells are responsible for the obstruction of outflow that results in ghost-cell glaucoma.

By gonioscopy, the angle may appear normal, but if there are many ghost cells in the anterior chamber, they may form a khaki-colored layer on the filtration portion of the TM, occasionally resembling a layer of butter. In more extreme cases, the ghost cells may fill the dependent angle. The tan or yellowish color distinguishes this accumulation from an exudate or hypopyon of inflammatory cells.

The main causes of ghost-cell glaucoma in our experience have been the following:

- Cataract extraction complicated by hemorrhage into the anterior chamber or vitreous cavity

- Blunt or penetrating trauma with hemorrhage into the anterior chamber or vitreous cavity

- Closed vitrectomy for removal of vitreous hemorrhage for the purpose of improving vision

Ghost-cell glaucoma can also result from extensive hyphema formation alone, but is most commonly associated with vitreous hemorrhage that acts as a reservoir for these cells to come into the anterior chamber after a subsequent interval of time.

DIAGNOSIS

The diagnosis of hemolytic or ghost-cell glaucoma should be suspected whenever hemorrhage into the vitreous cavity has occurred and has been followed within 3 or 4 weeks by elevated IOP in the range of 30 to 70 mm Hg, associated myriad very small cells circulating in the anterior chamber, with no conglomerate keratic precipitates (KPs) on the corneal endothelium. There may be a tan hyphema, sometimes mixed with red blood (Figure 45-1). When there has been trauma, gonioscopy may also show contusion-disruption of angle structures, but this should not distract attention from the importance of the fine cells in the aqueous humor. The diagnosis can be most securely established by aspirating the

aqueous humor from the anterior chamber and examining it immediately by phase-contrast microscopy without centrifuging, filtering, drying, or staining. Characteristically, no inflammatory cells are seen, but a rare macrophage may be found with innumerable erythrocyte ghost cells.

MECHANISM

Experiments by Campbell and colleagues[2,3,5] have provided evidence that permits one to explain the development of high IOP in this condition. Normal red blood cells are so pliable that they pass readily through spaces smaller than the ordinary diameter of these cells (that are presumably present in the outflow pathway), but when they degenerate to ghost cells, they lose this pliability and are unable to pass through the same small spaces. This has been well-demonstrated in vitro with standard micro-porous filters. Campbell has confirmed that fresh human red blood cells pass readily from the anterior chamber through the outflow system to the aqueous veins in enucleated normal human eyes, producing only a modest decrease in facility of aqueous outflow, and he has demonstrated that human erythrocyte ghosts differ from the fresh cells in being rigid and unable to pass from the anterior chamber through the aqueous outflow system.[2] Instead, they obstruct and cause a marked reduction in facility of aqueous outflow, leading to the elevation of IOP.

TREATMENT

Treatment may be medical or surgical, depending on the seriousness of the situation. If IOP is not high, it may respond to medical therapy (aqueous suppressant therapy). Although miotics have been used with occasional success in the past by presumably mechanically widening the outflow channels to allow egress, this also may be counterproductive as in any eye with inflammation. If the IOP can be kept down to the 30- to 40-mm Hg range with this treatment, the cornea is not edematous, and the patient is not in pain, the ghost cells may gradually clear in the course of some weeks (but remember the above potential contrary effect of corticosteroids) and the IOP may fall. However, if the amount of old hemorrhagic material in the vitreous is large, it may take too long to clear by slow diffusion forward into the anterior chamber and out the drainage system. When the IOP is in the 60- to 70-mm Hg range, it is rare for medical treatment to reduce the IOP sufficiently and surgical treatment is required. Systemic hyperosmotic agents usually help only temporarily. Surgical treatment is indicated also in those cases in which IOP in the 40 to 50 mm Hg range persists for weeks despite medical treatment. In eyes prone to retinal or optic nerve vascular occlusion, such as those with sickle cell anemia or trait, there is a much lower IOP threshold for surgical intervention (24 to 30 mm Hg).

The surgical treatment consists of making a small paracentesis in the cornea, draining the contents of the anterior chamber, and irrigating the anterior chamber with a physiologic saline solution to wash out as many of the ghost cells as possible. If the ghost cells have come from a hemorrhage in the anterior chamber with little or no hemorrhage into the vitreous cavity, this treatment can be very effective, but if the ghost cells come from a large reservoir of old hemorrhagic material in the vitreous cavity, usually a single evacuation and irrigation of the anterior chamber is insufficient for lasting control. After a few days, the anterior chamber commonly again contains myriad cells that have come from the vitreous chamber, the IOP is again high, and repeat evacuation and aspiration are required. In such cases, proceed to surgical vitrectomy rather than repeat anterior chamber irrigation. (Anterior chamber irrigation probably does not remove ghost cells from the interstices of the outflow pathway. Rather, it eliminates a future load of such cells from going into the TM and allows endogenous processes within this latter tissue to act to break down and remove the blood elements. It is this process that corticosteroids may interfere with within the outflow pathway tissue.)

Vitrectomy has been effective in a number of cases in removing the reservoir of old blood from the vitreous cavity, allowing the anterior chamber to clear and IOP to come down. Experience with vitrectomy suggests that, to be effective in relieving the glaucoma, it must include thorough irrigation of the vitreous cavity to leave behind as little of the old blood as possible.

This inference is drawn from a study[8] in which patients who had old hemorrhage in the vitreous cavity, but no glaucoma, were subjected to closed vitrectomy to improve vision. In some of these cases, glaucoma developed within 2 to 10 days after the procedure. This was associated with a flooding of the anterior chamber with ghost cells, presumably entering through some breach in the anterior hyaloid membrane. This complication occurred less frequently when thorough irrigation was performed to remove as much old blood as possible from the vitreous cavity. In cases of ghost-cell glaucoma precipitated by closed vitrectomies with less thorough irrigation, the IOP characteristically was greater than 40 mm Hg, sometimes higher than 60 mm Hg. Some of these cases were controlled medically and others required repeated irrigation of the anterior chamber. When only a small amount of the old blood remained in the vitreous cavity, there was less tendency for recurrence of glaucoma than when a larger reservoir of ghost cells was left in the vitreous cavity.

After vitrectomy, an increase of IOP can be produced in other ways. One must also consider the possibilities of corticosteroid glaucoma, lens-induced glaucoma, neovascular glaucoma, and obstruction of the outflow system by sickle cells in a patient with this disease.[9] However, persistent ghost-cell glaucoma has been the most commonly observed cause of an increase of IOP after vitrectomy.

If, despite these measures, there is re-accumulation of many cells in the anterior chamber and high IOP, other procedures must be considered. Cyclocryotherapy or newer ciliary destructive techniques have been effective in reducing the IOP in some cases, presumably by reducing the rate of aqueous formation.

The following case illustrates a typical course of ghost-cell glaucoma from contusion of the eye.

Case 45-1

A middle-aged man was struck in one eye by a block of wood, causing a small conjunctival laceration, moderate hyphema, and IOP below normal. Surgical exploration of the outer surface of the globe showed no rupture. In a few days, the hyphema spontaneously cleared from the anterior chamber. Gonioscopy showed contusion-disruption of angle structures superiorly, and the anterior chamber was abnormally deep superiorly, with a slight posterior subluxation of the upper portion of the lens. The pupil was not appreciably distorted and the lens was clear, but there was no fundus reflex due to extensive hemorrhage into the vitreous cavity. In about 2 weeks, the IOP became normal. In 3 weeks, the IOP was in the 60s with diffuse corneal edema, pain, and myriad fine cells in the anterior chamber, but no KPs. Although the eye did not appear inflamed, the cells were misinterpreted as a sign of "iritis," and anti-inflammatory treatment was started with atropine and frequent application of corticosteroid. Oral glycerin produced only transient reduction of IOP. After 2 or 3 days with fundamentally no change, the patient was seen by one of us. A presumptive diagnosis of ghost-cell glaucoma was made, and diagnostic aspiration of aqueous humor and therapeutic washing out of the anterior chamber were done. Phase-contrast microscopy of the aqueous humor immediately after removal from the anterior chamber showed innumerable ghost cells but no inflammatory cells or macrophages. For a day or two, IOP was normal, but soon more ghost cells leaked from the reservoir in the vitreous cavity to the anterior chamber, presumably through a defect in the anterior hyaloid membrane produced when the lens was subluxated, and the IOP increased again.

In contemplating the pathogenesis of various types of glaucoma and the mechanism by which they respond to various treatments and in thinking about how to evolve better treatments, it is interesting to consider that, both in ghost-cell glaucoma and in lens-induced glaucoma, there is a good clinical response to washing out the anterior chamber, provided that there is no reservoir of ghost cells or lens material to replenish what was washed out.[10] Usually in the following days, the IOP is normal, suggesting that the aqueous outflow system has become cleared of the obstructing material. Yet, when the conditions are reproduced experimentally in an excised human eye by introducing ghost cells or lens proteins[11] into the anterior chamber, clearly obstructing outflow of aqueous fluid from the anterior chamber, we find no immediate relief of the obstruction when we washout the anterior chamber. Therefore, in vivo, there must be some vital aid to clearing the outflow channels after the bulk of the material has been removed from the anterior chamber. Corticosteroids may interfere with these trabecular cellular processes. We wonder if macrophages are helping to clear the outflow system and whether there could be some advantage in stimulating their activity. Other therapeutic approaches might conceivably include use of enzymes to break down ghost cells or lens proteins to fragments that might more easily pass through the aqueous outflow system and obstruct it less.

HEMOSIDEROTIC GLAUCOMA

The discussion in this chapter has been limited to the acute problems posed by erythrocyte ghost cells; we have not considered the late consequence of leaving blood degenerating in the eye for a long time that may lead to a different condition called *hemosiderotic glaucoma*, which is usually diagnosed histologically after enucleation of a blind eye. That condition is characterized by degeneration of the TM with positive staining for iron.[12,13]

REFERENCES

1. Fenton RH, Zimmerman LE. Hemolytic glaucoma. *Arch Ophthalmol.* 1963;70:236-239.
2. Campbell DG, Simmons RJ, Grant WM. Ghost cells as a cause of glaucoma. *Am J Ophthalmol.* 1976;81:441-450.
3. Campbell DG, Essigmann EM. Hemolytic ghost cell glaucoma. Further studies. *Arch Ophthalmol.* 1979;97:2141-2146.
4. Campbell DG. Ghost cell glaucoma following trauma. *Ophthalmology.* 1981;88:1151-1158.
5. Lambrou FH Jr, Aiken DG, Woods WD, Campbell DG. The production and mechanism of ghost cell glaucoma in the cat and primate. *Invest Ophthalmol Vis Sci.* 1985;26:893-897.
6. Mansour AM, Chess J, Starita R. Nontraumatic ghost cell glaucoma—a case report. *Ophthalmic Surg.* 1986;17:34-36.
7. Frazer DG, Kidd MN, Johnston PB. Ghost cell glaucoma in phakic eyes. *Int Ophthalmol.* 1987;11:51-54.
8. Campbell DG, Simmons RJ, Tolentino FI, et al. Glaucoma occurring after closed vitrectomy. *Am J Ophthalmol.* 1977;83:63-69.
9. Wilensky JT, Goldberg MF, Alward P. Glaucoma after pars plana vitrectomy. *Trans Am Acad Ophthalmol Otolaryngol.* 1977;83:114-121.
10. Phelps CD, Watzke RC. Hemolytic glaucoma. *Am J Ophthalmol.* 1975;80:690-695.
11. Epstein DL, Jedziniak JA, Grant WM. Obstruction of aqueous outflow by lens particles and by heavy molecular weight soluble lens protein. *Invest Ophthalmol Vis Sci.* 1978;17:272-277.
12. Benson WE, Spaiter HF. Vitreous hemorrhage. *Surv Ophthalmol.* 1975;15:297-311.
13. Wollensak J. Phakolytisches und Hamolytisches Glaukom. *Klin Monatsbl Augenheilkd.* 1976;168:447-452.

Glaucoma Associated With Extraocular Venous Congestion (Increased Episcleral Venous Pressure)

Ian P. Conner, MD, PhD; Joel S. Schuman, MD, FACS; and David L. Epstein, MD, MMM

Increased episcleral venous pressure may be seen in the following clinical situations:

- Carotid-cavernous sinus fistulas and dural shunts
- Sturge-Weber syndrome
- An idiopathic type[1-5]

Glaucoma due to increased episcleral venous pressure is actually not uncommon. It is routine for clinicians to focus on the slit-lamp examination of the cornea, anterior chamber, or posterior segment and to perhaps overlook the presence of abnormally prominent episcleral veins. Routinely evaluating eyes with a penlight (see Chapter 5) can greatly assist in making the diagnosis in these red-eye glaucomas. Both the idiopathic type and that due to a subclinical dural shunt are underdiagnosed.

When an antiglaucoma therapy does not decrease the intraocular pressure (IOP), in addition to repeating gonioscopy, it is important to carefully re-examine the episcleral vessels. Recall that the IOP cannot be lowered below the episcleral venous pressure (see Chapter 3) without surgically bypassing the trabecular outflow system; therefore, the IOP remains elevated after initiation of medical therapy in this condition.

Anytime blood in Schlemm's canal is observed spontaneously in an eye with elevated IOP, elevated episcleral venous pressure should also be entertained. Imagine the case with an overfiltering bleb and associated hypotony—it is not uncommon to observe blood reflux into Schlemm's canal in this circumstance. This occurs because the episcleral venous pressure is higher than the IOP.

In many instances of elevated episcleral venous pressure, especially the idiopathic and Sturge-Weber types, fistulizing surgery is often performed because of the persistent elevation of IOP despite maximal tolerated medical therapy. The increased episcleral venous pressure causing the elevated IOP via the anterior segment is an indicator of an increase in orbital venous pressure. Thus, when such eyes are decompressed through the usual limbal incision for the filtration fistula, the transmitted elevation in choroidal venous pressure may result in transudation of fluid into the suprachoroidal space,[2] which then forces intraocular contents forward through the fistula. Prophylactic posterior sclerotomies performed before entry into the anterior chamber can diminish the severity of this occurrence and also the postoperative sequelae.[2] Smaller incision/excision trabeculectomy techniques with use of anterior chamber viscoelastics or maintainers should also be used.

INCREASED ORBITAL VENOUS PRESSURE

Increasing the venous pressure in the head and orbit causes the IOP to increase. Some of the pathophysiology of this relationship has been studied experimentally by Comberg and Pilz.[6] Clinically, the causes of elevation of venous pressure that are of particular significance to the eye include carotid-cavernous sinus fistula, thrombosis of orbital veins or cavernous sinus, dural arteriovenous shunts, endocrine exophthalmos,[7] pulmonary venous obstruction

Kahook MY, Schuman JS, eds.
Chandler and Grant's Glaucoma, Fifth Edition (pp 435-439).

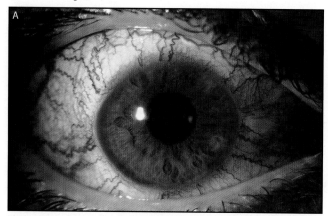
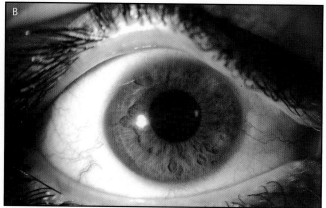

Figure 46-1. (A) Prominent episcleral veins, increased episcleral venous pressure, and glaucoma due to dural shunt. (B) The same eye appears normal with resolution of IOP elevation 4 weeks after neurosurgical closure of the shunt.

by tumors or cardiopulmonary disease, and obstruction of the superior vena cava. Congestive heart failure causes only a slight increase in IOP.[8]

The venous abnormalities of the head and orbit are often unilateral and affect only one eye, whereas compression of veins in the neck or chest usually affects both eyes. There are other conditions in which both the extraocular venous pressure and the IOP are elevated, but their exact mechanism for this elevation of venous pressure is as yet unclear. This includes certain cases of hemangioma with glaucoma (Sturge-Weber syndrome) and the particular combination of conspicuously dilated episcleral vessels with open-angle glaucoma, but without other demonstrated extraocular vasculopathy (that we have termed *idiopathic*) (Figure 46-1).

Signs and Symptoms

The signs and symptoms of thrombosis of orbital veins or arteriovenous fistula may have rapid onset, sometimes with pain on the same side of the head.[9] The episcleral veins appear dilated on the affected side. Chemosis and exophthalmos may develop within hours or days. The exophthalmos may be pulsating, and an orbital bruit may be appreciated if an arteriovenous fistula is present. The retinal veins may appear dilated on the same side. The IOP becomes elevated, most commonly to the mid-20s to mid-30s (mm Hg), and the ocular pulse is increased. These changes are most pronounced in cases of arteriovenous communication. If pressure is measured in the episcleral or orbital veins, the increase of IOP is about the same as the increase of venous pressure above its ordinary baseline of approximately 8 to 10 mm Hg.

A rare complication of elevated orbital venous pressure is shallowing of the anterior chamber on the affected side[10-12]; angle-closure glaucoma may result. The shallowing is attributable to increased venous volume leading to effusion in the posterior segment, in some cases visible as choroidal detachment.[10,11]

In rare cases of carotid-cavernous sinus fistula, not only may there be elevated orbital venous pressure, but the arterial blood supply to the eye may be partially obstructed and the rate of aqueous formation may be reduced. Then, the IOP may remain low despite elevated venous pressure. In rare instances, anterior segment ischemic necrosis has occurred under these circumstances.[13,14] The danger appears to be greatest when the arteriovenous fistula has been treated by occluding the feeding artery.

A further complication in cases of long-standing elevated venous pressure and reduced arterial supply is growth of new blood vessels on the iris and in the angle, leading potentially to neovascular glaucoma.[12,15]

In dural shunts (Figure 46-1A),[16] which are lower-pressure arteriovenous shunts than the carotid-cavernous fistula described previously, the signs and symptoms may be much more subtle. Patients may actually be unaware of their red eye. This is also true in the idiopathic variety of increased episcleral venous pressure. Also, many patients with Sturge-Weber syndrome, although fully aware of their facial hemangioma, do not appreciate well the episcleral involvement, which, as will be discussed, may not become prominent until the teenage years.

In most cases of elevated orbital venous pressure with secondary modest elevation of IOP, the angle remains open, and in most cases, the tonographic facility of outflow remains normal. In these cases, if the orbital venous pressure subsequently becomes normal, either spontaneously or as a result of treatment, the IOP returns to normal. However, when the facility of outflow is abnormal (as it often is in long-standing cases of increased episcleral venous pressure), glaucoma may persist even after venous pressure is normalized as though permanent damage has been done to the aqueous outflow system by the chronic elevation of episcleral venous pressure.[17] In cases of neovascularization and synechial closure of the angle, this persistent glaucoma is understandable, but the outflow system of eyes with open angles may also be affected as postulated by Weekers and Grieten.[18] This is a consideration that seems to us to deserve more study: Why would chronic elevation of episcleral venous pressure cause permanent trabecular meshwork (TM) dysfunction?

IDIOPATHIC ELEVATION OF EPISCLERAL VENOUS PRESSURE

To this point, we have mainly discussed elevations of IOP that are apparently secondary to abnormally high extraocular venous pressure and that can usually be relieved if the venous pressure can be reduced. There is another group of unusual cases[1-5,19] in which there is no recognized cause outside of the eye for elevation of venous pressure; these are thus termed *idiopathic cases*, but vessels on the globe are conspicuously large, and measurement shows the pressure in these vessels to be elevated to more than 30 mm Hg in some cases. Patients who have primary open-angle glaucoma have normal episcleral venous pressure.

This idiopathic variety of increased episcleral venous pressure is fascinating but poorly understood. It is likely underdiagnosed and needs to be considered in the differential diagnosis of refractory cases of open-angle glaucoma, as the external manifestations can be rather subtle. This condition can be either unilateral or bilateral. As this is a diagnosis of exclusion, these patients have intracranial imaging with no observed abnormality. Presumably, this condition must then be caused by some orbital[4] or periocular venous abnormality with increased pressure transmitted to both the episcleral and choroidal veins. Therefore, prophylactic posterior sclerotomies,[2] smaller incision/excision trabeculectomies, and anterior chamber viscoelastics or maintainers should be strongly considered at the time of fistulizing surgery in such patients, as in other glaucoma patients with elevated venous pressure.

STURGE-WEBER SYNDROME

A similar set of conditions can be found unilaterally or occasionally bilaterally in cases of hemangioma (Sturge-Weber syndrome) with open-angle glaucoma.[20-23] Patients with Sturge-Weber syndrome and glaucoma fall into 1 of the following 2 categories:

1. Those with congenital mesodermal angle abnormalities

2. Those with elevated episcleral (and orbital) venous pressure presumably due to the presence of orbital and periocular hemangiomas

In the first category, the onset of glaucoma is typically early in life with frequent buphthalmos, anisometropia with amblyopia, and advanced disc cupping when first detected. These patients are usually quite refractory to medical glaucoma therapy. Sometimes, the angle abnormality[24-26] may be accompanied (perhaps later in life) by the presence of dilated episcleral vessels with increased venous pressure.

AQUEOUS HUMOR DYNAMICS: A TRICK QUESTION
David L. Epstein, MD, MMM

A frequent trick question given to ophthalmology residents and students is, What is the tonographic outflow facility in a patient with elevated IOP due to increased episcleral venous pressure? There is a natural tendency to answer that outflow facility is abnormal because, obviously, the IOP is elevated. This is incorrect. Tonographic outflow facility, at least early in the disease process, can be, and is usually, normal despite the elevated IOP.

Consider the following: With a normal IOP of 16 mm Hg, there is a resistance decrease across the TM (the inverse of which is mathematically termed the outflow facility or C value) to the downstream collector channel (episcleral venous) pressure of 8 mm Hg. Assume that episcleral venous pressure is now suddenly elevated an additional 10 mm Hg to a value of 18, then the IOP would also increase 10 mm Hg to 26 mm Hg, even though the resistance across the TM is unchanged (ie, the C value remains normal).

We have studied this phenomenon in preliminary research using ophthalmic resident volunteers who, in performing a Valsalva maneuver, raised both measured episcleral venous pressure and IOP similarly millimeter for millimeter. For some residents, despite facial congestion during the attempted Valsalva maneuver, their episcleral venous pressure and IOP did not increase at all, whereas others did as described.

For completeness sake, the concept of pseudofacility[1] will also be described. In normal patients who had a blood pressure cuff placed around their neck and inflated, episcleral venous pressure became elevated but IOP increased to a slightly smaller degree. IOP usually increased within 1 mm Hg of the induced episcleral venous pressure elevation. This small difference between episcleral venous and IOP elevation was termed *pseudofacility* and indicated what was believed to be an induced decrease in aqueous humor formation in response to this elevation of eye pressure. The effect is small, and the overall phenomenon actually indicated that aqueous humor formation does not, in fact, self-regulate in response to the level of IOP. There are also no known feedback loops or anatomical connections that could allow such a regulatory process (other than a direct pressure effect on the fluid-secreting cells in the ciliary body).

REFERENCE
1. Kupfer C. Clinical significance of pseudofacility. Sanford R. Gifford Memorial Lecture. *Am J Ophthalmol.* 1973;75:193-204.

In the second category, there is no buphthalmos, etc, and, in fact, there is often a history of onset of a red eye and accompanying glaucoma in the teenage years, sometimes at menarche. If examined at that time, there is often high IOP but only early disc cupping, implying a later onset to the glaucoma (and perhaps also the episcleral venous prominence), as if something new were happening hemodynamically in the teenage years. Regardless, the glaucoma associated with Sturge-Weber syndrome, once observed, is commonly characterized by persisting high IOP, requiring filtration surgery.

TREATMENT

Standard medical antiglaucoma therapy is used first, especially the aqueous humor suppressants, which by their action can reduce the IOP downward toward the level of the (elevated) episcleral venous pressure. When the IOP is still high enough to damage the optic disc and visual field despite maximal tolerated medical treatment, surgery becomes necessary. Tonography in these long-standing cases, whether due to dural shunt, Sturge-Weber syndrome, or the idiopathic variety, shows subnormal facility of aqueous outflow, and accordingly there is little expectation that the glaucoma would be cured by reducing the venous pressure at this stage of the disease, even if it were possible to do it. Laser trabeculoplasty should be attempted and occasionally can be surprisingly effective when there is subnormal outflow facility. However, fistulizing surgery is required most commonly.

Fistulizing Surgery

A major complication of intraocular surgery in these cases is a tendency for the lens-iris diaphragm and ciliary body to push forward and flatten the anterior chamber when the anterior chamber is opened. In the postoperative period, there is a tendency for large choroidal detachments[2,24,27,28] to persist with an associated shallow or flat anterior chamber.

Prophylactic Posterior Sclerotomy

In patients who have had open-angle glaucoma and elevated episcleral venous pressure, and in certain patients with hemangioma and glaucoma, effusion of suprachoroidal fluid can begin during the fistulizing surgery itself, presumably in response to rapid reduction of IOP when the anterior chamber is opened.[2] The episcleral and vortex veins drain separate areas of the globe. However, we believe that the elevated episcleral venous pressure that we measure identifies an abnormal elevation of venous pressure that affects both the episcleral and choroidal venous system in these patients. The effusion can thus create pushing forward of the lens, ciliary processes, and iris. The risk of intraoperative anterior chamber shallowing can be reduced by initially performing posterior sclerotomies before entering the eye. This is done by making an incision through the sclera to the potential suprachoroidal space so that uveal effusion fluid can drain from the globe as it forms, rather than cause the anterior chamber to flatten.[2] This also appears to reduce the extent of postoperative choroidal detachment.

There does remain some controversy regarding the value of this maneuver,[29] and overall it is not routinely performed, but still it may provide some value in reducing the complications of surgery in eyes with abnormally high episcleral venous pressure.

OTHER BASIC ASPECTS

Aside from these practical clinical points, there are some intriguing basic aspects that deserve further thought and investigation. Measurements by DLE have shown that reducing the IOP by filtering surgery in the syndrome of open-angle glaucoma associated with elevated episcleral venous pressure does not change the episcleral venous pressure, and we therefore conclude that the pressure in these vessels must be determined by something other than the rate of outflow of aqueous humor. After successful filtration surgery, the aqueous humor is no longer constrained by the regular outflow system to enter the episcleral veins against venous back-pressure, but it is free to bypass this system and escape into the extravascular tissue at low IOPs.

One final intriguing aspect of the open-angle glaucoma associated with idiopathic elevated episcleral venous pressure is that in some cases no blood has been seen gonioscopically in Schlemm's canal either before or after surgery, despite the fact that the filtration operations have made the IOP considerably lower than the pressure in the episcleral veins on the surface of the globe. This suggests obstruction may occur within or beyond Schlemm's canal. This phenomenon may also be involved in the pathogenesis of the reduced aqueous humor outflow, which is commonly seen with chronic elevation of episcleral venous pressure.

REFERENCES

1. Radius RL, Maumenee AE. Dilated episcleral vessels and open-angle glaucoma. *Am J Ophthalmol.* 1978;86:31-35.
2. Bellows AR, Chylack LT, Epstein DL, et al. Intraoperative choroidal effusion during glaucoma surgery in patients with elevated episcleral venous pressure. *Arch Ophthalmol.* 1979;97:493-497.
3. Talusan ED, Fishbein SL, Schwartz B. Increased pressure of dilated episcleral veins with open-angle glaucoma. *Ophthalmology.* 1983;90:257-265.
4. de Keizer RJ. Secondary vascular glaucoma. *Doc Ophthalmol.* 1983;56:195-202.
5. Jorgensen JS, Guthoff R. The role of episcleral venous pressure in the development of secondary glaucomas [in German]. *Klin Monatsbl Augenheilkd.* 1988;193:471-475.
6. Comberg D, Pilz A. Der Augendruck als Funktion des Venendruckes. *Ber Dtsch Ophthalmol Ges.* 1961;63:332-336.
7. Aron-Rosa D, Morax PV, Aron JJ, et al. Exopthalmie oedemateuses endocriniennes et blocage circulatoire veineux orbitaire. Interet cles phlebographies. *Ann Ocul (Paris).* 1970;203:1-24.
8. Bettelheim H. Der episklerale Venendruck bei pulmonaler Hypertension. Ein Beitrag zur Frage des kardiogenen Glaukoms. *Graefes Arch Klin Exp Ophthalmol.* 1969;177:108-115.
9. Aron-Rosa D, Offret G, Ramee A, et al. La phlebographie orbitaire. *Bull Soc Ophthalmol Fr Numero Special.* 1967:1-36.
10. Blervacque A, Voillez M, Dufour D, et al. Role des troubles circulatoires orbito-caverneux dans la genese du soulevement retino-choroidien ante-rieur. *Bull Soc Ophthalmol Fr.* 1968;68:1056-1058.

11. Guerry D III, Harbison JW, Wiesinger H. Bilateral choroidal detachment and fluctuating proptosis secondary to bilateral dural arteriovenous fistula treated with transcranial orbital decompression with resolution: report of a case. *Trans Am Ophthalmol Soc.* 1975;73:64-73.

12. Fiore PM, Latina MA, Shingleton BJ, et al. The dural shunt syndrome. I. Management of glaucoma. *Ophthalmology.* 1990; 97:56-62.

13. Sanders MD, Hoyt WF. Hypoxic ocular sequelae of carotid-cavernous fistulae. *Br J Ophthalmol.* 1969;53:82-97.

14. Spencer WH, Thompson HS, Hoyt WF. Ischaemic ocular necrosis from carotid-cavernous fistula. *Br J Ophthalmol.* 1973;57:145-152.

15. Weiss DI, Shaffer RN, Nehrenberg TR. Neovascular glaucoma complicating carotid-cavernous fistula. *Arch Ophthalmol.* 1963;69:304-307.

16. Grove AS Jr. The dural shunt syndrome. Pathophysiology and clinical course. *Ophthalmology.* 1984;91:31-44.

17. Nordmann J, Lobstein A, Gerhard JP, et al. A propos cle 14 cas de glaucoma par hypertension veinuse d'origine extraoculaire. *Ophthalmology.* 1961;142(suppl):501-505.

18. Weekers R, Grieten J. Pathogenie et traitement de l'hypertension ocu-laire dans l'exophalmie par an.evrisme arterio-veineux. *Arch Ophtalmol (Pans).* 1965;25:531-536.

19. Rhee DJ, Gupta M, Moncavage MB, Moster ML, Moster MR. Idiopathic elevated episcleral venous pressure and open-angle glaucoma. *Br J Ophthalmol.* 2009;93(2):231-234.

20. Bessiere E, Verin P. Le tonogramme vasculaire. *Arch Ophthalmol (Paris).* 1965;25:449-458.

21. Phelps CD. The pathogenesis of glaucoma in Sturge-Weber syndrome. *Ophthalmology.* 1978;85:276-286.

22. Phelps CD, Thompson HS, Ossoinig KC. The diagnosis and prognosis of atypical carotid-cavernous fistula (red-eyed shunt syndrome). *Am J Ophthalmol.* 1982;93:423-436.

23. Jorgensen JS, Guthoff R. Sturge-Weber syndrome: glaucoma with elevated episcleral venous pressure [in German]. *Klin Monatsbl Augenheilkd.* 1987;191:275-278.

24. Christensen GR, Records RE. Glaucoma and expulsive hemorrhage mechanisms in the Sturge-Weber syndrome. *Ophthalmology.* 1979;86:1360-1366.

25. Cibis GW, Tripathi RC, Tripathi BJ. Glaucoma in Sturge-Weber syndrome. *Ophthalmology.* 1984;91:1061-1071.

26. Mwinula JH, Sagawa T, Tawara A, et al. Anterior chamber angle vascularization in Sturge-Weber syndrome. Report of a case. *Graefes Arch Clin Exp Ophthalmol.* 1994;232:387-391.

27. Iwach AG, Hoskins HD Jr, Hetherington J Jr, et al. Analysis of surgical and medical management of glaucoma in Sturge-Weber syndrome. *Ophthalmology.* 1990;97:904-909.

28. Bellows AR, Chylack LT Jr, Hutchinson BT. Choroidal detachment. Clinical manifestation, therapy and mechanism of formation. *Ophthalmology.* 1981;88:1107-1115.

29. Eibschitz-Tsimhoni M, Lichter PR, Del Monte MA, et al. Assessing the need for posterior sclerotomy at the time of filtering surgery in patients with Sturge-Weber syndrome. *Ophthalmology.* 2003;110(7):1361-1363.

47

Lens-Induced Glaucoma

Ian P. Conner, MD, PhD; Joel S. Schuman, MD, FACS; and David L. Epstein, MD, MMM

We use the term *lens-induced* glaucoma for the secondary open-angle glaucoma associated with leakage of lens proteins into the eye, from lens particles directly affecting the function of the trabecular meshwork (TM), or from phacoantigenic inflammation. Prior laboratory investigations have given insight into underlying mechanisms and offer a framework for understanding and classification.

PHACOLYTIC GLAUCOMA

History

The term *phacolytic* glaucoma was first proposed by Flocks and colleagues[1] as a type of secondary open-angle glaucoma of rapid onset associated with a leaking hypermature cataract. Subsequently, others have occasionally misused the term phacolytic as though it applied to all types of lens-induced glaucomas. Flocks and colleagues[1] believed that phacolytic glaucoma was attributable to obstruction of the intertrabecular spaces by macrophages distended with engulfed lens material and Morgagnian fluid that had escaped from the intact crystalline lens. Goldberg[2] popularized Millipore filtration for diagnostic identification of the macrophages in this condition but also suspected that the glaucoma was caused by blockage of the angle by both proteinaceous debris and macrophages. In recent years, the supposed role of macrophages in producing the glaucoma has been emphasized, and the possible obstruction of the TM by liberated lens material has been mentioned infrequently.

Mechanisms for the Glaucoma

Our laboratory investigations indicate that soluble lens proteins that leak from hypermature cataracts cause severe obstruction of aqueous outflow and that this is likely important in the pathogenesis of phacolytic glaucoma.[3]

In these experiments, heavy-molecular-weight lens protein, infused into the anterior chamber of enucleated human eyes in amounts similar to those found clinically in the aqueous humor of patients with phacolytic glaucoma, produced a severe obstruction of fluid outflow that increased with the length of the perfusion time. This obstruction was not relieved by simple irrigation of the anterior chamber, suggesting that dynamic mechanisms, perhaps involving macrophages, may be required in vivo to relieve such an obstruction.

Other experiments indicated that the aqueous outflow channels were also easily obstructed by particulate lens material. It was not determined what proportion of the lens particle obstruction was attributable to insoluble lens protein and what proportion to cell membrane fragments. This lens-particle glaucoma seems likely to be the predominant mechanism in early postoperative glaucoma due to retained lens cortex and to be less often involved in spontaneous phacolytic glaucoma. In some cases of phacolytic glaucoma, however, a hypermature lens may rupture either spontaneously or during surgery, and in such cases, glaucoma of acute onset may be due to a combination of both obstructing lens particles and soluble lens proteins.

Analogous to interference with outflow by lens proteins, we found that obstruction of outflow by serum proteins may be an important factor in open-angle glaucoma associated with uveitis.[4] In related experiments, infusion of human serum into enucleated human eyes produced a significant decrease in facility of outflow that likewise was not relieved by simple irrigation of the anterior chamber. Diluted serum caused greater obstruction upon perfusion than would be expected on the basis of viscosity alone. Lens depression, induced experimentally to mechanically simulate ciliary muscle contraction, improved the facility of outflow but did not alleviate the partial obstruction induced by serum. It is possible that normal serum components may become entrapped in the outflow channels and produce glaucoma.

Kahook MY, Schuman JS, eds.
Chandler and Grant's Glaucoma, Fifth Edition (pp 441-447).
© 2013 SLACK Incorporated.

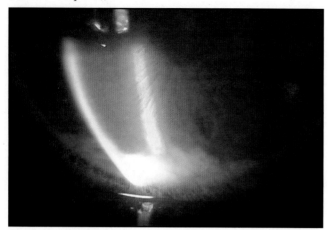

Figure 47-1. Leaking hypermature cataract with pseudohypopyon layering in the anterior chamber angle. (Reprinted with permission from Amina Malik, MD.)

Such serum obstruction may be a factor in glaucoma refractory to corticosteroid therapy in eyes with chronic uveitis (see Chapter 42), especially when there is little cellular reaction but persistent flare.

In phacolytic glaucoma, the role of macrophages is unclear, but they may be present simply as scavengers of lens material in the anterior chamber, clearing lens protein from the outflow pathways. In children, macrophages have been observed in the anterior chamber in the presence of lens material without causing elevation of IOP. Yanoff and Scheie[5] in particular described typical engorged macrophages, although perhaps fewer than in phacolytic glaucoma, in the anterior chamber fluid of children at the time of surgery for secondary cataracts, without evidence of glaucoma. Interestingly, D. K. Dueker (personal communication, 1977) has placed large numbers of rabbit macrophages, which have engulfed oil in the peritoneum, into the anterior chamber of rabbits and failed to observe any significant elevation of intraocular pressure (IOP).

Clinical Findings

In phacolytic glaucoma, there is typically rapid onset of pain and redness in the eye. IOP may become extremely high, even greater than 80 mm Hg in some cases. Corneal epithelial edema is usually present. The angle remains open and without visible abnormality. The lens usually shows hypermature or mature cataract, or rarely an immature cataract in which there is liquefaction of the posterior cortex. When seen with immature cataract, the glaucoma tends to be less acute in onset and not associated with such high IOP at presentation. Patches of white material, thought to be clusters of macrophages, may be seen on the anterior surface of the crystalline lens. In rare cases, the cataractous lens is dislocated into the vitreous cavity, either spontaneously or as a result of trauma.

Inflammatory precipitates, such as scattered cells or conglomerate keratic precipitates (KPs), may or may not be present on the corneal endothelium. Rarely in this condition have we seen what looked like KP in the anterior chamber angle. Cellular reaction in the anterior chamber can vary from mild to the appearance of a pseudohypopyon (Figure 47-1).[6] Usually, one sees circulating white particles that are significantly larger than white blood cells and that have been variously interpreted as very large cells[7,8] (presumably swollen macrophages), cellular aggregates, or small particles of lens material (likely aggregated insoluble lens protein).

Treatment

The eye in phacolytic glaucoma is typically recalcitrant to medical antiglaucoma and anti-inflammatory therapy. The IOP may be reduced considerably, but only temporarily, with beta-blockers, brimonidine, carbonic anhydrase inhibitors, and osmotic agents; usually the IOP rebounds and remains too high for adequate medical management. As a rule, patients with presumed phacolytic glaucoma will require cataract surgery for definitive treatment. This may be indicated emergently if the IOP does not respond from a dangerously high level in response to the initial medical treatment. The IOP usually returns to normal within a few days after cataract surgery.

Possible Laboratory Studies

Microscopic examination of anterior chamber fluid usually reveals engorged macrophages.[7,8] They are not often numerous and their number does not correlate with the severity of the glaucoma. Occasionally, there are no macrophages in the aspirated fluid, but in almost all cases, there is fine amorphous material in the anterior chamber fluid. Biochemical studies have identified heavy-molecular-weight lens protein in aqueous humor from all cases of phacolytic glaucoma so far examined for this material.[9]

The heavy-molecular-weight lens protein is not present in the aqueous humor of nonglaucomatous patients with ordinary cataracts or in patients with cataract and primary open-angle glaucoma. Biochemical analysis of anterior chamber fluid is potentially useful in the clinical diagnosis of phacolytic glaucoma. It is considered accepted practice in suspected cases to aspirate the aqueous humor and to obtain washings of the anterior chamber for microscopic search for macrophages and lens proteins (polymerase chain reaction [PCR] analysis for viral agents, eg, herpes simplex virus [HSV], varicella-zoster virus [VZV], and cytomegalovirus [CMV], is usually also performed if aqueous is aspirated). However, one can usually arrive at the correct diagnosis on purely clinical grounds.

Calcium oxalate crystals have also been found in the aqueous humor of certain patients with phacolytic glaucoma,[10] presumably liberated from the lens itself.

Understanding Lens-Induced Glaucomas

Ian P. Conner, MD, PhD and David L. Epstein, MD, MMM

A simple way to view these lens-induced glaucomas is to conceptualize that, with the exception of phacoantigenic glaucoma (previously termed *phacoanaphylaxis*), these entities exist as mechanical glaucomas that are due to the direct obstructive properties[1] of lens proteins in the case of a leaking but essentially intact crystalline lens or lens particles in the case of a grossly disrupted lens (free lens cortical material)—hence, the terms *lens protein glaucoma* (phacolytic) and *lens particle glaucoma*. In the former, it is the viscous heavy-molecular-weight lens proteins[2] present in advanced cataracts that leak into the anterior chamber that obstruct the TM, and in the latter the fragments of gross crystalline lens material.[1] The inflammatory macrophage-type cellular response is not itself viewed as impairing trabecular outflow and may actually help in clearing the liberated lens material from the outflow pathway. In fact, the presence of macrophages likely represents part of the spectrum of presentation of phacolytic glaucoma and is not truly necessary for the occurrence or diagnosis of this entity.[3]

With this construct, the treatment is fairly straightforward and consists of removing at least the continuing source of the lens material. In lens particle glaucoma, the free lens material is removed from the anterior chamber, and in lens protein glaucoma where there is a relatively intact cataractous lens, treatment consists of cataract surgery. Common presentations of lens particle glaucoma include postoperative, where fragments of lens material are unintentionally left in the eye, and post-traumatic when the lens capsule is violated. In the past, intracapsular cataract surgery was preferred for phacolytic (lens protein) glaucoma because there was usually a friable lens capsule (through which the lens proteins were leaking), commonly weak zonules, and typically a large, floppy capsular bag. This presented the potential for phacoanaphylaxis or other forms of severe inflammation should lens material containing these aggregated lens proteins be mixed with vitreous due to unexpected vitreous loss. (These heavy-molecular-weight lens proteins are normally concentrated in the crystalline lens nucleus and may be responsible for phacoanaphylaxis and severe complications that ensue when a nucleus is lost into the vitreous and allowed to remain.) However, this practice transitioned to extracapsular cataract surgery after several reports[4,5] with good results in patients with phacolytic glaucoma. In planned extracapsular cataract surgery, an adequately wide incision should be employed, with attention to potentially loose zonules and a friable capsule, with an adequate cortical clean-up. With advances in viscoelastic stabilization of the eye intraoperatively and improvements in phacoemulsification technique and efficiency, it is now usually possible to even avoid the extracapsular technique, although the surgeon should be prepared to convert to deliver the nucleus if phacoemulsification should prove inadequate. Attention should be placed especially on avoiding capsular tears and thus the mixing of the offending lens contents with the vitreous.

References

1. Epstein DL, Jedziniak JA, Grant WM. Obstruction of aqueous outflow by lens particles and by heavy-molecular-weight soluble lens proteins. *Invest Ophthalmol Vis Sci.* 1978;17:272-277.
2. Epstein DL, Jedziniak JA, Grant WM. Identification of heavy molecular weight soluble lens protein in aqueous humor in human phacolytic glaucoma. *Invest Ophthalmol Vis Sci.* 1978;17:398-402.
3. Mavrakanas N, Axmann S, Issum CV, Schutz JS, Shaarawy T. Phacolytic glaucoma: are there 2 forms? *J Glaucoma.* 2012;21(4):248-249.
4. Lane SS, Kopietz LA, Lindquist TD, et al. Treatment of phacolytic glaucoma with extracapsular cataract extraction. *Ophthalmology.* 1988;95:749-753.
5. Singh G, Kaur J, Mall S. Phacolytic glaucoma—its treatment by planned extracapsular cataract extraction with posterior chamber intraocular lens implantation. *Ind J Ophthalmol.* 1994;42:145-147.

Diagnosis

Diagnosis of phacolytic glaucoma can be made based on clinical findings alone, but aqueous sampling can aid significantly in making this diagnosis that should not be missed. If the diagnosis for an inflamed cataractous eye with considerably elevated IOP is in doubt, then the usual medical treatment for glaucoma secondary to inflammation is used: cycloplegics, topical corticosteroids, beta-blockers, brimonidine, carbonic anhydrase inhibitors, and oral osmotic agents if needed. This treatment may bring about a temporary improvement, but if the condition is secondary to phacolysis then we cannot cure it, and the elevated IOP will eventually require cataract surgery for definitive management.

Clinical Examples

The state of the cataract that may induce phacolytic glaucoma varies from case to case. Hypermature cataract in situ is usually responsible, but phacolytic glaucoma can also be caused by an immature cataract. We will discuss the differences in these circumstances.

Hypermature Cataract: Lens In Situ

The onset of glaucoma is usually rapid with IOP reaching very high levels, but occasionally the onset is more gradual. Unilateral severe glaucoma associated with a hypermature cataract with any or all of the signs already discussed is probably due to phacolysis and will not respond to medical measures; thus, treatment should consist of removing the cataract.

In cases associated with hypermature cataract, vision may be poor, light projection may be faulty, and some eyes appear to have no more than light perception. Regardless, cataract surgery should be performed after the IOP has been lowered as much as possible by medical means. In some eyes in which light projection was extremely poor preoperatively, useful vision has been obtained after cataract surgery. In previous decades, many such eyes were unnecessarily removed when the condition could have been completely relieved by cataract surgery. In neglected cases in which the IOP has been allowed to remain high so long that no useful vision is

Completely Dislocated Hypermature Cataract and Glaucoma

Ian P. Conner, MD, PhD; Joel S. Schuman, MD, FACS; and David L. Epstein, MD, MMM

Phacolytic glaucoma may occur after complete posterior dislocation of the lens into the vitreous cavity, either spontaneously or as a result of trauma. The completely dislocated lens may go through the stages of immature, mature, and hypermature cataract formation, just as if it were in the anatomic position. The diagnosis of phacolytic glaucoma in cases of completely posterior dislocation of the lens may not be obvious at first.

The glaucoma may develop acutely with a high IOP or have a more gradual onset. Even if the onset is gradual, the IOP eventually reaches high levels, despite intensive medical treatment. The diagnosis may be suspected because of the absence of any other obvious cause for such severe glaucoma, with the angle of the anterior chamber open. In these cases, one may also find a few cells in the aqueous that do not circulate freely, but only tremble on motion of the eye (this clinical point may reflect the presence of viscous lens proteins in the aqueous humor). The vitreous in these cases is usually almost completely liquefied, but vitreous strands in the posterior segment commonly have exudates present on them. Again, diagnostic paracentesis and examination of the anterior chamber fluid may be performed to help establish the correct diagnosis. If provisions for proper examination of anterior chamber fluid are not readily available, then one should again be able to make the diagnosis on purely clinical grounds. This is a glaucoma out of control despite intensive medical treatment, for which we can find no other cause.

The current standard of care includes vitreoretinal consultation and pars plana removal of such dislocated phacolytic lenses. However, it is interesting to note Chandler's methods of treating this condition before the availability of these techniques. Dr. Chandler writes:

> If the lens floats in the vitreous cavity and is not attached to the retina, the simplest method of removal is to make the usual incision for cataract extraction, do a sector iridectomy and inferior iridotomy, and irrigate the vitreous cavity, directing the stream of fluid toward the posterior pole of the globe as advised by Verhoeff.[1]

> The lens may immediately float up into the wound and be removed without difficulty. If the lens floats about freely during the irrigation, but will not come out, it is because it is attached to the retina by a strand of tissue. It can be removed with forceps, but this is not a wise policy, because in a case treated by Dr. Chandler, a hole was torn in the retina by this maneuver. Fortunately, the hole was treated and closed before the retina became detached. We have seen a safer method employed in a case in which the lens came well forward on irrigation of the vitreous chamber but would not come out. In this case, although the lens was held forward with forceps, the strand of tissue attached to the posterior surface of the lens was cut with scissors and then the lens was removed without further complications.

Reference

1. Verhoeff FH. A simple and safe method for removing a cataract dislocated into fluid vitreous. *Am J Ophthalmol.* 1942;25:725.

regained after cataract removal, the eye at least remains quiet and comfortable after removal of the cataract.

The following case illustrates how poor the vision can be in lens-induced glaucoma associated with a hypermature cataract in situ, yet how much vision can be regained and how strikingly glaucoma can be cured by removal of the cataract.

Case 47-1

A 69-year-old man had an injury to the left eye 28 years previously. He stated that vision in this eye was gone within 6 months after the injury. He had had no trouble with the eye until recently, when it became red and painful. He consulted an ophthalmologist who gave him acetazolamide. When seen by us, the right eye was normal in all respects. The left eye was exotropic, markedly injected with corneal clouding, normal anterior chamber depth, and light projection accurate only temporally. Because of the corneal edema, one could not adequately assess the anterior chamber except for depth. IOP was measured at 45 mm Hg. He was admitted to the hospital at once, and cataract extraction was planned. After the usual limbal incision, when the corneal flap was lifted, it could be seen that the lens had ruptured posteriorly and that only the capsule was present in the pupil. Alpha chymotrypsin was injected for zonulysis, and after 3 minutes, the capsule was removed with forceps. It then could be seen that the vitreous had a milky appearance. The vitreous chamber was irrigated and much of this milky material was washed out. No formed vitreous was seen. The convalescence was fairly stormy, but eventually the eye became quiet with very little vitreous opacity. The disc was found to be normal, corrected vision 20/30, and IOP normal without treatment.

Because the lens had actually ruptured in situ, the glaucoma may have resulted from direct obstruction by both liberated lens particles and soluble lens proteins.

Immature Cataract: Lens In Situ

Phacolytic glaucoma can also occur in exceptional instances in eyes with immature cataract with the vision as good as 20/50. In these extraordinary cases, there is presumably localized liquefaction of the posterior cortex. A diagnosis of phacolytic glaucoma due to immature cataract can be difficult to establish. The question arises: is this actually a case of uveitis with an immature cataract, or are the inflammation and secondary glaucoma attributable to the lens? One cannot be sure at the initial examination. Therefore, the usual treatment for glaucoma secondary to uveitis is instituted, including topical corticosteroids, cycloplegics, beta-blockers, brimonidine, and carbonic anhydrase inhibitors. Then, if in a period of weeks or months, despite vigorous medical treatment, the uveitis and glaucoma gradually worsen and IOP reaches high levels, one is justified in performing cataract surgery with a strong probability that the uveitis and the glaucoma will thereby be relieved. Diagnostic paracentesis before surgery may help establish the correct diagnosis by documenting the presence of typical engorged macrophages or high-molecular-weight lens protein.

Irvine and Irvine[11] describe a case in which the cataract was clinically immature, but pathologic examination of the lens revealed that the posterior cortex was completely liquefied just as in a hypermature cataract. Chandler[12] also published an example of phacolytic glaucoma induced by a clinically immature cataract and relieved by removal of the lens.

Biochemical analysis of the liquefied cortex of hypermature phacolytic lenses has indicated the presence of high levels of heavy-molecular-weight soluble lens protein. Such liquefied lens cortex contains aggregated rather than degraded lens proteins.

GLAUCOMA DUE TO RETAINED LENS CORTEX (LENS PARTICLE GLAUCOMA)

After planned or unplanned extracapsular cataract extraction (with or without phacoemulsification), or after traumatic injury to the lens capsule, a secondary open-angle glaucoma may develop (Figure 47-2). If not much cortical material is present, the usual methods of treatment for uveitis and secondary glaucoma may be employed, such as cycloplegics, corticosteroids, beta-blockers, brimonidine, and carbonic anhydrase inhibitors. This may suffice until the residual cortical material is completely absorbed, after which the inflammation subsides and the IOP falls. However, if by the usual treatment the inflammation is not quickly brought under control, and the IOP remains elevated, one should proceed without delay to remove the residual lens cortex.

If definitive treatment by removal of residual lens cortex is obviously necessary but is delayed too long, serious consequences may result, including persistent glaucoma due to peripheral anterior synechiae secondary to the continued inflammation. A dense inflammatory pupillary membrane may develop and may cause pupillary block. Cystoid macular edema may occur with loss of central vision. The retina may become detached as a result of inflammatory membranes that extend posteriorly and pull on the retina. Finally, there may be permanent edema of the cornea. Likewise, it is not known whether prolonged absorption of lens material, which must occur via the aqueous outflow channels, may result in outflow dysfunction and apparent open-angle glaucoma in later years. It has been postulated that this latter mechanism may play a role in the common occurrence of open-angle glaucoma that can follow pediatric cataract surgery.[13-17]

In view of the seriousness of these late complications, bold measures are justified in attempting to relieve the condition. If the previous cataract operation or injury has been recent,

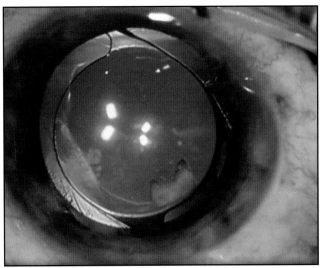

Figure 47-2. Fluffed-up lens cortical material in the anterior chamber that may obstruct the TM (lens particle glaucoma). This photograph was taken intraoperatively when the patient was taken back to the operating room for lens particle removal. The pupil was inadvertently dilated by the operating room staff; in most cases, it is advisable to constrict the pupil before re-entering the anterior chamber in order to minimize the possibility of losing the lens fragment posteriorly.

and there is a great deal of loose cortical material in the anterior chamber, it may easily be irrigated out. If operation is undertaken weeks or months after the onset of the trouble, cortical material may be trapped between membranes, either capsular or inflammatory. Anterior segment microvitrectomy instrumentation is often then useful in removing such residual lens material.

In glaucoma that develops months or years after extracapsular cataract extraction or after injury of the lens, it can be challenging to know which of several possible mechanisms may be most important, including the role of accompanying inflammatory cells. Indeed, the presence of macrophages may be acting to clear obstructing lens material, but may also contribute to the obstruction to aqueous outflow. We do know that severe obstruction can be produced by lens particles and by high-molecular-weight soluble lens proteins in the absence of inflammatory cells and that clinically washing out the anterior chamber or removing retained lens matter can dramatically alleviate the glaucoma, even in these later-onset cases.

We believe that the following case is an example of late lens-induced glaucoma from retained cortex, relieved by washing out the anterior chamber.

Case 47-2

A 53-year-old woman with hand motion vision in the right eye from an old retinal detachment had an unintentional extracapsular cataract extraction in the left eye during planned intracapsular cataract surgery. Convalescence was stormy, but final corrected vision was 20/30. In the upper half of the pupil, there was posterior capsule; the lower half was clear. The disc was normal. She was examined 9 years later, with a history that in recent weeks there had been episodes of profound loss of vision in the left eye. IOP in the left eye was 72 mm Hg, and after a gram of acetazolamide, it was 55 mm Hg. There was epithelial edema. Corrected vision after clearing the cornea with glycerin was 20/100, and to confrontation there was less than a 10-degree field. There were long stringy sheets of vitreous opacities that swirled around freely and obscured fundus details. They did not have the appearance of blood and did not resemble the exudative vitreous opacities that one sees in acute chorioretinitis. On gonioscopy, the view was hazy but the angle seemed wide and open except for focal synechiae. On the capsular membrane in the upper half of the pupil, there were many coarse whitish deposits, somewhat like KP, but irregular in size and shape. There were no deposits on the cornea.

After treatment with acetazolamide, epinephrine, glycerin, and systemic steroids, during 3 days, IOP varied from 17 mm Hg to more than 60 mm Hg. The cornea became clearer and, through the peripheral coloboma above and temporally, one could see a grayish substance that looked like lens material. With a working diagnosis of lens-induced glaucoma, surgery was performed. Through a beveled incision in the inferior cornea, all the aqueous possible was aspirated. Then, with another syringe filled with saline, by alternately depressing the plunger on the syringe and withdrawing it, the aqueous was thoroughly stirred up and, again, the aqueous was aspirated. Finally, the anterior chamber was irrigated with 10 mL of saline solution. During the irrigation, some rather coarse flecks of whitish material could be seen swirling in the anterior chamber. The 2 samples of fluid aspirated from the anterior chamber were examined under a glass slide within an hour by T. Kuwabara. There were isolated cells and sheets of cells that had every appearance of macrophages. All treatment, local and systemic, was discontinued. Postoperatively, the IOP remained 17 mm Hg or less.

One week later, corrected vision was 20/40, and by confrontation only the upper-nasal field was absent. The disc showed glaucomatous cupping. Two weeks later, the vitreous was practically clear except for a few fine stringy opacities; no exudates could be seen on the membrane; there were no cells or flare.

Several years after the irrigation of the anterior chamber, the eye still remained quiet with no cells or KP, the vitreous was clear, and IOP was 17 mm Hg without treatment. This case illustrates the point that the most important treatment goal in the management of lens particle glaucoma is removal of all solid and liquefied lens material from the eye. Modern techniques would include removal of lens material using automated IA or microvitrectomy if vitreous is involved, but the lesson from this case is instructive even today.

Sometimes, in patients with significant amounts of residual cortical material, many years after extracapsular or phacoemulsification cataract surgery, spontaneous liberation of lens particulate material into the anterior chamber may occur associated with elevation of IOP.[17-29] This material was presumably trapped by the IOL in the capsular bag, or more likely hidden in the ciliary sulcus until its translocation into the anterior chamber. This may also represent a form of lens particle glaucoma, although the inflammatory response to such liberated lens material may also be involved. Nevertheless, these cases respond favorably to removal of the liberated lens material.

We need to keep the entity of delayed lens-particle glaucoma in mind as the decades continue to pass for our patients who now have had modern extracapsular or phacoemulsification cataract surgery. Especially when first performed, residual cortical lens material was commonly left behind. This was the usual situation also for open-angle glaucoma eyes on chronic miotic therapy. From the preceding observations, it seems that sometimes with the passage of time the normal sequestration barriers that the eye employs to seal off such crystalline lens material may be subject to break-down, with resulting liberation of lens material into the anterior chamber and outflow pathway. Such lens material could also be immunogenic.[20] These possibilities should be remembered when evaluating patients who have unexplained glaucoma or uveitis many years or decades after extracapsular cataract surgery.

INTRAOCULAR PRESSURE ELEVATION FOLLOWING POSTERIOR CAPSULOTOMY WITH A NEODYMIUM:YTTIRUM-ALUMINUM-GARNET LASER

Within hours after seemingly uneventful posterior capsulotomy with the neodymium:yttrium-aluminum-garnet (Nd:YAG) laser, a dramatic elevation of IOP can occur.[21-23] IOP greater than 60 mm Hg has been observed and may persist for at least 24 to 36 hours. Needless to say, IOP should be carefully monitored after Nd:YAG laser capsulotomy, and significant elevations need to be treated. Most patients should receive at least a single drop of brimonidine at the time of YAG capsulotomy and high-risk patients (eg, those with known glaucoma or impaired trabecular outflow facility) should have closer follow-up. Based on our laboratory studies, we have wondered whether the mechanism in some of these cases involves a form of lens-particle or lens-protein glaucoma due to small fragments of lens material or soluble lens proteins that are liberated into the anterior chamber and pass into the angle[24] after this procedure. Other possibilities include inflammatory[25] or mechanical[26] effects within the eye following Nd:YAG laser energy absorption, or purported vitreous factors.[27]

PHACOANTIGENIC (PREVIOUSLY PHACOANAPHYLACTIC) GLAUCOMA

This rare type of glaucoma can be difficult to definitively diagnose in a living eye. The pathological criteria in enucleated eye specimens that distinguish it from phacolytic glaucoma have been well defined by Zimmerman[28] and by Perlman and Albert.[29] The immunologic response to lens protein involves a latent period or a previous sensitization to lens proteins. Normally, lens proteins are isolated within the lens capsule, and they must first escape before the sensitization process can begin. We suspect that a mixture of lens material and vitreous, which may occur as a result of vitreous loss during cataract extraction or trauma, may favor development of phacoanaphylaxis by retaining and slowly releasing the sensitizing lens proteins. We believe that phacoantigenic reactions (with or without glaucoma) can occur especially when an intact lens nucleus is lost into the vitreous.

The following 2 criteria must be satisfied before accepting a diagnosis of phacoantigenic glaucoma:

1. Polymorphonuclear leukocytes must be present in the aqueous or vitreous specimen

2. The circulating lens protein or particle content of the aqueous humor must be insufficient by itself to explain the glaucoma

The clinical presentation can be variable but usually involves anterior chamber cellular reaction, endothelial and sometimes capsular keratic precipitates, and often anterior vitritis.

From a practical standpoint, if this condition is suspected clinically, it is treated in the same manner as phacolytic glaucoma: by removal of the lens or lens matter.

REFERENCES

1. Flocks M, Littwin CS, Zimmerman LE. Phacolytic glaucoma: clinicopathologic study of 138 cases of glaucoma associated with hypermature cataract. *Arch Ophthalmol.* 1955;54:37-47.

2. Goldberg MF. Cytological diagnosis of phacolytic glaucoma utilizing Millipore filtration of the aqueous. *Br J Ophthalmol.* 1967;51:847-853.

3. Epstein DL, Jedziniak JA, Grant WM. Obstruction of aqueous outflow by lens particles and by heavy-molecular-weight soluble lens proteins. *Invest Ophthalmol Vis Sci.* 1978;17:272-277.

4. Epstein DL, Hashimoto JM, Grant WM. Serum obstruction of aqueous outflow in enucleated human eyes. *Am J Ophthalmol.* 1978;86:101-105.

5. Yanoff M, Scheie HG. Cytology of human lens aspirate. *Arch Ophthalmol.* 1968;80:166-170.

6. Bremond D, Ridings B, Devin F, et al. An uncommon clinical form of phakolytic glaucoma [French]. *Bull Soc Ophtalmol Fr.* 1989;89:853-856.

7. Ueno H, Tamai A, Iyota K, et al. Electron microscopic observation of the cells floating in the anterior chamber in a case of phacolytic glaucoma. *Jpn J Ophthalmol.* 1989;33:103-113.

8. Brooks AM, Grant G, Gillies WE. Comparison of specular microscopy and examination of aspirate in phacolytic glaucoma. *Ophthalmology.* 1990;97:85-89.

9. Epstein DL, Jedziniak JA, Grant WM. Identification of heavy molecular weight soluble lens protein in aqueous humor in human phacolytic glaucoma. *Invest Ophthalmol Vis Sci.* 1978;17:398-402.

10. Bartholomew RS, Rebello PF. Calcium oxalate crystals in the aqueous. *Am J Ophthalmol.* 1979;88:1026-1028.

11. Irvine SR, Irvine AR Jr. Lens-induced uveitis and glaucoma. II the phacotoxic reaction. *Am J Ophthalmol.* 1952;36:370-375.

12. Chandler PA. Problems in the diagnosis and treatment of lens-induced uveitis and glaucoma. *Arch Ophthalmol.* 1958;60:828-841.

13. Phelps CD, Arafat NI. Open-angle glaucoma following surgery for congenital cataracts. *Arch Ophthalmol.* 1977;95:1985-1987.

14. Simon JW, Mehta N, Simmons ST, Catalano RA, Lininger LL. Glaucoma after pediatric lensectomy/vitrectomy. *Ophthalmology.* 1991;98:670-674.

15. Parks MM, Johnson DA, Read GW. Long-term visual results and complications in children with aphakia: a function of cataract type. *Ophthalmology.* 1993;100:826-824.

16. Munoz M, Parrish RK, Murray TG. Open-angle glaucoma after pars plicata lensectomy and vitrectomy for congenital cataracts. *Am J Ophthalmol.* 1995;119:103-104.

17. Epstein DL. Diagnosis and management of lens-induced glaucoma. *Ophthalmology.* 1982;89:227-230.

18. Epstein DL. Lens-induced open-angle glaucoma. In: Ritch R, Shields MB, eds. *The Secondary Glaucomas.* St Louis, MO: CV Mosby Co; 1982:216-223.

19. Barnhorst D, Meyers SM, Myers T. Lens-induced glaucoma 65 years after congenital cataract surgery. *Am J Ophthalmol.* 1994;118:807-808.

20. Rosenbaum JT, Samples JR, Seymour B, Langlois L, David L. Chemotactic activity of lens proteins and the pathogenesis of phacolytic glaucoma. *Arch Ophthalmol.* 1987;105:1582-1584.

21. Terry AC, Stark WJ, Maumenee AE, et al. Neodymium-YAG laser for posterior capsulotomy. *Am J Ophthalmol.* 1983;96:716-720.

22. Channell MM, Beckman H. Intraocular pressure changes after neodymium-YAG laser posterior capsulotomy. *Arch Ophthalmol.* 1984;102:1024-1026.

23. Richter CU, Arzeno G, Pappas HR, et al. Intraocular pressure elevation following Nd:YAG laser posterior capsulotomy. *Ophthalmology.* 1985;92:636-640.

24. Flohr MJ, Robin AL, Kelley JS. Early complications following Q-switched neodymium: YAG laser posterior capsulotomy. *Ophthalmology.* 1985;92:360-363.

25. Lynch MG, Quigley HA, Green WR, Pollack IP, Robin AL. The effect of neodymium: YAG laser capsulotomy on aqueous humor dynamics in the monkey eye. *Ophthalmology.* 1986;93:1270-1275.

26. Aron-Rosa DS. Influence of picosecond and nanosecond YAG laser capsulotomy on intraocular pressure. *J Am Intraocul Implant Soc.* 1985;11:249-252.

27. Schubert HD, Morris WJ, Trokel SL, et al. The role of the vitreous in the intraocular pressure rise after neodymium-YAG laser capsulotomy. *Arch Ophthalmol.* 1985;103:1538-1542.

28. Zimmerman LE. Lens-induced inflammation in human eyes. In: Maumenee AE, Silverstein AM, eds. *Immunopathology of Uveitis.* Baltimore, MD: Williams & Wilkins; 1964.

29. Perlman EM, Albert DM. Clinically unsuspected phacoanaphylaxis after ocular trauma. *Arch Ophthalmol.* 1977;95:244-246.

48

Amyloidosis and Open-Angle Glaucoma

David L. Epstein, MD, MMM

Primary familial amyloidosis is a generalized systemic disease that may involve the eyes in a number of ways. Bilateral, often severe, open-angle glaucoma may develop in the third, fourth, or fifth decade of life, with progressive accumulation of amyloid vitreous opacities. These vitreous opacities may increase to the extent that vision is seriously impaired and the fundus cannot be seen. The opacities can also develop in the absence of glaucoma. Glaucoma in cases reported by Legrand et al,[1] Limon et al,[2] and Tsukahara and Matsuo[3] has been described as similar to pigmentary glaucoma or to open-angle glaucoma associated with exfoliation, in that there was pigment on the back of the cornea, a heavy accumulation of pigment in the trabecular meshwork (TM), and abnormal transillumination of the iris. In all cases, there were amyloid vitreous opacities. Deposition of amyloid fibrils in the TM has been described by Tsukahara and Matsuo[3] and Segawa[4] from electron microscopy of trabeculectomy biopsy specimens. Amyloid in this location may have an important role in the obstruction of aqueous outflow.

In a case of familial amyloidosis reported by Plane et al,[5] clinically, there was pigment in the angle and powdery material assumed to be amyloid in the vitreous and on the front surface of the lens, yet no glaucoma.

In a series of 70 patients older than 40 years of age with lattice corneal dystrophy as a manifestation of amyloid disease, Meretoja[6] diagnosed open-angle glaucoma in 23% but noted no vitreous changes.

In another report,[7] 17% of patients with vitreous amyloidosis (requiring vitrectomy) also required filtration surgery. There is a strong hereditary tendency in familial amyloidosis, and in any family in which there is hereditary glaucoma with pigment dissemination or vitreous opacities, all

members of the family should be examined for amyloidosis and open-angle glaucoma. Similarly, evidence of amyloidosis and open-angle glaucoma should be looked for in patients with lattice corneal dystrophy.[8]

Our experience with primary familial amyloidosis and glaucoma included the following 2 cases.

CASE 48-1

A 55-year-old woman had a strong family history of glaucoma (ie, mother, uncle, and brother). Her brother became blind from glaucoma and was said to have a great cloud of vitreous opacities. When he died, extensive amyloidosis was found at autopsy. She herself had been under treatment for glaucoma for several months, using 4% pilocarpine every 2 hours, epinephrine twice a day, eserine ointment at bedtime, and acetazolamide 250 mg 3 times daily. Despite this treatment, intraocular pressure (IOP) was right and left 52 mm Hg. Vision was right and left 6/9. The angles were wide open with ciliary band visible for 360-degrees. There was light brown pigment on the corneoscleral meshwork throughout, but the band was not as dark or broad as in pigmentary glaucoma. The right disc was almost totally cupped. In the right eye, the lower field was limited on the perimeter, absent entirely on the tangent screen. In the left eye, the cup was wide but within physiologic limits and the field was full.

A trephining was done on the right eye. Acetazolamide was discontinued postoperatively, and within 2 days the IOP in the left eye was 70 mm Hg despite intensive local medication. A trephining was done on the left eye. For several months, IOP ranged from 12 to 15 mm Hg in both eyes, and there appeared to be good functioning blebs, but opacities began to appear in the vitreous. These opacities

Kahook MY, Schuman JS, eds.
Chandler and Grant's Glaucoma, Fifth Edition (pp 449-450).
© 2013 SLACK Incorporated.

were not blood and did not resemble exudative opacities. These gradually increased until the fundi could not be seen. Nine months after operation, IOP was right 24 mm Hg, left 32 mm Hg, and the bleb in each eye, though unchanged in height and extent, now had a whitish opaque appearance. Only at the borders did the blebs appear thin and succulent. At first, IOP could be lowered substantially by digital pressure from below. This was done regularly by the patient. She was given pilocarpine 4% and epinephrine. Two years after the operations, IOP was right and left 27 mm Hg on pilocarpine and epinephrine, and it could not be lowered by digital pressure. An operation was done on both eyes and a thin flap was dissected to the limbus; the whitish tissue was excised, exposing the scleral opening. (The appearance of this whitened but still elevated bleb tissue was so different from the appearance of an ordinary scarred bleb that we assume it was infiltrated by amyloid, but unfortunately histologic studies were not performed on this tissue.)

During the following 9 months, IOP was 12 to 20 mm Hg and could always be lowered by digital pressure. However, within 2 years, there was gradual failure of filtration, and under the care of Richard J. Simmons, MD, the following procedures were done in succession: cyclocryotherapy in the right eye, combined cataract extraction and cyclodialysis on both eyes, another cyclodialysis on both eyes, and then another cyclocryotherapy on both eyes.

After the cataract extraction and cyclodialysis, vision was only counting fingers at a few feet in the better left eye due to vitreous opacities. Later, a vitrectomy was done on the left eye by Robert J. Brockhurst with restoration of good vision in this eye. Examination of the material removed by vitrectomy established that it contained amyloid. When last seen, IOP was right 22 mm Hg, left 11 mm Hg. Corrected vision, left 6/12.

CASE 48-2

A man aged 57, uncle of the patient in the preceding case, was first seen in 1944, with vision right faint hand motions, left counting fingers at 16 feet. IOP right 90 mm Hg, left 58 mm Hg. The anterior chambers were of good depth. In both eyes, there were deep corneal opacities near the limbus nasally and temporally and some near the pupil, but there were no vessels in the cornea. There were also many vitreous opacities, but the fundi could be seen. The right disc was totally cupped and atrophic; the left was similarly cupped but the nasal rim was intact. The left eye on the perimeter showed loss of slightly more than the lower nasal quadrant; on the tangent screen, there was a double Bjerrum scotoma isolating a small central island. With intensive miotic therapy, IOP in the left eye fell to 38 mm Hg. A filtering operation was done on this eye. During the next 7 months, IOP was usually in the mid-to-low 20s but could always be

softened by digital pressure, which the patient did regularly. Then, IOP rose to 35 mm Hg and a cyclodialysis was done. During the following 7 years, IOP was generally 13 to 17 mm Hg. The vitreous opacity gradually increased so that, at the last visit in 1952, fundus details could not be seen. Last vision recorded was 6/60.

The family history of amyloidosis proven in 2 members of this family and the gradual increase in vitreous opacity make it probable that the patient in Case 48-2 also suffered from amyloid disease. The good control of the glaucoma for more than 7 years after filtering operation and cyclodialysis is unusual in this disease. Our experience with these patients confirms the observation of others that intraocular amyloidosis is a very serious disorder.

A relationship between ocular amyloidosis and pseudo-exfoliation syndrome has been described by Meretoja and Tarkkanen,[9] on the basis of histologic evidence, suggesting that the pseudoexfoliation syndrome may be a form of amyloid disease. However, clinically, we have not noted vitreous opacities to be associated with pseudoexfoliation and glaucoma.

A recent report has implicated histopathologically the deposition of a cytoskeletal-modulating protein (gelsolin) product in ocular tissues in the Finnish familial form of systemic amyloidosis (Meretoja's syndrome).[10] The authors suggest that the amyloid deposits in the optic nerve might cause an increase in susceptibility of the optic nerve to cupping.

REFERENCES

1. Legrand J, Guenel J, Dubigeon M. Glaucome et opacification du vitre par amylose. *Bull Soc Ophthalmol Fr.* 1986;68:13-20.

2. Limon S, Rousselie F, Joseph E. A propos d'une observation familiale d'amylose vitréenne héréditaire associée à un glaucoma. *Arch Ophthalmol (Paris).* 1973;33:525-528.

3. Tsukahara S, Matsuo T. Secondary glaucoma accompanied with primary familial amyloidosis. *Ophthalmologica.* 1977;175:250-262.

4. Segawa K. The fine structure of the iridocorneal angle tissue in glaucomatous eyes (5). Glaucoma secondary to primary familial amyloidosis. *Jpn J Clin Ophthalmol.* 1976;30:1375-1380.

5. Plane C, Maupetit J, Colnet G, et al. Manifestations oculaires de l'amy-lose Portugaise de Corino de Andrade. *Bull Soc Ophthalmol Fr.* 1977;77:123-125.

6. Meretoja J. Comparative histological and clinical findings in eyes with lattice corneal dystrophy of two different types. *Ophthalmologica.* 1972;165:15-37.

7. Doft BH, Machemer R, Skinner M, et al. Pars plana vitrectomy for vitreous amyloidosis. *Ophthalmology.* 1987;94:607-611.

8. Starck T, Kenyon KR, Hanninen LA, et al. Clinical and histopathologic studies of two families with lattice corneal dystrophy and familial systemic amyloidosis (Meretoja syndrome). *Ophthalmology.* 1991;98:1197-1206.

9. Meretoja J, Tarkkanen A. Occurrence of amyloid in eyes with exfoliation. *Ophthalmic Res.* 1977;9:80-91.

10. Kivela T, Tarkkanen A, Frangione B, et al. Ocular amyloid deposition in familial amyloidosis, Finnish: an analysis of native and variant gelsolin in Meretoja's syndrome. *Invest Ophthalmol Vis Sci.* 1994;35:3759-3769.

49

Glaucoma in the Phakomatoses

Cynthia Mattox, MD and Priti Batta, MD

The phakomatoses (Table 49-1) are a diverse group of disorders. The categorization of many disorders under the heading of the phakomatoses has created controversy and confusion since the term was first introduced by Dutch ophthalmologist Jan van der Hoeve in the early 20th century.[1,2] Van der Hoeve first described tuberous sclerosis[3,4] (Bourneville's disease) and neurofibromatosis (von Recklinghausen's disease) as phakomatoses in his earliest publications on the subject, then later added von Hippel-Lindau[2] and Sturge-Weber syndrome.[4-6] The common denominator seemed to be the congenital nature of multisystem tumors. Jan van der Hoeve called them *phakomata* after the Greek name for motherspot, indicating the congenital nature of the conditions. Others later interpreted this to mean that the phakomatoses had a birthmark that indicated an underlying multi-organ condition.[7] In a more contemporary interpretation of the meaning behind grouping these diverse conditions, Hogan and Zimmerman[8] described the phakomatoses as disseminated hamartomas affecting the eye, central nervous system (CNS), skin, and internal organs. Hamartomas are tumorous masses that arise from tissue elements normally found at the site, as opposed to choristomas, which are tumors derived from elements not normally found at the site. Others[9] have proposed that the phakomatoses may be disorders of the regulation of paracrine growth factors.

Glaucoma is a common feature of encephalotrigeminal angiomatosis (Sturge-Weber syndrome) and is occasionally found in neurofibromatosis type 1 and von Hippel-Lindau disease. The other phakomatoses rarely have an associated glaucoma, although a secondary glaucoma may be present as a complication of the other ocular manifestations of the disease.

STURGE-WEBER SYNDROME (ENCEPHALOTRIGEMINAL ANGIOMATOSIS)

In 1860, Schirmer[10] described a patient with glaucoma and a facial angioma. Sturge[11] presented a case in 1879 of a child with a "port-wine stain" angioma involving half the face and head, with ipsilateral buphthalmos, congenital glaucoma, as well as seizure disorder. He also noticed the choroid of the involved eye was a darker red and hypothesized that the choroid was involved with a vascular lesion similar to the face. In 1922, Weber[12] reported the characteristic intracranial calcifications seen radiographically in patients with the syndrome and suggested the parallel streaks were a result of a meningeal angioma. The syndrome became known as the Sturge-Weber syndrome and in its full presentation includes a facial hemangioma, with an ipsilateral intracranial angioma, an ipsilateral choroidal hemangioma, and congenital glaucoma.[13] Incomplete forms occur, but all have the characteristic facial angioma or nevus flammeus. The syndrome has no racial or gender predilection. Unlike the other phakomatoses, Sturge-Weber does not have any identifiable hereditary pattern.

Systemic Findings

The facial angioma (Figure 49-1) is usually unilateral in the distribution of the first and second divisions of the trigeminal nerve. The lesion occurs bilaterally in 10% to 30% of cases.[14-16] It appears deep burgundy in color, and facial hypertrophy of varying degrees of the involved area occurs frequently. Histopathologically, the angioma is composed of dilated, telangiectatic capillaries lined by a single layer

Kahook MY, Schuman JS, eds.
Chandler and Grant's Glaucoma, Fifth Edition (pp 451-464).
© 2013 SLACK Incorporated.

TABLE 49-1. THE PHAKOMATOSES

Disorder	Heredity/Chromosomal Abnormalities	Systemic Involvement	Ocular Findings	Types of Glaucoma	Reference
Sturge-Weber syndrome	Sporadic	Facial angioma Leptomeningeal hemangioma	Hemangioma of lids, orbit, conjunctiva, iris, ciliary body, choroid	Incidence: develops in 30% to 70% of patients Congenital with buphthalmos (60%)	29
Klippel-Trenaunay-Weber syndrome	Sporadic	Facial hemangioma Hemangioma of extremities with hypertrophy	Orbital varices or hyper-trophy, conjunctival telan-giectasias, heterochromia iridis, choroidal angiomas, retinal varicosities or vascular tumors, disc anomalies	Later onset (40%) Incidence: less frequent than Sturge-Weber	49
Neurofibromatosis	Autosomal dominant, 100% penetrance, variable expressivity NF-1; chromosome 17; NF-2: chromosome 22	Cafe-au-lait spots, fib-roma molluscum plexi-form neurofibromas. Neurofibromas of the nerve roots or spinal cord, meningiomas, intracranial or spinal cord gliomas Acoustic neuromas in NF-2 Skeletal problems, pheochromocytomas	Neurofibromas of eyelids, conjunctiva, or orbit Absent greater wing of sphenoid bone Prominent corneal nerves Optic nerve glioma Lisch nodules Posterior subcapsular cataracts in NF-2	Incidence: 23% to 50% Congenital glaucoma with buphthalmos Childhood onset with ectropion uveae and iridogoniodysgenesis	71
von Hippel-Lindau disease	Autosomal dominant with incomplete penetrance Chromosome 3	Cerebellar hemangioblastoma Polycythemia Renal cell carcinoma	Retinal angioma	Incidence: low Occasional neovascu-lar glaucoma follow-ing exudative retinal detachment	81
Tuberous sclerosis	Autosomal dominant with high penetrance but variable expressivity Chromosome 9	Ash-leaf spots Adenoma sebaceum Seizures; infantile spasms Periventricular brain tumors	Astrocytic retinal hamartoma	Incidence: very rare Secondary complica-tion of total retinal detachment or neovascularization	95 96

(continued)

TABLE 49-1. THE PHAKOMATOSES (CONTINUED)

Disorder	Heredity/Chromosomal Abnormalities	Systemic Involvement	Ocular Findings	Types of Glaucoma	Reference
Ataxia telangiectasia	Autosomal recessive Chromosome 11	Progressive cerebellar ataxia Skin telangiectasias Hypoplasia of thymus gland Recurrent sinopulmonary infections	Conjunctival telangiectasias Abnormal extraocular movements and gaze disorders	Incidence: none	104
Wyburn-Mason syndrome	Sporadic	Ipsilateral facial angiomas Intracranial, ipsilateral arteriovenous malformation	Retinal arteriovenous malformation	Incidence: very rare Secondary complication of retinal ischemia	112
Linear nevus sebaceous syndrome	Sporadic	Congenital organoid nevi with benign and malignant transformation Ipsilateral central nervous system involvement	Coloboma or ptosis of ipsilateral upper eyelid Epibulbar dermoids; corneal scarring/neovascularization Colobomas of iris; ciliary body; choroid. Optic nerve hypoplasia; pallor; cupping	Incidence: extremely rare	119
Basal cell nevus syndrome	Autosomal dominant with variable penetrance	Basal cell epitheliomas	Orbital involvement by tumor; hypertelorism; congenital cataract; strabismus; optic nerve and choroidal coloboma; corneal leukoma	Incidence: extremely rare	128
Nevus of Ota	Sporadic	Oculodermal melanosis	Ipsilateral hyperpigmentation of sclera; conjunctiva; cornea; iris; choroid; angle structures Uveal and orbital malignant melanoma	Incidence: low Associated with increased pigmentation in the angle	133
Cutis marmorata telangiectatica congenital	Sporadic	Congenital persistent cutis marmorata; phlebectasia; telangiectasis; superficial ulcerations of skin	Ipsilateral congenital glaucoma	Incidence: 6 out of 65 reported cases Immature angle development as in primary congenital glaucoma	141

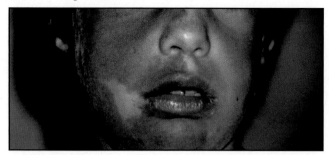

Figure 49-1. Sturge-Weber syndrome patient with characteristic "port-wine stain" facial hemangioma. (Reprinted with permission from David S. Walton, MD.)

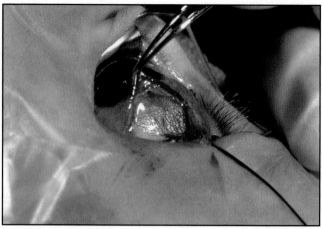

Figure 49-2. Episcleral hemangioma in a patient with glaucoma and Sturge-Weber syndrome. (Reprinted with permission from David S. Walton, MD.)

of endothelial cells in the dermis.[17] Some success has been achieved using laser therapy to diminish the appearance of the lesion.

A racemose leptomeningeal hemangioma is the intracranial lesion of Sturge-Weber syndrome. It is usually ipsilateral to the facial angioma and is located over the parieto-occipital region. Progressive calcification of the angioma occurs during childhood.[18] Adjacent atrophy of the underlying cerebral cortex is frequent and may result in varying degrees of intellectual deficit and mental retardation in about 60% of patients.[19] Contralateral focal motor seizures occur in 85% of patients and usually begin after the age of 1, but become more generalized with age.[19] Permanent hemiparesis, hemiplegia, and homonymous hemianopsia may occur as a consequence of the seizures.

Ophthalmic Manifestations

The lids, orbit, episclera (Figure 49-2), conjunctiva, iris, and ciliary body may be involved with a hemangioma. Although exceptions occur, if the upper eyelid is involved with hemangioma, there is intraocular involvement according to Anderson's rule.[18] The iris, if involved, will be hyperchromic in about 7% of cases.[20]

Choroidal hemangiomas are the most frequent ocular manifestation of Sturge-Weber syndrome. They have been found in 40% to 50% of patients upon pathologic examination.[21,22] In young children, the lesion may simply appear as a darker red choroidal hue in the ipsilateral eye, called the "tomato-catsup fundus."[23] However, as it slowly grows, it will appear as a mildly elevated, orange-yellow diffuse mass involving the posterior pole, and usually more than half the choroid. Histopathologically, the lesions are mixed-type hemangiomas, with elements of both capillary and cavernous hemangiomas.[24] Vision loss may occur in young adulthood due to a degeneration of the overlying choriocapillaris, retinal pigment epithelium, and photoreceptors.[17] Serous detachment of the retina can occur.

Glaucoma in Sturge-Weber Syndrome

Glaucoma develops in a reported 30% to 70% of Sturge-Weber syndrome patients. Approximately 60% present as congenital glaucomas with buphthalmos, whereas 40% present in later childhood or adulthood.[20,25] Usually, the upper eyelid is involved by the hemangioma. The most common presentation is unilateral and congenital, before the age of 2 years, on the side of the facial angioma. Bilateral glaucoma can occur, although usually in the presence of a bilateral facial hemangioma.

Many theories have been put forth to explain the mechanism of glaucoma in Sturge-Weber syndrome. Early theories proposed that abnormal sympathetic innervation might cause a loss of regulation of the normal uveal capillary bed, which then results in stasis and glaucoma.[26] Others[20,27,28] proposed that transudation of fluid from the choroidal hemangioma might cause congestion of the choroid or change the composition of aqueous. These theories have largely been disproven or discounted, as later studies[29-31] (discussed in the following text) revealed structural as well as functional alterations in Sturge-Weber eyes that seemed to correlate with development of glaucoma.

The congenital glaucoma that is associated with Sturge-Weber syndrome is usually associated with immature angle development, as in primary congenital glaucoma. Careful gonioscopic examination will reveal indistinct angle structures with a high iris insertion. Histopathologic specimens have shown changes consistent with developmental anomalies, such as poorly developed scleral spur, thickened uveal meshwork, and an anteriorly displaced iris root.[18,21,29,32-34] Others have found few structural angle abnormalities. Cibis and colleagues[30] examined 3 trabeculectomy specimens from 2 patients with Sturge-Weber syndrome, both of whom had episcleral hemangiomas; the overall architecture of the trabecular meshwork and Schlemm's canal were found to be well preserved.[30] However, the individual trabecular beams were thickened and showed signs of degeneration, which the authors proposed were primary changes associated with premature aging.

Weiss[29] proposed that glaucoma in Sturge-Weber syndrome was a result of 2 mechanisms. In clinical experience, the congenital glaucoma cases had anomalous-appearing angles as opposed to cases with later-onset glaucoma that had normal-appearing angles; evidence of episcleral or conjunctival angiomas was found in all patients examined. Weiss[29] proposed that increased episcleral venous pressure from the episcleral angioma contributed to the congenital glaucoma cases, in addition to an angle abnormality, whereas juvenile and adult-onset cases without angle malformations were secondary to the elevated episcleral venous pressure. Phelps,[31] and then Bellows and colleagues,[35] later measured episcleral venous pressure and found it elevated in patients with Sturge-Weber syndrome and glaucoma.

Management depends on the presentation of the glaucoma. Congenital cases and those with buphthalmos, implying congenital onset, can initially be managed surgically with goniotomy or trabeculotomy. The advantage of goniotomy/trabeculotomy over filtering surgery is the reduction in the risk of sudden intraoperative or prolonged postoperative hypotony that can precipitate choroidal effusions or suprachoroidal hemorrhages in these eyes. However, these procedures are frequently ineffective, and many eyes eventually require filtering surgery. The angle dysgenesis in Sturge-Weber syndrome is clinically indistinguishable from primary congenital glaucoma but the surgical success rate is lower. One retrospective review[34] of 30 cases (28 goniotomies and 2 trabeculotomies) found a surgical failure rate of 60%. Iwach and colleagues[25] found the stable interval of control after a single goniotomy to be only a median of 8 months in Sturge-Weber syndrome patients presenting before age 4 years of age. Interestingly, in these same patients, multiple goniotomies plus medical therapy allowed stability for almost 9 years. Olsen and colleagues[36] published a study of 16 Sturge-Weber syndrome eyes with early-onset glaucoma treated with one or more goniotomies or trabeculotomies; 10 of these patients had good control of IOP over a median of 5.4 years of follow-up. However, the majority of their patients required more than one surgical procedure for adequate control also. Mandal[37] has suggested performing combined trabeculotomy-trabeculectomy to address both mechanisms of early-onset glaucoma in Sturge-Weber. The addition of filtering surgery bypasses the elevated episcleral venous pressure that may be playing a secondary role in the pathogenesis of congenital glaucoma in these patients. In 10 of the patients described by Mandal who underwent primary combined trabeculotomy-trabeculectomy, all had good IOP control over a mean follow-up of 27.6 months.

Older patients are often managed with medical therapy for as long as possible, but in most cases medical therapy eventually fails. Laser trabeculoplasty was performed in 6 of 16 older-onset glaucoma eyes by Iwach and colleagues[25] and was effective in 5 of the 6 for approximately 2 years,

but such efficacy has unfortunately not been our experience. When surgical intervention is indicated, older patients are more likely to receive a trabeculectomy. The rationale for using trabeculectomy in the older patients stems from Weiss'[29] theory that the primary mechanism in these patients is increased episcleral venous pressure, rather than angle dysgenesis. The trabeculectomy will bypass the episcleral venous system, whereas goniotomy, trabeculotomy, or laser trabeculoplasty will not. Though it remains the treatment of choice for late-onset cases, the success rates of trabeculectomy have been variable in children, presumably due to their more vigorous healing response, causing scarring and thereby preventing adequate filtration. There have been limited reports[38,39] suggesting favorable success rates for filtering surgery with antimetabolites such as 5-fluorouracil and mitomycin C in children. However, a number of these patients developed bleb-related infections.[39] Glaucoma drainage implants have also been used in Sturge-Weber syndrome eyes. Budenz and colleagues[40] published their results on a 2-staged Baerveldt implant procedure in 10 Sturge-Weber eyes with late-onset glaucoma.[41] All displayed adequate IOP control over a mean follow-up of 35 months with no cases of intraoperative choroidal hemorrhage. Performing the surgery in 2 stages allows time for encapsulation of the implant plate prior to placement of the filtering tube into the anterior chamber. This prevents hypotony and will help to avoid the most dreaded complication of all filtration surgeries in eyes with elevated episcleral venous pressure: sudden massive intraoperative choroidal effusion or expulsive hemorrhage.[21,25,35,41] The rapid transudation of fluid from the intravascular to the extravascular space in the setting of sudden hypotony and increased venous pressure is thought to be responsible for the effusion. Bellows and associates[35] reported success in minimizing the intraoperative complications from the effusion by creating a posterior sclerotomy prior to entering the anterior chamber. A more recent study[42] suggests that the incidence of intraoperative or postoperative choroidal detachment or hemorrhage may not be as high as previously suggested and that prophylactic sclerotomies may be unnecessary. To help prevent potentially devastating hemorrhages and effusions, the IOP should be reduced as much as possible prior to surgery and controlled intraoperatively with viscoelastic or anterior chamber maintainers, and the postoperative period requires slow, controlled lowering of IOP to avoid their development after surgery.

KLIPPEL-TRENAUNAY-WEBER SYNDROME

In 1900, Klippel and Trenaunay[43] described a syndrome of cutaneous hemangioma of the extremities and face, with varicosities and hypertrophy of bone and soft tissues in the affected limb. Weber[44] later described the same disorder and reported the association of arteriovenous fistulas. Seizures, mental retardation, and cerebral hemangiomas may also occur in patients. Many features of this syndrome are similar to Sturge-Weber syndrome.

Ophthalmic Manifestations

Ophthalmic involvement is occasionally found and may include orbital varices or hypertrophy, conjunctival telangiectasias, heterochromia iridis, choroidal angiomas, retinal varicosities or vascular tumors, disc anomalies, and glaucoma with or without buphthalmos.[45-48] The glaucoma is associated with an ipsilateral facial hemangioma, but the incidence appears to be less frequent than in Sturge-Weber syndrome. One eye has been examined histopathologically and found to have an anomalous development of the anterior chamber angle.[49]

NEUROFIBROMATOSIS (VON RECKLINGHAUSEN'S DISEASE)

In a classic monograph by the German pathologist Freidrich Daniel von Recklinghausen in 1882, neurofibromatosis (NF) was described. NF is inherited as an autosomal dominant disease with nearly 100% penetrance but highly variable expressivity. Neuroectodermal elements of the skin, eyes, and central nervous system are involved with the development of hamartomas that grow in size and number throughout life. The hamartomas may be present at birth, later in childhood, or adulthood.

Two forms of NF are recognized. NF-1 is the classic form of von Recklinghausen's neurofibromatosis and is more common. The diagnosis of NF-1 is made if the patient has 2 or more of the following:

- Six or more café-au-lait macules over 5 mm in greatest diameter in prepubertal individuals, or over 15 mm in greatest diameter in postpubertal individuals

- Two or more neurofibromas of any type or 1 plexiform neurofibroma

- Freckling in axillary or inguinal regions

- Optic glioma

- Two or more Lisch nodules

- A distinctive osseous lesion such as sphenoid dysplasia or thinning of long bone cortex with or without pseudoarthrosis

- A first-degree relative with NF-1 by the above criteria[50]

NF-1 occurs at a frequency of about 1/3000 to 1/4000, with no known racial or gender predilection.[51,52] The NF-1 gene has been isolated on the long arm of chromosome 17 and encodes for a protein related to guanosine diphosphatase-activating protein (GAP).[53-55] GAP regulates another protein, Ras, that signals cells to grow. Mutation of the NF-1 gene is thought to inactivate the gene.[55]

NF-2, also called bilateral acoustic neurofibromatosis, was first described by Henneberg and Koch[56] in 1902. The National Institutes of Health (NIH) diagnostic criteria requires bilateral acoustic neuromas or a first-degree relative with NF-2 and a unilateral acoustic neuroma or 2 of the following: meningioma, glioma, schwannoma, neurofibroma, or presenile posterior subcapsular lens opacity.[50] NF-2 is present in only 1 out of 50,000 population. The NF-2 locus has been isolated to near the center of the long arm of chromosome 22, but the molecular genetics have not been elucidated yet.[57,58]

Systemic Findings

The skin is the most commonly involved organ in NF-1.[18] Café-au-lait spots are brown macules usually found on the trunk. Fibroma molluscum are isolated, pedunculated, pigmented nodules that are found to have enlarged cutaneous nerves, Schwann's cells, and connective tissue elements, histopathologically. Plexiform neurofibromas are groups of enlarged nerves with thickened perineural sheaths that may feel like a bag of worms on palpation. These lesions often appear or worsen around puberty and may increase in size and number with age. Hypertrophy of the involved areas may occur. NF-2 has very little skin involvement.

CNS tumors are common in both NF-1 and NF-2. CNS tumors in NF-1 and NF-2 include neurofibromas of the nerve roots or spinal cord, meningiomas, and intracranial or spinal cord gliomas. Acoustic neuromas in NF-2 usually present in the second or third decades when hearing loss, tinnitus, or balance problems are noted. In individuals with a family history of NF-2, early detection with screening tests is possible.

Skeletal problems in patients with NF-1 include rapidly progressive kyphoscoliosis and pseudoarthroses, or nonhealing fractures.[17] Pheochromocytomas are 10 times more common in patients with NF than the general population.[59] Other organs may be involved by hamartomas or malignant tumors.

Ophthalmic Manifestations

The eyelids are frequently involved by neurofibromas and may produce a characteristic S-shaped upper eyelid contour (Figure 49-3). Any of the other characteristic skin lesions may present in the eyelids or surrounding periorbital area and may develop in approximately 25% of patients.[60] Rarely, the conjunctiva or orbit may develop neurofibromas, while some patients have prominent corneal nerves visible on slit-lamp examination. The greater wing of the sphenoid bone at the orbital apex may be absent, allowing the frontal lobe to herniate into the orbital apex.

Optic nerve glioma has been reported to occur in 15% of NF-1 patients, although many are asymptomatic.[61,62] Optic nerve gliomas tend to grow slowly and extremely

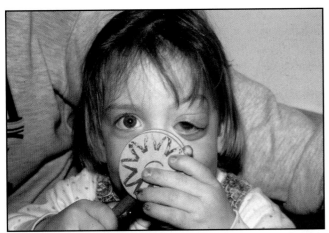

Figure 49-3. Patient with neurofibromatosis; characteristic S-shaped upper lid from neurofibroma, and buphthalmos from congenital glaucoma. (Reprinted with permission from David S. Walton, MD.)

rarely develop malignant transformation, although they can be very destructive locally. Optic nerve gliomas are the primary cause of visual loss in NF. Tumors that invade intracranially into the chiasm have a much poorer prognosis than optic nerve gliomas that involve the orbital portion of the optic nerve. Symptoms and signs of optic nerve glioma include decreased visual acuity, proptosis, strabismus, visual field loss, and optic atrophy. Contrast-enhanced computed tomography (CT) scanning or magnetic resonance imaging (MRI) will demonstrate enlargement and kinking of the optic nerve anywhere along its course and into the chiasmal region, although MRI may be able to detect intracanalicular and chiasmal masses better.[63]

Lisch nodules are melanocytic hamartomas of the iris and are found in more than 90% of NF-1 patients older than 5 years of age.[64] Patients younger than 2 years of age rarely have any Lisch nodules, and they are not present in unaffected first-degree relatives.[60,65] Lisch nodules are avascular, smooth, dome-shaped gelatinous nodules found on the iris surface. They may be mildly translucent to dark brown in color, ranging up to 2 mm in size.

NF-2 patients have a high incidence of posterior subcapsular cataract occurring at a young age.[66] This association has not been seen with NF-1. Choroidal hamartomas have been reported in a series of White NF patients but were not seen in Black patients.[60] Occasionally, retinal astrocytic hamartomas or combined retinal and retinal pigment epithelial hamartomas have been seen in patients with NF-1.

Glaucoma in Neurofibromatosis

Congenital glaucoma and glaucoma presenting somewhat later in childhood have been reported in cases of NF-1. The actual incidence of glaucoma in neurofibromatosis is unknown. Buphthalmos in the absence of elevated IOP has been reported as a manifestation of regional giantism.[67] Care must be taken to distinguish this condition from true congenital glaucoma in neurofibromatosis. Two presentations of glaucoma in neurofibromatosis are recognized.

Infants and toddlers have presented with unilateral buphthalmos and elevated IOP, usually with a plexiform neurofibroma formation of the upper eyelid and hemihypertrophy of the face (Francois syndrome), and are subsequently diagnosed with NF-1.[68,69] It is reported that glaucoma is present in 50% of eyes with a plexiform neurofibroma of the upper lid,[70] though more recently Morales and colleagues[71] report a rate of glaucoma of only 23% in patients with orbito-facial NF-1. In their study of 80 patients with NF-1, glaucoma presented only in patients with orbito-facial NF-1, and the majority were diagnosed with glaucoma prior to 3 years of age. Glaucoma in these patients was consistently associated with severe globe enlargement.

Several mechanisms for this congenital form of glaucoma have been suggested. Failure of the normal angle development, as in primary congenital glaucoma, has been implicated and is likely the most common cause of infantile-onset glaucoma in neurofibromatosis.[68,72] Quaranta and colleagues[73] looked at the angles of 42 young patients with NF-1 and found evidence of anteriorization of the iris insertion in 69%. Seventy-six percent had a very narrow or invisible ciliary body band. Only 3 of the patients had juvenile-onset glaucoma, and they had more severe angle dysgenesis. Infiltration of the angle by neurofibroma was documented by gonioscopy by Grant and Walton[72] and was found histopathologically by Francois. Progressive angle infiltration by neurofibroma may also cause later-onset glaucoma. Closure of the angle by diffuse involvement of the ciliary body and choroid has also been recognized and may also develop as a late complication.[68] Synechial angle closure from neovascularization has been reported in neurofibromatosis.[74]

The other presentation of glaucoma in neurofibromatosis is usually later in childhood in association with what appears to be a unilateral congenital ectropion uveae[75,76] (Figure 49-4). In a series of 8 patients with congenital ectropion uveae and glaucoma, 3 were found to have neurofibromatosis.[75] Congenital ectropion uveae is usually accompanied by ipsilateral ptosis, although not a palpable neurofibroma mass. The pupil may be mistaken as enlarged or irregular. On careful inspection, however, pigmented uveal tissue is found to overlie the iris surrounding the pupil. This tissue has been identified as hyperplasia of the iris pigment epithelium, not a true ectropion, and is usually unchanged in its appearance over time.[77] Glaucoma is strongly associated with congenital ectropion uveae; the mechanism for development of glaucoma in these cases is an iridogoniodysgenesis. Gonioscopic findings reveal a high, or anterior, iris insertion into the trabecular meshwork.[75,77]

Treatment of the glaucoma depends on the underlying mechanism. Congenital cases with abnormal angle development or infiltration are best managed by goniotomy or trabeculotomy initially and with trabeculectomy if those procedures fail. Cases presenting later in childhood may

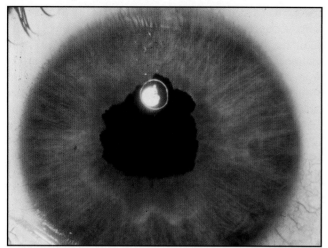

Figure 49-4. Congenital ectropion uveae in a patient with neurofibromatosis and glaucoma. (Reprinted with permission from David S. Walton, MD.)

be successfully managed medically or surgically. Because marked infiltration of the choroid or ciliary body may develop later in childhood, periodic gonioscopy is necessary to detect progressive angle closure.

VON HIPPEL-LINDAU DISEASE (RETINAL AND CEREBELLAR ANGIOMATOSIS)

In 1904, von Hippel published a seminal paper describing retinal angiomatosis in 2 patients. He later performed a pathologic examination and identified the lesion as a hemangioblastoma, naming the condition angiomatosis retinae. Lindau, in 1926, made the association of cerebellar hemangiomatous cysts in many patients with von Hippel's disease. The term *von Hippel-Lindau disease* is used when the disease involves the CNS and retina; when only the retina is involved, it is called *von Hippel disease*. Von Hippel disease is estimated to occur in one in 22,500 patients seen by ophthalmologists.[78] About 20% to 25% of cases are familial, inherited as an autosomal dominant trait with incomplete penetrance. Linkage analysis has mapped the gene for von Hippel-Lindau disease to the short arm of chromosome 3.[79]

Systemic Findings

The cerebellar hemangioblastoma tumor is the characteristic CNS lesion that occurs in an estimated two-thirds of von Hippel-Lindau cases.[80,81] These tumors are often resectable but recurrences may occur. Death may ensue due to neurologic effects of the tumor. The typical presentation is of headache, vertigo, or cerebellar signs developing in the third decade of life. Medullary and spinal hemangio-blastomas

are uncommon.[81] Polycythemia is associated with the CNS hemangioblastomas.[82]

Renal cell carcinoma occurs in about one-quarter of patients and may cause death from uremia or metastatic disease.[80,81] It is usually diagnosed in the fifth decade of life. Pheochromocytoma is associated with von Hippel-Lindau disease in various kindreds, and therefore, the reported frequency varies.[81,83] Renal and pancreatic cysts may also be present. Screening affected individuals and family members with CT or MRI of the head and abdomen may detect these lesions before the patient becomes symptomatic.[81]

Ophthalmic Manifestations

The retinal angioma is usually the first feature of the syndrome to be diagnosed as it tends to present in the second or third decade of life. Retinal angiomas are detected in about two-thirds of von Hippel-Lindau patients and are usually asymptomatic at the time of diagnosis.[81,83] The capillary-type angiomas are bilateral in about 50% and are usually located in the mid-periphery of the retina.[84-86] The tumor develops from a lesion as small as a diabetic microaneurysm into a reddish, elevated mass of 1- to 3-disc diameters in size. A single dilated tortuous feeder artery is paired with a similar-appearing vein, and there is arteriovenous shunting through the tumor.[87] If left untreated, the incompetent vascular endothelium of the tumor allows leakage and exudation to develop in the surrounding retina and ultimately leads to an exudative retinal detachment involving the posterior pole. The neovascular glaucoma that may occur is found in this end-stage setting. Treatment of the angioma can be accomplished with direct photocoagulation, diathermy, or cryotherapy of the lesion.[88]

The incidence of glaucoma in this condition is low and most commonly associated with neovascularization following exudative retinal detachment. Hardwig and Robertson,[81] in their report on 36 eyes, noted 3 of 13 eyes with poor vision due to glaucoma and an additional 4 eyes enucleated because of pain and blindness.

TUBEROUS SCLEROSIS (BOURNEVILLE'S DISEASE)

Tuberous sclerosis was first described in 1880 by Bourneville.[89] Vogt[90] later described the triad of epilepsy, adenoma sebaceum, and mental deficiency. Tuberous sclerosis has a prevalence of one in 10,000 to 15,000.[91,92] The disease is transmitted as an autosomal dominant trait with high penetrance but variable expressivity. Detection of gene carriers is possible using CT scanning and an evaluation of skin lesions.[93] Genetic linkage analysis has located the gene for tuberous sclerosis on the distal portion of the long-arm of chromosome 9.[94]

Systemic Findings

Ash-leaf spots on the skin detected by ultraviolet light are usually present at birth in at least 80% of affected patients and are considered diagnostic of tuberous sclerosis.[95,96] Adenoma sebaceum is the characteristic rash that appears after 2 years of age and is present in 83% of cases.[96] It appears as small, reddish-brown papules over the cheeks, nose, and chin, which are histologically angiofibromata.[18,33] These lesions may also affect the eyelids and conjunctiva. Shagreen patches and yellow plaques are found in about one-third of patients and are usually located over the lower back or the eyelids.

Seizures develop in 80% to 90% of patients. Infantile spasms are a common presentation of tuberous sclerosis, while later in childhood the seizures become more generalized.[19,97] Mental retardation occurs in 50% to 60% of patients.[19,96,97] The CNS effects are a result of benign periventricular brain tumors that become calcified (*brain stones*) and are seen on CT scan in about half of patients.[96] Renal cysts and hamartomas are also common.

Ophthalmic Manifestations

The most common associated ocular feature of tuberous sclerosis is an astrocytic retinal hamartoma, occuring singly or multiply in half of patients.[96] Multiple retinal hamartomas are diagnostic of the disease when present. The classic tumor is described as a translucent white mulberry-like lesion, calcified and located near the optic disc. These retinal tumors usually do not cause any associated visual or anatomic problems. Rarely, an exudative retinal detachment or vitreous hemorrhage may occur or the hamartoma may undergo cystic degeneration and mimic necrotizing retinitis.[98-100] The only association with glaucoma is as a rare secondary complication of a total retinal detachment or neovascularization.[95,101] Eagle and colleagues[102] described the histopathology of 2 tuberous sclerosis eyes with iris hamartomas; both eyes had peripheral anterior synechiae and florid iris neovascularization. Both eyes were enucleated secondary to a blind painful eye; one eye had IOP of 43 mm Hg prior to enucleation.

ATAXIA TELANGIECTASIA (LOUIS-BAR SYNDROME)

In 1941, Louis-Bar[103] reported a child with progressive cerebellar ataxia and telangiectasias of the skin and conjunctiva. In 1957, Boder and Sedgwick reported 7 cases and coined the name *ataxia telangiectasia*.[104]

This rare syndrome is inherited as an autosomal recessive trait. The search for one of the possible genes for ataxia telangiectasia has been narrowed to chromosome region 11q22 to 11q23 by linkage analysis.[105]

Systemic Findings

Progressive cerebellar ataxia is usually diagnosed in the first years of life. Progression occurs so that the patient is unable to walk and has difficulty with speech and responses by the first decade of life. Cerebellar atrophy is the characteristic lesion.[104]

The skin becomes involved with telangiectasias between the ages of 3 and 7 years. These are noted on the cheeks, nose, ears, palate, and ocular adnexae. Older patients develop telangiectasias of the skin of the neck, antecubital and popliteal areas, dorsal hands, and feet.[104]

Hypoplasia of the thymus gland may be seen, along with an increased susceptibility to recurrent sinus and pulmonary infections in approximately 85% of patients.[104] This is felt to be associated with an underlying immunological disorder.[106] Patients with ataxia telangiectasia have a greatly increased risk of developing a malignancy.[105]

Ophthalmic Manifestations

Conjunctival telangiectasias are seen in childhood in all patients, usually bilaterally. Abnormal extraocular muscle movements and gaze disorders are common.[107-109]

Glaucoma is not a reported feature of ataxia telangiectasia.

WYBURN-MASON SYNDROME

In 1943, Wyburn-Mason[110] published a review of all reported cases of retinal arteriovenous (AV) communications and emphasized the common association of intracranial arteriovenous communications in 81% of patients. Only a few of these patients had documented intracranial AV malformations, however. Subsequent studies[111,112] have placed the incidence of intracranial AV communication in patients with retinal AV malformations at 23% to 30%. The Wyburn-Mason syndrome is not hereditary and has no gender predilection.

Systemic Findings

Approximately half of patients have associated ipsilateral facial angiomas of variable appearance.[112] The intracranial AV malformation is unilateral, ipsilateral to the involved eye, and usually in the midbrain. Symptoms of headache and vomiting, often related to cerebral or subarachnoid bleeding from the lesion, develop in the second to third decades of life. Signs of hydrocephalus from obstruction of the cerebral aqueduct by an enlarging malformation may occur. Seizures are uncommon, but other neurologic deficits may result from the mid-brain lesion. Treatment is generally not undertaken due to the inaccessible location of the AV malformation.

Ophthalmic Manifestations

The AV communication in the retina typically involves the vessels in the temporal midperiphery. The lesion varies from an arteriolar or capillary plexus between an artery and vein to a direct communication through large, dilated, intertwined twisting vessels.[113] The retinal appearance remains stable, but vision loss may develop in the second to third decade of life, especially with the more severe malformations, and progress due to associated retinal involvement. The lesion may produce retinal or vitreous hemorrhage, nonperfusion of the retina, retinal edema, and exudation.[113] The vascular malformation may extend from the eye to the midbrain and cause compression of the optic nerve or visual pathway with resulting visual field defects. Symptomatic eyes may be treated with laser photocoagulation.[114] Proptosis is common, secondary to orbital AV malformation.[115]

Neovascular glaucoma has been reported in at least 2 patients, including a 4-year-old child who developed widespread retinal and choroidal ischemia secondary to central retinal vein occlusion.[116] At least 2 other cases of glaucoma related to elevated episcleral pressure have also been described.

LINEAR NEVUS SEBACEOUS SYNDROME (NEVUS SEBACEOUS OF JADASSOHN)

In 1932, Robinson[117] reported the linear nevus sebaceous syndrome, with a skin lesion as described by Jadassohn, in 4 patients. The syndrome consists of a triad of linear nevus sebaceous, seizure disorder, and mental retardation. There is no known hereditary association.

Systemic Findings

The skin lesions consist of congenital organoid nevi that progress through stages, beginning with underdevelopment of hair and sebaceous glands to massive development of sebaceous glands and papillomatous epidermoid hyperplasia.[118] Eventually, the nevus develops benign and malignant neoplasms.[119] Malignant transformation may occur in 10% to 35% of nevi.[118,120] Surgical excision is usually curative.

The syndrome may involve multiple other organ systems, including CNS, ophthalmic, skeletal, cardiovascular, and urogenital systems.[119] Ipsilateral CNS involvement is more likely when the epidermal nevi are found on the head.[121,122]

Ophthalmic Manifestations

Ophthalmic involvement is found in 68% of patients with the linear nevus sebaceous syndrome.[119] Involvement of the adnexa with a coloboma or ptosis of the upper eyelid is common. Epibulbar dermoids that appear firm, flat,

pink, and vascularized may involve the conjunctiva bilaterally in any location.[119] The cornea may be involved with partial or total vascularization, dermoid tumor, or scarring.[119] Unilateral and bilateral colobomas of the iris and ciliary body, choroid, and retina have been reported.[119] Optic nerve hypoplasia, optic disc pallor, and optic disc cupping also have been reported.[119]

Although glaucoma has not been specifically reported, 2 reports[122,123] have noted incomplete opening of the anterior chamber angle on pathologic examination.

BASAL CELL NEVUS SYNDROME

Basal cell nevus syndrome was described by Binkley and Johnson in 1951.[124] It is inherited as an autosomal dominant trait with variable penetrance. Multiple basal cell epitheliomas, which may be present at birth and enlarge during adolescence, develop over the eyelids and face, and occasionally on the trunk and neck, and may be locally invasive.[125-127] A characteristic dyskeratosis of the skin may occur in addition to bony abnormalities and neurologic and genital anomalies.[125] Variable ocular findings occur in 30% of cases.[128] Orbital involvement by tumor, hypertelorism, congenital cataract, strabismus, optic nerve and choroidal coloboma, corneal leukoma, and glaucoma have been reported in some patients.[127-130]

GLAUCOMAS ASSOCIATED WITH OTHER SKIN DISORDERS: NEVUS OF OTA (OCULODERMAL MELANOCYTOSIS, CONGENITAL OCULAR MELANOSIS)

The skin lesion in oculodermal melanosis or Nevus of Ota is a deeply pigmented, slate-gray appearance to the skin in the distribution of the first and second divisions of the trigeminal nerve. There is no known hereditary influence. It is common in Asian and Black patients.[131]

Ophthalmic Manifestations

Most patients with skin pigmentation have an ipsilateral hyperpigmentation of the globe that may include the sclera (Figure 49-5), conjunctiva, cornea, iris, and choroid. These patients are at risk for developing uveal and orbital malignant melanoma.[132] The scleral pigmentation is a muted bluish or slate-gray in color. Markedly increased pigmentation may be found in the angle structures of the involved eye. This finding may be seen without evidence of increased IOP, but open-angle glaucoma has been reported in several cases.[133-135] The glaucoma responds to management as a primary open-angle glaucoma.

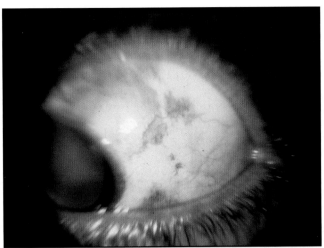

Figure 49-5. Characteristic bluish, slate-gray appearance of scleral pigmentation in a patient with oculodermal melanocytosis (Nevus of Ota).

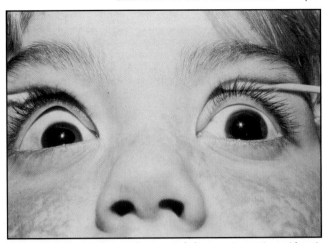

Figure 49-6. Buphthalmos and congenital glaucoma in a patient with cutis marmorata telangiectatica congenita. Note the telangiectatic, marbled appearance of the bilateral facial lesion that is more subtle than the nevus flammeus of Sturge-Weber syndrome. (Reprinted with permission from A. Robert Bellows, MD.)

CUTIS MARMORATA TELANGIECTATICA CONGENITA

Cutis marmorata telangiectatica congenita (CMTC) is a rare cutaneous vascular anomaly first described in 1922 by Lohuizen.[136] There is no known genetic pattern for CMTC. It is characterized by congenital persistent cutis marmorata, phlebectasia, telangiectasis, and superficial ulcerations, with slow clinical improvement during childhood.[137] The affected skin has a cutaneous marbling effect, deeper in color than in infants exposed to cold temperature (Figure 49-6). Regional involvement of the face, trunk, or extremities occurs in about half of the cases, while generalized involvement occurs in the remainder of patients.[138-141]

Ophthalmic Manifestations

Several cases of congenital glaucoma have been reported in the literature,[141] usually associated with ipsilateral facial involvement. We have seen 2 additional patients with congenital glaucoma who also had facial involvement. The associated glaucoma is related to immature angle development as in primary congenital glaucoma.[141] Increased episcleral venous pressure does not appear to occur in CMTC, as episcleral or conjunctival vascular changes were not found in the reported cases[141] or ours, nor was blood visible in Schlemm's canal on gonioscopy. However, a case report[142] describes an intraoperative suprachoroidal hemorrhage in a child with CMTC during a repeat trabeculectomy. The report described the involved eye as buphthalmic with an immature angle appearance on gonioscopy, without any vascular abnormality of the eye.[142] Glaucoma in CMTC can be managed with goniotomy or trabeculotomy initially, adding medical therapy as needed. However, the glaucoma in these patients can be difficult to control, with need for trabeculectomy or drainage implant surgery reported.

REFERENCES

1. Van der Hoeve J. Eye symptoms in phakomatoses. *Trans Ophthalmol Soc U K.* 1932;52:380-401.
2. Van der Hoeve J. Les phakomatoses de Bourneville, de Recklinghausen, et de von Hippel-Landau. *J Belge Neurolol Physicatr.* 1933;33:752-756.
3. Van der Hoeve J. Eye symptoms in tuberous sclerosis of the brain. *Trans Ophthalmol Soc U K.* 1920;40:329-334.
4. Van Der Hoeve J. Eye diseases in tuberous sclerosis of the brain and in Recklinghausen's disease. *Trans Ophthalmol Soc UK.* 1923;43:534.
5. Brouwer B, Van Der Hoeve J, Mahoney W. A fourth type of phakomatosis: Sturge-Weber syndrome. *Verh K Akad Wet Amst.* 1937;36:1.
6. Van der Hoeve J. Fourth type of phakomatosis. *Arch Ophthalmol.* 1937;18:679-682.
7. Duke-Elder S. Part 2, congenital deformities. In: *System of Ophthalmology. Normal and Abnormal Development.* St Louis, MO: CV Mosby; 1964:1153.
8. Hogan MJ, Zimmerman LE. *Ophthalmic Pathology: An Atlas and Textbook.* Philadelphia, PA: WB Saunders Co; 1962.
9. Kousseff BG. The phakomatoses as paracrine growth disorders (paracrinopathies). *Clin Genetics.* 1990;37:97-105.
10. Schirmer R. Ein Fall von Teleangiektasie. *Arch Ophthalmol.* 1860;7:119.
11. Sturge WA. A case of partial epilepsy apparently due to a lesion of one of the vasomotor centres of the brain. *Clin Soc Transoct.* 1879;12:162.
12. Weber FP. Right-sided hemi-hypotrophy resulting from right-sided congenital spastic hemiplegia with a morbid condition of the left side of the brain, revealed by radiograms. *J Neurol.* 1922;3:134-139.
13. Reese AB. *Tumors of the Eye.* New York, NY: Harper & Row; 1976.
14. Duke-Elder S, Jay B. *System of Ophthalmology: Diseases of the Lens and Vitreous; Glaucoma and Hypotony.* St Louis, MO: CV Mosby; 1969.
15. Shaffer RN, Weiss DI. *Congenital and Pediatric Glaucomas.* St Louis, MO: CV Mosby; 1970.
16. Peterman AF, Hayles AB, Dockerty MB, et al. Encephalotrigeminal angiomatosis: clinical study of 35 cases. *JAMA.* 1958;167:2169-2176.

17. Ebert EM, Albert DM. Phakomatoses. In: Albert DM, Jakobiec FA, eds. *Principles and Practice of Ophthalmology: Clinical Practice.* Philadelphia, PA: WB Saunders Co; 1994:3298-3328.

18. Font RL, Ferry AP. The phakomatoses. *Int Ophthalmol Clin.* 1972;12:1-50.

19. Beck RW, Hanno R. The phakomatoses. *Int Ophthalmol Clin.* 1985;25:97-116.

20. Alexander GL, Norman RM. *The Sturge-Weber Syndrome.* Bristol, England: John Wright & Sons; 1960.

21. Christensen GR, Records RE. Glaucoma and expulsive hemorrhage mechanisms in the Sturge-Weber syndrome. *Ophthalmology.* 1979;86:1360-1366.

22. Duke-Elder S, Perkins ES. *System of Ophthalmology: Diseases of the Uveal Tract.* St Louis, MO: CV Mosby; 1966.

23. Susac JO, Smith JL, Scelfo RJ. The "tomatoe-catsup" fundus in Sturge-Weber syndrome. *Arch Ophthalmol.* 1974;92:69-70.

24. Witschel H, Font RL. Hemangioma of the choroid. A clinico-pathologic study of 71 cases and a review of the literature. *Surv Ophthalmol.* 1974;20:415-431.

25. Iwach AG, Hoskins HD, Hetherington J, et al. Analysis of surgical and medical management of glaucoma in Sturge-Weber syndrome. *Ophthalmology.* 1990;97:904-909.

26. Cushing H. Cases of spontaneous intracranial hemorrhage associated with trigeminal naevi. *JAMA.* 1906;47:178.

27. Dunphy EB. Glaucoma accompanying nevus flammeus. *Trans Am Ophthalmol Soc.* 1934;32:143-152.

28. Tyson HH. Nevus flammeus of the face and globe. *Arch Ophthalmol.* 1932;8:365.

29. Weiss DI. Dual origin of glaucoma in encephalotrigeminal haemangiomatosis. *Trans Ophthalmol Soc UK.* 1973;93:477-493.

30. Cibis GW, Tripathi RC, Tripathi BJ. Glaucoma in Sturge-Weber syndrome. *Ophthalmology.* 1984;91:1061-1071.

31. Phelps CD. The pathogenesis of glaucoma in Sturge-Weber syndrome. *Ophthalmology.* 1978;85:276.

32. Barkan O. Goniotomy for glaucoma associated with nevus flammeus. *Am J Ophthalmol.* 1957;43:545-549.

33. Gass JD. The phakomatoses. In: Smith JL, ed. *Neurophthalmology.* St Louis, MO: CV Mosby; 1965.

34. Patrianakos TD, Nagao K, Walton DS. Surgical management of glaucoma with the Sturge-Weber syndrome. *Int Ophthalmol Clinics.* 2008;48:63-78.

35. Bellows AR, Chylack LT, Epstein DL, et al. Choroidal effusion during glaucoma surgery in patients with prominent episcleral vessels. *Arch Ophthalmol.* 1979;97:493.

36. Olsen KE, Huang AS, Wright MM. The efficacy of goniotomy/trabeculotomy in early-onset glaucoma associated with the Sturge-Weber syndrome. *J AAPOS.* 1998;2:365-368.

37. Mandal AK. Primary combined trabeculotomy-trabeculectomy for early-onset glaucoma in Sturge-Weber syndrome. *Ophthalmology.* 1999;106:1621-1627.

38. Snir M, Lusky M, Shalev B, et al. Mitomycin C and 5-fluorouracil antimetabolite therapy for pediatric glaucoma filtration surgery. *Ophthalmic Surg.* 2000;31:31-37.

39. Sidoti PA, Belmonte SJ, Liebmann JM, et al. Trabeculectomy with mitomycin-C in the treatment of pediatric glaucomas. *Ophthalmology.* 2000;107:422-429.

40. Budenz DL, Sakamoto D, Eliezer R, et al. Two-staged Baerveldt glaucoma implant for childhood glaucoma associated with Sturge-Weber syndrome. *Ophthalmology.* 2000;107:2105-2110.

41. Shihab ZM, Kristan RW. Recurrent intraoperative choroidal effusion in Sturge-Weber syndrome. *J Pediatric Ophthalmol Strabismus.* 1983;20:250-252.

42. Eibschitz-Tsimhoni M, Lichter PR, Del Monte MA, et al. Assessing the need for posterior sclerotomy at the time of filtering surgery in patients with Sturge-Weber syndrome. *Ophthalmology.* 2003;110:1361-1363.

43. Klippel M, Trenaunay P. Du naevus variqueux osteohypertrophique. *Arch Gen Med Paris.* 1900;3:611-672.

44. Weber FP. Angioma formation in connection with hypertrophy of limbs and hemi-hypertrophy. *Br J Dermatol.* 1907;19:231-235.

45. O'Connor PS, Smith JD. Optic nerve variant in the Klippel-Trenaunay-Weber syndrome. *Ann Ophthalmol.* 1978;10:131.

46. Brod RD, Shields JA, Shields CL, et al. Unusual retinal and renal vascular lesions in the Klippel-Trenaunay-Weber syndrome. *Retina.* 1992;12:355-358.

47. Limaye SR, Doyle HA, Tang RA. Retinal varicosity in Klippel-Trenaunay syndrome. *J Pediatr Ophthalmol Strabismus.* 1979;16:371-373.

48. Good WV, Hoyt CS. Optic nerve shadow enlargement in the Klippel-Trenaunay-Weber syndrome. *J Pediatr Ophthalmol Strabismus.* 1989;26:288-289.

49. Reynolds JD, Johnson BL, Gloster S, Biglan AW. Glaucoma and Klippel-Trenaunay-Weber syndrome. *Am J Ophthalmol.* 1988;106:495-496.

50. Neurofibromatosis. Conference statement. National Institutes of Health Consensus Development Conference. *Arch Neurol.* 1988;45:575-578.

51. Rasmussen SA, Friedman JM. NF1 gene and neurofibromatosis 1. *Am J Epidemiol.* 2000;151(1):33-40.

52. Friedman JM. Epidemiology of neurofibromatosis type 1. *Am J Med Genet.* 1999;89(1):1-6.

53. Barker D, Wright E, Nguyen K, et al. Gene for von Recklinghausen neurofibromatosis is in the pericentromeric region of chromosome 17. *Science.* 1987;236:1100-1102.

54. Seizinger BR, Rouleau GA, Ozelius LJ, et al. Genetic linkage of von Recklinghausen neurofibromatosis to the nerve growth factor receptor gene. *Cell.* 1987;49:589-594.

55. Xu G, O'Connell P, Viskochil D, et al. The neurofibromatosis type 1 gene encodes a protein related to GAP. *Cell.* 1990;62:599-608.

56. Henneberg K, Koch M. Ueber "centrale" Neurofibromatose und die Geschwülste des Kleinhirnbrückenwinkels (Acusticusneurome). *Arch Psy Nervenkr.* 1902;36(1)251-304.

57. Rouleau GA, Wertelecki W, Haines JL, et al. Genetic linkage of bilateral acoustic neurofibromatosis to a DNA marker on chromosome 22. *Nature.* 1987;329:246-248.

58. Rouleau GA, Haines JL, Bazanowski A, et al. A genetic linkage map of the long arm of human chromosome 22. *Genomics.* 1989;4:1-6.

59. DeAngelis LM, Kelleher MB, Post KD, et al. Multiple paragangliomas in neurofibromatosis. *Neurology.* 1987;37:129-133.

60. Lewis RA, Riccardi VM. von Recklinghausen neurofibromatosis. Incidence of iris hamartomata. *Ophthalmology.* 1981;88:348-354.

61. Lewis RA, Gerson LP, Axelson KA, et al. von Recklinghausen neurofibromatosis. II. Incidence of optic gliomata. *Ophthalmology.* 1984;91:929-935.

62. Listernick R, Charrow J, Greenwald MJ, Esterly NB. Optic gliomas in children with neurofibromatosis type 1. *J Pediatrics.* 1989;114:788-792.

63. Braffman BH, Bilaniuk LT, Zimmerman RA. The central nervous system manifestations of the phakomatoses on MR. *Radiol Clin North Am.* 1988;26:773-800.

64. Perry HD, Font RL. Iris nodules in von Recklinghausen's neurofibromatosis. Electron microscopic confirmation of their melanocytic origin. *Arch Ophthalmol.* 1982;100:1635-1640.

65. Lubs ME, Bauer M, Formas ME, et al. Iris hamartomas in the diagnosis of neurofibromatosis-1. *Int Pediatrics.* 1990;5:261.

66. Pearson-Webb MA, Kaiser-Kupfer MI, Eldridge R. Eye findings in bilateral acoustic (central) neurofibromatosis: association with presenile lens opacities and cataracts but absence of Lisch nodules [letter]. *N Engl J Med.* 1986;315:1553-1554.

67. Hoyt CS, Billson FA. Buphthalmos in neurofibromatosis: is it an expression of regional giantism? *J Pediatric Ophthalmol.* 1977;14:228-234.

68. Brownstein S, Little JM. Ocular neurofibromatosis. *Ophthalmology*. 1983;90:1595-1599.

69. Politi F, Sachs R, Barishak R. Neurofibromatosis and congenital glaucoma. A case report. *Ophthalmologica*. 1977;176:155-159.

70. Lieb WA, Wirth WA, Geeraets WJ. Hydrophthalmos and neurofibromatosis (von Recklinghausen). *Confin Neurol*. 1958;19:230-247.

71. Morales J, Chaudhry IA, Bosley TM. Glaucoma and globe enlargement associated with neurofibromatosis type 1. *Ophthalmology*. 2009;116:1725-1730.

72. Grant WM, Walton DS. Distinctive gonioscopic findings in glaucoma due to neurofibromatosis. *Arch Ophthalmol*. 1968;79:127-134.

73. Quaranta L, Semeraro F, Turano R, et al. Gonioscopic findings in patients with type 1 neurofibromatosis (von Recklinghausen disease). *J Glaucoma*. 2004;13:90-95.

74. Wolter JR, Butler R. Pigment spots of the iris and ectropion uveae with glaucoma in neurofibromatosis. *Am J Ophthalmol*. 1963;56:964-973.

75. Ritch R, Forbes M, Hetherington J Jr, et al. Congenital ectropion uveae with glaucoma. *Ophthalmology*. 1984;91:326-331.

76. Roth H, Shaffer RN. Neurofibromatosis and glaucoma. In: Bellows JG, ed. *Contemporary Ophthalmology*. Baltimore, MD: Williams & Wilkins; 1972:180-189.

77. Dowling J, Walton DS, Richardson TM, et al. Glaucoma with congenital ectropion uveae. *Ophthalmology*. 1985;92:912-921.

78. Pinkerton OD. Angioma of the retina; report of two cases with fundus photographs. *Am J Ophthalmol*. 1946;29:711.

79. Seizinger BR, Rouleau GA, Ozelius LJ, et al. von Hippel-Lindau disease maps to the region of chromosome 3 associated with renal cell carcinoma. *Nature*. 1988;332:268-269.

80. Maher ER, Yates JRW, Harries R, et al. Clinical features and natural history of von Hippel-Lindau disease. *QJ Med*. 1990;77:1151-1163.

81. Hardwig P, Robertson DM. von Hippel-Lindau disease: a familial, often lethal, multisystem phakomatosis. *Ophthalmology*. 1984;91:263-270.

82. Cramer F, Kimsey W. The cerebellar hemangioblastomas; review of 53 cases, with special reference to cerebellar cysts and the association of polycythemia. *Arch Neurol Psychiatry*. 1952;67:237-252.

83. Melmon KL, Rosen SW. Lindau's disease: review of the literature and study of a large kindred. *Am J Med*. 1964;36:595-617.

84. Welch RB. von Hippel-Lindau disease: the recognition and treatment of early angiomatosis retinae and the use of cryosurgery as an adjunct to therapy. *Trans Am Ophthal Soc*. 1970;66:367-424.

85. Nicholson DH, Green WR, Kenyon KR. Light and electron microscopic study of early lesions in angiomatosis retinae. *Am J Ophthalmol*. 1976;82:193-204.

86. Jakobiec F, Font RL, Johnson FB. Angiomatosis retinae: an ultrastructural study and lipid analysis. *Cancer*. 1976;38:2042-2056.

87. Haining WM, Zweifach PH. Fluorescein angiography in von Hippel-Lindau disease. *Arch Ophthalmol*. 1967;78:475-479.

88. Gass JDM. Treatment of retinal vascular anomalies. Symposium: retinal vascular disease. *Trans Am Acad Ophthalmol Otolaryngol*. 1977;83:432.

89. Bourneville DM. Sclerose tubereuse der circonvolutions cerebrales: idiotie et epilepsie hemiplegique. *Arch Neurol (Paris)*. 1880;1:91-91.

90. Vogt H. Zur Pathologie und pathologischen Anatomie der verschiedenen Idiotieformen. *Mschr Psychiat Neurol*. 1908;24:106-117.

91. Wiederholt WC, Gomez MR, Kurland LT. Incidence and prevalence of tuberous sclerosis in Rochester, Minnesota, 1950 through 1982. *Neurology*. 1985;35:600-603.

92. Hunt A, Lindenbaum RH. Tuberous sclerosis: a new estimate of prevalence within the Oxford region. *J Med Genet*. 1984;21:272-277.

93. Flinter FA, Neville BGR. Examining the parents of children with tuberous sclerosis. *Lancet*. 1986;2:1167.

94. Fryer AE, Chalmers A, Connor JM, et al. Evidence that the gene for tuberous sclerosis is on chromosome 9. *Lancet*. 1987;1:659-661.

95. Gomez MR. *Tuberous Sclerosis*. New York, NY: Raven Press; 1979.

96. Lagos JC, Gomez MR. Tuberous sclerosis: reappraisal of a clinical entity. *Mayo Clin Proc*. 1967;42:26-49.

97. Williams R, Taylor D. Tuberous sclerosis. *Surv Ophthalmol*. 1985;30:143-154.

98. Kroll AJ, Ricker DP, Robb RM, et al. Vitreous hemorrhage complicating retinal astrocytic hamartoma. *Surv Ophthalmol*. 1981;26:31-38.

99. Jost BF, Oik RJ. Atypical retinitis proliferans retinal telangiectasis, and vitreous hemorrhage in a patient with tuberous sclerosis. *Retina*. 1986;6:53-56.

100. Coppeto JR, Lubin JR, Albert DM. Astrocytic hamartoma in tuberous sclerosis mimicking necrotizing retinochoroiditis. *J Pediatr Ophthalmol Strabismus*. 1982;19:306-313.

101. Wolter JR, Mertus JM. Exophytic retinal astrocytoma in tuberous sclerosis. *J Pediatr Ophthalmol*. 1969;6:186.

102. Eagle RC, Shields JA, Shields CL, et al. Hamartomas of the iris and ciliary epithelium in tuberous sclerosis complex. *Arch Ophthalmol*. 2000;118:711-715.

103. Louis-Bar D. Sur un syndrome progressif cormprenant des télangiectasies capillaires cutanées et conjonctivales symétriques, à disposition naevoïde et des troubles cérébelleux. *Confin Neurol*. 1941;4:32-42.

104. Boder E, Sedgwick RP. Ataxia telangiectasia: familial syndrome of progressive cerebellar ataxia, oculocutaneous telangiectasia, and frequent pulmonary infection. *Pediatrics*. 1958; 21:526-554.

105. Gatti RA, Berkel I, Boder E, et al. Localization of an ataxia telangiectasia gene to chromosome llq22-23. *Nature*. 1988;336: 577-580.

106. Saxon A, Stevens RH, Golde DW. Helper and suppressor T-lymphocyte leukemia in ataxia telangiectasia. *N Engl J Med*. 1979;300:700-704.

107. Baloh RW, Yee RD, Boder E. Eye movements in ataxia-telangiectasia. *Neurology*. 1978;28:1099-1104.

108. Stell R, Bronstein AM, Plant GT, et al. Ataxia telangiectasia: a reappraisal of the ocular motor features and their value in the diagnosis of atypical cases. *Movement Disorders*. 1989;4:320-329.

109. Arman KF, Shalev B, Crawford TO, et al. Ocular manifestations of ataxia-telangiectasia. *Am J Ophthalmol*. 2002;134:891-896.

110. Wyburn-Mason R. Arteriovenous aneurysm of mid-brain and retina, facial naevi, and mental changes. *Brain*. 1943;66:163.

111. Bech K, Jenson OA. On the frequency of coexisting racemose haemangiomata of the retina and brain. *Acta Psychiatr Scand*. 1961;36:47-56.

112. Theron J, Newton TH, Hoyt WF. Unilateral retinocephalic vascular malformations. *Neuroradiology*. 1974;7:185.

113. Archer DB, Deutman A, Ernest JT, et al. Arteriovenous communications of the retina. *Am J Ophthalmol*. 1973;75:224-241.

114. Hopen G, Smith JL, Hoff JT, Quencer R. The Wyburn-mason syndrome: concomitant chiasmal and fundus vascular malformations. *J Clin Neurol Ophthalmol*. 1983;3:53-62.

115. Schmidt D, Pache M, Schumacher M. The congenital unilateral retinocephalic vascular malformation syndrome (Bonnet-Dechaume-Blanc syndrome or Wyburn-Mason syndrome): review of the literature. *Surv Ophthalmol*. 2008;53:227-249.

116. Effron L, Zakov ZN, Tomsak RL. Neovascular glaucoma as a complication of the Wyburn-mason syndrome. *J Clin Neuro Ophthalmol*. 1985;5:95-98.

117. Robinson S. Naevus sebaceous (Jadassohn): report of 4 cases. *Arch Dermatol*. 1932;26:663.

118. Mehregan AH, Pinkus H. Life history of organoid nevi. Special reference to the nevus sebaceous of Jadassohn. *Arch Dermatol*. 1965;91:574-588.

119. Katz B, Wiley CA, Lee VW. Optic nerve hypoplasia and the syndrome of nevus sebaceous of Jadassohn. A new association. *Ophthalmology*. 1987;94:1570-1576.

120. Domingo J, Helwig EB. Malignant neoplasms associated with nevus sebaceous of Jadassohn. *J Am Acad Dermatol.* 1979;1:545-556.

121. Baker RS, Ross PA, Baumann RJ. Neurological complications of the epidermal nevus syndrome. *Arch Neurol.* 1987;44(2):227-232.

122. Wilkes SR, Campbell RJ, Waller RR. Ocular malformation in association with ipsilateral facial nevus of Jadassohn. *Am J Ophthalmol.* 1981;92:344-352.

123. Schochot Y, Romano A, Barishak YR. Eye findings in the linear sebaceous nevus syndrome: a possible clue to the pathogenesis. *J Craniofac Genet Dev Biol.* 1982;2:289-294.

124. Binkley GW, Johnson HH Jr. Epithelioma adenoides cysticum: basal cell nevi, agenesis of the corpus callosum, and dental cysts. *Arch Dermatol Syph.* 1951;63:73-84.

125. Southwick GJ, Schwartz RA. The basal cell nevus syndrome: disasters occurring among a series of 36 patients. *Cancer.* 1979;44: 2294-2305.

126. Nerad JA, Whitaker DC. Periocular basal cell carcinoma in adults 35 years of age and younger. *Am J Ophthalmol.* 1988;106:723-729.

127. Markovits A, Quickert M. Basal cell nevus. *Arch Ophthalmol.* 1972;88:397-399.

128. Fehman S, Apt L, Roth A. The basal cell nevus syndrome. *Am J Ophthalmol.* 1974;78:222-228.

129. Gorlin RJ, Vickers RA, Kellen E, Williamson JJ. The multiple basal cell nevi syndrome. An analysis of a syndrome consisting of multiple nevoid basal-cell carcinoma, jaw cysts, skeletal anomalies, medulloblastoma, and hyporesponsiveness to parathormone. *Cancer.* 1965;18:89-104.

130. Kahn LB, Gordon W. Basal cell naevus syndrome—a report of a case. *S Afr Med J.* 1967;41:832-835.

131. Chan HH, Kono T. Nevus of Ota: clinical aspects and management. *Skinmed.* 2003;2(2):89-96.

132. Gonder JR, Shields JA, Albert DM. malignant melanoma of the choroid associated with oculodermal melanocytosis. *Ophthalmology.* 1981;88:372-376.

133. Teekhasaenee C, Ritch R, Rutnin U, Leelawongs N. Glaucoma in oculodermal melanocytosis. *Ophthalmology.* 1990;97:562-570.

134. Foulks GN, Shields MB. Glaucoma in oculodermal melanocytosis. *Ann Ophthalmol.* 1977;9:1299-1304.

135. Weiss DI, Krohn DL. Benign melanocytic glaucoma complicating oculodermal melanocytosis. *Ann Ophthalmol.* 1975,3:958.

136. Lohuizen C. Über eine seltene angeborene Hautanomalie (Cutis marmorata telangiectatica congenita). *Acta Derm Venereol.* 1922;3:202-211.

137. South DA, Jacobs AH. Cutis marmorata telangiectatica congenita. *Pediatrics.* 1978;93:944.

138. Spitzer MS, Szurman P, Rohrbach JM, Aisenbrey S. Bilateral congenital glaucoma in a child with cutis marmorata telangiectatica congenita: a case report. *Klin Monbl Augenheilkd.* 2007;224(1):66-69.

139. Miranda I, Alonso MJ, Jimenez M, Tomas-Barberan S, Ferro M, Ruiz R. Cutis marmorata telangiectatica congenita and glaucoma. *Ophthalmic Paediatr Genet.* 1990;11(2):129-132.

140. Murphy CC, Khong CH, Ward WJ, Morgan WH. Late-onset pediatric glaucoma associated with cutis marmorata telangiectatica congenita managed with Molteno implant surgery: case report and review of the literature. *J AAPOS.* 2001;11(5):519-521.

141. Sato SE, Herschler J, Lynch PJ, et al. Congenital glaucoma associated with cutis marmorata telangiectatica congenita: two case reports. *J Pediatr Ophthalmol Strabismus.* 1988;25:13-17.

142. Kremer I, Metzker A, Yassur Y. Intraoperative suprachoroidal hemorrhage in congenital glaucoma associated with cutis marmorata telangiectatica congenita. *Arch Ophthalmol.* 1991;109: 1199-1200.

Juvenile Open-Angle Glaucoma

Janey L. Wiggs, MD, PhD

Primary open-angle glaucoma (POAG) that develops in patients younger than 40 years of age has been called juvenile-onset POAG (JOAG) or early-onset POAG.[1-4] This disorder is less common than adult-onset POAG and typically is associated with severely elevated intraocular pressure (IOP) that frequently requires surgical therapy. Affected individuals have a clinically normal anterior segment, without features of anterior segment dysgenesis. The normal development of the angle structures in JOAG patients suggests that the elevation of IOP occurs as a consequence of a molecular abnormality that may be more amenable to gene-based therapies than the anatomically abnormal angle that is the consequence of defective ocular development.

The age of onset for JOAG is variable, and although the disease typically develops between 3 and 20 years of age, the disease can be first diagnosed decades later. Family history of glaucoma is frequently found in patients with JOAG; however, the age of onset may vary considerably among family members.[5] Juvenile glaucoma has been previously classified as true juvenile glaucoma, neglected infantile (congenital) glaucoma, presenile glaucoma, and angle-closure glaucoma. The discussion in this chapter refers to the form of juvenile glaucoma previously classified as true juvenile glaucoma. The disease process is characterized by a severe high-pressure glaucoma that can result in significant damage to the optic nerve leaving affected individuals with little useful vision early in life. Although early-onset glaucoma may be a component of chromosome syndromes and other systemic disorders,[6] there are no consistent systemic findings in patients with true JOAG.

Characteristic ocular features often include a high incidence of myopia.[7] Affected eyes do not show signs of buphthalmos. The cornea does not demonstrate breaks in Descemet's membrane. Gonioscopy typically shows a normal appearance to the angle structures. There is no evidence of increased pigment deposition in the angle or other findings consistent with the pigment dispersion syndrome. Some patients with JOAG may have an increased number of iris processes, some of which have an anterior insertion crossing the scleral spur and posterior trabecular meshwork (TM). However, this is not a consistently identified finding, and these patients do not have any of the other features of developmental glaucoma, including posterior embryotoxon.[1] JOAG patients do not have a Barkan membrane covering the angle as is typical of patients affected by congenital glaucoma. One histopathologic study[8] suggested that a thick compact tissue on the anterior chamber side of Schlemm's canal was present in 10 cases of juvenile glaucoma. In these 10 patients, the mechanism of glaucoma was postulated to be a developmental immaturity of the TM.[8] Other specific anatomical abnormalities have not been identified in patients with juvenile glaucoma.

Patients affected by JOAG may be successfully treated medically but frequently require surgical intervention for adequate IOP control. Medical treatment with latanoprost[9] has been shown to be particularly effective in JOAG patients. Patients have also been treated effectively by goniotomy,[10] trabeculectomy,[11] viscocanalostomy,[12] and valve implants.[13] For some JOAG patients with Myocilin mutations, genotype-phenotype correlations can help guide therapeutic decisions based on expected disease prognosis.

JOAG is commonly inherited as an autosomal dominant trait. The early onset of disease leads to the formation of large multigenerational families that are suitable for linkage analyses. Five of the 29 open-angle glaucoma genetic loci are primarily associated with JOAG: GLC1A, GLC1J, GLC1K, GLC1M, and GLC1N.[4,14-16] Myocilin is the gene located in the GLC1A region, and mutations in these genes account for 10% to 20% of cases of JOAG and also up to 5% of adult-onset POAG.[17-19] Disease-causing mutations (both early- and late-onset glaucoma) have been found primarily in the third axon that codes for the olfactomedin-like

Kahook MY, Schuman JS, eds.
Chandler and Grant's Glaucoma, Fifth Edition (pp 465–467).
© 2013 SLACK Incorporated.

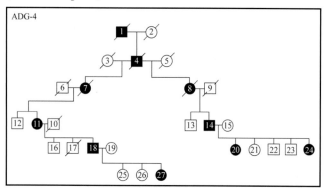

Figure 50-1. Juvenile glaucoma pedigree (ADG-4). Affected individuals are shown as solid circles (females) or squares (males). Deceased individuals not available for linkage analysis are indicated with slashes. All affected members of this pedigree have the Myocilin Pro370Leu mutation.

portion of the protein.[18-22] Mutations in the protein appear to cause misfolding of the nascent polypeptide chain, leading to accumulation of precipitated protein in the endoplasmic reticulum and subsequent cell death.[23-26] The loss of the Myocilin protein due to null alleles or gene deletion does not cause glaucoma.[27-29] A transgenic mouse containing one of the most severe human mutations (TYR437HIS) has a glaucoma phenotype.[30] Aggregation of mutant Myocilin has recently been shown to be inhibited in vitro by small molecule chemical chaperones,[31,32] a result that may lead to future therapies for individuals with glaucoma caused by Myocilin mutations.

Myocilin mutations may cause early- (before 10 years of age), middle- (between 10 and 30 years of age), and late-onset (older than 40 years of age) POAG. There are more than 50 different disease-associated Myocilin mutations, and the majority are missense changes rather than insertion/deletion mutations or nonsense mutations.[19] Families affected with glaucoma caused by a Myocilin mutation may have a consistent age of onset or may show significant intrafamilial variability. The penetrance of the condition is felt to be high, although formal penetrance studies have not been completed. Myocilin mutations that are consistently associated with severe early-onset disease include Pro370Leu[33,34] (Figure 50-1) and Tyr437His.[35] The Gln368Stop mutation is primarily associated with adult-onset (older than 40 yeras of age) disease.[36,37] Several mutations are associated with an intermediate phenotype[38] including the Thr377Met mutation.[39,40]

Myocilin is currently the only gene known to cause JOAG glaucoma, and the fact that mutations in this gene account for at most 10% of early-onset primary open-angle glaucoma cases[17,18] suggests that JOAG is a genetically heterogeneous disease and that other genes are likely to be responsible for this disorder. Genome-wide linkage studies have revealed new loci for JOAG: GLC1J (9q22)[4]; GLC1K (20p12)[4]; GLC1M (5q22)[16]; and GLC1N (15q).[15] The causative genes located in GLC1J and GLC1K have not yet been identified; however,

the size of the GLC1K locus has been refined.[41] An important candidate gene, neuregulin, has been excluded from GLC1M,[16] and the region defined by GLC1N contains the LOXL1 gene known to contribute to exfoliation syndrome.[15] Current evidence suggests that LOXL1 does not contribute to glaucoma independent of exfoliation syndrome and that another gene in this region is likely responsible for early-onset glaucoma.[42] GLC1I, a genomic region associated with early adult-onset POAG, is also located on chromosome 15 and may overlap with GLC1N.[43] The identification of new JOAG genes will help define the underlying pathophysiology of the condition as well as lead to the development of DNA-based screening tests and novel therapeutics.

REFERENCES

1. Turalba AV, Chen TC. Clinical and genetic characteristics of primary juvenile-onset open-angle glaucoma (JOAG). *Semin Ophthalmol.* 2008;23(1):19-25.
2. Wiggs JL, Del Bono EA, Schuman JS, Hutchinson BT, Walton DS. Clinical features of five pedigrees genetically linked to the juvenile glaucoma locus on chromosome 1q21-q31. *Ophthalmology.* 1995;102(12):1782-1789.
3. Wiggs JL, Damji KF, Haines JL, Pericak-Vance MA, Allingham RR. The distinction between juvenile and adult-onset primary open-angle glaucoma. *Am J Hum Genet.* 1996;58(1):243-244.
4. Wiggs JL, Lynch S, Ynagi G, et al. A genomewide scan identifies novel early-onset primary open-angle glaucoma loci on 9q22 and 20p12. *Am J Hum Genet.* 2004;74(6):1314-1320.
5. Wirtz MK, Samples JR, Choi D, Gaudette ND. Clinical features associated with an Asp380His Myocilin mutation in a US family with primary open-angle glaucoma. *Am J Ophthalmol.* 2007;144(1):75-80.
6. Saha K, Lloyd IC, Russell-Eggitt IM, Taylor DS. Chromosomal abnormalities and glaucoma: a case of congenital glaucoma associated with 9p deletion syndrome. *Ophthalmic Genet.* 2007;28(2):69-72.
7. Ko YC, Liu CJ, Chou JC, Chen MR, Hsu WM, Liu JH. Comparisons of risk factors and visual field changes between juvenile-onset and late-onset primary open-angle glaucoma. *Ophthalmologica.* 2002;216(1):27-32.
8. Tawara A, Inomata H. Developmental immaturity of the trabecular meshwork in juvenile glaucoma. *Am J Ophthalmol.* 1984;98:82-97.
9. Black AC, Jones S, Yanovitch TL, Enyedi LB, Stinnett SS, Freedman SF. Latanoprost in pediatric glaucoma--pediatric exposure over a decade. *J AAPOS.* 2009;13(6):558-562.
10. Yeung HH, Walton DS. Goniotomy for juvenile open-angle glaucoma. *J Glaucoma.* 2010;19(1):1-4.
11. Park SC, Kee C. Large diurnal variation of intraocular pressure despite maximal medical treatment in juvenile open angle glaucoma. *J Glaucoma.* 2007;16(1):164-168.
12. Stangos AN, Whatham AR, Sunaric-Megevand G. Primary viscocanalostomy for juvenile open-angle glaucoma. *Am J Ophthalmol.* 2005;140(3):490-496.
13. Wilson MR, Mendis U, Paliwal A, Haynatzka V. Long-term follow-up of primary glaucoma surgery with Ahmed glaucoma valve implant versus trabeculectomy. *Am J Ophthalmol.* 2003;136(3):464-470.
14. Stone EM, Fingert JH, Alward WL, et al. Identification of a gene that causes primary open angle glaucoma. *Science.* 1997;275(5300):668-670.
15. Wang DY, Fan BJ, Chua JK, et al. A genome-wide scan maps a novel juvenile-onset primary open-angle glaucoma locus to 15q. *Invest Ophthalmol Vis Sci.* 2006;47(12):5315-5321.

16. Fan BJ, Ko WC, Wang DY, et al. Fine mapping of new glaucoma locus GLC1M and exclusion of neuregulin 2 as the causative gene. *Mol Vis.* 2007;13:779-784.

17. Wiggs JL, Allingham RR, Vollrath D, et al. Prevalence of mutations in TIGR/Myocilin in patients with adult and juvenile primary open-angle glaucoma. *Am J Hum Genet.* 1998;63(5):1549-1552.

18. Fingert JH, Héon E, Liebmann JM, et al. Analysis of myocilin mutations in 1703 glaucoma patients from five different populations. *Hum Mol Genet.* 1999;8(5):899-905.

19. Hewitt AW, Mackey DA, Craig JE. Myocilin allele-specific glaucoma phenotype database. *Hum Mutat.* 2008;29(2):207-211.

20. Rozsa FW, Shimizu S, Lichter PR, et al. GLC1A mutations point to regions of potential functional importance on the TIGR/MYOC protein. *Mol Vis.* 1998;4:20.

21. Alward WL, Kwon YH, Khanna CL, et al. Variations in the myocilin gene in patients with open-angle glaucoma. *Arch Ophthalmol.* 2002;120:1189-1197.

22. Graul TA, Kwon YH, Zimmerman MB, et al. A case-control comparison of the clinical characteristics of glaucoma and ocular hypertensive patients with and without the myocilin Gln368Stop mutation. *Am J Ophthalmol.* 2002;134:884-890.

23. Joe MK, Sohn S, Hur W, Moon Y, Choi YR, Kee C. Accumulation of mutant myocilins in ER leads to ER stress and potential cytotoxicity in human trabecular meshwork cells. *Biochem Biophys Res Commun.* 2003;312(3):592-600.

24. Liu Y, Vollrath D. Reversal of mutant myocilin nonsecretion and cell killing: implications for glaucoma. *Hum Mol Genet.* 2004;13(11):1193-1204.

25. Vollrath D, Liu Y. Temperature sensitive secretion of mutant myocilins. *Exp Eye Res.* 2006;82(6):1030-1036.

26. Gould DB, Reedy M, Wilson LA, Smith RS, Johnson RL, John SW. Mutant myocilin nonsecretion in vivo is not sufficient to cause glaucoma. *Mol Cell Biol.* 2006;26(22):8427-8436.

27. Wiggs JL, Vollrath D. Molecular and clinical evaluation of a patient hemizygous for TIGR/Myocilin. *Arch Ophthalmol.* 2001;119:1674-1678.

28. Kim BS, Savinova OV, Reedy MV, et al. Targeted disruption of the myocilin gene (Myoc) suggests that human glaucoma-causing mutations are gain of function. *Mol Cell Biol.* 2001;21(22):7707-7713.

29. Lam DSC, Leung YF, Chua JK, et al. Truncations in the TIGR gene in individuals with and without primary open-angle glaucoma. *Invest Ophthalmol Vis Sci.* 2000;41:1386-1391.

30. Zhou Y, Grinchuk O, Tomarev SI. Transgenic mice expressing the Tyr437His mutant of human myocilin protein develop glaucoma. *Invest Ophthalmol Vis Sci.* 2008;49(5):1932-1939.

31. Burns JN, Orwig SD, Harris JL, Watkins JD, Vollrath D, Lieberman RL. Rescue of glaucoma-causing mutant myocilin thermal stability by chemical chaperones. *ACS Chem Biol.* 2010;5(5):477-487.

32. Jia LY, Gong B, Pang CP, et al. Correction of the disease phenotype of myocilin-causing glaucoma by a natural osmolyte. *Invest Ophthalmol Vis Sci.* 2009;50(8):3743-3749.

33. Shimizu S, Lichter PR, Johnson AT, et al. Age-dependent prevalence of mutations at the GLC1A locus in primary open-angle glaucoma. *Am J Ophthalmol.* 2000;130(2):165-177.

34. Zhuo YH, Wei YT, Bai YJ, et al. Pro370Leu MYOC gene mutation in a large Chinese family with juvenile-onset open angle glaucoma: correlation between genotype and phenotype. *Mol Vis.* 2008;14:1533-1539.

35. Fingert JH, Stone EM, Sheffield VC, Alward WL. Myocilin glaucoma. *Surv Ophthalmol.* 2002;47(6):547-561.

36. Angius A, Spinelli P, Ghilotti G, et al. Myocilin Gln368stop mutation and advanced age as risk factors for late-onset primary open-angle glaucoma. *Arch Ophthalmol.* 2000;118(5):674-679.

37. Allingham RR, Wiggs JL, De La Paz MA, et al. Gln368STOP myocilin mutation in families with late-onset primary open-angle glaucoma. *Invest Ophthalmol Vis Sci.* 1998;39(12):2288-2295.

38. Hewitt AW, Bennett SL, Richards JE, et al. Myocilin Gly252Arg mutation and glaucoma of intermediate severity in Caucasian individuals. *Arch Ophthalmol.* 2007;125(1):98-104.

39. Hewitt AW, Samples JR, Allingham RR, et al. Investigation of founder effects for the Thr377Met Myocilin mutation in glaucoma families from differing ethnic backgrounds. *Mol Vis.* 2007;13:487-492.

40. Wirtz MK, Samples JR, Toumanidou V, et al. Association of POAG risk factors and the Thr377Met MYOC mutation in an isolated Greek population. *Invest Ophthalmol Vis Sci.* 2010;51(6):3055-3060.

41. Sud A, Del Bono EA, Haines JL, Wiggs JL. Fine mapping of the GLC1K juvenile primary open-angle glaucoma locus and exclusion of candidate genes. *Mol Vis.* 2008;14:1319-1326.

42. Liu Y, Schmidt S, Qin X, et al. Lack of association between LOXL1 variants and primary open-angle glaucoma in three different populations. *Invest Ophthalmol Vis Sci.* 2008;49(8):3465-3468.

43. Allingham RR, Wiggs JL, Hauser ER, et al. Early adult-onset POAG linked to 15q11-13 using ordered subset analysis. *Invest Ophthalmol Vis Sci.* 2005;46(6):2002-2005.

SECTION *VIII*

LASER METHODS IN GLAUCOMA

51

Glaucoma Laser Surgery

Jeremy B. Wingard, MD and Joel S. Schuman, MD, FACS

Since the previous editions of this book, glaucoma laser surgery has progressed in several areas. Some of the most notable advances have been innovations in laser trabeculoplasty (LTP) and the technological advances of endoscopic cyclophotocoagulation (ECP) and excimer laser trabeculotomy. Additionally, lasers have remained useful for gonioplasty to shrink the iris away from the trabecular meshwork (TM) in cases of early peripheral anterior synechiae (PAS) or plateau iris; for laser suture lysis, to titrate intraocular pressure (IOP) after trabeculectomy; for treatment of failing blebs, to incise areas of episcleral or subconjunctival fibrosis; in instances of hypotony, to coagulate, scar, and induce inflammation in the conjunctiva, or to cause adhesion of the conjunctiva to the underlying episclera. Lasers are now rarely used for goniophotocoagulation, to ablate new blood vessels growing in the TM while waiting for panretinal photocoagulation to take effect; or for goniopuncture, in which the neodymium:yttrium-aluminum-garnet (Nd:YAG) laser is aimed at the TM to open channels into Schlemm's canal, in cases such as juvenile open-angle glaucoma and angle-recession glaucoma, in which a hyaline membrane is thought to obstruct outflow.[1-3]

An overview of glaucoma laser therapy is presented in Tables 51-1 and 51-2. Each of these applications is covered throughout the chapters of this section, "Laser Methods in Glaucoma." LTP, which has proven effective in postponing trabeculectomy, or in some cases eliminating the need for filtering surgery entirely, has been studied extensively since the fourth edition of this book.[4-15] Although the exact mechanism by which this procedure functions is still not known, insight has been gained into its workings and effects. In this way, realistic expectations allow the clinician to apply this technique in the appropriate settings and to anticipate the outcome of such treatment. The last decade has provided demonstrations of the comparative effectiveness of selective LTP (SLT) compared

with argon LTP, [6,9,12,13] and SLT has become the treatment of choice in many centers. Other wavelengths are available for performing LTP as well, the effects of which are relatively wavelength-independent. In fact, nearly any photocoagulator, including the argon, diode,[16,17] krypton, and continuous wave Nd:YAG laser (different from the Q-switched, pulsed Nd:YAG laser used for photodisruption), can be successfully employed for LTP. Recently, multipulse technologies, utilizing 100-μs pulses with a low-duty cycle, have been studied as a means to lower the total energy delivered to the TM in LTP.[18]

Since publication of the previous edition, the pulsed Nd:YAG laser has remained the preferred instrument for performing laser peripheral iridotomy (LPI). We have learned that such iridotomies are, in fact, more likely to retain their patency than those created with the argon laser.[19-24] Photocoagulators, such as those mentioned for LTP, have their place in LPI, as they coagulate blood vessels, thin the iris, and do not induce bleeding at the time of LPI; however, LPI is more efficient and long lasting when done with the Nd:YAG laser or with a combination of a photocoagulator and photodisruptor.[23,24]

When the fourth edition was published, laser cyclophotocoagulation (CPC) had just supplanted cyclocryotherapy (CCT) as the cyclodestructive procedure of choice in advanced glaucoma uncontrolled by maximal tolerated medical therapy. This modality remains a gentler means to reduce aqueous production and perhaps slightly increase outflow as compared with CCT. Contact trans-scleral Nd:YAG or diode laser CPC causes little postoperative discomfort but carries with it the same risks for hypotony and visual loss as CCT; therefore, laser CPC remains a procedure of last resort. Since the last edition, however, technology has emerged and developed that allows ECP, direct intraoperative diode laser application to the ciliary processes without the same degree of tissue destruction as trans-scleral CPC.[25-36] This relative

Kahook MY, Schuman JS, eds.
Chandler and Grant's Glaucoma, Fifth Edition (pp 471-475).
© 2013 SLACK Incorporated.

TABLE 51-1. GLAUCOMA LASER THERAPY		
Procedure	**Laser**	**Settings**
LTP	Argon green	50-μm spot; 0.1 s; 300 to 1000 mW; 35 to 50 spots over 180; Goldmann (Haag-Streit, Bern, Switzerland) or Ritch lens (Ocular Instruments, Bellevue, WA).
	Diode	50- to 75-μm spot; 0.1 s; 750 to 1250 mW; 35 to 50 spots over 180; Goldmann or Ritch lens.
	SLT	400-μm spot; 3 ns; 0.4 to 1.4 mJ/spot; 100 spots over 360; Latina SLT lens (Ocular Instruments).
Laser iridotomy	Nd:YAG	4 to 8 mJ; 1 to 3 applications; Abraham lens (Ocular Instruments).
	Argon green	Short pulse technique (dark-brown iris): 50-μm spot; 0.02 to 0.05 s; 1000 to 1500 mW; 20 to 50 spots; Abraham or Wise lens (Ocular Instruments). Long pulse technique (blue, hazel, or light-brown iris): 50-μm spot; 0.2 s; 1000 mW; 20 to 30 spots; Abraham or Wise lens.
Combined argon or diode and Nd:YAG laser iridotomy	Diode	50- to 75-μm spot; 0.05 to 0.1 s; 750 to 1250 mW; 20 to 50 spots; Abraham or Wise lens.
	Argon/diode: Nd:YAG	50-μm spot; 0.02 to 0.05 s; 1000 mW; 5 to 10 spots. 4 to 6 mJ; 1 to 3 bursts of 3 pulses per burst; Abraham lens.
Laser CPC	Contact cwNd:YAG	7 W; 0.7 s; 24 to 32 spots; probe centered 1.5 to 2 mm posterior to limbus; sapphire-tipped probe.
	Contact diode	3 W; 1.3 to 1.5 s; 18 spots; probe with automatic offset of 1.2 mm from limbus (G-Probe [Iridex, Mountain View, CA]).
	Endoscopic diode	Continuous wave energy, adjustable from 250 mW starting point; probe 2 mm from tissue (Endo Optiks [Little Silver, NJ] probe, available curved or straight).
Laser sclerectomy	Holmium	100 mJ/pulse; 20 to 30 pulses to perforate; side-firing fiberoptic.
	cwNd:YAG	10 to 12 W; 1.0 s; 2 to 5 spots to penetrate; synthetic sapphire tip.
Laser trabeculotomy	XeCl excimer	200-μm spot; 80 ns; 1.2 mJ/pulse; 8 spots separated by 500 μm.[38]
Laser gonioplasty	Argon; diode	200- to 500-μm spot; 0.2 to 0.5 s; 200 to 400 mW; 24 to 32 spots in far periphery; Goldmann lens.
Laser suture lysis	Argon; diode	50-μm spot; 0.01 s; 300 to 800 mW; 1 or more spots; Hoskins lens (Ocular Instruments).
Laser to conjunctiva (hypotony)	Argon; diode	Paint bleb with 2% fluorescein or methylene blue for argon; indocyanine green for diode laser. 200-μm spot; 0.5 s; 200 to 300 mW; 30 to 50 spots or more covering as much conjunctiva as possible.
Laser goniophotocoagulation	Argon	50-μm spot; 0.1 s; 1000 mW; sufficient spots to blanch vessel trunks.
Laser goniopuncture	Nd:YAG	5 to 7 mJ; 3 pulses per burst; fire through TM until bright-white of outer wall of Schlemm's canal is seen. Begin inferiorly as may get blood reflux. Open 1 to 2 clock-hours.

cwNd:YAG: continuous wave neodymium:yttrium-aluminum-garnet; 5-FU: 5-fluorouracil; SLT: selective laser trabeculoplasty; TM: trabecular meshwork; XeCl: xenon chloride.

Procedure	Preoperative	Postoperative
LTP	Brimonidine 0.1% to 0.2%	ALT: prednisolone acetate 1% qid for 4 days; then stop. Check IOP at 1 hour; 1 day; 1 week; and 4 to 6 weeks. SLT: topical NSAID may be given for discomfort (eg, ketorolac 0.5% qid as needed for 4 days). Check IOP at 1 hour; 2 weeks; and 6 to 8 weeks.
Laser iridotomy	Brimonidine 0.1% to 0.2%; pilocarpine 2% × 3	Prednisolone acetate 1% hourly for 1 day; then qid for 4 days; then stop. Check IOP at 1 hour; 1 day; 1 week; and 4 weeks. Gonioscopy at 1 and 4 weeks and dilation at 4 weeks.
Laser CPC	Brimonidine 0.1% to 0.2%; retrobulbar Lidocaine 2%/bupivacaine (Marcaine) 0.75%/hyaluronidase (Wydase) 150 units	Prednisolone acetate 1% qid and atropine 1% bid until inflammation subsides. Continue all preoperative antiglaucoma medications; with exception of miotics (may resume when eye quiet).
Laser trabeculotomy	Lidocaine 4%	Tobramycin-dexamethasone drops qid × 14 days.[38]
Laser gonioplasty	Brimonidine 0.1% to 0.2%; pilocarpine 2% × 3	Prednisolone acetate 1% hourly for 1 day; then qid for 4 days; then stop. Check IOP at 1 hour; 1 day; and 1 week. Gonioscopy and dilation at 1 week.
Laser suture lysis	Proparacaine 0.5%	Check IOP 1 hour after LSL. Do not cut more than 1 suture per day.
Laser to conjunctiva (hypotony)	Proparacaine 0.5%	Check IOP 1 hour; 1 day; and 1 week after procedure. If ineffective, may require repeat treatment or other intervention.
Laser goniophotocoagulation	Brimonidine 0.1% to 0.2%	Prednisolone acetate 1% hourly for 1 day; then qid for 4 days; then stop. Follow carefully for regression of vessels or regrowth.
Laser goniopuncture	Brimonidine 0.1% to 0.2%	Prednisolone acetate 1% hourly for 1 day; then qid for 4 days; then stop.

ALT: argon laser trabeculoplasty; IOP: intraocular pressure; LSL: laser suture lysis; NSAID: nonsteroidal anti-inflammatory drug; SLT: selective laser trabeculoplasty.

safety has led some practitioners to use ECP as a cyclodestructive procedure much earlier in the course of disease, although risks of hypotony and vision loss remain.[37]

Laser sclerectomy remains a technique in evolution. A variety of lasers have been investigated for this application, although randomized clinical trials are lacking to date. The prospect for this procedure is tantalizing: a minimally invasive means by which to perform filtering surgery with little or no conjunctival manipulation, perhaps even performed in the office. Recently, work has been completed in the related area of laser trabeculotomy, an attempt to treat the juxtacanalicular outflow obstruction believed to be the site of primary pathology in most open-angle glaucoma patients, without scleral perforation and therefore no filtering bleb. There has been one prospective, randomized study that shows promising results for ab interno laser trabeculotomy with the 308-nm xenon-chloride excimer laser.[38]

The list of miscellaneous procedures continues to grow as our experience with lasers increases. Gonioplasty is useful in eyes with angle closure despite a patent iridotomy, either to break PAS formed within the previous 6 months[39] or to thin the peripheral iris. Laser suture lysis allows titration of IOP in the early postoperative period but carries with it the risks of hypotony and conjunctival bleb leak (due to an inadvertent conjunctival burn). Laser treatment of the bleb tissue, using an absorbing dye such as 2% fluorescein, methylene blue, or indocyanine green, is effective in some cases of overfiltration with hypotony, inducing conjunctival contraction, scarring, and adhesion to the underlying sclera. Goniophotocoagulation, now rarely performed, can treat blood vessels encroaching on the TM in the postpanretinal photocoagulation period of neovascular glaucoma. In many settings, this technique has been replaced by intravitreal injection of vascular endothelial growth factor inhibitors, which have become widely available since the last edition of this text.

Each of these miscellaneous procedures requires the use of a photocoagulator, and each can be done with an argon or diode laser (or others). To incise tissue, as is necessary when treating a failing bleb or for goniopuncture, the pulsed Nd:YAG laser is needed. This is the same laser used for LPI or capsulotomy. Other pulsed lasers, such as the picosecond laser or excimer laser, although not widely available, can also be used for this task.

REFERENCES

1. Melamed S, Latina MA, Epstein DL. Neodymium:YAG laser trabeculopuncture in juvenile open-angle glaucoma. *Ophthalmology.* 1987;94(2):163-170.

2. Melamed S, Pei J, Puliafito CA, Epstein DL. Q-switched neodymium-YAG laser trabeculopuncture in monkeys. *Arch Ophthalmol.* 1985;103(1):129-133.

3. Epstein DL, Melamed S, Puliafto CA, Steinert RF. Neodymium:YAG laser trabeculopuncture in open-angle glaucoma. *Ophthalmology.* 1985;92(7):931-937.

4. Heijl A, Leske MC, Bengtsson B, et al. Reduction of intraocular pressure and glaucoma progression: results from the Early Manifest Glaucoma Trial. *Arch Ophthalmol.* 2002;120(10):1268-1279.

5. Hong BK, Winer JC, Martone JF, et al. Repeat selective laser trabeculoplasty. *J Glaucoma.* 2009;18(3):180-183.

6. Juzych MS, Chopra V, Banitt MR, et al. Comparison of long-term outcomes of selective laser trabeculoplasty versus argon laser trabeculoplasty in open-angle glaucoma. *Ophthalmology.* 2004;111(10):1853-1859.

7. Kramer TR, Noecker RJ. Comparison of the morphologic changes after selective laser trabeculoplasty and argon laser trabeculoplasty in human eye bank eyes. *Ophthalmology.* 2001;108(4):773-779.

8. Nagar M, Luhishi E, Shah N. Intraocular pressure control and fluctuation: the effect of treatment with selective laser trabeculoplasty. *Br J Ophthalmol.* 2009;93(4):497-501.

9. Russo V, Barone A, Cosma A, et al. Selective laser trabculoplasty versus argon laser trabeculoplasty in patients with uncontrolled open-angle glaucoma. *Eur J Ophthalmol.* 2009;19(3):429-434.

10. Goyal S, Beltran-Agullo L, Rashid S, et al. Effect of primary selective laser trabeculoplasty on tonographic outflow facility: a randomised clinical trial. *Br J Ophthalmol.* 2010;94(11):1443-1447.

11. Francis BA, Ianchulev T, Schofield JK, Minckler DS. Selective laser trabeculoplasty as a replacement for medical therapy in open-angle glaucoma. *Am J Ophthalmol.* 2005;140(3):524-525.

12. Damji KF, Bovell AM, Hodge WG, et al. Selective laser trabeculoplasty versus argon laser trabeculoplasty: results from a 1-year randomised clinical trial. *Br J Ophthalmol.* 2006;90(12):1490-1494.

13. Damji KF, Shah KC, Rock WJ, et al. Selective laser trabeculoplasty vs argon laser trabeculoplasty: a prospective randomised clinical trial. *Br J Ophthalmol.* 1999;83(6):718-722.

14. Chen TC. Brimonidine 0.15% versus apraclonidine 0.5% for prevention of intraocular pressure elevation after anterior segment laser surgery. *J Cataract Refract Surg.* 2005;31(9):1707-1712.

15. Latina MA, Sibayan SA, Shin DH, et al. Q-switched 532-nm Nd:YAG laser trabeculoplasty (selective laser trabeculoplasty): a multicenter, pilot, clinical study. *Ophthalmology.* 1998;105(11):2082-2088; discussion 9-90.

16. Agarwal HC, Poovali S, Sihota R, Dada T. Comparative evaluation of diode laser trabeculoplasty vs frequency doubled Nd:YAG laser trabeculoplasty in primary open angle glaucoma. *Eye (Lond).* 2006;20(12):1352-1356.

17. Chung PY, Schuman JS, Netland PA, et al. Five-year results of a randomized, prospective, clinical trial of diode vs argon laser trabeculoplasty for open-angle glaucoma. *Am J Ophthalmol.* 1998;126(2):185-190.

18. Fea AM, Bosone A, Rolle T, et al. Micropulse diode laser trabeculoplasty (MDLT): a phase II clinical study with 12 months follow-up. *Clin Ophthalmol.* 2008;2(2):247-252.

19. Latina MA, Puliafito CA, Steinert RR, Epstein DL. Experimental iridotomy with the Q-switched neodymium-YAG laser. *Arch Ophthalmol.* 1984;102(8):1211-1213.

20. Moster MR, Schwartz LW, Spaeth GL, et al. Laser iridectomy. A controlled study comparing argon and neodymium:YAG. *Ophthalmology.* 1986;93(1):20-24.

21. Pollack IP, Robin AL, Dragon DM, et al. Use of the neodymium:YAG laser to create iridotomies in monkeys and humans. *Trans Am Ophthalmol Soc.* 1984;82:307-328.

22. Richardson TM, Brown SV, Thomas JV, Simmons RJ. Shock-wave effect on anterior segment structures following experimental neodymium:YAG laser iridectomy. *Ophthalmology.* 1985;92(10):1387-1395.

23. Robin AL, Pollack IP. A comparison of neodymium:YAG and argon laser iridotomies. *Ophthalmology.* 1984;91(9):1011-1016.

24. Striga M, Curkovic T, Vukas Z. Combined technique of argon-laser and neodymium-YAG laser photocoagulation for narrow-or closed-angle glaucoma. *Acta Med Iugosl.* 1990;44(5):521-532.

25. Neely DE, Plager DA. Endocyclophotocoagulation for management of difficult pediatric glaucomas. *J AAPOS.* 2001;5(4):221-229.

26. Mora JS, Iwach AG, Gaffney MM, et al. Endoscopic diode laser cyclophotocoagulation with a limbal approach. *Ophthalmic Surg Lasers.* 1997;28(2):118-123.

27. Barkana Y, Morad Y, Ben-nun J. Endoscopic photocoagulation of the ciliary body after repeated failure of trans-scleral diode-laser cyclophotocoagulation. *Am J Ophthalmol.* 2002;133(3):405-407.

28. Lima FE, Magacho L, Carvalho DM, et al. A prospective, comparative study between endoscopic cyclophotocoagulation and the Ahmed drainage implant in refractory glaucoma. *J Glaucoma.* 2004;13(3):233-237.

29. Lin SC, Chen MJ, Lin MS, et al. Vascular effects on ciliary tissue from endoscopic versus trans-scleral cyclophotocoagulation. *Br J Ophthalmol.* 2006;90(4):496-500.

30. Al-Haddad CE, Freedman SF. Endoscopic laser cyclophotocoagulation in pediatric glaucoma with corneal opacities. *J AAPOS.* 2007;11(1):23-28.

31. Carter BC, Plager DA, Neely DE, et al. Endoscopic diode laser cyclophotocoagulation in the management of aphakic and pseudophakic glaucoma in children. *J AAPOS.* 2007;11(1):34-40.

32. Kahook MY, Lathrop KL, Noecker RJ. One-site versus two-site endoscopic cyclophotocoagulation. *J Glaucoma.* 2007;16(6):527-530.

33. Pantcheva MB, Kahook MY, Schuman JS, Noecker RJ. Comparison of acute structural and histopathological changes in human autopsy eyes after endoscopic cyclophotocoagulation and trans-scleral cyclophotocoagulation. *Br J Ophthalmol.* 2007;91(2):248-252.

34. Pantcheva MB, Kahook MY, Schuman JS, et al. Comparison of acute structural and histopathological changes of the porcine ciliary processes after endoscopic cyclophotocoagulation and transscleral cyclophotocoagulation. *Clin Experiment Ophthalmol.* 2007;35(3):270-274.

35. Yu JY, Kahook MY, Lathrop KL, Noecker RJ. The effect of probe placement and type of viscoelastic material on endoscopic cyclophotocoagulation laser energy transmission. *Ophthalmic Surg Lasers Imaging.* 2008;39(2):133-136.

36. Yip LW, Yong SO, Earnest A, et al. Endoscopic cyclophotocoagulation for the treatment of glaucoma: an Asian experience. *Clin Experiment Ophthalmol.* 2009;37(7):692-697.

37. Ahmad S, Wallace DJ, Herndon LW. Phthisis after endoscopic cyclophotocoagulation. *Ophthalmic Surg Lasers Imaging.* 2008;39(5):407-408.

38. Babighian S, Caretti L, Tavolato M, et al. Excimer laser trabeculotomy vs 180 degrees selective laser trabeculoplasty in primary open-angle glaucoma. A 2-year randomized, controlled trial. *Eye (Lond).* 2010;24(4):632-638.

39. Weiss HS, Shingleton BJ, Goode SM, et al. Argon laser gonioplasty in the treatment of angle-closure glaucoma. *Am J Ophthalmol.* 1992;114(1):14-18.

Laser Trabeculoplasty

Jeremy B. Wingard, MD and Joel S. Schuman, MD, FACS

Because the tissue between the anterior chamber and Schlemm's canal is the site of both normal resistance to aqueous humor outflow and abnormal resistance,[1] it was natural to attempt to penetrate this tissue with the laser and thus bypass the abnormality. However, similar to the results of Barkan's surgical goniotomy in adult open-angle glaucoma, only temporary lowering of intraocular pressure (IOP) was achieved with laser applications that attempted to penetrate to Schlemm's canal. Gaasterland and Kupfer[2] then demonstrated that heavy applications of argon laser energy to the trabecular meshwork (TM) can actually produce glaucoma in animals. After this demonstration, enthusiasm for laser therapy to the TM in glaucomatous eyes diminished.

We owe a great debt to Wise and Witter[3] for reintroducing laser treatment to the TM. Instead of attempting to penetrate the TM, they popularized circumferential, nonpenetrating applications to the tissue to produce small superficial scars. They hypothesized that this corrected a supposed mechanical sag of the tissue that they felt to be the basic defect in open-angle glaucoma. One can debate whether these authors were the first to apply such a laser method and whether this hypothesis is correct. It is clear, however, that they deserve much credit for advocating and promulgating this technique in the face of adverse laboratory data and for introducing the modern laser era of open-angle glaucoma therapy.

The results of Wise and Witter have been confirmed by many authors.[4-10] It is remarkable how consistent the results have been. Depending on the pretreatment IOP and type of glaucoma, an average of 6 to 10 mm Hg, or approximately 20%, pressure reduction can be expected. The best response is obtained in pseudoexfoliation glaucoma (PXF), whereas the poorest results tend to be in young patients with glaucoma.[10] Certain secondary glaucomas, such as uveitic glaucoma, also respond poorly, although occasional successes are reported. It seems worthwhile now to attempt laser trabeculoplasty (LTP) in almost all forms of open-angle glaucoma before embarking on filtration surgery. Further,

the availability of selective laser trabeculoplasty (SLT) obviates the need to treat less than 360 degrees of the angle, even in cases with poor prognosis, because the risk of worsening IOP with the laser is much lower than with argon laser trabeculoplasty (ALT).

Since the last revision of this text, SLT has been introduced into clinical practice.[11] As opposed to ALT, SLT employs short pulse durations (3 to 10 ns compared with 0.1 sec for ALT) and delivers significantly less total energy than ALT. The SLT unit is a Q-switched, frequency-doubled (532 nm) neodymium:yttrium-aluminum-garnet (Nd:YAG) laser with a spot size of 400 μm that affixes to a slit lamp. Comparative studies performed by Damji and colleagues showed equivalence between the 2 laser treatments in IOP reduction for open-angle glaucoma patients at both 6 months[12] and 12 months[13] of follow-up. This equivalence was verified during 5 years of retrospective follow-up by Juzych and colleagues.[14] Other lasers have been used for trabeculoplasty as well, with clinical IOP-lowering success demonstrated for diode LTP (0.1 sec duration, 50-μm spot size, power 700 to 1200 mW)[15] and micropulse diode laser trabeculoplasty (15% duty cycle with 100 pulses over a 0.2 sec application, 200-μm spot size, power 2 W).[16] The longest duration study of diode LTP (0.5 sec, 100-μm, 570 to 850 mW) showed equivalent IOP lowering compared with ALT at 5 years of follow-up.[17]

Depending on the indications for LTP, most patients who are uncontrolled before ALT need to maintain maximally tolerated medical therapy after laser treatment. For less severe glaucoma or in eyes with dramatic responses, some medications can be discontinued. The efficacy of LTP should be assessed 4 to 6 weeks after treatment. Shorter-term IOP measurements may be misleading.

The major risk of the procedure is acute IOP elevation, and although this risk seems lower with SLT than with ALT, it can be severe and can compromise vision. This should be monitored and treated appropriately. The magnitude

Kahook MY, Schuman JS, eds.
Chandler and Grant's Glaucoma, Fifth Edition (pp 477-485).
© 2013 SLACK Incorporated.

of IOP elevation after ALT has been reduced by the tendency to divide ALT treatment into 2 or 3 sessions, using 35 to 50 spots per session, with lower power settings than originally described. In addition, both SLT and ALT are routinely performed with the perioperative use of alpha-2 agonists, such as apraclonidine[18,19] or brimonidine.

Mechanistically, it is unclear how LTP works. It is possible that Wise's hypothesis is correct, but there are certain inconsistencies with this mechanical hypothesis. Treating smaller portions of the angle, rather than 360 degrees, often produces a disproportionally greater effect than would be anticipated mechanically. Also, the type of glaucoma that responds best to LTP, PXF, is the one type of glaucoma in which mechanical trabecular collapse is not believed to be involved; rather, it seems that accumulation of extracellular pseudoexfoliation material in the juxtacanalicular tissue is responsible for the increase in outflow resistance.[20] Histopathologic study in human autopsy eyes showed that ALT caused coagulative damage and disruption of the trabecular beam structure, whereas SLT did not cause these changes, suggesting that the 2 lasers may work differently.[21] More likely, it may be that ALT and SLT create their IOP-lowering effects similarly, but SLT does so without changing the structure of the TM, creating a margin of safety and also preserving the TM for the possibility of novel surgical treatment of Schlemm's canal in the future.

The effects of LTP on IOP seem to persist for years in most patients, although occasional patients demonstrate drift of IOP upward after 6 months. This seems especially common in exfoliation glaucoma (ie, is more material being deposited?) As a general rule, ALT maintains IOP control in 80% of eyes for 1 year, 50% for 5 years, and 30% for 10 years.[22] The largest long-term SLT study[14] shows slightly lower success over 5 years, but the ALT results in that study are identical, suggesting that SLT and ALT results probably follow the same trend. In addition to static IOP lowering, diurnal IOP fluctuation was demonstrated to improve at 6-month follow-up after SLT.[23] At 1 month of follow-up, tonographic outflow facility improved after either 180- or 360-degree SLT.[24]

Roughly 30% of eyes respond to retreatment with ALT[25] and we have observed some success with retreatment in some patients who initially demonstrated a good, but not long-lasting, response. (In contrast, no success has been observed with retreatment in those who failed to respond initially.) More importantly, no dramatic worsening of the glaucoma has been demonstrated in those who failed to respond to ALT retreatment on half the angle (with less than 50 applications), and subsequently, filtration surgery has been performed uneventfully. However, patients previously treated with ALT appear to respond better to subsequent SLT treatment than to repeat ALT,[12,26] and so we do not recommend repeat ALT in most situations. In addition, patients with prior successful SLT whose effect fails after 6 months may be treated successfully with repeat SLT.[27] We

have had success with this strategy in many patients and there does not appear to be an increased risk of treatment complications.

There are many unanswered questions about LTP. In open-angle glaucoma, it is not certain what the basic abnormality may be (nor is it known precisely how aqueous humor normally makes its way through the aqueous outflow system). Yet, it is clear that LTP works, at least for several years. It is also clear that ALT damages the angle in ways that SLT does not, resulting in destruction of TM tissue that has been demonstrated in a cynomolgus monkey[28] and has been shown in contradistinction to SLT-related damage in human autopsy eyes.[21] There is still the potential for long-term adverse effects (eg, downgrowth of endothelial cells from the cornea and hyalinization of the angle). (Some authors[3] have hypothesized that TM cells may normally act by contact inhibition to prevent this endothelial downgrowth.) It is likely that SLT provides a safety margin compared to ALT in this regard. It is obvious that because of the initial good results of LTP, it is now being applied to earlier stages of open-angle glaucoma. It could be reasonably asked whether LTP should be a substitute for all medical glaucoma therapy as initial treatment (see the discussion of the Glaucoma Laser Trial), and with the availability of the relatively low-risk SLT, this has become a somewhat popular trend. In a single study designed to assess the ability of SLT to provide a reduction in IOP-lowering medication use, a predefined IOP target was maintained while discontinuing an average of 2.0 medications at 6 months and 1.5 medications at 1 year,[29] supporting the idea that SLT could replace medications, at least early in the disease. This is a thought-provoking question that warrants further study, but given its overall safety, it seems reasonable to offer SLT at the diagnosis of most open-angle glaucomas in select patients, especially those who are predicted to have difficulty with follow-up or medication compliance.

It is interesting to compare the dose of laser energy used in ALT with the dose required to produce glaucoma in monkeys. Quigley and Hohman[30] have demonstrated that these differ by an approximate factor of 6. Given the much-lower total energy delivered and absence of detectable damage to the TM, this concern is diminished with SLT.

Wise[31] has stressed the importance of precise focusing of the laser and proper alignment of the instrument, both of which are quite appropriate in ALT. Although the SLT beam is much wider (400 μm compared to 50 to 100 μm for traditional ALT), it remains possible to inappropriately aim or focus the beam, thereby compromising the effectiveness of the laser and also risking iris or endothelial damage, depending on the direction of dislocation. It is likewise important that the actual power output of the laser be checked and calibrated periodically. Care and caution are necessary to avoid errors in LTP (Table 52-1).

TABLE 52-1. COMMON MISTAKES IN LASER TRABECULOPLASTY	
Error	**Solution**
Treatment too anterior	This results in ineffective ALT and may decrease the effectiveness of SLT. It is more common in the setting of Sampaolesi's line and a narrow angle (eg, pseudoexfoliation). Take care to perform gonioscopy prior to LTP to identify landmarks that can be used during the surgery.
Treatment too posterior	Posterior burns predispose to postoperative uveitis and PAS formation in ALT, although this is less likely with SLT. Careful gonioscopy, with identification of landmarks, avoids this problem.
Treatment too intense	Bursting bubbles during treatment indicate explosive tissue damage. The desired endpoint is just a blanching of the tissue or fine champagne bubbles in SLT. Excessive energy during LTP incites unwanted postoperative inflammation and PAS formation.
Treatment too light	If there is no tissue response with ALT, it is unlikely that there will be an IOP response. A blanching of the tissue should be seen with each spot and the power titrated to produce this effect. SLT power should be titrated at or just below the appearance of champagne bubbles with treatment. The diode laser is an exception, as there is generally no tissue response, regardless of the parameters employed.
Retreatment of previously treated angle	As discussed in the text, SLT performs better than ALT for retreatment of eyes previously treated with either ALT or SLT. Any untreated part of the angle, for example, after a prior 180-degree ALT treatment, may be treated safely.
Difficulty treating the horizontal angle, or when the angle appears too narrow	A simple means to gain access to a narrow appearing angle, or to the horizontal angle, is to have the patient look toward the goniomirror. This will have the effect of opening the angle for treatment.
Treating with an elliptical spot	It is important that the spot be round and sharp in order to deliver laser energy with maximum efficiency. A round spot can be achieved by keeping the goniolens perpendicular to the laser beam at all times; this will also achieve the sharpest focus on the tissue.
ALT: argon laser trabeculoplasty; IOP: intraocular pressure; LTP: laser trabeculoplasty; PAS: peripheral anterior synechiae; SLT: selective laser trabeculoplasty.	

HOW DO WE DO LASER TRABECULOPLASTY?

We are frequently questioned regarding our technique for LTP, a commonly performed procedure. In our center, SLT has replaced ALT almost completely, although we continue to see patients on referral who were recently treated with ALT. Therefore, we will describe our updated technique for ALT as well as our current protocol for SLT.

Following informed consent, the patient receives a drop of brimonidine 0.1% to 0.2% in the eye to be treated. Proparacaine 0.5% is placed in both eyes to anesthetize the treated eye, but also to decrease blinking in the contralateral eye, which can disrupt the treatment. A Goldmann 3-mirror lens (Haag-Streit, Bern, Switzerland) is applied for ALT, or the Latina SLT lens (Ocular Instruments, Bellevue, WA) is used for SLT, using a

hypromellose 0.3% gel as a coupling solution. Although this is our procedure, any goniolens with the user's choice of viscous coupling solution could be employed.

The angle, which was evaluated preoperatively, is again examined. If the angle is judged to be narrow preoperatively to an extent that would preclude LTP, laser iridectomy and gonioplasty, if necessary, are performed at least 1 week prior to LTP. A week is allowed to intervene between treatments to minimize the effect of inflammatory material and debris on scattering of the laser energy during LTP.

The decision of initial treatment zone is nuanced in ALT but we usually choose the temporal angle. The rationale is that if the ALT is ineffective and the patient requires filtering surgery, then the nasal angle is not directly involved by the ALT and the filtering surgery may be less likely to suffer bleb encapsulation from the prior ALT.[32] Alternately, the nasal angle may be treated first for the same reason, as the completion of the ALT (the second 180) then involves the temporal 180. If then the completion of the ALT is not successful, filtering surgery can ensue shortly after without the nasal angle having recent exposure to laser energy. Another tactic is to treat the inferior angle as the initial site as it is generally the widest area of the angle. This is acceptable but is not our practice. The single most important factor in deciding where to treat is consistency: if one treats the temporal angle first, one should always treat this area first. In this way, errors are avoided, and when the patient's chart cannot be found but the patient is to have his or her second ALT session, one knows that the temporal angle was the part treated previously.

We routinely carry out treatment for a full 360 degrees with SLT, although in select patients at high risk for an acute IOP spike, 180 degrees may be treated first. It remains important to maintain a consistent pattern so that if a treatment is interrupted for any reason, it will be clear where to begin at the next session.

The area to receive LTP is visualized in the goniolens and the 6 o'clock position is treated first. Additional burns are then made moving temporally in the mirror, treating more temporally inferiorly. It is crucial to remember that the mirror does not cross the image of the angle and that the more temporal portion in the mirror is indeed the more temporal part of the angle (see Figures 7-1 and 52-1). The goniolens is rotated clockwise in the right eye, or counterclockwise in the left eye, in order to keep the beam in the center of the goniomirror, to keep the spot round, and to deliver the most effective treatment with the least possible energy.

Approximately 50 spots are applied over 180 degrees, 8 or 9 spots per clock-hour. The laser settings for ALT are a 50-μm spot, 0.1-s duration, and the starting power is generally 600 mW. The surgical endpoint is a blanch or small bubble. If the bubble bursts, then the power setting is too high; if there is no blanch, the power is too low. Burns are placed at the junction of the anterior third and posterior two-thirds of the TM, in an effort to avoid injury to the filtering portion of the TM (Figure 52-2). Also, the more posterior the burn, the more likely inflammation and peripheral anterior synechiae (PAS) are to occur postoperatively.

SLT is continued for the second 180 degrees in almost all cases, as described above. The laser settings are 400-μm spot, 3-ns duration, and a starting power generally 0.6 mJ that may be titrated up or down in 0.1-mJ increments. The desired tissue effect is either a champagne bubble or just below the threshold that produces this effect. Large cavitation bubbles are not desired and the energy is titrated lower if these occur. The power setting may be varied during the procedure if necessary, which may occur if pigmentation is variable as one proceeds around the angle. Burns are placed across the entire TM, over which the aiming beam should be centered. Approximately 100 spots are required to provide a full, nonoverlapping treatment.

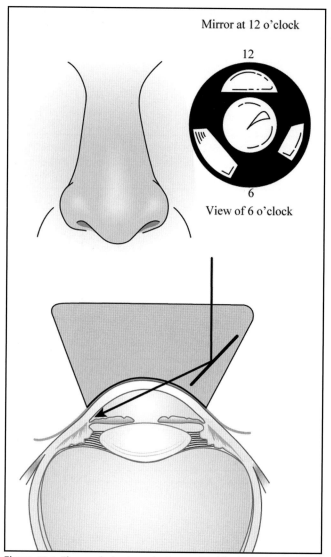

Figure 52-1. The parabola-shaped mirror at 12 o'clock, used to view and treat the angle, produces a view of the TM at 6 o'clock. The 12 o'clock position of the mirror permits treatment of the inferior TM with LTP.

Following ALT, the patient is given prednisolone acetate 4 times a day for 4 days, and then this drug is discontinued. Our SLT protocol is to use no postoperative drops routinely but to give a topical nonsteroidal anti-inflammatory drop if the patient experiences discomfort. The patient is examined after 30 to 60 minutes to ensure that an acute IOP elevation has not occurred. The follow-up intervals for ALT are then 1 day, 1 week, and 4 to 6 weeks; the efficacy is judged at the 4- to 6-week follow-up examination. For SLT patients, we generally follow-up at 2 weeks postoperatively unless there was an acute IOP rise in the first hour after treatment, in which case the patient is usually seen on the first postoperative day.

IMMEDIATE POST-LASER TREATMENT

Immediately after LTP, the patient may experience minor photophobia and irritation and examination may show

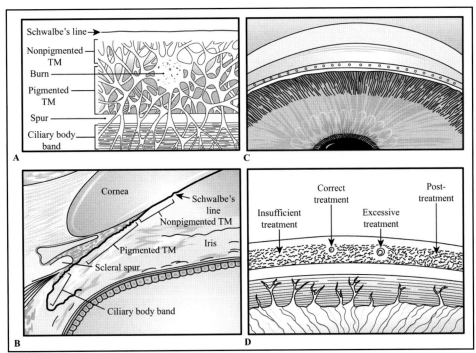

Figure 52-2. (A) ALT lesions are placed at the junction of the anterior one-third and posterior two-thirds of the TM. (B) This minimizes damage to the more posterior TM, which is the filtering portion, with access to Schlemm's canal. (C) Spots are placed 100 to 150 μm apart, such that 50 spots cover 180 degrees of the angle. (D) The endpoint is a blanch or small bubble. If a large bubble is seen or if the bubble bursts, then excessive energy is being delivered to the TM and the treatment power should be decreased.

conjunctival injection, ciliary flush, and anterior chamber cellular reaction. With ALT, topical steroids are prescribed over a 4-day period. The patient is free to ambulate without restriction. The principal short-term risk is acute IOP elevation, which should be monitored. Additional antiglaucoma therapy with oral carbonic anhydrase inhibitors (CAIs) or osmotics may be prescribed if necessary to control a spike in IOP. Data show that neither pretreatment with corticosteroids nor antiprostaglandin drugs reduces the magnitude of the acute post-ALT IOP elevation[33]; however, a single drop of preoperative brimonidine greatly diminishes the likelihood of postoperative acute IOP elevations.[34] Commercially available brimonidine 0.1% to 0.2% and apraclonidine 0.5% exhibit equal abilities to prevent acute IOP elevation after anterior segment laser surgery.[35]

POST-LASER VISITS

When we began using SLT in our clinics, it became apparent that the incidence of problems seen on postoperative day 1 was exceedingly low. We have therefore modified our pattern of follow-up visits relative to ALT, and unless there is an acute IOP elevation at 1 hour after SLT, the patient is not asked to return to the clinic for 2 weeks. In cases where the IOP is acutely elevated immediately following the laser treatment, it is wise to see patients sooner. The 2-week visit has become a safety check for anterior chamber inflammation

that, if seen, may prompt the initiation of steroid therapy until the inflammation can be controlled.

The ALT protocol is somewhat different given the higher energy delivered and associated increased risks of IOP elevation and inflammation in the near term. Following the patient's first ALT treatment in the first eye, it is wise to have the patient return 24 hours after treatment for evaluation. At all post-ALT visits, in addition to routine ophthalmological examination in which applanation tonometry and examination for anterior chamber inflammation are performed, the angle should be carefully examined with gonioscopy for signs of inflammatory exudates and beginning PAS formation. Such synechiae are not always benign, and when observed to be forming, steroid dosage should be increased. On the first day after ALT, occasionally, we have seen true inflammatory precipitates, keratic precipitates (KPs), on the TM.[36] At these sites, subsequent PAS to the TM have evolved, similar to organization of KPs in the angle in certain inflammatory glaucomas. (These must be differentiated, of course, from mere blanched areas, which are often still visible 24 hours after ALT but soon disappear.) After all, one is actually burning the TM and initiating an inflammatory reaction, which may be part of the mechanism for its efficacy. It is important to detect these inflammatory changes in the meshwork at an early stage in order to increase steroid therapy and attempt to prevent PAS that, when extending up to the meshwork in a substantial portion of the circumference, can result in impairment of outflow and in poorer glaucoma control.

Depending on the findings at the first post-ALT visit, the interval for the next visit is determined. For example, if IOP is elevated or if there are inflammatory signs in the angle, the patient should be seen in a few days. Otherwise, if this is the first laser treatment, the patient is seen within a week, at which time the above examination is repeated, including gonioscopy. Often, there is some IOP elevation at this time, which might relate to the laser healing process or to the steroid therapy, which has been discontinued after the first 4 or 5 days. SLT patients are routinely seen for their first post-laser visit at 2 weeks. If nothing adverse is detected, the patient is usually next seen 4 to 6 weeks later, at which time the efficacy of LTP (SLT or ALT) is truly assessed for the first time.

At this post-LTP visit, some IOP lowering is to be expected, usually more than half the ultimate total effect on outflow pressure (ie, IOP minus episcleral venous pressure). It is to be expected that the lower the starting IOP before the treatment, the less the absolute reduction in mm Hg for an equivalent effect. For example, with an episcleral venous pressure of 10 mm Hg, an IOP reduction from 20 to 15 mm Hg is equivalent to that from 30 to 20 mm Hg. Both represent a 50% decrease in outflow pressure. If no IOP reduction is manifest, it is unlikely that completing the remaining half of the angle, when applicable, will result in substantial IOP reduction, but there are notable exceptions to this. Further, if a complete 360-degree treatment has not produced any effect by this time, repeat treatment with either LTP modality is likely to fail, as discussed above.

Unless there has been actual worsening of IOP from the first half of ALT, or extensive PAS formation, the second half of the angle is treated. For the second half of treatment, one is tempted in such nonresponsive cases to alter the laser parameters somewhat (eg, in a pale meshwork to increase the power to higher levels to try to achieve bubble formation, or if fewer than 50 applications were made for the first half, to apply a full 50 applications to the second half). However, it is not certain that these maneuvers result in any improvement in efficacy. If the first half of LTP results in an adequate IOP decrease, it is justifiable not to perform the second half of treatment until a time when IOP drifts higher. In some patients, this has not yet happened, and only one-half of the angle has been treated. Especially if some PAS formation has occurred, even if not to meshwork but only to scleral spur, one should pause in patients with good responses before completing LTP therapy. Thus, gonioscopy should always be performed at this post-LTP visit.

It is curious that there is little correlation between the acute effects of LTP on IOP and the long-term efficacy. Patients with acute IOP elevation seem, at first glance, just as likely to show a long-term IOP improvement as those without such acute IOP elevation. This question has not been extensively studied, but it will be interesting to see whether some correlation between short-term and long-term IOP effects does, however, emerge.

It is important to state that, when some IOP decrease occurs with full LTP treatment, it is still necessary for the ophthalmologist to judge whether there has been sufficient lowering of IOP to obviate the need for filtration surgery. There seems to be a tendency, which to us is not at all justified, not to proceed with filtration surgery in patients with advanced glaucoma who have had LTP with minimal IOP lowering. For example, in a patient with a central island of vision due to glaucoma and an IOP of 30 mm Hg, if LTP lowers the IOP to only 25 mm Hg 1 month after full treatment, filtration surgery should be performed. A pressure of 25 is clearly too high for such a patient (an IOP in the low teens is required), and if such an IOP were encountered on maximum medical therapy, filtration surgery would have been proposed.

INDICATIONS

In almost all forms of open-angle glaucoma, LTP should be performed before embarking on filtration surgery. In young patients with juvenile open-angle glaucoma, or those with secondary inflammatory glaucomas, it is rare for LTP to be effective, but there are noteworthy exceptions. The risk/benefit ratio of LTP versus filtration surgery is such that it always seems justifiable to perform LTP prior to performing filtration surgery, especially when SLT is available. For those with unfavorable prognosis in whom there seems to be some potential for actual worsening of the glaucoma with LTP (such as in inflammatory glaucomas or young patients), it seems prudent not to attempt LTP. Some would argue that full LTP treatment in the whole angle should be performed prior to filtration surgery in all open-angle glaucoma patients; however, especially in cases with poor prognosis and definite chronic elevation of IOP after initial LTP, this does not seem warranted to us.

In aphakic and many pseudophakic eyes, the response to LTP, although often significant, seems less than in the phakic eye. (The reason for this is obscure; there does not seem to be any "mechanical" basis for this.) Pseudophakic eyes may behave no differently with respect to LTP response than do phakic eyes, although this point has been controversial.[37] There are no recent studies that adequately address this question, and there are no more concrete data regarding relative effectiveness of either ALT or SLT in phakic, aphakic, or pseudophakic patients than there were at last publication. Dreyer and Gorla[37] studied the effectiveness of ALT in pseudophakic eyes in a retrospective fashion using historical controls. An unpublished subgroup analysis (ARVO abstract, 2005) based on the data set by Damji and colleagues[13] has suggested that there is no difference between phakic and pseudophakic eyes in response to ALT or SLT. While these data suggest no difference in the effectiveness of LTP in pseudophakic and phakic eyes with primary open-angle glaucoma

(POAG), this problem deserves further investigation in a prospective study.

In patients with chronic angle-closure glaucoma with synechiae in the angle, we will always treat the open portions of the angle (if 3 or more hours are open) with LTP prior to embarking on filtration surgery. This is most often unsuccessful, but there are occasional gratifying exceptions.

All these discussions have concerned patients on maximum tolerated medical therapy who are facing filtration surgery. What is the role of LTP in replacing medical therapy for glaucoma? The Glaucoma Laser Trial, a study of 271 patients with POAG, attempted to answer these questions for ALT.[38,39] In this experiment, one eye received 360-degree ALT divided into 2 sessions separated by 1 month, while the other eye was treated with timolol. There was a series of medical steps that the medication-first eye could undergo for IOP control, from timolol to dipivefrin, to low-dose pilocarpine, to high-dose pilocarpine, to timolol and high-dose pilocarpine, to dipivefrin and high-dose pilocarpine, then to the ophthalmologist's discretion. The laser-first eye initially received no medications but was medically treated if necessary for IOP control.

Of the eyes treated with ALT, 44% were controlled on no medications, 70% were controlled with the addition of timolol, and 89% were controlled with ALT and medications, but no surgery. The medication-first eyes showed 30% controlled on timolol alone, 51% controlled on a single medication, and 66% controlled on multiple medications. These short-term, 2-year results indicate that ALT is efficacious in lowering IOP but that it is not a panacea.[38,39] Indeed, more than half the eyes treated with ALT first later required some sort of medical or surgical therapy. A further follow-up of 3.5 years examining visual field progression found little difference between the laser-first and medication-first groups, although the laser-first eyes performed slightly better on some measures of visual field function.[40]

ALT is a destructive procedure,[28] eliminating a portion of an already marginally functional TM. It may make future filtering surgery less likely to succeed and may predispose to bleb encapsulation following trabeculectomy.[32] For these reasons, we would place ALT in our armamentarium after conventional antihypertensive eye drops but before systemic CAIs and trabeculectomy.

The situation is different for our current LTP modality of choice, SLT. We are much more liberal in its application because of its low risk of complications, few side effects, and lack of observable intrinsic angle damage on histopathologic study and clinical follow-up exams. We believe that it is reasonable to offer SLT as initial therapy at diagnosis of almost any open-angle glaucoma, especially if there is a high risk of medication noncompliance or if failure to follow up is expected over the long term. As previously noted, SLT has been shown to reduce the need for medication use while maintaining a predefined goal IOP,[29] suggesting that SLT could be used at any point during the treatment of open-angle glaucoma prior to incisional surgery.

CONTRAINDICATIONS

Except for corneal opacification or total synechial closure of the angle, LTP should be attempted in at least a portion of the angle for uncontrolled glaucoma, as already discussed. We believe that documented long-term worsening of the glaucoma after the initial half-angle treatment is at least a relative contraindication to the completion of the treatment, as discussed in the previous section.

COMPLICATIONS

Long-Term Worsening of the Glaucoma

It must be remembered that approximately 3% of patients with open-angle glaucoma actually get worse following ALT,[6] although this rate has not been reported for SLT. This, of course, does not specifically refer to or include patients with acute IOP elevation shortly after the procedure. The mechanism for this sustained worsening is not known, but it possibly may relate to the destruction of meshwork tissue with the laser, with possible scar formation.[28]

Acute Pressure Elevation

Permanent visual loss is possible with extreme IOP elevation, even if relatively short lived. The IOP shortly after LTP needs to be monitored and treated.

Uveitis

Occasionally, uveitis is severe and needs to be vigorously treated to prevent synechiae formation.

Peripheral Anterior Synechiae

PAS relate more strongly to ALT and are rare if present at all following SLT. They are often described as being benign and extending only up to scleral spur. However, cases of extensive functional angle closure due to PAS have been documented following ALT. The appearance of the angle post-LTP needs to be carefully monitored and steroid dosage appropriately adjusted.

Corneal Burns

Occasionally, corneal epithelial opacities are encountered, but these heal within a few days without sequelae. Corneal endothelial burns are rare.

Hyphema

Hyphema is an uncommon complication, but it has been observed. As with most potential complications, this risk is much less of a concern with SLT than ALT. There seems to be 2 causes of hyphema after ALT. Occasionally, there are meandering normal vessels in the angle that are inadvertently disrupted by the laser energy. Treatment immediately consists of pressing the goniolens against the cornea to raise IOP and thus achieve hemostasis, or if the vessel is visible through the goniolens, to treat it directly with further ALT laser applications in order to coagulate it as in goniophotocoagulation. (This approach would be unlikely to succeed using the SLT laser, which does not have coagulative ability.) The other cause of hyphema is encountered when there is blood in Schlemm's canal and the laser energy penetrates deeply into the meshwork to the canal. Most patients with open-angle glaucoma do not have blood in Schlemm's canal (it is important to contemplate why this is so), but occasionally it is found, especially in patients with abnormally elevated episcleral venous pressure (eg, in association with a dural shunt). Treatment consists of raising IOP with goniolens pressure and/or tilting the lens to relieve compression at the limbus in the involved portion of the angle. It is this initial compression of limbal episcleral vessels with the goniolens that promotes blood reflux into the canal. One should avoid the temptation to increase the laser power further and treat the bleeding portion of the angle further (unless a blood vessel can be identified), for this simply may allow further penetration into the blood-filled canal. If hemostasis is obtained by these means, one can proceed to complete the LTP, but lower power settings should be chosen for the remaining portions of the angle. Usually, only a small amount of bleeding is encountered in such cases, but rarely significant hyphema has been observed with associated elevation of IOP.

The Unknown

In any procedure whose optimal parameters and long-term biological effects are not clearly known, we must all be diligent in looking for and documenting unexpected long-term consequences of our treatment.

A discussion of the mechanisms of action of LTP and the treatment of acute IOP elevation are covered in the following chapters.

REFERENCES

1.   Grant WM. Further studies on facility of flow through the trabecular meshwork. *Arch Ophthalmol.* 1958;60(4 pt 1):523-533.
2.   Gaasterland D, Kupfer C. Experimental glaucoma in the rhesus monkey. *Invest Ophthalmol.* 1974;13(6):455-457.
3.   Wise JB, Witter SL. Argon laser therapy for open-angle glaucoma. A pilot study. *Arch Ophthalmol.* 1979;97(2):319-322.
4.   Schwartz AL, Whitten ME, Bleiman B, Martin D. Argon laser trabecular surgery in uncontrolled phakic open angle glaucoma. *Ophthalmology.* 1981;88(3):203-212.
5.   Wilensky JT, Jampol LM. Laser therapy for open angle glaucoma. *Ophthalmology.* 1981;88(3):213-217.
6.   Thomas JV, Simmons RJ, Belcher CD 3rd. Argon laser trabeculoplasty in the presurgical glaucoma patient. *Ophthalmology.* 1982;89(3):187-197.
7.   Wise JB. Long-term control of adult open angle glaucoma by argon laser treatment. *Ophthalmology.* 1981;88(3):197-202.
8.   Odberg T, Sandvik L. The medium and long-term efficacy of primary argon laser trabeculoplasty in avoiding topical medication in open angle glaucoma. *Acta Ophthalmol Scand.* 1999;77(2):176-181.
9.   The Glaucoma Laser Trial (GLT) and glaucoma laser trial follow-up study: 7. Results. Glaucoma Laser Trial Research Group. *Am J Ophthalmol.* 1995;120(6):718-731.
10. Heijl A, Leske MC, Bengtsson B, et al. Reduction of intraocular pressure and glaucoma progression: results from the Early Manifest Glaucoma Trial. *Arch Ophthalmol.* 2002;120(10):1268-1279.
11. Latina MA, Sibayan SA, Shin DH, et al. Q-switched 532-nm Nd:YAG laser trabeculoplasty (selective laser trabeculoplasty): a multicenter, pilot, clinical study. *Ophthalmology.* 1998;105(11):2082-2088; discussion 9-90.
12. Damji KF, Shah KC, Rock WJ, et al. Selective laser trabeculoplasty v argon laser trabeculoplasty: a prospective randomised clinical trial. *Br J Ophthalmol.* 1999;83(6):718-722.
13. Damji KF, Bovell AM, Hodge WG, et al. Selective laser trabeculoplasty versus argon laser trabeculoplasty: results from a 1-year randomised clinical trial. *Br J Ophthalmol.* 2006;90(12):1490-1494.
14. Juzych MS, Chopra V, Banitt MR, et al. Comparison of long-term outcomes of selective laser trabeculoplasty versus argon laser trabeculoplasty in open-angle glaucoma. *Ophthalmology.* 2004;111(10):1853-1859.
15. Agarwal HC, Poovali S, Sihota R, Dada T. Comparative evaluation of diode laser trabeculoplasty vs frequency doubled Nd:YAG laser trabeculoplasty in primary open angle glaucoma. *Eye (Lond).* 2006;20(12):1352-1356.
16. Fea AM, Bosone A, Rolle T, et al. Micropulse diode laser trabeculoplasty (MDLT): a phase II clinical study with 12 months follow-up. *Clin Ophthalmol.* 2008;2(2):247-252.
17. Chung PY, Schuman JS, Netland PA, et al. Five-year results of a randomized, prospective, clinical trial of diode vs argon laser trabeculoplasty for open-angle glaucoma. *Am J Ophthalmol.* 1998;126(2):185-190.
18. Coleman AL, Robin AL, Pollack IP. Apraclonidine hydrochloride. *Ophthalmol Clin North Am.* 1989;2:97-108.
19. Robin AL. The role of apraclonidine hydrochloride in laser therapy for glaucoma. *Trans Am Ophthalmol Soc.* 1989;87:729-761.
20. Richardson TM, Epstein DL. Exfoliation glaucoma: a quantitative perfusion and ultrastructural study. *Ophthalmology.* 1981;88:968-980.
21. Kramer TR, Noecker RJ. Comparison of the morphologic changes after selective laser trabeculoplasty and argon laser trabeculoplasty in human eye bank eyes. *Ophthalmology.* 2001;108(4):773-779.
22. Shingleton BJ, Richter CU, Bellows AR, et al. Long-term efficacy of argon laser trabeculoplasty. *Ophthalmology.* 1987;94(12):1513-1518.
23. Nagar M, Luhishi E, Shah N. Intraocular pressure control and fluctuation: the effect of treatment with selective laser trabeculoplasty. *Br J Ophthalmol.* 2009;93(4):497-501.
24. Goyal S, Beltran-Agullo L, Rashid S, et al. Effect of primary selective laser trabeculoplasty on tonographic outflow facility: a randomised clinical trial. *Br J Ophthalmol.* 2010;94(11):1443-1447.
25. Richter CU, Shingleton BJ, Bellows AR, et al. Retreatment with argon laser trabeculoplasty. *Ophthalmology.* 1987;94(9):1085-1089.

26. Russo V, Barone A, Cosma A, et al. Selective laser trabeculoplasty versus argon laser trabeculoplasty in patients with uncontrolled open-angle glaucoma. *Eur J Ophthalmol.* 2009;19(3):429-434.

27. Hong BK, Winer JC, Martone JF, et al. Repeat selective laser trabeculoplasty. *J Glaucoma.* 2009;18(3):180-183.

28. Melamed S, Pei J, Epstein DL. Delayed response to argon laser trabeculoplasty in monkeys. Morphological and morphometric analysis. *Arch Ophthalmol.* 1986;104(7):1078-1083.

29. Francis BA, Ianchulev T, Schofield JK, Minckler DS. Selective laser trabeculoplasty as a replacement for medical therapy in open-angle glaucoma. *Am J Ophthalmol.* 2005;140(3):524-525.

30. Quigley HA, Hohman RM. Laser energy levels for trabecular meshwork damage in the primate eye. *Invest Ophthalmol Vis Sci.* 1983;24(9):1305-1307.

31. Wise JB. Errors in laser spot size in laser trabeculoplasty. *Ophthalmology.* 1984;91(2):186-190.

32. Richter CU, Shingleton BJ, Bellows AR, et al. The development of encapsulated filtering blebs. *Ophthalmology.* 1988;95(9):1163-1168.

33. Pappas HR, Berry DP, Partamian L, et al. Topical indomethacin therapy before argon laser trabeculoplasty. *Am J Ophthalmol.* 1985;99(5):571-575.

34. Barnebey HS, Robin AL, Zimmerman TJ, et al. The efficacy of brimonidine in decreasing elevations in intraocular pressure after laser trabeculoplasty. *Ophthalmology.* 1993;100(7):1083-1088.

35. Chen TC. Brimonidine 0.15% versus apraclonidine 0.5% for prevention of intraocular pressure elevation after anterior segment laser surgery. *J Cataract Refract Surg.* 2005;31(9):1707-1712.

36. Fiore PM, Melamed S, Epstein DL. Trabecular precipitates and elevated intraocular pressure following argon laser trabeculoplasty. *Ophthalmic Surg.* 1989;20(10):697-701.

37. Dreyer EB, Gorla M. Laser trabeculoplasty in the pseudophakic patient. *J Glaucoma.* 1993;2(4):313-315.

38. The Glaucoma Laser Trial. I. Acute effects of argon laser trabeculoplasty on intraocular pressure. Glaucoma Laser Trial Research Group. *Arch Ophthalmol.* 1989;107(8):1135-1142.

39. The Glaucoma Laser Trial (GLT): 2. Results of argon laser trabeculoplasty versus topical medicines. The Glaucoma Laser Trial Research Group. *Ophthalmology.* 1990;97(11):1403-1413.

40. The Glaucoma Laser Trial (GLT): 6. Treatment group differences in visual field changes. Glaucoma Laser Trial Research Group. *Am J Ophthalmol.* 1995;120(1):10-22.

Laser Trabeculoplasty

How Does It Work?

Daniel Cotlear, MD; Shlomo Melamed, MD; and Modi Goldenfeld, MD

Laser trabeculoplasty (LTP) is an effective treatment in patients with open-angle glaucoma either as primary therapy or as an adjunct to topical glaucoma medications.[1] The chromophore or target is melanin, which absorbs green light (wavelength of 532 nm) and results in a cascade that ultimately leads to a decrease in intraocular pressure (IOP). A decrease in IOP of up to 30% has been reported, although the effect may be temporary, lasting months to years.[2-5] Several types of lasers are currently used for trabeculoplasty, including argon, diode, titanium-sapphire laser, and double-frequency neodymium:yttrium-aluminum-garnet (Nd:YAG).[3,6-12]

In an attempt to maintain LTP's efficacy while minimizing the thermal damage and subsequent destruction of the trabecular meshwork (TM) and adjacent tissues, several technologies have been developed and gained popularity. However, argon laser trabeculoplasty (ALT) is still the most commonly used laser treatment for trabeculoplasty around the world[1-5] and is usually applied after maximally tolerated medical therapy has failed to control the IOP.[5] Although LTP is considered a very safe and effective method, its exact mechanism of action still remains unclear. We will discuss possible mechanisms of action relating to LTP and expand on the clinical use of this treatment modality.

ARGON LASER TRABECULOPLASTY

Clinical Observations Related to the Mechanism

Krasnov[13] initially described the potential of using laser to treat the TM to decrease IOP in 1973. This concept evolved into the currently used ALT, as described initially by Wise

and Witter in 1979,[2] that has become a standard method of treatment for medically uncontrolled open-angle glaucoma. ALT's efficacy and safety has been repeatedly confirmed by numerous studies.[6-15] Today, it is widely accepted that ALT reduces IOP in uncontrolled open-angle glaucoma patients,[16] with success rates of approximately 80% at 1 year, 50% at 5 years, and 33% at 10 years.[15]

The following observations reported in clinical studies of ALT may give some hints as to the mode of action of this procedure:

1. Increased outflow facility—tonography was performed in patients before and after ALT, and C (outflow) values were substantially increased after treatment.[10] A fluorophotometric study disclosed no effect on aqueous humor inflow.[17] From these studies, it was concluded that ALT mainly affects outflow facility, most probably through the TM—Schlemm's canal region.

2. Complete (360 degrees) versus partial (90 to 180 degrees) ALT treatments may be equally effective in IOP control. Additionally, low-dose[12] and low-power[18] ALT has also been observed to effectively control IOP in glaucoma patients. Such successful results of only minimal or partial treatment of the outflow system may suggest that a triggered biological process could be involved, affecting nonlasered regions as well.

Some subtypes of open-angle glaucoma are more responsive to ALT than others. Pseudoexfoliative glaucoma (PXF), primary open-angle glaucoma (POAG), and pigment dispersion glaucoma (PDG) are subtypes of glaucoma in which ALT appears to be most beneficial.[5] The common feature of these 3 diseases may be the wear-and-tear phenomenon. In this concept, particulate matter (PXF material, pigment, or some unknown protein or proteoglycan) is blocking the

Kahook MY, Schuman JS, eds.
Chandler and Grant's Glaucoma, Fifth Edition (pp 487-495).
© 2013 SLACK Incorporated.

HOW I DO LASER TRABECULOPLASTY

Claudia U. Richter, MD

LTP is performed to lower IOP after the clinical evaluation determines that the procedure is likely to benefit the patient. The preoperative assessment includes a slit-lamp examination to ensure that the cornea is clear enough to allow visualization of the angle, and gonioscopy to ascertain that the angle is open, without neovascularization or extensive peripheral anterior synechiae. Informed consent is obtained from the patient. Topical brimonidine is administered prior to the laser to minimize a post-laser IOP spike.[1] If the patient is already taking brimonidine or has an allergy, other topical antiglaucomatous medications may be used.[2] The patient is seated at the laser slit-lamp, adjusted to ensure the patient's comfort. While LTP is not typically a long procedure, a patient who is comfortable will move less, making the procedure easier for both the surgeon and the patient. Topical proparacaine is instilled and a mirrored gonioscopy lens filled with goniosolution is placed on the appropriate eye. The Goldmann 3-mirrored lens (Ocular Instruments, Bellevue, WA) is used for ALT and the Latina lens (Ocular Instruments) for SLT. The Ritch lens (Ocular Instruments) is helpful with the diode laser to reduce the 100-micron spot size to 71.4 microns. The mirror is rotated superiorly so the LTP begins at the 6 o'clock position.

A number of lasers currently are available to perform LTP and all are effective in reducing IOP. The type of laser used determines the laser settings, the target tissue, and the desired tissue response (Table 53-1).

Lasers with larger spot size (SLT and micropulse) require focusing on the entire TM and laser spots that are contiguous but not overlapping. Lasers with smaller spot size require focusing at the junction of the anterior and posterior TM and spacing equivalent to 3 laser spots between each applied treatment. While some ophthalmologists treat 360 degrees of the TM in one session, I typically treat only 180 degrees of TM in one session, hoping to minimize the risk of an IOP spike. I always treat the nasal TM at the first session and the temporal TM at the second.

Following the laser, an additional dose of brimonidine or other antiglaucomatous medication is instilled. The IOP is measured 1 hour after LTP. Patients are told to continue their usual glaucoma medications and are given a prescription for loteprednol 4 times a day for 5 days. Other topical steroids or nonsteroidal anti-inflammatory medications are effective in minimizing post-LTP iritis, but loteprednol is effective and seems to result in steroid-induced IOP elevations less frequently than other steroids in my patient population. No post-laser topical steroids or nonsteroidal anti-inflammatory medications are given after selective LTP. Patients are then seen 1 week and 6 weeks following LTP to ascertain response to therapy.

While LTP is a straight forward procedure, not getting lost in the angle during the procedure is important, particularly for ophthalmologists performing their first procedures. For this reason, gonioscopy prior to laser demonstrates any variations in angle appearance, such as synechiae, pigment, and blood vessels, that may be used as landmarks during the laser. Areas of increased pigmentation may require less laser energy. It is important to be able to distinguish Schwalbe's line, pigmented TM, scleral spur, and ciliary body band before beginning treatment.

Ease with LTP is facilitated by beginning treatment at the same position with every patient so the starting point and resultingly, the end point are always known. Also, remember to note (and write down if necessary) which way the contact lens will be rotated during the procedure so that the direction is not inadvertently reversed and the same area retreated. Finally, when the contact lens is rotated to treat additional portions of the TM, rotate the mirror so both treated and untreated areas are visible, using angle and iris landmarks if necessary, to prevent skipping areas or retreating areas of meshwork.

REFERENCES

1. Ren J, Shin DH, Chang HS, et al. Efficacy of apraclonidine 1% versus pilocarpine 4% for prophylaxis of intraocular pressure spike after argon laser trabeculoplasty. *Ophthalmology*. 1999;106:1135-1139.
2. Barnes SD, Campagna JA, Dirks MS, Doe EA. Control of intraocular pressure elevations after argon laser trabeculoplasty comparison of brimonidine 0.2% to apraclonidine 1.0%. *Ophthalmology*. 1999;196:2033-2037.
3. Pham H, Mansberger S, Brandt JD, Damji K, Ramulu PY, Parrish RK. Argon laser trabeculoplasty. The gold standard. *Surv Ophthalmol*. 2008;53:641-646.
4. Latina MA, de Leon JMS. Selective laser trabeculoplasty. *Ophthalmol Clin North Am*. 2005;18:409-419.
5. Fea AM, Bosone A, Rolle T, Brogliatti B, Grignolo FM. Micropulse diode laser trabeculoplasty (MDLT): a phase II clinical study with 12 months follow-up. *Clin Ophthalmol*. 2008;2:247-252.
6. Chung PY, Schuman JS, Netland PA, Lloyd-Muhammad RA, Jacobs DS. Five-year results of a randomized, prospective, clinical trial of diode vs argon laser trabeculoplasty for open-angle glaucoma. *Am J Ophthalmol*. 1998;126:185-190.

Table 53-1. Laser Types and Settings

Laser	Spot Size	Duration	Starting Power	Target	Desired Tissue Reaction
Argon[3]	50 µm	0.1 s	800 mW	Junction of pigmented and nonpigmented TM	Slight blanching or large bubble formation
Pascal	60 µm	0.1 s	500 mW	Junction of pigmented and nonpigmented TM	Slight blanching or large bubble formation
Selective[4]	400 µm	3 ns	0.8 mJ	Centered on the entire height of the TM	Tiny champagne bubbles
Micropulse[5]	300 µm	300 msec	2000 mW	Centered on the entire height of the TM	—
Diode[6]	100 µm	0.5 s	600 mW	Junction of pigmented and nonpigmented TM	Blanch or small bubble formation

trabecular spaces and is associated with a diminished number of trabecular cells.[19] Reduction in trabecular cellularity may subsequently result in adherence of trabecular beams and total collapse of the TM with increased resistance to aqueous flow. It is conceivable, then, that ALT may affect vital cellular processes related to this wear-and-tear phenomenon, and indeed several studies confirmed such an effect of ALT and will be described later in this chapter.[20-25] In contrast, other types of open-angle glaucoma are poorly responsive to ALT, such as aphakic/pseudophakic glaucoma, uveitic glaucoma, and juvenile glaucoma.[5]

Mechanical Theory of Argon Laser Trabeculoplasty

Wise and Witter[2] initially proposed this treatment, suggesting that mechanical shrinkage of the trabecular ring following ALT causes widening of the trabecular spaces with subsequent decrease in resistance to aqueous outflow and reduction of IOP. However, to date, no proof for such mechanical stretching of the trabecular sheets has been reported. It has been speculated that in glaucomatous eyes, where the trabecular beams are collapsed, the pattern of ALT may result in scarring of the lasered areas with widening of the trabecular spaces and Schlemm's canal due to traction of the beams in adjacent regions. However, in a study of 23 pairs of enucleated human eyes,[26] no significant change in the cross-sectional area of Schlemm's canal could be demonstrated after ALT. Because no accurate morphometric analysis has been done in glaucomatous eyes after ALT, the mechanical explanation for its effect still remains theoretical.

Biological Effect of Argon Laser Trabeculoplasty

ALT may be associated with triggering of a cascade of complex biological processes in the outflow system.[20-25,27,28]

The cellular theory proposes that in response to coagulative necrosis induced by the laser, there is migration of macrophages that phagocytose debris and thus clear the TM from obstruction.[29] Recently, an addition to the cellular theory has been suggested. This theory employs facts reported by Wang and colleagues,[30] who demonstrated that the TM endothelium shares a similar response to oxidative insults as the systemic endothelial cells and that inflammatory cytokines can play a role in glaucoma. Wang and colleagues[30] demonstrated that, in response to sublethal stress performed on TM cells, cytokines such as endothelial leukocyte adhesion molecule-1 (ELAM-1) are released into the aqueous and influence glaucomatous aqueous outflow pathways. Signals, such as laser energy, promote oxidative stress. The gene for ELAM-1 has receptors in its promoter region that respond to this type of stress, subsequently releasing and activating inflammatory cytokines, such as interleukin-1 (IL-1).

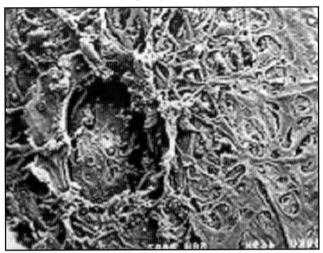

Figure 53-1. Scanning electron microscope image of TM after ALT showing localized and collateral injury to the tissue.

IL-1 in turn increases the formation of ELAM-1. Bradley and colleagues[31,32] have demonstrated that IL-1 increases outflow facility and showed that IL-1β and tumor necrosis factor-alpha mediate ALT-induced matrix metalloproteinases (MMP) expression. For the first time, it was shown that the humoral pathway can be as important as the mechanical one.

Although the Glaucoma Laser Trial[33] demonstrated the efficacy of ALT, follow-up studies[1,34] revealed that only 20% to 32% of treated patients remained controlled after 7 to 10 years post-treatment. The need for repeat laser therapy was evident, but the fact that ALT creates a scar in the treated TM (Figure 53-1) limited the possibility of repeated treatment. It could thus be inferred that, if the biologic treatment is true, the effects of such treatment are contradicted by the trauma incurred by using thermal energy to influence cytokine release.

Histopathology of Argon Laser Trabeculoplasty

In a series of electron-microscopy experiments performed in nonglaucomatous monkeys,[20,21,24] Melamed and colleagues described the acute and long-term cellular changes in the TM and Schlemm's canal in the treated eyes. Immediately after ALT, the common features of laser effect were coagulative necrosis, disruption of trabecular beams, and dispersion of tissue debris (Figure 53-2). Small fragments of tissue could be found throughout the trabecular spaces, accumulating in the juxtacanalicular region. This accumulation of debris might explain the IOP spike sometimes detected immediately after ALT (in up to 31% of ALT cases).[35] Many trabecular cells were rounded up, dislodged from their supportive beams, and some were very actively phagocytic, containing large phagosomes with an excessive

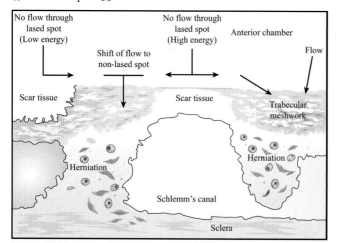

Figure 53-2. LTP results in regions of decreased flow where the actual laser lesions occur and areas of increased flow are visible as locations where the TM is herniated into Schlemm's canal. Note the arrows indicating areas of no flow, stretching and reopening the adjacent, untreated intertrabecular spaces.

amount of fibrillar material. After 4 weeks, the treated, lasered spots were detected as scarred regions with flattened beams. A cellular layer continuous with the corneal endothelium was found to cover these regions. The inner wall beneath these areas was flat with no giant vacuoles present. Rodrigues and colleagues[36] and Weber and colleagues[37] found similar changes in their studies of trabeculectomy specimens. Early changes consisted of disrupted trabecular beams and accumulation of fibrinous debris. Six months later, treated regions were scarred with a corneal endothelial sheet covering its surface, whereas nontreated regions appeared normal.[37]

In human eyes, ALT reduces IOP despite scarring of the lasered regions. In a tracer study[25] performed in monkeys by using cationized ferritin, the scarred lasered sites were observed to be impermeable to aqueous flow. Gaasterland and Kupfer[38] showed that confluent ALT results in chronic IOP elevation due to trabecular scarring (in fact, it is the best available method still in practice to create a model for glaucoma in monkeys). One might wonder how, despite all the incurred damage to and scarring of the TM, IOP is reduced after ALT. Several studies[20,22-25,39,40] may help in resolving this intriguing puzzle by suggesting some biological processes that might be initiated or enhanced by this therapy.

Enhanced Biological and Phagocytic Activity of Trabecular Cells

One of the main tasks of the trabecular cells is to act as the biological filter of the eye. Material obliterating the trabecular spaces is usually engulfed by phagocytes that later migrate away from the beams and the outflow system. After ALT, trabecular cells have been detected in various stages of enhanced biological and phagocytic activity.[20] This increased activity might have resulted from the absorption

of laser energy itself or could have been triggered by the debris of lasered tissue. It is conceivable that such an effect of ALT might explain its high success rate in the wear-and-tear glaucomas, where the presumed particulate matter blocking the trabecular spaces may be more efficiently removed by trabecular cells activated by ALT, with subsequent reduction of resistance to aqueous flow.

Structural Changes of Regions Adjacent to Lasered Sites

Four weeks after ALT, nonlasered regions adjacent to lasered spots demonstrated an array of significant structural changes.[21] These regions have wide-open intertrabecular spaces with herniations of the juxtacanalicular meshwork and inner wall of Schlemm's canal into and across its lumen. These herniations contain more vacuoles than in control eyes, suggesting an increased flow of aqueous humor. A tracer study[24] with cationized ferritin also suggested this with the demonstration of greater tracer deposition of untreated trabecular spaces, in contrast to nondeposition of tracer in adjacent treated and scarred areas. It was suggested that these changes are a compensatory response to ALT, allowing the aqueous blocked by the scarred spots to be shifted into less resistant trabecular routes, with the net effect of IOP reduction (see Figure 53-2).

Inflammatory Response Initiated by Argon Laser Trabeculoplasty

In humans, ALT usually stimulates an inflammatory response in the eye, requiring the use of anti-inflammatory agents.[8,9] In addition, the TM in monkeys was found to contain an abundance of inflammatory cells, such as lymphocytes, pigment-laden macrophages, and plasma cells.[21] Such trabeculitis may also be associated with decreased IOP through the release of mediators affecting aqueous outflow, similar to the cytokine-related stress response theories described previously.

Increased Cell Division After Argon Laser Trabeculoplasty

Further support for the importance of the biological response of the TM to ALT was given by a series of experiments evaluating cellular division after treatment.[22-24] Increased trabecular cell division after ALT has been shown in organ-cultured human eyes[22] as well as living cats[24] and monkeys.[39]

In organ-cultured human eyes, trabecular cell division and migration were studied by exposure to thymidine. Two days after ALT, nontreated areas of the TM disclosed a marked incorporation of thymidine into the nucleic DNA, indicating increased cellular division.[22,23]

In the organ-cultured human eyes, thymidine incorporation occurred predominantly in the anterior, nonfiltering region of the TM (which might represent Schwalbe's line cells). Two weeks later, the labeled cells were more concentrated in the lasered regions, suggesting active migration from the anterior trabeculum into the treated area. In the living cat model, DNA replication in the TM was also demonstrated in response to ALT,[25] although no accurate localization to the anterior trabecular region could be made. A significant increase in the mitotic index of trabecular cells in response to ALT was also confirmed by Dueker and colleagues[39] in the monkey model. Enhanced DNA synthesis, cell replication, and migration comprise a fundamental biological response of trabecular cells to ALT.

Alteration in Turnover or Synthesis of Glycosaminoglycans After Argon Laser Trabeculoplasty

The hypothesis that ALT causes the release of a factor that induces trabecular cell division or other cellular and extracellular actions away from the lasered site was tested by Ruddat and colleagues.[40] In this study, the levels of mRNA for a family of MMPs were measured in response to ALT. These enzymes are synthesized and secreted to release cells from their extracellular matrix, allowing their increased mobility. After ALT, the levels of mRNA were significantly increased, suggesting the release of media-borne signals by ALT, biologically affecting remote, nontreated trabecular regions. In addition, evidence for alteration of turnover or synthesis of glycosaminoglycans after ALT has been reported.[22]

Argon Laser Trabeculoplasty Summary

ALT is a widely accepted treatment modality for open-angle glaucoma. Despite its widespread use, we still lack a thorough understanding of its mode of action. With the support of numerous reported studies to date, the mechanical explanation for IOP reduction in glaucomatous eyes cannot be ruled out, but it may be too simplistic and awaits scientific confirmation. In contrast, several biological processes are triggered by ALT and may play an important role in altering outflow pathway conductivity. These biological processes in the TM include early increase in cell division, migration, and phagocytic activity and release of media-borne factors as well as alteration of glycosaminoglycans. Additional structural changes in lasered and adjacent nontreated regions affecting aqueous flow patterns are also considered. These concepts are summarized in Table 53-2.

ALT is the most commonly used method for trabeculoplasty around the world; however, it is associated with early anterior chamber reaction, local irritation, peripheral anterior synechiae (PAS) formation, and IOP spikes.[7,10,12] Scarring of the TM that is associated with ALT limits its effectiveness in subsequent applications.[7,12,14-17] For this reason, other laser modalities that have a theoretically lower likelihood of injuring tissues have been explored and will be discussed next.

SELECTIVE LASER TRABECULOPLASTY

Selective laser trabeculoplasty (SLT) was developed as a gentler method of IOP reduction without the scarring of the TM that occurs after ALT.[41] SLT utilizes a frequency-doubled Nd:YAG laser trabeculoplasty (Nd:YAG SLT) to target the pigmented cells of the TM without transfer of significant energy to the surrounding tissue. In this mechanism of action, no thermal damage is inflicted to adjacent cells in the TM.

In contrast to the mechanical theory of ALT (that causes coagulative damage to the TM, which results in collagen shrinkage → subsequent scarring of the TM → tightening of the meshwork in the area of each beam → and reopening the adjacent, untreated intertrabecular spaces) (see Figure 53-1),[2,42] the postulated mechanism in SLT is elective photothermolysis that enables the laser to precisely target intracellular melanin granules to activate individual cells while not disturbing adjacent nonpigmented cells. The activated cells release cytokines that trigger a targeted macrophage response to TM cells. The macrophages theoretically reactivate the TM and surrounding extracellular matrix, reducing fluid outflow resistance and lowering IOP.

In published studies,[43-49] SLT is considered to be relatively safe and as effective in lowering IOP as conventional ALT in patients with open-angle glaucoma, while also resulting in less ocular inflammation and fewer IOP spikes after treatment. There is a reported 30% incidence of elevations in IOP greater than 5 mm Hg with ALT compared to an incidence of less than 10% with SLT.[43]

Because of the lower chance of thermal injury and scarring to the targeted tissue, SLT has the potential (and as of yet unproven) benefit of repeatability.[29,43,44,50-52]

Mean reduction in IOP post-SLT has ranged from 2 to 14 mm Hg at 1 month and 3 to 6 mm Hg at 3 months to 5 to 7 mm Hg at 6 months. Five-year data sets have also shown that SLT could be as effective as ALT in lowering IOP in eyes with POAG receiving maximally tolerated medical therapy.[53]

The lack of trabecular scarring after SLT may allow repeated treatments in patients with previous ALT. SLT was developed in order to take advantage of the fact that cellular and humoral mechanisms can affect the outflow facility without creating a permanent scar in the TM.[29-32] The energy delivered by SLT is mostly absorbed by pigmented cells and is therefore spatially confined to the pigmented TM cells without incurring collateral thermal damage to adjacent nonpigmented TM cells and underlying trabecular beams. SLT uses a

TABLE 53-2. ARGON LASER TRABECULOPLASTY: HOW DOES IT WORK?	
Clinical Facts Related to ALT Pathophysiology	
ALT reduces IOP in glaucoma patients	
ALT causes an increase in outflow facility in glaucoma patients	
ALT has no effect on inflow of aqueous humor	
ALT of both 180 and 360 degrees of the angle are effective	
It takes 4 to 6 weeks for ALT to reach its maximal effect	
Low-dose and low-power ALT are equally effective	
Wear-and-tear glaucoma (PXF, POAG, and pigmentary glaucoma) respond better to ALT than other types of open-angle glaucoma)	
Mechanism of Action of ALT	
Two main mechanisms of IOP reduction by ALT may be involved:	
The mechanical theory (below left)	
The biological effect of ALT (below right)	
Indications for the Mechanical Theory	**Indications for the Biological Effect**
• Shrinkage of the inner trabecular ring • Separation of trabecular sheets and opening of aqueous channels • Traction on collapsing Schlemm's canal (not proven in enucleated human eyes)	• Signs of increased biological and phagocytic activity of some trabecular cells • Lasered regions are flat, with cellular sheet extending from corneal endothelium covering them; inner wall of Schlemm's canal is flat with no vacuoles present • Adjacent nonlasered regions disclosed herniations of juxtacanalicular meshwork into Schlemm's canal, containing an abundance of vacuoles • Tracer studies with cationized ferritin demonstrated no aqueous flow through lasered areas, with probable shift of flow through adjacent herniations • Alteration in turnover or synthesis of glycosaminoglycans • Increased trabecular cell division after ALT • Signs for release of media-borne factor affecting remote, nontreated trabecular areas • Induced inflammatory response (trabeculitis)
ALT: argon laser trabeculoplasty; IOP: intraocular pressure; POAG: primary open-angle glaucoma; PXF: pseudoexfoliation glaucoma.	

Q-switched, frequency-doubled 532-nm Nd:YAG laser with a short pulse duration of 3 ns. This modality limits the conversion of energy to heat, further minimizing the collateral tissue damage.[54] Histological studies[54] in human cadaver eyes after SLT reveal no evidence of coagulative damage or disruption of the corneoscleral or uveal trabecular beam structure (Figure 53-3). Because of the minimal cytologic damage, SLT offers 2 theoretical advantages: it may be repeatable and it may have a higher safety profile.[55] Latina and colleagues[56] were the first to establish the efficacy and safety of SLT by demonstrating a 70% response rate and a 5.8 mm Hg (23.5%) IOP-lowering effect of SLT. In addition, they demonstrated that SLT can be repeated after failed ALT without the risk of post-laser IOP spike. Other studies[57-59] confirmed these

findings. Melamed and colleagues[44] treated newly diagnosed glaucoma patients with SLT and demonstrated a mean IOP reduction of 7.7 mm Hg (30%) while also witnessing a lower incidence of postoperative pressure spikes.

Chen and colleagues[60] reported that the IOP-lowering effect of SLT was independent of previous ALT and that there is no difference between the effects of 25 spots on 90 degrees of TM versus 50 spots on 180 degrees of TM. SLT was also reported to cause significantly less pain and flare than ALT.[61] To date, no remarkable postoperative complications have been reported with SLT.

In conclusion, SLT is at least as effective as ALT in reducing IOP. SLT may be safer than ALT because it delivers less energy to the TM, causing fewer post-treatment IOP spikes.

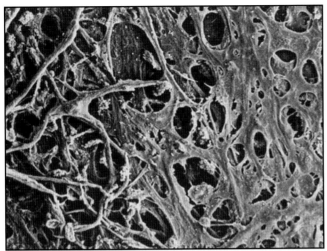

Figure 53-3. Scanning electron microscope image of TM after treatment with SLT showing no visible scar.

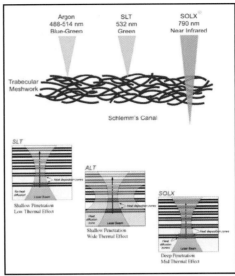

Figure 53-4. Multilayer optical model of TM effect of ALT versus SLT (adapted from Manns et al). Note the difference in the heat-diffusion zone, minimizing the collateral tissue damage. (Reprinted with permission from Garg A, Alio JL, eds. *Surgical Techniques in Ophthalmology: Glaucoma Surgery.* New Delhi, India: Jaypee Brothers; 2010.)

The lack of structural damage to the TM offers the possibility of retreatment following failed ALT. SLT should be considered as either a first- or second-line treatment in open-angle glaucoma patients with uncontrolled IOP.

Titanium-Sapphire Laser Trabeculoplasty

Titanium-sapphire laser trabeculoplasty (TiSLT) was developed in an attempt to improve the efficacy of existing modalities such as ALT and SLT. In a recent clinical study, TiSLT was noted to provide similar efficacy compared to ALT in reducing IOP.[62] The physical parameters of the Ti-Sapphire laser (wavelength of 790 nm; exposure time of 7 msec; and a spot size of 200 µm) are associated with deeper penetration into the TM, affecting tissues like the juxta-canalicular region and inner wall of Schlemm's canal (Figure 53-4). A study[63] comparing the histology of 3 different lasers (ALT, SLT, and TiSLT) in enucleated human eyes confirmed that TiSLT penetrates deeper with disruption of the inner wall of Schlemm's canal and that ALT showed the most tissue damage compared to TiSLT and SLT, which showed little anatomical change.

Micropulsed Diode Laser Trabeculoplasty

Micropulsed diode laser trabeculoplasty (MLT), like SLT, selectively targets pigmented TM cells to avoid collateral damage to adjacent nonpigmented cells. MLT delivers 100-µs pulses for a 0.2-s period at a 15% duty cycle (300-µs laser pulses), which allows the tissue to cool off and prevents the cell destruction. Unlike SLT, which is associated with localized photothermolysis, the interpulse separation of MLT is long enough to allow the temperature to return to baseline prior to the arrival of the next pulse and to prevent cumulative thermal rise.[64] As a consequence, MLT cannot theoretically produce micro-explosions, pigment dispersion, IOP spikes, and risk of IOP spikes in eyes with heavily pigmented TM.[65,66] MLT uses an 810-nm wavelength, which is not as efficiently absorbed by melanin as the shorter wavelengths used for ALT and SLT, also allowing MLT energy to penetrate to deeper tissues.

A 3-month prospective, comparative, randomized study[64] performed in 26 OAG patients randomized to treatment with either ALT or MLT has been found to induce a statistically significant IOP reduction comparable to ALT while post-laser treatment inflammation was clinically minimal and IOP spikes were not observed.

CONCLUSION

LTP is a proven method for decreasing IOP in several types of glaucoma. It may be used as primary therapy or as an adjunct after one or several topical drops have been used. While there are many theories as to why trabeculoplasty is effective at decreasing IOP, none have been definitively proven to date. Newer modalities of trabeculoplasty have been introduced over recent years and each offers unique theoretical benefits over traditional ALT. However, none of the modalities have been proven more effective in treating glaucoma compared to ALT and more studies are needed to both elucidate the mechanism of their action as well as to understand their utility in everyday clinical practice.

REFERENCES

1. Glaucoma Laser Trial Research Group. The Glaucoma Laser Trial (GLT) and Glaucoma Laser Trial Follow-up Study: 7. Results. *Am J Ophthalmol.* 1995;120(6):718-731.

2. Wise JB, Witter SL. Argon laser therapy for open angle glaucoma: a pilot study. *Arch Ophthalmol.* 1979;97(2):319-22.

3. Thomas JV, El-Mofty A, Hamdy EE, Simmons RJ. Argon laser trabeculoplasty as initial therapy for glaucoma. *Arch Ophthalmol.* 1984;102:702-703.

4. Horns DJ, Bellows AR, Hutchinson BT, Allen RC. Argon laser trabeculoplasty for open angle glaucoma: a retrospective study of 380 eyes. *Trans Ophthalmol Soc.* 1983;103(pt 3):288-296.

5. Thomas JV, Simmons RJ, Belcher CD 3rd. Argon laser trabeculoplasty in the presurgical glaucoma patient. *Ophthalmology.* 1982; 89:187-197.

6. Wise JB. Long term control of adult open-angle glaucoma by argon laser treatment. *Ophthalmology.* 1981;88(3):197-202.

7. Ruderman JM, Zweig KO, Wilensky JT, Weinreb RN. Effects of corticosteroid pretreatment on argon laser trabeculoplasty. *Am J Ophthalmol.* 1983;96:84-89.

8. Pappas HR, Berry DP, Partamian L, Hertzmark E, Epstein DL. Topical indomethacin therapy before argon laser trabeculoplasty. *Am J Ophthalmol.* 1985;99:571-575.

9. Weinreb RN, Robin AL, Baerveldt G, Drake MV, Blumenthal M, Wilensky J. Flurbiprofen pretreatment in argon laser trabeculoplasty for primary open angle glaucoma. *Arch Ophthalmol.* 1984;102:1629-1632.

10. Wilensky JT, Jampol LM. Laser therapy for open angle glaucoma. *Ophthalmology.* 1981;88:213.

11. Rouhiainen H, Terasvirta ME, Tuolinen EJ. The effect of some treatment variables on the results of trabeculoplasty. *Arch Ophthalmol.* 1988;106:611.

12. Wilensky JT, Weinreb RN. Low-dose trabeculoplasty. *Am J Ophthalmol.* 1983;95:423.

13. Krasnov MM. Laser puncture of anterior chamber angle in glaucoma. *Am J Ophthalmol.* 1973;75:674-678.

14. Klein HZ, Shields MB, Ernest JT. Two-stage argon laser trabeculoplasty in open angle glaucoma. *Am J Ophthalmol.* 1985;99:392.

15. Shingleton BJ, Richter CU, Dharma SK, et al. Long-term efficacy of argon laser trabeculoplasty. A 10-year follow-up study. *Ophthalmology.* 1993;100:1324-1329.

16. Ticho V, Nesher R. Laser trabeculoplasty in glaucoma: ten years evaluation. *Arch Ophthalmol.* 1989;107:844-846.

17. Yablonski ME, Cook DJ, Gray J. A fluorophotometric study of the effect of argon laser trabeculoplasty on aqueous humor dynamics. *Am J Ophthalmol.* 1985;99:579-582.

18. Shirakashi M, Iwatak NT. Long term efficacy of low power argon laser trabeculoplasty. *Arch Ophthalmol.* 1990;68:23-28.

19. Alvarado J, Murphy C, Juster R. Trabecular meshwork cellularity in primary open angle glaucoma and non-glaucomatous normals. *Ophthalmology.* 1984;91:564-579.

20. Melamed S, Pei J, Epstein DL. Short-term effect of argon laser trabeculoplasty in monkeys. *Arch Ophthalmol.* 1985;103:1546-1552.

21. Melamed S, Pei J, Epstein DL. Delayed response to argon laser trabeculoplasty in monkeys. *Arch Ophthalmol.* 1986;104:1078-1083.

22. Bylsma SS, Samples JR, Acott TS, Van Buskirk EM. Trabecular cell division after argon laser trabeculoplasty. *Arch Ophthalmol.* 1988;106:544-547.

23. Acott TS, Samples JR, Bradley JM, Bacon DR, Bylsma SS, Van Buskirk EM. Trabecular repopulation by anterior trabecular meshwork cells after laser trabeculoplasty. *Am J Ophthalmol.* 1989;107:1-6.

24. Melamed S, Pei J, Epstein DL. Alteration of aqueous humor outflow following argon laser trabeculoplasty in monkeys. *Br J Ophthalmol.* 1987;71:776-781.

25. Bylsma SS, Samples JR, Acott TS, Pirouzkar B, Van Buskirk EM. DNA replication in the cat trabecular meshwork after laser trabeculoplasty in vivo. *J Glaucoma.* 1994;3:36-43.

26. Van-Buskirk EM, Pond V, Rosenquist EC, Acott TS. Argon laser trabeculoplasty. Studies on mechanism of action. *Ophthalmology.* 1984;91:1005-1010.

27. Samples J. Effect of wavelengths on trabecular cell division after laser trabeculoplasty. *Invest Ophthal Vis Sci.* 1990;31(4):344.

28. Alvarado JA, Alvarado RG, Yeh RF, Franse-Carman L, Marcellino GR, Brownstein MJ. A new insight into the cellular regulation of aqueous outflow: how trabecular meshwork endothelial cells drive a mechanism that regulates the permeability of Schlemm's canal endothelial cells. *Br J Ophthalmol.* 2005;89(11):1500-1505.

29. Damji KF, Shah KC, Rock WJ, Bains HS, Hodge WG. Selective laser trabeculoplasty v argon laser trabeculoplasty: a prospective randomized clinical trial. *Br J Ophthalmol.* 1999;83:718-722.

30. Wang N, Chintala SK, Fini ME, Schuman JS. Activation of a tissue-specific stress response in the aqueous outflow pathway of the eye defines the glaucoma disease phenotype. *Nat Med.* 2001;7(3):304-309.

31. Bradley JM, Vranka J, Colvis CM, et al. Effect of matrix metalloproteinases activity on outflow in perfused human organ culture. *Invest Ophthalmol Vis Sci.* 1998;39:2649-2658.

32. Bradley JMB, Anderssohn AM, Colvis CM, et al. Mediation of laser trabeculoplasty-induced matrix metalloproteinase expression by IL-1ß and TNF. *Invest Ophthalmol Vis Sci.* 2000;41:422-430.

33. The Glaucoma Laser Trial (GLT). 2. Results of argon laser trabeculoplasty versus topical medicines. The Glaucoma Laser Trial Research Group. *Ophthalmology.* 1990;97:1403-1413.

34. Shingleton BJ, Richter CU, Dharma SK, et al . Long term efficacy of argon laser trabeculoplasty. *Ophthalmology.* 1993;100(9):1324-1329.

35. The Glaucoma Laser Trial. I. Acute effects of argon laser trabeculoplasty on intraocular pressure. Glaucoma Laser Trial Research Group. *Arch Ophthalmol.* 1989;107:1135-1142.

36. Rodrigues MM, Spaeth GL, Donahoo P. Electron microscopy of argon laser therapy in phakic open angle glaucoma. *Ophthalmology.* 1982;89:198-210.

37. Weber PA, Davidoff FH, McDonald C. Scanning electron microscopy of argon laser trabeculoplasty. *Ophthalmol Forum.* 1983;1:26-29.

38. Gaasterland D, Kupfer C. Experimental glaucoma in the Rhesus monkey. *Invest Ophthalmol Vis Sci.* 1974;14:455-457.

39. Dueker DK, Norberg M, Johnson DH, Tschumper RC, Feeney-Burns L. Stimulation of cell division by argon and Nd-YAG laser trabeculoplasty in cynomologous monkeys. *Invest Ophthalmol Vis Sci.* 1990;31:115-124.

40. Ruddat MS, Alexander JR, Samples JR, et al. Early changes in trabecular metalloproteinase mRNA levels in response to laser trabeculoplasty are induced by media borne factors. *Invest Ophthalmol Vis Sci.* 1989;30(suppl):280.

41. Alvarado JA. Selective laser trabeculoplasty: underlying mechanism. *Ophthalmol Manage.* 2002:1-8.

42. Reiss GR, Wilensky IT, Higginbotham El. Laser trabeculoplasty. *Surv Ophthalmol.* 1991;35:407-428.

43. Damji KF, Bovell AM, Hodgew G, et al. Selective laser trabeculoplasty versus argon laser trabeculoplasty: results from a 1-year randomised clinical trial. *Br J Ophthalmol.* 2006;90(12):1490-1494.

44. Melamed S, Ben Simon GJ, Levkovitch-Verbin H. Selective laser trabeculoplasty as primary treatment for open-angle glaucoma: a prospective, nonrandomized pilot study. *Arch Ophthalmol.* 2003;121:957-960.

45. Francis BA, Ianchulev T, Schofield JK, Minckler DS. Selective laser trabeculoplasty as a replacement for medical therapy in open-angle glaucoma. *Am J Ophthalmol.* 2005;140:524-525.

46. Latina MA, de Leon JM. Selective laser trabeculoplasty. *Ophthalmol Clin J North Am.* 2005;18:409-419.

47. Best UP, Domack H, Schmidt V. Long-term results after selective laser trabeculoplasty—a clinical study on 269 eyes [in German]. *Klin Monatsbl Augenheilkd.* 2005;222:326-331.

48. Gracner T, Pahor D, Gracner B. Efficacy of selective laser trabeculoplasty in the treatment of primary open-angle glaucoma [in German]. *Klin Monatsbl Augenheilkd.* 2003;220:848-852.

49. Stoiber J, Fernandez V, Lamar PD, et al. Trabecular meshwork alteration and intraocular pressure change following pulsed near-infrared laser trabeculoplasty in cats. *Ophthalmic Surg Lasers Imaging.* 2005;36:471-481.

50. Song J, Lee PP, Epstein DL, et al. High failure rate associated with 180 degrees selective laser trabeculoplasty. *J Glaucoma.* 2005;14(5):400-408.

51. Macias JM, Benitez-del-Castillo JM, Garcia-Sanchez J. Selective vs argon laser trabeculoplasty: hypotensive efficacy, anterior chamber inflammation, and postoperative pain. *Eye (Lond).* 2004;18(5): 498-502.

52. Zhao JC, Grosskreutz CL, Pasquale LR. Argon versus selective laser trabeculoplasty in the treatment of open angle glaucoma. *Int Ophthalmol Clin.* 2005;45(4):97-106.

53. Juzych MS, Chopra V, Banitt MR, et al. Comparison of long-term outcomes of selective laser trabeculoplasty versus argon laser trabeculoplasty in open-angle glaucoma. *Ophthalmology.* 2004;111(10):1853-1859.

54. Latina MA, Park C. Selective targeting of trabecular meshwork cells: In vitro studies of pulsed and CW laser interactions. *Exp Eye Res.* 1995;60:359-372.

55. Holz HA, Lim MC. Glaucoma lasers: a review of the newer techniques. *Curr Opin Ophthalmol.* 2005;16:89-93.

56. Latina MA, Sibayan SA, Shin DH, Noecker RJ, Marcellino G. Q switched 532-nm Nd:YAG, laser trabeculoplasty (selective laser trabeculoplasty): a multicenter pilot clinical study. *Ophthalmology.* 1998;105(11):2082-2088.

57. Mermound A, Herbort CP, Schnyder CC, Pittet N. Comparison of the effects of trabeculoplasty using the Nd:YAG laser and argon laser [in German]. *Klin Monatsbl Augenheilkd.* 1992;200:404-406.

58. Tabak S, de Waard PWT, Lemij HG, et al. Selective laser trabeculoplasty in glaucoma. *Invest Ophthalmol Vis Sci.* 1998;39:S472

59. Pirnazar JR, Kolker A, Wax M, et al. The efficacy of 532 nm laser trabeculoplasty. *Invest Ophthalmol Vis Sci.* 1998;39:S5.

60. Chen E, Golchin S, Blomindahl S. Comparison between 90 degrees and 180 degrees selective laser trabeculoplasty. *J Glaucoma.* 2004;13:62-65.

61. Martinez-de-Ia-Gasa JM, Garcia-Feijoo J, Castillo A, et al. Selective vs argon laser trabeculoplasty: hypotensive efficacy, anterior chamber inflammation, and postoperative pain. *Eye.* 2004;18: 498-502.

62. Goldenfeld M, Melamed S, Simon G, Ben Simon GJ. Titanium: sapphire laser trabeculoplasty versus argon laser trabeculoplasty in patients with open-angle glaucoma. *Ophthalmic Surg Lasers Imaging.* 2009;40(3):264-269.

63. Simon G, Lowery JA. Comparison of three types of lasers in laser trabeculoplasty in human donor eyes. Abstract presented at 2007 ASCRS Symposium, San Diego, CA.

64. Detry-Morel M, Muschart F, Pourjavan S. Micropulse diode laser (810 nm) versus argon laser trabeculoplasty in the treatment of open-angle glaucoma: comparative short-term safety and efficacy profile. *Bull Soc Belge Ophthalmol.* 2008;308:21-28.

65. Harasymowycz PJ, Papamatheakis DG, Latina M, De Leon M, Lesk MR, Damji KF. Selective laser trabeculoplasty (SLT) complicated by intraocular pressure elevation in eyes with heavily pigmented trabecular meshworks. *Am J Ophthalmol.* 2005;139(6):1110-1113.

66. Van de Veire S, Zeyen T, Stalmans I. Argon versus selective laser trabeculoplasty. *Bull Soc Belge Ophthalmol.* 2006;299:5-10.

54

Post-Laser Elevation of Intraocular Pressure

Marshall N. Cyrlin, MD

Many of the complications that can occur with traditional incisional surgery have been eliminated by anterior segment laser surgery for glaucoma and for postcataract surgery capsulotomy. Laser surgery has its own substantial risks. These include inflammation, hemorrhage, synechiae formation, and transient or prolonged intraocular pressure (IOP) elevation. Post-laser IOP elevations may be significant, particularly in the patient with pre-existing advanced glaucoma. IOP spikes, if undetected or untreated, can result in further visual loss or blindness.

MECHANISMS OF INTRAOCULAR PRESSURE ELEVATION

Argon laser for iridotomy (ALI) or trabeculoplasty (ALT) interacts with pigmented tissue through its coagulative effect. The laser can contract collagen (lower energies) or vaporize tissue with explosive force (higher energies). Laser treatment can result in the formation of vapor bubbles, pigment debris, and the release of prostaglandins, plasma, or fibrin that can reduce facility of outflow through the trabecular meshwork (TM) by mechanical obstruction or by inciting inflammation.

Selective laser trabeculoplasty (SLT) was developed as a more tissue-specific and possibly safer alternative to ALT. It is performed with a Q-switched, frequency-doubled, 532-nm neodymium:yttrium-aluminum-garnet (Nd:YAG) laser. The potential advantage of SLT over ALT to reduce the complications of laser trabeculoplasty (LTP) is based on its mechanism of selective photothermolysis. This mechanism allows for the selective absorption of short laser pulses to pigmented cells within the TM. This targeted treatment reduces collateral damage to the surrounding tissue of the TM and has been shown in histopathologic specimens to eliminate coagulative damage.[1,2] The lesser amount of tissue interaction and destruction from SLT would be expected to result in a lower incidence and magnitude of IOP elevations. In a study comparing treatments of 180 degrees of the angle with ALT versus SLT, the energy used for the treatment, discomfort during the treatment, and the immediate post-laser inflammation in the anterior chamber were significantly lower for SLT.[3]

Nd:YAG laser employed for iridotomy or capsulotomy exerts its physical effect on pigmented or nonpigmented tissue by photodisruption with the creation of an explosive, expanding plasma shockwave. IOP elevation may result from the previously noted mechanisms, as well as from hemorrhage or hyphema in the case of iridectomy, or from capsular or cortical debris in the case of capsulotomy.

INCIDENCE OF INTRAOCULAR PRESSURE ELEVATION

Postoperative elevation of IOP may commonly follow either ALI or Nd:YAG laser.[4,5] IOP elevation, which occurs within 2 hours post-laser in 96% of the cases, has been reported to have an incidence from 60% to 65% and a range from 1 to 38 mm Hg over pretreatment levels, with no significant difference found between the type of laser used, total energy employed, or the amount of resulting inflammation.[6,7]

IOP elevation after ALT may occur in approximately one-third[8] to one-half[9] of patients, is dependent on the treatment variables, and can be visually threatening if the optic nerve is already compromised by advanced glaucomatous optic atrophy.[10,11] The Glaucoma Laser Trial[12] evaluated the immediate post-laser IOP elevation in 271 eyes of patients with primary

Kahook MY, Schuman JS, eds.
Chandler and Grant's Glaucoma, Fifth Edition (pp 497-499).
© 2013 SLACK Incorporated.

open-angle glaucoma who were assigned to ALT as an initial treatment. The patients received 2 treatments, 1 month apart, to 180 degrees of the TM. The treatments were standardized as to power intensity (threshold of bubble formation) and to location (straddling the pigmented and nonpigmented anterior TM). IOPs were measured at 1 hour and 4 hours after each treatment session. Increases of IOP greater than 5 mm Hg occurred in 34% of eyes after one or both treatment sessions, and increases of greater than 10 mm Hg occurred in 12%. Only a small percentage of eyes had IOP rises greater than 5 mm Hg 4 hours after laser treatment without an elevation 1 hour after treatment. Eyes with increases of IOP after the first treatment were more likely to have increases after the second treatment. Of all of the parameters evaluated, only pigmentation of the TM was associated with IOP increases.[12] Other studies have found a greater incidence and severity of post-laser elevations of IOP from treatments of 100 burns delivered to 360 degrees than from 50 burns delivered to 180 degrees.[8,13]

Pressure elevations are similarly noted following SLT. An immediate post-SLT pressure spike accompanied by persistent anterior chamber reaction has been described and successfully treated medically.[14] In a large multicenter clinical trial, all cases of post-laser increased IOP responded to medical therapy.[15] Patients with previous ALT may be safely treated with SLT. However, patients with a history of previous ALT and eyes with heavy pigmentation have been reported to be at increased risk for post-laser IOP elevation.[16] Lowering the energy settings to result in only slight cavitation bubbling at the laser spot or reducing the number of laser spots may be helpful in preventing IOP elevations when treating heavily pigmented angles.

After Nd:YAG laser capsulotomy, IOP can rise within the first few hours and rarely may last for weeks or months.[17-20] The amount of laser energy delivered, pre-existing glaucoma, pre-laser elevated IOP, absence of an intraocular lens, or the sulcus fixation of a posterior chamber lens are additional risk factors.

MANAGEMENT

Preoperative pressure measurement and treatment with prophylactic medical therapy are tantamount in the prevention of IOP elevations after anterior segment laser surgery. Management continues with appropriate post-laser IOP monitoring and further medical treatment. Patients currently taking glaucoma medication should be instructed to take their medication before arriving for laser, or it should be administered on arrival. Baseline IOP measurements are taken before the laser treatment is performed. Routinely measure the IOP of the fellow eye to use as a control. Historically, pilocarpine, beta-blockers, oral carbonic anhydrase inhibitors (CAIs), oral osmotic agents, topical steroids, and nonsteroidal anti-inflammatory agents have been used with little or variable successes for either preoperative prophylaxis or post-laser treatment of IOP elevations.[10,21-27]

Apraclonidine hydrochloride, an alpha-2 adrenergic agonist that reduces the rate of aqueous formation, was the first medication to be significantly and reliably effective in reducing postoperative elevations of IOP following laser iridotomy, ALT, or Nd:YAG laser capsulotomy.[10,28-33] In a study of 261 eyes assigned to receive either apraclonidine 1%, pilocarpine 4%, timolol maleate 0.5%, dipivefrin 0.1%, or acetazolamide 250 mg both 1 hour before and immediately after 360-degree ALT, apraclonidine was the only medication to reduce the mean IOP significantly from baseline.[34] Only 3% of the apraclonidine eyes had elevations of IOP greater than 5 mm Hg, compared with 39% for acetazolamide, 38% for dipivefrin, 33% for pilocarpine, and 32% for timolol. Brimonidine 0.5%, another alpha-2 adrenergic, was also found to reduce the incidence of post-laser IOP elevation when administered either before or after ALT.[35,36] Increases in IOP greater than 10 mm Hg have been reported in 17% to 27% of laser iridotomy patients successfully managed with apraclonidine.[37,38]

Current prophylactic therapy dictates that the laser eye is pretreated with a drop of medication, preferably 0.5% apraclonidine or brimonidine 0.1% to 0.2%, either 30 to 60 minutes preoperatively and immediately postoperatively. The IOP should be measured again in both eyes at 1 and up to 2 hours after the laser. In cases of advanced glaucoma, a 3- or 4-hour post-laser pressure evaluation may be beneficial. Should the IOP become elevated 5 mm Hg or more from the baseline or should it reach a clinically unacceptable level, an additional drop of apraclonidine should be administered as well as any other topical miotic, beta-blocker, or CAIs that the patient is able to take.[39] For eyes unresponsive to the previous regimen or for more marked elevations of IOP in patients with advanced glaucoma, consider administering oral osmotic agents, if available, at a dose of at least 1 g/kg. Patients with significant elevations of post-laser IOP should be monitored until the IOP is reduced to a clinically acceptable level. They should be examined again the following day. Usually, the IOP will return to pretreatment levels or lower within 24 hours. A sustained increase in IOP may result in a very small percentage of patients following LTP and may require increased medical therapy or possibly surgery.

REFERENCES

1. Latina MA, Park C. Selective targeting of trabecular meshwork cells: in vitro studies of pulsed and CW laser interactions. *Exp Eye Res.* 1995;60:359-371.
2. Kramer TR, Noecker RJ. Comparison of the morphologic changes after selective laser trabeculoplasty and argon laser trabeculoplasty in human eye bank eyes. *Ophthalmology.* 2001;108:773-779.
3. Martinez-de-la-Casa J, Garcia-Feijoo J, Castillo A, et al. Selective vs. argon laser trabeculoplasty: hypotensive efficacy, anterior chamber inflammation, and postoperative pain. *Eye.* 2004;18:498-502.

4. Krupin T, Stone RA, Cohen BH, Kolker AE, Kass MA. Acute intraocular pressure response to argon laser iridotomy. *Ophthalmology.* 1985;92:922-926.

5. Taniguchi T, Rho SH, Gotoh Y, et al. Intraocular pressure rise following Q-switched neodymium:YAG laser iridotomy. *Ophthalmol Laser Ther.* 1987;2:99-104.

6. Robin AL, Pollack IP. A comparison of neodymium:YAG and argon laser iridotomies. *Ophthalmology.* 1984;91:1011-1016.

7. Moster MR, Schwartz LW, Spaeth GL, Wilson RP, McAllister JA, Poryzees EM. Laser iridectomy. A controlled study comparing argon and neodymium:YAG. *Ophthalmology.* 1986;93:20-26.

8. Weinreb RN, Ruderman J, Juster R, Zweig K. Immediate intraocular pressure response to argon laser trabeculoplasty. *Am J Ophthalmol.* 1983;95:279-286.

9. Krupin T, Kolker AE, Kass MA, et al. Intraocular pressure the day of argon laser trabeculoplasty in primary open angle glaucoma. *Ophthalmology.* 1984;91:361.

10. Robin AL. Medical management of acute post-operative intraocular pressure rises associated with anterior segment ophthalmic laser surgery. *Int Ophthalmol.* 1990;30:102-110.

11. Thomas JV, Simmons RJ, Belcher CD III. Complications of argon laser trabeculoplasty. *Glaucoma.* 1982;4:50-52.

12. The Glaucoma Laser Trial. I. Acute effects of argon laser trabeculoplasty on intraocular pressure. Glaucoma Laser Trial Research Group. *Arch Ophthalmol.* 1989;107:1135-1142.

13. Weinreb RN, Ruderman J, Juster R, Wilensky JT. Influence of the number of laser burns administered on the early results of argon laser trabeculoplasty. *Am J Ophthalmol.* 1983;95:287-292.

14. Lai JS, Chua JK, Tham CC, Lam DS. Five-year follow up of selective laser trabeculoplasty in Chinese eyes. *Clin Exp Ophthalmol.* 2004;32:368-372.

15. Latina MA, Tumbocon JA, Noecker RJ, et al. Selective laser trabeculoplasty (SLT): the United States prospective multicenter clinical trial results. *Invest Ophthalmol Vis Sci.* 2001;42:S546.

16. Harasymowycz PJ, Papamatheakis DG, Latina M, De Leon M, Lesk MR, Damji KF. Selective laser trabeculoplasty (SLT) complicated by pressure elevation in eyes with heavily pigmented trabecular meshwork. *Am J Ophthalmol.* 2005;139:1110-1113.

17. Channell MM, Beckman H. Intraocular pressure changes after neodymium-YAG laser posterior capsulotomy. *Arch Ophthalmol.* 1984;102:1024-1026.

18. Richter CU, Arzeno G, Pappas HR, Steinert RF, Puliafito C, Epstein DL. Intraocular pressure elevation following Nd:YAG laser posterior capsulotomy. *Ophthalmology.* 1985;92:636-640.

19. Keates RH, Steinert RF, Puliafito CA, Maxwell SK. Long-term follow-up of Nd:YAG laser posterior capsulotomy. *Ophthalmology.* 1985;92:636-638.

20. Demer JL, Koch DD, Smith JA, Knolle GE Jr. Persistent elevation in intraocular pressure after Nd:YAG laser treatment. *Ophthalmic Surg.* 1986;17:465-466.

21. Ruderman JM, Zweig KO, Wilensky JT, Weinreb RN. Effects of corticosteroid pretreatment on argon laser trabeculoplasty. *Am J Ophthalmol.* 1983;96:84-89.

22. Ofner S, Samples JR, Van Buskirk EM. Pilocarpine and the increase in intraocular pressure after trabeculoplasty. *Am J Ophthalmol.* 1984;97:647-649.

23. Hotchkiss ML, Robin AL, Pollack IP, Quigley HA. Nonsteroidal anti-inflammatory agents after argon laser trabeculoplasty. A trial with flurbiprofen and indomethacin. *Ophthalmology.* 1984;91:969-976.

24. Pappas HR, Berry DP, Partamian L, Hertzmark E, Epstein DL. Topical indomethacin therapy before argon laser trabeculoplasty. *Am J Ophthalmol.* 1985;99:571-575.

25. Cyrlin MN, Beckman H. Low-dose oral glycerin for the prevention of post-laser IOP elevation. *Invest Ophthalmol Vis Sci.* 1987;28(suppl):272.

26. Metcalfe TW, Etchells DE. Prevention of the immediate intraocular pressure rise following argon laser trabeculoplasty. *Br J Ophthalmol.* 1989;73:612-616.

27. Migliori ME, Beckman H, Channell MM. Intraocular pressure changes after neodymium-YAG laser capsulotomy in eyes pretreated with timolol. *Arch Ophthalmol.* 1987;105:473-475.

28. Robin AL, Pollack, IP, House B, Enger C. Effect of ALO 2145 on intraocular pressure following argon laser trabeculoplasty. *Arch Ophthalmol.* 1987;105:646-650.

29. Robin AL, Pollack IP, deFaller JM. Effects of topical ALO 2145 (p-aminoclonidine hydrochloride) on acute intraocular pressure rise following argon laser iridotomy. *Arch Ophthalmol.* 1987;105:1208-1211.

30. Brown RH, Stewart RH, Lynch MG, et al.. ALO 2145 reduces the intraocular pressure elevation after anterior segment laser surgery. *Ophthalmology.* 1988;95:378-384.

31. Pollack IP, Brown RH, Crandall AS, et al. Prevention of the rise in intraocular pressure following neodymium-YAG posterior capsulotomy using topical 1% ALO 2145. *Arch Ophthalmol.* 1988;106:754-757.

32. Yuen NS, Cheung P, Hui SP. Comparing brimonidine 0.2% to apraclonidine 1.0% in the prevention of intraocular pressure elevation and their pupillary effects following laser peripheral iridotomy. *Jpn J Ophthalmol.* 2005;48:89-92.

33. Chen TC. Brimonidine 0.15% versus apraclonidine 0.5% for the prevention of intraocular pressure elevation after anterior segment laser surgery. *J Cataract Refract Surg.* 2005;31:1707-1712.

34. Robin AL. Argon laser trabeculoplasty medical therapy to prevent the intraocular pressure rise associated with argon laser trabeculoplasty. *Ophthalmic Surg.* 1991;22:31-37.

35. Barnebey HS, Robin AL, Zimmerman TJ, et al. The efficacy of brimonidine in decreasing elevations in intraocular pressure after laser trabeculoplasty. *Ophthalmology.* 1993;100:1083-1088.

36. David R, Spaeth GL, Clevenger CE, et al. Brimonidine in the prevention of intraocular pressure elevation following argon laser trabeculoplasty. *Arch Ophthalmol.* 1993;111:1387-1390.

37. Kitazawa Y, Taniguchi T, Sugiyama K. Use of apraclonidine to reduce acute intraocular pressure rise following Q-switched Nd:YAG laser iridotomy. *Ophthalmic Surg.* 1989;20:49-52.

38. Hong C, Song KY, Park WH, Sohn YH. Effect of apraclonidine hydrochloride on acute intraocular pressure rise after argon laser iridotomy. *Korean J Ophthalmol.* 1991;5:37-41.

39. Dapling RB, Cunliffe IA, Longstaff S. Influence of apraclonidine and pilocarpine alone and in combination on postlaser trabeculoplasty pressure rise. *Br J Ophthalmol.* 1994;78:30-32.

55

Laser Peripheral Iridotomy

Lisa S. Gamell, MD; Timothy Saunders, MD; and Joel S. Schuman, MD, FACS

More than 4 decades ago, surgical iridotomy was the best available procedure for eyes with acute angle-closure glaucoma. Since that time, advances in laser technology and laser surgical techniques have allowed laser peripheral iridotomy (LPI) to emerge as the mainstay of treatment for most types of angle-closure glaucoma. Many deserve credit for early work on laser techniques for iridotomy,[1-5] but 2 major developments have contributed to the current application and efficacy of this method: the development of lasers with good optics, capable of delivering sufficient energy, and the development of a corneal contact lens with a plano-convex button, such as that developed by Robert Abraham (Figure 55-1) or that of James Wise, which improve energy delivery to the iris (Table 55-1).

In pupillary block, the most common type of angle-closure glaucoma, there is increased apposition of the iris to the lens at the pupillary border. This blocks the natural pathway of aqueous into the anterior chamber and out through the trabecular meshwork (TM). This causes peripheral anterior chamber shallowing and occlusion of the angle by the iris tissue and could ultimately lead to intraocular pressure (IOP) elevation. When this block occurs acutely, an acute angle-closure attack ensues. When the block is intermittent or gradual, IOP fluctuations may occur, leading to intermittent or chronic types of angle closure. In any of these scenarios, IOP elevation, posterior synechiae, and disc damage may occur.

By performing a laser iridotomy, a hole is created in the peripheral iris. This opening allows an alternate pathway for the flow of aqueous from the posterior chamber to the anterior chamber, bypassing the pupillary block. The equilibration of aqueous flow allows the iris to fall back into its natural position, no longer occluding angle structures. In many cases, as long as peripheral anterior synechiae (PAS) have not formed, LPI may be curative. This procedure can be performed safely, in the office, as an outpatient procedure. The proper indications and techniques will be described below.

This is a procedure that all ophthalmologists should be able to perform, as acute angle-closure glaucoma is one of the few ophthalmic emergencies and swift, accurate diagnosis and treatment can be sight-saving.

INDICATIONS

While LPI is clearly indicated in acute angle-closure glaucoma, there are several other situations where this procedure is beneficial as well. These settings include pupillary block with narrow, occludable angles, chronic angle-closure glaucoma, mixed mechanism glaucoma, imperforate surgical iridotomy, suspected malignant glaucoma, pupillary block after cataract surgery, prophylactic treatment of a fellow eye after an acute angle-closure attack, and nanophthalmos (Table 55-2).

Typically, acute angle-closure glaucoma is initially treated with medications to lower IOP. Ideally, the acute attack can be broken with medical therapy, and the laser iridotomy can be performed afterward when the eye is no longer acutely inflamed. In inflamed eyes, laser openings in the iris may close subsequently, necessitating a second treatment. If an iridotomy is attempted during an acute angle-closure attack, the argon laser is preferred because of the greater incidence of bleeding in these inflamed eyes. In eyes with a phacomorphic component, miotic agents should be used cautiously, as this may break the attack in some eyes, while causing a paradoxical reaction and worsening the attack in others. In the latter case, argon laser iridoplasty is very useful in breaking the attack.[1]

The safety profile and convenience of LPI have made it the preferred technique for most cases of acute angle closure. Even if it is suspected that the angle is extensively involved with PAS, an LPI should be done initially rather than filtration surgery, and the IOP and angle should be assessed after treatment. In combined-mechanism glaucoma, it eliminates the angle-closure component. In the past, we advocated surgical iridotomy (rather than medical therapy)

Kahook MY, Schuman JS, eds.
Chandler and Grant's Glaucoma, Fifth Edition (pp 501-510).
© 2013 SLACK Incorporated.

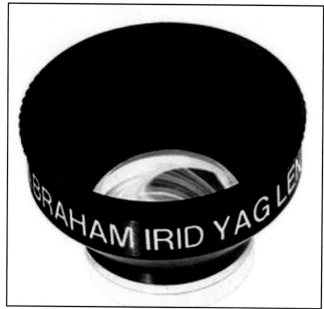

Figure 55-1. Abraham lens used for laser iridotomy. (Reprinted with permission from Ocular Instruments.)

TABLE 55-1. ADVANTAGES OF THERAPEUTIC CONTACT LENS USE IN THE PERFORMANCE OF A LASER IRIDOTOMY
Lens creates concentration of energy at the iris level
Lens acts as heat sink, decreasing corneal epithelial and endothelial burns
Lens acts as speculum, keeping lids apart
Lens provides limited control of ocular movement
Lens provides magnification of target site

TABLE 55-2. INDICATIONS FOR LASER PERIPHERAL IRIDOTOMY
Pupillary block with angle closure
Pupillary block with narrow, occludable angle
Chronic angle-closure glaucoma
Combined-mechanism glaucoma
Imperforate surgical iridotomy
Suspected malignant glaucoma
Fellow eye in acute angle-closure glaucoma
Pupillary block after cataract operation
Nanophthalmos

THE CHOICE OF IRIDOTOMY LENS

Joel S. Schuman, MD, FACS

We tend to favor the neodymium:yttrium-aluminum-garnet (Nd:YAG) laser Abraham iridotomy lens (Ocular Instruments, Bellevue, WA), as it has a 66-D plano-convex button that is both larger and easier to focus through than either the argon laser or Abraham iridotomy lens. The argon Abraham lens also has a 66-D button, but the button is smaller than the Nd:YAG laser version. This is because the cone angle of the argon laser is smaller than that of the Nd:YAG laser. (The cone angle is the angle created by the laser beam coming together to focus into a spot, which is the waist, or narrowest point of the beam. The smaller the cone angle, the easier it is to focus the laser, as the waist of the beam is present for a greater distance in space. This is why focus is so critical with the Nd:YAG laser, as there is only a very small area where the waist of the beam is present.) Because of the larger cone angle of the Nd:YAG laser, the Abraham lens for this instrument requires a bigger button. While this enables use of the lens with the Nd:YAG laser, it also facilitates its use with the argon or diode lasers.

The Wise lens, with its 103-D button, minifies the spot and magnifies the target to a greater extent than the Abraham lens, which is an advantage, as it concentrates the laser energy more; however, because of the higher power of the button, focus is more difficult with the Wise lens than with the Abraham. Many surgeons prefer the Wise lens because of its optical properties, while others favor the Abraham for its ease of use.

to treat eyes with angle closure and eyes with suspected combined-mechanism glaucoma. In fact, Paul Chandler had surgical peripheral iridotomy himself for the latter condition. Nowadays, LPI would be performed initially in most patients. Exceptions would be patients who could not cooperate at a slit-lamp or with the procedure while awake. Examples might include patients with Alzheimer's, other types of dementia, or developmental delay. In such cases where angle closure was suspected, an exam under anesthesia with a surgical peripheral iridotomy might be the optimal treatment.

However, what about the eye with a narrow angle with normal IOP and no PAS identified on indentation gonioscopy? In the past, we would follow such patients with repetitive dark-room tests, and if the results were negative, no iridotomy would be performed. Currently, we recommend performing an LPI in such patients. The risk/benefit ratio of LPI is such that, if an experienced observer were concerned that an angle appeared occludable, LPI is recommended. In this context, one should treat the patient as one would wish to be treated. It is seldom in medicine that any procedure is without risk, and the art and science of medicine involve balancing the benefits and risk of the disease with those of the treatment. Nonetheless, in experienced hands, the benefits of performing an LPI as a prophylactic measure to prevent acute or chronic angle closure in at-risk eyes far outweighs the risks. The most common risks include postoperative IOP spikes, inflammation, and localized hemorrhage. These can usually be minimized

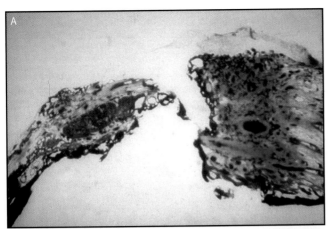

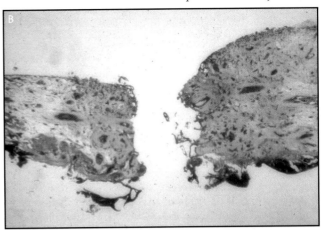

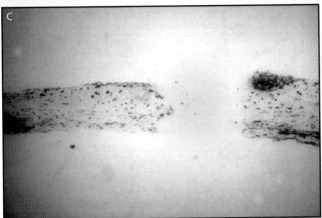

Figure 55-2. Argon (A), diode (B), and Nd:YAG (C) laser iridotomies. Note that iris pigment epithelium is intact up to the border of the argon and diode laser iridotomies, but is absent in the Nd:YAG laser iridotomy. This may account for the lower closure rate experienced with Nd:YAG laser iridotomy, as pigment migration and plugging accounts for most cases of closure.

by proper technique or managed medically in most cases. It is recommended with any laser procedure to check the IOP 1 hour after completion of the procedure, because the majority of postoperative IOP spikes occur during this time. There are few long-term risks or side effects of LPI that would be more devastating than if the patient did not have the procedure and went on to develop angle-closure glaucoma.

CONTRAINDICATIONS

In addition to the inability to position the patient at the slit-lamp, one should also be concerned about the presence of various corneal diseases and of a totally flat anterior chamber with iridocorneal touch. Nevertheless, we would recommend that consideration always be given to trying LPI initially, at least in 1 circumscribed area. We have successfully performed LPI in patients with interstitial keratitis and with posterior crocodile shagreen, although some endothelial damage did occur in the latter condition.

TECHNIQUE OF LASER IRIDOTOMY

There are several techniques that have been used to penetrate the iris and perform the procedure. Our favored

technique is described in the box "Technique of Laser Iridotomy" and involves the use of the Nd:YAG laser.

Time and experience have shown the value of photodisruption in LPI. While the argon (or diode) laser is a useful photocoagulator and may be used to thin the iris or coagulate blood vessels to prevent bleeding, the Nd:YAG laser is superior for the purpose of LPI. Iridotomies created with the Nd:YAG are both simpler to perform and longer lasting than those made by photocoagulation (Figure 55-2).[2-4]

ENLARGEMENT OF ARGON OR DIODE LASER IRIDOTOMY

It is also important that careful attention be given to this detail when enlarging the iris opening. One should attempt to treat the circumference of the opening rather than residual tissue or debris in the center of the opening. One often encounters, especially in blue irides, thin strands that bridge an iris opening but are resistant to coagulation. These are easy to sever with the Nd:YAG laser, but considerably more difficult to remove with a photocoagulator. If there is a patent iridotomy on either side of the strand, it should be left alone. If the strand is thinner than 50 µm, the center of the strand should be avoided, lest there be energy absorption by the crystalline lens, but instead the ends of the strand merging into the circumference of the opening can be treated if it is deemed important to break the strand. If there is an adequate opening in the iris to relieve pupillary block, even if it is irregular in shape or contains bridging strands, it is best left alone without additional (excessive) laser applications. On the other hand, one wants an opening sufficient in size to be able to see the underlying lens capsule before concluding the laser session.

TECHNIQUE OF LASER IRIDOTOMY

Lisa S. Gamell, MD

The concept behind a laser iridotomy is straightforward. A hole is put in the iris to relieve relative or absolute pupillary block and thus relieve iris bombé and angle-closure glaucoma. The hole can be made with any number of laser sources but most commonly argon, diode, Nd:YAG, or a combination of argon or diode and Nd:YAG lasers are used.

With all techniques, miotics should be used to constrict the pupil and thin the target tissue, and antiglaucoma medications should be used to prevent a post-laser pressure spike. An iridotomy lens should be used. The Nd:YAG laser Abraham-type iridotomy lens (Ocular Instruments, Inc) is an excellent choice. The contact lens increases the power density at the target site and additionally gives limited control over ocular movement. While the argon laser can be used for iridotomies in light or dark eyes, the Nd:YAG laser used alone is best with lighter eyes. The combined argon or diode and Nd:YAG laser technique can be used in almost all situations, but is excellent for dark eyes and in special situations, such as angle-closure attack eyes or pseudophakic pupillary block.

PRETREATMENT REGIMEN

- The vision and IOP are checked preoperatively.
- Pilocarpine 1% or 2% is given to cause pupillary constriction.
- Iopidine (apraclonidine) 0.5% or other alpha-agonist is given.
- About 30 minutes later, after pupillary constriction has occurred and the iris is immobile, the patient is seated at the laser, and a contact lens with methylcellulose is applied.

ARGON LASER TECHNIQUE

The technique with the argon laser, whether the long pulse technique in the lighter eye or the short pulse technique in the darker eye, is the same. The aiming beam is brought into focus at an appropriate spot on the iris surface at either 11 or 1 o'clock (12 o'clock is avoided to elude bubbles obstructing the view), and the laser is fired with the shots superimposed until a pigment flume is seen coming forward (smoke signal). When the anterior lens capsule is visible in the aiming beam, the iridotomy is complete.

Argon Parameters
Long pulse technique (for blue, hazel, or light brown eyes)
Time: 0.2 s
Power: 1000 mW
Spot Size: 50 μm
Number of Applications: 1 to 30
Short pulse technique (for dark brown eyes)
Time: 0.02 to 0.05 s
Power: 500 to 1000 Mw
Spot Size: 50 μm
Number of Applications: 25 to 100

NEODYMIUM:YTTRIUM-ALUMINUM-GARNET LASER TECHNIQUE

The iridotomy can be placed anywhere between 11 and 1 o'clock as bubbles are less of an issue. Try to avoid visible blood vessels. The spots of the aiming beam are brought into single, crisp focus aiming through the center of the contact lens button. The red aiming beams are then separated slightly, by advancing focus forward, to ensure focus into the iris stroma. The laser is fired; frequently, the iridotomy will be complete after the first burst. If not, sequential bursts are applied, taking care to avoid any injury to the anterior lens capsule.

Neodymium:Yttrium-Aluminum-Garnet Parameters
Energy: 3 to 6 mJ
Number of Applications: 1 to 10 bursts of 1 to 3 pulses per burst
Argon/Nd:YAG Technique

The argon laser is used to thin the iris so that approximately 20% of the tissue remains. It is done in identical fashion to the argon technique mentioned above using the 0.02 to 0.05 time settings. When this is accomplished, the laser is changed to the Nd:YAG mode, or the patient is moved to the Nd:YAG laser. The contact lens can usually be left in place and will not fall out. The Nd:YAG laser beam is then focused into the depth of the crater, and one shot will usually complete the iridotomy.

Argon/Neodymium:Yttrium-Aluminum-Garnet Parameters
For dark brown eyes, pseudophakic eyes, patients on anticoagulant therapy.
Argon thinning of the iris:
Time: 0.02 to 0.05 s
Power: 500 to 1000 mW
Spot Size: 50 μm
Number of Applications: 5 to 25
Nd:YAG perforation of the iris:
Energy: 3 to 6 mJ
Number of Applications: One or more bursts of 1 to 3 pulses per burst

POSTOPERATIVE MANAGEMENT

Following laser iridotomy, the IOP should be checked sometime during the first postoperative hour to be sure there is no IOP elevation. If the IOP is high and the optic nerve is at risk or has pre-existing damage, the IOP may be checked the next day; aqueous suppressants are prescribed as needed. In general, if the postoperative IOP is normal, the patient is seen 1 week later. During the first postoperative week, prednisolone acetate 1% is typically prescribed 4 times a day for 4 days (or longer in eyes with exuberant inflammation). At the postoperative week 1 visit, gonioscopy is performed to assess the success in opening the drainage angle. Topical steroids are routinely used 4 times a day for 3 days.

This is a modification of the techniques previously outlined in the Fourth Edition by C. Davis Belcher III, MD.

ENLARGEMENT OF NEODYMIUM:YTTRIUM-ALUMINUM-GARNET LASER IRIDOTOMY

Frequently, 1 or 2 bursts of 3 pulses per burst are all that is required to create a patent Nd:YAG laser iridotomy. If the LPI is patent, but the opening is small, the surgeon may wish to enlarge the opening. This is done by treating the edges of the iridotomy, using the same energy settings employed initially, but switching to only 1 pulse per shot. The edges of the iridotomy are chipped away, until the iridotomy is of a sufficient size to allow visualization of the underlying lens capsule, such that it is unlikely to close in the future. Intervening strands are easily severed with the Nd:YAG laser, but care should be taken to avoid blood vessels traversing the opening. Should a blood vessel be ruptured, gentle pressure applied through the goniolens is usually sufficient to arrest any bleeding. Such bleeding tends to be inconsequential and self-limited in any event.

A Second Iridotomy

After completing 1 iridotomy, or while waiting for pigment and debris from the first opening to clear from the overlying aqueous humor, a second iridotomy is sometimes initiated in the other upper quadrant, particularly in iris bombé or inflammatory pupillary block. Because only 1 iridotomy is required to cure pupillary block, if 1 of the 2 openings should close during the ensuing weeks, no further laser sessions will be required. This offers convenience to the patient, but must be weighed against the effect of additional applications of laser energy during the second iridotomy. Occasionally, iritis can develop after LPI, although this has resolved without sequelae in our experience. At the present time, we do 2 iridotomies only when 1 is likely to close, such as in iris bombé or inflammatory pupillary block.

Lens Opacities

One risk of this procedure is possible lens injury, either direct (from the laser itself) or indirect (due to reduced nourishment of the lens by circulating aqueous). The procedure should be planned with the purpose of avoiding any whitening of, or damage to, the lens underlying the treatment site. Sometimes, with the argon or diode laser, a small capsular whitening cannot be avoided, but one should strive to avoid this. Such capsular white areas do not appear to progress, but the implication that these are harmless may be misleading. The lens epithelium is the permeability barrier of the lens, and if there is epithelial-capsular injury, one would expect fluid shifts within the whole lens (possibly increasing nuclear sclerosis or posterior subcapsular changes) rather than merely a progression locally in the whitened areas of the lens epithelium.

It is extremely unusual to induce lens injury with the Nd:YAG laser; such injury manifests as a rupture in the lens capsule and should be avoided at all costs.

In argon or diode laser iridotomies, localized lens whitening occurs about one-third of the time, after the initial penetration through the iris pigment epithelium when the iris opening is enlarged.[5-7] When the lens capsule is exposed by opening the iris, it is vulnerable to laser injury if the subsequent applications are not fully absorbed by iris tissue. Another mechanism for lens whitening with photocoagulation is posterior displacement of pigment from the iris onto the anterior lens capsule during the iridotomy, with subsequent absorption of laser energy by this pigment through a patent iridotomy. It is therefore imperative that the surgeon recognize when the iridotomy is patent, in order to avoid thermal injury to the lens capsule in this manner.

Postoperative Visits

Week 1

The patient is usually seen 1 week after the LPI is performed. At that time, in addition to the routine ophthalmologic examination including measurement of visual acuity and applanation IOP, the status of the overlying corneal endothelium, anterior chamber reaction, and iridotomy patency are evaluated.

If at the postoperative week 1 visit the anterior chamber of the treated eye is quiet, then the fellow eye may be treated if necessary (Table 55-3). This saves the patient unnecessary visits to the office. Then, the patient may be seen 1 week later as well, and bilateral gonioscopy may be performed to assess the response to the procedure. Gonioscopy is always performed to be sure pupillary block has been relieved and to determine the extent of PAS. With a patent iridotomy and relative pupillary block now relieved, the iris should no longer be convex, but rather flat in contour.

Occasionally, one observes an apparently patent LPI, but pupillary block seems not to have been relieved. In such a case, one should suspect posterior sequestration of the iridotomy by adherence of the iris to the lens capsule. An additional LPI should then be performed. By performing the LPI as far peripherally as possible, one can usually avoid this situation.

TABLE 55-3. PERIOPERATIVE CARE: LASER IRIDOTOMY	
Preoperative	**Postoperative**
Apraclonidine 0.5%	Prednisolone acetate 1% every 2 hours for 1 day, then 4 times daily for 4 days, then stop.
Pilocarpine 2%	Check IOP at 1 hour, postoperative at 1 week and DFE when LPI complete (ie, if fellow eye needs to be done). Follow-up at 4 to 6 weeks to check patency if high-risk eye.

Often, an iridotomy created with the argon or diode laser, due to thermal coagulation necrosis in the adjacent tissue, will increase in size spontaneously after several weeks. If the iridotomy has closed, then an additional laser application should be performed. (If 2 LPIs were performed and 1 subsequently closes, however, no retreatment is required.) Such retreatments are often easily accomplished.

We are often asked about the smallest-sized iris opening that is acceptable following LPI. We suppose that the answer is 60 μm or greater. More importantly, however, one must be able to see the lens capsule through the iris opening and document relief of pupillary block by gonioscopy. Failing this, repeat treatment is indicated.

Long-Term Follow-Up

If the LPI is patent at the week 1 visit, the eye is quiet, and the angle is no longer occludable, follow-up can be determined on an individual basis. Once patent LPIs are present, the patient may be safely dilated, and a thorough evaluation of the optic nerve may be done. At this visit, gonioscopy should always be performed prior to and after pupillary dilation with a weak mydriatic to rule out the rare condition of plateau iris (see Chapters 25 and 26). Also, the crystalline lens should be carefully inspected with the pupil dilated, and routine retinal examination (including indirect ophthalmoscopy) should be performed. If needed, baseline disc photos and optical coherence tomography may be performed, along with subsequent visual field testing. Based upon the health of the optic nerve and any evidence of visual field loss, follow-up may be determined. We recommend that patients without residual glaucoma be next examined in 6 months and then yearly. More commonly than expected, some type of open-angle glaucoma seems to develop in patients with previous angle-closure glaucoma, for which such patients should always be followed.

With the use of the Nd:YAG laser for LPI, the risk of closure is small. In eyes at high risk for LPI closure, such as very small LPI or those with recurrent or pre-existing inflammation or silicone oil, a follow-up visit at 4 to 6 weeks may be indicated to check for LPI patency. If the iridotomy is

irregular, but pupillary block has been relieved, nothing further needs to be done. Needless touch-ups should be avoided. Performed in the aforementioned manner, a retreatment rate of approximately 20% with the argon or diode laser should be expected. The retreatment rate for Nd:YAG laser or combined argon or diode and Nd:YAG laser iridotomies is considerably lower.[7-13]

RESIDUAL GLAUCOMA

In patients with residual PAS or combined-mechanism glaucoma, IOP may, of course, continue to be uncontrolled after LPI. However, in addition to the almost immediate elevation of IOP that may occur following LPI, due to the open-angle mechanism described above, the IOP may be moderately elevated for several weeks to months due to a second ill-defined open-angle mechanism. Perhaps this relates to liberation of pigment or other debris, for often the inferior angle especially contains much more pigment after LPI. In any case, this is usually a temporary phenomenon. Therefore, for borderline or moderately uncontrolled residual open-angle glaucoma, it is best to wait if possible at least a month after LPI before deciding on further intervention, such as LTP or filtration surgery.

For residual PAS, especially if these are of suspected recent onset (less than 6 months or so), one may elect to perform iridoplasty or gonioplasty to separate these adhesions from the angle wall and open up potentially functional trabecular tissue.

COMPLICATIONS

While any serious complication of laser peripheral iridotomy is rare, a number of complications can occur, as described below and listed in Tables 55-4 and 55-5.

CORNEA

As mentioned previously, corneal endothelial whitening can occur with photocoagulation (argon, diode) due to energy absorption by the endothelium, necessitating prompt discontinuation of laser applications through this area. When so discontinued, these clouded endothelial areas disappear with time without residue, but we have heard of unusual cases in which permanent corneal edema has resulted. Corneal endothelial burns can be responsible for patient discomfort following the procedures. As already mentioned, we have observed endothelial blister formation (see Figure 55-2) in a patient with pre-existing posterior crocodile shagreen, which has so far persisted without apparent adverse effects on corneal clarity and function.

With the Nd:YAG laser, localized corneal edema can occur, due to disruption of the corneal endothelium overlying the site of the LPI, especially in eyes with very little space between the iris and the posterior surface of the cornea. These lesions tend

TABLE 55-4. COMMON ERRORS AND PROBLEMS IN LASER PERIPHERAL IRIDOTOMY	
Error or Problem	**Solution**
• Iridotomy not patent	• Make sure lens capsule is visible through iridotomy site at conclusion of procedure. "Smoke signal" is not enough!
• Pupil distorted at conclusion of LPI	• Inadequate miosis prior to procedure. Much more common with argon or diode LPI than with Nd:YAG laser. Will likely resolve with time.
• Diplopia	• Iridotomy made in palpebral fissure, or so peripheral that tear meniscus acts as prism, creating second image. If intolerable, patient can wear cosmetic contact lens, blocking light from LPI, but not pupil.
• Bleeding	• Choose correct laser; use argon, diode, or argon or diode plus Nd:YAG in patients on anticoagulants, with iris neovascularization.
• Difficulty in perforating the iris	• Use correct techniques for eye color and situation. • Use adequate miotics to thin and stabilize target. • Use contact lens.
• Closure of initially patent iridotomy	• Use argon or diode plus Nd:YAG or Nd:YAG to prevent closure and use Nd:YAG to reopen to prevent repeat occurrence.
• Pressure spike	• Use aggressive premedication to prevent pressure spikes, especially in eyes with compromised optic nerves and visual field deficits.

TABLE 55-5. COMPLICATIONS OF LASER IRIDOTOMY
Corneal burns
Uveitis
Transient elevation of the IOP
Lenticular opacities
Pigment dispersion
Retinal burns
Corectopia
Diplopia
Iris atrophy
Precipitation of malignant glaucoma
Failure to obtain iridotomy
Late closure of iridotomy
Posterior synechiae formation
Hemorrhage
Ciliochoroidal effusion

to be small and self-limited and resolve over time with adjacent corneal endothelial cells spreading to cover the defect.

Rarely, corneal epithelial burns can occur as with laser trabeculoplasty, but these clear without sequelae.

UVEITIS

A small amount of inflammation is to be expected following LPI, for which a few days' tapering course of topical steroids is routinely prescribed. Our routine regimen is prednisolone acetate every 2 hours the day of the LPI, followed by 4-times-a-day administration for 4 days, and then discontinuation of the drop. Occasionally, substantial iritis can occur, but this has always responded well to increased steroid therapy and has been short-lived in our experience. Nevertheless, one should always remember that, after all, we are ablating iris tissue with this procedure, and varying amounts of inflammation are to be expected.

ELEVATED INTRAOCULAR PRESSURE

This has been discussed previously. On the day of the procedure, additional antiglaucoma therapy may be prescribed, and the IOP should be monitored. A moderate, although often temporary, IOP elevation may persist for a month or so, which must be remembered when considering additional surgical intervention.

LENS INJURY

This has been discussed previously. Although the white epithelial capsular opacity often seen following argon or

One Technique for Laser Peripheral Iridotomy

Joel S. Schuman, MD, FACS

We are often asked for our technique for LPI that has been outlined in this chapter; however, what follows is a brief synopsis of our LPI method.

Following informed consent, the patient receives a drop of apraclonidine just prior to the procedure and a drop of pilocarpine 2%. When adequate miosis and akinesia of the pupil are achieved, the patient is seated at the laser. The Nd:YAG laser is set at 3 to 4 mJ, 3 pulses per burst. A drop of proparacaine 0.5% is instilled, and the Nd:YAG laser Abraham iridotomy lens is placed on the eye, using methylcellulose as the coupling solution. The patient is instructed to look straight ahead, and the lens is held perpendicular to the laser beam. The 2 or 4 spots of the Nd:YAG laser aiming beam are brought into a single spot by focusing the laser. If the spots cannot be brought together, it is due to malposition of the lens, which is moved slightly to join the beams.

The laser is then moved *slightly* toward the patient to defocus the beam just the smallest amount (Figure 55-3). The patient may see a flash or hear a pop, but should feel no pain and should not move. The laser is fired, and an iridotomy is often achieved with the first burst. If an iridotomy is not achieved, the focusing and firing procedure are repeated until a patent iridotomy is present.

If the iridotomy is small, it is enlarged by changing the laser setting to the single pulse mode and lowering the power, and the laser is aimed at the edges of the opening. The laser is fired until the iridotomy is of adequate size, generally about 200 µm.

The lens is removed, a drop of prednisolone acetate 1% is placed in the patient's eye, and the patient is asked to wait 1 hour. Following this, the IOP is checked, and the patient is told to instill prednisolone acetate 1% every 2 hours until bedtime and then 4 times a day for 4 days. The patient is seen 1 week later.

If the IOP is greatly elevated at 1 clock-hour postoperative, for example, 35 mm Hg or higher, or too high for a compromised optic nerve, additional IOP lowering meds and Diamox (acetazolamide), if necessary, are given in the office. The IOP is checked every 30 to 40 minutes until adequate control is achieved. If necessary, the patient is sent home on aqueous suppressants and is followed up in a day or 2 to ensure that the IOP is controlled.

The measures presented in this chapter are specific for Nd:YAG laser iridotomy, but the same principles apply for argon or diode laser iridotomy or for combined argon or diode and Nd:YAG

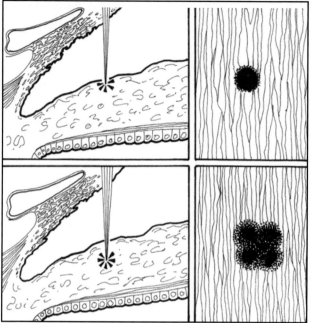

Figure 55-3. The top panel demonstrates sharp focus of the laser, with the 4 aiming beams joining to form a single spot when the laser is focused on the surface of the iris. The laser is defocused slightly posteriorly by moving it toward the patient, and the beams separate minimally (below panel). This is the optimal condition for Nd:YAG laser iridotomy, as it makes maximal use of the shock wave generated by the laser by focusing the laser slightly below the surface of the iris. Subsequent exposures are treated in the same manner, focusing slightly deep to the surface of the tissue, to maximize laser effect and minimize the number of shots necessary to create a patent iridotomy.

laser iridotomy. If a photocoagulator is used, either the short pulse technique, for dark brown irides (50-µm spot, 0.02 to 0.05 s, 1000 to 1500 mW, 20 to 50 spots, Abraham or Wise lens), or the long pulse technique, for blue, hazel, or light brown irides (50-µm spot, 0.2 s, 1000 mW, 20 to 30 spots, Abraham or Wise lens), is used. The laser is focused to a tight spot and fired repeatedly into the crater, creating an iridotomy. The LPI is complete only when the anterior lens capsule can be seen through the opening; a plume of pigment is not a signal that the procedure is finished.

diode LPI may not progress, evidence of fluid movement into the crystalline lens must be monitored. Lens injury represents the main unknown long-term potential complication of this procedure.

PIGMENT DISSEMINATION

The TM in the open portions of the angle frequently contains additional pigment after LPI. Possibly, this relates to the moderate IOP elevation that may occur for several weeks to months after the procedure. The long-term consequences of this pigment dissemination on the outflow pathways is not known.

RETINAL BURN

We have not observed this complication of photocoagulation of the iris, but it has been reported by others. Some protection may be gained by performing LPI far peripherally beyond the lens equator and by aiming obliquely rather than perpendicularly through the cornea.

CORECTOPIA

The pupil often becomes irregularly dilated toward the lasered quadrant when photocoagulation is used during the LPI procedure, but most often this returns to normal in a few days. Rarely has it persisted.

DIPLOPIA

Occasionally, patients will complain of diplopia or ghost imaging after LPI. It has been more commonly observed when LPI has been performed in the horizontal meridians or more centrally, but it is also surprising how many patients with such exposed laser openings do not notice such symptoms. By performing LPI in the upper quadrants and far peripherally where the iris openings are covered by the upper lid, such patient complaints can be minimized. Interestingly, some patients have diplopia despite an iridotomy well covered by the upper lid, which disappears when the lid is lifted away from the eye. This is presumably due to the prism effect of the tear meniscus of the upper lid.[14] Some advocate performing LPI at the 3 or 9 o'clock position to avoid this effect. LPIs in this position may, however, be a cosmetic issue. A study by Spaeth,[15] however, did not demonstrate a distinct advantage to fully exposed LPIs. Visual disturbances were found in 9% of eyes with completely covered LPIs, 26% with partially covered LPIs, and 18% with fully exposed LPIs.[16] We prefer to perform them between 11 and 1 o'clock, making sure they are peripheral enough to be fully covered by the upper lid.

IRIS ATROPHY

Iris atrophy is rare with modern LPI techniques. In the early days of LPI, when only low-power photocoagulators were available, a method called *hump-and-burn* was used to create the iridotomy. This resulted in a large area of collateral thermal damage to the iris surrounding the actual iridotomy. This area appeared intact at the time of the procedure, but several weeks later would thin and develop a lacy appearance, finally becoming atrophic and eventually resulting in a large iridotomy, often 2 to 3 times the size of the original opening.

MALIGNANT GLAUCOMA

This complication has been reported following LPI.[17] Perhaps not surprisingly, as the eyes most susceptible to malignant glaucoma are those eyes requiring LPI, the process of LPI itself can apparently precipitate an attack of malignant glaucoma. It is easy to differentiate malignant glaucoma from pupillary block, on the basis of lens position and axial anterior chamber depth (see Chapter 29).

FAILURE TO OBTAIN AN IRIDOTOMY

It is essential to always ensure that the iridotomy is patent, if possible through direct visualization of the anterior lens capsule. If the iridotomy is not patent, it is often a simple task, using the Nd:YAG laser, to perforate the iris through the partial-thickness iridotomy.

LATE CLOSURE OF IRIDOTOMY

Occasionally, especially in the case of iridotomies created with the argon or diode laser, the iridotomy will close late, after the first 4 to 6 weeks. In these cases, it is relatively easy to reopen the LPI with the Nd:YAG laser; or, if the occluding material is pigmented, the argon or diode laser can be used. As the Nd:YAG laser creates a large zone of iris pigment epithelial loss surrounding the iridotomy (see Figure 55-2), presumably due to its shock wave effect, and because pigment migration is the most common cause of late iridotomy closure, the Nd:YAG laser is preferred for this task.

POSTERIOR SYNECHIAE

Inflammation in the anterior segment can result in the formation of posterior synechiae. These are best avoided after LPI by dilating the pupil, when certain that the iridotomy is patent, at the 1- or 4-week follow-up visit.

HEMORRHAGE

This problem is almost unique to LPIs created using the Nd:YAG laser. Because the argon and diode lasers are photocoagulators, they function by absorption of the light energy and conversion of the energy to heat. This heat cauterizes the tissue as it burns a hole through the iris. The Nd:YAG laser creates optical breakdown of tissue, inducing a plasma that results in a cavitation bubble and shock wave that tears the tissue apart. The photodisruption does not heat the tissue, and any blood vessels ruptured therefore bleed. This bleeding is generally minimal and self-limited, but can be treated by gentle pressure on the eye applied through the contact lens. Once the bleeding has stopped, the contact lens is slowly removed from the eye, and no special precautions are necessary other than the usual postoperative regimen.

REFERENCES

1. Spaeth GL, Idowu O, Seligsohn A, et al. The effects of iridotomy size and position on symptoms following laser peripheral iridotomy. *J Glaucoma*. 2005;14(5):364-367.
2. Latina MA, Puliafito CA, Steinert RR, et al. Experimental iridotomy with the Q-switched neodymium-YAG laser. *Arch Ophthalmol*. 1984;102:1211-1213.
3. Robin AL, Pollack IP. A comparison of neodymiunr.YAG and argon laser iridotomies. *Ophthalmology*. 1984;91:1011-1016.
4. Pollack IP, Robin AL, Dragon DM, et al. Use of the neodymium:YAG laser to create iridotomies in monkeys and humans. *Trans Am Ophthalmol Soc*. 1984;82:307-328.
5. Pollack IP. Use of argon laser energy to produce iridotomies. *Trans Am Ophthalmol Soc*. 1979;77:674-706.
6. Pollack IP. Use of argon laser energy to produce iridotomies. *Ophthalmic Surg*. 1980;11:506-515.
7. Schuman JS, Jacobson JJ, Puliafito CA. Semiconductor diode laser peripheral iridotomy. *Arch Ophthalmol*. 1990;108:1207-1208.

8. Beckman H, Barraco R, Sugar S, et al. Laser iridectomies. *Am J Ophthalmol Soc.* 1971;77:674-706.

9. Ritch R, Liebmann J, Solomon IS. Laser iridectomy and iridoplasty. In: Ritch R, Shields MB, Krupin T, eds. *Glaucomas.* St. Louis, MO: CV Mosby; 1989:581-603.

10. Ritch R, Podos SM. Argon laser treatment of angle-closure glaucoma. *Perspect Ophthalmol.* 1980;4:129.

11. Moster MR, Schwartz LW, Spaeth GL, et al. Laser iridectomy. A controlled study comparing argon and neodymium:YAG. *Ophthalmology.* 1986;93:20-24.

12. Jacobson JJ, Schuman JS, El Khoumy H, et al. Diode laser peripheral iridectomy. *Int Ophthalmol Clin.* 1990;30:120-122.

13. Beckman H, Sugar HS. Laser iridectomy therapy of glaucoma. *Arch Ophthalmol.* 1973;90:453.

14. Weintraub J, Berke SJ. Blurring after iridotomy. *Ophthalmology.* 1992;99:479-480.

15. Spaeth GL, Idowu O, Seligsohn A, et al. The effects of iridotomy size and position on symptoms following laser peripheral iridotomy. *J Glaucoma.* 2005;14(5):364-367.

16. Cashwell LF, Martin TJ. Malignant glaucoma after laser iridectomy. *Ophthalmology.* 1992;99:651-658.

17. Liebmann JM, Ritch R. Laser surgery for angle closure glaucoma. *Semin Ophthalmol.* 2002;17(2):84-91.

Cyclodestruction

Mina B. Pantcheva, MD and Joel S. Schuman, MD, FACS

Cyclodestructive surgery is a procedure of last resort. It is used to lower intraocular pressure (IOP) by decreasing aqueous production. Glaucoma occasionally is refractory to conventional medical and surgical treatment and requires destruction of the ciliary body to bring the IOP to a level adequate for the preservation of optic nerve tissue and vision. Filtration surgery is usually preferable to cyclodestructive procedures, as filtration surgery attacks the cause of the glaucoma, lowering the IOP by improving aqueous outflow, while cyclodestructive procedures tend to have more complications than filtering surgery and do not treat the root of the problem. Several techniques have been used to destroy the ciliary processes.

HISTORICAL PERSPECTIVE

The first reports of destruction of the ciliary body in order to lower IOP were by Weve[1] in 1933, using diathermy. Penetrating diathermy was used by Vogt[2] in 1936 and was reported again by Stocker in 1945,[3] by Lachman and Rochwell[4] in 1953, and by Nesterov and Egorov[5] in 1983. The principle was the ablation of the ciliary body by the heat caused by the diathermy procedure.[6] A report by Walton and Grant[7] in 1970 revealed low success rates for this procedure, as well as significant hypotony, and led to the gradual abandonment of cyclodiathermy. Nonpenetrating diathermy has been investigated by several investigators; however, both penetrating and nonpenetrating diathermy appear to cause significant scleral damage in addition to the effect on the ciliary body.[4,8-14] Haik and colleagues[15] used beta irradiation to induce ciliary ablation, but this was cataractogenic. Cyclo-electrolysis was described in 1949 by Berens and associates,[16] but did not gain favor, as the technique did not represent a significant advantage over cyclodiathermy. [6]

Freezing to destroy the ciliary body was suggested in 1950 by Bietti,[17] and, in 1964, Polack and de Roetth[18] and McLean and Lincoff[19] reported on the use of this technique in rabbits and in humans. This procedure was called cyclocryotherapy (CCT), and de Roetth[20,21] later showed long-term effectiveness of CCT in lowering IOP. CCT was adopted quickly, as it was felt to be less destructive and more predictable than penetrating cyclodiathermy.[22] Bellows and Grant[23,24] reported that CCT was especially useful in advanced, inadequately controlled glaucoma, particularly in aphakic eyes. CCT had limited success in treating neovascular glaucoma; however, this glaucoma subtype was notoriously difficult to manage with any means, and reports of IOP control using CCT were variable.[25,26] A major complication noted with CCT was phthisis, rates of which varied from 0% to 12% or more. Visual loss was also a significant complication, with rates up to 67% of treated eyes.[23-29] The use of xenon arc panretinal photocoagulation in combination with CCT resulted in good IOP control and no phthisis after 2.5 years, according to Nissen and colleagues[30]; there was no control group in this study.

Ultrasound has been used to cause focal ciliary body destruction since its description by Purnell and associates[31] in 1964 for that purpose. Perhaps the greatest proponent of this technique has been Coleman, who has reported significant pressure lowering with ultrasound, proposing a mechanism of ciliary body destruction, thinning of scleral collagen, and separation of the ciliary body from the sclera.[32-35] Several reports have supported these findings, both clinically[36] and in animal models.[37-39]

Finally, Freyler and Scheimbauer[40] noted that partial cyclectomy could control end-stage glaucoma in some cases, although the phthisis rate was 10% to 15%.

CYCLOPHOTOCOAGULATION

The first form of cyclophotocoagulation (CPC) was performed not with a laser, but with the xenon arc photocoagulator. Trans-scleral xenon arc CPC was reported by Weekers and colleagues[41] in 1961. Unfortunately, this technique

Kahook MY, Schuman JS, eds.
Chandler and Grant's Glaucoma, Fifth Edition (pp 511-522).
© 2013 SLACK Incorporated.

offered no clear advantage over other treatment modalities, and it was not until 1971 that the use of the laser for CPC was introduced. Lee and Pomerantzeff[42] suggested trans-pupillary CPC, but Shields[22] showed that this procedure produced only limited success, due to the small amount of ciliary process that could be visualized through the pupil. Shields[22,43] found that the argon laser could be used for laser endoscopic cyclophotocoagulation (ECP) with good results. Uram[44-46] has shown excellent results for ECP using a diode laser coupled to a fiberoptic endoscope.

A less invasive means of CPC is via the trans-scleral route, and in 1972, Beckman and colleagues[47] described trans-scleral CPC using a ruby laser. In a 10-year follow-up of 241 patients treated with trans-scleral CPC with the ruby laser, 62% were found to have an IOP of 5 to 22 mm Hg.[48,49] The greatest success was in aphakic eyes, and the highest phthisis rates were in neovascular glaucoma patients (10% compared to 7% overall and a 17% incidence of hypotony overall).

Until recently, despite good results with CPC, the cyclodestructive treatment of choice in patients with glaucoma refractory to medical and surgical treatment has been CCT. This was due to the limited availability of the ruby laser; however, the excellent results shown for neodymium:yttrium-aluminum-garnet (Nd:YAG) and diode laser CPC have revolutionized this therapeutic modality. The Nd:YAG and diode lasers have several advantages over the ruby and neodymium lasers. Longer wavelengths provide good scleral penetration with less backscatter than shorter wavelengths.[50-52] Both the Nd:YAG and diode lasers have excellent absorption by melanin within the ciliary body. Nd:YAG and diode lasers are present in many medical centers, and contact Nd:YAG lasers may be found in many general hospitals, as they have many uses outside of ophthalmology. Diode lasers can be used as photocoagulators for laser trabeculoplasty,[53-55] laser iridectomy,[56-58] retinal photocoagulation, endophotocoagulation, and trans-scleral retinopexy.[59-68] Diode lasers are compact, portable, lightweight, air or electrically cooled, and use standard current. Finally, the Nd:YAG and diode lasers offer an inexpensive means by which to perform CPC compared to the ruby laser.

INDICATIONS AND CASE SELECTION FOR TRANS-SCLERAL LASER CYCLOPHOTOCOAGULATION

Laser CPC is a destructive procedure. It is a therapeutic modality of last resort, useful in advanced glaucoma, in which the IOP is uncontrolled despite maximum tolerated medical treatment, in eyes that have failed filtering surgery or are likely to fail future filtering surgery. This includes eyes in which filtering surgery has a high risk, such as aphakic glaucoma, neovascular glaucoma, glaucoma

after penetrating keratoplasty, or in eyes with very low visual potential. CPC destroys tissue, lowering IOP by the destruction of the ciliary body, decreasing the amount of aqueous humor produced. Hypotony can result from overly aggressive treatment, because inadequate functional ciliary body remains, while an insufficient treatment will not produce adequate lowering of IOP. The therapeutic window is relatively narrow in cyclodestructive procedures, especially in light of the fact that aqueous outflow tends to be compromised in eyes undergoing this type of surgery.

Other possible risks of cyclodestructive surgery include pain, inflammation, chronic hypotony with macular edema, vitreous hemorrhage, and phthisis. While CPC may produce fewer side effects than other cyclodestructive procedures, these risks persist and tend to make CPC a treatment of last resort in the management of advanced glaucoma.

A patient to undergo CPC should have IOP that is uncontrolled despite maximum tolerated treatment and 1 of the following:

- Failed prior filtration surgery or the expectation that further glaucoma filtering surgery will fail

- Glaucoma that is likely to fail filtering surgery (neovascular, inflammatory, postpenetrating keratoplasty, post-scleral buckling) or is a high risk for complications of filtering surgery (vitrectomized aphakic eye)

- Poor visual acuity, such that the eye is being treated with CPC to maintain comfort and prevent visual loss

- The patient is not a surgical candidate for filtering surgery for general medical reasons

TRANS-SCLERAL LASER CYCLOPHOTOCOAGULATION

Trans-scleral laser CPC may be performed either with a fiberoptic touching the eye (contact) or through the air (noncontact).

CONTACT

Laboratory Studies

Contact trans-scleral Nd:YAG laser cyclophotocoagulation (CYC) was first reported by Brancato and colleagues[69] in 1987. They studied the effects of CYC on Chinchilla rabbits. Federman and colleagues,[70] that same year, as well as Peyman and colleagues[71] in 1987 and Schubert and Federman[72,73] in 1989, in addition to Latina and coauthors in 1989,[74] each studied CYC lesions in rabbit ciliary bodies. The lesions appeared on postoperative day 1 to be 1-mm white well-demarcated spots.[69,74] Thermal injury occurred in the ciliary body stroma, with coagulation necrosis of the ciliary pigmented and nonpigmented

TABLE 56-1. SUCCESS RATES IN 4 SUBTYPES OF GLAUCOMA PRESENT IN PATIENTS TREATED WITH CONTACT TRANS-SCLERAL ND:YAG LASER CYCLOPHOTOCOAGULATION			
	Ranges in mm Hg		
	3 to 25	3 to 22	3 to >19
Primary open-angle glaucoma	78% (35/45)	68% (32/47)	60% (28/47)
Neovascular glaucoma	43% (10/23)	39% (9/23)	39% (9/23)
Glaucoma in aphakia or pseudophakia	76% (52/69)	69% (49/71)	63% (45/71)
Postpenetrating keratoplasty	70% (7/10)	60% (6/10)	50% (5/10)

This article was published in *Ophthalmology,* 99, Schuman JS, Bellows AR, Shingleton BJ, et al, Contact transscleral Nd:YAG laser cyclophotocoagulation: midterm results, 1089-1094, Copyright Elsevier 1992.

epithelia; there was no significant scleral damage.[69,74] Four-week follow-up demonstrated atrophy, fusion, and fibrosis of the ciliary processes.[73,74] In some cases, the ciliary process was covered with a fibrous membrane, with abnormal ciliary epithelium, pigment epithelial proliferation, and focal epithelial interruptions.[69,73,74] Areas of scleral compression and hypercellularity occurred, but there was no scleral thermal damage present.[73] Epithelial regeneration following CYC did not occur, according to van der Zypen and colleagues,[75,76] indicating that the vascular network remained atrophic in the ciliary body. Similar lesions have been noted using the diode laser in the contact mode in rabbit eyes.[77,78]

Pulsed CYC results in lesions similar to noncontact transscleral Nd:YAG laser cyclophotocoagulation (NCYC).[79] The coagulative lesions seen with CYC do not occur in this setting; rather, blistering lesions are noted.

CYC performed in human cadaver eyes causes coagulation to occur in the ciliary body, with disruption of the ciliary pigmented and nonpigmented epithelium.[80] Allingham and colleagues[80] showed that optimal probe placement is with the anterior edge of the contact probe 0.5 to 1 mm posterior to the limbus. More posterior placement results in lesions in the pars plana, while more anterior placement causes iris burns. The optimal power setting was found to be 7 to 9 watts, with 5 watts creating only minimal coagulation necrosis of the ciliary body and 11 watts causing a striking loss of anatomic integrity of the ciliary process. No scleral damage was noted at this power setting. Exposure time was optimized at 0.7 s.[80] Brancato and colleagues[81] showed in vivo in eyes destined for enucleation due to choroidal melanoma that only 2 J of energy were needed to create lesions in the ciliary body using placement similar to that described above; however, in another paper, Brancato and colleagues[82] showed that higher energy levels produce better clinical results.

Contact diode laser cyclophotocoagulation (CDC) in human cadaver eyes induced similar epithelial coagulation necrosis and thermal coagulation of the ciliary stroma and vasculature. Energy levels were 3 to 5 J.[83]

Clinical Studies

In 116 eyes of 114 patients followed for a minimum of 1 year after treatment with CYC, Schuman and colleagues[84] in 1992 found that 75% of eyes achieved an average final IOP of 25 mm Hg or less, 66% had 22 mm Hg or less, and more than 50% of the eyes treated achieved a final IOP of 19 mm Hg or less (Table 56-1). The major complications noted were hypotony and visual loss. Nine eyes (8%) had a final IOP less than 3 mm Hg, with an IOP of 0 mm Hg in 6 eyes. Seventeen of 36 eyes (47%) with an initial visual acuity of 20/200 or better lost 2 or more Snellen lines. Nineteen eyes, all with an initial visual acuity of counting fingers or worse, progressed to no light perception. Retreatment was required in 31 eyes (27%).[84] The findings were similar to that group's earlier report[85] in 1990, studying 160 treatments in 140 eyes of 136 patients. The interesting finding in comparing these 2 studies was that the success rates remained similar, but the rate of complications increased over time.[84,85]

Brancato and colleagues[82] reported on CYC in 23 patients, using less energy and fewer spots. The success rate in this case was somewhat lower than that reported by Schuman,[84] and retreatment was required in 57% of eyes.

The contact diode laser has been used clinically for CPC and was approved for this procedure by the US Food and Drug Administration in 1994. Gaasterland and colleagues[86] performed a multicenter clinical study of 30 eyes in 30 patients and noted results nearly identical to those encountered with CYC. The treatment parameters for CDC, however, called for less energy and fewer spots than CYC, and the fact that similar clinical results could be achieved using these parameters suggested that CDC resulted in a larger area of tissue destruction per spot. Further, Carassa and colleagues,[87] using CDC, noted a 50% IOP lowering in 12 eyes of 12 patients, with 16 spots over 360 degrees, using 2.5 watts for 1.5 s (3.75 J).

Noncontact Cyclophotocoagulation

Laboratory Studies

Noncontact Nd:YAG laser CYC (NCYC) preceded CYC historically; however, it has proven to be a modality resulting in more inflammation and pain postoperatively than CYC. CYC, therefore, is generally preferred to NCYC in treating patients. Wilensky and colleagues[88] reported NCYC in rabbits in 1985. Reports[52,89-94] on histopathology of the laser lesions and the use of the technique in patients followed shortly after.

Fankhauser and colleagues[95] demonstrated NCYC lesions in the ciliary body of human cadaver eyes using 6 to 7 J aiming the spot 0.5- to 1-mm posterior to the limbus with maximum defocusing and a 20-msec pulse. Hampton and Shields[96] showed that optimum parameters for treatment were an energy level of 8 J delivered 1.5-mm posterior to the limbus with maximum defocusing. They showed histologic damage to the iris when the beam was aimed more anteriorly and pars plana lesions when the beam was aimed more posteriorly. No differences were seen when the energy was delivered tangentially versus perpendicular to the sclera. Later studies[97,98] noted that a specialized contact lens could increase the efficiency and accuracy of laser delivery. Hampton and Shields[96] found that tissue damage with NCYC differed from that seen with CYC: the destruction of the ciliary epithelium was accompanied by the creation of a blister-like space, and coagulation necrosis was not present. Similar findings have been seen *in vivo* in blind human eyes treated with NCYC just prior to enucleation for pain. In these cases, the blister-like space was filled with eosinophilic material.[99]

NCYC in rabbits resulted in the acute destruction of the ciliary epithelium and the associated vessels, with subsequent atrophy of the ciliary processes 1 to 2 months after injury.[52,89,90] The laser energy was absorbed by melanin; no histopathologic changes were seen in albino rabbits.[100]

Unlike the effects seen with NCYC, noncontact transscleral diode laser cyclophotocoagulation (NCDC) resulted in a thermal ciliary body lesion.[101] Hennis and colleagues[102] demonstrated thermal effects in the ciliary body with as little as 900 mJ energy with NCDC, using a spot size of 100 to 500 μm, with the beam 0.5-mm posterior to the limbus, defocused 1-mm posteriorly. In a study comparing CDC and NCDC in living rabbits using the same laser for both treatments, Shepps and colleagues[101] reported that 50% more energy was needed to create the same lesion with NCDC as compared to CDC. This is consistent with the findings on scleral light scattering presented by Vogel and colleagues.[51] In comparing NCDC to NCYC and CCT in cadaver eyes, Assia and colleagues[103] found that all were effective in ciliary body destruction, and none damaged the crystalline lens.

Clinical Studies

Cyrlin and colleagues[93] reported in 1985 that 60% to 70% of patients treated with NCYC had an IOP between 5 and 22 mm Hg at 6 to 12 months follow-up, using 8 J of energy, with 32 spots. In 1986, Schwartz and Moster[104] found that 20 of 29 treated eyes (69%) had final IOPs of 22 mm Hg or less and noted 1 questionable case of phthisis, with an average 32-week follow-up. Devenyi and colleagues[94] used 40 spots at 1.8 to 3.0 J for 20 msec placed 2 to 3 mm posterior to the limbus with maximum defocusing and found that 11 of 24 eyes developed an IOP of 21 mm Hg or less and that neovascular glaucoma eyes did somewhat worse than others. While this study[94] with 8.8 months average follow-up, had no cases of phthisis, in a subsequent study on the same patient population, Trope and Ma[105] reported a phthisis rate of 10.7% and a 30% rate of visual loss, when the patients were followed for an average of 21.9 months.

Klapper and colleagues[106] reported that 86% of treated eyes achieved an IOP between 5 and 22 mm Hg, with a mean decrease in IOP of 68%, with an average follow-up of 6 months. This study used 32 spots at 3.5 to 4.5 J for 20 msec placed 2- to 3-mm posterior to the limbus with maximum defocusing.

Hampton and colleagues[107] reported on 100 NCYC treatments and noted severe pain in 13.5%, severe inflammation in 28%, a retreatment rate of 25%, and visual loss in 50%. Wright and colleagues[108] noted that a majority of 35 eyes treated required further intervention, or lost vision if followed long enough, and that 31% of eyes lost 2 or more lines of vision or light perception over the 3-year follow-up period of the study.

Hennis and Stewart[109] found a 30% reduction in IOP over a 6-month follow-up with a single NCDC treatment in 14 eyes, using 1.2 watts for 0.99 s (1.2 J) with 40 to 45 applications of a 100-μm spot placed 1-mm posterior to the limbus and defocused 1-mm posteriorly. Similar to NCYC, conjunctival burns occurred with NCDC, as well as anterior chamber inflammation.

Maus and Katz[110] found severe hypotony, flat anterior chamber, and serous choroidal detachment after NCYC in 3 patients, all of whom had previous filtering surgery; 2 of the patients were African American. Fiore and colleagues[111] reported focal scleral thinning following NCYC in one patient. Hardten and Brown[112] reported malignant glaucoma following NCYC in one eye, as did Wand, Schuman, and Puliafito.[113] Blomquist and colleagues[114] showed that NCYC could damage intraocular lens (IOL) haptics in cadaver eyes at energy levels higher than those used clinically; Lim and colleagues[115] failed to damage IOL haptics with CYC. Subretinal fibrosis and lens subluxation, while reported with CCT,[116,117] have not been found with Nd:YAG or CDC.

Sympathetic ophthalmia is a controversial finding in association with CPC. Reports of this complication have been in eyes having previous trauma or other ocular procedures,[118,119] and the relationship between CPC and sympathetic ophthalmia is uncertain.[120] Sympathetic ophthalmia has been described following CCT,[121] as well as after helium ion irradiation followed by CCT.[122]

CYCLOPHOTOCOAGULATION VERSUS OTHER CYCLODESTRUCTIVE PROCEDURES

As a treatment of last resort, CCT was an effective means to control IOP in eyes refractory to all other forms of treatment. Bellows and Grant showed that the IOP could be lowered in advanced, uncontrolled glaucoma, especially in aphakia, with CCT.[23,24] Nevertheless, phthisis occurred in up to 12% of patients and visual loss in two-thirds of CCT treated eyes; this relegated CCT to the role of a treatment of last resort.[23-27] Trans-scleral laser CPC destroys less tissue than CCT, with similar effects on IOP in rabbits, as demonstrated by Higginbotham et al.[123] NCYC may be as effective as CCT clinically, but produces fewer complications, as shown by Suzuki and colleagues.[124] Further, NCYC was demonstrated in an uncontrolled retrospective study,[125] to be superior to drainage implant surgery. Noureddin and colleagues[125] found that while both procedures lowered IOP, serious complications such as retinal detachment, expulsive hemorrhage, phthisis, and endophthalmitis were much more common in the tube-treated group. In addition, the incidence of visual loss among tube-treated eyes was higher than in eyes treated with NCYC. Both groups had similar postoperative IOPs reported.[125]

CONTACT VERSUS NONCONTACT CYCLOPHOTOCOAGULATION

There are several differences between CYC and NCYC. CYC is performed with the patient supine, while NCYC is done with the patient at the slit-lamp. The contact laser is portable and can be used in remote locations, such as the operating room with the patient under general anesthesia, with relative ease. NCYC uses more energy, and significantly more power, than CYC and results in more inflammation and pain postoperatively than CYC.[52,82,85,94,104,106,107]

CYC, NCYC, CDC, and NCDC all center the laser beam approximately 1.5-mm posterior to the limbus.[52,80,83,96] With the laser delivered via fiberoptic, as in CYC and CDC, the anterior edge of the probe is offset from the limbus to achieve beam placement. With the noncontact techniques, the laser is aimed approximately 1.5-mm posterior to the limbus. Schuman and colleauges[84,85,126] did not find any clinical differences in CYC treatments performed with the beam centered 1.5-, 2.0-, or 2.5-mm posterior to the limbus. Schubert,[127] however, showed that NCYC and CYC lesions

performed with the beam centered 3.0-mm posterior to the limbus caused lesions in the pars plana. He demonstrated that these lesions resulted in an increase in outflow facility,[128] and this report was supported by Pham-Duy, who also showed that CCT increased outflow facility while transiently reducing aqueous flow.[129] These studies, however, were limited by blood-aqueous barrier disruption following CCT. Higginbotham and colleagues[130] demonstrated ciliary epithelial destruction in proportion to the degree of CCT, with consequent proportional effects on IOP and aqueous flow; however, outflow facility was not studied. CYC has been shown to increase uveoscleral outflow in rabbits, possibly by an effect mediated by prostaglandins.[131] In work by Schmidt and colleagues,[131] when IOP returned to normal, uveoscleral flow returned to baseline as well.

Contact CPC appears to have several advantages over the noncontact modality. A longer exposure time is used for CYC as compared to NCYC. The histopathological change in CYC is coagulative necrosis, whereas explosive damage is seen with NCYC.[73,80,96,97] With regard to the diode laser, both modalities use long exposure times; however, 50% more energy is required with NCDC to achieve the same lesion seen with CDC.[101] In comparing the diode and Nd:YAG lasers, the diode laser has the advantage of greater absorption by melanin and nearly equivalent scleral transmission when the sclera is compressed as it is for contact CPC.[51] The diode laser offers greater convenience and economy compared to the Nd:YAG laser. Anecdotally, there is less pain and inflammation with CYC as opposed to NCYC, which is most likely related to the histopathological changes noted above. The CYC unit is portable, is present in many general hospitals, and is therefore more available than the NCYC unit. The diode unit, with its multitude of uses in ophthalmology, affords even greater flexibility to the ophthalmologist, as well as potentially greater availability. Any of the above CPC techniques offer a titratable treatment that is generally well-tolerated by the appropriately selected patient.

GLAUCOMA SUBTYPE AND THE PIGMENT EFFECT

Glaucoma subtype may be important in the response to CPC. Neovascular glaucoma, difficult to treat with any modality, responds least well of the glaucoma subtypes to cyclodestruction,[23,26] and eyes with neovascular glaucoma have the most severe and greatest number of complications (inflammation, pain, and visual loss). Neovascular glaucoma eyes have less IOP response to CPC as well, although the difference in IOP response does not achieve statistical significance.[84,85]

While aphakic eyes respond better to CCT than phakic eyes, this is not seen with CYC.[24,84] Aphakic eyes do have less inflammation than others. CPC seems to be an effective means of controlling IOP in eyes following penetrating keratoplasty.[85,123-134]

TABLE 56-2. LASER CYCLOPHOTOCOAGULATION TECHNIQUE
Continue all preoperative glaucoma medications prior to treatment
Informed consent
Laser operational
Retrobulbar or peribulbar anesthesia
Patient recumbent for contact CPC; sitting for noncontact treatment
Laser settings • Contact Nd: YAG: 7 watts, 0.7 s • Contact diode: 3 watts, 1.3 s • With contact treatment, if pops are heard with 3 consecutive spots, decrease power by 0.5 watts • Noncontact Nd:YAG: 4 to 8 J; 20 msec exposure (thermal mode); maximum offset is at position 9
Treatment parameters • Nd:YAG: 32 spots over 360 degrees; 8 spots per quadrant, sparing 3 and 9 o'clock • Diode: 18 spots over 270 degrees, sparing inferonasal quadrant
Spot location • Contact Nd:YAG: anterior edge of probe 0.5- to 1.0-mm posterior to limbus. Measure with calipers. Press gently with probe during treatment throughout exposure, keeping the handpiece perpendicular to the sclera. Maintain contact throughout energy delivery. • Contact diode: with G-Probe, place edge of handpiece at limbus, which centers fiberoptic 1.2-mm posterior to limbus. With each subsequent spot, the radial edge of the handpiece overlaps the previous spot, producing 18 spots over 270 degrees. Press gently with probe during treatment throughout exposure, keeping the handpiece perpendicular to the sclera. Maintain contact throughout energy delivery. • Noncontact Nd:YAG: center beam 1.0- to 1.5-mm posterior to limbus, using calipers to measure for each spot; alternately, keeping the aiming beam in the center of a 3.0-mm slit beam placed with one edge on the limbus produces a displacement of 1.5 mm from the limbus.
CPC: cyclophotocoagulation; Nd:YAG: neodymium:yttrium-aluminum-garnet.

Intraocular pigment is a significant factor in the response to cyclodestruction, and in subsequent complications. This has been seen with CCT, as noted by de Roetth,[21] and Cantor et al[100] noted this in studying NCYC in pigmented and albino rabbits. Schubert and Federman[73] reported this phenomenon in relation to CPC, as well. Coleman and colleagues[135] found the pigment effect in cadaver eyes and in monkeys, and Schuman and colleagues[85] described this finding in relation to CYC. Eyes with more pigment may require less energy for the same level of cyclodestruction than less heavily pigmented eyes, as the pigment acts as a chromophore, absorbing the light energy and converting it to heat, with greater tissue damage at the same energy level in eyes with more pigment.

OPERATIVE TECHNIQUE

The treatment technique for laser CPC is shown in Table 56-2. All glaucoma medications are continued prior to laser treatment. Written informed consent is obtained,

and retrobulbar or peribulbar anesthesia is administered. The contralateral eye is patched, and the patient lies supine. A lid speculum is placed upon the eye receiving treatment, and surgeon and assistants wear protective eyeglasses (blocking 1064 nanometers for the Nd:YAG laser and 800 nanometers for the diode laser). Patients with neovascular glaucoma and non-White patients may develop fewer complications if treated with less power than that called for in the standard protocol (5 to 6 watts instead of 7 watts for CYC, 2 to 2.5 watts instead of 3 watts for CDC); however, this has not been systematically evaluated to date. For CYC, studies have evaluated the use of 32 spots (8 spots per quadrant), sparing the 3 and 9 o'clock meridians. CDC has used 18 spots over 270 degrees. Fewer spots may be used, and Schuman and colleagues found no difference in the results of CYC with 24 versus 32 spots, either for IOP effects or for complications. The probe is centered 1.5-mm posterior to the limbus[84] (for CYC, the anterior edge of the probe is placed 0.5- to 1-mm posterior to the limbus) (Figure 56-1). The

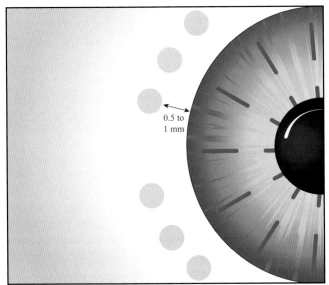

Figure 56-1. Distance of application from limbus for cyclophotocoagulation. Noncontact spots should be centered 1.0- to 1.5-mm posterior to limbus (not shown). With contact trans-scleral Nd:YAG cyclophotocoagulation, the anterior edge of the probe should be placed 0.5- to 1.0-mm posterior to the limbus (as illustrated).

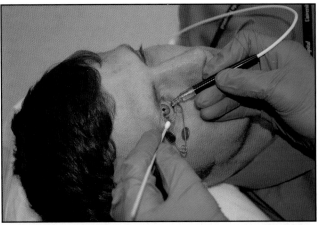

Figure 56-2. Patient is supine for treatment. A lid speculum is placed in the eye to be treated, and the probe is held perpendicular to the sclera. Contact between the probe and the eye is maintained throughout energy delivery.

offset from the limbus may be measured with calipers. The probe is gently pressed against the eye and kept perpendicular to the sclera, and contact with the eye is maintained throughout laser energy delivery (Figure 56-2).

Power, duration, number of applications, distance from the limbus, total energy delivered, and treatment pattern are documented.

POSTOPERATIVE CARE

The treated eye is patched for 6 hours after CPC following the instillation of prednisolone acetate 1% and atropine sulfate 1%. Prednisolone acetate 1% is applied 4 times a day, and atropine sulfate 1% is given twice a day; both are tapered as the inflammation subsides. All preoperative glaucoma medications are continued with the exception of miotics, which may be reinstituted as the inflammation is reduced. The IOP should be checked postoperatively at 1 day and 1 week, and thereafter depending on the patient's clinical response.

RETREATMENT

At times, patients require retreatment due to inadequate response to CPC. This may be performed at 1 month postoperatively.[126] All parameters are identical to that for the initial treatment. There is no limit to the number of times that retreatment may be performed; however, each retreatment increases the possibility of phthisis.

ENDOSCOPIC CYCLOPHOTOCOAGULATION

The laser unit for ECP incorporates a diode laser that emits pulsed continuous wave energy of 810 nm, a 175-W xenon light source, a helium-neon laser aiming beam, and video camera imaging that can be recorded. All 4 elements are transmitted via fiberoptics to a 20-gauge probe that is inserted intraocularly. The main unit is compact and portable with controls for adjusting laser power and duration on the console, and a foot pedal controlling the laser firing with the actual duration of each treatment determined by how long the pedal is depressed.

Laboratory Studies

Two studies[136,137] have compared the histologic effects of trans-scleral CDC and ECP. Lin and colleagues[136] studied the acute and late effects of CDC and ECP on the histology and ciliary blood flow in rabbits. CDC caused severe disruption of the ciliary processes and iris root and substantial reduction of their blood flow up to 1 month after treatment. In contrast, ECP caused localized shrinkage of the processes and initial reduction in blood flow with partial reperfusion by 1 month. It was speculated that the partial return of blood flow may partially account for the lack of hypotony and phthisis with ECP. Pantcheva and colleagues[137] observed acute histologic changes in human autopsy eyes after ECP and CDC. Tissue treated with CDC showed pronounced tissue disruption of the ciliary body muscle and stroma, ciliary processes, and both pigmented and nonpigmented ciliary epithelium. ECP-treated tissue exhibited contraction of the ciliary processes with disruption of the ciliary body epithelium, sparing of the ciliary

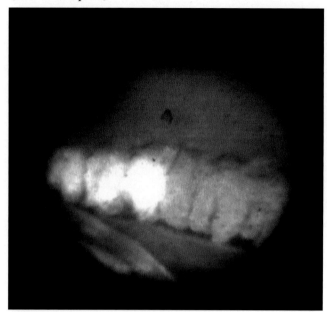

Figure 56-3. ECP—the treated ciliary processes are shrunken and white in contrast to the adjacent nontreated ciliary processes.

body muscle, and less architectural disorganization. The sclera was not affected by either laser treatment. Compared with CDC, ECP seemed to be a more selective form of CPC, resulting in less tissue disruption while achieving the goal of destroying ciliary body epithelium.

Clinical Studies

Chen and colleagues reported that 61 of 68 treated eyes (90%) achieved an IOP of 21 mm Hg or less followed for an average of 12.9 months.[138] The mean number of glaucoma medications used by each patient was reduced from 3.0 ± 1.3 preoperatively to 2.0 ± 1.3 postoperatively ($p < 0.0001$). There were no cases of hypotony, phthisis, or sympathetic ophthalmia. Uram[139] reported on 10 patients with combined ECP, phacoemulsification, and IOL implantation. After an average follow-up of 19.2 months, the mean IOP was reduced 57%.

In a randomized prospective study of combined cataract and glaucoma surgery, Gayton and colleagues[140] compared the efficacy and safety profiles of concurrent trabeculectomy versus ECP. With an average follow-up of 2 years, the success rate in maintaining IOP below 19 mm Hg without medication was 42% in the trabeculectomy group and 30% in the ECP group.

Neely and Plager[141] treated 36 eyes of 29 pediatric patients with various childhood glaucomas. After 19 months of average follow-up, 12 eyes (34%) remained successfully treated with IOP less than 21 mm Hg (with or without medication) after the initial ECP, and 15 eyes (43%) were successfully controlled with 1 or more ECP treatments (mean of 1.42 procedures). Significant complications occurred in 4 eyes and included 2 retinal detachments, 1 case of chronic hypotony,

and 1 patient who progressed from hand movement vision to no light perception (unclear etiology).

In a randomized trial comparing ECP with Ahmed valve (New World Medical, Rancho Cucamonga, CA) surgery for refractory glaucoma, Lima and colleagues[142] found the 2 procedures effective in reducing IOP. The success rates (IOP 6 to 20 mm Hg with or without topical medications) by Kaplan-Meier analysis were 70.6% and 73.5% for the Ahmed (mean follow-up of 19.82 months) and ECP (mean follow-up of 21.29 months) groups, respectively. Overall, there were more complications in the Ahmed valve group.

Complications associated with ECP included the following in the largest series to date: fibrin exudate in 24%, hyphema in 12%, cystoid macular edema in 10%, vision loss of 2 lines or more in 6%, and choroidal detachment in 4%.[138] Other reported serious complications include retinal detachment and hypotony, although most of these were in pediatric cases.[141] Although not reported in the literature, endophthalmitis and choroidal hemorrhage are potential severe complications, owing to the intraocular nature of the surgery.[143] No cases of sympathetic ophthalmia have yet been identified in relation to ECP, but malignant glaucoma was encountered in 1 case after an initially unremarkable post-ECP course.[138] One case of phthisis was reported by Ahmad and colleagues[144] after a single session of ECP in an adult patient.

OPERATIVE TECHNIQUE

The main approach to reach the ciliary processes is via a limbal or a pars plana entry.

In the limbal approach, after dilation of the pupil with cyclopentolate 1% and phenylephrine 2.5%, a paracentesis is created, and the ciliary sulcus is filled with viscoelastic agent in order to expand it. A 2.2-mm keratome is then used to enter into the anterior chamber at the temporal limbus. A 20-gauge probe is inserted through the incision and into the posterior sulcus. At this time, the ciliary processes are viewed on the monitor, and treatment can begin. The laser is set at continuous-wave, and energy settings are 0.25 to 0.8 W. Approximately a 180-degree span of ciliary processes are photocoagulated (more area can be treated if a curved probe is used). Laser energy is applied to each process until shrinkage and whitening occur. Ciliary processes are treated individually or in a painting fashion across multiple processes (Figure 56-3). If excessive energy is used, the process explodes (or pops) with bubble formation, leading to excessive inflammation and breakdown of the blood-aqueous barrier. After the nasal 180 degrees of ciliary processes are treated, a separate incision is created at the nasal limbus in a similar fashion as above. The temporal processes are then photocoagulated for a total of up to 360 degrees, if so desired. Before closure of the wounds, viscoelastic is removed from the anterior chamber with irrigation and aspiration.

The same laser settings are used in the pars plana approach, which requires an infusion port to be inserted through the inferior pars plana. Two entries are created for vitrectomy and illumination supratemporally and supranasally. Only a limited anterior vitrectomy is performed to allow adequate and safe access to all of the ciliary processes. The ECP probe can be inserted through each superior entry for treatment of the opposite 180 degrees of processes. There may be a few superior processes that cannot be accessed because the entry ports are not exactly 180 degrees opposite to each other.

POSTOPERATIVE CARE

In all patients, whether under local or general anesthesia, retrobulbar bupivacaine is administered before or at the end of the surgery to minimize postoperative pain. Sub-Tenon's injection of 1 mL of triamcinolone (40 mg/mL) also may be given for inflammation. On postoperative day 1, patients are placed on a regimen of topical antibiotics, steroids, nonsteroidal anti-inflammatory agents, cycloplegics, and their preoperative glaucoma medications except for miotics and prostaglandin analogs because these may exacerbate intraocular inflammation or its sequelae. Antibiotics are discontinued after 1 week, and the steroids, nonsteroidal anti-inflammatory agents, and cycloplegics are tapered as inflammation subsides. Glaucoma medications are removed according to the IOP requirements. Administration of acetazolamide during the evening of surgery may be used to prevent a spike in IOP from underlying glaucoma, inflammation, or possible retained viscoelastic.

CONCLUSION

Laser CPC offers the opportunity to control IOP in eyes refractory to other forms of medical and surgical treatment. While CPC is restricted to patients with the most advanced glaucoma, this therapeutic modality is the current state-of-the-art in cyclodestructive procedures, a treatment that has moved from cyclodiathermy through CCT to trans-scleral and ECP.

REFERENCES

1. Weve H. Die Zyklodiatermie das Corpus ciliare bei Glaukom. *Zentralbl Ophthalmol.* 1933;29:562-569.
2. Vogt A. Versuche zur intraokularen Druckherabsetzung mittels Diater-mieschadigung des Corpus cilare (Zyklodiatermiestichelung). *Klin Monatsbl Augenheilkd.* 1936;97:672-677.
3. Stocker F. Response of chronic simple glaucoma to treatment with cyclodiathermy puncture. *Arch Ophthalmol.* 1945;34:181-189.
4. Lachman B, Rochwell P. Follow-up study of 39 patients with glaucoma treated with cyclodiathermy. *Arch Ophthalmol.* 1953;50:265-266.
5. Nesterov A, Egorov E. Transconjunctival penetrating cyclodiathermy in glaucoma. *J Ocular Ther Surg.* 1983:216-217.
6. Sheppard L. Retrociliary cyclodiathermy versus retrociliary cyclo-electrolysis: effects on the normal rabbit eye. *Am J Ophthalmol.* 1958;46:27-37.
7. Walton D, Grant W. Penetrating cyclodiathermy for filtration. *Arch Ophthalmol.* 1970;83:47-48.
8. Pham L, Wang Y, Wang N, et al. Experimental nonpenetrating transscleral cyclodiathermy in rabbits. *Ophthalmic Surg Lasers.* 1996;27:301-307.
9. Berens C. Glaucoma surgery. *Arch Ophthalmol.* 1955;54:548-563.
10. Oosterhuie J, Brihaye M, De Haan A. A comparative study of experimental transscleral cryocoagulation by solid carbon dioxide and diathermocoagulation of the retina. *Ophthalmologica.* 1968;156:38-76.
11. Swan D, Christensen L. Ocular changes induced by diathermy in the treatment of retinal detachment. *Trans Am Ophthalmol Soc.* 1954;52:65.
12. deGuillebon H, Eng D, Ishii Y. Scleral changes during diathermy application. *Arch Ophthalmol.* 1970;83:752-759.
13. deGuillebon H, Eng D, Elzeneiny I. Electrical impedance of ocular coats during diathermy applications, voltage and time of application. *Arch Ophthalmol.* 1970;83:489-503.
14. Elzeneiny I, deGuillebon H, Eng D. Scleral damage in diathermy. *Am J Ophthalmol.* 1970;69:754-762.
15. Haik G, Breffeilh L, Barbar A. Beta irradiation as a possible therapeutic agent in glaucoma: an experimental study with the report of a clinical case. *Am J Ophthalmol.* 1948;31:945-952.
16. Berens C, Sheppard L, Duel A Jr. Cycloelectrolysis for glaucoma. *Trans Am Ophthalmol Soc.* 1949;47:364-380.
17. Bietti G. Surgical intervention on the ciliary body: new trends for the relief of glaucoma. *JAMA.* 1950;142:889-897.
18. Polack F, de Roetth A. Effect of freezing on the ciliary body (cyclocryotherapy). *Invest Ophthalmol.* 1964;3:164.
19. McLean J, Lincoff H. Cryosurgery of the ciliary body. *Trans Am Ophthalmol Soc.* 1964;62:385.
20. de Roetth A. Cryosurgery for the treatment of glaucoma. *Trans Am Ophthalmol Soc.* 1965;63:189.
21. de Roetth A. Cryosurgery for the treatment of advanced simple glaucoma. *Am J Ophthalmol.* 1968;66:1034.
22. Shields MB. Cyclodestructive surgery for glaucoma: past, present, and future. *Trans Am Ophthalmol Soc.* 1985;83:285-303.
23. Bellows AR, Grant WM. Cyclocryotherapy in advanced inadequately controlled glaucoma. *Am J Ophthalmol.* 1973;75:679.
24. Bellows AR, Grant WM. Cyclocryotherapy of chronic open-angle glaucoma in aphakic eyes. *Am J Ophthalmol.* 1978;85:615-621.
25. Feibel R, Bigger J. Rubeosis iridis and neovascular glaucoma: evaluation of cyclocryotherapy. *Am J Ophthalmol.* 1972;74:862-867.
26. Krupin T, Mitchell K, Becker B. Cyclocryotherapy in neovascular glaucoma. *Am J Ophthalmol.* 1978;86:24-26.
27. Brindley G, Shields M. Values and limitations of cyclocryotherapy. *Graefes Arch Clin Exp Ophthalmol.* 1986;224:545-548.
28. Benson M, Nelson M. Cyclocryotherapy: a review of cases over a 10-year period. *Br J Ophthalmol.* 1990;74:103-105.
29. Gross R, Feldman R, Spaeth G, et al. Surgical therapy of chronic glaucoma in aphakia and pseudophakia. *Ophthalmology.* 1988;95:1195-1201.
30. Nissen O, Schiodte S, Kessing S. Panretinal xenonphotocoagulation combined with cyclocryotherapy in the treatment of severe glaucoma. *Acta Ophthalmol (Copenh).* 1989;67:652-656.
31. Purnell E, Sokollu A, Torchia R, et al. Focal chorioretinitis produced by ultrasound. *Invest Ophthalmol.* 1964;3:657-664.
32. Coleman D, Lizzi F, Driller J, et al. Therapeutic ultrasound in the treatment of glaucoma: I. Experimental model. *Ophthalmology.* 1985;92:339-346.
33. Coleman D, Lizzi F, Driller J, et al. Therapeutic ultrasound in the treatment of glaucoma: II. Clinical applications. *Ophthalmology.* 1985;92:347-353.

34. Coleman D, Lizzi F, Silverman R, et al. Treatment of glaucoma with high-intensity focused ultrasound. *Ophthalmology.* 1986;93:831.

35. Margo C. Therapeutic ultrasound. Light and electron microscopic findings in an eye treated for glaucoma. *Arch Ophthalmol.* 1986;104:735-738.

36. Haut J, Colliac JP, Falque L, et al. Indications and results of Sonocare (ultrasound) in the treatment of ocular hypertension. A preliminary study of 395 cases. *Ophtalmologie.* 1990;4(2):138-141.

37. Finger P, Smith P, Paglione R, et al. Transscleral microwave cyclodestruction. *Invest Ophthalmol Vis Sci.* 1990;31:2151-2155.

38. Finger P, Moshfeghi D, Smith P, et al. Microwave cyclodestruction for glaucoma in a rabbit model. *Arch Ophthalmol.* 1991;109:1001-1004.

39. Valtot F, Kopel J, Le M. Principles and histologic effects of the treatment of hypertension with focused high-intensity ultrasound. *Ophtalmologie.* 1990;4:135-137.

40. Freyler H, Scheimbauer I. Excision of the ciliary body (Sautter procedure) as a last resort in secondary glaucoma. *Klin Monatsbl Augenhielkd.* 1981;179:473-477.

41. Weekers R, Lavergne G, Watillion M, et al. Effects of photocoagulation of ciliary body upon ocular tension. *Am J Ophthalmol.* 1961;52:156-163.

42. Lee P-F, Pomerantzeff O. Transpupillary cyclophotocoagulation of rabbit eyes: an experimental approach to glaucoma surgery. *Am J Ophthalmol.* 1971;71:911-920.

43. Shields MB. Intraocular cyclophotocoagulation. *Transactions of the Ophthalmological Societies of the United Kingdom.* 1986;105(pt 2):237-241.

44. Uram M. Ophthalmic laser microendoscope ciliary process ablation in the management of neovascular glaucoma. *Ophthalmology.* 1992;99(12):1823-1828.

45. Uram M. Laser endoscope in the management of proliferative vitreoretinopathy. *Ophthalmology.* 1994;101(8):1404-1408.

46. Uram M. Diode laser endocyclodestruction [letter]. *Ophthalmic Surg.* 1994;25(4):268-269.

47. Beckman H, Kinoshita A, Rota AN, et al. Transscleral ruby laser irradiation of the ciliary body in the treatment of intractable glaucoma. *Trans Am Acad Ophthalmol Otolaryngol.* 1972;76(2):423-436.

48. Beckman H, Sugar HS. Neodymium laser cyclocoagulation. *Arch Ophthalmol.* 1973;90(1):27-28.

49. Beckman H, Waelterman J. Transscleral ruby laser cyclocoagulation. *Am J Ophthalmol.* 1984;98:788-795.

50. Rol P, Niederer P, Durr P, et al. Experimental investigations on the light scattering properties of the human sclera. *Lasers Light Ophthalmol.* 1990;3:201-221.

51. Vogel A, Dlugos C, Nuffer R, et al. Optical properties of human sclera and their significance for trans-scleral laser use. *Fortschritte der Ophthalmologic.* 1991;88(6):754-761.

52. Fankhauser F, van der Zypen E, Kwasniewska S, et al. Transscleral cyclophotocoagulation using a neodymium YAG laser. *Ophthalmic Surg.* 1986;17(2):94-100.

53. Chung PY, Schuman JS, Netland PA, et al. Five-year results of a randomized, prospective, clinical trial of diode vs argon laser trabeculoplasty for open-angle glaucoma. *Am J Ophthalmol.* 1998;126(2):185-190.

54. Brancato R, Carassa R, Trabucchi G. Diode laser compared with argon laser for trabeculoplasty. *Am J Ophthalmol.* 1991;112:50-55.

55. McHugh D, Marshall J, Ffytche J, et al. Diode laser trabeculoplasty for primary open angle glaucoma and ocular hypertension. *Br J Ophthalmol.* 1990;74:743.

56. Jacobson J, Schuman J, el Khoumy H, et al. Diode laser peripheral iridectomy. *Int Ophthalmol Clin.* 1990;30:120-122.

57. Schuman J, Jacobson J, Puliafito C. Semiconductor diode laser peripheral iridotomy. *Arch Ophthalmol.* 1990;108:1207-1208.

58. Emoto I, Okisaka S, Nakajima A. Diode laser iridotomy in rabbit and human eyes. *Am J Ophthalmol.* 1992;113:321-327.

59. Balles M, Puliafito C, D'Amico D, et al. Semiconductor diode laser photocoagulation in retinal vascular disease. *Ophthalmology.* 1990;97:1553-1561.

60. Brancato R, Pratesi R, Leoni G, et al. Histopathology of diode and argon laser lesions in rabbit retina. A comparative study. *Invest Ophthalmol Vis Sci.* 1989;30:1504-1510.

61. Duker J, Federman J, Schubert H, et al. Semiconductor diode laser endophotocoagulation. *Ophthalmic Surg.* 1989;20:717-719.

62. Jennings T, Fuller T, Vukich J, et al. Transscleral contact retinal photocoagulation with an 810-nm semiconductor diode laser. *Ophthalmic Surg.* 1990;21:492-496.

63. McHugh J, Marshall J, Ffytche T, et al. Initial clinical experience using a diode laser in the treatment of retinal vascular disease. *Eye.* 1989;3(pt 5):516-527.

64. Peyman G, Naguib K, Gaasterland D. Trans-scleral application of a semiconductor diode laser. *Lasers Surg Med.* 1990;10:569-575.

65. Puliafito C, Deutsch T, Boll J, et al. Semiconductor laser endophotocoagulation of the retina. *Arch Ophthalmol.* 1987;105:424-427.

66. Sato Y, Berkowitz B, Wilson C, et al. Blood-retinal barrier breakdown caused by diode vs argon laser endophotocoagulation. *Arch Ophthalmol.* 1992;110:277-281.

67. Suh J, Miki T, Obana A, et al. Effects of indocyanine green dye enhanced diode laser photocoagulation in non-pigmented rabbit eyes. *Osaka City Med J.* 1991;37:89-106.

68. Wallow I, Sponsel W, Stevens T. Clinicopathologic correlation of diode laser burns in monkeys. *Arch Ophthalmol.* 1991;109:648-653.

69. Brancato R, Leoni G, Trabucchi G, et al. Transscleral contact cyclophotocoagulation with Nd:YAG laser CW: experimental study on rabbit eyes. *Int J Tissue Reactions.* 1987;9(6):493-498.

70. Federman J, Ando F, Schubert H, et al. Contact laser for transscleral photocoagulation. *Ophthalmic Surg.* 1987;18:183-184.

71. Peyman GA, Katoh N, Tawakol M, et al. Transscleral and intravitreal contact Nd:YAG laser application. An experimental study. *Retina.* 1987;7(3):190-197.

72. Schubert HD, Federman JL. The role of inflammation in CW Nd:YAG contact transscleral photocoagulation and cryopexy. *Invest Ophthalmol Vis Sci.* 1989;30(3):543-549.

73. Schubert HD, Federman JL. A comparison of CW Nd:YAG contact transscleral cyclophotocoagulation with cyclocryopexy. *Invest Ophthalmol Vis Sci.* 1989;30(3):536-542.

74. Latina MA, Patel S, de Kater AW, et al. Transscleral cyclophotocoagulation using a contact laser probe: a histologic and clinical study in rabbits. *Lasers Sur Med.* 1989;9(5):465-470.

75. van der Zypen E, England C, Fankhauser F, et al. Cyclophotocoagulation in glaucoma therapy. *Int Ophthalmol.* 1989;13(1-2):163-166.

76. van der Zypen E, England C, Fankhauser F, et al. The effect of transscleral laser cyclophotocoagulation on rabbit ciliary body vascularization. *Graefes Arch Clin Exp Ophthalmol.* 1989;227(2):172-179.

77. Brancato R, Leoni G, Trabucchi G, et al. Histopathology of continuous wave neodymium: yttrium aluminum garnet and diode laser contact transscleral lesions in rabbit ciliary body. A comparative study. *Invest Ophthalmol Vis Sci.* 1991;32(5):1586-1592.

78. Schuman JS, Jacobson JJ, Puliafito CA, et al. Experimental use of semiconductor diode laser in contact transscleral cyclophotocoagulation in rabbits. *Arch Ophthalmol.* 1990;108(8):1152-1157.

79. Iwach AG, Drake MV, Hoskins HD Jr, et al. A new contact neodymium:YAG laser for cyclophotocoagulation. *Ophthalmic Surg.* 1991;22(6):345-348.

80. Allingham RR, de Kater AW, Bellows AR, et al. Probe placement and power levels in contact transscleral neodymium. YAG cyclophotocoagulation. *Arch Ophthalmol.* 1990;108(5):738-742.

81. Brancato R, Leoni G, Trabucchi G, et al. Probe placement and energy levels in continuous wave neodymium-YAG contact transscleral cyclophotocoagulation. *Arch Ophthalmol.* 1990;108(5):679-683.

82. Brancato R, Giovanni L, Trabbuchi G, et al. Contact transscleral cyclophotocoagulation with Nd:YAG laser in uncontrolled glaucoma. *Ophthalmic Surg.* 1989;20:547-551.

83. Schuman JS, Noecker RJ, Puliafito CA, et al. Energy levels and probe placement in contact transscleral semiconductor diode laser cyclophotocoagulation in human cadaver eyes. *Arch Ophthalmol.* 1991;109(11):1534-1538.

84. Schuman JS, Bellows AR, Shingleton BJ, et al. Contact transscleral Nd: YAG laser cyclophotocoagulation. Midterm results. *Ophthalmology.* 1992;99(7):1089-1094; discussion 1095.

85. Schuman JS, Puliafito CA, Allingham RR, et al. Contact transscleral continuous wave neodymium:YAG laser cyclophotocoagulation. *Ophthalmology.* 1990;97(5):571-580.

86. Gaasterland D, Abrams D, Belcher C, et al. A multicenter study of contact diode laser transscleral cyclophotocoagulation in glaucoma patients. *Invest Ophthalmol Vis Sci.* 1992;33(suppl):1019.

87. Carassa R, Trabucchi G, Bettin P, et al. Contact transscleral cyclophotocoagulation (CTCP) with diode laser: a pilot clinical study. *Invest Ophthalmol Vis Sci.* 1992;33(suppl):1019.

88. Wilensky JT, Welch D, Mirolovich M. Transscleral cyclocoagulation using a neodymium:YAG laser. *Ophthalmic Surg.* 1985;16(2):95-98.

89. England C, van der Zypen E, Fankhauser F, et al. Ultrastructure of the rabbit ciliary body following transscleral cyclophotocoagulation with the free-running Nd:YAG laser: preliminary findings. *Lasers Ophthalmol.* 1986;1:61-72.

90. Gross R, Smith J, Font R, et al. Transscleral Nd:YAG laser cycloablation in rabbits. *Invest Ophthalmol Vis Sci.* 1986;27(suppl):253.

91. Devenyi RG, Trope GE, Hunter WH. Neodymium-YAG transscleral cyclocoagulation in rabbit eyes. *Br J Ophthalmol.* 1987;71(6):441-444.

92. Moster M, Schwartz L, Cantor L, et al. Treatment of advanced glaucoma with Nd:YAG laser cyclodiathermy. *Invest Ophthalmol Vis Sci.* 1986;27(suppl):253.

93. Cyrlin M, Beckman H, Czedik C. Neodymium:YAG transscleral cyclocoagulation for severe glaucoma. *Invest Ophthalmol Vis Sci.* 1985;26(suppl):253.

94. Devenyi R, Trope G, Hunter W, et al. Neodymium:YAG transscleral cyclocoagulation in human eyes. *Ophthalmology.* 1987;94:1519-1522.

95. Fankhauser F, Kwasniewska S, van der Zypen E. Experimental and clinical use of the thermal mode neodymium:YAG laser. *Klin Monatsbl Augenheilkd.* 1987;191:169-173.

96. Hampton C, Shields MB. Transscleral neodymium-YAG cyclophotocoagulation. A histologic study of human autopsy eyes. *Arch Ophthalmol.* 1988;106(8):1121-1123.

97. Shields M, Blasini M, Simmons R, et al. A contact lens for transscleral Nd:YAG cyclophotocoagulation. *Am J Ophthalmol.* 1989;108:457-458.

98. Simmons RB, Blasini M, Shields MB, et al. Comparison of transscleral neodymium:YAG cyclophotocoagulation with and without a contact lens in human autopsy eyes. *Am J Ophthalmol.* 1990;109(2):174-179.

99. Blasini M, Simmons R, Shields MB. Early tissue response to transscleral neodymium: YAG cyclophotocoagulation. *Invest Ophthalmol Vis Sci.* 1990;31(6):1114-1118.

100. Cantor L, Nichols D, Katz J, et al. Neodymium-YAG transscleral cyclophotocoagulation. The role of pigmentation. *Invest Ophthalmol Vis Sci.* 1989;30:1834-1837.

101. Shepps G, Schuman J, Wang N, et al. Noncontact versus contact semiconductor diode laser transscleral cyclophotocoagulation in rabbits. *Invest Ophthalmol Vis Sci.* 1991;32(suppl):8611.

102. Hennis HL, Assia E, Stewart WC, et al. Transscleral cyclophotocoagulation using a semiconductor diode laser in cadaver eyes. *Ophthalmic Surg.* 1991;22(5):274-278.

103. Assia EI, Hennis HL, Stewart WC, et al. A comparison of neodymium: yttrium aluminum garnet and diode laser transscleral cyclophotocoagulation and cyclocryotherapy. *Invest Ophthalmol Vis Sci.* 1991;32(10):2774-2778.

104. Schwartz L, Moster M. Neodymium:YAG laser transscleral cyclodiathermy. *Ophthalmic Laser Ther.* 1986;1:135-141.

105. Trope G, Ma S. Mid term effects of Nd:YAG transscleral cyclocoagulation in glaucoma. *Ophthalmology.* 1990;97:73-75.

106. Klapper R, Wandel T, Donnenfeld E, et al. Transscleral neodymium: YAG thermal cyclophotocoagulation in refractory glaucoma, a preliminary report. *Ophthalmology.* 1988;95:719-722.

107. Hampton C, Shields M, Miller K, et al. Evaluation of a protocol for transscleral cyclophotocoagulation in 100 consecutive patients. *Ophthalmology.* 1990;97:910-917.

108. Wright M, Grajewski A, Feuer W. Nd:YAG cyclophotocoagulation: Outcome of treatment for uncontrolled glaucoma. *Ophthalmic Surg.* 1991;22:279-283.

109. Hennis HL, Stewart WC. Semiconductor diode laser transscleral cyclophotocoagulation in patients with glaucoma. *Am J Ophthalmol.* 1992;113(1):81-85.

110. Maus M, Katz L. Choroidal detachment, flat anterior chamber and hypotony as complications of Nd:YAG laser cyclophotocoagulation. *Ophthalmology.* 1990;97:69-72.

111. Fiore P, Melamed S, Krug J. Focal scleral thinning after transscleral Nd:YAG cyclophotocoagulation. *Ophthalmic Surg.* 1989;20: 215-216.

112. Hardten D, Brown J. Malignant glaucoma after Nd:YAG cyclophotocoagulation [letter]. *Am J Ophthalmol.* 1991;111:245-247.

113. Wand M, Schuman J, Puliafito C. Malignant glaucoma after contact transscleral Nd:YAG laser cyclophotocoagulation. *J Glaucoma.* 1993;2(2):110-111.

114. Blomquist P, Gross R, Koch D. Effect of transscleral neodymium:YAG cyclophotocoagulation on intraocular lenses. *Ophthalmic Surg.* 1990;21:223-226.

115. Lim E, Solomon K, Van Meter W, et al. Continuous wave transscleral Nd:YAG laser: a postmortem study of probe placement and destructive effects on tissue, transscleral sutured lenses and capsular bag fixated lenses. *Invest Ophthalmol Vis Sci.* 1992; 33(suppl):1268.

116. Kao S, Morgan C, Bergstrom T. Subretinal fibrosis following cyclocryotherapy. Case report. *Arch Ophthalmol.* 1987;105:1175-1176.

117. Pearson P, Baldwin L, Smith T. Lens subluxation as a complication of cyclocryotherapy. *Ophthalmic Surg.* 1989;20:445-446.

118. Bechrakis NE, Muller-Stolzenburg NW, Helbig H, et al. Sympathetic ophthalmia following laser cyclocoagulation. *Arch Ophthalmol.* 1994;112:80-84.

119. Edward D, Brown S, Higginbotham E, et al. Sympathetic ophthalmia following Nd:YAG cyclotherapy. *Ophthalmic Surg.* 1989;20:544-546.

120. Minckler D. Does Nd:YAG cyclotherapy cause sympathetic ophthalmia? *Ophthalmic Surg.* 1989;20:543.

121. Sabates R. Choroiditis compatible with the histopathologic diagnosis of sympathetic ophthalmia following cyclocryotherapy of neovascular glaucoma. *Ophthalmic Surg.* 1988;19:176-182.

122. Fries P, Char D, Crawford J, et al. Sympathetic ophthalmia complicating helium ion irradiation of a choroidal melanoma. *Arch Ophthalmol.* 1987;105:1561-1564.

123. Higginbotham EJ, Harrison M, Zou XL. Cyclophotocoagulation with the transscleral contact neodymium: YAG laser versus cyclocryotherapy in rabbits. *Ophthalmic Surg.* 1991;22:27-30.

124. Suzuki Y, Araie M, Yumita A, et al. Transscleral Nd:YAG laser cyclophotocoagulation versus cyclocryotherapy. *Graefes Arch Clin Exp Ophthalmol.* 1991;229:33-36.

125. Noureddin B, Wilson-Holt N, Lavin M, et al. Advanced uncontrolled glaucoma: Nd:YAG cyclophotocoagulation or tube surgery. *Ophthalmology.* 1992;99:430-437.

126. Schuman JS, Puliafito CA. Laser cyclophotocoagulation. *Int Ophthalmol Clin.* 1990;30:111-119.

127. Schubert HD. Noncontact and contact pars plana transscleral neodymium:YAG laser cyclophotocoagulation in postmortem eyes. *Ophthalmology.* 1989;96:1471-1475.

128. Schubert HD, Agarwala A, Arbizo V. Changes in aqueous outflow after in vitro neodymium: yttrium aluminum garnet laser cyclophotocoagulation. *Invest Ophthalmol Vis Sci.* 1990;31:1834-1838.

129. Pham-Duy T. Cyclocryotherapy in chronic glaucoma. *Fortschr Ophthalmol.* 1989;86:214-220.

130. Higginbotham E, Lee D, Bartels S, et al. Effects of cyclocryotherapy on aqueous humor dynamics in cats. *Arch Ophthalmol.* 1988;106:396-403.

131. Schmidt K, Lee P, Bhuyan D, et al. The role of prostaglandins (PGs) and uveoscleral outflow (Fu) in the reduction of intraocular pressure (IOP) after contact transscleral Nd:YAG laser cyclophotocoagulation (CYC) in pigmented rabbits. *Invest Ophthalmol Vis Sci.* 1992;33(suppl):1269.

132. Zaidman G, Wandel T. Transscleral YAG laser photocoagulation for uncontrollable glaucoma in corneal patients. *Cornea.* 1988;7:112-114.

133. Levy NS, Bonney RC. Transscleral YAG cyclocoagulation of the ciliary body for persistently high intraocular pressure following penetrating keratoplasty. *Cornea.* 1989;8:178-181.

134. Cohen EJ, Schwartz LW, Luskind RD, et al. Neodymium:YAG laser transscleral cyclophotocoagulation for glaucoma after penetrating keratoplasty. *Ophthalmic Surg.* 1989;20:713-716.

135. Coleman A, Jampel H, Javitt J, et al. Transscleral cyclophotocoagulation of human autopsy and monkey eyes. *Ophthalmic Surg.* 1991;22:638-643.

136. Lin SC, Chen MJ, Lin MS, et al. Vascular effects on ciliary tissue from endoscopic versus trans-scleral cyclophotocoagulation. *Br J Ophthalmol.* 2006;90:496-500.

137. Pantcheva MB, Kahook MY, Schuman JS, et al. Comparison of acute structural and histopathological changes in human autopsy eyes after endoscopic cyclophotocoagulation and trans-scleral cyclophotocoagulation. *Br J Ophthalmol.* 2007;91:248-252.

138. Chen J, Cohn RA, Lin SC, et al. Endoscopic photocoagulation of the ciliary body for treatment of refractory glaucomas. *Am J Ophthalmol.* 1997;124:787-796.

139. Uram M. Combined phacoemulsification, endoscopic ciliary process photocoagulation, and intraocular lens implantation in glaucoma management. *Ophthalmic Surg.* 1995;26:346-352.

140. Gayton JL, Van De Karr M, Sanders V. Combined cataract and glaucoma surgery: trabeculectomy versus endoscopic laser cycloablation. *J Cataract Refract Surg.* 1999;25:1214-1219.

141. Neely DE, Plager DA. Endocyclophotocoagulation for management of difficult pediatric glaucomas. *J AAPOS.* 2001;5:221-229.

142. Lima FE, Magacho L, Carvalho DM, et al. A prospective, comparative study between endoscopic cyclophotocoagulation and the Ahmed drainage implant in refractory glaucoma. *J Glaucoma.* 2004;13:233-237.

143. Lin SC. Endoscopic and transscleral cyclophotocoagulation for the treatment of refractory glaucoma. *J Glaucoma.* 2008;17:238-247.

144. Ahmad S, Wallace DJ, Herndon LW. Phthisis after endoscopic cyclophotocoagulation. *Ophthalmic Surg Lasers Imaging.* 2008;39:407-408.

57

Laser Peripheral Iridoplasty

Lisa S. Gamell, MD and Cristan M. Arena, MD

Argon laser iridoplasty (also called *gonioplasty*) was first described by Hager in 1973, who used the procedure to coagulate the iris base and deepen a narrow angle. Since that time, it has been described to widen the angle in a variety of syndromes. Typically, the contraction burns are applied to the peripheral iris with an argon laser, thereby thinning the peripheral iris tissue. The iris then shrinks away from the angle structures, ideally fostering outflow.

Iridoplasty can be performed when a laser peripheral iridotomy (LPI) is not possible, in eyes that have a narrow angle despite the presence of a patent iridotomy, in eyes with narrow angles due to mechanisms other than pupillary block, or in the presence of narrow angles with peripheral anterior synechiae (PAS).

In this chapter, each of these indications will be described in detail, as will contraindications, technique, postoperative management, and postoperative complications.

INDICATIONS

Acute Angle Closure

One of the first things learned in residency is that LPI is the definitive treatment for primary acute angle-closure glaucoma (PACG) because it reverses pupillary block. However, in order to perform this procedure in a more facile manner, it is necessary to break the attack by first lowering intraocular pressure (IOP). This allows the edematous cornea to clear, but also allows for patient comfort. Breaking an attack of PACG is usually accomplished both with topical ocular hypotensives and systemic medication, such as carbonic anhydrase inhibitors and/or hyperosmotics.

Argon laser peripheral iridoplasty (ALPI) is valuable in that it can open the angle mechanically in PACG resistant to medical therapy. During an attack, iris is apposed to the trabecular meshwork (TM). Iridoplasty can contract the iris adequately to pull it away from the meshwork.[1] In addition, a recent prospective trial that randomized patients to either immediate ALPI or conventional systemic medical therapy (acetazolamide and mannitol) revealed that ALPI can be an effective alternative to conventional medical therapy in lowering IOP in PACG.[2] Furthermore, argon laser iridoplasty may be successful in treating angle-closure glaucoma unrelieved despite a patent laser iridotomy.[3]

It should be stressed that the definitive procedure to break pupillary block once IOP is controlled and the cornea is clear is indeed LPI.

Chronic Angle Closure

Chronic angle-closure glaucoma (CACG) may develop in 2 ways. The first is in eyes that have suffered an attack of PACG and residual angle closure leads to PAS formation. The second is in eyes with angles that slowly narrow over time, usually asymptomatically, and IOP rises slowly as the angle is compromised. The latter is more common.[4]

In patients who have suffered an attack of PACG and have residual angle closure and PAS, iridoplasty can be used. If PAS are of less than 1-year duation, there is a 50% chance of restoring outflow function to the affected portion of the angle, but best results are achieved if PAS have been present for less than 6 months. Anecdotal evidence suggests that PAS of up to 1-year duration can be broken with iridoplasty.[5] This has not been reproducible, and iridoplasty is rarely successful if the PAS have been present for more than 1 year. These may require surgical intervention, such as goniosynechialysis.[6,7]

In those patients with the second type of CACG, the intial procedure performed should be LPI. However, occasionally, LPI alone is insufficient to open the angle and prevent apposition. In this situation, laser peripheral iridoplasty is a useful adjunct to open the angle. Areas of apposition may be successfully treated as iris contraction mechanically pulls open

Kahook MY, Schuman JS, eds.
Chandler and Grant's Glaucoma, Fifth Edition (pp 523-527).
© 2013 SLACK Incorporated.

the angle, thus helping to prevent PAS formation. Iridoplasty may be successful even after the development of PAS.[5]

Lens-Induced Angle Closure

Angle-closure glaucoma can be the result of the size or position of the lens. Iridoplasty can be used in eyes with narrow angles from gradually enlarging lenses without significant visual dysfunction. This can delay the need for lens extraction; however, if the cataract is visually significant or the angle is unresponsive to iridoplasty, cataract extraction should be performed.

In conditions such as phacomorphic glaucoma or anterior subluxation of the lens, lens extraction is indeed the definitive treatment needed. Nevertheless, like other types of angle-closure glaucoma, corneal edema and inflammation may preclude this procedure. In eyes that do not respond to medical therapy and laser iridotomy, iridoplasty can be used to eliminate appositional closure until such time as cataract surgery can be performed.[6]

Plateau Iris Syndrome

Plateau iris describes an abnormal iris configuration in which angle-closure glaucoma occurs without pupillary block. Plateau iris configuration describes the gonioscopic appearance of a closed angle but flat iris plane and deep central anterior chamber. Abnormal ciliary processes are most often responsible for this condition. On ultrasound biomicroscopy, the ciliary processes are anteriorly positioned and shortened, which in turn result in a more anterior insertion of the iris and crowding of the angle. Most of these cases may be treated with LPI. Plateau iris syndrome results when such an angle is persistently narrow despite a patent iridotomy, resulting in IOP elevation after pupillary dilation.[8]

Miotics such as pilocarpine may be initially effective in keeping the angle open, but over time, synechiae may still develop. Iridoplasty can help prevent synechial angle closure in these patients.[9]

Laser Trabeculoplasty

Laser peripheral iridoplasty can be used to pull the iris away from the TM and increase visibility, thus permitting laser trabeculoplasty.[1,6]

Nanophthalmos

Nanophthalmos is a rare condition in which an otherwise normal eye has a small volume, small equatorial diameter, and small corneal diameter. The lens is normal in size, however, which results in shallowing of the anterior chamber and narrowing of the angle. The condition has been described to follow certain stages. In stage 1, the angle is narrow, and IOP is normal. In stages 2 and 3, the angle appears more narrow and becomes partially closed. Once stage 4 is reached, angle closure is present, and IOP is elevated but controllable with medications. At stage 5, synechial angle closure is present, and IOP is no longer controllable with medications. Early LPI is the treatment of choice, preferably in stage 1 or 2, to prevent angle closure. If the angle continues to narrow or remains narrow despite a patent iridotomy, laser iridoplasty is used to open the angle. It may be repeated if necessary. In addition, once stage 3 or 4 is reached, iridioplasty may be a useful adjunct to iridotomy. If a nanophthalmic eye reaches stage 5, it will most likely need surgery to control IOP. Therefore, given the complications of surgery in nanophthalmos, such as choroidal effusion and serous retinal detachment, early diagnosis and aggressive treatment with LPI and iridoplasty are of utmost importance.[1,6]

Topiramate-Induced Angle Closure

Topiramate was first approved by the Food and Drug Administration as an antiepileptic in partial-onset seizures and primary generalized tonic-clonic seizures in 1996. In 2004, it received approval for the prophylaxis of migraine headaches. With this indication, use of topiramate increased.

Topiramate has been associated with a syndrome in which supraciliary effusion causes anterior displacement of the lens-iris diaphragm, with resultant acute myopia and secondary angle closure. Symptoms typically occur within 1 month of initiating therapy. In contrast to PACG, which is rare in individuals younger than 40 years, secondary angle-closure glaucoma associated with topiramate has been reported in pediatric patients as well as adults. Furthermore, while bilateral primary acute angle-closure glaucoma is rare, topiramate usually affects both eyes.[10]

First and foremost, topiramate must be discontinued. Pilocarpine is contraindicated in this situation, as it can promote further anterior displacement of the lens-iris diaphragm. Topical and oral medications to lower IOP are initiated, and cycloplegic agents can be used in an attempt to shift the lens-iris diaphragm posteriorly. It is important to note that pupillary block does not play a role in this situation; thus, a LPI would be unsuccessful in breaking the attack.

There have been reported cases of laser peripheral iridoplasty being effective in topiramate-associated bilateral acute angle-closure glaucoma. In one series, the IOP was markedly reduced and the anterior chamber deepened after several hours of ineffective medical therapy in 4 patients.[11] Another report demonstrated ALPI to open the angle within 1 hour after treatment.[12]

Vitreoretinal Procedures

Certain vitreoretinal procedures, such as scleral buckling and panretinal photocoagulation, can lead to ciliary body edema. Ciliary body edema causes anterior lens displacement and narrowing of the angle. Iridoplasty can be used to treat angle closure in these situations.[6]

Uveitis-Induced Angle Closure

One case has been reported in the European literature of a patient with uveitic acute closure who responded to ALPI after medical treatment and laser iridotomy failed to break the attack. In this situation, iridoplasty broke posterior synechiae, opened the angle, and reduced the IOP.[13]

CONTRAINDICATIONS

Poor Visualization

In PACG, the cornea is often edematous, precluding an adequate view of the iris to allow for laser treatment, both iridotomy and iridoplasty. In this case, laser treatment of any kind may further damage the cornea.

Flat Anterior Chamber

Similarly, peforming iridoplasty in the setting of a flat anterior chamber can result in endothelial burns and irreparable corneal damage.

Synechial Angle Closure

Peripheral iridoplasty is most effective in treating PAS that have been present for less than 6 months and is rarely successful if the PAS have been present for more than a year. Although success of iridoplasty in breaking PAS present for up to 1 year has been described, most have not experienced such success.

TECHNIQUE OF LASER PERIPHERAL IRIDOPLASTY

A topical anesthetic, such as proparacaine or tetracaine, is administered. Pilocarpine 2% is used to stretch the iris, and an alpha-adrenergic agent, either apraclonidine 0.5% or brimonidine 0.2%, is also applied to minimize the chance of postoperative IOP spikes.

Two techniques for performing laser peripheral iridoplasty have been described. One is a direct technique, using a lens such as an Abraham or center of a Goldmann, to apply laser energy to the peripheral iris. The other is an indirect technique, using a single-mirror goniscopy lens to direct the laser toward the peripheral iris.

Argon Laser Peripheral Iridoplasty

The argon laser is the usual laser of choice when performing laser peripheral iridoplasty. Most offices have an argon laser, which has many other uses, such as LPI. The step-by-step technique in Table 57-1 describes the appropriate settings for the argon laser.

PRACTICAL CONSIDERATIONS FOR
ARGON LASER PERIPHERAL IRIDOPLASTY

Lisa S. Gamell, MD

In many patients with occludable angles after laser iridotomy, there may be some component of phacomorphic block occurring due to the increased thickness of the cataractous lens. Certainly, in patients with visually significant cataracts, who are viable candidates for surgery, a reasonable choice might be to proceed with cataract surgery; this would relieve the phacomorphic component, and hopefully restore functional angle anatomy, as long as PAS have not formed (Figures 57-1 and 57-2).

In patients who are poor surgical candidates, or in whom cataracts are not yet visually significant—and where the benefits do not outweigh the risks of surgery—ALPI is a reasonable option for treating residual angle closure. It is preferable to treat with ALPI before PAS formation is apparent. Note, however, that if IOP starts to rise despite medical therapy or angle anatomy is seriously compromised, then lens extraction should be seriously considered.

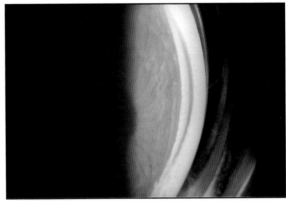

Figure 57-1. Gonioscopic view of closed angle prior to phacoemulsification.

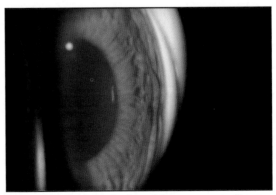

Figure 57-2. Gonioscopic view of the same eye as Figure 57-1 after phacoemulsification revealing an opening of the angle.

TABLE 57-1. TECHNIQUE FOR LASER PERIPHERAL IRIDOPLASTY	
Step 1	Obtain informed consent; include discussion of the following: • Pain/discomfort • Inflammation • Increased intraocular pressure • Change in iris/pupil appearance • Ineffectiveness/need for retreatment
Step 2	Pretreat with • Anesthetic • Pilocarpine 2% • Alpha-adrenergic agent • Wait approximately 20 to 30 minutes for drops to take effect.
Step 3	Argon laser settings: • Power—300 to 500 mW • Spot size—300 to 500 um • Duration—300 to 500 msec
Step 4	Place a viscous coupling agent on the lens of your choice (eg, Abraham, single-mirror gonioscopy lens, Goldmann)
Step 5	Treat entire peripheral iris titrating laser power to cause visible contraction of iris tissue without bubble formation or pigment release
Step 6	• Remove lens and clean the patient's eye • Give a second drop of your chosen alpha-adrenergic agent and a drop of prednisolone acetate 1% • Recheck intraocular pressure in 1 hour • Send the patient home with prednisolone acetate 1% 4 times a day for 4 days • Follow-up in 1 week

Adapted from Kahook MY, Noecker RJ. Iridoplasty: advice on appropriate technique. *Glaucoma Today.* July/August 2006:34-36.

PERSONAL TECHNIQUE
Lisa S. Gamell, MD

Before any laser procedure, obtain informed consent, and check the vision and pressure on the day of the visit. Preoperatively, we give iopidine 0.5% and pilocarpine 2% in the eye to be treated. We also mark the eye by placing a piece of paper tape with an "x" on it on the forehead over the eye to be treated. Once the pupil is constricted—about 30 minutes after the drops are given—Proparacaine is given, and the procedure may begin.

We typically use the direct technique with an Abraham lens and a coupling medium (eg, goniosol). When using the Abraham lens, one can use the nonfocusing area of the lens or the focusing button. Bear in mind that if you use the focusing button, less energy will be necessary. It is important to remember that the endpoint for ALPI is contraction of the iris tissue, not charring of tissue. If the shots are leaving visible burns on the iris, the power must be turned down. Treatment spots may be spaced about 1 to 1.5 burn widths apart, anywhere from 6 to 8 per quadrant.

Typical settings on the Argon Green laser are typically a 500-μm spot, 500 mW, and 500 msec (or 0.5 s) duration. Using the "fives" as a starting point makes it easy to remember. In a deeply pigmented iris, the energy will be readily absorbed, so less energy may be needed. In addition, when using the focusing button of the Abraham lens, the starting energy may be lower—around 200 or 250 for example. In a lightly pigmented iris, higher energy settings will be needed and can be titrated until a proper endpoint tissue response is noted.

When using the direct technique, it is important to position the aiming beam as far peripheral on the iris as possible. The beam may even overlap the peripheral edge of the lens onto the limbus. Remember, due to total internal reflection, the laser will not reach the angle of the eye. But by positioning the aiming beam in the far periphery, contraction burns are more likely to be effective in contracting the iris and thinning the more problematic portions of iris tissue.

After rinsing the coupling medium out of the eye at the end of the procedure, we give another drop of iopidine 0.5% and then wait 1 hour to check the IOP. The patient is sent home on prednisolone acetate 1% 4 times daily for 4 days and is seen in 1 week. At the 1-week visit, gonioscopy is performed, and the angle is reassessed. If there are still occludable areas present, the procedure may be repeated once any anterior chamber inflammation has abated. If there are a few areas with PAS of less than 6 months duration by our best estimation, then the indirect approach may be used with a Goldmann lens for a more specific, tailored treatment.

The angle may be reassessed every 3 to 6 months, depending upon the severity of the angle closure, IOP, and disc damage.

Diode Laser Peripheral Iridoplasty

Diode laser peripheral iridoplasty has been shown to be safe and effective as the first-line treatment of an acute attack of PACG (MK Khambaty, DW Richards, unpublished data).[14]

Krypton Laser Peripheral Iridoplasty

A pilot study has suggested krypton (red) laser iridoplasty of blue eyes to be a viable alternative to argon (blue-green) laser peripheral iridoplasty. The theory behind this is that red light should be more readily absorbed in blue eyes, but prospective studies are needed.

Postoperative Management

Immediately after the procedure, a drop of topical steroid and alpha-adrenergic agent is given. Topical steroids are continued 4 to 6 times a day for 3 to 5 days. IOP is also monitored postoperatively, with measurement at 1 hour being the optimum time frame. If IOP is elevated, it should be treated accordingly.

Gonioscopy should be performed at approximately 1 week postoperatively to evaluate effectiveness and determine need for retreatment. IOP should also be measured at subsequent visits.

Complications

Iritis

A mild iritis may occur, which typically responds to topical corticosteroids.

Intraocular Pressure Spike

As with most laser procedures, a transient rise in IOP may occur, which can be managed with topical ocular hypotensives. The patient's IOP should be checked approximately 1 hour after treatment.

Corneal Endothelial Burn

Corneal endothelial burn can be avoided by not using the procedure in eyes with severe corneal edema and/or flat anterior chambers.

Persistent Angle Closure

Gonioscopy needs to be followed at regular intervals for recurrence of appositional closure, and retreatment should be given as necessary. This is most often from a growing lens, as described in the section "Lens-Induced Angle Closure."

References

1. Ritch R, Liebman JM. Argon laser peripheral iridoplasty. *Ophthalmic Surg Lasers.* 1996;26:289-300.
2. Lam DS, Lai JS, Tham CC, Chua JK, Poon AS. Argon laser peripheral iridoplasty versus conventional systemic medical therapy in treatment of acute primary angle-closure glaucoma: a prospective, randomized, controlled trial. *Ophthalmology.* 2002;109(9):1591-1596.
3. Weiss HS, Shingleton BJ, Goode SM, Bellows AR, Richter CU. Argon laser gonioplasty in the treatment of angle-closure glaucoma. *Am J Ophthalmol.* 1992;114:14-18.
4. American Academy of Ophthalmology. Chronic angle closure. In: *Glaucoma.* Vol 10. San Francisco, CA: Author; 2006-2007:126-127.
5. Wand M. Argon laser gonioplasty for synechial angle closure. *Arch Ophthalmol.* 1992;110:363-367.
6. Ritch R, Tham CC, Lam DS. Argon laser peripheral iridoplasty (ALPI): an update. *Surv Ophthalmol.* 2007;52(3):279-288.
7. Tarongoy P, Ho CL, Walton DS. Angle-closure glaucoma: the role of the lens in the pathogenesis, prevention, and treatment. *Surv Ophthalmol.* 2009;54(2):211-225.
8. Allingham RR, et al. Plateau iris. In: Allingham RR et al, ed. *Shields' Textbook of Glaucoma.* 5th ed. Philadelphia, PA: Lippincott Williams & Wilkins; 2005:313.
9. Ritch R, Tham CC, Lam DS. Long-term success of argon laser peripheral iridoplasty in the management of plateau iris syndrome. *Ophthalmology.* 2004;111(1):104-108.
10. Zalta AH, Smith RT. Peripheral iridoplasty efficacy in refractory topiramate-associated bilateral acute angle-closure glaucoma. *Arch Ophthalmol.* 2008;126(11):1603-1605.
11. Sbeity Z, Gvozdyuk N, Amde W, Liebmann JM, Ritch R. Argon laser peripheral iridoplasty for topiramate-induced bilateral acute angle closure. *J Glaucoma.* 2009;18(4):269-271.
12. Mansouri K, Ravinet E. Argon-laser iridoplasty in the management of uveitis-induced acute angle-closure glaucoma. *Eur J Ophthalmol.* 2009;19(2):304-306.
13. Kahook MY, Noecker RJ. Iridoplasty: advice on appropriate technique. *Glaucoma Today.* 2006:34-36.
14. Lai JS, Tham CC, Chua JK, Lam DS. Immediate diode laser peripheral iridoplasty as treatment of acute attack of primary angle closure glaucoma: a preliminary study. *J Glaucoma.* 2001;10(2):89-94.

GLAUCOMA SURGERY

58

What to Say to Glaucoma Patients Prior to Filtration Surgery

Mahmoud A. Khaimi, MD

Patients who face glaucoma filtering surgery often have a variety of questions regarding the need for surgery, goals of the operation, and likely outcome (Table 58-1). Because the main goal of filtering surgery is to reduce intraocular pressure (IOP) and preserve vision rather than improve vision, this should be carefully discussed preoperatively. Not infrequently, it may be necessary to briefly review the pathophysiology of glaucoma and how it causes vision loss. New therapies and the use of adjunctive antimetabolites, such as mitomycin C, should be discussed comprehensively, including their indications, use, risks, and benefits. An additional point of discussion, if indicated, is whether cataract surgery should be performed as a staged procedure or as a combined operation.

What follows is a stylized exchange between a patient and her ophthalmologist regarding planned glaucoma filtering surgery. Although it is not practical to address all of the questions raised in this discussion with each patient prior to filtering surgery, we strongly feel that it is in the best interests of all concerned to have a well-informed and prepared patient prior to embarking on the surgical management of glaucoma.

Mrs. Smith is a 65-year-old African American woman with primary open-angle glaucoma (POAG) in both eyes, diagnosed approximately 4 to 5 years previously. Despite maximally tolerated medical and laser therapy, the patient's IOP is 30 mm Hg in the right eye. The left eye pressure is 18 mm Hg and is currently being treated with a prostaglandin analog. The patient's visual acuity is 20/60 in the left eye with correction of $-1.75 + 0.75$ X 165 and $20/30^{-2}$ OS with correction of $-1.00 + 1.00$ X 10. Relevant family history includes a sister who has undergone laser trabeculoplasty (LTP) treatment and a glaucoma filtering procedure for glaucoma, and Mrs. Smith's mother was on drops for glaucoma in the 2 years just prior to her death at age 74. Mrs. Smith is also being treated for mild essential hypertension, which is presently controlled with one drug therapy.

Dr. Khaimi: "Mrs. Smith, as we have discussed on many occasions, glaucoma is a very serious and chronic condition, which is a leading cause of blindness."

Mrs. Smith: "Yes, Dr. Khaimi, I have been so afraid of losing my vision. I have tried very hard to use the medicines as you have prescribed, and I still can see to sew, to drive, and to do most things."

Dr. Khaimi: "Fortunately, glaucoma does not affect the central vision until the very end stages of the disease; yet, you do appear to have damage in both eyes. Actually, from the time of diagnosis, the right eye has evidenced rather significant damage from the appearance of the optic nerve and as well from the visual field, which we have previously discussed is the test that evaluates the function of the optic nerve."

Mrs. Smith: "Is my left eye also damaged?"

Dr. Khaimi: "At least from the appearance of the optic nerve and a suggestion of early changes on the visual field, it also evidences damage. Fortunately, however, there have been no advanced changes or threatening findings on the visual field. The concern presently is with the pressure being too high in the right eye."

Mrs. Smith: "But I thought that the pressures had come down significantly! How low does the pressure need to be?"

Dr. Khaimi: "Actually, your pressure had responded and initially, for a year or so, was adequately reduced. We don't really know exactly what the safe pressure level is for people in general. It is a very individual consideration with the pressure goal for each patient's glaucoma being different and perhaps even different for each eye of each patient. Because the damage in your right eye is significantly greater than would appear in the left eye, it would be reasonable to understand

Kahook MY, Schuman JS, eds.
Chandler and Grant's Glaucoma, Fifth Edition (pp 531-535).
© 2013 SLACK Incorporated.

TABLE 58-1. POINTS TO DISCUSS BEFORE FILTRATION SURGERY

Glaucoma
How it causes vision loss
Why reducing IOP is beneficial
Treatment alternatives
Combined cataract surgery
Goals of filtering surgery
Reduce IOP
• Preserve vision
• Potential for vision improvement (if any)
• Reduce medications
• Risks and benefits
Filtering surgery
• Anesthesia
• Description of surgery
• Length of surgery
• Antimetabolites
• Postoperative course
○ Medications
○ Eye shield
○ Activity restrictions
○ Vision changes
○ Frequency of eye exams
• Common complications
○ Hypotony
○ Elevated IOP (postoperative)
○ Choroidal effusion or hemorrhage
○ Cataract
• Cosmetic factors (eyelid, bleb)
• Success rate
• Risk of endophthalmitis
Preoperative instructions
• Discontinue aspirin and nonsteroidal anti-inflammatory drug
Glaucoma medications (discontinue prior to surgery)

was considered in the normal range, glaucoma-type damage to the optic nerves has still occurred. Such patients are felt to have normal or low-pressure glaucoma in that the optic nerve has some peculiar sensitivity to even 'normal' levels of pressure. It would seem that we need your pressures at a very low level in the right eye, perhaps high single digits or low teens on a continuous basis, and at 18 or so in the left eye."

Mrs. Smith: "But I thought that we had gotten the pressure to a safe level! The pressure in the right eye had been in the teens after the laser. Has the laser stopped working again? We seem to have gotten a really good effect from the original laser and some help from the one retreatment 2 years later. Can't we try the laser again?"

Dr. Khaimi: "Often, laser will work very well, especially in certain types of glaucoma. We have talked many times about your glaucoma and have also discussed that LTP can be highly effective, especially initially and even with a retreatment. However, over time, POAG tends to be progressive, and ultimately there will be little to gain from repeated treatments with the laser."

Mrs. Smith: "Well, is there any alternative other than surgery?"

Dr. Khaimi: "As you know, we have had to use oral Diamox in an effort to obtain better control of your eye pressures. Unfortunately, despite initiating systemic therapy, your right eye's pressure is still uncontrolled."

Mrs. Smith: "By the way, I felt awful on the 2 tablets twice a day and still seem to have no energy. I just don't feel like myself."

Dr. Khaimi: "Well, I am sure it is difficult to get through the day feeling that you have no energy, and this is one more reason why we have evolved to the point of needing to discuss surgery. You will likely not be able to tolerate the oral medications for much longer, and stopping this medication will lead to a further increase in your pressure. Glaucoma filtering surgery is designed to create a new pathway for the fluid in your eye, which is not effectively draining through your eye's natural drain system."

Mrs. Smith: "Yes, we have talked about surgery in the past. But, what exactly is involved with glaucoma filtering surgery? Do you place a tube in my eye? It seems that I have heard or read about drainage devices being placed in an eye."

Dr. Khaimi: "There are glaucoma drainage devices that are used and inserted in some eyes that have glaucoma. Typically, however, glaucoma drainage devices are used in patients with more advanced forms of glaucoma, in patients who have not responded to conventional filtering surgery, or in those who have certain significant risk factors, such as inflammation in the eye or significant scar tissue formation from previous eye surgery."

Mrs. Smith: "What actually do you do? Do you put me to sleep? Will the surgery be painful?"

Dr. Khaimi: "Actually, the surgery is performed under local anesthesia. You will be given preoperative sedation so that you

that the right eye pressure must be reduced to a much lower level than the left eye pressure. In some patients with pressures at even 20 to 22 mm Hg or lower, which previously are relaxed, and you will be kept sedated and comfortable for the procedure. A member of the anesthesia staff will be monitoring your vital systems, and it is unlikely that you will have any life-threatening problems. It will be necessary to use a local anesthetic to inject medicine around your eye to put the pain and motor fibers to sleep so that your eye will not move and you will have no discomfort during the surgery. The method for using local anesthesia to put the eye to sleep is quite similar to that which is performed for a dental procedure.

"The surgery is very delicate and involves creating a controlled opening, which will allow fluid to escape from the eye. It is somewhat like creating a manhole cover with stitches around the edges of the cover so that fluid can flow out around the edges of the cover. A medication called mitomycin C is placed on certain parts of the eye at the time of surgery, and this medication has been shown to have local effects in preventing scar formation and enhancing the drainage of fluid from the eye. An additional outer layer of tissue known as the conjunctiva will then be sewn over the draining fluid, which will help allow the fluid to spread out and away from the inside of the eye."

Mrs. Smith: "Will I feel this filter or be able to see it?"

Dr. Khaimi: "Yes, often, there will be a small raised, localized area of tissue, like a little bubble or bleb, which will be hidden under the upper lid. It is likely that you could see it in a mirror with the lid elevated, and it may be that you will have an awareness or sensation of a raised area under your lid with blinking and lid movement."

Mrs. Smith: "How long will the surgery take?"

Dr. Khaimi: "The time required for the surgery will vary with each patient. Sometimes, the tissue dissection can be more difficult due to the conjunctiva being thinner, or there can be prominent blood vessels and a bit more localized bleeding in certain patients, thus requiring more time for the surgery. So, do not let the time be a concern, although usually the surgery lasts approximately 30 to 45 minutes once we start."

Mrs. Smith: "Will I see better or differently after the surgery?"

Dr. Khaimi: "It's good that you asked about your vision, as there are several important considerations. As you have commented on several occasions, your vision has been variable and at times somewhat blurred."

Mrs. Smith: "Yes, and my night vision has been poor for some time. I have even stopped driving at all after sunset because things are so dark. I also have had difficulty reading, and I seem to need more light to be able to read the newspaper."

Dr. Khaimi: "These symptoms, as we have discussed before, are related to both the maturing cataract and the worsening of your glaucoma in your right eye. The goal of filtering surgery is to lower your eye pressure in efforts to halt the progression of your glaucoma. Glaucoma surgery is not done to improve your vision but is needed to keep your present vision from progressively getting worse. Remember that loss of vision due to glaucoma is irreversible, and hopefully, glaucoma surgery will lower your eye pressure to a safe and protective range, whereby you will no longer have further loss of vision."

Mrs. Smith: "Is the surgery reasonably safe? Could my vision be worse or even possibly could I go blind?"

Dr. Khaimi: "In every way, I want to reassure you that the chances are very minimal that you would have any major problem that would affect your vision significantly. Patients who undergo any type of intraocular surgery can experience some degree of accelerated cataract formation. Because you already have a cataract related to your age, it is likely that your cataract could significantly progress over time, requiring removal of the cataract. And, one must acknowledge that, however small the risk, you could develop an infection or have a hemorrhage that could result in loss of some or all vision in your eye and possibly even have to have the eye removed. Because glaucoma patients typically have variable eye pressure, which affects the vessels in the retina and back of the eye, they are at greater risk for developing spontaneous bleeds than are patients who do not have glaucoma and are merely undergoing cataract surgery. While complications are not likely during the surgery, they can still happen, and it is important to realize that before deciding on the surgery."

Mrs. Smith: "Are there any other complications or problems that may occur and that I need to know about?"

Dr. Khaimi: "During the early postoperative period, your filtering site can drain too much fluid from the eye, which can result in the front part of the eye shallowing and subsequently in the lens moving forward and possibly even touching the back surface of the cornea. Occasionally, if too much fluid is draining from the eye, you can get swelling in the back of the eye that leads to some loss of vision. If the process does not respond to tight patching of the eye or certain medications that we use in these circumstances, then an additional surgical procedure may be required."

Mrs. Smith: "What type of surgical procedure, and would it be very risky to have this surgery?"

Dr. Khaimi: "Yes, unfortunately there is rather moderate risk with each additional surgical intervention; yet, the procedure is usually able to be performed without significant additional complications. Should there be excess fluid drainage from the eye in the early postoperative period that warrants correction, then we would need to return to surgery again under local anesthesia to perform a procedure in which the fluid is drained from the choroid and the chamber is deepened. A small incision will have been placed into the anterior chamber through the cornea, and this incision site will be used for filling the chamber with fluid, which will allow deepening of the chamber and thus normalizing the distance between the cornea and the lens. At the same time, a small incision will be made just back from the edge of the cornea over the site of fluid accumulation, which will allow drainage of the fluid from the choroid and thus will also assist with deepening the chamber and reducing the excessive filtration of fluid. It can happen that the incision in the tissue overlying the choroid could result in a significant hemorrhage or possibly even a tear of the retina. There could also be more accelerated cataract formation, which develops over several days or perhaps over several months, thus necessitating removal of the cataract."

Mrs. Smith: "Well, you have indicated that I already have a cataract. Why aren't we removing the cataract at the same time I'm to undergo the glaucoma surgery so that all is done at one time?"

Dr. Khaimi: "I am glad that you mentioned this, Mrs. Smith. It certainly is possible that a combined cataract-glaucoma procedure could be performed with insertion of an implant, and often this type of combined procedure is performed very successfully. Your cataract is mature enough to seriously consider this option. Often, glaucoma filtering surgery is combined with cataract surgery and lens implant because glaucoma surgery can cause the cataract to progress. If this were the case, one would have to go back to the operating room to take out the cataract at a later point. Therefore, if a patient has moderate cataract formation, I typically suggest proceeding with a combined procedure in order to avoid another surgical procedure later on and to address the cataract that is currently present."

Mrs. Smith: "That makes sense. I really don't think I would want to go through a second operation if it could be avoided. Earlier, while describing the glaucoma filtering procedure, you mentioned the use of mitomycin C to prevent scarring."

Dr. Khaimi: "Yes, numerous studies have indicated a significant benefit in using certain types of adjunctive medications know as antimetabolite agents, such as mitomycin C or 5-fluorouracil, during glaucoma filtering surgery. Mitomycin C is applied at the time of surgery to a very localized area, which can, as I had mentioned, have local effects in preventing scar formation and enhancing filtration."

Mrs. Smith: "Are there any dangers with using these drugs? Are both drugs considered to be safe to use in the eye?"

Dr. Khaimi: "Both drugs are very powerful agents that interfere with the activity of cells that cause scar tissue formation. Yet, these drugs can also result in defective healing with resultant separation of the wound, defects in the filter site itself with leakage and flattening of the bleb, and can be dangerous to the internal aspects of the eye if they inadvertently get into the interior of the eye. Yet, much information has been gathered about these drugs, and we have become very skilled at using them in appropriate doses for our desired effect. It also must be mentioned that a very thin filtering bleb may develop after use of these drugs, and with time the eye can overfilter with the pressure becoming too low. The filtering bleb itself can become too thin, resulting in leakage and prompting the need to have the area resutured

and possibly revised. If indeed the pressure becomes too low on an extended basis, then the eye can become soft with stretch marks developing in the central retina or the macular area with some damaging effect from the hypotony. If the pressure is not adequately reduced or is too high in the early postoperative period, whether a primary filtering procedure is done or a combined cataract-filtering procedure, then the laser can be used to cut one of the stitches in the edge of the "manhole cover" to allow more fluid to be released from the eye, thus lowering the pressure. Usually, there are no problems with performing the laser. One must be aware that the laser being performed through the conjunctiva or outer layer of tissue could result in a hole being created, which would leak and thus require suturing or patching. I must also mention that adjunctive antimetabolites have been shown to increase the lifetime risk of eye infection and that any potential signs of infection, such as eye redness, pain, or discharge, must be addressed immediately."

Mrs. Smith: "Well, it seems that we have decided what to do about the right eye. Do you feel comfortable that my left eye is in a stable situation?"

Dr. Khaimi: "Actually, I have some concern that there has been damage of the optic nerve. There also are early changes in the visual field, and the pressure is at a borderline level even now while on an oral medication, which we will need to discontinue for the filtering surgery. It is our usual practice to discontinue the oral Diamox because it affects both eyes, and the effect is that of reducing flow in the eye, which results in lower pressures. Once the filter is created, it is necessary that fluid flow through the opening in order to maintain the patency and to assist with the filter becoming established and reducing the eye pressure. Thus, it would be potentially harmful to the success of the surgery to be on the oral medication."

Mrs. Smith: "But, what about the pressure in my left eye?"

Dr. Khaimi: "It is likely that the pressure will increase once you are off of the Diamox, and the pressure would then be at a level that would be unsafe. We can add a second pressure-lowering drop to hopefully avoid this problem. Another consideration would be to keep you on your topical pressure-lowering drop and to perform LTP to reduce the pressure to a safer level in the left eye by the time of the surgery for the right eye, which is to be done in the next few weeks. We will definitely pay close attention to your left eye while we are following the postoperative course of your right eye."

Mrs. Smith: "After surgery on my right eye, will I still have to use my glaucoma drops?"

Dr. Khaimi: "No. You will immediately stop taking your glaucoma drops that you were on in your right eye prior to surgery and start postoperative drops the day after your surgery. On your postoperative day 1 visit, I will take the patch and shield off your operated eye and check your vision and pressure. I will also carefully examine your eye. You will then be instructed on how to properly take your postoperative drops. You will be placed on a topical steroid on a somewhat frequent basis in the right eye in order to quiet the inflammation from the surgery to prevent scarring of the filter. You will use a topical antibiotic drop to prevent infection. You will also be placed on a combination antibiotic and steroid ointment to be used at bedtime. In some cases, you might need a drop that dilates your pupil and helps in cases where the eye pressure might be too low early on. This drop can cause your vision to be blurry early on but is helpful in specific situations."

Mrs. Smith: "Are there any restrictions after surgery?"

Dr. Khaimi: "Yes. I ask all my patients to avoid bending, lifting, and any strenuous activity for several weeks after surgery. I also instruct all my patients to protect the operated eye by wearing their original glasses or the protective eyewear we give out in the postoperative kit. Finally, I instruct all my patients to wear a shield over the operated eye at bedtime for at least 2 weeks postoperatively."

Mrs. Smith: "Dr. Khaimi, I want to thank you for discussing this surgery and my various options and the risks of this procedure as I have had great concern about my vision. Actually, I should tell you that my mother was nearly completely blinded by her glaucoma because she avoided glaucoma surgery at all costs because she was terrified of surgery."

Dr. Khaimi: "Mrs. Smith, there is risk with everything that we do. The greatest risk in glaucoma is not controlling the pressure and not being appropriately aggressive, because untreated glaucoma and inadequately reduced pressure results in loss of all vision as it did with your mother. What I would want you and your family to know and to understand is that we are partners in this process and that no matter what may occur, we will deal with problems and situations as they come up. Meanwhile, we will be confident that things will go well and that we can achieve control of your pressure and preserve your vision."

59

Filtering Surgery in the Management of Glaucoma

Mahmoud A. Khaimi, MD and Marcos Reyes, MD

Glaucoma filtration surgery is performed to provide an alternative route for aqueous humor efflux from the anterior chamber and past the diseased trabecular meshwork (TM) to a space external to the eye. Aqueous then collects underneath the conjunctiva and Tenon's capsule, an area known as the bleb, to be carried away by blood vessels and transudation past the bleb wall. The desired result is to decrease the intraocular pressure (IOP) to a lower level that would slow down or halt the progression of axonal loss that is characteristic of glaucomatous optic neuropathy.

Embarking on incisional surgery for the treatment of glaucoma is a major decision made between patient and physician (Table 59-1). Typically, this becomes a viable management alternative after medical and laser treatment have failed to reduce IOP to the desired level. Indications for advancing therapy are progressive glaucomatous optic nerve with characteristic cupping of the nerve and/or visual field loss or uncontrolled elevation of IOP that has a high likelihood of producing optic nerve damage. Many techniques and procedural variations have been developed to bypass the diseased TM. In the past, unguarded or full-thickness surgery was primarily used.[1] However, the incidence of postoperative hypotony, with its associated complications, was extremely high. Since that time, our understanding of surgical approaches has evolved, and our techniques have improved to include partial-thickness surgery with the use of adjunctive antimetabolites. Today, guarded filtration surgery, also commonly referred to as partial-thickness trabeculectomy, is the primary operation performed for the surgical management of glaucoma. What follows is a discussion of the various concerns that must be taken into account when deciding on and performing filtration surgery.

PREOPERATIVE ASSESSMENT

Many factors contribute to the final outcome of filtration surgery. In some cases, the risk factors for failure can be modified or reduced by taking specific courses of action before and during filtration surgery.

With the exception of highly myopic patients, younger patients are at increased risk for filtration failure. The younger the patient, the greater the risk.[2] Other risk factors for filtration failure include diabetes,[2] higher preoperative IOP,[2] African American ancestry,[3] neovascularization,[3] uveitis,[3] and prior failed surgery.[3] A concerted effort to reduce pre- and postoperative scarring and inflammation is imperative. Intra- and/or postoperative antimetabolite therapy increases the success rate of all filtration surgery and especially in those with the above risks.[4-7] Those patients who are elderly have memory difficulties or physical handicaps require additional attention and education. Discussing the perioperative process with family or other support people or occasionally consulting with social services may be necessary. It is crucial to establish that the patient will be able to care for him- or herself or be cared for before surgery is undertaken. The patient and appropriate family members must understand that the postoperative care is just as important as the surgery itself and that, without adequate care, the surgery can ultimately end in failure and perhaps potentially lead to adverse postoperative issues such as prolonged uveitis, posterior synechiae, and cystoid macular edema.

Other considerations relate to the preoperative ocular status (Table 59-2). Hyperopic eyes, particularly those that are very small (axial length < 21 mm) frequently have an axially shallow anterior chamber. There may be a history of chronic

Kahook MY, Schuman JS, eds.
Chandler and Grant's Glaucoma, Fifth Edition (pp 537-554).
© 2013 SLACK Incorporated.

TABLE 59-1. INDICATIONS FOR FILTERING SURGERY
Progressive visual field loss or optic nerve cupping despite maximally tolerated medical and or laser therapy
Uncontrolled intraocular pressure that could lead to progressive visual field loss or optic nerve cupping
Inability to achieve intraocular pressure (usually low teens) in patients with visual field loss approaching fixation (unable to follow for progression)

TABLE 59-2. SPECIAL PREOPERATIVE CONSIDERATIONS
Hyperopic eyes
1. More prone to shallow or flat anterior chambers postoperatively
2. In chronic angle-closure eyes, there is an increased risk of malignant glaucoma
3. Consider tighter scleral flap closure to avoid postoperative hypotony and shallow/flat anterior chamber
Pseudophakic (postoperative) eyes
1. Check conjunctival mobility prior to choosing a filter site
2. Use caution when creating scleral flap through old cataract wound incision (risk of avulsion of scleral flap)
3. Perform anterior vitrectomy for vitreous in the anterior chamber
4. Use antimetabolites (mitomycin C or 5-fluorouacil)

angle closure. These eyes are prone to postoperative shallow or flat chambers or, more rarely, malignant glaucoma. Such complications can be reduced by using tighter scleral flap closure to guard against postoperative hypotony and by minimizing intraoperative hypotony by use of anterior chamber maintainers or viscoelastics. Preoperatively, every eye should be evaluated for conjunctival mobility, especially with a history of prior surgery. Special care should be taken in the vicinity of scleral incisions or where vitreous may be present near the planned sclerectomy site. A scleral flap may be difficult to create and at risk for amputation in eyes that have undergone previous surgery. Proper preoperative planning for placement of the scleral flap will allow the careful surgeon to mitigate these issues.

TOPICAL AND SYSTEMIC MEDICATIONS

Factors that increase pre- and postoperative inflammation should be reduced. One of these factors is the use of preoperative glaucoma medications. Generally speaking, topical and oral glaucoma medications may be continued until the day of surgery. Topical medications, such as beta-blockers, may be stopped 24 to 48 hours before filtration surgery. In patients taking timolol, it has been shown that aqueous humor production begins to increase to baseline levels only after 3 to 4 days.[8] Though currently this may not be performed routinely, historically, surgeons found it to be advantageous to try to promote aqueous humor production in patients undergoing filtration surgery to reduce the incidence of postoperative hypotony.

Preoperative steroids may be useful in those patients with uveitic glaucoma where inflammation poses an increased risk for surgical failure. This approach needs to be individualized for each patient. The use of topical steroids such as prednisolone acetate 1% every 2 hours 24 to 48 hours before filtration surgery may be useful. Some surgeons find a short course of perioperative oral corticosteroids to be of benefit in those patients with a history of severe uveitis or in those with active inflammation needing urgent surgery. Preoperative systemic steroids can produce a wide variety of serious adverse effects and should only be used in selected cases and after consultation with an internist or uveitis specialist.

Systemic medications may also influence the outcome of filtration surgery. Anticoagulants and antiplatelet agents can add significantly to complications during and after filtration surgery. Excessive bleeding encountered during surgery may produce increased postoperative bleeding and scarring, which will make laser suture lysis of the trabeculectomy flap increasingly difficult and, at times depending on the severity, impossible. These medications also increase the risk of suprachoroidal hemorrhage.[9] Stopping all use of aspirin, aspirin-containing compounds, and nonsteroidal anti-inflammatory agents just before surgery is desirable, if medically safe. It may be helpful to instruct the patient to use only acetaminophen compounds only for the time prior to and immediately after surgery. In cases where blood-thinning agents are used long-term for prophylaxis of specific medical conditions, it is advisable to consult with the patient's internist before changing or withholding these medications. In many cases, it is possible to stop these for 1 to 2 weeks.

Coumadin is another commonly encountered anticoagulant. This medication has also been associated with increased risk of bleeding during and after surgery, and in general we recommend discontinuation of Coumadin (Warfarin) 3 days prior to surgery and resuming it after surgery.[10]

These interventions described should always be considered within their clinical context. Adjusting systemic medications should only be entertained after consultation with the patient's internist. In patients with far advanced optic nerve disease, where even short-term elevations of IOP may be hazardous to the patient, caution should be used when altering the medical regimen. On the other hand, reducing intraoperative and postoperative bleeding, inflammation, and scarring are important to long-term surgical success.

BASIC SURGICAL TECHNIQUE

Glaucoma filtration surgery is typically performed in either the superonasal quadrant or directly superior. This approach leaves a relatively undisturbed superotemporal quadrant if additional glaucoma surgery is required, such as a repeat filtration surgery or the use of a glaucoma drainage device.

What follows is a view of the step-by-step approach to modern guarded filtration surgery. It should become apparent that each step in the process of performing this surgery must be carefully considered.

Anesthesia

Retrobulbar anesthesia with lidocaine, bupivacaine, and hyaluronidase is effective for the majority of cases. Additional blocks that are used for lid akinesia, such as the modified van Lint or O'Brian, are often not necessary for filtering surgery. Retrobulbar anesthesia is preferred over peribulbar anesthesia that inflates the conjunctiva, rendering surgical dissection more difficult.

In cases in which extensive and/or numerous previous surgeries have been performed, obtaining satisfactory local anesthesia may prove problematic, and carefully monitored conscious sedation or general anesthesia maybe required. This is particularly true where prior scleral buckling surgery has been performed. In these cases, peribulbar scarring may prevent adequate anesthesia despite multiple injections. In such complex cases, good communication between the surgeon and the anesthesiologist is key to achieving a good anesthetic outcome.

Traction Sutures

Retracting the eye inferiorly is useful because surgery is usually performed in a superior quadrant.

The traditional approach is to use a superior corneal bridle suture. In this case, a 6-0 or 7-0 Vicryl (Ethicon, Inc, Somerville, NJ) or silk suture on a spatulated needle is passed through clear, mid-stromal cornea approximately 1 mm from the limbus for approximately 2 to 2.5 mm. Gentle traction on the suture ensures its integrity prior to taping or clamping the suture to the inferior drape or having an assistant hold during the case. An alternative approach is to place an inferior corneal bridle suture. In this instance, the mid-stromal corneal suture is placed 1-mm above the inferior limbal margin. The suture is then placed beneath the inferior lid speculum. Gentle traction on the suture depresses the eye. In either case, it is essential that the suture does not pass into the anterior chamber, which produces a persistent aqueous leak at the suture site, hypotony, and a shallow anterior chamber during surgery, increasing the

difficulty of the procedure and making mitomycin C (MMC) application hazardous.

An alternative approach is to use a superior rectus bridle suture for surgical exposure. The assistant gently sweeps the superior conjunctiva toward the limbus as the surgeon grasps the superior rectus muscle with 0.5-mm forceps. Using a 4-0 silk suture on a tapered needle, the surgeon places the suture beneath the superior rectus tendon. The suture is drawn superiorly and is clamped to the drape.

Corneal bridle sutures produce wide exposure of the superior conjunctiva. Additionally, inflammation or bleeding from manipulating the superior rectus and tenting of the conjunctiva in this region is avoided, making closure of the conjunctival flap easier. A potential disadvantage is the small area of corneal epithelial disruption at the suture site; however, this area is usually re-epithelialized within 24 to 48 hours after surgery in the vast majority of patients.

Paracentesis

Placement of a paracentesis during filtration surgery just before the sclerotomy is essential. Most surgeons also wait until after application and rinsing of antifibrotic agent before making the paracentesis, thereby avoiding the risk, however small, of the medication entering the anterior chamber. A paracentesis permits the surgeon to gain access to the anterior chamber throughout the procedure. The paracentesis also allows the surgeon to reform the anterior chamber, test the function of the sclerectomy, check the relative seal of the scleral flap, and fill the conjunctival bleb to test for leaks at the end of the procedure. In cases where the IOP is very high, the paracentesis can be used early in the case to bring the IOP down gently, which prevents the eye pressure from rapidly plummeting when the sclerectomy is performed later in the procedure. Avoiding rapid decompression of the eye may help prevent the development of intraoperative suprachoroidal hemorrhage.

The paracentesis is typically placed temporally. It should be beveled, which makes the wound self-sealing. A side port blade of the surgeon's preference can be used. The blade is oriented tangential to the pupil to reduce the chance of lens injury. The orientation of the paracentesis and location should be carefully kept in mind by the surgeon for future access. A frustrating and not infrequent occurrence is the inability of the surgeon to locate the entrance. This problem can be easily alleviated by having the scrub technician paint the blade used for paracentesis with a marking pen. When the paracentesis is then performed the epithelial entrance to the paracentesis is marked for the duration of the case and usually for the next 24 hours. Another frequent problem is successfully cannulating the paracentesis. This problem is compounded in the presence of a soft eye. The inclination to force a cannula through the paracentesis is tempting but futile. Suffice it to say, this approach does not work. Gently cannulating the paracentesis site in the correct orientation is essential to gain

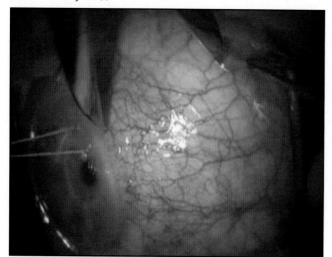

Figure 59-1. Limbus-based conjunctival-Tenon's flap. The conjunctival incision is made 8 to 10 mm from the limbus.

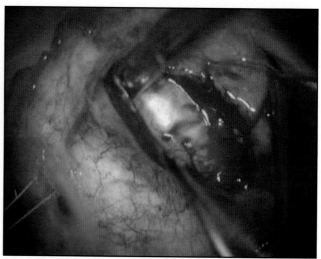

Figure 59-2. The conjunctival-Tenon's flap is dissected anteriorly with a combination of blunt and sharp dissection.

access to the anterior chamber. Additionally, it is important that the internal opening (endothelial side) is of adequate size. It is wise to cannulate the paracentesis immediately after it is made to ensure its patency rather than discover later that it is nonfunctional when it is needed and the eye is hypotonous. Although the paracentesis wound is usually self-sealing, it is important to check for a leak at the end of the case. If the paracentesis wound is leaking at the end of the case, then gentle hydration of the wound is recommended to obtain a water-tight seal. Placement of a 10-0 Nylon suture will be required if there is a persistent leak.

Creation of the Conjunctival Flap

The surgical management of the conjunctiva in filtering surgery is crucial to the long-term surgical outcome. This tissue will ultimately function as a fluid flow resistor. If IOP is to be in the normal range postoperatively, subconjunctival fibrosis,[11] the most common cause of filtration failure, must be minimized. Therefore, excessive tissue manipulation should be avoided. Only nontoothed forceps should be used on this tissue.

The conjunctival flap may be either limbus- or fornix-based. Glaucoma surgeons have been divided as to which technique (fornix- versus limbal-based) they have adopted into their practice. There are strong advocates on either side, and in fact, some surgeons perform both techniques. We have found that both techniques have their advantages and disadvantages, and both have been found to be successful.[12] Some advocate that limbal-based flaps tend to leak less and provide a lower postoperative IOP, where others suggest that fornix-based procedures are easier to perform and less assistant-dependent. Fornix-based flaps may also be necessary in cases where there is significant peri-limbal scarring from previous surgical procedures. However, in our experience, careful conjunctival dissection and advancement during

limbus-based surgery can still be successfully performed in an eye with conjunctival scarring.

Limbus-Based Flap

Limbus-based conjunctival flaps are less likely to leak postoperatively and, therefore, may be less likely to flatten and scar down. Usually, the postoperative posterior limit of the filtering bleb is demarcated by the conjunctival closure site (however, with diffuse application of an antimetabolite such as MMC, the posterior limit of the bleb can often be the conjunctival closure site). Therefore, it is necessary to make the initial incision through the conjunctiva as posterior as possible. A minimum of 8 mm is advisable (Figure 59-1). A Castroviejo caliper can be used to ensure that one does not enter the conjunctiva too anteriorly, because once done, the surgeon is committed. Once the conjunctiva is incised, Tenon's fascia in turn is grasped and incised. This process continues until the episclera is visualized. The conjunctival wound should be lengthened to approximately 2 clock hours. The conjunctiva and Tenon's tissue should only be incised when in the grasp of a forceps and while they are raised over the episclera. This precaution reduces the likelihood of accidentally incorporating a rectus muscle with these tissues, which is more likely to occur in cases where scarring from previous surgery is present or in some elderly individuals in which the superior rectus muscle has become more floppy and less apposed to the sclera.

The conjunctival-Tenon's fascia flap is bluntly dissected to the limbus (Figure 59-2). If only a conjunctival flap is used, the bleb may subsequently become too thin. Meticulous hemostasis using tapered tip cautery is essential to prevent blood from collecting in the subconjunctival space where it can create adhesions between conjunctiva and episclera postoperatively. Caution to avoid too much cautery that could lead to burning of tissue and promotion of postoperative scarring

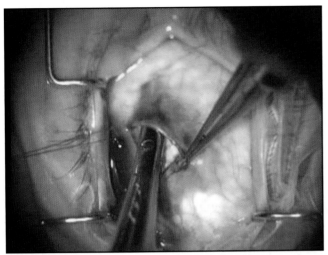

Figure 59-3. Fornix-based conjunctival-Tenon's flap. After the peritomy is made, a conjunctival flap is formed with a combination of sharp and blunt dissection.

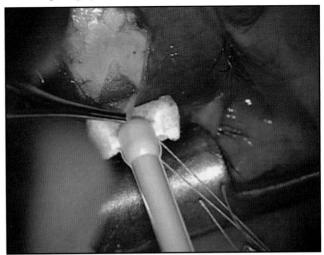

Figure 59-4. Scleral flap. The scleral flap is one-half to two-thirds scleral thickness and should extend into clear cornea.

should guide the surgeon as to the extent of cautery needed. Hydrodissection can be employed in cases where postoperative scarring is present from prior surgery. Hydrodissection helps define regions of conjunctival adhesion to the episclera. These sites are particularly prone to the development of buttonholes during blunt dissection and require gentle, deliberate sharp dissection. A blunt-tipped Westcott scissors is used to carry the dissection through the insertion of Tenon's fascia (approximately 0.5- to 0.75-mm posterior to the limbus) to the insertion of the conjunctiva, which is about 0.5 mm onto clear cornea.

Fornix-Based Flap

Fornix-based conjunctival flaps are initiated with a 1.5 to 2 clock hour limbal peritomy. Blunt dissection is carried posteriorly using a blunt-tipped Westcott scissors through the insertion of Tenon's fascia (Figure 59-3). Hydrodissection may be useful to define areas of subconjunctival scarring when present. Blunt dissection is then carried posteriorly and laterally as far as the Westcott scissors can reach to obtain the most diffuse bleb possible. A common mistake during this step is to limit dissection to the area immediately posterior to the limbus. Success in achieving a shallow and diffuse bleb is enhanced with meticulous care in reaching a far-reaching nasal, temporal, and posterior dissection plain.

Tenon's Capsule

The utility of performing a tenonectomy is still debated. Some surgeons find it aids in visualization of the sutures for lysis postoperatively; however, studies[13,14] comparing a partial tenonectomy to no tenonectomy have shown comparable IOP reduction with either technique. If a tenonectomy is performed, it is generally easier using a limbus-based

technique; however, with the fornix-based approach, it may be useful to remove at least the leading edge of Tenon's fascia prior to suturing the flap to the limbus postoperatively. This helps to prevent wicking of aqueous through the flap and aids the conjunctival epithelium in healing and anchoring to the limbal stroma.

Creating a Scleral Flap

The sclera is an excellent barrier to fluid flow, and therefore the scleral flap should not be considered a porous tissue that will function as a fluid filter in the mature bleb. Rather, the scleral flap, if adequately sutured, is a temporary resistor to the flow of aqueous through the sclerotomy site in the early postoperative period that reduces the incidence of hypotony. The shape of the scleral flap is of little consequence as long as the flap completely covers the sclerectomy. Our preference is to make a triangular flap 3.5 mm × 3.5 mm × 3.5 mm. A 15-degree blade can be used to create the margins of the flap as the globe is held in place with a 0.12-mm forceps. The flap is dissected anteriorly in a lamellar fashion with the same 15-degree blade, although some surgeons prefer a Beaver blade No. 57 or 69 blade (Beaver, Waltham, MA).

The flap thickness should be at least one-half to two-thirds of the scleral thickness. Otherwise, the flap may be difficult to close or may avulse or tear during manipulation. The dissection is carried forward well beyond the gray line and into clear cornea, if possible (Figure 59-4). It is important to create a flap that is hinged as far forward as possible to ensure that the entry site for the sclerectomy is well anterior of the scleral spur and ciliary body. A paracentesis is then made, and the anterior chamber is filled with viscoelastic or balanced salt solution prior to creating the sclerectomy to prevent shallowing of the anterior chamber.

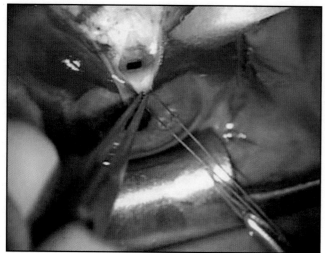

Figure 59-5. A Kelly-Descemet punch is used to create a 1.5-mm sclerectomy. The sclerectomy should extend to the scleral spur.

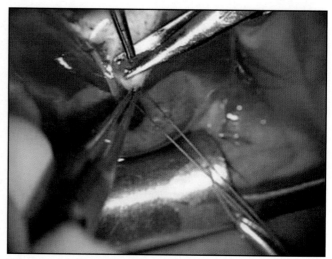

Figure 59-6. Iridectomy. Mini Westcott scissors are used to cut the iris as it is gently retracted through the sclerectomy.

Sclerectomy

The sclerectomy is created by excising a block of tissue at the corneoscleral junction with the tissue punch or with scissors; each approach has its advocates. In either case, the anterior chamber is entered at the anterior-most point adjacent to the scleral flap with a 15-degree blade or other suitable sharp knife. If a block of tissue is to be excised, two radial incisions are made approximately 1.5- to 2-mm apart using Vannas scissors centered under the scleral flap. The block, now hinged posteriorly, is retracted posteriorly and excised with Vannas scissors. Frequently, the TM can be viewed directly while employing this procedure, which reduces the likelihood of bleeding as a result of inadvertent cutting into the ciliary body. Alternatively, a sclerectomy can be made with a Kelly-Descemet punch. Two to 3 punches may be required to make a sclerectomy of adequate size (Figure 59-5). The punch is technically easier to use. However, bleeding from small vessels in the angle is more common. Gentle cautery of small bleeders can be performed under direct visualization and preferably prior to making the iridectomy. In order to stop persistent bleeding, epinephrine 1:100,000 solution (sterile and unpreserved) can be used. If the iris balloons forward through the surgical opening at any time during the construction of the sclerectomy, a small radial snip of the iris with Vannas scissors can deflate the ballooning by allowing aqueous to escape and the iris to fall back into the anterior chamber. Completion of the sclerectomy with less concern of iris incarceration in the tissue punch can then be performed.

Iridectomy

A peripheral iridectomy is performed to prevent obstruction of the sclerectomy by the iris. It should be larger than the sclerectomy in all dimensions. Performing an iridectomy in a deliberate and careful manner is essential to prevent the undesired challenge of revising an inadequate iridectomy, which is difficult to do and can be hazardous. The iridectomy should be wide at its base but should not extend too far anteriorly, because this can result in monocular diplopia. The assistant should gently retract the scleral flap to permit an unobstructed view of the sclerectomy. The surgeon grasps the iris 0.5 mm from its root with 0.12-mm or Calibri forceps in the surgeon's nondominant hand. The peripheral iris is retracted radially through the sclerectomy. The Vannas or Mini Westcott scissors, in the surgeon's dominant hand, are opened enough to encompass the retracted iris (Figure 59-6), and in one smooth cut, the iridotomy is made. The iris is reposited with a stream of balanced salt or by closing and gently massaging over the scleral flap. Forceps are never used, as they may cause lens injury or vitreous loss. Upon completion of the iridectomy, the surgeon should have a view of the ciliary processes and, occasionally, the lens equator. If iris remnants or ciliary processes occlude the sclerectomy, these should be excised only with great caution. It is exceedingly easy to damage the lens or hyaloid face. Deepening the anterior chamber adjacent to the sclerectomy with viscoelastic material or balanced salt solution through the paracentesis is a useful maneuver to give the surgeon working space in these situations.

SCLERAL FLAP CLOSURE

The scleral flap should be closed tightly enough to prevent postoperative hypotony. It is generally easier to cut or release sutures when the IOP is higher than desired than to deal with the complications related to prolonged low postoperative IOP. The flap is closed with interrupted 10-0 Nylon sutures. A 3-1-1 knot buries well and secures the flap adequately. Usually, 3 to 5 sutures are used to close a triangular flap (Figure 59-7), and 2 to 4 sutures are used for a rectangular flap. Once the flap is secured, it is wise to reform the anterior chamber through the paracentesis with balanced salt solution and bring the eye up to an adequate intraocular pressure. In this way, the integrity and function

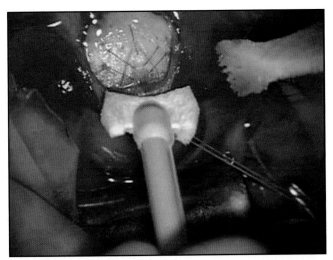

Figure 59-7. The scleral flap is closed with 10-0 nylon sutures. Scleral flap function is assessed with a Weck-cell sponge after the anterior chamber is filled with balanced salt solution.

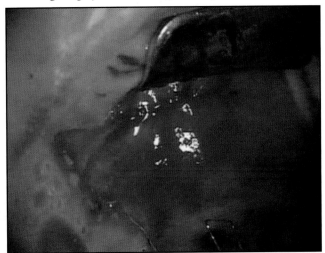

Figure 59-8. Running closure of conjunctival wound with absorbable 8-0 suture on a tapered needle. Finished appearance is shown.

of the scleral flap can be assessed using a Weck-cell sponge. If the IOP and anterior chamber depth are maintained with slow oozing of aqueous humor, then scleral flap closure is usually adequate. However, if aqueous humor flows freely and the anterior chamber shallows, additional sutures are required. On the other hand, if the IOP is high and aqueous does not flow through the flap, sutures should be loosened or removed and replaced. If aqueous humor still does not flow, it may be necessary to reopen the scleral flap and inspect the sclerectomy to ensure it is not obstructed.

Conjunctival Closure

Water-tight conjunctival closure using nontoothed forceps is necessary to create an elevated filtering bleb. Tissues should be brought to apposition only. Tight sutures cheesewire, or tear through the tissue, postoperatively, creating a leaky, inflamed wound. Meticulous closure of the conjunctiva can save many postoperative hours dealing with the complications related to poorly closed wounds.

Limbus-Based Flap Closure

Limbus-based flaps are closed in a variety of ways. However, most surgeons currently favor the use of running conjunctival closures with 8-0 or 9-0 absorbable suture (eg, Vicryl) on a blood vessel (bv) needle. Beginning on the side of surgeon's dominant hand, the Tenon's fascia is closed with a running suture followed by the conjunctiva in the same manner. It is useful to lock the running suture every second to third throw to provide water-tight closure. Care should be taken not to take large bites of the anterior Tenon's or conjunctiva, as this may cause the wound to migrate anteriorly and create unwanted tension on the limbal conjunctiva. After closure of conjunctiva (Figure 59-8), the wound is checked with a Weck-cell for water-tight closure. At this point, many

surgeons irrigate the anterior chamber until a small bleb forms. This is to ensure adequate flow is established.

Fornix-Based Flap Closure

Fornix-based flaps can be closed in a water-tight manner as well. Closure with winged sutures using nylon or Vicryl at either end of the conjunctival flap may position the leading edge of the flap over the limbus but may not offer a water-tight closure in the early postoperative period. This can produce a lower, more circumscribed bleb postoperatively and delay the use of 5-fluorouracil (5-FU) if it is needed. If conjunctival wing sutures prove inadequate for water-tight closure of a fornix-based flap, three or four long mattress sutures are placed at the limbus using 10-0 nylon or 8-0 to 10-0 Vicryl on a spatulated needle. The suture should be placed through mid-stromal cornea. In order to avoid cheesewiring, the sutures should not be tied too tightly. Typically, the sutures become buried in conjunctival tissues and cause no postoperative discomfort. Exposed nonabsorbable sutures are removed after wound healing has occurred.

Some surgeons have used other techniques that may help to decrease the incidence of early postoperative bleb leaks in fornix-based flaps. Débriding a 1- to 1.5-mm zone of limbal corneal epithelium by gentle abrasion with a knife or by using cautery promotes adhesion of the conjunctival flap to the corneal stroma. Trimming Tenon's fascia from beneath the leading edge of the conjunctival flap may help to prevent wicking of aqueous humor under the anterior flap edge.

Fluorescein testing for bleb leaks should be performed at the conclusion of fornix-based surgery. This can be done after the anterior chamber has been reformed with balanced salt solution and the bleb has been inflated. Either 2% fluorescein sodium solution or a saturated fluorescein strip is placed on the conjunctival closure covering this region in dense orange. A leak is readily apparent as an area of greenish flow in a sea of orange. If a bleb leak is detected, it should be closed with a single suture or a horizontal mattress suture and the wound rechecked with fluorescein. A beveled paracentesis site rarely leaks; however, if a persistent leak does occur, a single interrupted 10-0 Vicryl or nylon suture should be placed.

Conjunctival Buttonholes

Buttonholes can generally be avoided by meticulous handling of the conjunctiva with nontoothed forceps. Where they are more likely to occur is where there is conjunctival scarring from previous surgery or trauma, or where excessive traction has been used in an attempt to improve exposure of the surgical site. If a large buttonhole is found that overlies the filter site early in the case, the surgeon should consider relocating the filter to the adjacent quadrant.

It is frequently best to repair buttonholes after completing the planned filtration surgery. By delaying it to the end of operation, it is less likely that the conjunctival repair will be weakened. However, where there is a buttonhole, the surgeon must be especially cautious not to extend it during the operative procedure.

The manner of repair depends on the location of the buttonhole. If the edges of the buttonhole are within the conjunctiva, a horizontal mattress suture that includes both conjunctival margins and Tenon's fascia is effective. Absorbable 10-0 Vicryl suture on a tapered vascular needle is preferred. When closed, the inner conjunctival wound margins should be well-apposed.

If the buttonhole is located at the limbus where no conjunctiva is available on the corneal side of the buttonhole, a horizontal mattress suture is placed that includes peripheral cornea and the edges of the conjunctiva. Prior to closing the buttonhole, the peripheral corneal epithelium may be abraded or removed by gentle cautery to promote adhesion of the conjunctiva to the cornea. A 10-0 nylon suture on a tapered needle or an absorbable suture can be used. Tapered needles are fragile and bend easily. However, if the needle is grasped closer to the point, it is usually possible to pass the needle through the superficial cornea.

Once the conjunctival flap closure is complete, the anterior chamber is filled with balanced salt solution, and the bleb is elevated. Water-tight closure of the buttonhole repair and the conjunctival wound is tested with fluorescein.

Conclusion

At the conclusion of filtering surgery, subconjunctival dexamethasone phosphate 5 mg is injected opposite the site of the filtering bleb. Injectable antibiotics can be used, but some surgeons feel it may increase postoperative inflammation. Cycloplegics (eg, atropine 1%, homatropine 5%, or scopolamine 0.25%) are used if the patient is still phakic or has a shallow chamber to begin with. This is followed by a combination steroid/antibiotic ointment (eg, Tobradex or Maxitrol), which is then applied. The eye is then gently patched and an eye shield applied.

IMMEDIATE POSTOPERATIVE MANAGEMENT

The postoperative period following glaucoma filtering surgery is frequently challenging (see Chapter 60). This is largely because surgery is only the initial step in a long process that culminates in an alternative functional drain for aqueous humor. In order to be successful, the surgeon must frustrate the natural healing process while attending to fluctuations of IOP in the operated eye and not infrequently the fellow eye as well. Due to the number of events transpiring in this period, frequent examinations are required.

The Fellow Eye

Postoperatively, there could be changes in the medical regimen that may affect the IOP in the fellow eye. This would be the case if a patient had uncontrolled IOP in both eyes that necessitated the use of an oral carbonic anhydrase inhibitor (CAI) prior to performing surgery in one eye. In this scenario, the benefit of continued oral CAI to protect the nonsurgical eye must be balanced against the risk of hypotony or failure of the newly created filtering site in the surgical eye. It might be beneficial or even necessary to proceed with surgery in the second eye soon after the surgery in the first eye.

Unintentional noncompliance may occur due to major changes in the patient's drug regimen. A medication chart is very useful for patients who may be taking half a dozen different drops with varying dosing schedules. Having patients describe how they are actually taking their medication can be illuminating as well. On rare occasion, topical steroids in the operated eye may produce a crossover effect on IOP in the fellow eye.[15-17] This is due to ocular venous absorption of topical medications bypassing the first-pass effect of liver enzymes that orally administered medications encounter. This phenomenon via application of ophthalmic steroids is not universally agreed upon,[18] but given the possibility of a response it is essential to monitor postoperative IOP in both eyes following unilateral surgery.

If the IOP reaches unsafe levels in the fellow eye, the surgeon must advance therapy accordingly. The introduction of additional topical medications may be useful. Laser intervention or filtration surgery may ultimately be necessary. Although the prospect of additional surgery is stressful to the patient, it is important to prevent progressive optic nerve damage from occurring in the fellow eye during this time period.

Antiproliferative Therapy
for Filtration Surgery

**Mahmoud A. Khaimi, MD; Marcos Reyes, MD; and
David A. Lee, MD, MS, MBA, FACS, FARVO**

The purpose of glaucoma filtration surgery is to bypass the pathological obstruction of the outflow channels of the eye in order to decrease the IOP to a level low enough to prevent progressive damage to the optic nerve. Glaucoma filtration surgery does not directly address the causes of the abnormalities in aqueous humor outflow and cure glaucoma. However, it does lower the IOP by a more physiological mechanism than by decreasing the inflow of aqueous humor into the eye as is done by many of the topical and systemic antiglaucoma medications. It is arguable whether glaucoma filtration surgery should be performed early in the treatment of glaucoma, even before the use of antiglaucoma medications. The surgical treatment of glaucoma does have its risks that may be greater than those from medical therapy.

A major risk of glaucoma filtration surgery is failure due to obstruction of drainage of aqueous humor through the surgical site. This obstruction is most commonly due to the normal ocular wound healing response to surgical injury. The end result is formation of scar tissue, which blocks the passage of aqueous humor from the surgical area. Conditions that may increase the risk of failure of glaucoma filtration surgery include previously failed glaucoma surgery, aphakia or pseudophakia, uveitis, neovascularization, youth, or an African American ethnic background.

To improve the success of glaucoma filtration surgery and limit scar tissue formation, it is important to understand the basic mechanisms of the wound-healing response. The wound-healing response is essential to the survival of all living organisms and has evolved over millions of years. It is a complex and time-limited series of events that begin when tissue is injured.[1] The initial event is coagulation and vasoconstriction to stop the bleeding. This is immediately followed by inflammation with the entry of white blood cells into the injured area and the release of enzymes and cytokines to prevent infection and initiate the wound-healing process. Epithelial cells, macrophages, and fibroblasts migrate into the injured area to begin closure of the wound and tissue repair. Granulation tissue forms and is composed of vascular endothelial cells that deliver a new blood supply to nourish the rapidly dividing fibroblasts. These events occur within the first several days following injury. Over the following weeks, as the inflammatory process subsides, the fibroblasts produce and secrete collagens and other extracellular matrix proteins that are the major components of scar tissue. The collagen becomes cross-linked, and remodeling occurs as the scar tissue matures over the following months and the wound healing process concludes. The remaining scar tissue that is impermeable to aqueous humor causes failure of glaucoma filtration surgery.

Tissue culture and animal models have been used to better understand and control the complex wound-healing process. Tissue culture models can quantitatively study isolated aspects of fibroblastic activity (attachment, migration, proliferation, and extracellular matrix protein synthesis) relatively rapidly and inexpensively. However, the immune and vascular systems important to wound healing cannot be accurately duplicated in tissue culture. The most commonly used animals to model glaucoma filtration surgery and ocular wound healing are monkeys and rabbits because of similarities in ocular size and anatomy to human eyes. However, both of these animal species have a more rapid and aggressive ocular scarring reaction following glaucoma filtration surgery than humans, and the results in an animal model may not be totally applicable to humans. Both tissue culture and animal models have been used to test the efficacy, safety, and proper concentrations of wound healing inhibitory agents before their use in human eyes.

Many attempts have been made to minimize the scarring and improve the success of glaucoma filtration surgery including modifications of surgical technique, drainage devices, and medications. Various medications can affect the different stages of the wound-healing process. Some of the earliest and most commonly used agents were topical corticosteroids that inhibit the initial ocular inflammatory response following surgery. These agents are very efficacious, but are frequently not sufficient to prevent the scar tissue growth that causes surgical failure. Antiproliferative agents that inhibit the growth of living cells have been used for the treatment of cancer for many years and for the prevention of ocular scar formation for more than 10 years. They have been used to treat proliferative vitreoretinopathy as well as to prevent scarring after glaucoma filtration surgery.

The first antiproliferative agent used following glaucoma filtration surgery was 5-FU.[2] It was later used intraoperatively and then followed by weekly injections. This agent acts selectively during the synthesis phase of the cell cycle to inhibit DNA synthesis. The metabolites of 5-FU are even more potent than the original drug in inhibiting cell proliferation. This agent was originally administered as a subconjunctival injection following surgery at a dose of 5 mg in 0.5 mL twice daily in the first postoperative week and once a day in the second postoperative week, for a maximum total dose of 105 mg. The subconjunctival injections were given with a 30-gauge needle 180 from the surgical site after local anesthesia was induced using a cotton pledget soaked with proparacaine or cocaine. This regimen was found to significantly improve the success rate of glaucoma filtration surgery in eyes at high risk for failure from 26% in the standard treatment group to 51% in the 5-FU treatment group after 3 years of follow-up. Complications from this treatment include corneal epithelial defects, conjunctival wound leaks, and bleb ruptures. The frequency and amounts of 5-FU have been titrated according to clinical response, and lower doses (ranging from a total amount of 17.5 to 62.5 mg given in 2 to 12 injections) may be as effective as the original regimen with fewer adverse side effects.

MMC is almost 100 times more potent than 5-FU in inhibiting fibroblast proliferation and is not cell cycle specific, inhibiting DNA-dependent RNA synthesis. It may also have antiangiogenic effects on blood vessels and toxicity to the ciliary epithelium and its nerve supply. These effects may account for the conjunctival avascularity and hypotony seen after MMC is used during glaucoma filtration surgery. This agent is usually administered at the time of surgery using a Weck-cell sponge saturated with 0.2 to 0.5 mg/mL of MMC and placed between the sclera and conjunctival flap for 1 to 5 minutes.[3] The sponge is then removed, and the exposed area is irrigated with 15 to 250 mL of balanced salt solution to minimize toxic effects. Complications from mitomycin C are similar to 5-FU and also include chronic hypotony and maculopathy.

Other antiproliferative agents are currently under investigation that may be safer, more potent, or more specific for the cells actively involved in the wound-healing process. A key challenge is to find an agent, or more likely a group of agents, which selectively acts on those cells that produce or assist in the production of scar tissue and

(continued)

(continued)

physiologically regulates their behavior. Perhaps the most promising agents are cytokines or antibodies to cytokine receptors that are able to affect collagen synthesis without interfering with other normal cellular activities.[4] After these agents are identified, there is the further challenge of delivering them to their intended site of action at the most effective concentration and at the proper duration. Novel drug delivery systems include liposomal-based delivery systems[5,6] and synthetic polymers of various shapes and sizes. An ideal system would provide nontoxic, localized, and sustained delivery of the agent(s) of choice in a properly timed sequence, and it would eventually disappear to avoid any foreign-body complications.

Understanding and addressing the basic mechanisms of the ocular wound-healing response are the best ways to improve the success and safety of glaucoma filtration surgery.

REFERENCES

1. Tahery MM, Lee DA. Pharmacologic control of wound healing in glaucoma filtration surgery. *J Ocul Pharmacol.* 1989;5:155-179.

2. The Fluorouracil Filtering Surgery Study Group. Three-year follow-up of the fluorouracil filtering surgery study. *Am J Ophthalmol.* 1993;115:82-92.

3. Chen CW, Huang HT, Bair JS, et al. Trabeculectomy with topical application of mitomycin-C in refractory glaucoma. *J Ocul Pharmacol.* 1990;6:175-182.

4. Nguyen KD, Hoang AT, Lee DA. Transcriptional control of human Tenon's capsule fibroblast collagen synthesis in vitro by gamma-interferon. *Invest Ophthalmol Vis Sci.* 1994;35:3064-3070.

5. Maigenen F, Tilleul P, Billardon C, et al. Antiproliferative activity of a liposomal delivery system of mitoxantrone on rabbit subconjunctival fibroblasts in an *ex-vivo* model. *J Ocular Pharmacol Ther.* 1996;12(3):289-298.

6. Mietz H, Welsand G, Krieglstein GK, et al. Gene therapy to modulate wound healing following trabeculectomy: transfection of Tenon fibroblasts with oligonucleotides. *Invest Ophthalmol Vis Sci.* 2003;44.

Postoperative Medications

Topical steroids improve intermediate and long-term postoperative IOP control after filtering surgery, although no additional benefit has been demonstrated with the use of systemic prednisone.[19] Prednisolone acetate 1% is administered every 1 to 2 hours to reduce postoperative inflammation and scarring. Steroids are tapered over 8 to 12 weeks according to the patient's clinical response, although occasionally they are continued for longer periods of time for persistent inflammation.

Cycloplegics (atropine 1% or scopolamine 0.25%) can be used twice a day for 2 to 3 weeks after surgery to help maintain anterior chamber depth and prevent synechiae in phakic eyes. Antibiotics are given over a shorter duration (2 weeks) than topical steroids. An antibiotic ointment at bedtime is all that is necessary.

ANTIFIBROTIC AGENTS

Antimetabolites, primarily MMC and 5-FU, have played a crucial role in improving the postoperative surgical success in both primary open-angle and high-risk glaucoma cases. MMC and 5-FU act by decreasing postoperative subconjunctival fibrosis, the most common cause of filtration surgery failure. 5-FU, a pyrimidine base analog, is incorporated into replicating strands of RNA and DNA. MMC, an antineoplastic antibiotic, acts as an alkylating agent that blocks DNA and protein synthesis leading to cell death. MMC is approximately 100 times more potent than 5-FU on a weight-for-weight basis[20] and has emerged as the leading adjunctive antimetabolite for glaucoma filtering surgery.

5-Fluorouracil

5-FU was the first chemotherapeutic agent to be successfully used to reduce filter failure in high-risk surgical cases.

The original regimen consisted of 5-mg subconjunctival injections (0.5 mL) twice daily for 1 week followed by once-daily injections for an additional week.[21] Complications of 5-FU use include corneal toxicity, bleb leaks, and postoperative hypotony. An increased incidence of postoperative endophthalmitis may also occur.[22,23] Fewer injections maintain surgical success while decreasing the incidence of toxic side effects.[24,25] The use of 5-FU in primary filtration surgery clearly increased operative success.[26,27]

The use of adjunctive 5-FU is also indicated when there are signs of impending bleb failure. These include increased vascularization around the bleb site, particularly in those cases where the bleb is becoming marginated and cystic, or there is decreasing microcyst formation, or flattening of the bleb. Frequent injections of 5-FU are needed when these signs appear to be increasing. Injections 2 to 3 times a week may suffice if initiated early in the course of bleb failure.

If frequent injections of 5-FU are anticipated or there are concerns about corneal toxicity, a large-diameter therapeutic contact lens can reduce toxic effects of this drug and promote patient comfort.[28] Pain from 5-FU injections is of brief duration but can be substantial; therefore, it is important to apply adequate topical anesthesia when injecting 5-FU. Placing a small rolled pledget of cotton or holding a cotton-tipped applicator that has been saturated with 4% lidocaine in the inferior fornix works well. Applying a drop of phenylephrine 2.5% to 5% to the eye prior to the injection will constrict conjunctival vessels and reduce subconjunctival bleeding, which can be brisk.

5-FU can also be used intraoperatively in a manner similar to MMC.[29] In this case, after conjunctival dissection, a sponge saturated with 5-FU solution (50 mg/mL) is placed on bare sclera for 5 minutes. The surgical site is then irrigated with balanced salt solution, and then the process is repeated with another application of the 5-FU solution for another 5 minutes. The area is again rinsed with balanced salt solution, and the remainder of the operation is completed in the usual manner. 5-FU was very beneficial in improving the success rate of filtration surgery, but MMC was found to be much more efficacious.[30,31]

Mitomycin C

MMC is used intraoperatively to reduce postoperative subconjunctival scarring, thus reducing the need for or eliminating multiple postoperative subconjunctival injections of 5-FU. When compared to 5-FU, MMC produces less corneal toxicity.[31,32] However, a severe dose-dependent complication from MMC administration is long-term postoperative hypotony with associated maculopathy.[33-35] The hypotony is usually due to overfiltration through avascular thin-walled filtering blebs. However, aqueous hypo-secretion secondary to ciliary body toxicity may play a role in some cases.[36]

The concentration of MMC employed and the duration of application during glaucoma filtration surgery varies in the literature.[31,33-35,37-39] The concentration of MMC used in clinical studies to date has varied from 0.2 to 0.5 mg/mL. The duration of exposure has also varied from 2 to 5 minutes.[40] In order to reduce the risk of long-term hypotony with maculopathy, a protocol has been reported that adjusts the duration of MMC exposure according to risk factors of the individual patient.[39]

Because MMC can be highly toxic to the corneal endothelium and tissues of the anterior segment,[41,42] it should be applied in a controlled manner to bare sclera prior to entering the eye. A cellulose or cut end of a Weck-cell sponge that has been saturated with MMC is applied to bare sclera. (We recommend diffuse application of MMC in order to decrease the incidence of high avascular localized blebs and to promote low diffuse filtering blebs.) After the exposure period, the sponge is removed, and the surgical site is thoroughly irrigated with balanced salt solution (15 mL). The remainder of the surgical procedure is completed in the usual manner.

It is not necessary to alter the suture material used for conjunctival closure when using MMC. Absorbable 8-0 or 9-0 sutures (Vicryl) perform well whether 5-FU or MMC is employed. Conjunctival closure, as usual, must always be meticulous to avoid postoperative bleb leaks.

Scleral Flap Suture Release

Laser suture lysis is a technique that allows the surgeon to modify scleral flap aqueous humor outflow resistance postoperatively.[43-45] By so doing, the scleral flap can be closed more tightly intraoperatively, thus reducing the occurrence of postoperative hypotony and its attendant complications.

Suture lysis is performed sequentially, that is, 1 suture at a time. The time interval between cutting sutures can be from hours to days, depending on the response. Suture lysis can be performed as early as 1 week after filtering surgery and as far out as 18 weeks after surgery,[46] in which some cases still developed hypotony.[47] The time frame for suture lysis with

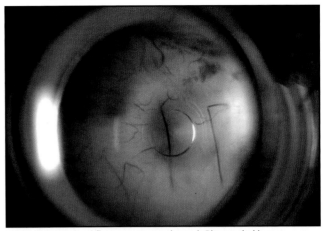

Figure 59-9. Scleral flap suture seen through Blumenthal lens.

the use of postoperative 5-FU does not seem to be substantially altered from that where no 5-FU has been used.

After application of topical anesthesia, a Zeiss (Ocular Instruments, Bellevue, WA), Hoskins (Ocular Instruments), or Blumenthal lens (Volk Optical Inc, Mentor, OH) is used to flatten the bleb overlying the scleral flap. By placing the lens over the peripheral cornea first and gently sliding the lens toward the scleral flap, there is less stress on the conjunctival wound (for fornix-based conjunctival flaps, the approach is reversed). The lens may need to be held in place for a short period of time (usually under a minute) to compress the bleb tissues and to improve the view of the suture before laser application (Figure 59-9). An argon red or green or comparable wavelength is used with settings of 240 to 300 mW, 0.1 s, and a 50-μm spot size. Argon red is useful if subconjunctival hemorrhage or pigmentation is present because of its reduced absorption by these substances. The suture should clearly separate when successfully cut. If there is no clear separation of the suture, it wasn't cut or it was not functionally closing the scleral flap. Additional sutures may need to be cut in the latter situation. Occasionally, a cut end stands vertically inside the bleb after lysis. We, therefore, always recommend cutting the suture at its 2 ends in order to prevent this from occurring. Releasable sutures, a method to remove scleral flap sutures at the slit-lamp, can be used to circumvent the need for a laser. Blood, Tenon's fascia, conjunctival pigmentation, or fibrovascular tissue can obstruct the view of the suture and frustrate the surgeon's ability to release the flap by laser suture lysis. Additionally, the conjunctiva can be buttonholed by the laser, or stresses to the bleb can create wound leaks, both of which may produce hypotony and increased risk of bleb-related endophthalmitis. Sometimes, there may not be ready availability of a laser.

Methods have been developed for sutures that can be released at the slit-lamp. The main advantages of these techniques are the relative ease of suture removal and the lack of bleb manipulation. One or more sutures can be placed to produce a water-tight scleral flap. The time frame for suture removal is similar to that described above for laser suture lysis. However, scar tissue may be incorporated within the releasable knot after 10 to 14 days, thus preventing its removal. If the suture breaks or cannot be released, the suture can still usually be cut with a laser. After pulling or lysing a suture, it is important to judge the patency of the flap using digital pressure or the Carlo Traverso maneuver (pressure using a cotton applicator adjacent to but outside the flap boundary)[48] to see if there is an elevation in the bleb after suture lysis.

THE FAILED FILTER

Unfortunately, even surgery performed and followed in the most meticulous manner may fail. Failure occurs when aqueous humor meets elevated resistance between the sclerectomy and the conjunctival epithelium. The most common cause of filter failure is subconjunctival (episcleral) fibrosis. If intervention is made early, filter failure can be avoided in many instances. This includes strict adherence to the postoperative topical anti-inflammatory drop regimen, early digital compression, and the use of 5-FU injections. In some cases, the sclerectomy is blocked by iris, vitreous, or lens material. In others, the scleral flap may become fibrosed. A Tenon's cyst can form, which is a fluid-filled cavity lined internally by fibrous tissue. Revision filtration surgery can be successful in selected cases. Revision surgery is especially likely to succeed when a filtering bleb was functional for months or years prior to failure. In many cases, the filtration site is quiet, and the procedure can be performed without producing the usual amount of postoperative inflammation. Additionally, revision surgery conserves conjunctiva for future filtration surgery if it should become necessary. In any case, the failed filter requires careful examination prior to embarking on revision surgery in order to define the cause of failure. Once the cause of failure is known, the optimal surgical approach can be determined.

Conjunctival mobility can be assessed with a sterile moistened cotton-tipped swab after topical anesthesia has been applied. In regions where the conjunctiva is tightly adherent to the episclera and little conjunctival movement can be demonstrated, it is unlikely that revision surgery will succeed. If the conjunctiva overlying the previous filter site is mobile, surgical revision is more likely to be successful. This technique should always be used in the initial evaluation to examine the conjunctiva prior to embarking on filtration surgery in cases where there has been previous surgery or trauma.

Gonioscopy is performed to assess patency of the sclerectomy. Membranes, iris, or lens remnants may cover or occlude the internal sclerectomy. It is possible to reopen the sclerectomy with Nd:YAG or argon laser in selected cases.[49-53]

Anesthesia considerations are identical to primary filtration surgery.

Internal Surgical Revisions

Internal revision of the failed filter is most likely to succeed in cases where the filtering bleb was functional for a period of months or years. The bleb conjunctiva is freely mobile. The site of the obstruction is at the level of the sclerectomy and/or scleral flap. This approach entails opening the sclerectomy and scleral flap with the use of a cyclodialysis spatula, needle knife, cautery, or trephination.[54]

A beveled paracentesis is made through clear cornea. The paracentesis is angled toward the sclerectomy site. The anterior chamber is then filled with viscoelastic in order to maintain the chamber and protect the lens in phakic eyes. Under gonioscopic visualization, a 0.5-mm cyclodialysis spatula is guided through the sclerectomy into the subconjunctival space. The goniolens is removed when the tip of the instrument is visualized in the subconjunctival space. Episcleral attachments are broken by forcefully sweeping the spatula in an arc-like fashion. Aqueous humor typically fills the bleb during this maneuver, demonstrating restored patency of the sclerectomy.

In some cases, a needle or thermal cautery may be required to restore patency of the sclerectomy.[55] In order to avoid perforating the conjunctiva, balanced salt solution is injected subconjunctivally to elevate the bleb prior to probing the sclerectomy site. A coaxial endodiathermy can be used to recannulate obstructed sclerectomies. A needle can restore patency of the sclerectomy. However, cautery enlarges the sclerectomy by producing collagen shrinkage around and away from the probe. This may prevent recurrent closure of the sclerectomy.

This may also be combined with external needle revision (see "External Surgical Revision"), resulting in good surgical success.[56]

External Surgical Revision

In cases of bleb failure resulting from an elevated thick-walled encapsulated bleb (Tenon's cyst) or from advanced episcleral fibrosis causing a flat bleb, a needling procedure[57] may be used in an attempt to successfully revise the original filtering surgery. This is performed using a tuberculin syringe to draw up 0.1 mL of sterile nonpreserved 1% lidocaine and 0.1 mL of 0.4 mg/mL MMC. This gives a final concentration of 0.2 mg/mL of MMC. Under sterile technique in the operating room or at the slit-lamp, the diluted MMC is injected subconjunctivally in the superotemporal quadrant far from the failed bleb. If at the slit-lamp, massage the MMC, through the closed eyelid, toward the site of the initial surgery until the area is flat. If in the operating room, one may use a cotton-tipped applicator on the conjunctiva to accomplish this flattening. A 25- or 27-gauge needle on a TB syringe or a 1.0-mm side-port blade is then inserted subconjunctivally far from the bleb and away from the area of the MMC. The needle is then advanced until reaching the failed bleb (Figure 59-10), and the sharp edges are used to break up scar tissue, lift the flap,

TABLE 59-3. COMMON ERRORS AND PROBLEMS IN FILTERING SURGERY	
Short conjunctival flap (limbus-based flap)	Reduces potential filtration area and increases likelihood of postoperative failure. Initiate conjunctival flap at least 8 mm from the limbus.
Toothed forceps for conjunctival manipulation	Use of nontoothed forceps and gentle handling of tissues reduces buttonholes and postoperative inflammation.
Thin or small scleral flap	The scleral flap should be at least half total scleral thickness and large enough to functionally cover the sclerectomy site to prevent prolonged postoperative hypotony.
Paracentesis too small, cannot be found, or cannot be cannulated	To cannulate easily, a paracentesis must have a large internal (endothelial) opening and known location and orientation (test paracentesis before continuing case).
Iridectomy imperforate or too small	The iridectomy must be patent and extend to the posterior sclerectomy margins (so one can see the red reflex or ciliary processes). Extreme caution must be used to enlarge a small iridectomy to avoid vitreous loss.
Sclerectomy site too far posterior	Excessive bleeding or occlusion of the sclerectomy by the ciliary body can be avoided by making the initial anterior chamber entry site as far anterior as possible (well into the limbal gray-blue zone). Cautery should be performed cautiously for bleeding.
Sclerectomy site too close to lateral scleral flap margin	The scleral flap must completely cover the sclerectomy; otherwise, resistance to aqueous flow will be low, and hypotony will result.
Occlusion of the sclerectomy by ciliary processes	Particularly seen in small hyperopic eyes. An anterior sclerectomy site is helpful. Ciliary processes can be gently cauterized, grasped with 0.12 forceps and excised with Vannas scissors if necessary.
Vitreous loss through sclerectomy site	Fortunately a rare complication. A meticulous Weck-cell vitrectomy can salvage the bleb. Postoperative hypotony with a shallow anterior chamber must be avoided (to prevent posterior vitreous from entering the sclerectomy site).
Scleral flap closure (too tight or too loose)	With irrigation through the paracentesis, fluid should flow slowly with a maintained anterior chamber depth.
Conjunctival wound leak	Wound leaks can be reduced by meticulous wound closure and testing with fluorescein.

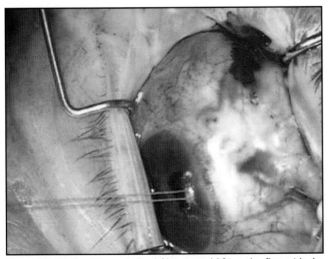

Figure 59-10. Breaking episcleral fibrosis and lifting the flap with the side-port blade.

and enter the anterior chamber through the sclerotomy site in order to reinstate aqueous flow. Success is accomplished when the bleb reforms or becomes more diffuse after injecting BSS into the anterior chamber through a previously formed paracentesis. The conjunctival entry sites may be closed with a suture or hand-held cautery.

CONCLUSION

The process of glaucoma filtration surgery is a challenge to the ophthalmic surgeon (Table 59-3). Meticulous technique combined with careful and close observation are required throughout the perioperative period. Managing

Externalized Releasable Sutures in Filtering Surgery

Murray A. Johnstone, MD and Annisa L. Jamil, MD

Externalized releasable sutures have several benefits in comparison with laser suture lysis. The first is avoidance of need for laser access, scheduling, and cost. The second is the lack of a need for compression of the conjunctiva with a lens; this avoids issues of pain, inflammation, and the risk of disrupting the limbal adhesion of fornix-based flaps. A third benefit is lack of a need for suture visualization. Inability to visualize the suture is common with laser suture lysis when the overlying conjunctiva is thickened, edematous, or contains blood; these are situations where the ability to release the suture early is of special importance. A fourth benefit is the absence of the risk of perforation of the conjunctival flap, a special concern with laser suture lysis in the presence of blood. Conjunctival perforations are of greater significance after mitomycin treatment because of the tendency of perforations to be persistent in tissue devoid of the normal fibroblast population.

Externalized Releasable Suture Techniques

Surgeons have described alternative types of externalized releasable sutures to close the scleral flap in trabeculectomy. The first, described by Wilson,[1] involved use of a horizontal mattress suture that passes from the edge of the rectangular scleral flap, beneath the conjunctival reflection, to the surface of the cornea (Figure 59-11). Another technique described by Shin[2] uses a slip knot at the apex of a triangular scleral flap, with the suture end then brought to the surface of the conjunctiva. Cohen and Osher[3] reported the use of a slip knot at the apex of the triangular flap, with the suture end then passed beneath the corneal reflection to rest on the surface of the cornea. A modification uses two of the same type of slip knot sutures in the corners of a rectangular scleral flap.

A technique that we have used in more than 3000 trabeculectomies since 1984 involves placement of compression sutures directly over the scleral flap. The compression or tamponading effect occurs because the scleral flap is not pinned down at its corners by short interrupted sutures. The flap is loosely anchored posteriorly by a single, horizontal mattress suture that passes through the posterior corners of the flap (Figures 59-12 and 59-13). This mattress suture combines with the releasable suture to create a web of nylon over the anterior surface of the flap and a V-shaped area of compression just behind the sclerotomy site (Figures 59-14 and 59-15). The surface arrangement allows the flap to function as a valve-like device. The long runs of nylon in the web are free to stretch as IOP increases, permitting the flap to elevate slightly and release aqueous into the bleb. As the IOP decreases, the active elastic recoil in the nylon sutures pushes the flap back to its position in the scleral bed, preventing excessive filtration.

This technique generally provides satisfactory filtration while preventing a substantial reduction in chamber depth.[4] In a series[5] of primary trabeculectomies, mean first day postoperative IOP grouped by week varied from 8.3 to 11.2 mm Hg during the first 6 weeks after surgery. Sufficient anterior chamber shallowing to cause iridocorneal apposition was seen in eight of 230 (3.4%) eyes. No anterior chambers had persistent shallowing beyond the first 2 weeks, and there were no axially flat chambers.

A modification of the technique involves the use of an additional releasable horizontal suture over the flap. The second suture further safeguards against a shallow chamber, overfiltration, and hypotony (Figures 59-16 and 59-17).

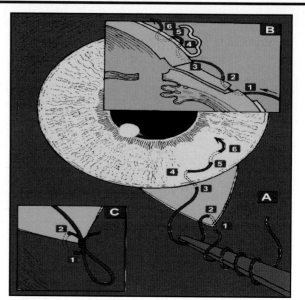

Figure 59-11. Example of a horizontal mattress suture.

Suture Release Timing

Suture release is generally delayed for 2 to 6 weeks or longer after surgery in eyes with an acceptably low IOP or if IOP can be lowered easily with digital pressure. Early suture release may increase the incidence of complications and does not generally appear to improve the long-term results in eyes with acceptable initial control.

In patients who have received antimetabolites, the interval in which suture release increases the risk of hypotony is extended and should be delayed beyond 2 weeks whenever possible. In a recent study involving antimetabolites, with use of the scleral flap tamponade suture and digital pressure, only 6% of eyes required suture release within the first 2 weeks after surgery.[5]

Tezel and colleagues also found that the use of antifibrotics in trabeculectomies with releasable sutures extended the period during which suture release is effective.[6]

The concept of placing multiple sutures with subsequent control of IOP by incremental suture release is appealing. However, tight closure with multiple short sutures at the incision edges tends to force earlier suture release. In addition, there is often a single key or cardinal suture that causes most of the IOP-lowering effect. It is not possible to know whether the key or cardinal suture will be the first, an intermediate, or the last suture cut. Because of the unpredictability of the effect of releasing any individual suture, it is appropriate to be cautious with suture release whether one or multiple sutures have been placed.

Valuable indicators of the ability to release sutures without causing persistent hypotony are the need for progressively more digital pressure to cause distention of the bleb, clearly defined margins limiting the extent of lateral dissection and elevation of the bleb with digital pressure, and a subtle line of finely arborizing vessels completely outlining the margins of the bleb. Recurrent bleb flattening despite repeated digital pressure and generalized bleb vascularity are additional useful factors in deciding the timing of suture release.

When the externalized compression suture over the scleral flap and the externalized horizontal mattress suture are used in combination, the sutures tend to act in a self-adjusting fashion. Suture removal is not done as long as IOP remains in a satisfactory range. If IOP becomes

(continued)

(*continued*)

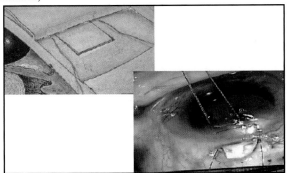

Figure 59-12. Placement of the first releasable suture.

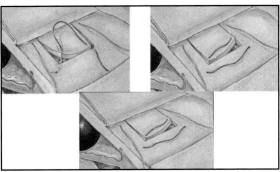

Figure 59-13. Placement of the posterior horizontal mattress suture through the scleral flap.

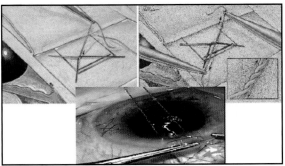

Figure 59-14. V-shaped area of compression of the scleral flap created by the releasable suture and posterior horizontal suture (arrow).

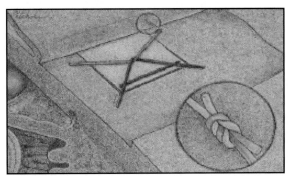

Figure 59-15. The releasable suture is then tied, and the knot is rotated into the cornea.

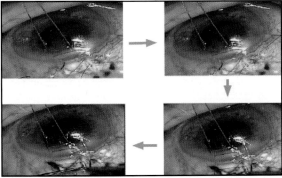

Figure 59-16. Placement of the second releasable suture.

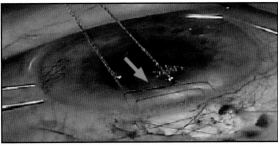

Figure 59-17. Placement of a second horizontal suture (arrow).

elevated and does not respond to digital pressure, the horizontal mattress suture may be removed anytime after surgery. Release of the X-shaped compression suture is preferably delayed for 2 weeks after surgery. Pressure elevation is managed with digital pressure as necessary to mobilize the scleral flap, and medications may also be temporarily added. Fortunately, because of the self-adjusting nature of the scleral flap compression sutures, the need for earlier suture release is very rare.

Conclusion

Releasable suture techniques increase our ability to avoid the profound hypotony and aqueous runoff associated with shallow and flat anterior chambers. The use of releasable sutures raises new questions related to optimizing suture placement techniques and finding additional clinical clues to assist in identifying the optimal timing of suture release.

References

1. Wilson RP. Technical advances in filtration surgery. In: McAllister JA, Wilson RP, eds. *Glaucoma.* Boston, MA: Butterworths; 1986:243-250.
2. Shin DH. Removable-suture closure of the lamellar scleral flap in trabeculectomy. *Ann Ophthalmol.* 1987;19:51-53,55.
3. Cohen J, Osher RH. Releasable suture in filtering and combined surgery. *Ophthalmol Clin North Am.* 1988;1:187-197.
4. Johnstone MA, Wellington DP, Ziel CJ. A releasable scleral-flap tamponade suture for guarded filtration surgery. *Arch Ophthalmol.* 1993;111(3):398-403.
5. Johnstone MA, Ziel CJ. Releasable scleral flap tamponade suture to control IOP and chamber depth after filtering surgery. *Invest Ophthalmol Vis Sci.* 1995;36(4):411.
6. Tezel G, Kolker A, Kass M, Wax M. Late removal of releasable sutures after trabeculectomy or combined trabeculectomy with cataract extraction supplemented with antifibrotics. *J Glaucoma.* 1998;7:75-81.

How to Handle Mitomycin C

David P. Tingey, BA, MD, FRCSC

The use of mitomycin C (MMC) intraoperatively for glaucoma filtration procedures requires a relatively small volume of a very potent and expensive chemotherapeutic agent. This raises issues of safety and cost.

MMC is packaged as 5 mg of powder contained in a 10-cc amber glass vial. It is also available in a 20-mg vial. It must be reconstituted by adding the necessary amount of sterile water for the desired concentration. The vial is then shaken and allowed to stand at room temperature until the powder is dissolved completely. The concentration of mitomycin used by most surgeons during filtration surgery ranges from 0.2 mg/mL to 0.5 mg/mL. Adding 10 cc of sterile water to the 5-mg vial gives a final concentration of 0.5 mg/mL. For lower concentrations of mitomycin, the solution must be removed and further diluted to the desired concentration. Reconstitution may be carried out in the operating room for immediate use, or it may be done preoperatively in the pharmacy.

The stability of MMC is pH-dependent.[1] Acidic pH will rapidly inactivate MMC. Sterile water or sterile 0.9% sodium chloride solution diluents can range in pH from 4 to 7. Diluents having a pH in the lower range may contribute to instability.[2] During and after reconstitution, the solution must be handled with great care in the operating room. Direct exposure to skin or eyes as well as inhalation of aerosolized solution is to be avoided. All personnel handling MMC must have appropriate protective eyewear, operating room mask, and gloves. If the MMC is being reconstituted in the operating room, a specialized vial cap such as the Oncoline (Chemo Pin) may be used to prevent aerosolization. The desired quantity of reconstituted MMC (eg, 1or 2 cc) is placed in a sterile container within the sterile field. Mitomycin degrades after prolonged exposure to light, and it should be covered from light once it is out of the vial awaiting use. After use, all materials must be handled as biohazardous waste and disposed of via the appropriate institutional biohazardous waste methods.

For centers performing a large volume of surgery with MMC, a single reconstituted vial may be used on consecutive cases over a short period of time. Reconstituted MMC is stable for 7 days if stored at room temperature (25°C) and for 14 days under refrigeration (4°C) according to the product insert; however, the actual stability for practical use may be longer.[3]

For less frequent use, it would be ideal to store the reconstituted solution for some time. It has been shown that MMC 0.5 mg/mL demonstrates greater than 85% inhibition of fibroblast proliferation measured by titrated thymidine uptake even after being stored at room temperature for 6 weeks.[4] McMenemy and colleagues studied the effect of lower concentrations of MMC (0.1 mg/mL and 0.2 mg/mL) on fibroblast proliferation after storage using a Coulter counter method. They suggested that it is feasible to store MMC at 0°C to 5°C for up to 4 weeks with negligible loss of activity.[5] A comparison of the effect of fresh MMC versus stored mitomycin on bleb survival in rabbits suggested that MMC that has been stored for up to 2 months is as effective as fresh mitomycin C in prolonging bleb life and lowering intraocular pressure.[6]

There is preliminary evidence that storage beyond the manufacturer's recommended duration still affords effectiveness, but this is unproven in human subjects. In addition, issues of sterility with prolonged storage at room temperature and 4°C have not been addressed. However, prolonged storage at room temperature might be the only option for some remote third world settings without refrigeration. MMC 0.5 mg/mL in sterile water for injection USP has less than a 10% loss of potency for up to 52 weeks when stored at -20°C in amber glass vials. It may be frozen and thawed for up to 17 cycles and still retain its potency according to one manufacturer.[2] One study indicated that MMC reconstituted at 0.6 mg/mL in normal saline and stored in plastic bags at -20°C showed a significant loss of potency, which the authors felt was due to crystallization. At -30°C, there was no significant loss of potency over a 4-week period.[7] Some authors have recommended that, after reconstitution with sterile water, small aliquots of MMC in the desired concentrations be aseptically transferred in a laminar-airflow hood to sterile vials or syringes, appropriately sealed, and frozen at -20°C for single use.[1] Several subsequent studies looking at this issue have also shown favorable results with refrigeration.

Velpandian and colleagues studied the stability of extemporaneously prepared ophthalmic formulation by examining the stability of mitomycin at three different concentrations while stored at three different temperatures of 25°, 4°, or -70°C and at 3 different pH values of 6, 7, and 8. High-performance liquid chromatography indicated that the mitomycin degradation is high in acidic pH at room temperature relative to higher pH and cooler storage temperatures. In spite of this degradation, flow cytometry revealed that degraded mitomycin can still retain its antiproliferative activity even after degradation.[8]

Different methods of long-term storage were also examined by Georgopoulos and colleagues who stored various concentrations of mitomycin at 22°C, 4°C, and -20°C for durations varying from 30 minutes to 180 days. Mitomycin activity was investigated by a microagar diffusion method (bioassay). They concluded that dissolved mitomycin C can be stored in the refrigerator for up to 3 months without significant activity loss. They recommended against storage at room temperature.[9]

The ability of mitomycin C to inhibit fibroblast proliferation was used as a comparison between fresh mitomycin and mitomycin stored for as long as 18 months at either 4° or -20° by authors Hu, Chen, and Oda. The inhibition rate was 88% using fresh mitomycin, and it was reduced to 73% after storage for 18 months at 4°C. They did find a significant decline in potency down to 68% when stored at -20°C.[10]

Francoeur and colleagues from the University of Montreal surveyed 21 North American hospitals and found that the preparation methods of six of the hospitals (28%) resulted in unstable solutions underscoring the importance of storage temperature and buffering.[11]

As alluded to previously, there is little correlation of in vitro activity preservation after long-term mitomycin storage with its in vivo clinical efficacy. Chen and colleagues reported on their results of mitomycin trabeculectomy using long-term stored mitomycin in a West Indian population. They concluded that long-term stored mitomycin may be a beneficial adjunctive treatment in initial trabeculectomy in this population.[12] Unfortunately, the study population was small, reporting on only 10 eyes with no randomized control group.

In summary, the extemporaneous preparation and storage of mitomycin aliquots for later use appears to be a safe and cost-effective method of using this adjunctive intraoperative medication for trabeculectomy.

References

1. Fiscella RG, Proffitt DF, Weisbacker CA. Stability of mitomycin for ophthalmic use. *Am J Hosp Pharm.* 1994;49:2438-2440.

(continued)

(continued)

2. Dorr RT. University of Arizona. Unpublished report provided by Bristol-Myers Squibb Medical Information Services; 1994.
3. Bristol Laboratories. Mitomycin for injection package insert. Evansville, IN; May 1990.
4. Tingey DP, Hooper PL, Woo E, et al. Stability of Mitomycin C after reconstitution. Poster Presentation, American Academy of Ophthalmology, Annual Meeting, October 1994.
5. McMenemy MG, Lahiri-Munir D, King RT, et al. Effect of storage on antifibroblastic activity of mitomycin C. *Invest Ophthal Vis Sci.* 1994;35:425.
6. Henderson PR, Karp K, Higginbotham EJ, et al. Evaluation of the efficacy of stored mitomycin-C as adjunctive therapy in glaucoma filtration surgery in rabbits. *Invest Ophthal Vis Sci.* 1994;35:1425.
7. Stolk LM, Fruijtier A, Umans R. Stability after freezing and thawing of solutions of mitomycin C in plastic minibags for intravesical use. *Pharmaceutisch Weekblad Scientific Edition.* 1996;8:286-288.

8. Velpandian T, Saluja V, Ravi AK, et al. Evaluation of the stability of extemporaneously prepared ophthalmic formulation of mitomycin C. *J Ocul Pharmacol Ther.* 2005;21(3):217-222.
9. Georgopoulos M, Vass C, Vatanparast Z, Wolfsberger A, Georgopoulos A. Activity of dissolved mitomycin C after different methods of long-term storage. *J Glaucoma.* 2002;11(1):17-20.
10. Hu D, Chen PP, Oda D. The effect of mitomycin C after long-term storage on human Tenon's fibroblast proliferation. *J Glaucoma.* 1999;8(5):302-305.
11. Francoeur AM, Assalian A, Lesk MR, et al. A comparative study of the chemical stability of various mitomycin C solutions used in glaucoma filtering surgery. *J Glaucoma.* 1999;8(4):242-246.
12. Chen PP, Basich FM, Khadem E. Trabeculectomy with long-term-stored mitomycin C in West Indian population. *Ophthalmologica.* 1998;212(6):404-406.

and supporting the patient through this process can be a daunting task at times; however, a successful outcome is highly gratifying to both the patient and the surgeon and is definitely worth the effort.

REFERENCES

1. Simmons RJ. Filtering operations. In: Epstein DL, ed. *Chandler and Grant's Glaucoma.* 3rd ed. New York, NY: Lea & Febiger; 1986:425-426.
2. AGIS Investigators, The Advanced Glaucoma Intervention Study (AGIS): 11. risk factors for failure of trabeculectomy and argon laser trabeculoplasty. *Am J Ophthalmol.* 2002;134(4):481-498.
3. Phillips B, Krupin T. The risk profile of glaucoma filtration surgery. *Curr Opin Ophthalmol.* 1999;10(2):112-116.
4. Three-year follow-up of the fluorouracil filtering surgery study. *Am J Ophthalmol.* 1993;115:82-92.
5. Palmer SS. Mitomycin as adjunct chemotherapy with trabeculectomy. *Ophthalmology.* 1991;98:317-321.
6. Mermoud A, Salmon JF, Murray AD. Trabeculectomy with mitomycin C for refractory glaucoma in blacks. *Am J Ophthalmol.* 1993;116:72-78.
7. Prata JA Jr, Neves RA, Minckler DS, et al. Trabeculectomy with mitomycin C in glaucoma associated with uveitis. *Ophthalmic Surg.* 1994;25:616-620.
8. Schlect LP, Brubaker RF. The effects of withdrawal of timolol in chronically treated glaucoma patients. *Ophthalmology.* 1988;95:1212-1216.
9. Law SK, Song BJ, Yu F, Kurbanyan K, Yang TA, Caprioli J. Hemorrhagic complications from glaucoma surgery in patients on anticoagulation therapy or antiplatelet therapy. *Am J Ophthalmol.* 2008;145(4):736-746.
10. Cobb CJ, Chakrabarti S, Chadha V, et al. The effect of aspirin and warfarin therapy in trabeculectomy. *Eye.* 2007;21:598-603.
11. Mietz H, Arnold G, Kirchhof B, Diestelhorst M, Krieglstein GK. Histopathology of episcleral fibrosis after trabeculectomy with and without mitomycin C. *Graefes Arch Clin Exp Ophthalmol.* 1996;234(6):364-368.
12. Kohl DA, Walton DS. Limbus-based versus fornix-based conjunctival flaps in trabeculectomy: 2005 update. *Int Ophthalmol Clin.* 2005;45(4):107-113.
13. Miller KN, Blasini M, Shields MB, Ho CH. A comparison of total and partial tenonectomy with trabeculectomy. *Am J Ophthalmol.* 1991;111:323-326.

14. Kapetansky FM. Trabeculectomy, or trabeculectomy plus tenectomy: a comparative study. *Glaucoma.* 1980;2:451-453.
15. Amba SK, Jain IS, Gupta SD. Topical corticosteroid and intraocular pressure in high myopia. I. Study of pressure response. *Indian J Ophthalmol.* 1973;21:102-107.
16. Armaly MF. The heritable nature of dexamethasone induced ocular hypertension. *Arch Ophthalmol.* 1966;75:32-35.
17. Schwartz B. The response of ocular pressure to corticosteroids. *Int Ophthalmol Clin.* 1996;6(4):929-989.
18. Palmberg PF, Mandell A, Wilensky JT, et al. The reproducibility of the intraocular pressure response to dexamethasone. *Am J Ophthalmology.* 1975;80(5):844-856.
19. Starita RJ, Fellman RL, Spaeth GL, et al. Short and long-term effects of postoperative corticosteroids on trabeculectomy. *Ophthalmology.* 1985;92:938-946.
20. Yamamoto T, Varani J, Soong KH, et al. Effects of 5-fluorouracil and MMC on cultured rabbit subconjunctival fibroblasts. *Ophthalmology.* 1990;97:1204-1210.
21. The Fluorouracil Filtering Surgery Study Group. Three-year follow-up of the Fluorouracil Filtering Surgery Study. *Am J Ophthalmol.* 1993;115:82-92.
22. Wolner B, Liebmann JM, Sassani JW, et al. Late bleb-related endophthalmitis after trabeculectomy with adjunctive 5-fluorouracil. *Ophthalmology.* 1991;98:1053-1060.
23. Rockwood EJ, Parrish RK II, Heuer DK, et al. Glaucoma filtering surgery with 5-fluorouracil. *Ophthalmology.* 1987;94:1071-1078.
24. Weinreb RN. Adjusting the dose of 5-fluorouracil after glaucoma filtering surgery to minimize the side effects. *Ophthalmology.* 1987;94:564-570.
25. Krug JH, Melamed S. Adjunctive use of delayed and adjustable low-dose 5-fluorouracil in refractory glaucoma. *Am J Ophthalmol.* 1990;109:412-418.
26. Ophir A, Ticho U. A randomized study of trabeculectomy and subconjunctival administration of fluorouracil in primary glaucomas. *Arch Ophthalmol.* 1992;110:1072-1075.
27. Liebmann JM, Ritch R, Marmor M, et al. Initial 5-fluorouracil trabeculectomy in uncomplicated glaucoma. *Ophthalmology.* 1991;98:1036-1041.
28. Beckman RL, Sofinski SJ, Greff LJ, et al. Bandage contact lens augmentation of 5-fluorouracil treatment in glaucoma filtration surgery. *Ophthalmic Surg.* 1991;22:563-564.
29. Dietze PJ, Feldman RM, Gross RL. Intraoperative application of 5-fluorouracil during trabeculectomy. *Ophthalmic Surg.* 1992;23:662-665.
30. Katz GJ, Higginbotham EJ, Lichter PR, et al. Mitomycin C versus 5-fluorouracil in high-risk glaucoma filtering surgery: extended follow-up. *Ophthalmology.* 1995;102:1263-1269.

31. Skuta GL, Beeson CC, Higginbotham EJ, et al. Intraoperative mitomycin versus postoperative 5-fluorouracil in high-risk glaucoma filtering surgery. *Ophthalmology.* 1992;99:438-444.

32. Lee DA, Hersh P, Kersten D, et al. Complications of subconjunctival 5-fluorouracil following glaucoma filtering surgery. *Ophthalmic Surg.* 1987;18:187-190.

33. Chen C-W. Enhanced intraocular pressure controlling effectiveness of trabeculectomy by local application of MMC. *Trans Asia-Pacific Acad Ophthalmol.* 1983;9:172-177.

34. Chen C-W, Huang H-T, Sheu M-M. Enhancement of IOP control effect of trabeculectomy by local application of anticancer drug. *Acta XXV Concilium Ophthalmologicum (Rome).* 1986;2:1487-1491.

35. Chen C-W, Huang H-T, Bair JS, et al. Trabeculectomy with simultaneous topical applications of mitomycin C in refractory glaucomas. *J Ocul Pharmacol.* 1990;6:175-182.

36. Kirchhof B, Diestelhorst M. The effect of mitomycin C on the aqueous humor dynamics in glaucomatous eyes. *Invest Ophthalmol Vis Sci.* 1993;34(suppl):815-817.

37. Kitazawa Y, Suemori-Matsushita H, Yamamoto T, et al. Low-dose and high-dose mitomycin trabeculectomy as an initial surgery in primary open-angle glaucoma. *Ophthalmology.* 1993;100: 1624-1628.

38. Neelakantan A, Rao BS, Vijaya L, et al. Effect of the concentration and duration of application of mitomycin C in trabeculectomy. *Ophthalmic Surg.* 1994;25:612-615.

39. Shields MB, Scroggs MW, Sloop CM, et al. Clinical and histopathologic observations concerning hypotony after trabeculectomy with adjunctive mitomycin C. *Am J Ophthalmol.* 1993;116:673-683.

40. Megevand GS, Salmon JF, Scholtz RP, Murray AD. The effect of reducing the exposure time of mitomycin C in glaucoma filtering surgery. *Ophthalmology.* 1995;102:84-90.

41. Derick RJ, Pasquale L, Quigley HA, Jampel H. Potential toxicity of mitomycin C. *Arch Ophthalmol.* 1991;109:1635.

42. Seah SK, Prata JA Jr, Minckler DS, et al. Mitomycin-C concentration in human aqueous humour following trabeculectomy. *Eye.* 1993;7:652-655.

43. Hoskins HD Jr, Migliazzo C. Management of failing filtering blebs with the argon laser. *Ophthalmic Surg.* 1984;15:731-733.

44. Savage JA, Simmons RJ. Staged glaucoma filtration surgery with planned early conversion from scleral flap to full-thickness operation using the argon laser. *Ophthalmic Laser Therapy.* 1986;1:201-210.

45. Savage JA, Condon GP, Lytle RA, Simmons RJ. Laser suture lysis after trabeculectomy. *Ophthalmology.* 1988;95:1631-1638.

46. Pappa KS, Derick RJ, Weber PA, et al. Late argon laser suture lysis after mitomycin C trabeculectomy. *Ophthalmology.* 1993;100(8):1268-1271.

47. Pappa KS, Derick RJ, Weber PA, et al. Late argon suture lysis after mitomycin C trabeculectomy. *Ophthalmology.* 1993;100:1268-1271.

48. Spaeth G. *Ophthalmic Surgery: Principles and Practice.* 3rd ed. Philadelphia, PA: Saunders; 2003:282.

49. Ticho U, Irvy M. Reopening of occluded filtering blebs by argon laser photocoagulation. *Am J Ophthalmol.* 1977;84:413.

50. Van Buskirk EM. Reopening filtration fistulas with the argon laser. *Am J Ophthalmol.* 1982;94:1-3.

51. Cohn HC, Aron-Rosa D. Reopening blocked trabeculectomy sites with the YAG laser. *Am J Ophthalmol.* 1983;95:293-294.

52. Kurata F, Krupin T, Kolker AE. Reopening filtration fistulas with transconjunctival argon laser photocoagulation. *Am J Ophthalmol.* 1984;98:340-343.

53. Latina MA, Rankin GA. Internal and transconjunctival neodymium: YAG laser revision of late failing filters. *Ophthalmology.* 1991;98:215-221.

54. Shihadeh WA, Ritch R, Liebmann JM. Rescue of failed filtering blebs with ab interno trephination. *J Cataract Refract Surg.* 2006;32:918-922.

55. Lytle RA, Simmons RJ. Internal revision in glaucoma filtration surgery. Scientific Poster 79, American Academy of Ophthalmology Annual Meeting, Las Vegas, NV, October 8-12, 1988.

56. Pasternack JJ, Wand M, Shields MB, et al. Needle revision of failed filtering blebs using 5-Fluorouracil and a combined ab-externo and ab-interno approach. *J Glaucoma.* 2005;14(1):47-51.

57. Shetty RK, Wartluft L, Moster MR. Slit-lamp needle revision of failed filtering blebs using high-dose mitomycin C. *J Glaucoma.* 2005;14(1):52-56.

60

Postoperative Management Following Filtration Surgery

Mahmoud A. Khaimi, MD and Marcos Reyes, MD

The role of trabeculectomy in achieving control of glaucoma is well-established.[1] Management of the patient following filtration surgery for glaucoma is the most important step in obtaining long-term success in control of intraocular pressure (IOP) and preservation of vision. Advances in surgical techniques, careful patient selection, recognition of high-risk patients, the common use of antimetabolites that are used intraoperatively, postoperatively, or both, and awareness of the early signs of bleb compromise have all improved long-term surgical success rates.

The intraoperative advances that have evolved since the introduction of the operating microscope for almost all glaucoma surgery have clearly enhanced the exact technique of tissue manipulation and alignment. Serious problems, such as failure to recognize a thin fragment of Descemet's membrane, which were not easily assessed with loupes, are more easily recognized using the operating microscope. The advent of microsurgical instrumentation, extremely sharp blades and scissors, precise cautery or diathermy (electrocautery), delicate tissue handling, and fine suture materials have resulted in improved surgical techniques that enhance the possibility of surgical success.

The recognition and management of early postoperative complications, including wound leaks, choroidal detachment, flat chambers, and compromised blebs, have been facilitated by the absolute necessity of examining patients with the slit-lamp biomicroscope and indirect ophthalmoscopy with attention to the finest details of recently operated eyes.

Recognizing a satisfactory postoperative bleb appearance and overall ocular course is essential. Recognizing impending bleb failure and ultimate loss of IOP control is critical to successful postoperative management following filtration surgery. The early observations of bleb compromise with vascular injection and inflammation of Tenon's capsule and the episclera are important. Observing a diffusely quiet and noninflamed bleb with tiny microcysts and an IOP in the high single digits or low teens is the ultimate goal of all glaucoma surgeons. However, recognizing a slight but definitive vascular ingrowth into the base of the bleb, decreased size and evidence of flattening of a previously functioning bleb, and a gradual IOP increase alerts the surgeon that bleb failure is occurring. Intervention at this stage is absolutely critical to long-term bleb survival. There are many techniques and options available to the surgeon at this time; frequent postoperative visits are necessary to institute the appropriate techniques to shepherd the bleb through this critical time.

In the late stages of bleb evolution when the ocular condition is stable and the IOP is controlled, the risk of infection and late aqueous leaks must be adequately conveyed to the patient and the patient's family. A delay in follow-up examination when early bleb infection or early endophthalmitis is present could result in blindness. Alerting the patient to the symptoms and signs of infection and/or leak is an absolute necessity and is the surgeon's responsibility. The symptoms and signs of ocular infection should be reviewed at all patient visits, and the patient should be encouraged to seek ophthalmic assessment at the earliest suggestion of ocular infection.

PREVENTION OF COMPLICATIONS

The discontinuation of topical agents that may create vascular congestion and ocular inflammatory reactions can be considered 3 to 5 days preoperatively. Although less commonly used currently, phospholine iodine can cause alterations in vascular permeability that persists intraoperatively.

- 555 -

Kahook MY, Schuman JS, eds.
Chandler and Grant's Glaucoma, Fifth Edition (pp 555-566).
© 2013 SLACK Incorporated.

Evidence of lid infection or inflammation should be treated before filtration surgery is contemplated. Patients with underlying uveitis should be receiving topical corticosteroids preoperatively with or without a course of oral steroids (physician dependent), and those with neovascular glaucoma should have undergone an adequate course of panretinal photocoagulation to decrease the fibrovascular reactive state. More recently, intravitreal injection of antivascular endothelial growth factor (VEGF) medication have been shown to more quickly and dramatically reduce the neovascularization and should be considered in all cases of neovascularization in addition to panretinal photocoagulation. These carefully planned preoperative steps aid in promoting the successful outcome of filtration surgery.

Gentle handling of ocular tissues is an integral part of the surgical management of glaucoma patients. Using smooth or cusped forceps when handling conjunctiva and Tenon's capsule prevents multiple tiny perforations and prevents the crushing of tissue that occurs with toothed or serrated forceps, both of which can promote the release of inflammatory mediators that increase scarring.[2]

The immediate use of hemostasis with unipolar diathermy or wet-field bipolar cautery is essential to prevent blood and blood products that stimulate inflammation from permeating the periocular space. When blood is absorbed by Tenon's tissue, it often can be removed only by excision. Immediate cautery is advised to minimize blood in the subconjunctival space when bleeding occurs.

Additional intraoperative therapeutic modalities have become an essential part of filtration surgery to minimize postoperative complications, particularly fibrosis, scarring, and bleb failure. The common use of mitomycin C in concentrations ranging from 0.2 to 0.4 mg/cc for 1 to 5 minutes has become a routine adjunct to glaucoma filtering surgery, and it is the rare case in which it is not used.[3-7] Although now less commonly used, 5-fluorouracil (5-FU) was the initial antimetabolite tested and used to prevent postoperative fibrosis. Studies[8] showed the use of postoperative 5-FU also decreased the failure rate of patients when used in a standard protocol or with modifications.[9,10] The long-term complications of antimetabolite usage are late bleb thinning resulting in chronic leaks, an increased incidence of blebitis, bleb-related endophthalmitis, and the potential of bleb necrosis and sloughing. Efforts to minimize these potential complications have included decreased application time of antimetabolites, decreased concentration of applied antimetabolite, and more diffuse application of antimetabolite at the time of surgery.

Efforts to achieve tight trabeculectomy flap closure with subsequent laser suture lysis or a releasable suture that provides firm flap apposition and better control of aqueous egress result in a high proportion of well-formed anterior chambers and reasonable early postoperative IOPs. This suturing technique combined with meticulous conjunctival closure (as in the example of a limbal-based trabeculectomy closure whereby a single running-locking closure or double closure involving Tenon's capsule first and a conjunctival closure second) has been facilitated with fine-tapered needles and absorbable suture material (Vicryl, Ethicon, Inc, Somerville, NJ). The capacity to reduce wound leaks with tight conjunctival closure has resulted in significantly fewer flat anterior chambers with hypotony and subsequent choroidal detachment, and fewer prolonged flat anterior chambers.

EARLY POSTOPERATIVE MANAGEMENT

The critical period of postoperative management of filtration surgery occurs in the following 3 phases:

1. The early postoperative course of approximately 1 to 7 days

2. The mid-postoperative course, between 1 week and 3 months

3. The late postoperative course, 3 months and longer

On the first postoperative day, routine assessments are made of the anterior chamber depth; the character, extent, and elevation of the bleb; conjunctival wound closure and integrity; IOP; and the posterior pole.

Assessment of Flat Anterior Chamber

Wound Leaks

When a shallow or flat anterior chamber is present during the first postoperative week, wound leaks are often responsible. The wound leak is almost always accompanied by a low IOP (0 to 6 mm Hg) and must be evaluated with a moistened fluorescein strip used to paint both the conjunctiva of the bleb and the conjunctival wound. A 2% solution of fluorescein can also be used. With the patient looking down, the 2% fluorescein is applied to the conjunctival surface in the region of the conjunctival incision and the entire surface of the bleb. Using either the fluorescein strip or the 2% solution, the physician must immediately examine this region with a cobalt blue filter on a standard biomicroscope. A leak is present if cascading darker aqueous with fluorescent edges is observed as the fluid runs from the wound leak. This is popularly called a positive Seidel test. The entire bleb surface should then be methodically examined, with particular attention to the area of the conjunctival wound and the area over the sclerectomy. A large buttonhole or a very tiny bleb perforation can result in significant aqueous flow and profound anterior chamber shallowing.

When a leak is detected, some advocate the use of aqueous suppressants, beta-blockers, and/or carbonic anhydrase inhibitors (CAIs). These agents decrease aqueous flow and allow conjunctival epithelial cells to slide to seal or diminish the leak. The use of a firm pressure patch is a time-honored remedy for a flat anterior chamber associated with a wound leak. However, this therapy can exacerbate lenticular-corneal

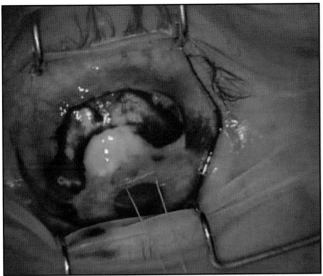

Figure 60-1. Conjunctival advancement. Limbus-to-limbus dissection of the vascular conjunctiva at the border of the leaking avascular bleb.

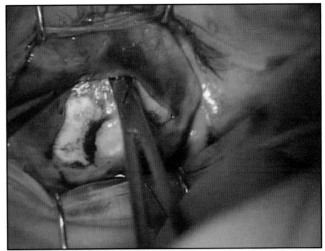

Figure 60-2. Conjunctival advancement. Complete posterior undermining of Tenon's to achieve mobile conjunctiva.

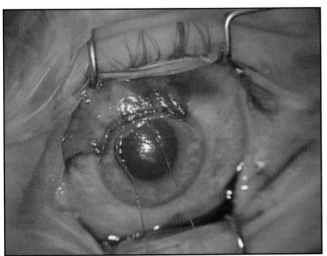

Figure 60-3. Conjunctival advancement. End closure using the Weis closure designed for fornix-based closures.

touch and can even precipitate the active development of lens opacification.

If the leak is still present after 1 or 2 days of aqueous suppressant therapy and the chamber remains shallow, suturing the leak under biomicroscopic observation with the appropriate microvascular needle (9-0 Vicryl) can effectively close the leak and re-establish the normal anterior chamber architecture. If a wound leak persists despite these efforts, and no improvement is observed, a definitive operating room procedure involving deepening of the anterior chamber, choroidal tap if necessary, and wound repair or complete bleb revision may be indicated.

Management of Wound Leaks Wound leaks that develop in thin conjunctival tissue close to the limbus and sclerectomy site can be effectively managed in many different ways. If the leak is small, topical antibiotics, artificial tear

therapy (±topical lubricating or antibiotic ointment), and observation, alone or in combination with aqueous suppressant, may be adequate. In other cases, a large, soft contact lens (18 to 24 mm) that serves to tamponade the leak may be necessary.[11,12] The contact lens may be left in place for up to 10 to 14 days. The rigid glaucoma (Simmons) shell is most effective when used early in managing friable conjunctival tissue with multiple holes. Autologous tissue glues[13] have also been reported to be a useful adjunct and a nonsurgical alternative to managing wound leaks. If the wound does not close after a trial period of conservative therapy, then surgical closure is recommended. Surgical revision usually consists of conjunctival advancement (Figures 60-1 through 60-3),[14] conjunctival rotational flap (Figures 60-4 and 60-5), or if needed a conjunctival autograft.[15] The use of amniotic membrane[16] to assist in the surgical revision of a persistent wound leak has also been reported to be another option; however, its use has not matched the success rate of conjunctival advancement.

Choroidal Detachment

If the anterior chamber is shallow or flat with a normal or low IOP and no demonstrable wound leak, choroidal detachment (Figure 60-6) should be considered. Fluid collects in the suprachoroidal space and results in forward movement of the lens iris diaphragm with anterior chamber shallowing and flattening.[17,18] The serous effusion is easily recognized when the pupil is dilated and mound-like elevations of the peripheral retina and choroid are seen. The most common clinical scenario is an IOP reading below 6 mm Hg, a shallow anterior chamber, no lenticular-corneal touch, and large choroidal effusions. In the absence of a significant indication to perform surgical drainage (choroidal tap), choroidal detachment can be treated conservatively with cycloplegic-mydriatics, topical steroids, and observation. If there is evidence of corneal edema and lenticular-corneal touch as well as a failing bleb, increasing inflammation, rising IOP, and retinal apposition *kissing*

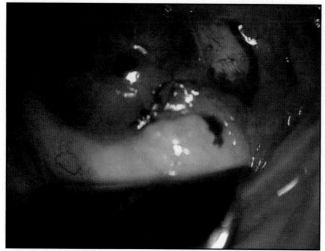

Figure 60-4. Conjunctival flap pedicle. (Reprinted with permission from Donald U. Stone, MD.)

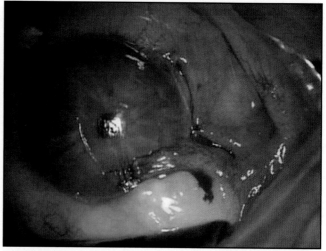

Figure 60-5. Conjunctival flap closure. (Reprinted with permission from Donald U. Stone, MD.)

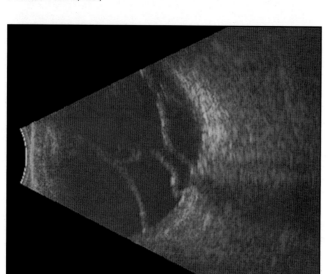

Figure 60-6. Large kissing choroidal effusions.

choroidals (see Figure 60-6), then drainage of the suprachoroidal space and anterior chamber reformation are advised.[17]

In the absence of indications to drain the suprachoroidal space, the anterior chamber gradually deepens as the suprachoroidal fluid is absorbed when the IOP rises to more normal levels (Table 60-1). Observation and medical management are usually effective in treating this disorder.

Suprachoroidal Hemorrhage

A much more serious complication of filtration surgery is the development of a suprachoroidal hemorrhage. This often dramatic complication usually occurs within the first week after filtration surgery and is usually associated with postoperative hypotony. (Note that in effort to prevent this occurrence, cycloplegics should be initiated whenever there is hypotony from any cause [eg, leak, overfiltration, or inflammation]). A suprachoroidal hemorrhage is heralded by the

sudden onset of severe pain that is diagnostic when associated with profound choroidal detachment, a shallow anterior chamber, and a highly elevated IOP.[19,20] After the acute event, the eye frequently becomes inflamed. The patient may have an inordinate amount of pain before the blood is drained from the suprachoroidal space. A waiting period of 7 to 10 days following a suprachoroidal hemorrhage is advised for the fibrinolytic response of fluid to liquefy the clot and allow for more effective evacuation of the suprachoroidal space and retinal and choroidal flattening.[21] The risk of suprachoroidal hemorrhage is greater in patients with nanophthalmos, glaucoma associated with increased episcleral venous pressure (eg, Sturge-Weber syndrome), high myopia, aphakia, or pseudophakia, and in vitrectomized patients, in the presence of elevated blood pressure, advanced arteriosclerosis, bleeding disorders, and following the hypotony associated with tube-shunt surgery. At the time of suprachoroidal fluid drainage, using vitrectomy techniques with the instillation of air, intraocular expandable gases, or silicone oil are all options available if deemed appropriate by the retina surgeons to decrease the incidence of rebleeding and to tamponade the choroid and retina in their anatomic positions. Inflation of the bleb and evaluation of wound leaks should be performed during evacuation of the suprachoroidal space.

Pupillary Block

Pupillary block is another cause for formation of a peripherally shallow or flat anterior chamber in the early postoperative period. Pupillary block may occur in the presence of normal or elevated IOP. The inability of aqueous to pass from the posterior to anterior chamber results in the forward movement of the peripheral iris and closure of the drainage channel. Pupillary block occurs when there is a peripheral iridectomy that is not patent, when there are adhesions of the iris to the lens (posterior synechiae) with resultant iris bombé, or with an anterior chamber

TABLE 60-1. INDICATIONS FOR CHOROIDAL TAP	
Lens-cornea touch (axially flat anterior chamber)	Choroidal tap should be performed within 24 hours of lens-cornea touch.
Corneal edema	Associated with very shallow anterior chamber.
Prolonged peripherally flat anterior chamber (>5 days)	In the absence of anterior chamber deepening.
Appositional or kissing choroidals	Choroidal tap should be performed within 24 to 48 hours.
Prolonged hypotony, low bleb (>7 days) with a moderate to large choroidal effusion	

PERFORMING A CHOROIDAL TAP
R. Rand Allingham, MD

A choroidal tap is performed to reform the anterior chamber and drain suprachoroidal fluid (effusion or blood in the case of a suprachoroidal hemorrhage). If the eye is extremely soft, we prefer to use a peribulbar block. Local anesthetic is placed subconjunctivally in the quadrants to either side and the furthest away from the filtering bleb.

If the original paracentesis cannot be found or cannulated, a new beveled paracentesis is made. The paracentesis should be made slowly with a very sharp blade in order to avoid a rapid entry into the anterior chamber, which could result in damage to the iris or lens. Grasping the horizontal rectus muscle on the same side as the paracentesis with a 0.5-mm forcep can help stabilize the eye and reduce corneal wrinkling while performing the paracentesis. Using a 27-gauge cannula, the anterior chamber is reformed with balanced salt solution. The cannula tip must be through the cornea and in the anterior chamber before infusing fluid to prevent the stripping of Descemet's membrane.

A horizontal conjunctival incision is made 3 to 6 mm from the limbus in the inferonasal or inferotemporal quadrant (away from the filtering bleb). Small blood vessels are gently cauterized prior to making the sclerotomy. The 2- to 3-mm radial sclerotomy is centered 3 to 4 mm from the limbus. We prefer to use a No. 15 Bard-Parker (Katena Eye Instruments, Denville, NJ) or No. 67 Beaver blade (Beaver, Waltham, MA) to make the sclerotomy because they are sharp enough to incise the sclera, but not so extremely sharp as to cut through the choroid on contact. Sharper blades can be used, but there is increased risk of penetrating the choroid and inadvertently entering the vitreous cavity. Clear to yellowish-tinged fluid often drains spontaneously once the incision is carried into the suprachoroidal space. Once the fluid flow slows, the tip of a 0.5- to 1.0-mm cyclodialysis spatula can be carefully inserted into the suprachoroidal space in a circumferential direction (parallel to the limbus). The spatula is removed and reinserted in the opposite direction. The anterior chamber is reformed periodically when the eye softens. The eye should not be allowed to become too soft in order to reduce the possibility of suprachoroidal hemorrhage. This cycle of anterior chamber reformation and fluid drainage is repeated until no further fluid drains from the sclerotomy. The anterior chamber is then reformed with special emphasis on reforming the filtering bleb. The eye pressure required to elevate the filtering bleb may be quite high to break conjunctival adhesions to episclera.

Once the anterior chamber has been reformed and the choroidal effusions have been drained, the sclerotomy openings are left open, and the conjunctiva is closed with 10-0 absorbable suture. Subconjunctival dexamethasone phosphate 8 to 12 mg is injected inferiorly. Atropine and antibiotic ointment are applied to the eye. The eye is gently patched and an eye shield placed.

---

lens (without a peripheral iridectomy) that prevents aqueous movement into the anterior chamber. Therapy with cycloplegic-mydriatics sometimes resolves pupillary block. However, a laser iridectomy is curative and advisable. In the presence of localized compartments of block, multiple iridectomies are suggested.

Malignant Glaucoma

The final differential diagnostic category of a shallow to flat anterior chamber during the early postoperative period is characterized by an IOP elevated to the high-normal or much higher levels and is associated with malignant glaucoma or aqueous misdirection.[22] Aqueous misdirection results from posterior movement of aqueous into the vitreous cavity that forces the vitreous forward with resultant lens-iris diaphragm displacement and closure of the drainage channel angle. Hyperopic eyes with chronic angle closure following filtration surgery are most at risk. However, pseudophakic or aphakic eyes with an impermeable anterior hyaloid face are also at risk of developing this uncommon symptom complex.[23]

Malignant glaucoma may respond to medical management with CAIs (oral or topical), mydriatic-cycloplegics, and beta-blocking agents with re-establishment of the anterior chamber and an IOP decrease. If medical management is not successful, yttrium-aluminum-garnet (YAG) laser disruption of the anterior hyaloid face and posterior capsule can immediately and effectively deepen the anterior chamber and lower the IOP.[24] If phakic patients do not respond to medical therapy, the neodymium (Nd):YAG laser may be attempted if a view of the ciliary processes can be obtained through a peripheral iridectomy or dilated pupil. This view is often difficult to obtain, and injury to the crystalline lens can occur. Surgical therapy for aqueous misdirection is penetration or removal of the anterior hyaloid face and penetration of the posterior vitreous with aspiration of liquid vitreous with a needle or vitreous cutting instrument.[25]

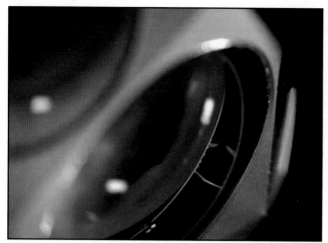

Figure 60-7. Iris incarceration of the sclerectomy site.

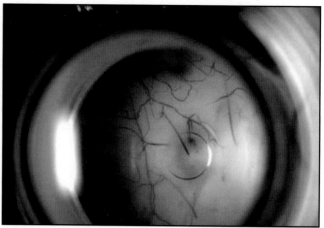

Figure 60-8. Scleral flap suture status post-laser suture lysis. Laser energy is applied to either the posterior or anterior end of the suture.

Early Bleb Evaluation

Careful observation of the bleb in the early postoperative period is extremely important. A diffuse nonvascular, slightly elevated bleb with diffuse microcysts and an appearance of succulence that involves a superior portion of the globe is an encouraging observation following filtration surgery. Recognizing blood under the bleb, a flat vascularized bleb, or a very localized elevated bleb[26] during the early postoperative period is a very poor prognostic sign and requires aggressive management. Little can be done for blood under the bleb, but blood and blood products that seal the trabeculectomy flap or hyphema and a blood clot in the sclerectomy respond dramatically to an intracameral or subconjunctival injection of tissue plasminogen activator (tPA). Dosages from 6 to 25 µg (10 µg/0.l cc) have been documented, but lower doses[27,28] such as 12.5 µg or less are recommended to avoid hyphema. This procedure can be done at the biomicroscope through a paracentesis and can be repeated if necessary.[29] The frequent use of topical steroids and cycloplegics can minimize the inflammatory response that occurs when blood is present in the subconjunctival or intraocular space.

If the bleb is flat and vascularized and the anterior chamber is formed with a normal or elevated IOP, obstruction of aqueous flow into the bleb is likely. Determining the site of obstruction is essential, and gonioscopy is the most effective method of evaluating the internal structures that are obstructed. Gonioscopy is essential for evaluating all postoperative bleb complications because the obstruction site can only be determined by careful examination. If there is evidence of obstruction by a Descemet's flap, iris (Figure 60-7), ciliary body, or vitreous, laser intervention is often helpful. The argon laser can remove pigmented uveal tissue or blood products from the sclerectomy site. In other situations, an Nd:YAG laser can remove clear membranes or cut adherent uveal tissue that is not amenable to argon laser therapy.

When the sclerectomy site is patent, attention needs to be directed to the episcleral ocular surface. The most common site of obstruction to aqueous outflow is at the level of the episclera in the region of the trabeculectomy flap. Gentle digital pressure can result in the bleb filling with aqueous and adequate aqueous flow into the bleb. If digital pressure does not result in bleb elevation, laser suture lysis is the next step.

Cutting a single radial suture with the argon laser using the Hoskins, Blumenthal, or other similar suture lysis lenses encourages flow. With the advent of intraoperative antimetabolites, it is advisable to cut only one suture at a time, because overfiltration can result when multiple sutures are released. Some physicians are hesitant to do laser suture lysis on the first or second postoperative days, especially those who perform fornix-based filters in order to promote healing of the conjunctival wound and ensure a leak-free seal. Often, if the postoperative pressure is not too high, laser suture lysis is reserved for postoperative week 1. However, if the IOP is dangerously high and optic nerve integrity is threatened, the physician should proceed without delay to laser suture lysis as a means to quickly lower the pressure. (In the case of fornix-based filters, the limbal conjunctival wound should then be carefully checked for any subsequent wound leaks.) The utility of laser suture lysis diminishes with time. In the rare case in which no adjunctive antimetabolites were used during filtering surgery, laser suture lysis should be performed within 1 week and at a more aggressive pace in order to prevent early scarring. When adjunctive mitomycin C is employed, then suture lysis (Figure 60-8) or release can be performed within 1 week and up to 3 or more months[30] after surgery. Releasable sutures with more than one arm can be effectively altered by performing laser suture lysis on the posterior extent of the releasable suture, thus elevating the back of the flap while maintaining tension on the anterior portion of the flap. This gradual release of the flap helps prevent a sudden decrease in IOP and helps maintain anterior chamber depth. It should be kept in mind that laser suture lysis may produce complications, such as hypotony, conjunctival wound leaks, or hyphemas.

In the early postoperative period, focal pressure with a cotton-tipped swab (Carlo Traverso maneuver),[31] muscle hook, or digital pressure adjacent to the scleral flap can sometimes gape the scleral flap and allow aqueous to dissect and elevate the bleb. This technique is less useful after actual subconjunctival fibrosis has occurred.

MID-POSTOPERATIVE COURSE FOLLOWING FILTRATION SURGERY (1 WEEK TO 3 MONTHS)

Following filtration surgery, it is ideal to maintain the IOP between the high single digits to low mid-teens (7 to 12) with a low diffuse superonasally placed bleb. Low diffuse conjunctival elevation with minimal vasculature, multiple fine microcysts, nonthin-walled conjunctiva, and indistinct margins are the hallmarks of a well-functioning and long-lived filtration bleb. It is advisable to observe the bleb and peribleb region critically throughout this time period. Subtle vascular ingrowth patterns, flattening of a previously elevated bleb, development of a Tenon's cyst, subtle thickening of the bleb, and a rising IOP should alert the surgeon to potential problems. It is important for the patient to continue taking anti-inflammatory medications during this mid-postoperative period until all signs of inflammation have disappeared. The use of topical steroids must be predicated upon the inflammatory response of the episclera, not the anterior chamber.

In addition to topical anti-inflammatory agents, subconjunctivally injected 5-FU can help diminish postfiltration inflammation. The administration of 5 mg of 5-FU into the subconjunctival space can decrease the vascular proliferative process and result in a quiet functioning bleb (see Chapter 59). Postoperative subconjunctival injections of mitomycin C, though not routine nor widely practiced, have also been tried, with success, in patients with failing filtering surgery.[32,33]

Recognizing a Failing Bleb

Recognizing a failing bleb during the mid-postoperative period following filtration surgery is key to salvaging the operative results. Progressive management of a compromised or failing bleb is essential to long-term success. Occasionally, the bleb may appear to be unchanged from week to week. However, if the IOP is gradually rising from single digits to the mid-teens and higher, bleb failure is in progress. The signs of impending bleb failure are often subtle and identified late in the course so that therapy is less effective. An inflamed, flat bleb that has lost its succulence and is surrounded by blood vessels has a very grim prognosis. The high, thick-walled, highly domed elevation of an encapsulated Tenon's cyst is also a problematic prognostic sign.

Managing a failing bleb should begin the moment failure is suspected. If there is evidence of iris (see Figure 60-7), Descemet's membrane, fibrin, or vitreous blocking the sclerectomy, laser intervention or even surgical removal of the obstruction may be necessary. Suture lysis, especially in those patients where intraoperative adjunctive mitomycin C has been used, may be effective even months after filtration surgery. Repeat gonioscopy at this time is essential to assess the patency of the sclerectomy.

Topical anti-inflammatory medications including steroids and cycloplegic-mydriatic agents should be prescribed in increased frequencies. Frequent application of topical steroids (every 2 hours) is advised during the early part of this period involving the maturation of the filtration bleb and then slowly tapered weekly.

Digital Pressure

Some physicians elect to perform digital pressure at this time and also teach this technique to their patients. There are many techniques that have been developed for applying digital pressure, but it is essential to evaluate the pressure response following the application of digital pressure to a recently filtered eye. The surgeon is advised to apply digital pressure with the index finger to either the inferior or superior portion of the globe while observing the anterior chamber and appearance of the bleb at the slit-lamp. (Note that if digital pressure is applied to the superior globe, it should be done temporal to the scleral flap. Caution is advised not to disrupt the limbal conjunctival wound in fornix-based filters.) With these precautions, exact, effective properly applied pressure can be evaluated. If the IOP decreases and the patient can master this maneuver, the digital pressure technique should be taught to the patient or a person available to perform this technique at home.

The technique generally used is as follows. Instruct the patient to look up and nasal and then to identify the infra-orbital rim with his or her index finger. The patient should place the soft fingerprint portion of the index finger against the inferior aspect of the globe through the lower lid with pressure directed inward and upward for a count of 10 s. If this maneuver results in a lowering of the IOP by 3 mm Hg or more, the patient is encouraged to perform this maneuver once daily depending on individual needs.

Each time the patient is examined, the IOP should be measured, and the patient should be requested to perform digital pressure in the manner in which he or she performs at home. Not infrequently, a refresher course is necessary. When digital pressure effectively lowers the IOP acutely, the surgeon should establish how long after the procedure the pressure remains in an acceptable range. Once the bleb has been salvaged, the patient can gradually taper the daily repetitions of the technique.

Tenon's Cyst

When Tenon's capsule adheres to the episclera near the operative site, a high-domed, smooth, 2-layered bleb forms that is impervious to aqueous humor and is an extension of the anterior chamber, with a resultant IOP elevation. With time and IOP management, this barrier often becomes less dense, and the IOP stabilizes at a safe level. However, not infrequently, when IOP elevation associated with a Tenon's cyst cannot be tolerated by a severely compromised optic nerve, additional therapy is necessary.[34-36] As stated earlier, needling of Tenon's cysts at the slit-lamp can effectively penetrate the fibrous barrier and encourage filtration. A more extensive surgical revision (ie, excising the fibrovascular membrane) also may be necessary.[35,36]

When a Tenon's cyst is identified, introducing topical pressure-lowering therapy may decrease the IOP. Adding digital pressure can break the cicatrix responsible for the pressure elevation. If these noninvasive techniques are ineffective, a bleb needling procedure or glaucoma surgery will be necessary.

Needling the Bleb

When there is bleb failure in the early to mid postoperative period, needling the bleb can be a useful intervention in addition to medical treatment. Common methods[37,38] include a sharp needle (25 to 30 gauge) on a tuberculin syringe with either 0.1 mL lidocaine 1% (or 0.2 mL bupivacaine) with or without epinephrine combined with 0.1 mL of mitomycin C 0.4 mg/mL (final concentration of 0.2 mg/mL). Whether performed in the operating room or at the slit-lamp, the procedure is the same. After topical proparacaine is applied, the needle is inserted into the subconjunctival space approximately 5 to 10 mm from the scleral flap, and the solution is injected, elevating the conjunctiva. Then, as the conjunctiva elevates, the needle is advanced until the tip of the needle is inside the filtering bleb. The needle is then advanced into the anterior chamber through the sclerectomy site to ensure its patency. No further fluid is injected once the needle is within the bleb. If there is a fibrous capsule, the needle can be used to create several openings. The location of the needle tip must be kept in mind at all times to prevent cutting blood vessels or perforating the globe or bleb. This procedure can be remarkably effective when used within a few days of the conjunctiva adhering to the episclera. However, it is less effective after the bleb capsule has become thick and firmly adherent.

Alternatively, bleb needling can be performed using a 1.2-mm side-port or microvitreoretinal (MVR) blade. After anesthetizing the conjunctiva as stated above, a cotton tip is then used to roll and disperse the anesthetic/antimetabolite solution in the direction of the scleral flap. The side-port or MVR blade is then inserted 5 to 8 mm from the bleb opposite to the site of injected antimetabolite and is advanced toward the scleral flap. The blade is used in a similar fashion to the sharp needle described above to break away fibrous adhesions, elevate the scleral flap, and enter the anterior chamber.

Progressive Bleb Failure

If all efforts at medical and minimally invasive surgical management are unsuccessful, the possibility of bleb revision or reoperation in an adjacent site should be considered (see Chapter 59). Internal bleb revision may be effective if a blunt spatula is passed into the sclerectomy and used to break any adhesions present. This technique is most effective during the first 2 to 3 months following filtration surgery. It is also most effective and least likely to cause problems when blood vessels in this area are minimal. Topical vasoconstrictors can be very important in decreasing the chance of bleeding during manipulation of the bleb associated with internal revision. Wet-field cautery to coagulate bleeding vessels intraoperatively has been helpful.

If there is marked scarring and a thick-walled, highly vascularized bleb is present, external revision may be more effective. As discussed above, a bleb needling procedure can be used. Even in a late postoperative course, a needle procedure can be an effective and a minimally invasive surgical option[39,40] prior to attempting another filtering procedure or placement of a drainage device. When there is significant inflammation, extremely friable conjunctiva, or densely bound down tissues, an adjacent, nonoperated site should be used to create a new area for filtration.

Hypotonous Maculopathy

One of the most serious recognized complications, primarily associated with the use of MMC and 5-FU, is the development of hypotonous maculopathy.[41-44] This complication is characterized by a low IOP (usually less than 6 mm Hg) with associated swelling of the macula often accompanied by choroidal and retinal folds. There is a dose- and time-related component, but the high-risk patient is often young and highly myopic. Early interventions that have been suggested include pressure patching with eye pads, placement of an oversized bandage contact lens,[45] YAG laser of conjunctival vessels to induce intrableb bleeding,[46] YAG laser combined with viscoelastic,[47] or direct cautery application to the bleb. Resuturing the flap transconjunctivally[48] (Figure 60-9), using bleb compression sutures,[49] or obliterating the bleb have also been suggested. In addition, the use of autologous blood injected into the bleb has been advocated.[44,50]

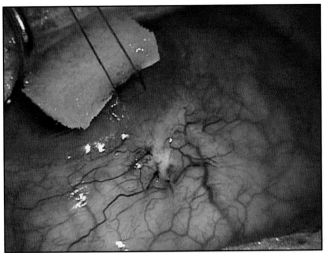

Figure 60-9. Transconjunctival suturing of an overfiltering trabeculectomy. (Reprinted with permission from Steven R. Sarkisian Jr, MD.)

LATE POSTOPERATIVE MANAGEMENT AFTER FILTRATION SURGERY

Infection

The ideal course following filtration surgery is to control the IOP below the anticipated target pressure. In phakic patients, the bleb that is identified with successful control of IOP often is diffuse, slightly elevated, avascular, succulent, and superiorly placed with no visible boundaries. Also, the bleb manifests delicate microcysts and is not particularly thin-walled. Unfortunately, the development of the ideal bleb is difficult to achieve, and all permutations of this bleb description are possible. The advent of subconjunctival application of antimetabolites (mitomycin C [MMC] and 5-FU specifically) has increased the success rate of trabeculectomy. However, with that success has come the inherent risk of localized, avascular, leak-prone filtering blebs. With severely avascular blebs and/or bleb leakage comes the risk of bleb infection and its associated devastating ocular complications.

Bleb infection, or blebitis, and bleb-related endophthalmitis are the most serious complications following successful filtration surgery. The surgeon must instruct his or her patients about the symptoms and signs of bleb infection and insist that the patient be seen immediately if these symptoms develop. The incidence of bleb infection was not well-established before the advent of antimetabolites, but may range between 2% and 5%. In the current era of adjunctive antimetabolite use with MMC, there has certainly been a higher incidence of bleb-related endophthalmitis when a full-thickness, thin-walled bleb is present.[51,52]

We instruct our patients and members of the patient's family that ocular inflammation characterized by a red eye with purulent discharge, localized discomfort, and even subtle alterations of vision may be the earliest signs of a bleb infection, and the patient must be examined promptly. It is not uncommon to have a bleb leak precede a definitive infection,[53,54] so that the onset of profound tearing or ocular discharge should be reported to an ophthalmologist. There is clinical evidence to suggest that blebs placed inferiorly have a higher incidence of endophthalmitis than blebs placed under the upper lid.[55] Attention and therapy should be directed toward treating blepharitis and recurrent conjunctivitis in patients with filtering blebs.

When a patient with a suspected bleb infection is examined, there is often a definitive vascular response at the base of the bleb that creates a peribleb halo of blood vessels, which may be the earliest sign of bleb infection. It is helpful to use 2% fluorescein to stain the bleb to recognize subtle leaks and visible epithelial defects that may be the site of bacterial penetration. An increase in the haziness of a previously clear bleb or frank pus in the bleb (otherwise known as a bleb with a hypopyon) may be the extremes noted when evaluating the bleb for infection. The anterior chamber may have a significant cellular response and even hypopyon indicating endophthalmitis. In phakic or pseudophakic eyes, the vitreous cavity may not be involved, and drastic surgical intervention may not be necessary. However, with visualization of inflammatory cells in the vitreous cavity or ultrasonographic evidence[56] to indicate vitreous involvement, immediate vitrectomy and administration of intravitreal antibiotics is advised.

When blebitis or bleb involvement with anterior chamber reaction is recognized, the immediate and aggressive use of topical antibiotics with or without topical steroids and cycloplegics is indicated. A culture of the bleb surface, conjunctiva, and aqueous leak should be obtained prior to the use of antibiotics. An aggressive course of topical antibiotics should be introduced. Most commonly prescribed by glaucoma physicians is a fourth-generation fluoroquinolone with or without additional antibiotics as well as a bactericidal ointment applied at bedtime.[57] Following 24 to 48 hours of intensive topical antibiotic therapy, prednisolone acetate 1% can be prescribed every 2 to 4 hours if improvement is noted.

When an infected bleb is associated with moderate to severe anterior chamber inflammation including fibrin, it is common to treat the case as endophthalmitis. Some physicians also use the presence of a hypopyon to prompt endophthalmitis treatment. Currently, the most advised treatment is a vitreous tap and injection with vancomycin and ceftazidime with or without dexamethasone.[58] The decision to proceed directly to vitrectomy should be a decision made between a consulted retina specialist and the glaucoma surgeon, and is often based upon the severity of findings. Common organisms found in bleb-related infections depend upon whether it is early or late in the postoperative course and include *Staphylococcus* species (*S epidermidis* more than *S aureus*) and highly infectious organisms such as *Streptococcus* and *Haemophilus influenza*.[58-62] However, many other organisms, including gram-negative organisms, have been identified.[63] The use of

Mahmoud A. Khaimi, MD; Marcos Reyes, MD; and R. Rand Allingham, MD

TREATMENT OF HYPOTONOUS MACULOPATHY

Hypotonous maculopathy secondary to antifibrotic therapy in the glaucoma filter patient should be treated in a step-wise fashion.

1. Medications should be reviewed with the patient. Unbeknownst to the physician, the patient may still be taking glaucoma medications in the hypotonous eye. If the patient is taking systemic CAIs for the fellow eye, it may be possible to switch to topical dorzolamide instead. Topical beta-blockers used in the fellow eye may also be stopped due to the known contralateral effect.[1,2] Topical steroids should be stopped. The use of medications that "irritate" the bleb (eg, gentamicin) are of little benefit.

2. Contact lens trial. The use of large-diameter contact lenses, in our experience, has not been effective where a large diffuse bleb is present. In cases where there is a single leaking site, they can be used effectively.

3. Autologous blood injection into the bleb is another option. An approach similar to that described by Nuyts and colleagues[3] proceeds as follows. The anterior chamber is filled with viscoelastic in order to prevent blood from flowing through the sclerectomy and entering the anterior chamber. One cc of blood is drawn from the patient's arm in a sterile manner. A sterile 27-gauge needle is used to inject the blood. The needle enters the subconjunctival space approximately 7 to 8 mm away and is carefully moved to the center of the bleb. The bleb is inflated with blood (approximately 0.1 to 0.2 cc). Postoperatively, the patient is seen the next day. Elevated IOP is reduced by paracentesis, if necessary. The patient is then seen weekly. The procedure can be repeated.

4. Surgical management. In patients where autologous blood injection has failed, we revise the bleb. If possible, we attempt transconjunctival flap closure with interrupted 10-0 nylon sutures (Figure 60-9). The scleral flap can also be closed after takedown of the conjunctiva if a transconjunctival view is not possible. If the sclera is friable or insufficient, donor sclera can be used to close the sclerectomy site. Occasionally, the conjunctiva over the flap is so fragile that it must be resected in its entirety. In these cases, surrounding conjunctiva is mobilized and brought over the filter site and sutured to the limbus with the Wise closure technique[4] or use of horizontal mattress sutures. In rare cases, conjunctiva must be harvested from the inferior fornix. Despite extensive tissue manipulation, many of these patients do well with long-term functioning blebs. Postoperatively, patients are treated in the same manner as other filter patients.

5. Coexisting cataract. In patients with hypotonous maculopathy who have a cataract (pre-existing or one that developed postoperatively), inflammation from cataract surgery alone often increases IOP and improves visual acuity. In general, the bleb should not be revised in conjunction with cataract surgery in these cases.

REFERENCES

1. Vela MA, Campbell DG. Hypotony and ciliochoroidal detachment following pharmacologic aqueous suppressant therapy in previously filtered patients. *Ophthalmology.* 1985;92:50-57.
2. Geyer O, Neudorfer M, Lazar M. Recurrent choroidal detachment following timolol therapy in previously filtered eye. Choroidal detachment post filtering surgery. *Acta Ophthalmol (Copenh).* 1992;70:702-703.
3. Nuyts RMMA, Greve EL, Geijssen HC, Langerhorst CT. Treatment of hypotonous maculopathy after trabeculectomy with mitomycin-C. *Am J Ophthalmol.* 1994;118:322.
4. Wise JB. Mitomycin-compatible suture technique for fornix-based conjunctival flaps in glaucoma filtration surgery. *Arch Ophthalmol.* 1993;111(7):992-997.

prophylactic antibiotics[64] after filtering surgery has not been commonly performed; however, some glaucoma surgeons may elect to keep patients who have thin avascular blebs with a history of bleb leak or blebitis on a long-term topical antibiotic ointment used at bedtime. Ointment is preferred over topical drops in these cases because it serves to both lubricate the eye as well as provide antimicrobial coverage.

With early intervention, aggressive treatment as mentioned above, and particularly with nonvirulent pathogens, filtering blebs can be salvaged. The critical elements are the immediate examination of the patient and institution of appropriate therapy.

Cataract Formation

When the development of a flat anterior chamber and early profound hypotony were common, the incidence of cataract formation was thought to be between 20% and 30%.[65] More recently, with adoption of trabeculectomy and laser suture lysis, the development and progression of cataract formation is less. However, despite these improved surgical techniques, cataract formation remains a significant problem. Cataracts develop in 22% to 47% of patients after trabeculectomy surgery.[65-67] The risk of cataract formation increases with age, presence of exfoliation, when air is used to reform the anterior chamber, and in cases where hypotony occurs postoperatively.[68,69]

When a cataract becomes visually significant, small-incision phacoemulsification with intraocular lens implantation has resulted in effective visual rehabilitation and preservation of functioning filtering blebs.[70-73] With the diminution of intra- and postoperative complications, the use of phacoemulsification combined with glaucoma surgery[74-76] has improved vision and controlled the IOP with a reduction or discontinuation of medication. The gratitude expressed by a patient who has improved vision and a diminished need for long-term antiglaucoma medications has been a recognized benefit of these newer surgical advances with improvement in the patient's quality of life.

Late Bleb Failure

Despite a perfect operation and a very successful early, mid, and late postoperative course with a functioning filtering bleb and low IOP, a small percentage of patients will have constant wound modification and a definite incidence of late bleb failure. This can be a frustrating situation for both the patient and the surgeon. Frequently, the next sensible treatment is restarting topical therapy in a step-wise fashion until maximum medical therapy is reached. There is no consensus on which intraocular pressure-lowering medication is best to start first after failed trabeculectomy, but many physicians advocate aqueous suppressants.

When a failing bleb no longer responds to maximum medical therapy, either bleb revision, filtration in an area with virgin conjunctiva, or a glaucoma drainage device is considered. We have found that, in these difficult recalcitrant cases, the most effective subsequent surgical approach is repeat filtration surgery if the conjunctiva superiorly is amenable.

CONCLUSION

The range of emotions in the postoperative period after glaucoma surgery can vary immensely from elation to frustration because we as surgeons invest ourselves in each patient and his or her surgery, and we desire and strive for a perfect outcome. Although we may wish to, we do not control anything after our patients leave the office. We hope they understand and follow through on all instructions, as medication compliance and healing correctly is half the battle in glaucoma.

Besides patient compliance, the most important insurance for long-term success is intensive clinical observation postoperatively. At each visit, evaluation of the bleb structure and anterior chamber combined with intraocular pressure measurement will guide the astute surgeon to the correct course of action. Recognition of early, mid, and late changes in bleb status and initiating a planned response to each can prevent failure of the bleb and impending serious complications. A solid base of knowledge can be an excellent guide to helping us recognize those small important changes. Success likely cannot be achieved 100% of the time with glaucoma surgery, but intimate technical knowledge and increased experience can help enhance clinical decision-making and promote improved surgical success.

REFERENCES

1. Watson PG, Grierson I. The place of trabeculectomy in the treatment of glaucoma. *Ophthalmology,* 1981;88:175-196.
2. Skuta GL, Parrish RK. Wound healing in glaucoma filtering surgery. *Surv Ophthalmol.* 1987;32:149-70.
3. Chen C-W. Enhanced intraocular pressure controlling effectiveness of trabeculectomy by local application of mitomycin-C. *Trans Asia-Pacific Acad Ophthalmol.* 1983;9:172-176.
4. Skuta GL, Beeson CC, Higginbotham EJ, et al. Intraoperative mitomycin vs. postoperative 5-FU in high risk glaucoma filtering surgery. *Ophthalmology.* 1992;99:438-444.
5. Palmer SS. Mitomycin as adjunct chemotherapy with trabeculectomy. *Ophthalmology.* 1991;98:317-321.
6. Katz GJ, Higginbotham EJ, Lichter PR, et al. Mitomycin versus 5-fluorouracil in high-risk glaucoma filtering surgery: extended follow-up. *Ophthalmology.* 1995;102:1263-1269.
7. Mirza GE, Karaküçük S, Dogan H, Erkiliç K. Filtering surgery with Mitomycin-C in uncomplicated (primary open angle) glaucoma. *Acta Ophthalmol (Copenh).* 1994;72:155-161.
8. Rockwood EJ, Parrish RK II, Heuer DK, et al. Glaucoma filtering surgery with 5-fluorouracil. *Ophthalmology.* 1987;94:1071-1078.
9. Weinreb RN. Adjusting the dose of 5-fluorouracil after filtration surgery to minimize side effects. *Ophthalmology.* 1987;94:564.
10. Goldenfeld M, Krupin T, Ruderman JM, et al. 5-Fluorouracil in initial trabeculectomy. A prospective, randomized, multicenter study. *Ophthalmology.* 1994;101:1024-1029.
11. Blok MD, Kok JH, van Mil C, Greve EL, Kijlstra A. Use of the Megasoft bandage lens for treatment of complications after trabeculectomy. *Am J Ophthalmol.* 1990;110:264-268.
12. Shoham A, Tessler Z, Finkelman Y, Lifshitz T. Large soft contact lenses in the management of leaking blebs. *CLAO J.* 2000;26:37-39.
13. Asrani SG, Wilensky JT. Management of bleb leaks after glaucoma filtering surgery: use of autologous fibrin tissue glue as an alternative. *Ophthalmology.* 1996;103:294-298.
14. Wise JB. Mitomycin-compatible suture technique for fornix-based conjunctival flaps in glaucoma filtration surgery. *Arch Ophthalmol.* 1993;111(7):992-997.
15. Wadhwani RA, Bellows AR, Hutchinson BT. Surgical repair of leaking filtering blebs. *Ophthalmology.* 2000;107(9):1681-1687.
16. Budenz DL, Barton K, Tseng SCG. Amniotic membrane transplantation for repair of leaking glaucoma filtering blebs. *Am J Ophthalmol.* 2000;130:580-588.
17. Bellows AR, Chylack LT, Hutchinson BT. Choroidal detachment: clinical manifestation, therapy and mechanism of formation. *Ophthalmology.* 1981;88:1107-1115.
18. Brubaker RF, Pederson JE. Ciliochoroidal detachments. *Surv Ophthalmol.* 1983;27:281-289.
19. Gressel MG, Parrish RK, Heuer DK. Delayed nonexpulsive suprachoroidal hemorrhage. *Arch Ophthalmol.* 1984;102:1757-1760.
20. Givens K, Shields MB. Suprachoroidal hemorrhage after glaucoma filtering surgery. *Am J Ophthalmol.* 1987;103:689-694.
21. Lambrou FH, Meredith TA, Kaplan HG. Secondary surgical management of expulsive choroidal hemorrhage. *Arch Ophthalmol.* 1987;105:1195-1198.
22. Chandler PA, Simmons RJ, Grant WM. Malignant glaucoma, medical and surgical treatment. *Am J Ophthalmol.* 1968;66:492-502.
23. Dueker D. Ciliary-block glaucoma: differential diagnosis and management. *J Glaucoma.* 1994;3:167-169.
24. Epstein DL, Steinert RF, Puliafito CA. Nd:YAG therapy to the anterior hyaloid in aphakic malignant (ciliovitreal block) glaucoma. *Am J Ophthalmol.* 1984;98:137-143.
25. Lois N, Wong D, Groenewald C. New surgical approach in the management of pseudophakic malignant glaucoma. *Ophthalmology.* 2001;108(4):780-783.
26. Scott DR, Quigley HJ. Medical management of a high bleb phase after trabeculectomies. *Ophthalmology.* 1988;95:1169-1173.
27. Smith MF, Doyle JW. Use of tissue plasminogen activator to revive blebs following intraocular surgery. *Arch Ophthalmol.* 2001;119(6):809-812.
28. Lundy DC, Sidoti P, Winarko T, et al. Intracameral tissue plasminogen activator after glaucoma surgery. Indications, effectiveness, and complications. *Ophthalmology.* 1996;103(2):274-282.
29. Tripathi RC, Tripathi BJ, Bornstein S, et al. Use of tissue plasminogen activator for rapid dissolution of fibrin and blood clots in the eye after surgery for glaucoma and cataract in humans. *Drug Dev Res.* 1992;27:147-159.
30. Aykan U, Bilge AH, Akin T, et al. Laser suture lysis or releasable sutures after trabeculectomy. *J Glaucoma.* 2007;16(2):240-245.
31. Spaeth G. *Ophthalmic Surgery: Principles and Practice.* Philadelphia, PA: Saunders; 2003:282.

32. Lester M, Ravinet E, Mermoud A. Postoperative subconjunctival mitomycin-C injection after non-penetrating glaucoma surgery. *J Ocul Pharmacol Ther.* 2002;18(4):307-312.

33. Apostolov VI, Siarov NP. Subconjunctival injection of low-dose Mitomycin-C for treatment of failing human trabeculectomies. *Int Ophthalmol.* 1996-1997;20(1-3):101-105.

34. Richter CU, Shingleton BJ, Bellows AR, et al. The development of encapsulated filtering blebs. *Ophthalmology.* 1988;95:1163-1168.

35. Peterson JE, Smith SG. Surgical management of encapsulated filtering blebs. *Ophthalmology.* 1985;92:955-958.

36. Shingleton BJ, Richter CU, Bellows AR, et al. Management of encapsulated filtration blebs. *Ophthalmology.* 1990;97:63-68.

37. Feldman RM, Tabet RR. Needle revision of filtering blebs. *J Glaucoma.* 2008;17(7):594-600.

38. Shetty RK, Wartluft L, Moster MR. Slit-lamp needle revision of failed filtering blebs using high-dose mitomycin C. *J Glaucoma.* 2005;14(1):52-56.

39. Perucho-Martínez S, Gutiérrez-Díaz E, Montero-Rodríguez M, et al. Needle revision of late failing filtering blebs after glaucoma surgery [in Spanish]. *Arch Soc Esp Oftalmol.* 2006;81(9):517-522.

40. Müller M, Pape S, Kusserow C, Hoerauf H, Laqua H. [Late needling with 5-fluorouracil when scarring of filtering bleb seems imminent] [Article in German]. *Ophthalmologe.* 2007;104(4):305-310.

41. Stampfer RL, McMenemy MG, Lieberman MF. Hypotonous maculopathy after trabeculectomy with subconjunctival 5-fluorouracil. *Am J Ophthalmol.* 1992;114:544-553.

42. Seah SK, Prata JA Jr, Minckler DS, Baerveldt G, Lee PP, Heuer DK. Hypotony following trabeculectomy. *J Glaucoma.* 1995;4:73-79.

43. Shields MB, et al. Clinical and histopathologic observations concerning hypotony after trabeculectomy with adjunctive mitomycin-C. *Am J Ophthalmol.* 1993;116:673-683.

44. Nuyts RMMA, Greve EL, Geijssen HC, Langerhorst CT. Treatment of hypotonous maculopathy after trabeculectomy with mitomycin-C. *Am J Ophthalmol.* 1994;118:322-331.

45. Smith MF, Doyle JW. Use of oversized bandage soft contact lenses in the management of early hypotony following filtration surgery. *Ophthalmic Surg Lasers.* 1996;27:417-421.

46. Kahook MY, Schuman JS, Noecker RJ. Trypan blue-assisted neodymium:YAG laser treatment for overfiltering bleb. *J Cataract Refract Surg.* 2006;32(7):1089-1090.

47. Ascaso FJ, Loras E, Cristobal JA. Combination of Nd:YAG laser-induced subconjunctival bleeding and intracameral viscoelastic injection to treat hypotony maculopathy. *Ophthalmic Surg Lasers.* 2002;33:504-507.

48. Maruyama K, Shirato S. Efficacy and safety of transconjunctival scleral flap resuturing for hypotony after glaucoma filtering surgery. *Graefes Arch Clin Exp Ophthalmol.* 2008;246(12):1751-1756.

49. Chen PP, Takahashi Y, Leen MM, Bhandari A, Li Y, Mills RP. The effects of compression sutures on filtering blebs in rabbit eyes. *Ophthalmic Surg Lasers.* 1999;30:216-220.

50. Wise JB. Treatment of chronic postfiltration hypotony by intrableb injection of autologous blood. *Arch Ophthalmol.* 1993;111:827-830.

51. Jampel HD, Quigley HA, Kerrigan-Baumrind LA, et al. Risk factors for late-onset infection following glaucoma filtration surgery. *Arch Ophthalmol.* 2001;119:1001-1008.

52. Mac I, Soltau JB. Glaucoma-filtering bleb infections. *Curr Opin Ophthalmol.* 2003;14(2):91-94.

53. Sharan S, Trope GE, Chipman M, Buys YM. Late-onset bleb infections: prevalence and risk factors. *Can J Ophthalmol.* 2009;44(3):279-283.

54. Soltau JB, Rothman RF, Budenz DL, et al. Risk factors for glaucoma filtering bleb infections. *Arch Ophthalmol.* 2000;118:338-342.

55. Wolner B, Liebmann JM, Sassani JW, Ritch R, Speaker M, Marmor M. Late bleb-related endophthalmitis after trabeculectomy with adjunctive 5-fluorouracil. *Ophthalmology.* 1991;98:1053-1060.

56. Dacey MP, et al. Echographic findings in infectious endophthalmitis. *Arch Ophthalmol.* 1994;112:1325-1333.

57. Reynolds AC, Skuta GL, Monlux R, Johnson J. Management of blebitis by members of the American Glaucoma Society: a survey. *J Glaucoma.* 2001;10(4):340-347.

58. Prasad N, Latina MA. Blebitis and endophthalmitis after glaucoma filtering surgery. *Int Ophthalmol Clin.* 2007;47(2):85-97.

59. Mandelbaum S, Forster RK, Gelender H, Culbertson W. Late-onset endophthalmitis associated with filtering blebs. *Ophthalmology.* 1985;92:964-972.

60. Ciulla TA, Beck AD, Topping TM, Baker AS. Blebitis, early endophthalmitis, and late endophthalmitis after glaucoma-filtering surgery. *Ophthalmology.* 1997;104:986-995.

61. Greenfield DS, Suner IJ, Miller MP, et al. Endophthalmitis after filtering surgery with mitomycin. *Arch Ophthalmol.* 1996;114:943-949.

62. Song A, Scott IU, Flynn HW Jr, et al. Delayed-onset bleb-associated endophthalmitis: clinical features and visual acuity outcomes. *Ophthalmology.* 2002;109:985-991.

63. Brown RH, Yang LH, Walker SD, Lynch MG, Martinez LA, Wilson LA. Treatment of bleb infection after glaucoma surgery. *Arch Ophthalmol.* 1994;112:57-61.

64. Wand M, Quintiliani R, Robinson A. Antibiotic prophylaxis in eyes with filtration blebs: survey of glaucoma specialists, microbiological study, and recommendations. *J Glaucoma.* 1995;4(2):103-109.

65. Lamping K, Bellows AR, Hutchinson BT, Afran SI. Long-term evaluation of initial filtration surgery. *Ophthalmology.* 1986;93:91-101.

66. Vesti E. Development of cataract after trabeculectomy. *Acta Ophthalmologica.* 1993;71:777-781.

67. Asamoto A, Yablonski ME. Post-trabeculectomy anterior subcapsular cataract formation induced by anterior chamber air. *Ophthalmic Surg.* 1993;24:314-319.

68. Akato SK, Goulstine DB, Rosenthal AR. Long-term post trabeculectomy intraocular pressures. *Acta Ophthalmol.* 1992;70:312-316.

69. Tornquest G, Drolsum LK. Trabeculectomies. A long-term study. *Acta Ophthalmol.* 1991;69:450-454.

70. Popovic V, Sjostrand J. Long-term outcome following trabeculectomy: I. Retrospective analysis of intraocular pressure regulation and cataract formation. *Acta Ophthalmol.* 1991;69:299-304.

71. Stewart WC, Krinkley CMC, Carlson AN. Results of trabeculectomy combined with phacoemulsification versus trabeculectomy combined with extracapsular cataract extraction in patients with advanced glaucoma. *Ophthalmic Surg.* 1994;25:621-627.

72. Wishart PK, Austin MW. Combined cataract extraction with trabeculectomy: Phacoemulsification compared with extracapsular technique. *Ophthalmic Surg.* 1993;24:814-821.

73. Lyle WA, Jin JC. Comparison of 3- and 6-mm incision in a combined phacoemulsification and trabeculectomy. *Am J Ophthalmol.* 1991;111:189-196.

74. Tsai HY, Liu CJ, Cheng CY. Combined trabeculectomy and cataract extraction versus trabeculectomy alone in primary angle-closure glaucoma. *Br J Ophthalmol.* 2009;93(7):943-948.

75. Hsu CH, Obstbaum SA. Technique and outcome of combined phacoemulsification and trabeculectomy. *Curr Opin Ophthalmol.* 1998;9(2):9-14.

76. Casson RJ, Salmon JF. Combined surgery in the treatment of patients with cataract and primary open-angle glaucoma. *J Cataract Refract Surg.* 2001;27(11):1854-1863.

61

The Management of Coexisting Cataract and Glaucoma

Carla I. Bourne, MD; Bradford J. Shingleton, MD; and Joel S. Schuman, MD, FACS

Cataract and glaucoma are common entities that frequently coexist, especially in older individuals. The management of either requires consideration of both, particularly when surgical intervention is contemplated. The decision for cataract or glaucoma surgery, or combined cataract and glaucoma surgery, necessitates evaluation of the need for visual rehabilitation and the urgency of intraocular pressure (IOP) control.

Cataract surgery is considered when the patient complains of deterioration of vision to a point where it interferes with the ability to read, write, and perform other activities of daily living and when examination of the patient's eye reveals cataract as the source of some or all of these visual complaints. The surgeon must recall, however, when determining the cataract's functional effect, that a small cataract may have a disproportionately large effect in the glaucomatous eye, especially in the presence of compromised visual field.

Glaucoma subtype, IOP control, current ocular hypotensive therapy, and the severity of glaucomatous optic nerve damage each has an impact on the decision regarding the role of glaucoma surgery in the patient with cataract. History of prior laser trabeculoplasty (LTP), laser iridectomy, or incisional glaucoma surgery are factors involved in the surgical decision-making for these patients. It may also be difficult to determine the extent of glaucomatous damage due to the impact of the cataract on optic nerve examination and visual field testing.

There are other factors that need to be considered when dealing with simultaneous management of cataract and glaucoma. These include whether 1 or 2 surgical procedures are warranted and if performing 2 procedures, which should be done first (Table 61-1). Both short- and long-term planning is essential in order to determine if a filter or nonfilter procedure would meet goals to prevent disease progression

and what would be the most suitable intraocular lens (IOL) implant given other ocular pathology. This detailed evaluation is necessary as the risks and complications are greater with cataract surgery in glaucomatous eyes than in nonglaucomatous eyes.

Surgery in glaucomatous eyes involves special considerations. Conjunctival scarring from previous surgery increases the difficulty of conjunctival dissection and increases the risk of conjunctival tear or buttonhole. Altered conjunctiva due to chronic glaucoma medication use or topical allergy may compromise conjunctival mobilization and lead to increased bleeding. A small pupil due to long-term use of miotics and a shallow anterior chamber in highly hyperopic/nanophthalmic eyes increases the difficulty of capsulorrhexis and phacoemulsification. Significant anterior synechiae may preclude anterior chamber IOL implantation. Eyes with pseudoexfoliation have weak zonular attachments, which increase the risk of zonular dialysis and vitreous loss during surgery. A high preoperative IOP, with a rapid reduction in IOP at the time of surgical entry into the eye, predisposes to suprachoroidal hemorrhage. The incidence of cystoid macular edema may increase after cataract surgery in eyes on multiple glaucoma medications. This may be most apparent in eyes on prostaglandin agonists that have complicated surgery with violation of the posterior capsule and vitreous loss.

SURGICAL OPTIONS

Cataract Surgery Alone

Glaucomatous eyes with visually significant cataract in which the IOP is well controlled on 1 or 2 medications can be considered for cataract extraction alone. Additional indications are presented in Figure 61-1. Studies

- 567 -

Kahook MY, Schuman JS, eds.
Chandler and Grant's Glaucoma, Fifth Edition (pp 567-578).
© 2013 SLACK Incorporated.

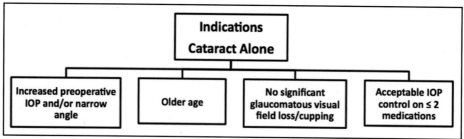

Figure 61-1. Indications for cataract surgery alone.

TABLE 61-1. KEY POINTS: SURGICAL OPTIONS FOR THE MANAGEMENT OF COEXISTING CATARACT AND GLAUCOMA
Cataract Surgery Alone
Combined Cataract and Glaucoma Surgery
Trabeculectomy
○ Separate site incisions
○ Single-site incision
Alternative Glaucoma Procedures
Two-Staged Cataract and Glaucoma Surgery
Glaucoma surgery followed by cataract extraction
Cataract surgery followed by glaucoma surgery

TABLE 61-2. ADVANTAGES AND DISADVANTAGES OF CATARACT SURGERY ALONE
Advantages
Restores vision promptly
Single procedure
Technically easiest—short surgical time
Facilitates postoperative assessment of optic nerve and visual field
Opportunity for later glaucoma procedure if needed
Small-incision phacoemulsification can yield improved long-term IOP control
Disadvantages
Early postoperative IOP elevation
Reduced long-term IOP control compared to combined surgery
Future filtration surgery success is potentially compromised if conjunctiva is violated
Postoperative IOP results are variable
No change in diurnal IOP fluctuation

have demonstrated that small-incision phacoemulsification can yield improved long-term IOP control. Shingleton and colleagues[1] showed a statistically significant IOP decrease of 1.8 ± 3.5 mm Hg 5 years after cataract surgery alone. Issa and colleagues[2] suggested that IOP reduction after cataract surgery is greatest in eyes with higher IOP and narrower angles preoperatively. Poley and colleagues[3] reported significantly greater IOP reduction in glaucomatous and nonglaucomatous eyes with higher preoperative IOPs. Mean IOP reduction approached 10 mm Hg in eyes with preoperative IOPs higher than 28 mm Hg. Shingleton and colleagues[4] confirmed significantly greater IOP reduction in pseudoexfoliation eyes with higher preoperative IOP. It must be noted that a long-term decrease in glaucoma medication requirement has not been substantiated and by year 5, most eyes require a return to preoperative medication levels.[1,5,6] If cataract surgery alone is performed, it is best to approach the eye from the temporal aspect to preserve superior conjunctiva if filtration surgery is needed in the future. Standard phacoemulsification techniques are used. We recommend the use of nonsteroidal anti-inflammatory drops preoperatively to decrease the risk of postoperative cystoid edema, and we do not routinely stop glaucoma medications preoperatively.

LTP can also be considered in conjunction with cataract surgery in eyes with borderline control of IOP. It can be performed prior to or after cataract surgery. LTP may be slightly more effective in phakic eyes, but clinically significant IOP reduction can also be achieved in pseudophakic eyes.[7,8]

During the preoperative evaluation, the advantages and disadvantages of cataract surgery alone must be weighed because IOP spikes may occur in both the early and long-term postoperative periods (Table 61-2). This can be due to retained viscoelastic, trabecular meshwork (TM) damage, collapse in the area of incision, residual pigment or cortical debris, breakdown of blood-aqueous barrier, and corticosteroid use. This is particularly important for patients with significant glaucomatous optic atrophy who might not be able to tolerate significant IOP elevation, even for a short time.

As early as 1 hour postoperatively, there have been reports of IOP elevation as high as 13.4 mm Hg in normal eyes,[9] and in glaucomatous eyes, there is tendency for this to be a greater and more frequent increase. IOP elevation may peak in the 2- to 8-hour range after cataract surgery,[10,11] and the elevation may extend into the first postoperative day.

TABLE 61-3. STRATEGIES TO MANAGE THE SMALL PUPIL
Vigorous preoperative dilation regimen
Intracameral medications
Nonpreserved epinephrine in infusion
Lidocaine + epinephrine (Shugarcaine)
Intracameral phenylephrine
Release of posterior synechiae and removal of pupillary membranes
Viscoelastic pupil expansion
Pupil expansion devices
Iris hooks (Figure 61-2)
Pupil ring expanders (eg, Malyugin ring) (Figure 61-3)
Manual manipulation techniques (not for IFIS)
Bimanual iris stretch
Multiple sphincterotomies

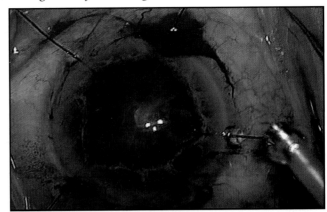

Figure 61-2. Iris hooks for pupil expansion.

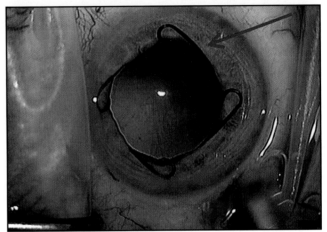

Figure 61-3. Malyugin ring (Microsurgical Technology, Redman, WA) for pupil expansion.

Shingleton and colleagues[12] reported that 8.1% of normal eyes compared with 15.6% of glaucomatous eyes had IOPs of higher than 30 mm Hg on postoperative day 1 following uncomplicated cataract surgery. Prophylactic use of aqueous suppressants, alpha-agonists, and miotics at the time of surgery can help moderate postoperative IOP elevation but there is no consensus of opinion as to which medicine, if any, is more efficacious.[13-16] If IOP elevation is of particular concern postoperatively, as may be the case in a patient with significant disc damage, IOP should be checked on the day of surgery. If significant IOP elevation occurs, we favor release of aqueous via the paracentesis and reinstitution of aqueous suppressants and alpha-agonists, as needed. Aqueous release is done at the slit-lamp under topical anesthesia and with sterile precautions. It is important to recheck the IOP 15 to 30 minutes after aqueous release as the IOP can respike, necessitating a repeat tap.[17]

At the other extreme, early hypotony (30 minutes postoperatively) can also infrequently occur, complicating healing if prolonged. Fortunately, when transient, it has not been shown to increase susceptibility to choroidal effusion, hemorrhage, or infection.[18]

Special Situations Impacting Cataract Surgery in the Glaucoma Patient

Small Pupil Management

A poorly dilating pupil presents special challenges for the cataract surgeon and is a common occurrence in the glaucoma patient. It can be associated with long-term miotic use, older age, alpha-blocking agents, pseudoexfoliation,

pupillary membranes, iridoschisis, anterior segment dysgenesis, noniatrogenic/iatrogenic trauma, and a poor preoperative dilation regimen. Table 61-3 provides an outline of strategies for managing a small pupil during cataract surgery (Figures 61-2 and 61-3).

Intraoperative Floppy Iris Syndrome

Intraoperative floppy iris syndrome (IFIS) is a well-documented issue due to use of alpha₁-blocking agents including tamsulosin (Flomax), terazosin (Hytrin), doxazosin (Cardura), alfuzosin (Uroxatral), saw palmetto (herbal remedy), psychotropic drugs (mianserin—antidepressant), and antihypertensives (prazosin, guanadrel [Hylorel], labetolol). It may also occur with Finasteride, which acts by inhibiting type II-5 reductase. Discontinuing the medications may improve but not eliminate IFIS, and it may occur with Flomax discontinued 1 or more years before cataract surgery. Variable incidence of complications has been documented,[19] but the intraoperative findings of poor dilation, floppy iris, iris prolapse, and progressive miosis have been reported to be as high as 63%.[20] Management is similar as for a poorly dilating pupil with the incorporation of special phacoemulsification techniques (Table 61-4).

TABLE 61-4. PHACOEMULSIFICATION TECHNIQUES IN INTRAOPERATIVE FLOPPY IRIS SYNDROME
Clear-cornea incision construction (long and anterior)
Soft-shell technique with viscoelastic
Gentle hydrodissection
Healon 5 with low-flow parameters
Phacoemulsification below anterior capsule
Nucleus flip/phaco above iris plane
Avoid infusion directed at level of iris plane
Biaxial microincisional cataract surgery

TABLE 61-5. CLUES TO ZONULE WEAKNESS IN PSEUDOEXFOLIATION
Preoperative
• Anterior chamber depth asymmetry
• Phacodonesis/iridodonesis/lens subluxation
• Visibility of lens equator on eccentric gaze
• Decentered nucleus on primary gaze
• Iridolenticular gap
• Changes in contour of lens periphery
• < 2.5 corneal thickness axial depth
Intraoperatively
• Pseudoelastic capsule (Figure 61-4)
• Anterior chamber depth instability
• Limited nucleus rotation
• Dramatic lens position shift

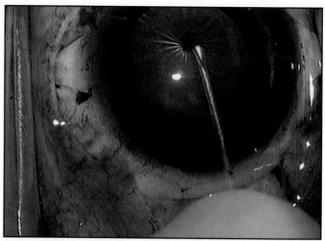

Figure 61-4. Pseudoelastic capsule in pseudoexfoliation.

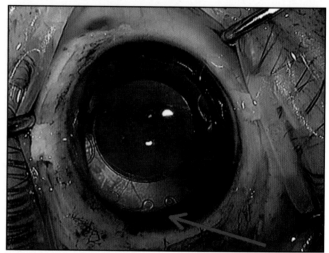

Figure 61-5. Capsular tension ring in pseudoexfoliation.

Pseudoexfoliation Syndrome

Zonule weakness may present in up to 2.5% of pseudo-exfoliation (PXE) eyes and may lead to a higher rate of complicated surgery necessitating vitrectomy.[4,21-23] Preoperative and intraoperative clues to zonule weakness are presented in Table 61-5 and Figure 61-4.

When anticipating the possibility of dealing with an unstable nucleus due to zonule weakness, the surgeon may consider a posterior limbal incision or scleral flap to enable an easy transition to extracapsular cataract extraction (ECCE), if required. Effective hydrodissection is critical to achieve free rotation of the nucleus within the capsular bag and to minimize extension of aspiration forces to the capsular equator during phacoemulsification. Capsule retractors, capsule tension rings (Figure 61-5), or capsule retaining segments can be used to distribute forces and to oppose capsule constriction and zonule separation during phacoemulsification.

Anterior chamber, iris sutured, or scleral sutured IOLs may be required if capsule/zonule support is inadequate.

Crowded Anterior Chamber

As mentioned previously, patients with narrow angles may benefit the most from cataract extraction by opening of the angle with resultant decline in IOP in nonsynechial angle closure.[2] With synechiae present, intraoperative gonio-synechialysis at the completion of cataract surgery can be performed to aid results.[24,25]

Nanophthalmic and high hyperopic patients often have deep set eyes, small orbits, tight lids, high lens/eye volume ratio, small corneas, thick sclera, and miotic pupils, leading to potentially complicated surgery. Because of space constraints, surgeons may consider using a small-volume anesthetic block with external compression. Keratome entry into the anterior chamber should be anterior to avoid iris prolapse. Healon V (Alcon Laboratories, Fort Worth, TX) can be effective in maintaining anterior chamber depth and flattening the

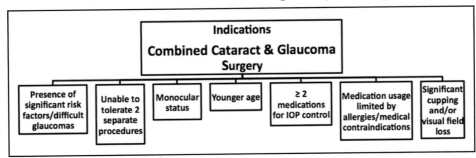

Figure 61-6. Indications for combined cataract and glaucoma surgery.

lens/iris contour. It may be necessary to perform a pars plana vitrectomy or vitreous tap to achieve a satisfactory anterior chamber depth that will permit safe creation of a capsulorrhexis. Pupil support devices are often helpful. Following completion of the cataract surgery, intraoperative gonioscopy is indicated to assess for residual angle closure that might be amenable to intraoperative goniosynechialysis. Postoperatively, these eyes are at a higher risk for aqueous misdirection.

Angle-Closure Glaucoma

Effective IOP reduction in acute angle-closure glaucoma has been documented with primary phacoemulsification and IOL implantation.[26-29] In some cases, IOP elevation and vision improvement may be achieved with fewer interventions by this approach than by the more conventional program of initial medical therapy followed by laser iridectomy and subsequent cataract surgery.

Combined Cataract and Glaucoma Surgery

Cataract and glaucoma surgery is commonly performed in the same session in those eyes with visually significant cataract coupled with glaucoma that is advanced, poorly controlled, or requires multiple medications. Combined surgery can also be performed to reduce the risk of an IOP spike following cataract surgery in eyes with severely compromised optic nerves, where such an IOP spike increases the risk for further loss of visual field. Other indications are presented in Figure 61-6. The combined procedure offers the advantage of relatively rapid visual recovery and reasonable control of IOP. Visual rehabilitation is generally faster than with a 2-stage procedure, and control of IOP, especially with the use of antimetabolites, approaches that of filtering surgery alone.

Combined surgery, however, is more time-consuming and technically challenging than cataract surgery alone. With greater potential complications, combined procedures require more intensive postoperative care. Combined cataract and trabeculectomy surgery can be performed via separate or single incisions. Studies indicate that IOP control is essentially equivalent for each approach.[30-35] Advantages

TABLE 61-6. ADVANTAGES AND DISADVANTAGES OF COMBINED CATARACT AND TRABECULECTOMY SURGERY
Advantages
Restores vision promptly
Single procedure
Decreased glaucoma medication requirements
Good early intraocular pressure control
Better long-term intraocular pressure control than phacoemulsification alone
Antimetabolite use—potential for achieving lower intraocular pressure
Multiple glaucoma surgical options
Facilitate postoperative nerve evaluation and visual field assessment
Disadvantages
Increased intraoperative and postoperative complications
Longer surgical time
More intensive postoperative care requirements
Glaucoma meds often needed postoperatively

and disadvantages of combined cataract and glaucoma surgery are listed in Table 61-6.

Separate Site Incisions

In this approach, cataract surgery is typically performed first via a temporal incision followed by the surgeon's preferred technique for superior trabeculectomy with or without antimetabolite. A 10-0 nylon suture should be placed at the cataract incision to maintain chamber stability during the trabeculectomy phase and to facilitate postoperative manipulation of the developing filtration bleb.

An alternative approach is to begin with the trabeculectomy portion superiorly, completing placement and removal of antimetabolite and creation of the partial-thickness sclera flap prior to phacoemulsification from the temporal aspect. The sclerectomy, iridectomy, and flap closure are

TABLE 61-7. ADVANTAGES AND DISADVANTAGES OF SEPARATE INCISIONS APPROACH FOR COMBINED SURGERY
Advantages
• Clear cornea/limbal approach—minimizes conjunctival manipulation
• More comfortable phacoemulsification position for a majority of cataract surgeons
• Small amount of with-the-rule astigmatism induced
• Good for against-the-rule astigmatism
Disadvantages
• Longer operative time than combined surgery via single incision

TABLE 61-8. COMBINED CATARACT AND GLAUCOMA SURGERY USING OTHER GLAUCOMA PROCEDURES
Glaucoma drainage devices
Ex-PRESS mini glaucoma shunt
Nonpenetrating deep sclerectomy
• Viscocanalostomy
• Canaloplasty
Trabectome
Endoscopic cyclophotocoagulation
Ab interno opening into Schlemm's canal
Suprachoroidal shunt

then completed superiorly in a standard fashion after the cataract is removed.

Single-Site Incision

Single-site incision is simple, safe, fast, and effective but potentially less comfortable for the temporally oriented phaco surgeon[36-38] (Table 61-7). Both limbal-based and fornix-based conjunctival flaps are effective for lowering IOP, bleb development, improving vision, and decreasing the need for glaucoma medications. The trabeculectomy portion, with or without an antimetabolite, is performed in a standard manner. The conjunctival and scleral flaps are typically mobilized first, along with antimetabolite application as indicated, followed by phacoemulsification and IOL implantation via an incision underneath the scleral flap. Sclerectomy, peripheral iridectomy, and conjunctival closure are then performed in typical fashion to complete the case.

The issue of peripheral iridectomy in combined procedures is somewhat controversial. Studies[39,40] have shown that the absence of an iridectomy in combined procedures may not increase the incidence of pupillary block or sclerectomy obstruction, and creation of an iridectomy slightly increases the incidence of hyphema. Surgical iridectomy is recommended in any eye with a shallow anterior chamber or one predisposed to angle closure.

When performing combined phacotrabeculectomy without intraoperative antimetabolite via a single incision, one study[38] reported that at 1 year there is an average decrease in IOP of 5 mm Hg and 75% of patients have decreased need for additional glaucoma medication. IOP reduction is sustained at 3 years but there is increased need for medications to maintain IOP. The addition of intraoperative antimetabolite, such as mitomycin C, can

improve results,[35] with Jin and colleagues[41] reporting an average decline in IOP by 8 mm Hg sustained at 30 months postoperatively.

Combined Cataract and Glaucoma Surgery: Alternative Glaucoma Procedures

Many other glaucoma procedures can be combined simultaneously with cataract surgery (Table 61-8). The surgeon's choice should be based on familiarity with the procedure, realistic expectations of postoperative IOP, and potential complications of the procedure. Because many of these techniques are recent innovations, data from large randomized studies are limited.

Glaucoma Drainage Device

Combined phacoemulsification and glaucoma drainage device (GDD) surgery provides good visual rehabilitation and control of IOP, with a low incidence of complications.[42-45] Standard techniques are employed, and all types of GDDs can be used (eg, Molteno [Molteno Ophthalmic Ltd, Dunedin, New Zealand], Ahmed [New World Medical, Rancho Cucamonga, CA], Baerveldt [Abbott Medical Optics, Santa Ana, CA], and Krupin [E Benson Hood Laboratoy, Pembroke, MA]). A GDD may be a better alternative to a trabeculectomy in cases of prior failed trabeculectomy, active uveitic or neovascular glaucoma, prominent ocular surface disease, or in any case where bleb development may be problematic.

Ex-PRESS Mini Glaucoma Shunt

The Ex-PRESS Mini Glaucoma Shunt (Alcon Laboratories, Fort Worth, TX) is a small metal shunt placed under a partial-thickness scleral flap. Benefits of the implant may include similar IOP results to trabeculectomy with reduced early postoperative hypotony[46] and minimization of inflammation because no sclerectomy or iridectomy is performed. There is no consensus as to the efficacy, but Kanner and colleagues[47] reported that when combined with phacoemulsification, success rates at 3 years were as high as 95.6%. As a primary procedure with mitomycin C, De Feo and colleagues[48] report success rates of 78% for a postoperative IOP less than 18 mm Hg and 70% for an IOP less than 15 mm Hg. Postoperative management is similar to that of traditional trabeculectomy, including bleb needling and 5-fluorouracil supplementation as needed.

Nonpenetrating Deep Sclerectomy

Viscocanalostomy can be performed by a wide variety of techniques (Figure 61-7). In general, combined viscocanalo-plasty procedures tend to yield higher postoperative IOPs than combined phacotrabeculectomies, even though some studies have noted equal results.[49] However, it has a better postoperative safety profile than phacotrabeculectomies, particularly as it relates to hypotony, and IOP reduction is typically better than phacoemulsification alone.[50]

Canaloplasty (iScience Interventional, Menlo Park, CA), a modification of viscocanalostomy, involves 360-degree circumferential dilation of Schlemm's canal with a microcatheter, coupled with placement of a 10-0 Prolene suture to place tension on the TM. Canaloplasty is associated with greater IOP reduction than viscocanalostomy. One combined phaco/canaloplasty study[51] reported a mean IOP reduction of 8 mm Hg at 1 year with a significant decrease in glaucoma medication requirements and minimal complications.

Trabectome

The Trabectome (NeoMedix Corp, Tustin, CA) works by ablating the juxtacanalicular aspect of the inner wall of the TM while keeping the outer wall of Schlemm's canal and the collector channels intact. The presumed reduction in resistance to aqueous outflow lowers IOP. One of the main benefits is that the procedure spares conjunctiva for future filtering procedures if needed. Francis and colleagues[52] reported on 304 eyes undergoing combined Trabectome and phacoemulsification. They noted a mean IOP decrease of 4.5±2.9 mm Hg 1 year postoperatively with a decrease in the need for glaucoma medications. Transient blood reflux was noted to be the most frequent complication, suggesting a safer complication profile than trabeculectomy.

Endocyclophotoablation

Ciliary body endophotocoagulation offers the benefit of sparing the conjunctiva and avoiding creation of a filtration bleb.[53] In addition, the chronic inflammation common with external cycloablative approaches appears to be much less.[54,55] Compared to cataract surgery alone, combined phaco endocyclophotoablation (ECP) may have a similar IOP-lowering effect, but a greater reduction in need for postoperative glaucoma medications.

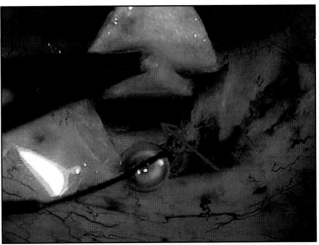

Figure 61-7. Deep sclerectomy flap with Schlemm's canal exposed.

Ab Interno Opening Into Schlemm's Canal

The Glaukos iStent (Glaukos Corp, Laguna Hills, CA) trabecular micro-bypass stent is currently undergoing clinical trials in the United States.[56] Factors that make it favorable include delivery of the stent ab interno through the previously completed cataract incision, which spares conjunctiva and decreases trauma to the eye from additional incisions. The stent, visualized via gonioprism, is advanced through the TM and is implanted into Schlemm's canal, where it creates a pathway for aqueous humor to drain directly from the anterior chamber into Schlemm's canal.

Interim studies[57] are promising with a reduction of 4.4 mm Hg seen 1-year postoperatively following combination surgery with phacoemulsification. This is in comparison to preliminary results[56] where IOP reduction was 5.7 mm Hg at 6 months. Future studies will provide better indications of the long-term efficacy and complications.

Ab interno trabeculostomy using an excimer laser to create an opening into Schlemm's canal has been employed with success outside the United States.

Suprachoroidal Shunt

The Solx gold shunt (SOLX, Waltham, MA) is a thin 24-karat gold shunt with channels through its body that is placed into the suprachoroidal space via an anterior chamber approach and a sclerotomy. Laser to the portion in the anterior chamber may provide titration of IOP over time.

Pilot results showed an average decrease of 9 mm Hg at 11.7 months, with hyphema being the most common complication.[58] Potential difficulties include fibrous encapsulation preventing posterior flow of aqueous in the suprachoroidal space.[59] Other suprachoroidal shunts of various configurations are in the developmental state.

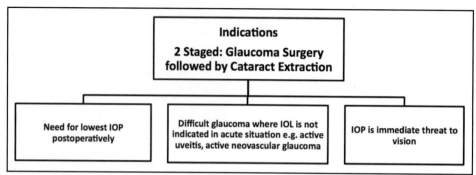

Figure 61-8. Indications for 2-staged approach to management of cataract and glaucoma surgery followed by cataract extraction.

TABLE 61-9. ADVANTAGES AND DISADVANTAGES OF 2-STAGED APPROACH TO MANAGEMENT OF CATARACT AND GLAUCOMA
Advantages
• Best for immediate intraocular pressure control
• Possibly best for long-term intraocular pressure control
• Opportunities for glaucoma enhancement at time of cataract surgery
Disadvantages
• Two stages: long delay in recovery
• Loss of intraocular pressure control after cataract operation
• Cataract surgery in presence of bleb is more challenging

Two-Staged Cataract and Glaucoma Surgery

Glaucoma Surgery Followed by Cataract Extraction

In eyes with advanced glaucomatous damage with profound cupping of the optic nerve and extensive visual field loss, where the IOP is poorly controlled despite maximum-tolerated medical treatment or where there is an urgent need to control the IOP, filtering surgery alone, followed at a later date by cataract extraction, may be the best option (Figure 61-8). While antimetabolites have altered the success rate associated with combined procedures, certain eyes may warrant filtering surgery first, with cataract extraction reserved for a later date. This is especially true in eyes with severely compromised optic nerves that are at a high risk for filter failure (eg, eyes that have undergone prior intraocular surgery, eyes with active neovascular or inflammatory glaucoma, eyes of young individuals, and eyes of African Americans).

Filtering surgery preceding cataract extraction may obviate the need for cataract surgery itself if the patient's lens opacities are visually significant only because of miotic use. The discontinuation of miotics after glaucoma surgery may lead to an improvement in visual function. Advantages of 2-stage surgery are listed in Table 61-9.

There are disadvantages to the 2-stage approach (see Table 61-9). This technique subjects the patient to 2 surgical procedures with 2 recovery periods, each requiring frequent office visits. The patient may have reduced vision for a prolonged time period while waiting for the second stage of cataract surgery. Finally, secondary cataract surgery may cause the previously created filter to fail. Cataract extraction after filtering surgery can be expected to elevate IOP postoperatively.[60-62]

Studies[63] have shown that trabeculectomy can increase the rate of cataract formation by up to 78%, especially if there is increased inflammation or a flat anterior chamber. In young patients with a mean age of 43.7 years, Adelman and colleagues[64] reported that 24% will undergo cataract extraction within a mean time of 26 months. These results also pertain to tube shunt procedures. Given the expectations of subsequent cataract surgery, superonasal filter placement permits easier access for later cataract operation. If required, it is best to delay cataract surgery as long as possible after glaucoma surgery, preferably 3 to 6 months to allow as much time as possible for the bleb to become established.

With the subsequent cataract surgery, technical considerations are similar to standard cataract surgery alone with some important caveats. The surgeon must proceed with an awareness of potential endothelial cell loss following the previous trabeculectomy. Preoperative Honan balloon (The Lebanon Corp, Lebanon, IN) or external compression should be avoided to reduce the chance for excessive hypotony. Anterior chamber keratome entry should be as far away from the bleb as possible—usually temporal or inferotemporal. Careful attention to infusion bottle height is important to avoid excessive anterior chamber deepening. Suture closure of the keratome entry site is favored to permit early and vigorous postoperative manipulation of the pre-existing filtration bleb, if needed. It is appropriate to

TABLE 61-10. CONSIDERATIONS FOR THE HYPOTONOUS EYE
Phacoemulsification more difficult
Paracentesis
Capsulorrhexis
Corneal striae
Nuclear cracking
IOL power calculation: Issue of axial length
Hypotonous eye → shorter eye (up to 3 mm) less than normal state
Base IOL calculation on axial length approximately midway between presumed prehypotony and actual hypotony axial lengths
Immersion ultrasound most accurate
IOP elevation after cataract surgery
May be enough to reduce maculopathy changes
Autologous blood injection at the time of phaco to limit bleb function
Bleb revision/pericardium graft/Palmberg suture

Cataract Surgery Followed by Glaucoma Surgery

In the pseudophakic eye, where glaucoma surgery is needed because topical medication or LTP have been unsuccessful in controlling IOP, considerations for subsequent intervention are similar to glaucoma surgery alone. All procedures can be considered—filter, GDD, nonpenetrating surgery, and cyclophotocoagulation (CPC). Particular attention should be paid to the conjunctival status because adherent, scarred conjunctiva makes filter survival less likely. This is also true for eyes with vitreous in the anterior chamber. In the setting of mobile conjunctiva and intact posterior capsule without anterior vitreous prolapse, success for filtration surgery in pseudophakic eyes can approach that of phakic eyes.[67] In eyes with moderately scarred conjunctiva, GDD surgery may be preferable. In eyes with densely adherent conjunctiva precluding conjunctival flap mobilization, CPC by an endoscopic or external route may be indicated. External CPC can be associated with a higher rate of visual loss than other procedures,[68] but if power, duration, and number of applications are reduced, hypotony, chronic inflammation, and visual loss may be reduced.

Special Considerations in Glaucoma Patients

Neodymium:Yttrium-Aluminum-Garnet Laser Capsulotomy

In patients with glaucoma, preoperative and postoperative IOP evaluation is important because of the potential of IOP elevation after laser capsulotomy. During the first hour after capsulotomy, as many as 20% of patients may have an IOP elevation of more than 5 mm Hg and 3% will have a spike of more than 10 mm Hg.[69]

Anterior capsule contraction (phimosis) is more common in pseudoexfoliation eyes. At the first sign of such annular anterior capsule change, the Nd:YAG laser can be used to perform anterior capsule relaxing incisions in a cruciate pattern to reduce capsule contraction and potential IOL displacement.

Intraocular Lens Choices

Improved IOL design and material have led to smaller phacoemulsification incisions, improved biocompatibility, and better refractive outcomes following cataract extraction.

Current-generation silicone, acrylic, and polymethylmethacrylate IOLs are all uveal biocompatible with minimal tendency for IOL deposits when the IOL is implanted within the capsular bag.[70] Capsule compatibility is also similar for all current-generation IOLs, although the incidence of anterior capsule contraction and posterior capsule opacification may be slightly higher with silicone IOLs. This may be of

confirm sclerectomy patency and bleb elevation at the end of the case.

Surgical techniques may vary based on the preoperative IOP and status of the bleb. If the IOP is too high, consideration can be given to adding internal or external revision of the bleb at the time of phacoemulsification. All other types of combined glaucoma procedures are also possible. If the IOP is too low (Table 61-10), autologous blood injection or surgical bleb revision may be added to supplement the slight increase in IOP anticipated with the cataract surgery itself. An additional important caveat must be appreciated in hypotonous eyes undergoing cataract surgery. Hypotony typically results in a shortening of the axial length of the eye compared to pre-existing nonhypotonous levels. Cataract surgery leads to increased IOP and a corresponding increase in axial length. IOL power calculation must take this factor into account.

Improvement in vision can be anticipated in most eyes undergoing cataract surgery in the presence of a filtering bleb. IOP tends to increase by a moderate (1 to 2 mm Hg) amount and glaucoma medication requirements tend to remain stable.[65] Factors associated with bleb compromise and loss of IOP control after cataract surgery include preoperative IOP levels higher than 10 mm Hg, increased iris manipulation, young age, postoperative IOP spike, pre-existing uveitis, and cataract surgery within 6 months of the filter.[66]

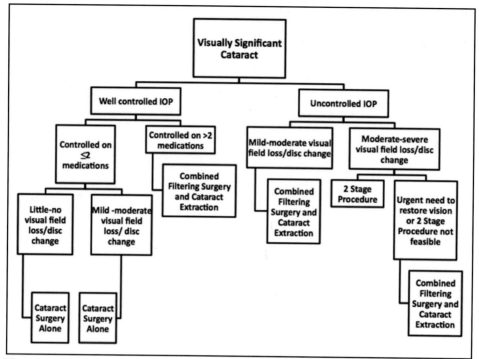

Figure 61-9. Clinical decision making in an eye with coexisting cataract and glaucoma.

special importance for pseudoexfoliation eyes where anterior capsule phimosis is more common and may predispose to IOL subluxation.

Aspheric IOLs alter spherical aberration and may improve contrast sensitivity. This may be beneficial for glaucoma patients who often have reduced contrast sensitivity even in early stages of the disease. However, decentered aspheric IOLs may actually magnify spherical aberration, so it may be appropriate to consider neutrally aspheric IOLs or spherical IOLs in pseudoexfoliation or trauma patients where capsule support may be compromised and IOL centration is a potential problem. Anterior chamber IOLs, iris-sutured, sulcus-fixated, or scleral-sutured IOLs may be indicated in these patients.

Glaucoma patients desire the same options in vision rehabilitation as nonglaucoma patients undergoing cataract surgery. This includes consideration of vision with reduced dependence on glasses. Monovision, achieved by IOL or contact lens correction, can be offered to glaucoma patients. Contact lenses are best avoided in patients with filtration blebs in order to minimize the risk of external infection. Some surgeons may consider multifocal or accommodating IOLs in glaucoma patients. This may be a reasonable consideration in patients with mild, well-controlled glaucoma without significant optic nerve damage or visual field compromise. However, because glaucoma is a progressive disease, a currently acceptable patient for a multifocal IOL may be problematic in the future.

Multifocal IOLs reduce image quality in part because diffractive interference reduces overall transmission of light and the subsequently transmitted light divides between distance and near foci. This is rarely a problem in a healthy eye. However, in a glaucomatous eye with reduced contrast sensitivity due to optic neuropathy, this may potentially compromise visual function.[71,72]

Accommodating IOLs do not reduce contrast sensitivity and thus may be better suited for glaucoma patients who desire relative spectacle/contact lens independence. Of special note with accommodating IOLs is the requirement for adequate capsule support. Patients with zonular weakness due to pseudoexfoliation or trauma are not good candidates for accommodating IOLs. Indeed, multifocal IOLs are also contraindicated in eyes with zonular weakness due to the need for stable centration.

Pupil size variability, astigmatism related to filtration blebs, and hypotony maculopathy can also magnify the potential deleterious effect on image quality caused by multifocal and accommodating IOLs. These factors must be taken into consideration by surgeons weighing IOL options in their glaucoma patients.

CONCLUSION

The ophthalmic surgeon should not be rigid about indications for any of the surgical options available to patients with cataract and glaucoma (Figure 61-9). The art and science of medicine must enter the decision-making process with the surgical plan individualized for each patient based on the general guidelines noted in this chapter. This is especially true as surgical techniques are constantly evolving and providing the means to produce earlier restoration of good visual acuity and more effective control of IOP.

REFERENCES

1. Shingleton BJ, Pasternack JJ, Hung JW, O'Donoghue MW. Three and five year changes in intraocular pressures after clear corneal phacoemulsification in open angle glaucoma patients, glaucoma suspects, and normal patients. *J Glaucoma*. 2006;15(6):494-498.

2. Issa SA, Pacheco J, Mahmood U, Nolan J, Beatty S. A novel index for predicting intraocular pressure reduction following cataract surgery. *Br J Ophthalmol*. 2005;89(5):543-546.

3. Poley BJ, Lindstrom RL, Samuelson TW, Schulze R Jr. Intraocular pressure reduction after phacoemulsification with intraocular lens implantation in glaucomatous and nonglaucomatous eyes: evaluation of a causal relationship between the natural lens and open-angle glaucoma. *J Cataract Refract Surg*. 2009;35(11):1946-1955.

4. Shingleton BJ, Laul A, Nagao K, et al. Effect of phacoemulsification on intraocular pressure in eyes with pseudoexfoliation: single-surgeon series. *J Cataract Refract Surg*. 2008;34(11):1834-1841.

5. Vizzeri G, Weinreb RN. Cataract surgery and glaucoma. *Curr Opin Ophthalmol*. 2010;21(1):20-24.

6. Shrivastava A, Singh K. The effect of cataract extraction on intraocular pressure. *Curr Opin Ophthalmol*. 2010;21(2):118-122.

7. Shingleton BJ, Richter CU, Dharma S, et. al. Long-term efficacy of argon laser trabeculoplasty—10-year follow-up. *Ophthalmology*. 1993;100:1324-1329.

8. Brown RH, Shingleton BJ, Johnstone M, et al. Glaucoma laser treatment parameters and practices of ASCRS members—1999 survey. American Society of Cataract and Refractive Surgery. *J Cataract Refract Surg*. 2000;26(5):755-765.

9. Rainer G, Menapace R, Schmid KE, et al. Natural course of intraocular pressure after cataract surgery with sodium chondroitin sulfate 4%-sodium hyaluronate 3% (Viscoat). *Ophthalmology*. 2005;112(10):1714-1718.

10. Ahmed IK, Kranemann, Chipman M, Malam F. Revisiting early postoperative follow-up after phacoemulsification. *J Cataract Refract Surg*. 2002;29:100-108.

11. Thirumalai B, Baranyovits PR. Intraocular pressure changes and the implications on patient review after phacoemulsification. *J Cataract Refract Surg*. 2003;29:504-507.

12. Shingleton BJ, Rosenberg RB, Teixeira R, O'Donoghue MW. Evaluation of intraocular pressure in the immediate postoperative period after phacoemulsification. *J Cataract Refract Surg*. 2007;33(11):1953-1957.

13. Levkovitch-Verbin H, Habot-Wilner Z, Burla N, et al. Intraocular pressure elevation within the first 24 hours after cataract surgery in patients with glaucoma or exfoliation syndrome. *Ophthalmology*. 2008;115(1):104-108.

14. Unal M, Yücel I. Effect of bimatoprost on intraocular pressure after cataract surgery. *Can J Ophthalmol*. 2008;43(6):712-716.

15. Borazan M, Karalezli A, Akman A, Akova YA. Effect of antiglaucoma agents on postoperative intraocular pressure after cataract surgery with Viscoat. *J Cataract Refract Surg*. 2007;33(11):1941-1945.

16. Kir E, Cakmak H, Dayanir V. Medical control of intraocular pressure with brinzolamide 1% after phacoemulsification. *Can J Ophthalmol*. 2008;43(5):559-562.

17. Hildebrand GD, Wickremasinghe SS, Tranos PG, Harris ML, Little BC. Efficacy of anterior chamber decompression in controlling early intraocular pressure spikes after uneventful phacoemulsification. *J Cataract Refract Surg*. 2003;29:1087-1092.

18. Shingleton BJ, Wadhwani RA, O'Donoghue MW, Baylus S, Hoey H. Evaluation of intraocular pressure in the immediate period after phacoemulsification. *J Cataract Refract Surg*. 2001;27(4):524-527.

19. Chang DF, Braga-Mele R, Mamalis N, et al. ASCRS Cataract Clinical Committee ASCRS White Paper: clinical review of intraoperative floppy-iris syndrome. *J Cataract Refract Surg*. 2008;34(12):2153-2162.

20. Chang DF, Campbell JR. Intraoperative floppy iris syndrome associated with tamsulosin. *J Cataract Refract Surg*. 2005;31(4):664-673.

21. Hyams M, Mathalone N, Herskovitz M, et al. Intraoperative complications of phacoemulsification in eyes with and without pseudoexfoliation. *J Cataract Refract Surg*. 2005;31(5):1002-1005.

22. Shingleton BJ, Crandall AS, Ahmed II. Pseudoexfoliation and the cataract surgeon: preoperative, intraoperative, and postoperative issues related to intraocular pressure, cataract, and intraocular lenses. *J Cataract Refract Surg*. 2009;35(6):1101-1120.

23. Jehan FS, Mamalis N, Crandall AS. Spontaneous late dislocation of intraocular lens within the capsular bag in pseudoexfoliation patients. *Ophthalmology*. 2001;108(10):1727-1731.

24. Shingleton BJ, Chang MA, Bellows AR, Thomas, AV. Surgical goniosynechialysis for angle-closure glaucoma. *Ophthalmology*. 1990;97(5):551-556.

25. Teekhasaenee C, Ritch R. Combined phacoemulsification and goniosynechialysis for uncontrolled chronic angle-closure glaucoma after acute angle-closure glaucoma. *Ophthalmology*. 1999;106(4):669-674; discussion 674-675.

26. Jacobi PC, Dietlein JS, Cala C, Engels B, Krieglstein GK. Primary phacoemulsification and intraocular lens implantation for acute angle-closure glaucoma. *Ophthalmology*. 2002;109(9):1597-1603.

27. Lam DS, Leung DY, Tham CC, et al. Randomized trial of early phacoemulsification versus peripheral iridotomy to prevent intraocular pressure rise after acute primary angle closure. *Ophthalmology*. 2008;115(7):1134-1140.

28. Imaizumi M, Takaki Y, Yamashita H. Phacoemulsification and intraocular lens implantation for acute angle closure not treated or previously treated by laser iridotomy. *J Cataract Refract Surg*. 2006;32(1):85-90.

29. Jacobi PC, Dietlein JS, Cala C, Engels B, Krieglstein GK. Primary phacoemulsification and intraocular lens implantation for acute angle-closure glaucoma. *Ophthalmology*. 2002;109:1597-1603.

30. Buys YM, Chipman ML, Zack B, Rootman DS, Slomovic AR, Trope GE. Prospective randomized comparison of one- versus two-site phacotrabeculectomy two-year results. *Ophthalmology*. 2008;115(7):1130-1133.e1.

31. Shingleton BJ, Price RS, O'Donoghue MW. Comparison of 1-site versus 2-site phacotrabeculectomy. *J Cataract Refract Surg*. 2006;32(5):799-802.

32. El Sayyad F, Helal M, El-Maghraby A, Khalil M, El-Hamzawey H. One site versus 2-site phacotrabeculectomy: a randomized study. *J Cataract Refract Surg*. 1999;25:77-82.

33. Wyse T, Meyer M, Ruderman JM, et al. Combined trabeculectomy and phacoemulsification: a one-site vs. a two-site approach. *Am J Ophthalmol*. 1998;125:334-339.

34. Bayer A, Erdem U, Mumcuoglu T, Akyol M. Two-site phacotrabeculectomy versus bimanual microincision cataract surgery combined with trabeculectomy. *Eur J Ophthalmol*. 2009;19(1):46-54.

35. Jampel HD, Friedman DS, Lubomski LH, et al. Effect of technique on intraocular pressure after combined cataract and glaucoma surgery: an evidence-based review. *Ophthalmology*. 2002;109(12):2215-2224.

36. Shingleton BJ, Chaudhry IM, O'Donoghue MW, et al. Phacotrabeculectomy: limbus-based versus fornix-based conjunctival flaps in fellow eyes. *Ophthalmology*. 1999;106(6):1152-1155.

37. Cagini C, Murdolo P, Gallai R. Longterm results of one-site phacotrabeculectomy. *Acta Ophthalmol Scand*. 2003;81(3):233-236.

38. Shingleton BJ, Kalina PH. Combined phacoemulsification, intraocular lens implantation, and trabeculectomy with a modified scleral tunnel and single-stitch closure. *J Cataract Refract Surg*. 1995;21(5):528-532.

39. Shingleton BJ, Chaudhry IM, O'Donoghue MW. Phacotrabe-culectomy: peripheral iridectomy or no peripheral iridectomy? *J Cataract Refract Surg.* 2002;28:998-1002.

40. Manners TD, Mireskandari K. Phacotrabeculectomy without peripheral iridectomy. *Ophthalmic Surg Lasers.* 1999;30(8):631-635.

41. Jin GJ, Crandall AS, Jones JJ. Phacotrabeculectomy: assessment of outcomes and surgical improvements. *J Cataract Refract Surg.* 2007;33(7):1201-1208.

42. Shin DH, Iskander NG, Ahec JA, et al. Long-term filtration and visual field outcomes after primary glaucoma triple procedure with and without mitomycin C. *Ophthalmology.* 2002;109:1607-1611.

43. Chung AN, Aung T, Wang JC. Surgical outcomes of combined phacoemulsification and glaucoma drainage implant surgery for Asian patients with refractory glaucoma with cataract. *Am J Ophthalmol.* 2004;137(2):294-300.

44. Nassiri N, Nassiri N, Sadeghi Yarandi S, Mohammadi B, Rahmani L. Combined phacoemulsification and Ahmed valve glaucoma drainage implant: a retrospective case series. *Eur J Ophthalmol.* 2008;18(2):191-198.

45. Hoffman KB, Feldman RM, Budenz DL, et al. Combined cataract extraction and Baerveldt glaucoma drainage implant: indications and outcomes. *Ophthalmology.* 2002;109(10):1916-1920.

46. Maris PJ Jr, Ishida K, Netland PA. Comparison of trabeculectomy with Ex-PRESS® miniature glaucoma device implanted under scleral flap. *J Glaucoma.* 2007;16(1):14-19.

47. Kanner EM, Netland PA, Sarkisian SR Jr, Du H. Ex-PRESS® miniature glaucoma device implanted under a scleral flap alone or combined with phacoemulsification cataract surgery. *J Glaucoma.* 2009;18(6):488-491.

48. De Feo F, Bagnis A, Bricola G, Scotto R, Traverso CE. Efficacy and safety of a steel drainage device implanted under a scleral flap. *Can J Ophthalmol.* 2009;44(4):457-462.

49. Kobayashi H, Kobayashi K. Randomized comparison of the intraocular pressure-lowering effect of phacoviscocanalostomy and phacotrabeculectomy. *Ophthalmology.* 2007;114:905-914.

50. Park M, Tanito M, Nishikawa M, Hayeshi K, Chihera E. Combined viscocanalostomy and cataract surgery compared with cataract surgery in Japanese patients with glaucoma. *J Glaucoma.* 2004;13:55-61.

51. Shingleton B, Tetz M, Korber N. Circumferential viscodilation and tensioning of Schlemm canal (canaloplasty) with temporal clear corneal phacoemulsification cataract surgery for open-angle glaucoma and visually significant cataract: one-year results. *J Cataract Refract Surg.* 2008;34(3):433-440.

52. Francis BA, Minckler D, Dustin L, et al. Trabectome Study Group. Combined cataract extraction and trabeculotomy by the internal approach for coexisting cataract and open-angle glaucoma: initial results. *J Cataract Refract Surg.* 2008;34(7):1096-1103.

53. Gayton JL, Van Der Karr MA, Sanders V. Combined cataract and glaucoma surgery: trabeculectomy vs. endoscopic laser cycloablation. *J Cataract Refract Surg.* 1999;25:1214-1219.

54. Uram M. Ophthalmic laser microendoscope endophotocoagulation. *Ophthalmology.* 1992;99(12):1829-1832.

55. Murthy GJ, Murthy PR, Murthy KR, Kulkarni VV. A study of the efficacy of endoscopic cyclophotocoagulation for the treatment of refractory glaucomas. *Indian J Ophthalmol.* 2009;57:127-132.

56. Spiegel D, García-Feijoó J, García-Sánchez J, Lamielle H. Coexistent primary open-angle glaucoma and cataract: preliminary analysis of treatment by cataract surgery and the iStent trabecular micro-bypass stent. *Adv Ther.* 2008;25(5):453-464.

57. Spiegel D, Wetzel W, Neuhann T, et al. Coexistent primary open-angle glaucoma and cataract: interim analysis of a trabecular micro-bypass stent and concurrent cataract surgery. *Eur J Ophthalmol.* 2009;19(3):393-399.

58. Melamed S, Simon GB, Goldenfeld M, Simon G. Efficacy and safety of gold micro shunt implantation to the supraciliary space in patients with glaucoma: a pilot study. *Arch Ophthalmol.* 2009;127(3):264-269.

59. Minckler DS, Hill RA. Use of novel devices for control of intraocular pressure. *Exp Eye Res.* 2009;88(4):792-798.

60. Rebolleda G, Munoz-Negrete FJ. Phacoemulsification in eyes with functioning filtering blebs: a prospective study. *Ophthalmology.* 2002;109:2248-2255.

61. Klink J, Schmitz B, Lieb WE, et al. Filtering bleb function after clear cornea phacoemulsification: a prospective study. *Br J Ophthalmol.* 2005;89(5):597-601.

62. Zaltas M, Schuman J, Shingleton B, et al. Cataract extraction following filtering surgery. *Invest Ophthalmol Vis Sci.* 1994;35(ARVO suppl):1420.

63. The AGIS Investigators. The advanced glaucoma intervention study, 8: risk of cataract formation after trabeculectomy. *Arch Ophthalmol.* 2001;199:1771-1780.

64. Adelman RA, Brauner SC, Afshari NA, Grosskreutz CL. Cataract formation after initial trabeculectomy in young patients. *Ophthalmology.* 2003;110:625-629.

65. Shingleton BJ, O'Donoghue MW, Hall PE. Results of phacoemulsification in eyes with preexisting glaucoma filters. *J Cataract Refract Surg.* 2003;29:1093-1096.

66. Chen PP, Weaver YK, Budenz DL, Feuer WJ, Parrish RK II. Trabeculectomy function after cataract extraction. *Ophthalmology.* 1996;105:1928-1935.

67. Shingleton BJ, Alfano C, O'Donoghue MW, Riviera J. The efficacy of glaucoma filtration surgery in pseudophakic patients with or without conjunctival scarring. *J Cataract Refract Surg.* 2004;30:2504-2509.

68. Pokroy R, Greenwald Y, Pollack A, Bukelman A, Zalish M. Visual loss after transscleral diode laser cyclophotocoagulation for primary open-angle and neovascular glaucoma. *Ophthalmic Surg Lasers Imaging.* 2008;39(1):22-29.

69. Barnes EA, Murdoch IE, Subramanian S, et al. Neodymium: Yttrium–Aluminum–Garnet capsulotomy and intraocular pressure in pseudophakic patients with glaucoma. *Ophthalmology.* 2004;111:1393-1397.

70. Samuelson TW, Chu YR, Kreiger RA. Evaluation of giant-cell deposits on foldable intraocular lenses after combined cataract and glaucoma surgery. *J Cataract Refract Surg.* 2000;26:817-823.

71. Teichman JC, Ahmed II. Intraocular lens choices for patients with glaucoma. *Curr Opin Ophthalmol.* 2010;21(2):135-143.

72. Kumar BV, Phillips RP, Prasad S. Multifocal intraocular lenses in the setting of glaucoma. *Curr Opin Ophthalmol.* 2007;18(1): 62-66.

62

Aqueous Shunting Procedures

Sarwat Salim, MD, FACS and Malik Y. Kahook, MD

Aqueous shunting procedures were introduced by Molteno and colleagues[1-4] in 1968 to treat refractory glaucomas. In the initial design, an 8.5-mm² acrylic plate was attached to an acrylic tube to allow the formation of a bleb, with free communication to the anterior chamber that could not shrink to an area less than that of the plate. This device successfully controlled intraocular pressure (IOP) in many patients who were otherwise poor surgical candidates. However, problems related to early postoperative hypotony from overfiltration and late IOP increases resulting from fibrous encapsulation of the filtering bleb limited the usefulness of this procedure.

During the past 40 years, design modifications and improvements in surgical techniques have led to greater success and lower complication rates with the Molteno implant (IOP Inc, Costa Mesa, CA, and Molteno Ophthalmic Ltd, Dunedin, New Zealand). In addition, other glaucoma drainage devices (GDD) have been introduced and offer unique features designed to facilitate implantation, improve IOP control, and reduce acute postoperative hypotony.

CURRENT GLAUCOMA DRAINAGE DEVICES

Available GDD differ in size, shape, and composition material. One fundamental feature distinguishing various types is the presence or absence of a valve in the implant. The valved or flow-restrictive devices allow only unidirectional flow from the anterior chamber to the subconjunctival space with a minimum opening pressure. Examples of valved devices include the Ahmed glaucoma valve (AGV; New World Medical, Inc, Rancho Cucamonga, CA) and Krupin valve (production discontinued). The nonvalved or open-tube or nonrestrictive devices provide passive flow in both anterograde and retrograde direction. Examples of nonvalved devices include the Molteno, Baerveldt (Abbott Medical Optics, Santa Ana, CA), Shocket, and Eagle Vision

(Eagle Vision Inc, Memphis, TN) implants. Because non-valved devices offer no flow restriction, additional measures, to be discussed later, are undertaken intraoperatively and postoperatively to prevent hypotony. Table 62-1 provides a summary of commercially available devices with their respective characteristics.

Molteno Implant

The Molteno implant is a nonvalved device consisting of a silicone tube with an internal diameter of 0.33 mm and an outer diameter of 0.63 mm and is connected to either a rigid polypropylene or a flexible silicone plate. Single-plate (area 137 mm²) and double-plate implants (area 274 mm²) are available.

A dual-chamber, single-plate implant that incorporates a pressure ridge on the upper surface of the episcleral plate has been introduced in an effort to reduce immediate postoperative hypotony and related complications. The double-plate implants are available in right and left models and consist of 2 plates connected by a 10-mm silicone tube. The double-plate implant has been shown to provide improved IOP control because of its larger surface area but is also associated with a higher rate of postoperative hypotony.[5]

Recently, the third-generation Molteno 3 implants have been introduced in both single-plate and double-plate models (Figures 62-1 and 62-2). These newer devices have a lower profile as the height of the original ridge has been reduced and its shape modified from a triangular to elliptical appearance. These modifications are expected to decrease the incidence of postoperative hypotony and improve IOP long-term control.

Shocket Tube: Anterior Chamber Tube to Encircling Band

The anterior chamber tube to encircling band (ACTEB) implant consists of a silastic tube connected to a #20 band

Kahook MY, Schuman JS, eds.
Chandler and Grant's Glaucoma, Fifth Edition (pp 579-594).
© 2013 SLACK Incorporated.

TABLE 62-1. COMMERCIALLY AVAILABLE GLAUCOMA DRAINAGE DEVICES			
Valved Implants			
Type	Model	Size	Material
Ahmed Implant			
Single plate	S2	184 mm^2	Polypropylene
Pediatric size	S3	96 mm^2	Polypropylene
Double plate	B1	364 mm^2	Polypropylene
Single plate	FP7	184 mm^2	Silicone
Pediatric size	FP8	96 mm^2	Silicone
Double plate	FX1	364 mm^2	Silicone
Pars plana	PS2	184 mm^2	Polypropylene
Pars plana (pediatric)	PS3	96 mm^2	Polypropylene
Pars plana	PC7	184 mm^2	Silicone
Pars plana pediatric)	PC8	96 mm^2	Silicone
Nonvalved Implants			
Baerveldt Implant			
Single plate	103-250	250 mm^2	Silicone
Single plate	101-350	350 mm^2	Silicone
Pars plana	102-350	350 mm^2	Silicone
Eagle Vision Implant	EG365	365 mm^2	Silicone
Molteno Implant			
Single plate	S1	137 mm^2	Polypropylene
Single plate/ridge	D1	137 mm^2	Polypropylene
For microphthalmic eyes	M1	50 mm^2	Polypropylene
Double plate	R2/L2	274 mm^2	Polypropylene
Double plate/ridge	DR2/DL2	274 mm^2	Polypropylene
Molteno 3/single plate	GS	175 mm^2	Polypropylene
Molteno 3/double plate	GL	230 mm^2	Polypropylene

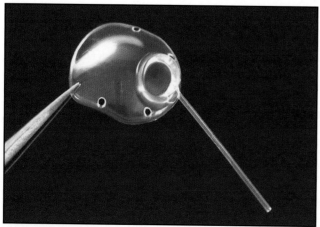

Figure 62-1. Single-plate Molteno. (Reprinted with permission from IOP Inc and Molteno Ophthalmic Ltd.)

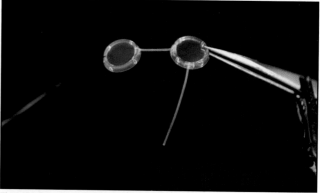

Figure 62-2. Double-plate Molteno. (Reprinted with permission from IOP Inc and Molteno Ophthalmic Ltd.)

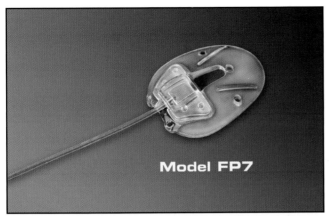

Figure 62-3. Ahmed glaucoma valve (model FP7). (Reprinted with permission from New World Medical, Inc.)

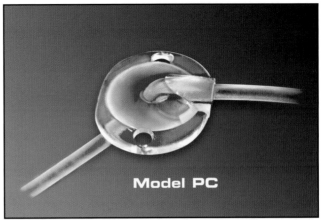

Figure 62-4. Pars plana clip. (Reprinted with permission from New World Medical, Inc.)

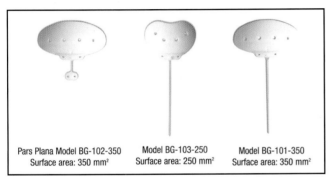

Figure 62-5. Different models of the Baerveldt implant. (Reprinted with permission from Abbott Medical Optics.)

360 degrees in length (surface area: 350 to 450 mm²). The band, placed under 2 or more rectus muscles, creates a reservoir for aqueous drainage. Surgical outcomes with the Shocket tube shunts have been compared to double-plate Molteno implants. Although the encircling band provides a larger surface area for aqueous drainage, the final IOP was reported to be lower than with the Molteno implants.[6,7]

Krupin Valve With Disc

The Krupin valve with disc is no longer being manufactured, but is mentioned for historical purposes; it was the first device to incorporate a unidirectional and pressure-sensitive slit valve (opening pressure 11 mm Hg; closing pressure 9 mm Hg) that served to maintain anterior chamber depth and IOP in the immediate postoperative period. The Krupin valve with disc consisted of a silastic tube with an internal diameter of 0.38 mm connected to an oval silicone plate measuring 13 mm × 18 mm and was 1.75-mm thick.

Ahmed Glaucoma Valve

The AGV is a valved implant consisting of a silastic tube with an outer diameter of 0.63 mm and an inner diameter of 0.30 mm, is connected to a silicone sheet valve, and is held in an elliptical polypropylene or silicone plate (Figure 62-3).

The pressure-sensitive valve consists of 2 opposed silastic sheets that separate to allow aqueous flow at an IOP between 8 and 12 mm Hg. One of the earlier studies[8] assessed the pressure-flow characteristics of various GDD in vitro and in vivo in rabbits. Both the Ahmed and Krupin valves functioned as flow-restricting devices, but a true valve function for these was not elucidated. Subsequent studies,[9,10] however, demonstrated a consistent valve behavior for the AGV, and IOP was regulated within a desired range by decreasing or increasing resistance as a function of flow.

Single-plate (area 184 mm²) and double-plate (area 364 mm²) implants are available. A pars plana clip allows insertion of the tube into the pars plana in aphakic or pseudophakic eyes after complete vitrectomy (Figure 62-4). Smaller-size implants are also available for pediatric use. However, most surgeons use a normal-size implant in children with the expected growth of a child's eye and to achieve better long-term IOP control.

Baerveldt Implant

The Baerveldt implant consists of a silicone tube with an internal diameter of 0.30 mm and an external diameter of 0.64 mm and is connected to a 1-mm thick barium-impregnated plate that allows radiographic identification. The plates are available with surface areas of 200 mm² (20 × 13 mm) and 350 mm² (32 × 14 mm). The pars plana variant consists of a 350-mm² plate with the silicone tube attached to a small silicone episcleral plate with an angled cannula to be inserted through a sclerostomy into the pars plana. This special Hoffman elbow provides a watertight closure that may not be achieved with insertion of the standard tube. All Baerveldt plates consist of 4 fenestrations on the body of the implant to allow fibrous capsule growth between the anterior conjunctival surface and posterior scleral walls (Figure 62-5). These fenestrations are intended to reduce the height of the resulting bleb to lessen the mass effect on the adjacent extraocular muscles and to minimize ocular motility disturbances.

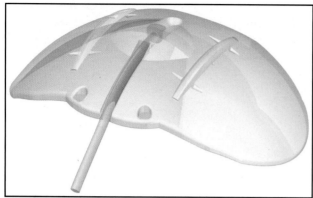

Figure 62-6. Eagle Vision implant. (Reprinted with permission from Eagle Vision Inc.)

TABLE 62-2. SURGICAL INDICATIONS FOR GLAUCOMA DRAINAGE DEVICES
Previously failed trabeculectomy
Conjunctival scarring from previous intraocular surgeries precluding trabeculectomy: previous keratoplasty or retinal surgery
Neovascular glaucoma
Aphakic/pseudophakic glaucoma
Traumatic glaucoma
Uveitic glaucoma
Congenital/juvenile glaucoma
Iridocorneal endothelial syndrome
Epithelial downgrowth
Primary surgery in patients with high risk of trabeculectomy complications

Eagle Vision Implant

The Eagle Vision implant is a nonvalved device with an explant area of 365 mm² (model EG365). Its larger surface area and a more posterior tube placement are designed to increase aqueous flow and promote a posterior bleb. The flexible silicone plate facilitates better globe contour, and added dorsal ridges allow a low bleb profile (Figure 62-6).

1. Preoperative Considerations

2. Patient Selection

GDD are typically reserved for patients with severe uncontrolled glaucoma who have failed previous glaucoma surgery. In addition, the devices appear to be advantageous as a primary procedure in patients with a high likelihood of trabeculectomy failure, including neovascular and uveitic glaucomas.[11-17] Their role in managing congenital and developmental glaucomas has increased exponentially.[18-24] Additional indications include traumatic glaucoma, aphakic and pseudophakic glaucoma, postkeratoplasty glaucoma, and other secondary glaucomas.[25-28] In eyes with useful remaining vision, these devices may be preferable to cyclodestructive procedures that are associated with a high rate of visual loss and phthisis bulbi. Recently, interest has increased in using these devices as a primary surgical procedure for uncontrolled primary open-angle glaucoma (POAG). A randomized, prospective clinical trial comparing trabeculectomy to tube surgery is ongoing, and the preliminary results will be discussed later in this chapter. Table 62-2 provides a summary of indications for inserting GDD.

Clinical Examination

Careful preoperative examination and planning are essential for successful surgical outcomes. Clinicians should assess mobility of the conjunctiva to determine the best quadrant for drainage implant insertion. Attention should be paid to areas of scleral thinning in patients with collagen vascular diseases and especially in children with buphthalmos.

These situations require extra caution and special needles when anchoring the plates to the sclera to avoid perforation. The cornea should be examined for arcus senilis, which may impair visualization and misguide tube insertion into the anterior chamber. If corneal endothelial damage is present, a pars plana tube insertion may be preferred. If there is significant corneal decompensation in the presence of a cataract, a triple procedure may be required. The iris should be inspected under high magnification to detect neovascularization to consider preoperative use of antivascular endothelial growth factor (anti-VEGF) agents to minimize intraoperative and postoperative bleeding. Anterior chamber depth should be assessed to determine if tube insertion in the anterior chamber would be safe without touching the iris or cornea. The lenticular status of the eye should be noted. The tube may be placed in the sulcus in a pseudophakic eye or pars plana in an aphakic, vitrectomized eye. In an eye with a cataract, a combined surgery may be considered. Gonioscopy should be performed to determine the locations of peripheral anterior synechiae (PAS), which are commonly seen in neovascular, uveitic, or traumatic glaucoma, and neovascularization of the angle in eyes with neovascular glaucoma. PAS-free sites should be marked in the chart for correct position of the tube intraoperatively. If PAS are low-lying, the tube may be entered anteriorly to these in the false angle. If PAS are very anteriorly placed, an iridectomy may be required intraoperatively to facilitate tube insertion. Alternatively, a tube in the sulcus or pars plana may be planned.

Selection of Glaucoma Drainage Device

For a beginning surgeon, valved devices may be preferred as the surgical technique is simpler with localization to one quadrant without manipulation of the adjacent rectus muscles. IOP control in the early postoperative period is more predictable with these devices because of flow-restricting mechanisms.

In eyes with a high likelihood of suprachoroidal hemorrhage, including those with aphakia, previous vitrectomy, uncontrolled blood pressure, use of anticoagulants, or very high IOP preoperatively, valved implants may be safer by minimizing dramatic IOP fluctuations.

In patients with poor compliance with postoperative medication use and follow-up visits, valved implants may be preferred because they usually require less postoperative follow-up and care.

The amount of conjunctival scarring may determine the size of the implant and available area for a single-plate versus double-plate device.

The most important factor determining the type of implant selected is the target IOP, both in the short-term and long-term. Early IOP control is determined by the presence or absence of a valve in an implant as the tube offers no resistance to aqueous flow. The valved devices provide more immediate IOP control and a lower rate of hypotony. Because nonvalved devices are often occluded with a stent or ligature suture, the postoperative IOP is unchanged and requires continuation of all preoperative medications until the fibrous capsule forms. With all devices, long-term IOP control depends on the surface area of the implant, which determines bleb size, tissue response to the implant, and thickness of the fibrous capsule controlling percolation of aqueous humor through the bleb wall. There is some suggestion[29] that earlier exposure of aqueous humor to the developing capsule may interfere with long-term IOP control. If this is indeed true, then 1-stage or 2-stage insertion of nonvalved devices may be preferable to valved devices to avoid immediate flow of aqueous humor to the plate.

Plate material has been studied in various studies to determine its influence on final IOP, as it may affect tissue reaction and the degree of bleb encapsulation. Ayyala and colleagues[30,31] demonstrated more inflammation with the polypropylene plate (Molteno implant) than with the silicone plate (Krupin implant) when inserted subconjunctivally in rabbits. Two retrospective studies[32,33] compared AGV silicone (model FP7) and polypropylene (model S2) and reported similar results with both models in terms of IOP control, final visual acuity, and postoperative antiglaucoma medications. In one of these studies,[32,33] the silicone valve was associated with fewer serious complications. The AGV silicone and polypropylene material has also been investigated in a prospective, multicenter, comparative series[34] that reported improved final IOP control with the silicone model compared with the polypropylene model. The investigators observed more Tenon's cysts in the polypropylene group.

Plate size of various implants has been investigated to determine its influence on the final IOP. Heuer and colleagues[5] reported improved IOP control with the Molteno

double-plate when compared with the single-plate in a prospective study assessing outcomes in aphakic and pseudophakic glaucoma. In a retrospective study,[35] the double-plate Molteno demonstrated lower mean IOP when compared with the single-plate AGV, 13.3 ± 5.1 mm Hg versus 19 ± 5.8 mm Hg ($p = 0.009$), respectively, at 24 months. In a prospective study comparing 350-mm^2 and 500-mm^2 Baerveldt implants, Lloyd and colleagues[36] reported statistically comparable results with respect to IOP control, visual acuity, and complications. In another prospective study comparing 350-mm^2 and 500-mm^2 Baerveldt implants, Britt and colleagues[37] found better IOP control with the 350-mm^2 Baerveldt implant than with the 500-mm^2 model. These studies indicate that size of the implant does matter, but to a limited extent. Further studies are warranted to determine which one of these variables—size, shape, or composition—is most likely to affect the long-term success of GDD.

Anesthetic Considerations

The choice of anesthesia for inserting a glaucoma drainage device depends on the presence of other medical comorbidities, the cooperation level of the patient, and the comfort of the surgeon. The most commonly used anesthesia is a peribulbar or retrobulbar block, which provides both akinesia and anesthesia. A sub-Tenon's injection is also a good alternative. Topical or intracameral anesthesia is usually not sufficient because of manipulation of extraocular muscles with some implants. General anesthesia may be reserved for patients with claustrophobia, altered mental status, or history of poor cooperation with local anesthesia in previous surgeries.

SURGICAL TECHNIQUE

Implantation of a GDD requires careful attention to detail at every step of the procedure to improve results and minimize postoperative complications. For a one-plate implant, a fornix-based or limbus-based conjunctival incision is created, extending for 90 degrees to 110 degrees centered between 2 rectus muscles. Implantation of the plate is easier with a fornix-based flap; however, the conjunctival closure is more involved. If a fornix-based conjunctival flap is created, 1 or 2 radial relaxing incisions are usually required to allow adequate exposure for insertion of the plate. A corneal or scleral suture can be placed to improve exposure in the working quadrant (Figure 62-7). With the conjunctiva and Tenon layers retracted away from the globe to expose bare sclera, the implant is positioned between 2 rectus muscles so that the anterior edge is approximately 8 to 10 mm posterior to the limbus (Figure 62-8). Larger implants (Baerveldt) are inserted with the long axis directed toward the apex of the orbit and then rotated horizontally so that the tube points directly toward the anterior chamber and the wings of the implant are under the rectus muscles. A muscle hook should be used to identify and mark muscle insertions for proper positioning of the plate between or under the muscles. If a

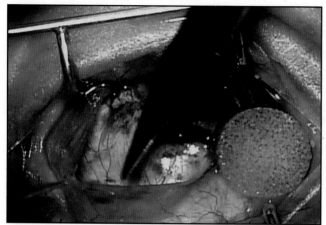

Figure 62-7. 7-0 silk scleral traction suture.

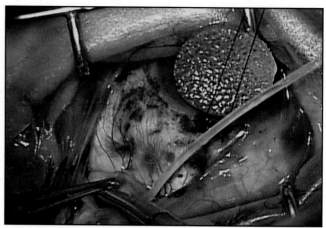

Figure 62-8. Anchorage of plate to sclera using an 8-0 nylon suture.

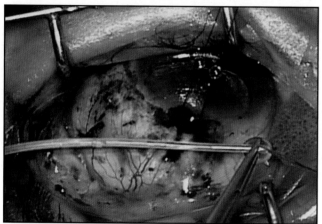

Figure 62-9. Priming of a valved implant.

2-plate implant is used, one plate is positioned in each of 2 quadrants. The tube connecting the 2 plates may be passed under or over the intervening rectus muscle. With all valved implants, the tube should be primed with balanced salt solution with a 30-gauge cannula prior to the plate anchorage to ensure that the valve leaflets are not fused after sterilization techniques (Figure 62-9). The tube of the nonvalved implant should be irrigated as well to ensure its patency.

Once the implant has been appropriately positioned, each plate is secured to the globe with 2 nonabsorbable sutures (8-0 or 9-0 nylon sutures on a spatulated needle). The suture knots should be rotated into the fixation eyelets to prevent erosion through the conjunctiva. Secure attachment to the underlying sclera is essential to prevent anterior, posterior, or lateral migration of the implant during the postoperative period. Inadequate scleral fixation may also lead to retraction of the tube from the anterior chamber or expulsion of the entire plate from the subconjunctival space.

After the plate is attached to the globe, the tube is laid across the cornea and cut with sharp scissors to create a beveled edge with the opening toward the cornea. The tube should extend approximately 2.5 to 3 mm into the anterior chamber to minimize the risk of tube-cornea touch or retraction out of the anterior chamber. A 23-gauge needle is used to create a track through which the tube is inserted into the anterior chamber just anterior and parallel to the iris (Figure 62-10A). Occasionally, insertion of the tube through the scleral track is difficult. A well-beveled tube end (30 degrees to 45 degrees, bevel up) and nontoothed forceps simplify this step. Alternatively, a tube inserter (New World Medical, Inc) is available to facilitate this maneuver (Figure 62-10B). After the tube has been inserted into the anterior chamber, its position is checked carefully to ensure that there is no tube-cornea touch or iris incarceration (Figure 62-10C). If the tube is malpositioned, a new entry track should be created to the side of the original track through which the tube should be reinserted. If the original entry site is leaking, the scleral opening should be sutured closed to maintain anterior chamber depth intraoperatively and to avoid postoperative overfiltration and hypotony. The tube may be secured to the sclera a few millimeters anterior to the plate with an 8-0 Vicryl suture (some surgeons prefer an 8-0 or 9-0 nylon suture). This suture helps to stabilize the tube and should not be tight; otherwise, it will restrict flow in valved devices.

The tube is covered to prevent its erosion through the conjunctiva. Patch graft materials include processed pericardium, sclera, fascia lata, dura, or cornea. Usually, a 6-mm × 6-mm patch graft is used to provide good coverage. The graft is positioned to overlay the tube insertion site into the anterior chamber, and the limbal edge is thinned to avoid an overhanging bleb that can lead to Dellen formation. The patch graft should be secured to the globe with interrupted sutures at the anterior corners by using either 8-0 Vicryl or nylon sutures (Figure 62-11). Recently, fibrin glue has been shown to be an effective, although expensive, substitute for sutures and was reported to reduce surgical time and postoperative inflammation.[38] Additional studies are needed to understand its role further. All suture ends should be buried beneath the scleral graft to prevent them from later eroding through the conjunctiva. If the patch graft material is not

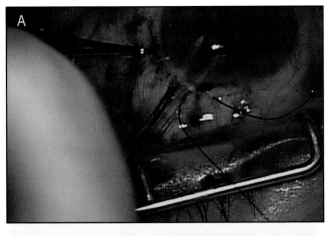

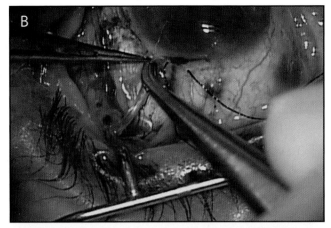

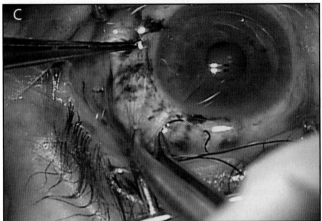

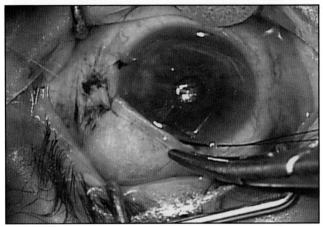

Figure 62-10. (A) Twenty-three-gauge needle entry. (B) Insertion of tube with tube inserter. (C) Correct position of tube.

Figure 62-11. Securing Tutoplast to the sclera with an 8-0 Vicryl suture.

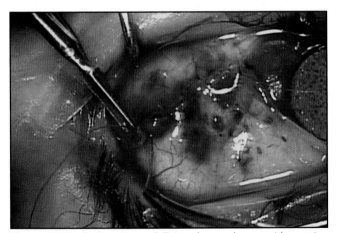

Figure 62-12. Conjunctiva and Tenon layers closure with running 8-0 Vicryl suture.

available, a partial-thickness scleral flap can be constructed. The needle track and tube entry are done under this flap. The flap is then sutured with 10-0 nylon sutures.

After the patch graft has been placed, the conjunctiva and Tenon layers are pulled over the plate, tube, and patch graft and are secured into place with an 8-0 Vicryl suture (Figure 62-12). In some cases, the monofilament 9-0 Vicryl suture is preferred because of its higher tensile strength and finer vascular needle to prevent buttonholes when handling thin conjunctiva. Prior to conjunctival closure, some surgeons cauterize the limbal margin of the cornea to remove the epithelium and to provide a bed to facilitate the attachment of the conjunctiva during the healing process. Wing sutures at both ends of the peritomy are recommended to approximate the conjunctiva at the limbus. A locked running Vicryl suture is useful in closing the radial relaxing incision.

At the end of the operation, the eye should be inspected to ensure that the implant plate, patch graft, and intraocular portion of the tube are in a good position. Fluorescein drops or strips can be used to inspect the conjunctiva for leaks. Any buttonholes found in the conjunctiva should be closed with a 9-0 Vicryl suture. At the conclusion of the procedure, a subconjunctival injection of antibiotic and steroid is given.

Modifications to Prevent Hypotony With Nonvalved Implants

Internal Tube Occlusion (Stent)

Aqueous drainage through a nonvalved device can be regulated in the early postoperative period by passing a 4-0 or 5-0 Prolene or nylon suture through the lumen of the implant tube.[39] The stent suture is brought out through the tube, over the implant plate, and is placed with its free end in an adjacent subconjunctival quadrant (Figure 62-13). Once the fibrous capsule around the plate has formed, the stent suture is removed at the slit-lamp under local anesthesia and the aqueous humor can flow freely into the fibrous capsule that has formed around the implant plate. Although this technique is effective in preventing early postoperative hypotony, immediate postoperative IOP elevations from tube occlusion may make early suture removal necessary, increasing the risk of hypotony, shallow chamber, and related complications.

External Tube Occlusion (Ligature)

The flow of aqueous humor through a nonvalved device can also be restricted by placing a suture ligature around the external aspect of the tube.[40,41] The external occlusion may be accomplished using a nonabsorbable 7-0 suture with a releasable knot or a 7-0 or 8-0 absorbable Vicryl suture tied around the tube. Alternatively, a 9-0 nylon or 10-0 Prolene suture may be used to ligate the tube inside the anterior chamber to allow for later suture lysis with the argon laser. The remnant of this suture remains in the anterior chamber. Similar to an internal occluding suture, release of an external ligating suture is usually performed 4 to 6 weeks postoperatively, which allows time for a fibrous capsule to form around the plate to provide resistance to aqueous flow when the suture is released. Because of this prolonged delay before the IOP is reduced, this technique is poorly suited for patients with exceedingly high pressures during the preoperative period. Attempts to tie the ligature sutures at different tensions to create a titrated aqueous flow rate are unpredictable and may result in under- or overfiltration. Some surgeons create venting slits anterior to the ligature suture with either a needle or a knife for aqueous drainage, thereby allowing immediate IOP control in the early postoperative period.

Two-Stage Procedure

To prevent postoperative hypotony, a shunt procedure may be performed in 2 stages.[2] In the first stage, the plate is attached to the globe and the tube is left in the subconjunctival space without entering the eye. Four to 6 weeks later, after

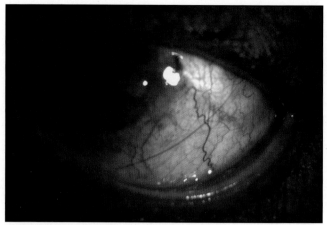

Figure 62-13. Prolene stent in an inferior fornix for a nonvalved implant.

a capsule has formed around the implant, the conjunctiva is opened and the tube is inserted into the anterior chamber to complete the procedure. A major disadvantage of this procedure is that it does not reduce IOP until the second stage is complete, making it poorly suited for eyes with extremely high IOP in the preoperative period. Combining the first stage of the operation with a trabeculectomy in an adjacent quadrant allows for immediate IOP control and provides time for capsule formation around the plate. In this procedure, the second stage of the procedure is performed when the trabeculectomy fails and IOP increases.

Pars Plana Insertion

The tube of the GDD is most commonly placed in the anterior chamber. However, the tube may also be placed in the sulcus in a pseudophakic eye or in the pars plana in a vitrectomized eye. This procedure can be accomplished using 1 of 2 options: a Pars Plana Clip (Model PC, New World Medical, Inc), which can be used with any drainage device, or Hoffman elbow, that is mounted on a Baerveldt 350-mm² implant (Abbott Medical Optics, Inc). The plate is secured to the sclera as described above. A 21-gauge needle is inserted through the sclera approximately 3 mm from the limbus in a pseudophakic eye and 3.5 mm from the limbus in a phakic eye. The needle should be angled parallel to the iris plane for proper positioning of the tube through this track. The tube should be of adequate length (4 to 5 mm) to allow visualization through the pupil. The tube can be secured and ligated, and the rest of the procedure can be completed as described above. The clip or the elbow portion should be secured to the sclera using nonabsorbable sutures. Pars plana models reduce the incidence of tube-related anterior segment complications, especially in the setting of a shallow anterior chamber, penetrating keratoplasty, or concomitant need for retina surgery; however, the eye must be completely vitrectomized to avoid occlusion of the tube with the vitreous.[42]

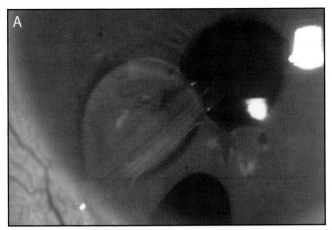 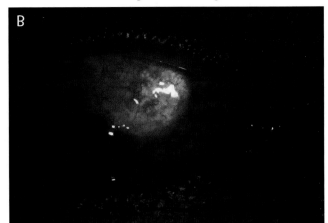

Figure 62-14. (A) Inferior Ahmed glaucoma valve with silicone oil around the tube. (B) Silicone oil under superior conjunctiva.

SITE OF IMPLANTATION

With the exception of the 2-plate implants, most glaucoma implants are placed in a single quadrant. Whenever possible, single-plate implants should be placed in the superotemporal quadrant. This area provides the easiest access for the surgeon to implant the plate and is least likely to produce motility disturbances. Implantation of a large-plate aqueous shunt in the superonasal quadrant has been associated with Brown's superior oblique tendon syndrome.[43] Substantial hypertropias and limitations of downgaze have been reported with inferior implantation of a 2-plate Molteno and the Krupin valve with disc.[44] If severe conjunctival scarring necessitates the placement of an inferior or superonasal shunt, the possibility of ocular motility disturbance and diplopia should be discussed with the patient. Using a smaller plate implant may be less likely to cause a muscle imbalance; however, the risk of strabismus must be weighed against the better IOP control, which is often achieved with a larger or multiple plate implants. In eyes containing silicone oil, the implant is placed in the inferior quadrant to minimize loss of oil, which is lighter than aqueous and floats up (Figure 62-14).

ROLE OF ANTIFIBROSIS AGENTS

Molteno[3] was the first to suggest that the success rate of aqueous shunting procedures could be improved by adding antifibrosis therapy. Molteno used a combination of epinephrine, atropine, topical steroids, oral steroids, and colchicine to reduce postoperative scarring and bleb fibrosis in an attempt to increase the success rate of his procedure. Because of the high frequency of systemic side effects associated with this regimen, it is rarely used today.

Using antimetabolites with improved success in trabeculectomy led to considerable interest in using these agents with GDDs. One early study[45] indicated that patients receiving mitomycin C at the time of glaucoma implant surgery had lower final IOP, required fewer postoperative medications, and had less pronounced hypertensive phases; however, the duration of the postoperative hypotensive phase was prolonged and was associated with an increase in choroidal effusions, flat anterior chambers, and other postoperative complications. However, subsequent studies have not shown these agents to be effective. Two retrospective studies[46,47] reported no benefit of intraoperative use of mitomycin C with Baerveldt implants. Two prospective randomized trials[48,49] studied the effectiveness of intraoperative use of mitomycin C with Molteno and AGV implantation. Neither trial demonstrated a higher success rate with intraoperative mitomycin C in terms of final IOP, visual acuity, and number of antiglaucoma medications required postoperatively. In addition, concern has been raised that antifibrosis agents may lead to exposure of the underlying implant because of thinning of the overlying issues, thereby increasing the risk of infection.[50] Therefore, antifibrosis agents are not used with insertion of GDD.

POSTOPERATIVE COURSE

Following glaucoma drainage implant surgery, the patient is seen on postoperative day 1, and attention is paid to the tube position and wound architecture. A topical antibiotic and steroid are started 4 times daily and are continued for 4 to 6 weeks. Initial follow-up is at 1 week and the frequency of visits depends on the clinical status of the eye. For valved implants, preoperative glaucoma medications are discontinued to prevent hypotony. For nonvalved implants, the glaucoma medications are usually continued until a fibrous capsule forms around the plate, at which point the ligature suture may spontaneously open. If further IOP lowering is required, the stent can also be removed.

COMPLICATIONS AND MANAGEMENT

Aqueous shunting procedures can be associated with various postoperative complications. The surgeon should be aware of the common complications and their management before undertaking these procedures. Judicious preoperative planning and meticulous surgical technique are keys to successful outcomes. Careful attention to plate and tube placement, use

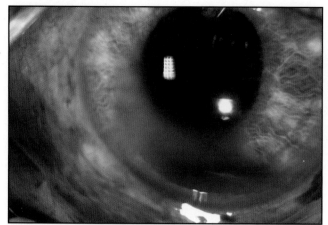

Figure 62-15. Hyphema after Ahmed glaucoma valve.

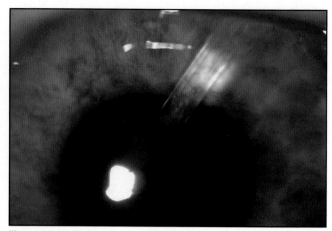

Figure 62-16. Occluded tube with blood.

of an appropriately fashioned patch graft, careful conjunctival closure, and use of a hypotony-preventing surgical modification or implant will minimize these problems. The early postoperative complications of aqueous shunt procedures are similar to other filtration procedures, including flat chambers, hypotony, and suprachoroidal hemorrhage.[3,5,11,36]

Hypotony

Hypotony and its related sequelae, choroidal effusions or suprachoroidal hemorrhage, are more commonly observed with the nonvalved drainage devices. Early postoperative hypotony usually results from wound leak, inflammation, incomplete occlusion of the tube, or larger venting slits with nonvalved implants. Valved implants usually reduce but do not eliminate hypotony. Hypotony with valved implants may result from overfiltration. Fluid may leak around the tube if a large-size needle is used to make the track or if the track is inadvertently extended as the needle is pulled out of the eye. It is important to stabilize the eye well when guiding the needle to make the track, and effort should be made to avoid lateral movement with the needle. Hypotonous eyes are conservatively managed as long as the anterior chamber depth is maintained. If there is lenticular-corneal touch, then a viscoelastic should be injected to reform the anterior chamber. Associated choroidal effusions are generally treated with corticosteroid and cycloplegic agents. If these measures fail, surgical revision may be required.

Valve Malfunction

This is a rare complication. All valved devices should be primed at the time of the surgery, as sterilization techniques may lead to adhesion of the valve membranes that prevents flow to the plate.[51] In addition, careful surgical handling during insertion is required to prevent damage to the plastic rivets holding the valve and to avoid creating gaps between the valve cover and valve body junction, which may be responsible for secondary fibrovascular ingrowth and late-onset distal occlusion and failure of the device.[52]

Hyphema

Hyphema may occur following procedures performed on eyes with neovascular glaucoma (Figure 62-15). However, the hyphema is typically small and clears spontaneously with no adverse effect on the outcome of surgery. It is seen less commonly now with the preoperative use of anti-VEGF agents.

Scleral Perforation

Scleral perforation is a rare complication during anchorage of the plate to the sclera. Care must be taken in buphthalmic eyes and eyes with collagen vascular diseases where there may be localized or diffuse areas of scleral thinning. These situations require rapid identification and immediate treatment to preserve remaining vision.

Tube-Related Problems

Care should be taken to place the tube in the anterior chamber correctly. The usual distance for tube insertion from the limbus is 0.5 to 1.5 mm. If the tube is placed too anteriorly, it will cause decompensation of the corneal endothelium. If the tube is placed too posteriorly, it will cause inflammation by rubbing on the iris and may also result in cataract formation if it touches the anterior lens capsule. If, in the operating room, the tube is found to be malpositioned, it should be removed. The needle track should be closed with interrupted 10-0 nylon sutures to maintain anterior chamber depth intraoperatively and prevent hypotony postoperatively. A new track should be created for tube reinsertion.

If the tube is inadvertently cut too short, either an angiocatheter or tube extender can be used to obtain the desired length.[53]

Tube block from blood (Figure 62-16), vitreous, fibrin, or iris incarceration in the early postoperative period can occur. A neodymium:yttrium-aluminum-garnet (Nd:YAG) laser may be helpful in some cases,[54] whereas in others, a return trip to the operating room to clear the tube end may be required, especially in eyes with retained vitreous that may necessitate vitrectomy. In cases with suspected incomplete vitrectomy, kenalog can be used to guide vitrectomy and ascertain that there is no remaining vitreous prior to tube insertion. If the tube is clogged by a blood clot, tissue plasminogen activator (0.1 to 0.2 mL of 5 to 20 μg) may be beneficial to dissolve the clot. Tube obstruction because of kinking of the tube has been reported after pars plana AGV insertion.[55] The obstruction was treated with a pars plana clip. The pars plana clip has a smooth surface, thereby avoiding tube kinking, and can be used with any glaucoma drainage device that is being considered for pars plana insertion. Alternatively, a Baerveldt implant with a Hoffman elbow is also available for pars plana insertion.

Tube retraction and anterior migration are more commonly seen in children. As the eye grows, the tube may retract or touch the corneal endothelium. Retracted tubes can be lengthened with tube extenders or, alternatively, can be placed in the pars plana. Anterior migration of the tube can be fixed by shortening its length and with a more posterior reinsertion.

Tube Erosion and Endophthalmitis

Tube erosion usually results from conjunctival melting near the limbus overlying the tube and may be related to poor patch graft preparation or placement; however, even without these factors, melting of the conjunctiva and patch graft occur over time and result in tube exposure (Figure 62-17). Replacing the patch graft and mobilizing a conjunctival sliding graft may be useful in repairing these defects. If conjunctival advancement is not sufficient, a conjunctival autograft should be obtained from another quadrant to cover the tube and patch graft. An exposed tube or plate is considered an ocular emergency requiring prompt surgical intervention to prevent endophthalmitis. The risk of endophthalmitis has been reported to be more common in children.[56]

Migration or Expulsion of the Plate

These are seen less commonly than are tube migration and tube erosion. Migration and expulsion usually result from placing the plate too anteriorly. A caliper should be used during surgery to assess correct distance from the limbus, and correct sutures should be used to secure the plate to the sclera.

Corneal Decompensation

Poor tube placement with lens-cornea touch or persistent flat chamber from hypotony may result in corneal edema. In eyes that have undergone penetrating keratoplasty, the risk of graft failure in eyes that develop a flat chamber postoperatively is high.[25,57-59] The use of valved and stented implants that better maintain the anterior chamber depth reduces this complication. Alternatively, placing the tube in pars plana helps to avoid corneal or graft decompensation.

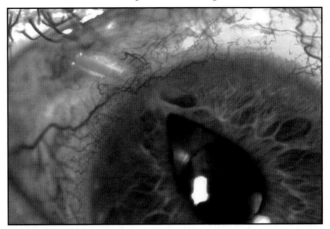
Figure 62-17. Exposed tube.

Overhanging Bleb

If the patch graft is too thick or the plate is too anterior, an overhanging bleb may be created, resulting in chronic Dellen formation and ocular irritation. This complication is best prevented by appropriate plate and patch graft placement during surgery.

Strabismus

Extraocular muscle imbalance with devastating diplopia may also occur and is particularly common in cases of inferior implant placement. This imbalance usually results from a mass effect of the plate and the surrounding bleb on adjacent extraocular muscles. Therefore, this appears to be more common in drainage devices with larger-diameter plates.[60-62] Other possible causes include Faden or posterior fixation suture effect induced by scarring under the rectus muscles, entrapment of superior oblique muscle, or fat fibrosis syndrome because of inadvertent manipulation of orbital fat.[63,64] With superonasal insertion of drainage devices, a pseudo-Brown's syndrome may occur.[43,65] Diplopia secondary to drainage devices is difficult to treat, and various treatment options include prisms, muscle surgery, or even removal of the drainage implant.

Hypertensive Phase

Hypertensive phase is characterized by elevated IOP, typically in the 30- to 50-mm Hg range, occurring anywhere between 1 and 6 weeks postoperatively. This condition has been reported after inserting all types of drainage devices, but more common with valved implants.[35,66] In eyes with hypertensive phase, the tube does not appear to be occluded by any of the methods described above, and elevated IOP is presumably secondary to a thick-walled bleb over the plate of the implant, which decreases permeability of the aqueous humor through the conjunctiva. In terms of etiology of this entity, some patient-related risk factors have been proposed,[67] including male gender, prior trabeculoplasty, prior conjunctival surgery, use of preoperative beta-blockers, or the type of glaucoma (neovascular or uveitic glaucoma, in particular); however, their potential influence needs to be evaluated further. In terms of implant-related factors, the incidence of hypertensive phase appears to be higher with valved implants than with nonvalved implants, smaller-size implants with less available surface area for filtration, or polypropylene plates rather than silicone plates.[31,32,34,68] Treatment options for hypertensive phase include medical therapy, digital massage, bleb needling with or without 5-fluorouracil, and possible surgical excision of the bleb.[68,69] When all these measures fail, a second drainage implant or cyclodestructive procedure may be considered.

CLINICAL OUTCOMES

GDD have been shown to provide effective IOP control in eyes that have failed prior surgery or have a poor prognosis for standard filtration surgery.[5,12,19,25,36,70] At 2 years of follow-up, most studies indicated overall success rates of 50% to 80% with the outcome depending on the type of glaucoma present and the type of implant selected.

Molteno Implant

The success rates with the Molteno implant have been reported to be 74% at 33 months and 57% with a mean follow-up of 44 months.[71,72] In the latter study,[72] linear attrition of success was demonstrated over 5 years by Kaplan-Meier curves; the highest success was observed in the uveitic glaucoma group; and no difference was noted in outcomes based on single- versus double-plate design and single-stage versus 2-stage surgery.[72] In contrast, Heuer and colleagues[5] reported more effective IOP control with double-plate implantation compared with single-plate implantation, 71% versus 46%, respectively, at 2 years. IOP reduction was found to be effective with the pressure-ridge Molteno implants, but occurrence of postoperative hypotony appeared to be unpredictable.[70,73]

Krupin Valve

The Krupin eye valve filtering surgery study group[74] evaluated this device in 50 eyes with various types of glaucomas. At mean follow-up of 25 months, IOP was 19 mm Hg or lower in 80% of the eyes, 59% of which were without adjunctive antiglaucoma medications. In a smaller retrospective study[75] of 25 eyes, surgical success was reported to be 84% and 66% at 6 and 12 months, respectively.

Ahmed Glaucoma Valve

Both retrospective and prospective studies have reported clinical outcomes with AGV. In a multicenter, prospective study[76] of 60 eyes with intractable glaucoma, the cumulative probability of success was found to be 78% at 1 year. In a follow-up study,[77] the investigators, using the original cohort

of patients, reported cumulative probabilities of success at 1, 2, 3, and 4 years to be 76%, 68%, 54%, and 45%, respectively, when corneal complications were included in the definition of failure. When corneal complications were excluded from the definition of failure, the cumulative probabilities of success at 1, 2, 3, and 4 years were 87%, 82%, 76%, and 76%, respectively. In a larger retrospective study[78] of 159 eyes, the cumulative probability of success was 87% at 1 year and 75% at 2 years.

Baerveldt Implant

In a multicenter, retrospective study[79] of 103 eyes receiving various models of Baerveldt implant, the surgical success, defined as IOP less than 22 mm Hg and greater than 5 mm Hg without additional glaucoma surgery, was 71.8% at almost 1 year and 60% at 2 years of follow-up. In another retrospective study using the Baerveldt 250-mm^2 model in 108 eyes, the mean postoperative IOP at the final visit was 15.8±7.6 mm Hg on antiglaucoma medications, and the Kaplan-Meier surgical success rate was 0.79 at 24 months (n=61).[80] Trible and Brown[46] reported the results of the Baerveldt 350-mm^2 model with and without use of antimetabolites in 46 eyes. While IOP control was comparable to previously reported studies, no additional benefit was observed with the use of antimetabolite agents. In a study[36] comparing the results of the 350-mm^2 and 500-mm^2 Baerveldt implants, the intermediate-term results were comparable with respect to IOP control and final visual acuity, but patients who received the larger implant required significantly fewer postoperative medications to maintain an adequate IOP.

Comparative Studies of Various Glaucoma Drainage Devices

A few retrospective studies have compared clinical outcomes of AGV versus Baerveldt implants.[81-83] Of these, the larger series[83] consisted of 118 eyes with a follow-up of 48 months, at which time the final success in terms of IOP control was reported to be comparable in both groups: 62% for the Ahmed group and 64% for the Baerveldt group (p=0.84). The postoperative complications differed in the 2 groups, with hypotony-related issues in the Baerveldt group and hypertensive crisis in the Ahmed group requiring antiglaucoma medications.[83] These studies had limitations given their retrospective designs in that the study groups were not similar: the eyes undergoing Ahmed valve implantation had higher preoperative IOP in one study,[83] and the mean age at implantation was significantly different in another study,[82] although this study found a higher success rate with Baerveldt than with Ahmed: 83% versus 67%, respectively, at 42 months.

Double-plate Molteno was compared to AGV in a retrospective, case-control study[35] with 30 subjects in each arm. At 24 months follow-up, mean IOP was 13.3±5.1 mm Hg in the Molteno group and 19.0±5.8 mm Hg in the AGV group

($p = 0.009$). This study[35] also reported a high incidence of postoperative hypotony in the nonvalved group and hypertensive crisis in the valved group.

The Ahmed Baerveldt Comparison Study (ABC) is a multicenter, randomized, prospective clinical trial[84,85] that recently completed recruitment. The preliminary results of this trial were presented at the annual meeting of the American Glaucoma Society in 2010. Two hundred and seventy-six subjects with uncontrolled glaucoma received either an AGV (model FP7) or a Baerveldt implant (model 350 mm²). The majority of the recruited subjects had either POAG or neovascular glaucoma. Forty-two percent of the subjects had previously failed trabeculectomy. The mean baseline IOP was 30 mm Hg. Failure was defined as an IOP greater than 21 mm Hg and less than 6 mm Hg, less than 20% IOP reduction from baseline, repeat surgery, or loss of light perception. At 1 year, the mean IOP was $15.4 \pm .5$ mm Hg in the Ahmed group and 13.2 ± 6.8 mm Hg in the Baerveldt group ($p = 0.007$). The cumulative probability of failure was 16.4% and 12.3% in the AGV and Baerveldt groups, respectively. The Baerveldt group required more surgical interventions postoperatively.

Surgical Outcomes in Refractory or Difficult Glaucomas

Using different models in controlling IOP in eyes with neovascular glaucoma, Sidoti and colleagues[14] assessed the effectiveness of the Baerveldt implant. The life-table success rates were 79% and 56% at 12 and 18 months, respectively. Although there were no significant differences noted between various models in terms of percentage of postoperative IOP reduction or complication rates, the postoperative visual loss was reported to be common in these eyes as a result of underlying disease. In another study,[12] IOP control was reported to be adequate to keep the eyes comfortable, but the visual outcome of patients with neovascular glaucoma was determined primarily by underlying disease process with diabetic patients doing significantly better than did patients with a central retinal vein occlusion.

Both AGV and Baerveldt implants have been shown to be effective in controlling IOP in uveitic eyes.[15-17] In a retrospective, noncomparative case series, Da Mata and colleagues[15] reported a cumulative probability of success of 94% at 1 year after AGV implant. In this series, all patients had uveitis controlled prior to surgery with immunomodulatory therapy, which may have contributed to the high success rate. Using different models of the Baerveldt implant, Ceballos and colleagues[16] reported a similar cumulative life-table success rate of 91.7% at 24 months. The AGV implant was found to be moderately successful when long-term results were reported for eyes with uveitic glaucoma.[17] The qualified success rates were 57% and 39% at 1 and 4 years, respectively. At 4 years, 74% of the patients required adjunctive glaucoma therapy to control IOP.

The AGV was shown to be very effective in treating medically uncontrolled IOP after pars plana vitrectomy and silicone oil injection for complicated retinal detachments. IOP was reduced from a mean of 44 ± 11.8 mm Hg before surgery to 14 ± 4.2 mm Hg at the most recent follow-up after surgery ($p < 0.001$). The number of glaucoma medications reduced after surgery was also statistically significant.[86]

Coleman and colleagues[26] reported clinical outcomes of AGV in eyes with prior or concurrent penetrating keratoplasty. The cumulative probabilities of success at 12 and 20 months were $75.4\% \pm 8.2\%$ and $51.5\% \pm 11.4\%$, respectively. Ayyala and colleagues[28] compared trabeculectomy with mitomycin C, glaucoma drainage device implantation with both valved and nonvalved implants, and Nd:YAG laser cyclophotocoagulation to manage intractable glaucoma after penetrating keratoplasty. No differences were found among the 3 glaucoma procedures in terms of final IOP control and graft failure. The laser-treated group tended to have higher incidence of graft failure, glaucoma failure, and loss of vision, but these results were not statistically significant. GDDs have also been reported to be effective in glaucoma associated with keratoprosthesis.[27]

GDDs are increasingly being used in pediatric glaucoma, which is often refractory to conventional medical and surgical therapy.[18-24] Billson and colleagues[18] reported favorable outcomes in developmental glaucomas using 2-stage implantation of the Molteno implant where final IOP with adjunctive glaucoma medications was less than 21 mm Hg in 78% of the cases. Coleman and colleagues[21] evaluated AGV in pediatric glaucoma cases and reported cumulative probabilities of success at 12 and 24 months to be $77.9\% \pm 8.8\%$ and $60.6\% \pm 13.7\%$, respectively. Englert and colleagues[22] reported AGV to be effective in refractory pediatric glaucoma cases, even in eyes with previous cycloablative procedures. Budenz and colleagues[23] evaluated the Baerveldt implant in childhood glaucoma associated with Sturge-Weber syndrome and concluded that 2-stage Baerveldt surgery was both effective and safe in these children. At average follow-up of 35 months, all 10 eyes had IOPs less than 21 mm Hg on medications without the need for additional glaucoma surgery.

Comparative Studies of Glaucoma Drainage Devices and Trabeculectomy

Wilson and colleagues[87] compared short and intermediate results of trabeculectomy and AGV in a randomized clinical trial and reported statistically lower mean IOP with trabeculectomy than with AGV at weeks 6 to 15 and months 11 to 13. The cumulative probability of success was 83.6% for the trabeculectomy group and 88.1% for the AGV ($p = 0.43$) group. There was no significant difference in complication rates between the 2 groups, but the AGV group required more glaucoma medications postoperatively. The same investigators subsequently reported the long-term results of these 2 procedures.[88] The cumulative probabilities of success at months 41 to 52 were 68.1% for the trabeculectomy group and 69.8% for the AGV group ($p = 0.86$). Adjunctive medication requirement was also comparable in both groups with longer follow-up.

Gedde and colleagues[89,90] have been investigating the clinical outcomes of nonvalved tube shunt, specifically the Baerveldt 350 mm², and standard trabeculectomy with mitomycin C in a multicenter, randomized clinical trial. A total of 212 eyes were enrolled with IOP ≥ 18 mm Hg and ≤ 40 mm Hg. The main outcome measures were IOP, visual acuity, and reoperation for glaucoma. At 1-year follow-up, IOP control was good in both groups with slightly lower pressures in the Baerveldt group. The mean IOP was 12.7 ± 3.9 mm Hg in the trabeculectomy group and 12.4 ± 3.9 mm Hg in the Baerveldt group ($p = 0.73$). The cumulative probability of failure during the first year was 3.9% in the Baerveldt group and 13.5% in the trabeculectomy group ($p = 0.17$). Intraoperative complications occurred in 7% of the Baerveldt group and 10% of the trabeculectomy group ($p = 0.59$). Postoperative complications were more common in the trabeculectomy group than in the Baerveldt group—57% versus 34%, respectively. Adjunctive glaucoma medications were required more in the Baerveldt group. Longer follow-up of this study will elucidate further details on IOP control and other variables with these 2 commonly performed glaucoma surgeries.

CONCLUSION

GDDs are designed to divert aqueous humor from the anterior chamber to an external reservoir, where a fibrous capsule forms about 4 to 6 weeks after surgery and regulates flow. These devices are available in different sizes, materials, and design with the presence or absence of an IOP-regulating valve. The nonvalved devices include the Molteno, Baerveldt, Shocket, and Eagle Vision implants. The most commonly used valved implant is the AGV. The decision to choose a particular type depends on a patient's underlying characteristics in terms of preoperative IOP and optic nerve status, desired long-term IOP control, and the surgeon's comfort and preference. Careful preoperative screening and planning along with meticulous surgical technique help minimize postoperative complications. These devices have shown success in controlling IOP in eyes with complicated secondary glaucomas, such as uveitic glaucoma and neovascular glaucoma, young patients, eyes with previously failed filters, and eyes with insufficient conjunctiva because of scarring from prior surgical procedures or injuries. The ongoing tube versus trabeculectomy and Ahmed–Baerveldt comparison studies will provide further information with respect to long-term IOP control achieved with these devices when compared with glaucoma filtration surgery and between valved and nonvalved devices, respectively.

REFERENCES

1. Molteno AC, Straughan JL, Ancker E, et al. Long tube implants in the management of glaucoma. *S Afr Med J.* 1976;50:1062-1066.
2. Molteno ACB, Biljon GV, Ancker E. Two-stage insertion of glaucoma drainage implants. *Trans Ophthal Soc.* 1979;31:17-26.
3. Molteno ACB. New implant for drainage in glaucoma: clinical trial. *Br J Ophthalmol.* 1979;53:606-615.
4. Molteno ACB. The optimal design of drainage implants for glaucoma. *Trans Ophthal Soc.* 1981;33:39-41.
5. Heuer DK, Lloyd MA, Abrams DA, et al. Which is better? One or two? A randomized clinical trial of single-plate versus double-plate Molteno implantation for glaucoma in aphakia and pseudophakia. *Ophthalmology.* 1992;99:1512-1519.
6. Wilson RP, Cantor L, Katz LJ, et al. Aqueous shunts: Molteno versus Shocket. *Ophthalmology.* 1992;99:672-676.
7. Smith MF, Sherwood MB, McGorray SP. Comparison of the double-plate Molteno drainage implant with the Shocket procedure. *Arch Ophthalmol.* 1992;110:1246-1250.
8. Prata JA Jr, Mermoud A, LaBree L, et al. In vitro and in vivo flow characteristics of glaucoma drainage implants. *Ophthalmology.* 1995;102:894-904.
9. Francis BA, Cortes A, Chen J, et al. Characteristics of glaucoma drainage implants during dynamic and steady-state flow conditions. *Ophthalmology.* 1998;105:1708-1714.
10. Eisenberg DL, Koo EY, Hafner G, et al. In vitro flow properties of glaucoma implant devices. *Ophthalmic Surg Lasers.* 1999;30:662-667.
11. Brown RD, Cairns JE. Experience with the Molteno long tube implant. *Trans Ophthalmol Soc UK.* 1983;103:297-312.
12. Mermoud A, Salmon JF, Alexander P, et al. Molteno tube implantation for neovascular glaucoma: long term results and factors influencing outcome. *Ophthalmology.* 1993;100:897-902.
13. Hill RA, Nguyen QH, Baerveldt G, et al. Trabeculectomy and Molteno implantation for glaucomas associated with uveitis. *Ophthalmology.* 1993;100:903-908.
14. Sidoti PA, Dunphy TR, Baerveldt G, et al. Experience with the Baerveldt glaucoma implant in treating neovascular glaucoma. *Ophthalmology.* 1995;102:1107-1118.
15. Da Mata A, Burk SE, Netland PA, et al. Management of uveitic glaucoma with Ahmed glaucoma valve implantation. *Ophthalmology.* 1999;106:2168-2172.
16. Ceballos EM, Parrish RK, Schiffman JC. Outcome of Baerveldt glaucoma drainage implants for the treatment of uveitic glaucoma. *Ophthalmology.* 2002;109:2256-2260.
17. Papadaki TG, Zacharopoulos IP, Pasquale LR, et al. Long-term results of Ahmed glaucoma valve implantation for uveitic glaucoma. *Am J Ophthalmol.* 2007;144:62-69.
18. Billson F, Thomas R, Aylward W. The use of two-stage molten implants in developmental glaucoma. *J Ped Ophthalmol Strabismus.* 1989;26:3-8.
19. Munoz M, Tomey KF, Traverso C, et al. Clinical experience with the Molteno implant in advanced infantile glaucoma. *J Ped Ophthalmol Strabismus.* 1991;28:68-72.
20. Netland PA, Walton DS. Glaucoma drainage implants in pediatric patients. *Ophthalmic Surg.* 1993;24:723-729.
21. Coleman AL, Smyth RJ, Wilson RM, et al. Initial clinical experience with the Ahmed glaucoma valve implant in pediatric patients. *Arch Ophthalmol.* 1997;115:186-191.
22. Englert JA, Freedman SF, Cox TA. The Ahmed valve in refractory pediatric glaucoma. *Am J Ophthalmol.* 1999;127:34-42.
23. Budenz DL, Sakamoto D, Eliezer R, et al. Two-staged Baerveldt glaucoma implant for childhood glaucoma associated with Sturge-Weber syndrome. *Ophthalmology.* 2000;107:2105-2110.

24. Djodeyre MR, Calvo JP, Gomez JA. Clinical evaluation and risk factors of time to failure of Ahmed glaucoma valve implant in pediatric patients. *Ophthalmology.* 2001;108:614-620.

25. Beebe WE, Starita RJ, Fellman RL. The use of the Molteno implant and anterior chamber tube shunt to encircling band for the treatment of glaucoma in keratoplasty patients. *Ophthalmology.* 1990;97:1414-1422.

26. Coleman AL, Mondino BJ, Wilson MR, et al. Clinical experience with the Ahmed glaucoma valve implant in eyes with prior or current penetrating keratoplasties. *Am J Ophthalmol.* 1997;123:54-61.

27. Netland PA, Terada H, Dohlman CH. Glaucoma associated with keratoprosthesis. *Ophthalmology.* 1998;105:751-757.

28. Ayyala RS, Pieroth L, Vinals AF, et al. Comparison of mitomycin C trabeculectomy, glaucoma drainage device implantation, and laser neodymium: YAG cyclophotocoagulation in the management of intractable glaucoma after penetrating keratoplasty. *Ophthalmology.* 1998;105:1550-1556.

29. Schwartz KS, Lee RK, Gedde SJ. Glaucoma drainage implants: a critical comparison of types. *Curr Opin Ophthalmol.* 2006;17:181-189.

30. Ayyala RS, Harman LE, Michelini-Norris B, et al. Comparison of different biomaterials for glaucoma drainage devices. *Arch Ophthalmol.* 1999;117:233-236.

31. Ayyala RS, Michelini-Norris B, Flores A, et al. Comparison of different biomaterials for glaucoma drainage devices: part 2. *Arch Ophthalmol.* 2000;118:1081-1084.

32. Mackenzie PJ, Schertzer RM, Isbister CM. Comparison of silicone and polypropylene Ahmed glaucoma valves: two-year follow-up. *Can J Ophthalmol.* 2007;42:227-232.

33. Brasil MVOM, Rockwood EJ, Smith S. Comparison of silicone and polypropylene Ahmed glaucoma valve implants. *J Glaucoma.* 2007;16:36-41.

34. Ishida K, Netland PA, Costa VP, et al. Comparison of polypropylene and silicone Ahmed glaucoma valves. *Ophthalmology.* 2006;113:1320-1326.

35. Ayyala RS, Zurakowski D, Monshizadeh R, et al. Comparison of double-plate Molteno and Ahmed glaucoma valve in patients with advanced uncontrolled glaucoma. *Ophthalmic Surg Lasers.* 2002;33:94-101.

36. Lloyd MA, Baerveldt G, Fellenbaum PS, et al. Intermediate-term results of a randomized clinical trial of the 350 versus the 500 mm^2 Baerveldt implant. *Ophthalmology.* 1994;101:1456-1464.

37. Britt MT, LaBree LD, Lloyd MA, et al. Randomized clinical trial of the 350-mm^2 versus the 500-mm^2 Baerveldt implant longer term results. Is bigger better? *Ophthalmology.* 1999;106:2312-2318.

38. Malik MY, Noecker RJ. Fibrin glue-assisted glaucoma drainage device surgery. *Br J Ophthalmol.* 2006;90:1486-1489.

39. Egbert PR, Lieberman MF. Internal suture occlusion of the Molteno glaucoma implant for the prevention of postoperative hypotony. *Ophthalmic Surg.* 1989;20:53-56.

40. Hoare Nairne JE, Sherwood D, Jacob JSH, et al. Single stage insertion of the Molteno tube for glaucoma and modifications to reduce postoperative hypotony. *Br J Ophthalmol.* 1988;72:846-851.

41. El-Sayyad F, El-Maghraby A, Helal M, et al. The use of releasable sutures in Molteno glaucoma implant procedures to reduce postoperative hypotony. *Ophthalmic Surg.* 1991;22:82-84.

42. Joos KM, Lavina AM, Tawansy KA, et al. Posterior repositioning of glaucoma implants for anterior segment complications. *Ophthalmology.* 2001;108:279-284.

43. Ball SF, Ellis GS, Herrington RG, et al. Browns superior oblique tendon syndrome after Baerveldt implant. *Arch Ophthalmol.* 1992;110:1368.

44. Christman LM, Wilson ME. Motility disturbances after Molteno implants. *J Ped Ophthalmol Strabismus.* 1992;29:44-48.

45. Gross FJ. Six month success of Krupin valve with and without Mitomycin-C in the treatment of complicated glaucomas. *Invest Ophthalmol Vis Sci.* 1994;35(suppl):1422.

46. Trible JR, Brown DB. Occlusive ligature and standardized fenestrations of a Baerveldt tube with and without antimetabolites for early postoperative intraocular pressure control. *Ophthalmology.* 1998;105:2243-2250.

47. Irak I, Moster MR, Fontanarosa J. Intermediate-term results of Baerveldt tube shunt surgery with mitomycin C use. *Ophthalmic Surg Laser Imaging.* 2004;35:189-196.

48. Cantor L, Burgoyne J, Sanders S, et al. The effect of mitomycin C on Molteno implant surgery: a 1-year randomized, masked, prospective study. *J Glaucoma.* 1998;7:240-246.

49. Costa VP, Azuara-Blanco A, Netland PA, et al. Efficacy and safety of adjunctive mitomycin C during Ahmed glaucoma valve implantation: a prospective randomized clinical trial. *Ophthalmology.* 2004;111:1071-1076.

50. Parrish R, Minckler D. Late endophthalmitis-filtering surgery time bomb? *Ophthalmology.* 1996;103:1167-1168.

51. Feldman RM, El-Harazi SM, Villanueva G. Valve membrane adhesion as a cause of Ahmed glaucoma valve failure. *J Glaucoma.* 1996;6:10-12.

52. Hill RA, Pirouzian A, Liaw LH. Pathophysiology of and prophylaxis against late Ahmed glaucoma valve occlusion. *Am J Ophthalmol.* 2000;129:608-612.

53. Sarkisian SR, Netland PA. Tube extender for revision of glaucoma drainage implants. *J Glaucoma.* 2007;16:637-639.

54. Tessler Z, Jluchoded S, Rosenthal G. Nd:YAG laser for Ahmed tube shunt occlusion by the posterior capsule. *Ophthalmic Surg Lasers.* 1997;28:69-70.

55. Netland PA, Schuman S. Management of glaucoma drainage implant tube kink and obstruction with pars plana clip. *Ophthalmic Surg Lasers Imaging.* 2005;36:167-168.

56. Tarbak AAA, Shahwan SA, Jadaan IA, et al. Endophthalmitis associated with the Ahmed glaucoma valve implant. *Br J Ophthalmol.* 2005;89:454-458.

57. Sherwood MB, Smith MF, Driebe WT Jr, et al. Drainage tube implants in the treatment of glaucoma following penetrating keratoplasty. *Ophthalmic Surg.* 1993;24(3):185-189.

58. McDonnell PJ, Robin JB, Schanzlin DJ, et al. Molteno implant for control of glaucoma in eyes after penetrating keratoplasty. *Ophthalmology.* 1988;95(3):364-369.

59. Lloyd MA, Sedlak T, Heuer DK, et al. Clinical experience with the single-plate Molteno implant in complicated glaucomas. Update of a pilot study. *Ophthalmology.* 1992;99(5):679-687.

60. Smith SL, Starita RJ, Fellman RL, et al. Early clinical experience with the Baerveldt 350 mm^2 glaucoma implant and associated extraocular muscle imbalance. *Ophthalmology.* 1993;100:914-918.

61. Munoz M, Parrish RK. Strabismus following implantation of Baerveldt drainage devices. *Arch Ophthalmol.* 1993;111:1096-1099.

62. Dobler-Dixon AA, Cantor LB, Sondhi N, et al. Prospective evaluation of extraocular motility following double-plate Molteno implantation. *Arch Ophthalmol.* 1999;117:1155-1160.

63. Christmann LM, Wilson ME. Motility disturbances after Molteno implants. *J Ped Ophthalmol Strabismus.* 1992;29:44-48.

64. Munoz M, Parrish RK. Prospective evaluation of extraocular motility following double-plate Molteno implantation. *Arch Ophthalmol.* 1999;117:1155-1160.

65. Ventura MP, Vianna RN, Souza Filho JP, et al. Acquired Brown's syndrome secondary to Ahmed valve implant for neovascular glaucoma. *Eye.* 2005;19:230-232.

66. Ayyala RS, Zurakowski D, Smith JA, et al. A clinical study of the Ahmed glaucoma valve implant in advanced glaucoma. *Ophthalmology.* 1998;105:1968-1976.

67. Johnson SM. Encapsulated filtering blebs after glaucoma shunt surgery. In: Schacknow PN, Samples JR, eds. *The Glaucoma Book.* New York, NY: Springer; 2010:824-826.

68. Nouri-Mahdavi K, Caprioli J. Evaluation of the hypertensive phase after insertion of the Ahmed glaucoma valve. *Am J Ophthalmol.* 2003;136:1001-1008.

69. Smith M, Geffen N, Alasbali T, et al. Digital ocular massage for hypertensive phase after Ahmed valve surgery. *J Glaucoma.* 2010;19:11-14.

70. Freedman J. Clinical experience with the Molteno dual-chamber single-plate implant. *Ophthalmic Surg.* 1992;23:238-241.

71. Price FW, Wellenmeyer M. Long-term results of Molteno implants. *Ophthalmic Surg.* 1995;26:130-135.

72. Mills RP, Reynolds A, Emond MJ, et al. Long-term survival of Molteno glaucoma drainage devices. *Ophthalmology.* 1996;103: 299-305.

73. Gerber SL, Cantor LB, Sponsel WE. A comparison of postoperative complications from pressure-ridge Molteno implants versus Molteno implants with suture ligation. *Ophthalmic Surg Lasers.* 1997;28:905-910.

74. The Krupin eye valve filtering surgery study group. Krupin eye valve with disk for filtration surgery. *Ophthalmology.* 1994;101: 651-658.

75. Fellenbaum PS, Almeida AR, Minckler DS, et al. Krupin disk implantation for complicated glaucomas. *Ophthalmology.* 1994;101:1178-1182.

76. Coleman AL, Hill R, Wilson MR, et al. Initial clinical experience with the Ahmed glaucoma valve implant. *Am J Ophthalmol.* 1995;120:23-31.

77. Topouzis F, Coleman AL, Choplin N, et al. Follow-up of the original cohort with the Ahmed glaucoma valve implant. *Am J Ophthalmol.* 1999;128:198-204.

78. Huang MC, Netland PA, Coleman AL, et al. Intermediate-term clinical experience with the Ahmed glaucoma valve implant. *Am J Ophthalmol.* 1999;127:27-33.

79. Siegner SW, Netland PA, Urban RC. Clinical experience with the Baerveldt glaucoma drainage implant. *Ophthalmology.* 1995;102:1298-1307.

80. WuDunn D, Phan ADT, Cantor LB, et al. Clinical experience with the Baerveldt 250-mm^2 glaucoma implant. *Ophthalmology.* 2006;113:766-772.

81. Syed HM, Law SK, Nam SH, et al. Baerveldt-350 implant versus Ahmed valve for refractory glaucoma: a case-controlled comparison. *J Glaucoma.* 2004;13:38-45.

82. Wang JC, See JL, Chew PT. Experience with the use of Baerveldt and Ahmed glaucoma drainage implants in an Asian population. *Ophthalmology.* 2004;111:1383-1388.

83. Tsai JC, Johnson CC, Kammer JA, et al. The Ahmed shunt versus the Baerveldt shunt for refractory glaucoma II: longer-term outcomes from a single surgeon. *Ophthalmology.* 2006;113:913-917.

84. Budenz DL, Barton K, Feuer WJ, et al. Treatment outcomes in the Ahmed Baerveldt Comparison (ABC) Study after one year of follow-up. 2011;118(3):443-452.

85. Barton K, Budenz DL, Gedde SJ, et al. Surgical complications in the Ahmed Baerveldt Comparison (ABC) Study during the first year of follow-up. 2011;118(3):435-442.

86. Al-Jazzaf AM, Netland PA, Charles S. Incidence and management of elevated intraocular pressure after silicone oil injection. *J Glaucoma.* 2005;14:40-46.

87. Wilson MR, Mendis U, Smith SD, et al. Ahmed glaucoma valve implant vs. trabeculectomy in the surgical treatment of glaucoma: a randomized clinical trial. *Am J Ophthalmol.* 2000;130:267-273.

88. Wilson MR, Mendis U, Paliwal A, et al. Long-term follow-up of primary glaucoma surgery with Ahmed glaucoma valve implant versus trabeculectomy. *Am J Ophthalmol.* 2003;136:464-470.

89. Gedde SJ, Schiffman JC, Feuer WJ, et al. Treatment outcomes in the tube versus trabeculectomy study after one year of follow-up. *Am J Ophthalmol.* 2007;143:9-22.

90. Gedde SJ, Herndon LW, Brandt JD, et al. Surgical complications in the tube versus trabeculectomy study during the first year follow-up. *Am J Ophthalmol.* 2007;143:23-31.

63

Cyclodialysis

David L. Epstein, MD, MMM

Cyclodialysis[1] performed in an eye rendered previously aphakic or as part of a combined intracapsular cataract operation[2] used to be a frequently performed glaucoma procedure. Although the success was only in the 30% to 40% range, it was a fairly quick procedure with a rapid postoperative recovery. It has fallen into disuse with the advancement in techniques of combined cataract/filtration surgery (see Chapter 61), but perhaps it deserves further evaluation in pseudophakic eyes with good central visual acuity that are not suitable for filtration surgery, prior to consideration of a laser ciliodestructive procedure (which has some risk of inducing cystoid macular edema and decreased central acuity). Some have proposed combination surgery of cyclodialysis with extracapsular cataract surgery.[3]

The mechanism of intraocular pressure (IOP) lowering with cyclodialysis is likely due to increased outflow into the nonconventional outflow pathway[4,5] via the surgically created cleft as has previously been described (see Chapters 2 and 3), although some have thought that the procedure also acts to decrease the rate of aqueous humor formation.[6] The technique of the surgical procedure will be described in this chapter.

SYNDROME OF SUDDEN CLOSURE OF A CYCLODIALYSIS CLEFT

One of the unfortunate complications that sometimes occurred in some of the "successes" with the cyclodialysis surgical procedure was ocular hypotony.[7] But, in addition, what was occasionally also observed was a syndrome of a sudden high IOP if the cyclodialysis cleft was suddenly closed. Often, the IOP observed in this syndrome would far exceed the preoperative IOP levels for a day or so. The mechanism for this phenomenon was believed to involve the fact that when the cyclodialysis cleft was functioning, aqueous humor was flowing not into the trabecular meshwork (TM), but into the cleft. When the cleft closed, the TM, having been previously underperfused and underutilized, temporarily offered substantially more resistance to aqueous outflow than prior to surgery. It is noteworthy that an early explanation of this phenomenon was made by Goldmann.[8] There have been histological studies of experimentally produced hypoperfusion of the TM, which demonstrated increased proteinaceous material extracellularly in the outflow pathway, as well as other structural changes.[9] Such an acute underperfusion syndrome of the TM theoretically might also occur after filtration surgery if the fistula were to suddenly close due to iris incarceration or blood, for example. Clinically, this sudden cleft closure syndrome lasted only 1 to 2 days, after which there was return to baseline glaucoma status (likely continued poor control).

Patients who were postoperative from cyclodialysis procedures would routinely be maintained on miotics indefinitely in order to cause ciliary muscle contraction, and therefore both to pull the ciliary body further away from the separated scleral spur and to narrow the ciliary body ring (see Chapter 29) and thus expand the potential fluid space beneath the sclera. Sometimes, sympathomimetic drugs such as phenylephrine were used in addition to miotics to contract the iris dilator muscle because it was felt that this action might, by increasing iris tone, act with coexisting cholinergic miotics to move the iris away from the cleft. Also, sympathomimetic drugs may cause weak contraction of the ciliary muscle.[10]

A common situation that precipitated the sudden cleft closure syndrome was when the patient was dilated for fundoscopy with a cycloplegic drug. Presumably, the cycloplegic drug caused relaxation of ciliary muscle tone and dilatation of the ciliary body ring (see Chapter 29), and this outward movement of the ciliary body could close the space between the ciliary body and sclera, which represented the cleft.

Kahook MY, Schuman JS, eds.
Chandler and Grant's Glaucoma, Fifth Edition (pp 595-600).
© 2013 SLACK Incorporated.

MYSTERY DIAGNOSIS

David L. Epstein, MD, MMM

I was once presented with the following case: A patient had just undergone trabeculectomy, performed elsewhere, for uncontrolled IOP in the 20s. On the first postoperative day, the IOP was 6 mm Hg, but there was no obvious bleb. On day 2, the IOP had suddenly increased to 60 mm Hg, which was much higher than it ever had been before. The angle was described as being open. One drop of 1% pilocarpine was placed in the eye and the IOP decreased to 9 mm Hg.

This patient proved to have an inadvertent cyclodialysis cleft as a result of the trabeculectomy, but it is important for the reader to realize that when trabeculectomy was first introduced as a surgical technique, it was common to extend the sclerectomy posteriorly and excise the scleral spur.[1] If one reads the early literature after the development of the procedure of trabeculectomy, there is often much confusion about the absence of blebs despite good IOP results in many patients (we believe now that this was likely due to having produced a cyclodialysis rather than a filter in such patients; maybe cyclodialysis is not such a bad operation after all!). Trabeculectomy originally was conceptualized to remove diseased TM and allow aqueous humor to flow into the cut ends of Schlemm's canal.[2] This does not, in fact, happen as the cut-ends of the canal collapse.[3] Regardless, there would be little potential anyway for resulting circumferential flow of aqueous humor in Schlemm's canal as the outflow pathway functions in a segmental manner[4,5] (see Chapter 3). Thus, this was not the first time, nor likely the last, that a procedure designed to work by one mechanism actually worked by another. Trabeculectomy functions really as a guarded filtering procedure in which, under a scleral flap, a fistula is created to the subconjunctival space.[6]

The key to the mystery diagnosis in this case was the sudden occurrence of a high IOP far above baseline postoperatively despite an open angle and the super-response to pilocarpine that actually resulted in the reopening of the cleft rather than a mechanical tension on the TM. (The first suspicion from the history, of course, was that with such a pilocarpine effect, the patient might have developed angle closure that was relieved with this weak miotic therapy or perhaps suffered a miotic-related retinal detachment, but this proved not to be the case.) Likely, in this case (and others), the routine use of a cycloplegic drug post-trabeculectomy may have precipitated the sudden cleft closure syndrome.

REFERENCES

1. Watson PG. Surgery of the glaucomas. *Br J Ophthalmol.* 1972; 56:299-306.
2. Cairns JE. Trabeculectomy. Preliminary report of a new method. *Am J Ophthalmol.* 1968;66:673-679.
3. Spencer WH. Histologic evaluation of microsurgical glaucoma techniques. *Trans Am Acad Ophthal Otol.* 1972;76:389-397.
4. Van Buskirk EM, Grant WM. Lens depression and aqueous outflow in enucleated primate eyes. *Am J Ophthalmol.* 1973;76:632-640.
5. Rosenquist RC, Epstein DL, Melamed S, Johnson M, Grant WM. Outflow resistance of enucleated human eyes with two different perfusion pressures and different extents of trabeculotomy. *Curr Eye Res.* 1989;8:1233-1240.
6. Grant WM. Symposium: microsurgery of the outflow channels. *Trans Am Acad Ophthalmol Otolaryngol.* 1972;76(2):398-404.

INADVERTENT CYCLODIALYSIS CLEFTS

Nowadays, one encounters cyclodialysis clefts mostly as inadvertent complications resulting from trauma (see Chapter 43) or after anterior segment surgery.[11-16] Sometimes, some of the newer scleral tunneling techniques[16] in cataract surgery may inadvertently cause this separation of the ciliary body from the scleral wall.

How should such inadvertent cyclodialyses be treated? Building upon what we have learned from the above, a trial of cycloplegics, initially short-acting agents but later daily atropine or scopolamine, should be attempted first. This failing (the cleft), if small, may be therapeutically closed sometimes by applying argon laser gonioplasty-type applications to the visible scleral wall of the cleft, with perhaps a few applications to the peripheral iris in the same area.[17-20] What one is really trying to do is cause inflammation to potentially encourage adhesion of the ciliary body back to the sclera. Therefore, minimal to no steroids should be used and cycloplegics should be maintained after argon laser treatment. Because the sclera is white and does not absorb the energy well (which is why the peripheral iris is sometimes also treated nonspecifically to encourage inflammation), and because there are likely nerves in the sclera, this is an uncomfortable procedure for the patient, and likely it should be performed in multiple smaller sessions. This argon laser procedure is not ideal and often fails. It probably is fruitless to attempt this procedure in the presence of a large cleft.

It is noteworthy in contemplating the limited efficacy of laser applications in closing clefts to realize that neodymium:yttrium-aluminum-garnet (Nd:YAG) laser applications have been reported to reopen a cleft![21]

The next alternative that I have had good success with is to treat the sclera external to the cleft with 2 rows of cyclocryotherapy ([CCT]; full freeze applications for 30 to 60 s each). One's goal is to totally overlap the circumferential extent of the cleft (eg, 1 to 3 hours of the limbus). The efficacy of this modality is felt to be by the induced inflammation that the procedure causes. Retrobulbar anesthesia is necessary, but the postoperative morbidity is much less than after the standard 6 clock-hour CCT for antiglaucoma therapy. However, one must also be prepared to deal with the high IOP of the sudden cleft closure syndrome should this procedure be successful.

Finally, as a last resort, some have described direct suturing[22-26] of the ciliary body back to the sclera, preferably under a scleral flap (Figure 63-1). Laser endophotocoagulation has also been described.[27]

One of the major problems in treating an inadvertent cleft is the difficulty in identifying the exact location of the cleft gonioscopically. In these cases, the anterior chamber is usually somewhat shallow because of the accumulating suprachoroidal fluid, and the iris therefore can

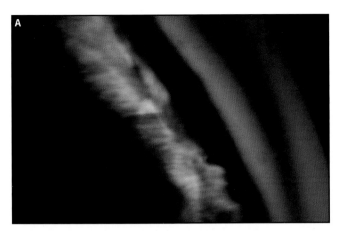
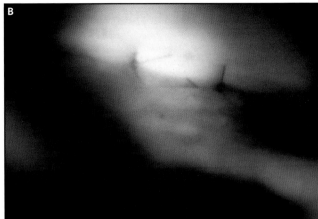

Figure 63-1. (A) Large cyclodialysis cleft visible gonioscopically that occurred following blunt trauma from a handball. Patient developed an IOP of 0 to 2 mm Hg and hypotonous maculopathy. (B) After cycloplegics and laser failed to close the cleft, the ciliary body was resutured to the sclera. IOP was maintained in the mid-teens following 1 to 2 days of IOPs in the 40s in the immediate postoperative period. Visual acuity was restored to a level of 20/25.

hide the area of the cleft. In this situation, one can deepen the anterior chamber with viscoelastic to identify the site of the cleft, and then perform one's therapy. I recommend always looking carefully at the 12 o'clock meridian because it is a common site of occurrence. An excellent noninvasive technique for identification and assessment of the cleft is the use of the ultrasound biomicroscope. The size and location of the cleft can thus be clearly mapped.

SURGICAL TECHNIQUE OF CYCLODIALYSIS FOR INTENDED ANTIGLAUCOMA THERAPY

The technique of cyclodialysis is simple. The first step in the operation should be to make a beveled paracentesis incision in the lower cornea with a Wheeler-type knife (British Quality Standard, Great Britain). A conjunctival incision is made radially in one quadrant, centered equidistant between rectus muscles 4 or 5 mm from the limbus. A circumferential scleral incision 4 to 5 mm from the limbus is made with a blunt-tipped knife such as a No. 67 Beaver (Beaver, Waltham, MA) or No. 15 Bard-Parker blade (Katena Eye Instruments, Denville, NJ), separating scleral fibers fully down to ciliary body but being careful not to penetrate it. A blunt-tipped cyclodialysis spatula[28] is then introduced into the suprachoroidal space with the dorsal surface of the spatula hugging the inner surface of the sclera. It is then passed toward the anterior chamber at the horizontal or vertical meridian. It is often useful to grasp the scleral wound with a Colibri forceps (Medetz, Dallas, PA) and elevate it as the spatula passes, hugging the inner (elevated) aspect of sclera, until the tip of the spatula is seen in the anterior chamber (as it passes just below the scleral spur). The spatula is then swept from the extreme position with the tip at the horizontal (or

vertical) meridian to a position with the tip straight ahead in the anterior chamber, being careful to avoid the corneal endothelium. The spatula is then withdrawn, staying within the suprachoroidal space, toward the scleral wound. It is then passed again as previously but toward the other extreme position (ie, the vertical [or horizontal] meridian), and the process is repeated.

For example, in a right eye, if the scleral incision is made inferonasally at the half past 4 o'clock position, the spatula is initially introduced into the anterior chamber at 3 o'clock then swept to half past 4 o'clock, partially withdrawn, then reintroduced into the anterior chamber at 6 o'clock with sweeping to half past 4 o'clock. With the spatula passed in this way from extreme toward the center rather than vice versa, false passages in the ciliary body are avoided. Following removal of the spatula, the anterior chamber should be entered via the paracentesis site and the chamber filled with an air bubble to firm the eye and achieve hemostasis. Hemorrhage frequently occurs, but unless it is massive, it apparently does not materially influence the result of the operation. Cyclodialysis is especially risky from the standpoint of hemorrhage if the eye is considerably inflamed at the time of operation. If hemorrhage is severe during operation, it can nearly always be stopped by quickly filling the anterior chamber with a large bubble of air. When it is apparent that the hemorrhage has stopped, the air can be removed, and at least some of the blood can be irrigated out of the anterior chamber. Then, at the end of the operation, the anterior chamber can be filled with saline solution or a bubble of air.

Hemorrhage can be reduced by use of viscoelastic[29] in the anterior chamber and possibly in the cleft space, but the potential for a severe postoperative secondary trabecular open-angle glaucoma needs to be remembered[30] should the cleft not function.

COMPLICATIONS

Damage to Angle Structures and Closure of the Cleft

In the region of the dialysis, the ciliary muscle is torn from the corneoscleral meshwork and from the scleral spur, and if a cleft does not form, the situation may be similar to what is seen after severe contusion of the globe with angle deformity (see Chapter 43). The portion of the angle where the cyclodialysis has been done may not function as well as other portions of the angle due to the absence of ciliary muscle tension in the affected segment. Cholinergic miotics should not be effective on (open-angle) TM function in the affected segment, and similar to the action of cycloplegics to elevate IOP on an open-angle mechanism in some primary open-angle glaucoma patients (see Chapters 3 and 25), intrinsic outflow function also may be adversely affected. However, it is important to realize that traumatic angle recession results in secondary open-angle glaucoma more from the direct contusion and damage to the TM[31] at the time of injury rather than the loss of ciliary muscle tone.

Thus, if the cleft closes or fails to form, the glaucoma is usually more difficult to control medically postoperatively than it is preoperatively. For this reason, it is wise not to dialyze too large an area. If 3 or 4 clock-hours are dialyzed, the chances of success are as good as if 6 to 12 clock-hours are dialyzed. If the cleft closes and the operation has to be repeated, it had best be done in the same area so as not to injure other portions of the angle if the cleft again closes. Cases have been observed in which half the circumference was dialyzed at the first operation, and when no cleft formed, the operation was repeated, dialyzing the remaining half. Then, when the cleft closed, the IOP reached high levels, as much as 80 mm Hg, with all the symptoms of acute glaucoma.

The continued use of miotics after cyclodialysis, especially the stronger miotics plus 5% phenylephrine, favors the formation and maintenance of an open cleft. Strong miotics should be used routinely and indefinitely in aphakic or pseudophakic eyes. In the uncommon circumstance when cyclodialysis is performed in a phakic eye, however, one must be more cautious because of the possibility of extensive formation of posterior synechiae. In phakic eyes, it is best not to begin miotic treatment until slit-lamp examination indicates that the anterior segment is entirely quiet, with the possible exception of eyes with a sector coloboma of the iris.

Eyes have been observed in which, after cyclodialysis, there was an adequate cleft with a low IOP, then weeks or months later, the cleft suddenly closed and IOP rose to very high levels. This situation was discussed previously in this chapter.

Corneal Damage

Descemet's membrane can be injured by the cyclodialysis spatula, but this is usually without sequelae.

Postoperative Hemorrhage

Severe hemorrhage occurring in the postoperative period may be a serious complication. In the first place, it greatly lessens the chance of ultimate success of the operation.

Furthermore, the hemorrhage itself may cause an acute rise in IOP. It may be controlled with aqueous humor suppressants, but in some cases, oral glycerin or intravenous mannitol is necessary. In some cases, one must open the eye and irrigate the blood from the anterior chamber. The redder the eye at the time of surgery, the greater the risk of hemorrhage at the time of operation or later. In any case in which cyclodialysis is planned, the operation should be deferred if at all possible until the eye is reasonably quiet. Viscoelastic can be injected into the anterior chamber at the time of the procedure to minimize hyphema, but viscoelastics themselves commonly produce a temporary severe secondary open-angle glaucoma[30] (see Chapter 39).

Hypotony

One of the most unfortunate and undesirable complications of cyclodialysis is extreme hypotony. IOP may be too low to register. There may be extensive separation of the ciliary body and the choroid, which may reach the macula and impair visual acuity. Papilledema is sometimes seen. Furthermore, very soft, phakic eyes often develop cataract within a year or 2 after cyclodialysis.

When a cyclodialysis cleft is open, there is always some separation of the ciliary body with a layer of fluid between ciliary body and sclera. Apparently, it is the circumferential extent of this separation of the ciliary body that determines the level of IOP. In one case of Chandler and Maumenee,[6] after a weak solution of fluorescein was injected into the anterior chamber, the sclera was opened 180 degrees away from the site of operation where presumably the cleft was. Fluorescein-stained fluid escaped through the wound, proving that a 360-degree separation of the ciliary body was present. The eye in this case was mushy soft.

In eyes in which the extent of separation of the ciliary body is limited to a small area, there is little or no reduction of IOP. In one of Chandler and Maumenee's cases,[6] there was a wide-open cleft from 11 o'clock to 1 o'clock. When the sclera was opened at 3 o'clock and a cyclodialysis spatula was passed upward, fluid was encountered only when the tip of the spatula reached the region of the cleft, demonstrating a limited separation of the ciliary body confined to the region of the cleft itself, insufficient to lower the IOP significantly.

In cases in which IOP is not unusually low after cyclodialysis (ie, of the order of 15, 20, or 25 mm Hg) but is considerably lower than before operation, it is presumed that there is separation of the ciliary body of a considerably lesser extent than 360 degrees. The extent of separation of the ciliary body necessary to give the ideal level of IOP is unknown, but it is probably of the order of one-half the circumference.

The degree of hypotony and separation of the ciliary body and choroid apparently bears no relation to the length or width of the cleft in the angle that is observed gonioscopically. In some cases, no sign of a cleft can be seen gonioscopically, but IOP is low, and we know that there is, in fact, a cleft even if we cannot see it.

I know of no technique of doing cyclodialysis to prevent the extreme hypotony that occurs in certain cases. Theoretically, one might partially close the cleft by penetrating cyclodiathermy or CCT in cases with extreme hypotony, but again, one has little control over this procedure. It may be completely ineffective on the one hand or completely effective on the other hand, closing the cleft and bringing about a return of high IOP.

Flat Anterior Chamber

In the immediate postoperative period following cyclodialysis, the anterior chamber may shallow, especially peripherally, associated with the induced choroidal separation. This can result in peripheral anterior synechiae formation and ultimate worsening of the glaucoma should there be late failure of the cleft. This usually transient shallowing of the chamber is not rare but it may be unsuspected because of the lowering of IOP from the cleft formation.

Special attention to this possibility should be made postoperatively, and gonioscopy should be performed if peripheral anterior chamber shallowing is observed. Frequent topical steroids may retard synechiae formation, but drainage of suprachoroidal fluid and reformation of the anterior chamber may be required, especially in combined cataract surgery (in which the potential for permanent peripheral anterior synechiae is even greater because of the presence of the fresh cataract wound).

CONCLUSION

Of all operations for the relief of glaucoma, cyclodialysis yields the least predictable results and it is the least amenable to improvement by variations in surgical technique. For these reasons, we believe cyclodialysis should be employed only in aphakic eyes or in eyes in which 2 or more conventional filtering operations have failed. Due to the unpredictability of the results, we believe cyclodialysis is not a good choice as a primary procedure in open-angle glaucoma.

REFERENCES

1. Boke H. Zur Geschichte der Zyklodialyse. *Klin Monatsbl Augenheilkd.* 1990;197(4):340-348.
2. Shields MB, Simmons RJ. Combined cyclodialysis and cataract extraction. *Ophthalmic Surg.* 1976;7(2):62-73.
3. Montgomery D, Gills JP. Extracapsular cataract extraction, lens implantation and cyclodialysis. *Ophthalmic Surg.* 1980;11(5):343-347.
4. Toris CB, Pederson JE. Effect of intraocular pressure on uveoscleral outflow following cyclodialysis in the monkey eye. *Invest Ophthalmol Vis Sci.* 1985;26(12):1745-1749.
5. Pederson JE. Ocular hypotony (review). *Trans Ophthalmol Soc UK.* 1986;105(pt 2)220-226.
6. Chandler PA, Maumenee AE. A major cause of hypotony. *Trans Am Acad Ophthalmol Otolaryngol.* 1961;2:609-618.
7. Shaffer RN, Weiss DL. Concerning cyclodialysis and hypotony. *Arch Ophthalmol.* 1962:25-31.
8. Goldmann H. Klinische Studien zum Glaucom-problem. *Ophthalmologica.* 1953;125:16-21.
9. Lütjen-Drecoll E. Functional and electron microscopic changes in the trabecular meshwork remaining after trabeculectomy in cynomolgus monkeys. *Invest Ophthalmol.* 1974;13(7):511-524.
10. Garner LF, Brown B, Baker R, et al. The effect of phenylephrine hydrochloride on the resting point of accommodation. *Invest Ophthalmol Vis Sci.* 1983;24(4):393-395.
11. Meislik J, Herschler J. Hypotony due to inadvertent cyclodialysis after intraocular lens implantation. *Arch Ophthalmol.* 1979;97(7):1297-1299.
12. Davenport WH, Brown RH, Lynch MG. Hypotony after rotation of an intraocular lens haptic into a cyclodialysis cleft. *Am J Ophthalmol.* 1986;101(6):736-737.
13. Terry SA. Cyclodialysis cleft following holmium laser sclerostomy, treated by argon laser photocoagulation. *Ophthalmic Surg.* 1992;23(12):825-826.
14. Aminlari A. Inadvertent cyclodialysis cleft. *Ophthalmic Surg.* 1993;24(5):331-335.
15. Small EA, Solomon JM, Prince AM. Hypotonous cyclodialysis cleft following suture fixation of a posterior chamber intraocular lens. *Ophthalmic Surg.* 1994;25(2):107-109.
16. Maffett MJ, O'Day DM. Cyclodialysis cleft following a scleral tunnel incision. *Ophthalmic Surg.* 1994;25(6):387-388.
17. Joondeph HC. Management of postoperative and post-traumatic cyclodialysis clefts with argon laser photocoagulation. *Ophthalmic Surg.* 1980;11(3):186-188.
18. Harbin TS Jr. Treatment of cyclodialysis clefts with argon laser photocoagulation. *Ophthalmology.* 1982;89(9):1082-1083.
19. Partamian LG. Treatment of a cyclodialysis cleft with argon laser photocoagulation in a patient with a shallow anterior chamber. *Am J Ophthalmol.* 1985;99(1):5-7.
20. Ormerod LD, Baerveldt G, Sunalp MA, et al. Management of the hypotonous cyclodialysis cleft. *Ophthalmology.* 1991;98(9):1384-1393.
21. Fellman RL, Starita RJ, Spaeth GL. Reopening cyclodialysis cleft with Nd:YAG laser following trabeculectomy. *Ophthalmic Surg.* 1984;15(4):285-288.
22. Shea M, Mednick EB. Ciliary body reattachment in ocular hypotony. *Arch Ophthalmol.* 1981;99(2):278-281.
23. Demeler U. Refixation of the ciliary body after traumatic cyclodialysis. *Dev Ophthalmol.* 1987;14:199-201.
24. Kuchle M, Naumann GO. Direkte Zyklopexie bei Zyklodialyse mit persistierendem Hypotonie-syndrom. *Fortschr Ophthalmol.* 1990;87(3):247-251.
25. Metrikin DC, Allinson RW, Snyder RW. Transscleral repair of recalcitrant, inadvertent, postoperative cyclodialysis cleft. *Ophthalmic Surg.* 1994;25(6):406-408.

26. Klemm M, Winter R. Reversible translimbal suture fixation of the ciliary body in treatment of ocular persistent hypotonia after surgical cyclodialysis. *Ophthalmologic.* 1994;91(5):694-696.

27. Alward WL, Hodapp EA, Parel JM, et al. Argon laser endophotocoagulator closure of cyclodialysis clefts. *Am J Ophthalmol.* 1988;106(6):748-749.

28. Simmons RJ, Kimbrough RL. A modified cyclodialysis spatula. *Ophthalmic Surg.* 1979;10(2):67-68.

29. Alpar JJ. Sodium hyaluronate (Healon) in cyclodialysis. *CLAO J.* 1985;11(3):201-204.

30. Berson FG, Patterson mm, Epstein DL. Obstruction of aqueous outflow by sodium hyaluronate in enucleated human eyes. *Am J Ophthalmol.* 1983;95:668-672.

31. Herschler J. Trabecular damage due to blunt anterior segment injury and its relationship to traumatic glaucoma. *Trans Am Acad Ophthalmol Otolaryngol.* 1977;83(2):239-248.

64

Surgical Peripheral Iridectomy

David L. Epstein, MD, MMM

The second edition of *Lectures on Glaucoma* makes the following statement:

> The first edition of *Lectures on Glaucoma* contained a detailed description of our preferred technique for doing a peripheral iridectomy. Peripheral iridectomy has become one of the commonly used operations for angle-closure glaucoma. All ophthalmic surgeons are capable of performing the operation well and have developed their own preferred technique. Suturing the wound is now almost universally practiced. For these reasons, we have decided to omit a detailed discussion of technique of iridectomy in this edition.

Since the advent of laser iridectomy, it is now rare for ophthalmology residents to perform a surgical peripheral iridectomy. Yet, as alluded to previously, there are certain situations when it is not possible to employ a laser technique (eg, cloudy cornea) when the ophthalmologist should be able to perform a surgical iridectomy. We should also not forget that there are areas of the world where lasers are not yet available.

Therefore, a few aspects of this surgical technique—often called the most underrated operation in ophthalmology—are presented in this chapter.

TECHNIQUE OF SURGICAL PERIPHERAL IRIDECTOMY

Either a limbal- or fornix-based flap is prepared over approximately 1.5 clock-hours in one of the upper quadrants in order to save the other quadrant for possible future filtration surgery (Figure 64-1). The superotemporal quadrant is usually preferred for iridectomy so that, if cataract formation were to occur after a subsequent superonasal quadrant filtering operation, the cataract could be removed more easily from the side rather than from below. We usually prefer a fornix-based flap due to its better limbal exposure.

The key to the operation is the incision. For this purpose, a somewhat rounded knife blade, such as a Beaver No. 67 (Beaver, Waltham, MA) or Bard-Parker No. 15 (Katena Eye Instruments, Denville, NJ), is preferred to enter the eye so that it will slide over the iris without perforating it. A sharp blade is best avoided because it is apt to make a small hole in the iris and the iris will then not spontaneously prolapse. The incision must be perpendicular, clean, and wide enough so that the iris will spontaneously prolapse and will easily reposit. An irregular incision will catch iris tissue and prevent repositioning. In making the incision, when one gets the first gush of aqueous humor, one should not immediately withdraw the knife (as is instinct) but should continue to enlarge the opening to a full clock-hour. One is more confident in doing this with a rounded rather than a sharp blade.

It is important to do this operation outside the eye rather than to reach inside to grasp the iris. If the incision is wide enough (and the iris is not penetrated by the knife), gentle pressure on the posterior lip of the wound will allow the pressure in the posterior chamber to spontaneously prolapse the iris into the wound, where it should be firmly grasped and cleanly cut. The cut iris tissue is inspected for pigment epithelium to ensure that full thickness of the iris has been excised. Then, the iris is reposited by exerting a sweeping motion with the irrigator tip across the limbal incision. No instrument is placed into the eye. Repositing the iris is often the most difficult part of the procedure. Preoperative pilocarpine will often aid in this.

After the iridectomy is performed, iris is often present in the wound. The gentle sweeping pressure of the irrigating tip allows some aqueous humor to escape and the iris to fall back inside the eye. Sometimes, this can also be accomplished by applying a small amount of pressure directly on the posterior lip of the wound or by gently separating the anterior and posterior lips with forceps. The iris is often boggy in eyes with acute angle closure and tends to get hung up in irregular incisions, especially if they are not of adequate size.

Kahook MY, Schuman JS, eds.
Chandler and Grant's Glaucoma, Fifth Edition (pp 601-603).
© 2013 SLACK Incorporated.

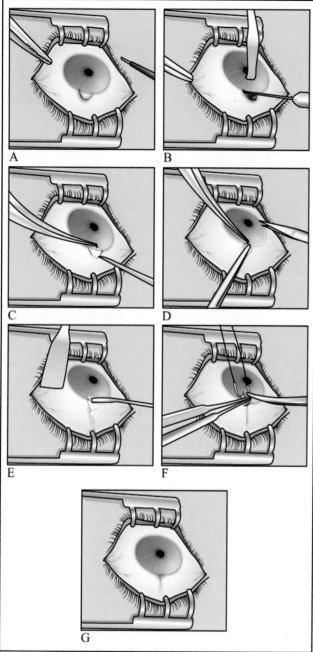

At the end of the procedure, the pupil should be round and the iridectomy opening visualized inside the eye. Otherwise, if the iridectomy is caught in the wound, pupillary block will not be relieved. The flap may be closed by a variety of methods. A useful closure approach is to incorporate conjunctiva in the single suture used to close the limbal incision (Figure 64-1F and G).

Surgical peripheral iridectomy is often a quick, straightforward procedure. However, there are numerous pitfalls that often relate to a suboptimal incision and subsequent problems with iris prolapse and repositioning.

POSTOPERATIVE CARE

A single dressing may be used, but in most cases no dressing is required. A combination of local steroid and antibiotic drops 3 or 4 times a day and 5% phenylephrine drops twice a day are begun on the day of operation and are continued until there are no inflammatory signs in the anterior segment, usually 2 to 3 weeks. One must make sure that the pupil dilates readily. If there is evidence of iritis, short-acting cycloplegics, such as cyclopentolate or tropicamide, are employed.

COMPLICATIONS

A flat or very shallow anterior chamber without elevation of intraocular pressure (IOP) is probably always due to a wound leak. The suture may have been placed too deeply, or it may not have been tied tightly. Of course, a wound leak is more apt to occur if no suture is used. A shallow or flat anterior chamber after peripheral iridectomy calls for prompt intervention. Iridectomy was chosen instead of some other operation because preoperatively, the angle was in large part capable of opening, and one must not allow the previously open angle to become closed by peripheral anterior synechiae (PAS) as a result of prolonged absence of the anterior chamber. There is much more urgency in the prompt reformation of the anterior chamber after a peripheral iridectomy than after a filtering operation. The wound should be promptly explored. The original suture or sutures should be removed, because they may have been improperly placed. Then, new sutures are placed until one can be sure that the wound is tight. After peripheral iridectomy, a flat or shallow anterior chamber and elevated IOP most likely indicates the development of malignant glaucoma (see Chapter 29).

If the iridectomy includes only the stroma of the iris and the pigment epithelium is left behind, then of course the operation will be completely without effect. When the iridectomy is done, one must make sure that there is posterior pigment epithelium on the piece of iris excised. If in the postoperative period it is discovered that the pigment epithelium in the peripheral coloboma is intact, it can generally be easily opened with an argon laser.

Figure 64-1. Technique of surgical peripheral iridectomy. (A) A fornix-based conjunctival flap is prepared with scissors. A knife with a rounded tip is brought forward to make the incision (B), which is perpendicular, clean, and accomplished by a slight rolling motion. After the first gush of aqueous, the incision is slightly extended and is then inspected (C). The anterior lip may be grasped with Colibri forceps, while the iris forceps gently depress the posterior lip (D) so that iris is spontaneously prolapsed into the wound where it is grasped with the iris forceps and is smoothly cut with fine scissors at the wound margin. No instruments should be placed inside the eye. The iris is reposited by a sweeping motion of the irrigator tip across the limbal incision (E). The pupil is observed to be round and the iridectomy patent. The wound and conjunctiva may be then closed by a variety of methods. Shown in (F) and (G) is the technique of incorporating the flap in which the posterior arm of a double-armed suture, having already been placed through the limbal wound, is passed a few millimeters posterior to the edge of the conjunctiva, and then the anterior arm of the same suture is placed (F) through the anterior edge and is then tied (G).

The incision should never be more than 1.5 mm from the limbus. If it is too posterior, a piece of ciliary body may be excised instead of iris. One cannot be sure that the operation has been properly performed unless a peripheral iris coloboma is clearly visible at the end of the operation. If some uveal tissue has been excised, but at the end of the operation, with the pupil round and central, no iris coloboma can be seen, one may think of reopening the wound, introducing forceps, grasping the peripheral iris, and doing a proper iridectomy. However, this entails significant risk of injury to the lens. It is better in such cases to suture the original wound and repeat the operation in another area.

Elevated IOP and haziness of the cornea may be noted in the immediate postoperative period. This does not need to cause great concern if the anterior chamber is of normal depth and a definite coloboma of the iris is present. Gonioscopy should be performed to determine whether the angle is, in fact, open or closed. The Zeiss lens is readily used in such postoperative eyes. If the angle is closed, then in the presence of a normal axial anterior chamber depth, plateau iris syndrome needs to be considered. Routine mydriatic/cycloplegic drops should be discontinued and weak pilocarpine therapy initiated. It is curious that, in the immediate postoperative period, certain cases of apparent plateau iris syndrome (see Chapter 26) that demonstrate angle closure with cycloplegic therapy will fail to do so again when rechallenged several months later. Such patients need to be followed long-term, but it seems as if certain patients may demonstrate angle closure with pupillary dilatation only as a temporary postoperative phenomenon, perhaps due to iris swelling.

Another cause of IOP elevation postoperatively is the presence of extensive pre-existing PAS.

Sometimes, IOP is temporarily elevated after surgical iridectomy due to an ill-defined open-angle glaucoma mechanism, which may relate to cycloplegic therapy, inflammation, or other unknown factors, but which can be managed conservatively with aqueous humor suppressants.

Posterior synechiae can be avoided in most cases by the routine use of phenylephrine along with local steroids beginning on the day of operation, but cycloplegics should be used where iritis develops.

Paul A. Chandler wrote:

Within a day or 2 after surgical iridectomy, when the eye is being treated with topical corticosteroid and periodic dilation of the pupil with phenylephrine to prevent formation of posterior synechiae, in rare instances there is a recurrence of acute glaucoma. This has happened in cases in which the attempt at iridectomy failed to produce a functional hole through the iris, owing to inadvertently leaving the pigment layer of the iris intact or to unintentionally incarcerating the iridectomy coloboma in the wound. The usual solution is to perform a laser iridectomy or, failing this, to go back promptly and do a proper iridectomy at a different site. However, if the intact iris pigment layer is visible in an easily accessible location and is bulging forward because of unrelieved pupillary block, it can usually be easily disrupted with the argon laser.

In doing a surgical peripheral iridectomy for angle-closure glaucoma, we may feel sure that we have excised uveal tissue, but in some cases no coloboma is visible. Did we really excise a piece of iris in the extreme periphery, or a piece of ciliary body? What should we do at this point? We cannot be certain that there is a real coloboma. One alternative is to introduce forceps that are toothless and without sharp points to grasp the iris, pull it out of the wound, and excise a piece. This is risky; however, suppose there is, in fact, a small peripheral coloboma of the iris. When forceps are introduced, there is great danger of injuring the lens. In one case, the lens was injured by this maneuver by Dr. Paul A. Chandler with rapid development of cataract. It was decided that never again would we introduce forceps in such a case. Instead, we have used the following course in patients in whom at the end of the operation no coloboma was visible. The anterior chamber is formed with saline solution, the suture is tied, and the entire operation is repeated, then and there, at another site.

I recall the case of a physician on whom a peripheral iridectomy was being done. At the end of the procedure, no coloboma was visible and the operation was promptly repeated at another site. There was then a visible coloboma. At the end of the procedure, the physician patient inquired how the operation had gone. The answer had to be, "The operation went very well, but I had to do it twice!"

65

Schlemm's Canal Surgery for Glaucoma Management

Steven R. Sarkisian Jr, MD and Marcos Reyes, MD

Schlemm's canal is named after German anatomist Friedrich Schlemm (1795-1858).[1] He noticed this previously uncharacterized structure in 1827 in the postmortem eye of a man who had hanged himself. What he saw was a circular structure at the limbus filled with blood, presumably from the mechanism of death. After meticulous dissection, he found he could cannulate the structure with a bristle. He believed he had discovered a new blood vessel and originally described it as a part of the ocular vasculature.

It was later found that this structure was not a blood vessel belonging to the venous system but rather a canal integral in the drainage of aqueous fluid.[1] Amazingly, his discovery was purely based upon macroscopic assessment.[2] This finding was impressive in his attention to detail and use of excellent dissection technique. We have known about Schlemm's canal for more than 100 years but our understanding of its physiology still evolving.

PHYSIOLOGY

Schlemm's canal is a continuous 360-degree structure found just posterior to the limbus. Its diameter varies from 190 to 370 μm. The canal is not a perfect tube-like structure, and it can and does, on occasion, change in and out of a plexus-like anatomy in its course around the anterior chamber.[3] Schlemm's canal can be thought of as having an inner and outer wall. The inner wall is comprised of 2 parts: the outermost layer of the trabecular meshwork ([TM]; juxtacanalicular meshwork) and the endothelium of Schlemm's canal. Aqueous fluid percolates through the TM and the inner wall of Schlemm's canal before entering the canal. Aqueous then flows into collector channels, which are found in the outer wall of Schlemm's canal within the sclera, draining aqueous into the deep scleral venous plexus.

It is here that the aqueous begins to mix with venous blood as it flows to the external superficial sclera venous vessels.

INTRODUCTION

Glaucoma has many causes but in primary open-angle glaucoma (POAG), the juxtacanalicular meshwork is thought to be the primary area of resistance to aqueous flow.[4] Most methods of glaucoma surgery focus on bypassing the blocked TM through the creation of a fistula (trabeculectomy) or by placing a drainage shunt (ie, Baerveldt [Abbott Medical Optics, Abbott Park, IL] or Ahmed [New World Medical, Rancho Cucamonga, CA]) to drain fluid to a distant plate sutured to the sclera. Trabeculectomy is a penetrating surgery because a permanent fistula (or filter) is created from the anterior chamber to the external subconjunctival space. This technique, although reliable and proven over the last half of the 20th century, has inherent risks associated with its design. Several of the known risks and complications of penetrating glaucoma filtering surgery include blebitis, hypotony, bleb dysesthesia, bleb leak, and endophthalmitis.

Given these known risks of penetrating surgery, new nonpenetrating surgical techniques are gaining favor. Some of these ideas involve augmenting the natural percolation of aqueous fluid from Schlemm's canal or its peripheral collecting channels without entering the anterior chamber. A few new devices are attempting to bypass the TM or remove it completely. These new techniques require an intimate knowledge of Schlemm's canal anatomy, its location, and surrounding structures. New instruments and devices are required for each technique, in addition to precise meticulous surgical dissection. In this chapter, we will discuss the most common of these new techniques detailing the surgical

Kahook MY, Schuman JS, eds.
Chandler and Grant's Glaucoma, Fifth Edition (pp 605-609).
© 2013 SLACK Incorporated.

approach, pearls for success, as well as a review of existing literature.

SURGICAL TECHNIQUES

Nonpenetrating Deep Sclerectomy

Though not a completely new idea, nonpenetrating deep sclerectomy (NPDS) has changed dramatically over the past 50 years. The first documented success was in the late 1950s by Edward Epstein in South Africa after he found oozing in the area over Schlemm's canal after deep excision of a pterygia.[5]

The surgery Epstein devised consisted of 180 degrees of deep sclerectomy in the area over Schlemm's canal that he then covered with conjunctiva.[5] This approach resulted in a functioning bleb, which lasted for a few months but then scarred over. In the late 1960s, Krasnov[6] performed a fistulizing procedure of Schlemm's canal by removing the outer portion of the canal (sinusotomy). This was performed only in the category of patients that, they felt, had obstruction of intrascleral collectors.[7] In the late 1980s, another group of Russian physicians documented success with NPDS[8] and also pioneered the use of a lyophilized porcine collagen implant under the superficial flap as a space maintainer to obtain lower intraocular pressure (IOP).

The traditional NPDS consists of dissection of a superficial sclera flap the size of which is surgeon-dependent. Underneath this superficial flap, a deeper flap is dissected (the deep sclerectomy) until there is only a thin layer of sclera above the uvea, usually seen as a bluish hue. This flap is extended anteriorly including corneal stroma until aqueous humor is seen percolating through a window of thin trabeculo-Descemet's membrane. This deep sclerectomy, including the outer wall of Schlemm's canal, is removed en bloc fashion. At this point, one can use a collagen implant sutured to the sclera floor, popularly known as the Aquaflow implant (Staar Surgical Co, Monrovia, CA), or leave the area empty as studies have shown equal success with and without the implant. The superficial flap is sutured closed with several sutures and the conjunctiva is closed in the normal fashion based on surgeon preference.[8,9]

This procedure effectively creates a scleral lake into which aqueous can percolate, thereby lowering the pressure without a bleb. The absence of a bleb likely results in a decrease of complications, such as infection (blebitis or endophthalmitis), bleb dysesthesia, and other issues associated with traditional penetrating procedures. In one study with 6-year postoperative follow-up, the data showed reasonable success. The mean preoperative IOP was 24.47 mm Hg ± 5.92 (SD), and after 6 years, there was an average lowering of 33.73% ± 20.9% with the mean IOP of 15.81 mm Hg ± 3.79 (SD).[10] There are few studies prospectively comparing the NPDS approach to that of traditional

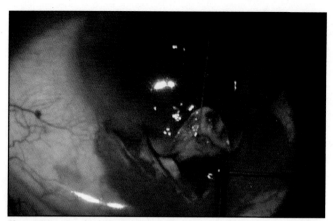

Figure 65-1. Canaloplasty procedure. The red LED light can be seen in the canal at 9 o'clock. (Reprinted with permission from Richard A. Lewis, MD.)

trabeculectomy, and this procedure remains accessible (due to surgical training) to only a handful of surgeons. Typically, a very low IOP is not achieved with this technique; however, this may be a beneficial procedure for less advanced glaucoma when a pressure of 15 to 16 mm Hg is targeted.

Canaloplasty

Canaloplasty was first described by Dr. Roger Stegmann and his team out of the Medical University of South Africa (Johannesburg). From astute observations made during NPDS surgery, Stegmann began methodically altering his surgical technique until he developed a procedure he named *viscocanalostomy*, which became a precursor to canaloplasty. Viscocanalostomy was developed in various stages during the 1990s.[11] The final leap in innovation was unveiled at the 2005 annual American Society of Cataract and Refractive Surgery (ASCRS) meeting where Stegmann[12] shared the results of his newest stage of development, a 360-degree microcanaloplasty, now popularly named canaloplasty.

The initial approach for this procedure is similar to NPDS. A superficial sclera flap is made first, followed by the creation of a second deeper scleral flap (aka deep sclerectomy), which is then extended over Descemet's membrane to create a window. Once the canal is correctly identified and exposed, the iScience (iScience Interventional, Menlo Park, CA) microcatheter is inserted into a surgical opening in the canal (Figure 65-1). The catheter has a blinking red tip so its location is known at all times. It also allows you to inject viscoelastic material through the catheter to reach the tip, aiding in its advance through Schlemm's canal. By slowly advancing the catheter through the entire canal with occasional injections of viscoelastic material, the 360-degree journey can be accomplished with full assurance that you are in the canal at all times using the blinking red light as a guide. Once the tip has reached the opening in Schlemm's canal, a 9-0 or 10-0 Prolene (Ethicon, Inc, Somerville, NJ) suture is tied to it, and the catheter is slowly withdrawn, pulling

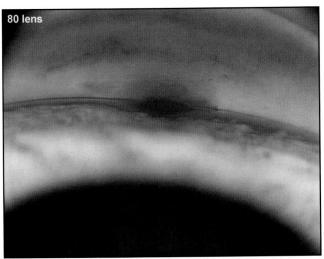

Figure 65-2. Gonioscopic photograph of the Prolene suture in the canal after canaloplasty. (Reprinted with permission from Richard A. Lewis, MD.)

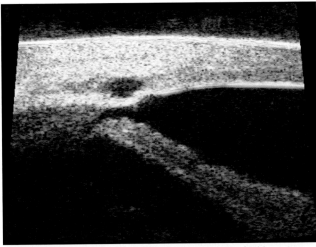

Figure 65-3. Anterior segment ultrasound photograph of Schlemm's canal seen dilated 2 years after canaloplasty. The Prolene suture can be seen in the lower left of the dilated canal. (Reprinted with permission from Richard A. Lewis, MD.)

the suture all the way around to encircle the entire inner wall of the canal. The suture is then tied to itself with a slip knot, which can be locked after the suture is tightened with enough tension to pull the TM inward (Figures 65-2 and 65-3). The superficial flap and then conjunctiva are sutured closed, tight enough to prevent leakage and bleb formation.

The initial pilot study of 33 patients presented at ASCRS in 2005 reported a mean IOP of 15.2 mm Hg±4.7 (SD) at 6 months.[11] Further studies by Lewis and colleagues[13] have shown additional long-term promise. In their case series of 127 eyes of 127 patients, the mean IOP at 24 months was 16.0 mm Hg±4.2 (SD) down from a baseline of 23.6 mm Hg±4.8 (SD). Glaucoma medication usage also dropped from a baseline of 1.9±0.8 to 0.5±0.8. The results were even more impressive with combined canaloplasty and cataract surgery, which is surprising given that traditional trabeculectomy and cataract surgery, in our hands, usually results in a higher pressure than trabeculectomy alone. With combined canaloplasty and cataract surgery, Lewis and colleagues[13] reported a mean IOP of 13.4±4.0 mm Hg and 0.2±0.4 medications down from a baseline IOP of 23.1±5.5 mm Hg and 1.7±1.0 medications. This appears to be an excellent choice for patients with early glaucoma with mild to moderate defects. Further studies are ongoing to evaluate long-term maintenance of low IOP.

Trabectome

The trabectome was developed by Drs. George Baerveldt and Don Minckler out of the University of California–Irvine.[14] It is a device that excises a ~60-degree strip of TM and inner wall of Schlemm's canal, creating a permanent cleft in the meshwork. It requires a good gonioscopic view of an open angle. Essentially, this device is a free-standing electrocautery unit applied to the angle to excise the inner wall of the canal and TM (Figure 65-4).

In the operating room, the patient's head is turned away from the eye having surgery, and after appropriate prepping and draping, a gonioscopy lens is used to ensure adequate view of the drainage angle. The lens is then removed and a 1.6-mm keratotomy incision is made. The device is inserted partially toward the opposite TM when a gonioscopic view is again obtained. Once a good view is established, the insulated foot plate is advanced to contact the TM and then is moved in an arc-like fashion either clockwise or counter-clockwise to engage the footplate into Schlemm's canal (Figure 65-5). The device is continually moved and the TM is simultaneously cauterized and aspirated. This is performed for approximately 30 degrees in one direction and then brought back to the starting position rotated to the opposite direction and then again engaged in the TM to begin the same process for another, approximately, 30 degrees. The cleft created by the procedure can be visualized with anterior segment ultrasound (Figure 65-6).

Results from the initial case series[15] showed a mean postoperative pressure of 16.3±2.0 mm Hg at 12 months from preoperative IOPs of 28.2 mm Hg±4.4 (SD). A follow-up larger case series of 1127 patients showed a total mean IOP decrease among trabectome-only cases of 40%, from a preoperative IOP of 25.7 mm Hg±7.7 (SD) to a postoperative IOP of 16.6 mm Hg±4.0 (SD) at 24 months. In the phacoemulsification-trabectome combination cases, the IOP decreased 18% from a preoperative IOP of 20.0 mm Hg±6.2 (SD) to a postoperative IOP of 15.9 mm Hg±3.3 (SD). The main intraoperative complication was reflux bleeding with development of hyphema, and there was a 7.8% failure rate.[16] This approach also shows promise as another method of treatment for

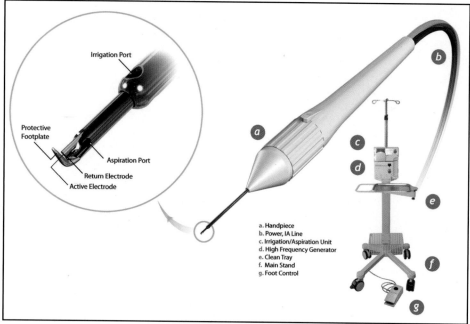

Figure 65-4. The trabectome device. (Reprinted with permission from Brian A. Francis, MD, MS.)

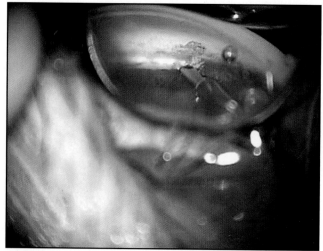

Figure 65-5. Gonioscopic photograph of the trabectome procedure demonstrating counterclockwise ablation. (Reprinted with permission from Brian A. Francis, MD, MS.)

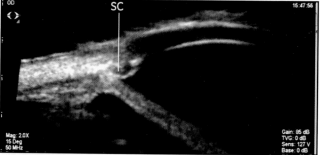

Figure 65-6. Anterior segment ultrasound photograph of Schlemm's canal seen after the trabectome procedure. The cleft in the canal wall can be seen adjacent to the anterior chamber. (Reprinted with permission from Brian A. Francis, MD, MS.)

glaucoma with mild visual field defect and has been commonly performed in tandem with cataract surgery. Further studies are ongoing to evaluate long-term pressure control.

Ab Interno Canal Surgery and the Future

We are currently in a time of surgical innovation in glaucoma therapy, with the focus of most new technology being on channeling aqueous humor to Schlemm's canal. There are several devices in various stages of the Food and Drug Administration (FDA) approval process at the time of this publication; however, there is one that is FDA approved for use now. This new development is the Glaukos istent (Glaukos Corp, Laguna Hills, CA). It is a 1.0-mm × 0.5-mm microbypass stent with a 0.12-mm lumen inserted through the TM into Schlemm's canal under gonioscopic view. It bypasses the TM providing direct access to Schlemm's canal. In a 12 month study comparing istent implantation combined with cataract surgery to cataract surgery alone, 66% of patients in the combined group achieved a decrease in IOP greater than or equal to 20%, compared to a 48% decrease in the cataract surgery group alone. The criterion for success was an IOP of less than or equal to 21%; 75% of the combined group were successful compared to 50% of the cataract surgery group alone. This is approved for mild to moderate glaucoma patients. One major advantage of this approach, similar to that of trabectome, is the preservation of the conjunctiva in case further invasive surgeries, such as trabeculectomy, are needed in the future.

One other canal stent of note in the FDA approval process is the Hydrus (Ivantis Inc, Irvine, CA).[17] It functions much like the istent; however, due to the longer length of the Hydrus, it is hypothesized that the postoperative IOP should be even lower. The innovation of microinvasive glaucoma surgery is altering the glaucoma treatment algorithm; moreover, the evidence demonstrating the efficacy and advantages of these procedures will likely be the debate of our generation.

Conclusion

One can envision future surgical techniques using Schlemm's canal, including other forms and varieties of stents, or perhaps even nanotechnology applications that may alter not only the canal but also the collector channels that, if obstructed, limit the distal flow of aqueous beyond the canal. Among the limitations of canal surgery, the potential for distal obstruction may prove to be the most significant barrier to achieving normal, physiologic IOP in many patients with glaucoma. At this time, there does not seem to be any canal-based procedure that can achieve the low pressures possible with traditional trabeculectomy, but these approaches are still in their infancy. Perhaps we will find that each new approach holds a particular place in our surgical armamentarium, which can be tailored to the needs of each individual patient.

References

1. Rust, JN. *Theoretisch-praktisches Handbuch der Chirurgie mit Einschlub der syphilitischen un Augenkrankheiten.* Berlin: Enslin; 1830:332-338.
2. Winkelmann A. Schlemm, the body snatcher? *Ann Anat.* 2008;190(3):223-229.
3. Rohen JW, Rentsch FJ. Morphology of Schlemm's canal and related vessels in the human eye [in German]. *Albrecht Von Graefes Arch Klin Exp Ophthalmol.* 1968;176(4):309-329.
4. Johnson MC, Kamm RD. The role of Schlemm's canal in aqueous outflow from the human eye. *Invest Ophthalmol Vis Sci.* 1983;24:320-325.
5. Epstein E. Communications fibrosing response to aqueous: its relation to glaucoma. *Br J Ophthalmol.* 1959;43:641-647.
6. Krasnov MM. Externalization of Schlemm's canal (sinusotomy) in glaucoma. *Br J Ophthalmol.* 1968;52:157-161.
7. Kozlov VI, Bagrov SN, Anisimova SY, et al. *Non penetrating deep sclerectomy with collagen.* IRTC "Eye Microsurgery," Moscow: RSFSR Ministry of Public Health; 1990;3:44-46.
8. Fyodorov SN, Kozlov VI, Timoshkina NT, et al. Nonpenetrating deep sclerectomy in open angle glaucoma. *Ophthalmosurgery.* 1990;3:52-55.
9. Demailly E, Lavat R, Kretz G, et al. Non-penetrating deep sclerectomy (NPDS) with or without collagen device (CD) in primary open-angle glaucoma: middle-term retrospective study. *Int Ophthalmol.* 1997;20:131-140.
10. Lachkar Y, Neverauskiene J, Jeanteur-Lunel MN, et al. Nonpenetrating deep sclerectomy: a 6-year retrospective study. *Eur J Ophthalmol.* 2004;14(1):26-36.
11. Stegmann R, Pienaar A, Miller D. Viscocanalostomy for open-angle glaucoma in black African patients. *J Cataract Refract Surg.* 1999;25:316-322.
12. Stegmann R. 360 Microcanalostomy of Schlemm's canal in POAG. Paper presented at the 2005-2006 Annual ASCRS symposium; Washington, DC. 2005.
13. Lewis RA, Wolff KV, Tetz M. Canaloplasty: circumferential viscodilation and tensioning of Schlemm canal using a flexible microcatheter for the treatment of open-angle glaucoma in adults. Two-year interim clinical study results. *J Cataract Refractive Surg.* 2009;35:814-824.
14. Minckler DS, Baerveldt G, Alfaro MR, et al. Clinical results with the trabectome, a novel surgical device for treatment of open-angle glaucoma. *Trans Am Ophthalmol Soc.* 2006;104:40-50.
15. Minckler DS, Baerveldt G, Alfaro MR, et al. Clinical results with the trabectome for treatment of open-angle glaucoma. *Ophthalmology.* 2005;112:962-967.
16. Minckler D, Mosaed S, Dustin L, et al. Trabectome (trabeculectomy-internal approach): additional experience and extended follow-up. *Trans Am Ophthalmol Soc.* 2008;106:149-160.
17. Camras LJ, Yuan F, Fan S, et al. A novel Schlemm's canal scaffold increases outflow facility in a human anterior segment perfusion model. *Invest Ophthalmo Vis Sci.* 2012;53(10):6115-6121.

66

Suprachoroidal Approach to Glaucoma Surgery

Ramesh S. Ayyala, MD, FRCS(E), FRCOphth(Lon); Farhan A. Irshad, MD; and Iqbal "Ike" K. Ahmed, MD, FRCSC

Surgical approaches to the suprachoroidal space range from traditional procedures aimed at draining fluid from the suprachoroidal space (blood or transudate) to implantation of newer devices that drain aqueous humor into the space as a means of controlling elevated intraocular pressure (IOP). The novel devices that access the suprachoroidal space, either from an ab externo or an ab interno approach, are still in early development and evidence-based medicine is lacking. We will cover the more traditional aspects of the suprachoroidal space as it relates to glaucoma in this chapter and only touch on the basics of the novel devices toward the end of this chapter.

Basic Anatomy

The suprachoroidal space is a potential space between the choroid and the sclera. It is limited anteriorly by the attachment of the longitudinal ciliary muscle to the scleral spur and posteriorly by the scleral aperture of the optic nerve. This space is not continuous and is segmented by the outward passage of the vortex veins, by the perforating short posterior ciliary arteries, and the loose attachment of the choroid to the sclera.

Basic Physiology

Transmural pressures in the choroidal circulation are affected by the same hydrostatic and oncotic pressures found throughout the peripheral vasculature. In the setting of increased blood pressure or low IOPs, this transmural pressure rises, leading to the passage of transudative serum from choroidal vessels into the suprachoroidal space. Transudative

fluid and the large molecule proteins it is associated with create its own oncotic pressure, drawing further fluid into the suprachoroidal space.

Surgical Problems Encountered in the Space

The following are problems that may be encountered during surgery:

- Collection of fluid in this space (either protein-rich fluid as in choroidal effusion or blood-mixed fluid as in choroidal hemorrhage) is usually located posterior to the ora serrata. This usually occurs in the immediate postoperative period with hypotony after glaucoma filtration surgery. Collection of fluid pushes the choroid/retina complex inward in a segmental fashion because of the outward passage of the vortex veins. Thus, indirect ophthalmoscopy or ultrasound scan will reveal the effusion as a dark-brown translucent dome-shaped elevation involving 1 to 4 quadrants on indirect ophthalmoscopy. Significant effusion can result in kissing choroids and compromise vision.

- Detachment of the longitudinal ciliary muscle to the scleral spur (cyclodialysis) can result in direct communication between the anterior chamber and the suprachoroidal space (cleft), which results in increased flow of aqueous humor into the suprachoroidal space and hypotony. The cleft can be visualized directly on gonioscopy as a dark area of detachment at the root of the iris with the white undersurface of the sclera visible or using high-frequency ultrasound.

Kahook MY, Schuman JS, eds.
Chandler and Grant's Glaucoma, Fifth Edition (pp 611-617).
© 2013 SLACK Incorporated.

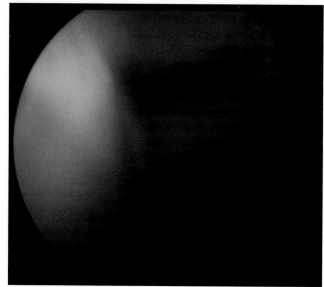

Figure 66-1. Choroidal effusion.

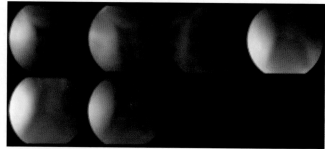

Figure 66-2. Kissing choroidal effusions.

- Redirection of the aqueous humor into the suprachoroidal space via artificial communication channels (ie, shunts and stents) can reduce and control the IOP.

Choroidal Effusion

Choroidal effusion (Figure 66-1) is a collection of protein-rich fluid in the suprachoroidal space in response to hypotony following glaucoma filtration surgery. This is more likely to occur in patients with altered choroidal vascular dynamics and obese patients.

Hypotony could be the result of overfiltration or a leaky bleb. Ciliary body detachment can occur following anterior migration of the ciliary body, resulting in decreased aqueous secretion, worsening of hypotony, and shallowing of the anterior chamber.

Patients can present with painless loss of vision or shadows in the peripheral visual fields. Conservative treatment includes topical steroids alongside cycloplegic agents along with a course of low-dose oral steroids (20 to 30 mg prednisolone on a tapering regimen over 2 to 3 weeks).

SLIT-LAMP PROCEDURES

Leaky blebs should be addressed by suturing the bleb at the slit-lamp. A flat anterior chamber should be addressed immediately with an injection of a highly cohesive viscoelastic substance, such as Healon GV (Abbott Medical Optics, Santa Ana, CA). This can be done at the slit-lamp under topical anesthesia. The resultant anterior chamber deepening and increase in IOP achieved with this procedure may also be helpful in treating choroidal effusions, effectively squeezing the effusion from the suprachoroidal space.

A highly cohesive viscoelastic injection (0.1 cc) (Healon GV or Healon 5) into the anterior chamber can also be tried to decrease choroidal effusions by a squeegee-type of mechanism.

Indications for surgical intervention include shallow to flat anterior chamber, decrease in vision with kissing choroidals (Figure 66-2), or effusions persisting longer than 6 to 8 weeks. Flat anterior chambers are among the most common reasons for choroidal effusion drainage. When conservative management (often with frequent topical corticosteroids and cycloplegia) fails to resolve persistent choroidals, choroidal effusion drainage is indicated. Furthermore, prophylactic posterior sclerotomies are often indicated in high-risk individuals prone to develop choroidal effusions following glaucoma or other ocular surgeries.

ANESTHESIA

Choroidal drainage can be performed under topical anesthesia supplemented by subconjunctival injection of preservative-free lidocaine 1% mixed with preservative-free epinephrine 1:1000 (7.5 cc of lidocaine with 2.5 cc of epinephrine). Injection of this combination achieves several things, including regional anesthesia, control of bleeding, and dissection of the subconjunctival space with minimal trauma.

TECHNIQUE

The procedure is performed in the operating room using the operating microscope. Following the placement of the lid speculum, the anterior segment is examined under the microscope. The anterior chamber depth, shape, location, and presence of the bleb are noted. The absence of red reflex under the scope indicates the presence of significant choroidal effusion.

Because the bleb is usually present in the superior limbal area in glaucoma patients, the preferred location for the surgery is the inferior temporal or nasal quadrants. Either via a paracentesis or using a 30-gauge needle (my preferred technique), 0.1 to 0.2 cc of viscoelastic substance is injected into the anterior chamber. This will deepen the anterior chamber and increase the IOP to facilitate the surgery. It is important to maintain the IOP higher than 20 mm Hg throughout the surgery, both to facilitate complete escape of the choroidal fluid through the sclerostomy and to prevent the occurrence of hemorrhage during the procedure. This is achieved by using an anterior chamber maintainer (alternatively, one can use a 23-gauge butterfly needle that is connected to a bottle held as high as possible).

A 7-0 Vicryl traction suture (Ethicon, Inc, Somerville, NJ) is placed to the 6 o'clock limbus and the eye is rotated superiorly. Limbal peritomy is performed in the inferior temporal quadrant followed by the sub-Tenon's injection of a lidocaine-epinephrine mixture. Posterior dissection is performed in the same plane using Westcott scissors. Hemostasis is achieved by using underwater cautery. Approximately 4-mm posterior to the limbus, a 4-mm radial sclera incision is performed using a 15-degree blade. The dissection is carried gently deeper until the suprachoroidal space is entered. Careful dissection can be ensured by having the assistant hold the lips of the incision apart using 0.12 forceps. Injury to the choroid should be avoided. As soon as the suprachoroidal space is entered, straw-colored fluid is seen to exit the incision. The lips of the incision are parted to facilitate further escape of the fluid. As the choroidal effusion escapes, the IOP decreases, unless the pressure is maintained using the chamber maintainer as described above. This procedure is repeated until all of the fluid escapes. Similar incision can be performed in the inferior nasal quadrant should the patient have significant effusion in that quadrant. As the effusion decreases, the pupillary reflex turns red. This can be confirmed with indirect ophthalmoscopy. The sclerotomy incision is left open to weep. The conjunctiva is secured back to the limbus using either a 10-0 nylon or Vicryl suture. We prefer to inject 0.1 to 0.3 cc of viscoelastic into the anterior chamber at the end of the procedure to maintain the IOP around 20 mm Hg. The bleb should also be examined to make sure that a leaky bleb does not exist.

Postoperative care consists of frequent application of a topical steroid along with cycloplegics for at least a month. Less than 5% of the choroidal effusions recur. Recurrence may be significant enough to require repeat drainage. If this were to happen, we prefer to close the scleral flap of the trabeculectomy operation with additional transconjunctival sutures to decrease the aqueous outflow at the end of the choroidal effusion drainage.

If combined with another surgical procedure, posterior sclerotomy should always be performed first as it decreases the amount of plasma proteins, inflammatory exudates, and fluid accumulation in the suprachoroidal space during surgery. As a result, even with lowering of IOP during surgery, there is less accumulation of fluid driven by osmotic pressure. It should also be noted that the technique for posterior sclerotomy is the same whether the procedure is performed for choroidal effusion drainage or for a suprachoroidal hemorrhage.

POSTOPERATIVE COMPLICATIONS

Complications include cataract formation, recurrence of choroidal effusions, and rarely retinal detachment and endophthalmitis. Usually, choroidal detachments are known to resolve completely within 6 weeks of a posterior sclerotomy. WuDunn and colleagues noted a success rate of 77% per drainage procedure. Cataracts are known to be a frequent complication after drainage of choroidal effusions and may be related to either reduced aqueous humor circulation around the lens or to lens-corneal touch. One study by WuDunn and colleagues noted a 77% cataract development rate in phakic eyes after choroidal effusion drainage.[1] Other complications associated with drainage of choroidal detachments include hyphema, vitreous hemorrhage, retinal tear or detachment, and recurrent suprachoroidal hemorrhage. As with any other ocular surgery, endophthalmitis remains a concern but rates are comparable to other ophthalmic procedures.

SPECIAL SITUATIONS

High-risk groups include nanophthalmic and hyperopic eyes as well as individuals who have previously developed effusions. As a result, scleral windows are often performed prophylactically in nanophthalmic eyes during other ocular surgeries to avoid potential complications. Patients with uveal effusion syndrome have both thick sclera and elevated episcleral venous pressure (EVP) that often necessitates prophylactic sclerotomy. In addition, patients with raised EVP are prone to develop both intraoperative and postoperative choroidal effusions. This includes patients with Sturge-Weber syndrome, carotid cavernous fistulas, choroidal hemangioma, and dural sinus shunts.[2,3]

Aside from scleral windows, key preventative steps include small incision size, precise attention to adequate and full-time pressurization of the eye, and avoidance of any anterior chamber shallowing using bimanual techniques during anterior segment procedures.

SUPRACHOROIDAL HEMORRHAGE

Suprachoroidal hemorrhage usually occurs during or in the immediate postoperative period following glaucoma filtration surgery. It occurs as a result of an initial effusion or separation of the choroid from the sclera with associated rupture of the choroidal blood vessels leading to collection of blood in the suprachoroidal space. As opposed to choroidal effusion, which is painless, suprachoroidal hemorrhage is associated with severe pain.[4,5]

Intraoperative Suprachoroidal Hemorrhage

If the patient complains of severe pain in the middle of surgery, one should suspect suprachoroidal hemorrhage. The anterior chamber tends to become shallow with the increase in the IOP along with the appearance of a rapidly increasing dark shadow in the fundus with alteration of the red reflex. As soon as the diagnosis is suspected, one should stop further intraocular manipulation and close the wound. The diagnosis can be confirmed by indirect ophthalmoscopy and ultrasound. Once the diagnosis is confirmed, the quadrant with the maximum hemorrhage should be identified. A sclerotomy may be performed as described above in that quadrant to drain out the blood. Drainage of even small quantities of blood will help decrease the pain and resolve the hemorrhage faster.

Suprachoroidal Hemorrhage in the Postoperative Period

Patients with a past history of multiple intraocular surgeries, aphakia with poorly controlled glaucoma, and older patients on blood thinners with uncontrolled hypertension are at higher risk of developing hemorrhage. Patients often present with sudden onset of ocular pain following a Valsalva maneuver. Examination will reveal decreased vision, elevated IOP, and shallow to flat chamber. Fundus exam will demonstrate dark shadows in the periphery. Ultrasound examination will demonstrate the presence of blood with high internal reflectivity. Because the blood clots soon after the bleeding, it is not possible to drain it until the blood clot begins to breakdown. Initial treatment is directed toward achieving symptomatic relief and consists of topical and systemic glaucoma medications to control elevated IOP, topical and systemic steroids to decrease inflammation, cycloplegic agents to deepen the chamber, and pain medications to control the pain. The indications for surgery include continued pain, kissing choroidal detachments, persistent shallow to flat chamber, and decrease in vision. Drainage of a suprachoroidal hemorrhage is similar to the drainage of effusions, typically performed after clot liquefaction (10 to 14 days).

CYCLODIALYSIS CLEFT REPAIR

Indications

Cyclodialysis clefts are the result of trauma. The cleft is created by the disinsertion of the longitudinal ciliary muscle from the scleral spur. This could be secondary to blunt trauma, such as fist or ball injury, or could be an unwanted complication of a surgical procedure such as the 25-gauge vitrectomy. It usually presents with very low IOPs and decreased vision. Diagnosis is confirmed by careful gonioscopy and high-frequency ultrasound. These clefts can usually be observed for resolution over 6 to 8 weeks. Various measures, including cycloplegia, injection of viscoelastics, Argon laser treatment, and cryotherapy, can be used to treat a cyclodialysis cleft. If these measure fail, however, incisional surgery should be attempted in order to prevent complications associated with intractable hypotony, including hypotony maculopathy. It should be noted that cyclodialysis cleft creation

has been used in the past for treatment of POAG, although results have often been unpredictable.

Surgical Technique

Various surgical techniques exist for repair of cyclodialysis clefts. Three common methods will be discussed here, including direct cyclopexy, cross-chamber cyclopexy, and iris base fixation techniques. For each technique, it is important to begin with the injection of viscoelastic material in the anterior chamber. This allows for the globe to become more rigid and also allows for better direct visualization of the cleft. Once visualized, the extent of the cleft should be marked using cautery or a marking pen for later reference. Next, it is necessary to create a limbus-based conjunctival peritomy adjacent to the cleft.

Direct Cyclopexy Technique

Originally described by Naumann, the direct cyclopexy technique has the benefit of direct visualization of the disinsertion of the ciliary body and scleral spur and thus allows the most anatomically precise closure of the cleft. However, this technique is also the most complex, and as such, comprehensive understanding of angle anatomy is required.[6]

After sufficient viscoelastic material is injected into the anterior chamber, a rectangular scleral flap at 60% scleral depth is created 4-mm radial to the limbus. The flap should extend at least 2 mm beyond the edge of the cyclodialysis cleft. Once the flap is dissected, a full-thickness incision through the bed of the dissection should be made about 1.5-mm posterior to the limbus. This incision should allow entry into the cleft and release of aqueous. Using 10-0 nylon sutures on a tapered vascular blood vessel needle, the ciliary body should be sutured directly to the sclera. Each suture should first pass through the anterior lip of the wound, then through the ciliary muscle, and finally out through the posterior lip of the scleral wound.

The sutures should only be tied after all have been placed in the appropriate areas. Cryotherapy can then be applied to the base of the scleral wound to enhance the adhesion of the sclera to the ciliary body. Next, the scleral flap is closed using 10-0 nylon, and, finally, the conjunctiva is closed.

Cross-Chamber Cyclopexy Technique

The cross-chamber cyclopexy technique, developed by Metrikin,[7] requires an aphakic or pseudophakic eye and is derived from the principles of suturing posterior chamber intraocular lenses (IOLs). It is also less technically challenging than the previously described technique. In this procedure, a 1- to 2-mm corneal keratotomy is made exactly 180 degrees opposite the location of the cyclodialysis cleft. This can be accomplished with a super-sharp blade. Once again, viscoelastic material should be injected to help maintain a formed anterior chamber. Next, a 27-gauge needle is inserted ab externa through the sclera located 1.5-mm posterior to the limbus at one end of the cleft. This needle is then passed through the ciliary sulcus between the iris and posterior chamber IOL. A 10-0 double-armed polypropylene suture on a straight needle is then threaded into the opening of this needle by inserting it through the previously made keratotomy site. The 27-gauge needle is subsequently pulled out of the eye along with the straight needle of the polypropylene suture. Next, this needle is reinserted into the sclera located 3-mm adjacent to the original entry site. The second arm of the polypropylene suture is then passed into the barrel of the needle before it is extracted from the eye again.

The 2 ends of the suture are then pulled tight, thus firmly bringing the ciliary body up against the wall of the sclera and closing the cyclodialysis cleft. The suture is tied and the knot is buried. This procedure is then repeated along the length of the entire cleft as often as necessary. Once again, cryotherapy is applied to the base of the sclera to promote and maintain further adhesion. After closure of the conjunctiva and corneal keratotomy, any remaining viscoelastic material should be removed from the anterior chamber.

Iris Base Fixation Technique

The iris base fixation procedure was developed by Mills et al[8] and is considered to be easier than the previously described techniques for cyclodialysis repair. Because it tends to create peripheral anterior synechiae (PAS), it is usually more appropriate for closure of smaller and shorter clefts.

Once again, a 1- to 2-mm keratotomy is made through the peripheral cornea; however, this incision is made 1-mm anterior to the limbus, adjacent to the location of the cleft. Next, a 60% thickness rectangular scleral flap is fashioned overlying the area of the cleft. One arm of a 10-0 nylon suture on a curved needle is then passed through the keratotomy, catching peripheral iris before exiting through the scleral bed, 1-mm posterior to the limbus. This procedure is then repeated with the other arm of the suture at a distance of 1 mm from the first bite. This suture is pulled tight, which often causes the pupil to peak as the peripheral iris is brought into contact with the scleral wall. Additional mattress sutures are placed along the peripheral iris to cover the entire length of the cleft. The scleral flap is closed using 10-0 nylon suture. The conjunctival peritomy is then closed. Any remaining viscoelastic material should be removed from the anterior chamber.

Postoperative Care

Atropine is used for at least 2 to 4 weeks following each of the previously described techniques. Steroids should generally be avoided because postoperative inflammation will help promote closure of the cyclodialysis cleft. It can sometimes take up to a few weeks before closure of the cleft occurs. Upon closure of the cleft, an IOP spike can sometimes occur. This is best treated with aqueous suppressants. Prophylactic hypotensive agents should never be used in this situation.

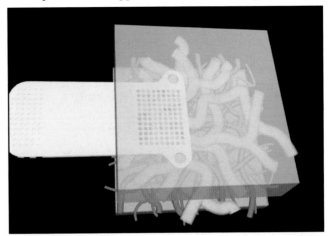

Figure 66-3. Schematic of the gold shunt. (Reprinted with permission from SOLX, Inc.)

Complications

Complications from cyclodialysis repair are rare but can include persistent hypotony, decreased vision, postoperative pressure spikes, PAS formation, and cataract development.

Novel Suprachoroidal Drainage Devices

A known pressure difference between the anterior chamber and suprachoroidal space of approximately 4 mm Hg creates a negative pressure gradient toward this space. This gradient increases with increasing IOP and increases from the limbal region to the optic nerve.[9] New ab interno and ab externo devices have been introduced recently with the SOLX gold shunt (Figure 66-3; SOLX, Inc, Waltham, MA) representing the ab externo technique and the Cypass (Transcend Medical, Menlo Park, CA) and iStent Supra (Glaukos Corp, Laguna Hills, CA) representing 2 versions of ab interno suprachoroidal devices. At this time, data are lacking for the ab interno devices and we are awaiting the publication of clinical trials to better understand the efficacy of such devices. We do know a little more about the ab externo device (SOLX) and will expand on this technique below.

DEEP LIGHT GLAUCOMA TREATMENT SYSTEM

The Deep Light Glaucoma Treatment System is a shunt that was developed by SOLX. It is a gold microshunt that attempts to reduce IOP without formation of a bleb.[10] It contains many microtubules that form a channel and bridge the anterior chamber to the suprachoroidal space and ultimately control the outflow. This gold shunt is a flat, 24-karat gold implant that is 3 mm wide, 6 mm long, and about the thickness of a human hair. The aqueous from the anterior chamber

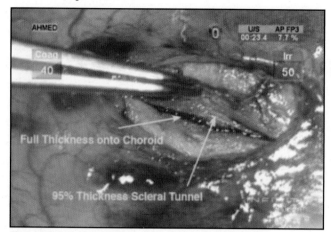

Figure 66-4. Surgical implantation of the gold shunt.

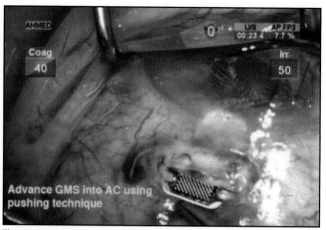

Figure 66-5. Proper positioning of the gold shunt using the pushing technique.

is directed through the minute channels and exits the shunt directly into the suprachoroidal space. The pressure gradient, which naturally exists between the anterior chamber and suprachoroidal space, creates a constant flow of aqueous through the gold shunt.

Surgical Technique

Implantation of the gold shunt involves a 4-mm fornix-based conjunctival incision (Figure 66-4). A 3.5-mm scleral cutdown (vertical scleral incision) is created 2-mm posterior to the limbus. A dissection is carried out to the depth where the choroid is visible through a thin layer of sclera. A scleral pocket at 95% depth is created, which is directed anteriorly toward the scleral spur. The vertical cutdown incision is deepened into the choroidal space, and viscoelastic material can be administered. An incision is made into the anterior chamber at the level of the scleral spur through the previously created pocket. The gold shunt is then inserted through the scleral incision into the anterior chamber using a push-then-pull technique. The posterior tabs should be left during the scleral cutdown. In order to position the shunt into the suprachoroidal space, the 2 posterior lateral tabs of the device are tucked into the suprachoroidal space using a sharp 27-gauge needle. Positioning and movement of the shunt can be assisted by slightly depressurizing the eye to relax the choroid and open up the supraciliary space (Figure 66-5).

Intraoperative gonioscopy can be done to confirm proper positioning of the shunt in the anterior chamber (Figure 66-6). Most of the anterior drainage openings should be visible, but no posterior drainage holes should be seen. In order to ensure watertight closure, 4 or 5 interrupted 10-0 nylon sutures are used to close the overlying scleral wound. A 10-0 Vicryl suture is used to close the conjunctiva.

Noecker and Schuman[11] performed a study to evaluate the efficacy of IOP reduction by the gold shunt. Seventy-six

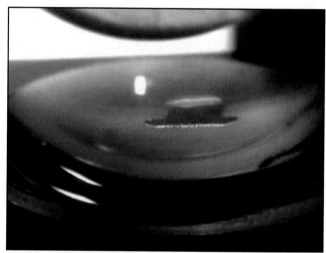

Figure 66-6. Gonioview of the gold shunt.

eyes affected by POAG were implanted with the shunt and were followed for 2 years. The mean preoperative IOP was 27.7 ± 5.9 mm Hg. The mean postoperative IOP at 1 year was 19.7 ± 7.9 mm Hg in 50 eyes and 19.7 ± 3.3 mm Hg at 2-year follow-up in 18 eyes.

Simon[12] performed a similar study with 76 implanted eyes and evaluated the results after 2 years. He found that the preoperative IOP average was 27.7 ± 5.9 mm Hg with the mean in 50 eyes at 19.7 ± 7.9 after 1 year. After 2 years, 18 eyes had a mean pressure of 17.4 ± 3.3 mm Hg. These initial results revealed that IOP reduction can be achieved without the formation of a filtration bleb, but more studies will need to be completed in order to validate this finding.

Complications

Complications seen to date with the shunt include anterior chamber inflammation, hyphema, hypotony, and blurred vision. All are transient and are considered minor complications. The frequency of serious adverse events appears to be rare.

For patients who have had a poor response to subconjunctival filtration or have developed a significant amount of fibrosis, suprachoroidal shunts, such as the SOLX gold shunt, may be a good alternative.

REFERENCES

1. WuDunn D, Ryser D, Cantor LB. Surgical drainage of choroidal effusions following glaucoma surgery. *J Glaucoma.* 2005;14(2):103-108.
2. Chen TC. *Surgical Techniques in Ophthalmology: Glaucoma Surgery.* Philadephia, PA: WB Saunders; 2008:207-215.
3. Spaeth GL. *Ophthalmic Surgery: Principles and Practice.* 3rd ed. Philadelphia, PA: Saunders; 2003:383-387, 409-412.
4. Bhagat N, Zarbin M. Drainage of choroidal detachments. In: Dunn JP, Langer PD, eds. *Basic Techniques of Ophthalmic Surgery.* San Francisco, CA: American Academy of Ophthalmology; 2009:279-282.
5. Kwon OW, Kang SJ, Lee JB, Lee SC, Yoon YD, Oh JH. Treatment of suprachoroidal hemorrhage with tissue plasminogen activator. *Ophthalmologica.* 1998;212:120-125.
6. Naumann GOH, Volcker HE. Direct cyclopexy for persisting hypotony syndrome due to traumatic cyclodialysis. In: Koch DD, Parke DW, Paton D, eds. *Current Management in Ophthalmology.* New York, NY: Churchill Livingstone; 1983:143-150.
7. Metrikin DC, Allinson RW, Snyder RW. Transscleral repair of recalcitrant, inadvertent, postoperative cyclodialysis cleft. *Ophthalmic Surg.* 1994;25:406-408.
8. Stewart JFG, Leen MM, Mills RP. Identification and management of cyclodialysis clefts. In: Lindquist TD, Lindstrom RL, eds. *Ophthalmic Surgery.* 5th ed. Chicago, IL: Mosby-Year Medical; 1996.
9. Emi K, Pederson JE, Toris CB. Hydrostatic pressure of the suprachoroidal space. *Invest Ophthalmol Vis Sci.* 1989;30(2):233-238.
10. Melamed S, Ben Simon GJ, Goldenfeld M, Simon G. Efficacy and safety of gold micro shunt implantation to the supraciliary space in patients with glaucoma: a pilot study. *Arch Ophthalmol.* 2009;127(3):264-269.
11. Noecker R, Schuman JS. Paper 22 presented at the American Glaucoma Society Meeting, 2007.
12. Simon G. Suprachoroidal shunts. New surgical approach in glaucoma. In: Garg A, Alio JL, eds. *Glaucoma Surgery.* New Delhi, India: Jaypee Brothers Medical Publishers; 2010.

Treatment of Occludable Angles and Angle Closure With Cataract Extraction

Michael A. Alunni, MD and Garry P. Condon, MD

Clinical studies from the past have well documented the effect of cataract extraction (eg, phacoemulsification and extracapsular cataract extraction) on intraocular pressure (IOP), anterior chamber depth (ACD), and angle opening width in the normal eye and in eyes with primary open-angle glaucoma (POAG).[1-4] Studies[1-4] have shown that phacoemulsification alone can effectively lower IOP by 2 to 5 mm Hg in patients with open angles with or without glaucoma. These studies have shown promising results and indicate that cataract extraction may be a powerful tool for IOP management in patients diagnosed with POAG.

The benefit of cataract extraction in eyes with angle closure and, to a lesser extent, occludable angles has also been evaluated and can be a viable treatment option. We identify these conditions and discuss the postoperative effect of cataract removal.

OCCLUDABLE ANGLES

The International Society of Geographical and Epidemiological Ophthalmology (ISGEO) have recently identified[5,6] eyes with narrow iridocorneal angles or occludable angles as primary angle-closure suspects (PACS). These eyes carry a long-term risk of poor visual outcomes and can be considered in the preglaucomatous stage because of the likelihood for progression to primary angle-closure glaucoma (PACG) over time.[5,6]

Clinically, classification of the angle varies widely and relies on practitioner skill and technique. Gonioscopy remains the gold standard, and for the purposes of this chapter, we will define the angle based on the Shaffer grading system, which describes the relationship between the trabecular

meshwork (TM) and iris. With this system, an occludable angle is present if a grading of slit, Grade 1, or Grade 2 is observed (Table 67-1). The presence of appositional closure, peripheral anterior synechiae (PAS), increased segmental TM pigmentation, a history of previous angle closure, anterior chamber depth less than 2 mm, and family history of angle closure also suggest that an angle is occludable and should be identified as such.[7,8]

We know that occludable angles carry the risk of progression to angle closure, which can cause extreme elevations in IOP and subsequent irreversible damage to the optic nerve, iris, lens, corneal endothelium, and TM.[9] The mechanism of elevated IOP is typically through pupillary block and, therefore, treatment modalities have been targeted to alleviate this event.[10,11] However patients diagnosed with occludable angles typically have not experienced pupillary block, and management of these patients is guided by prevention.

The cornerstone of prophylactic management for angle closure remains laser peripheral iridotomy (LPI). This procedure creates an alternate route for aqueous flow from the posterior chamber into the anterior chamber, allowing the iris to move posteriorly and free the TM from occlusion.[8] The IOP-lowering effect of LPI can be profound in cases of true angle closure and have been shown to significantly increase the angle width and decrease IOP in both angle closure and occludable angles.[12] However, LPI has not been shown to have a significant effect on ACD in these patients.[12] Because a shallow ACD can predispose an eye to angle closure, this needs to be considered when approaching the patient with potentially occludable angles.

It has been well documented that eyes with occludable angles also have shallower ACDs when compared to eyes

Kahook MY, Schuman JS, eds.
Chandler and Grant's Glaucoma, Fifth Edition (pp 619-622).
© 2013 SLACK Incorporated.

Shaffer	Degrees	Comments
4	35 to 40	Wide open angle in which all structures were visible up to the iris root and its attachment to the anterior ciliary body.
3	20 to 35	Wide open angle up to the scleral spur. In grades 3 and 4, no risk of angle closure existed.
2	20	Angle was narrow with visible trabecular meshwork. In this angle width, a possible risk of closure existed.
1	10	Occurred when the angle was extremely narrow up to the anterior trabecular meshwork and the Schwalbe's line, with a high risk of probably closure.
0	0	The angle was closed with iridocorneal contact and no visibility of the anterior chamber angle structures.

TABLE 67-1. GRADE SYSTEM ACCORDING TO SHAFFER GONIOSCOPIC CLASSIFICATION

with open angles.[13-15] The shallower ACD in this group is due to anatomical predisposition, steeper curvature of the anterior lens surface, narrower chamber angle, more anterior positioned ciliary bodies (plateau iris), more anteriorly located lens, and genetic predetermination.[14-16] In addition, mean intraocular lens (IOL) thickness was also shown to be greater in those eyes with occludable angles when compared to normal eyes.[13,14] The growth of the lens, as occurs in cataract development, leads to a progressive anterior chamber shallowing rate of 0.35 to 0.50 mm in 50 years.[17] Therefore, we know that increasing anteroposterior diameter of the crystalline lens throughout life results in gradual decrease in ACD and volume in all eyes.

Cataract extraction alone can lower IOP, increase ACD, and widen the angle in normal eyes and those with POAG as mentioned before.[1-4] Patients with occludable angles and lens opacities or visually significant cataracts should be strongly considered as appropriate surgical candidates for cataract extraction. The steeper curvature and anterior position of the crystalline lens in these eyes, which contribute to the risk of angle closure, are easily amenable to surgery with current phacoemulsification and foldable IOL techniques but not LPI. LPI remains the standard of therapy; however, ACD is not significantly affected in eyes with occludable angles. LPI also does not address the visual limitations caused by the developing cataract and carries the potential complication for lenticular damage and subsequent cataract development.

The decision to perform cataract extraction on a patient with occludable angles is dependent on the clinical presentation. In these cases, LPI and cataract removal are both intended for the purposes of prophylactic treatment against angle closure. Both can lower IOP and widen the anterior chamber angle; however, cataract removal has a more profound influence on increasing the ACD. With the proven benefits of cataract extraction, including improved visual outcomes, this approach may become a standard of care in patients with occludable angles with cataracts or in patients with occludable angles refractory to LPI.

ANGLE CLOSURE

Primary angle closure (PAC) can be categorized into 2 groups: acute primary angle closure (APAC) and chronic primary angle-closure glaucoma (CPACG).[5] These conditions are characterized by elevated IOP. APAC is considered a common ophthalmic emergency that requires immediate intervention and treatment to prevent glaucomatous optic nerve damage,[18] whereas CPACG is the leading cause of blindness in cases of primary angle-closure glaucoma (PACG).[19-21] Many treatment modalities are available in approaching patients with these conditions including cataract extraction.

The definitive treatment in PAC, especially in APAC, remains performing an LPI but this may not be possible in the acute setting. The initial treatment then is aimed at rapidly reducing IOP to alleviate symptoms of pain and prevent further irreversible damage to ocular tissues.[9] This is typically achieved with topical IOP-lowering medications, oral acetazolamide, and systemic hyperosmotic agents, such as mannitol. The drawback to these therapies is that they may fail to effectively reduce IOP in many cases, and the systemic medications can have serious systemic side effects.

Anterior chamber (AC) paracentesis is also an option in the emergent setting of APAC. AC paracentesis offers the advantage of rapid IOP reduction as well as instantaneous symptom relief.[22] Rapid IOP control also limits the extent of ocular tissue damage resulting from elevated IOP. APAC typically presents with corneal edema, which can make performing LPI a complex task; however, AC paracentesis can improve corneal clarity and facilitate laser iridotomy. AC paracentesis is limited by its inability to maintain lowered IOP over an extended period of time and, therefore, topical and systemic medications need to be used in conjunction with this procedure. Patients with APAC also tend to present with shallow anterior chambers, which can lead to iris and lens/capsular damage if these structures are breached by a paracentesis knife.[22]

Argon laser peripheral iridoplasty (ALPI) can also be used to mechanically open up the angle in cases of APAC and has long been used in cases of medically resistant APAC.[23] ALPI involves the placement of a ring of contraction burns on the peripheral iris to contract the iris stroma near the angle. This mechanically pulls open the closed angle, allowing aqueous to flow through the TM and reduce IOP. This allows the eye time to become quiet with lowered IOP before definitive treatment with laser iridotomy can be performed.[24] ALPI has also been thought to reduce the duration of appositional angle closure and thus the formation of PAS in cases of APAC.[25] This would potentially help reduce the risk of progression to CPACG; however, this is outcome is still being investigated.

Once IOP has been controlled in APAC, the goal of treatment is to prevent recurrence of acute attacks and avoid progression to CPACG. The ideal treatment should be aimed at eliminating pupillary block that would prevent future attacks and widening the angle and breaking appositional closure to prevent the development of CPACG. Traditionally, the treatment of choice is LPI. Although this therapy has been shown to reduce elevated IOP and break attacks of APAC, it is unclear whether this prevents recurrence of angle-closure attacks. Moreover, the ability of LPI to prevent progression to CPACG has been shown to be limited. Despite initial success with LPI, some studies have shown that as many as half of these patients go on to develop persistently elevated IOP.[26] This can be the result of extensive residual appositional closure, TM damage, formation of PAS as a result of inflammation, or prolonged angle closure during the acute attack.[27] With this in mind, alternative treatments need to be identified that address these outcomes.

Evidence suggests the important role of the crystalline lens in angle configuration.[13-15,17,27,28] The lens can narrow the angle by displacing the peripheral iris anteriorly, a situation which becomes more pronounced in the presence of a cataractous lens. The thickness of a cataractous lens can also contribute to pupillary blockade in predisposed eyes. Therefore, cataracts may be a major contributing factor in angle closure, because many patients presenting with PAC are elderly and have concomitant cataracts. Cataract extraction as a treatment modality for APAC and CPACG has been widely performed. In PAC, the underlying pathophysiology of elevated IOP is mechanical closure of the angle. Several mechanisms can be involved in angle closure; however, pupillary blockade appears to be the most important inciting incident.[10] The mechanism by which cataract extraction effectively treats PAC is not well understood; however, it is believed that relieving pupillary block and opening the anterior chamber angle play a large role.[29]

As in cases of POAG, cataract extraction offers the benefit of lowering the IOP, increasing the ACD, and widening the angle in PAC. A study by Hayashi and colleagues[28] found that the width and the depth of the anterior chamber angle in eyes with PACG increased significantly after cataract extraction and IOL implantation and became similar to that in eyes with POAG and in normal eyes. The decrease in IOP seen in the postoperative period may be attributed to these findings. It has been shown that early phacoemulsification with foldable IOL implantation significantly reduces the risk of IOP rise in patients after abortion of APAC when compared to conventional LPI and ALPI.[30] As mentioned above, recurrence of high IOP with LPI seems to be secondary to residual angle closure. Cataract extraction is more effective at dealing with residual angle closure by deepening the anterior chamber, widening the angle, and attenuating the anterior positioning of the ciliary processes.[30] This allows for greater aqueous outflow and IOP reduction over a longer period of time.

Another advantage of cataract extraction when compared to LPI and ALPI is the significant difference in the mean number of glaucoma medications needed to control IOP. After cataract extraction, patients with PAC require fewer topical medications than those treated with the laser modalities.[30] Also, patients receiving LPI have an increased risk of developing visually significant cataracts, especially posterior subcapsular cataracts, which will ultimately necessitate removal to improve vision.[31]

Although cataract extraction is effective in lowering IOP, widening the angle, and increasing ACD, patients with APAC tend to have better IOP outcomes than patients with CPACG. This is thought to be a result of more TM damage and formation of PAS in CPACG.[32] The presence of PAS then becomes a confounding variable in determining how effective cataract extraction will be in the long-term control of IOP. It has been suggested by Lai and colleagues[33] that the resolution of PAS in PAC after cataract surgery is due to viscodissection as well as positive flushing pressure and suction during lens and cortical removal. In any case, the presence of PAS postoperatively may significantly reduce the effect of cataract extraction on IOP; however, short-term IOP decrease is still significant.

With these considerations in mind, future improvements on treating PAC need to be evaluated. The effect of cataract extraction with implantable IOLs is an effective approach to reducing IOP, increasing ACD, and widening the angle in patients with PAC. These postoperative results were significant enough that Gunning and Greve[34] advocated cataract extraction with IOL implantation alone in the treatment of angle-closure glaucoma, as they found it resulted in IOP reduction to the same extent as traditional glaucoma filtering surgery with fewer complications. This technique has proven advantages over conventional laser therapies, namely LPI. However, cataract extraction in eyes with PAC is much more technically challenging than standard cataract surgery. Poor pupillary dilation, corneal edema, and weakened zonules are just some of the obstacles that a surgeon might face in dealing with PAC. The optimal timing for cataract surgery in these cases remains unclear, and it may be beneficial to quiet the eye with medication and laser prior to intraocular surgery. Goniosynechiolysis may also be another effective approach in treating extensive PAS and improving postoperative IOP in patients with both types of PAC as long as the TM is viable. With the advances in phacoemulsification and the relative safety of the procedure, cataract extraction in patients with PAC and concomitant cataract is a compelling clinical intervention.

REFERENCES

1. Sihota R, Gupta V, Agarwal HC, Pandey RM, Deepak KK. Comparison of symptomatic and asymptomatic, chronic, primary angle-closure glaucoma, open angle glaucoma, and controls. *J Glaucoma.* 2000;9:208-213.

2. Jahn CE. Reduced intraocular pressure after phacoemulsification and posterior chamber intraocular lens implantation. *J Cataract Refract Surg.* 1997;23:1260-1264.

3. Tong JT, Miller KM. Intraocular pressure change after sutureless phacoemulsification and foldable posterior chamber lens implantation. *J Cataract Refract Surg.* 1998;24:256-262.

4. Schwenn O, Dick HB, Krummernauerf R, Krist R, Pfeiffer N. Intraocular pressure after small incision cataract surgery: temporal sclerocorneal versus clear corneal incision. *J Cataract Refract Surg.* 2001;27:421-425.

5. Foster PJ, Buhrmann R, Quigley HA, Johnson GJ. The definition and classification of glaucoma in prevalence surveys. *Br J Ophthalmol.* 2002;86:238-242.

6. He M, Foster PJ, Johnson GJ, Khaw PT. Angle-closure glaucoma in East Asian and European people. Different diseases? *Eye.* 2006;20:3-12.

7. Epstein DL, Allingham RR, Schuman JS, eds. *Chandler and Grant's Glaucoma.* 4th ed. Baltimore, MD: Williams & Wilkins; 1997.

8. Shields MB. *Textbook of Glaucoma.* 4th ed. Philadelphia, PA: Williams & Wilkins; 2000.

9. Tessler DR, Yassur Z. Long-term outcome of primary acute angle closure glaucoma. *Br J Ophthalmol.* 1985;69:261-262.

10. Wang N, Wu H, Fan Z. Primary angle closure glaucoma in Chinese and Western populations. *Chin Med J (Engl).* 2002;115:1706-1715.

11. Robin AL, Pollack IP. Argon laser peripheral iridotomies in the treatment of primary angle closure glaucoma: long-term follow-up. *Arch Ophthalmol.* 1982;100:919-923.

12. He M, Friedman DS, Ge J, et al. Laser peripheral iridotomy in primary angle-closure suspect: biometric and gonioscopic outcomes: The Liwan eye study. *Ophthalmology.* 2007;114:494-500.

13. Panek WC, Christensen RE, Lee DA, Fazio DT, Fox LE, Scott TV. Biometric variables in patients with occludable anterior chamber angles. *Am J Ophthalmol.* 1990;110:185-188.

14. Lee DA, Brubaker RF, Ilstrup DM. Anterior chamber dimensions in patients with narrow angles and angle closure glaucoma. *Arch Ophthalmol.* 1984;102:46-50.

15. George R, Paul PG, Baskaran M, et al. Ocular biometry in occludable angles and angles closure glaucoma: a population based survey. *Br J Ophthalmol.* 2003;87:339-402.

16. Tornquist R. Shallow anterior chamber in acute glaucoma: a clinical and genetic study. *Acta Ophthalmol.* 1953;39:1-74.

17. Smith P. On the growth of crystalline lens. *Trans Ophthalmol Soc UK.* 1883;3:99.

18. Lai JS. Epidemiology of acute primary angle closure glaucoma in the Hong Kong Chinese population: prospective study. *Hong Kong Med J.* 2001;7:118-123.

19. Foster PJ, Baasanhu J, Alsbirk PH, et al. Glaucoma in Mongolia. A population based survey in Hovsgol Province, Northern Mongolia. *Arch Ophthalmol.* 1996;114:1235-1241.

20. Dandona L, Dandona R, Mandal P, et al. Angle closure glaucoma in an urban population in southern India. The Andhara Pradesh Eye Disease Study. *Ophthalmology.* 2000;107:1710-1716.

21. He M, Foster PJ, Ge J, et al. Prevalence and clinical characteristics of glaucoma in adult Chinese: a population-based study in Liwan District, Guangzhou. *Invest Ophthalmol Vis Sci.* 2006;47(7):2782-2788.

22. Lam DS, Chua JK, Tham CC, Lai JS. Efficacy and safety of immediate anterior chamber paracentesis in the treatment of acute primary angle closure glaucoma: a pilot study. *Ophthalmology.* 2002;109:64-70.

23. Ritch R, Liebmann JM. Argon laser peripheral iridoplasty. *Ophthalmic Surg Lasers.* 1996;27:289-300.

24. Ritch R. Argon laser treatment for medically unresponsive attacks of angle closure glaucoma. *Am J Ophthalmol.* 1982;94:197-204.

25. Lai JS, Tham CC, Chua JK, et al. To compare argon laser peripheral iridoplasty (ALPI) against systemic medications in treatment of acute primary angle closure glaucoma: mid-term results. *Eye.* 2006;20:309-314.

26. Aung T, Ang LP, Chan SP, Chew PT. Acute primary angle-closure: long-term intraocular pressure outcome in Asian eyes. *Am J Ophthalmol.* 2001;131:7-12.

27. Yeung BY, Ng PW, Chiu TY, et al. Prevalence and mechanism of appositional angle closure in acute primary angle closure after iridotomy. *Clin Experiment Ophthalmol.* 2005;33:478-482.

28. Hayashi K, Hayashi H, Nakao F, Hayashi F. Changes in anterior chamber angle width and depth after intraocular lens implantation in eyes with glaucoma. *Ophthalmology.* 2000;107:698-703.

29. Gunning FP, Greve EL. Lens extraction for uncontrolled angle-closure glaucoma: long-term follow-up. *J Cataract Refract Surg.* 1998;24:1347-1356.

30. Lam DS, Leung DY, Tham CC, et al. Randomized trial of early phacoemulsification versus peripheral iridotomy to prevent intraocular pressure rise after acute primary angle closure. *Ophthalmology.* 2008;115:1134-1140.

31. Lim LS, Husain R, Gazzard G, Seah SK, Aung T. Cataract progression after prophylactic laser peripheral iridotomy: potential implications for the prevention of glaucoma blindness. *Ophthalmology.* 2005;112:1355-1359.

32. Zhuo YH, Wang M, Li Y, et al. Phacoemulsification treatment of subjects with acute primary angle-closure and chronic angle-closure glaucoma. *J Glaucoma.* 2009;18:646-651.

33. Lai JS, Tham CC, Chan JC. The clinical outcomes of cataract extraction by phacoemulsification in eyes with primary angle-closure glaucoma and co-existing cataract: a prospective case series. *J Glaucoma.* 2006;15:47-52.

34. Gunning FP, Greve EL. Lens extraction for uncontrolled angle-closure glaucoma: long-term follow-up. *J Cataract Refract Surg.* 1998;24:1347-1356.

68

Pediatric Glaucoma

Richard W. Hertle, MD, FAAO, FACS, FAAP

In the more than 20 years that I have been caring for infants, children, and families of patients with glaucoma, I have learned that this is one of the most devastating group of eye diseases. It not only severely affects the developing visual system, but also forever changes the lives of the patient's family. Repeated visits to the physician, hospital, operating room, and social support systems as well as the frequent need for medication administration results in significant stress to the families. If a physician decides to assist with the care of these patients, an understanding of the chronicity, complexity, and unique social challenges of this group of patients is needed.

Glaucoma in infancy and childhood constitutes a rare but sight-threatening and heterogeneous group of diseases. It has been estimated that an average ophthalmologist in general practice will encounter a new case of childhood glaucoma about once every 5 years.[1] While patients with childhood glaucomas make up less than 0.1% of ophthalmic patients, they constitute 2% to 15% of populations in institutions for the blind.[1] Intraocular pressure (IOP) control is only a small part of the battle to preserve vision in children with glaucoma. The most common reason for visual loss is amblyopia complicated by optic nerve and lens damage, corneal opacification, and ametropia.[2,3]

The pathogenesis of glaucoma in childhood and the responses of the child's eye to this disorder are often very different from those seen in older patients. Specialized information and techniques for the evaluation and care of children with glaucoma are therefore required. In addition, successful management of the childhood glaucoma patient requires cooperation and support from the entire family, not only from the patient. Because systemic disorders do not infrequently coexist with glaucoma in children, and because most of these patients will require one or more general anesthetics during the management of their glaucoma, the ophthalmologist should work closely with his or her pediatric colleagues in the care of children with glaucoma.

CLASSIFICATION

Although many classification schemes have been devised to categorize the various childhood glaucomas, their subdivision into primary and secondary mechanisms can be clinically useful. Primary glaucomas are those resulting from an intrinsic disease of the aqueous outflow pathways and are often genetic in origin. Secondary glaucomas, by contrast, result from disease originating in other regions of the eye or body[4-6] (Table 68-1). Both primary and secondary glaucoma may be associated with significant systemic conditions often requiring additional consultation.

CLINICAL MANIFESTATIONS

Symptoms and Signs

Infants and young children with glaucoma usually present for ophthalmologic evaluation because the pediatrician or parents have noted something unusual about the appearance of the patient's eyes or behavior. Often, corneal opacification and/or enlargement (a response to elevated IOP) are the signs that signal glaucoma in the infant (Figures 68-1 and 68-2). At other times, the child's glaucoma may manifest itself as one or more of the classic triad of findings: epiphora, photophobia, and blepharospasm. Photophobia and epiphora result from corneal edema (often with associated breaks in Descemet's membrane). The baby may be noted to withdraw from light or to bury his or her head against the parent or bedding to prevent exposure to light. Even indoors, the infant may show an apparent reluctance to face upward and may mistakenly be considered shy. Blepharospasm may be yet another manifestation of photophobia, often accompanying epiphora, but without the mucoid discharge so often seen in congenital nasolacrimal duct obstruction[7-9] (Figure 68-3).

Kahook MY, Schuman JS, eds.
Chandler and Grant's Glaucoma, Fifth Edition (pp 625-659).
© 2013 SLACK Incorporated.

TABLE 68-1. CHILDHOOD GLAUCOMAS: A CLASSIFICATION SCHEME

I. Primary glaucoma
  A. Congenital open-angle glaucoma
  B. Congenital glaucoma associated with iris defects
  C. Juvenile glaucoma
  D. Primary glaucomas associated with systemic or ocular abnormalities
    1. Associated with systemic abnormalities
      a. Axenfeld-Rieger syndrome (iridocorneal goniodysgenesis)
      b. Chromosomal disorders
        i) Trisomy 13 (13-15 Trisomy)
        ii) Trisomy and partial deletions of chromosome 18
        iii) Turner syndrome
        iv) Chromosome 6 (ring syndrome and translocations)
      c. Congenital rubella
      d. Cutis marmorarta telangiectasia congenita
      e. Fetal alcohol syndrome
      f. Hepatocerebrorenal (Zellweger) syndrome
      g. Infantile glaucoma associated with mental retardation and paralysis
      h. Kniest syndrome
      i. Marfan syndrome
      j. Michel syndrome
      k. Mucopolysaccharidosis
      l. Neurofibromatosis (NF-I)
      m. Nonprogressive hemiatrophy
      n. Oculocerebrorenal (Lowe) syndrome
      o. Oculodentodigital syndrome
      p. Open-angle glaucoma associated with microcornea and absent frontal sinuses
      q. Prader-Willi syndrome
      r. Rubinstein-Taybi (broad-thumb) syndrome
      s. Stickler syndrome
      t. Sturge-Weber syndrome
      u. Warburg syndrome (skeletal dysplasia)
    2. Associated with ocular abnormalities
      a. Aniridia
      b. Anterior chamber staphyloma
      c. Axenfeld-Rieger syndrome
      d. Congenital ectropion uveae
      e. Congenital hereditary endothelial dystrophy
      f. Congenital microcoria with myopia
      g. Congenital ocular melanosis
      h. Familial iris hypoplasia
      i. Idiopathic or familial elevated episcleral venous pressure
      j. Peters syndrome
      k. Posterior polymorphous dystrophy
      l. Sclerocornea

II. Secondary glaucoma
  A. Traumatic glaucoma
    1. Acute onset
      a. Angle concussion
      b. Hyphema
    2. Late-onset with angle recession
    3. Arteriovenous fistula
  B. Glaucoma secondary to intraocular neoplasm
    1. Retinoblastoma
    2. Juvenile xanthogranuloma
    3. Leukemia
    4. Melanoma
    5. Melanocytoma
    6. Iris rhabdomyosarcoma
    7. Aggressive iris nevus
  C. Uveitic glaucoma
    1. Open-angle
    2. Angle closure
      a. Synechial angle closure
      b. Iris bombé with pupillary block
  D. Lens-induced glaucoma
    1. Subluxation-dislocation and pupillary block
      a. Marfan syndrome
      b. Homocysteinuria
    2. Spherophakia and pupillary block
    3. Phacolytic
  E. Aphakic glaucoma after congenital cataract surgery
    1. Lens material blockage of TM
    2. Pupillary block
    3. Chronic open-angle
  F. Steroid-induced glaucoma
  G. Neovascular glaucoma
    1. Retinoblastoma
    2. Coats' disease
    3. Medulloepithelioma
    4. Familial exudative vitreoretinopathy
  H. Secondary angle-closure glaucoma
    1. Retinopathy of prematurity
    2. Microphthalmos
    3. Nanophthalmos
    4. Retinoblastoma
    5. Persistent hyperplastic primary vitreous
    6. Congenital pupillary iris-lens membrane
    7. Aniridia
    8. Iridoschisis
    9. Cornea plana
    10. Cystinosis
  I. Glaucoma with increased episcleral venous pressure
  J. Glaucoma secondary to intraocular infection
    1. Acute recurrent toxoplasmosis
    2. Acute herpetic iritis

Adapted from Walton DS. Glaucoma in infants and children. In: Nelson B, Calhoun JH, Harley RD, eds. *Pediatric Ophthalmology.* 3rd ed. Philadelphia, PA: WB Saunders; 1991:175-176.

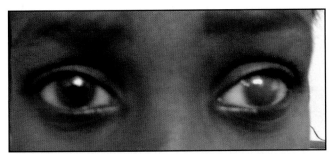

Figure 68-1. Child with bilateral anterior segment dysgenesis and secondary glaucoma with right eye status postfiltering surgery and corneal transplantation and left eye showing corneal clouding due to decompensation from the dysgenesis and untreated glaucoma.

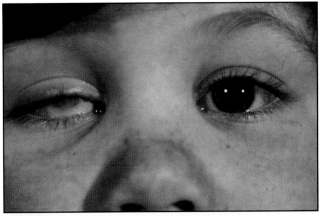

Figure 68-2. Unilateral untreated microphthalmia, sclerocornea, cornea plana, glaucoma, and ptosis.

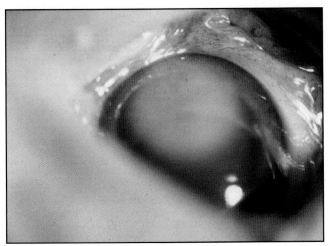

Figure 68-3. Corneal clouding in an infant with mucopolysaccharidosis and normal IOP.

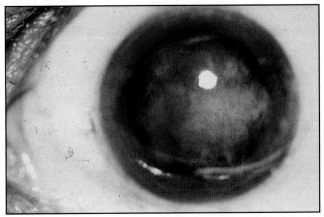

Figure 68-4. Corneal clouding in a child with corneal amyloidosis (lattice dystrophy) and normal IOP.

In children older than 1 year of age, glaucoma usually induces fewer overt signs and symptoms. Children with glaucoma developing between 1 and 4 years of age may not be correctly diagnosed unless glaucoma is suspected from other accompanying ocular or systemic abnormalities.

Children older than 4 years of age with glaucoma most frequently seek examination for decreased distance acuity related to myopia. Significant astigmatism and anisometropia are often also present. An exception to the relatively asymptomatic presentation of glaucoma in older children is secondary glaucoma presenting with an acute rise in IOP to levels sufficient to cause nauseating eye pain, headaches, and even colored haloes around lights (as seen with adults having angle-closure glaucoma). In these children, sudden-onset glaucoma may be the result of traumatic hyphema or of angle-closure glaucoma from lens dislocation or cicatricial retinopathy of prematurity. Less frequently, acute glaucoma develops secondary to other processes.[10,11]

DIFFERENTIAL DIAGNOSIS

The manifestations of epiphora, photophobia, and blepharospasm are not unique to infantile glaucoma and also can occur as a result of nasolacrimal duct obstruction, ocular

inflammation (uveitis), and corneal injury (eg, abrasion). Corneal edema or opacification may occur in the setting of storage diseases (eg, mucopolysaccharidoses, cystinosis), corneal dystrophies (eg, congenital hereditary endothelial dystrophy or posterior polymorphous dystrophy), birth trauma (with resultant Descemet's tears), and congenital anomalies (eg, sclerocornea, Peters' anomaly) (Figures 68-4 and 68-5). Isolated corneal enlargement occurs in megalocornea and high axial myopia. Although other nonglaucomatous eye conditions may share one or more signs with childhood glaucoma, care must be taken to rule out glaucoma in each of these cases. For example, glaucoma may complicate uveitis and has been reported in the setting of storage disease, corneal dystrophy, congenital anomalies such as Peter's anomaly, and megalocornea (Figure 68-6). Glaucoma may also occur coincident with congenital nasolacrimal duct obstruction.[12,13]

Rarely, a child may present after infancy with findings suggestive of primary infantile glaucoma, yet have normal IOP. Spontaneous cure in cases of mild primary infantile glaucoma has been described, but remains a diagnosis of exclusion.[14,15]

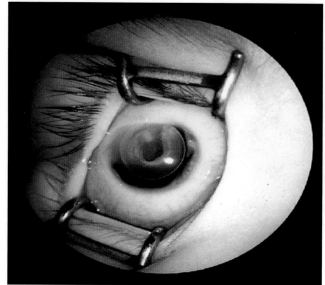

Figure 68-5. Microphthalmic eye of an infant with a complex anterior segment malformation consisting of partial sclerocornea, cornea plana, microcornea, aniridia, cataract, lenticulocorneal adhesion, irido-trabeculo dysgenesis, and glaucoma.

OCULAR EXPANSION

The neonatal globe is distensible and enlarges in response to elevated IOP. Stretching may occur in all parts of the infant eye, including the cornea, anterior chamber angle structures, sclera, optic nerve, scleral canal, and lamina cribrosa.[16-18] The normal horizontal corneal diameter at birth ranges from 9.5 to 10.5 mm (mean 10 mm), enlarging about 0.5 to 1.0 mm in the first year of life (Table 68-2).[18,19] Under 1 year of age, diameters of 12 to 12.5 mm are suggestive of glaucoma, and a measurement of 13 mm or more at any time in childhood strongly suggests abnormality, as does asymmetry in corneal diameter between eyes in a child. Whereas the cornea may enlarge because of elevated IOP until only the age of approximately 3 years, the sclera may deform in response to increased IOP until approximately 10 years of age. Progressive myopia and astigmatism are therefore often seen in older children with glaucoma.[18]

Elevated IOP stretches and sometimes breaks Descemet's membrane, resulting in acute localized corneal edema followed by deposition of new basement membrane into hyaline ridges (called Haab's striae). These permanent striae are usually fairly horizontal and rarely occur in corneas less than 12.5 mm in horizontal diameter or in children older than 2 years (Figure 68-7). In contrast, breaks in Descemet's membrane arising from obstetrical trauma (usually involving use of forceps) tend to have a more vertical orientation and to present at birth.[20,21]

Ultrasonography has been used to record changes in the axial length of eyes in infants with infantile glaucoma. Compared with corneal diameter, however, axial length seems less helpful in the evaluation of glaucomatous infant eyes.[22-24]

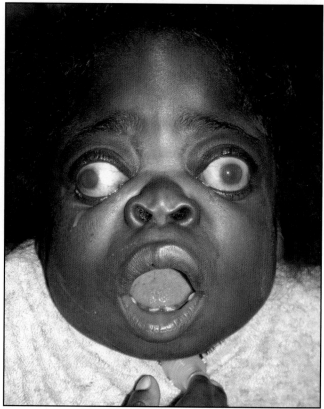

Figure 68-6. Toddler with bilateral corneal clouding and craniofacial characteristics of mucopolysaccharidosis (Hurler syndrome) and normal IOP.

OPTIC NERVE CUPPING

Optic nerve cupping occurs as a result of elevated IOP in childhood glaucoma, but its course (in infants and young children) may be quite different from that seen with adult glaucoma patients. In children with advanced glaucoma, as in adults, loss of neuroretinal rim tissue occurs, especially at the vertical poles of the disc, and the optic cup may extend to the disc margins.[15,25,26] In very young patients, one more often sees generalized enlargement of the optic cup with preservation of an intact neuroretinal rim. This pattern of symmetric cupping has been attributed to stretching of the optic canal and backward bowing of the lamina cribrosa in these young patients.[15] While this type of optic nerve cupping can occur early and quite rapidly in infants with glaucoma, dramatic reversal of cupping may occur with normalization of IOP (Figures 68-8 through 68-11).[15]

Large size of the optic nerve cup and asymmetry of cupping between fellow eyes is suggestive but not definite evidence of glaucoma. Illustratively, the cup/disc ratio exceeded 0.3 in 68% of 126 eyes with primary infantile glaucoma examined by Shaffer and Hetherington,[27] but in only 2.6% of 936 normal newborn eyes examined by Richardson.[28] Richardson also reported marked optic cup asymmetry in only 0.6% of normal eyes in his series, contrasted with 89% noted for infants with monocular glaucoma.[28]

TABLE 68-2. CORNEAL DIAMETER AND AXIAL LENGTH IN CHILDREN: NORMAL AND GLAUCOMATOUS EYES				
	Corneal Diameter (horizontal, in mm)		Axial Length (by ultrasound, in mm)	
Age	Normal	Glaucoma Suspected	Normal	Glaucoma Suspected
Term (newborn)	9.5 to 10.5	11.5	16 to 7	>20
1 year	10 to 11.5	>12 to 12.5	– 20	>22.5
2 years	11 to 12	>12.5	21	>23
Older child	12	>13	24	>25

Adapted from Consultation section. Cataract surgical problem. *J Cataract Refract Surg.* 2003;29:2261-2268; Tabbara KF, Ross-Degnan D. Blindness in Saudi Arabia. *JAMA.* 1986;255:3378-3384; and Taylor RH, Ainsworth JR, Evans AR, Levin AV. The epidemiology of pediatric glaucoma: the Toronto experience. *J AAPOS.* 1999;3:308-315.

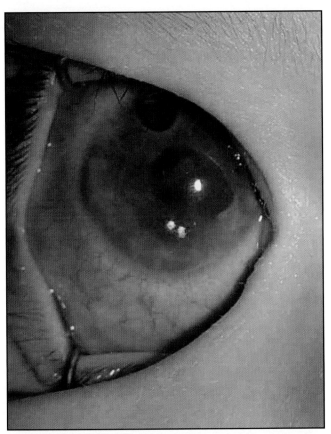

Figure 68-7. Eye of child with glaucoma after successful surgical pressure reduction showing persistent central corneal opacities due to scarring from Haab's striae.

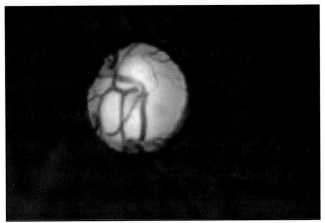

Figure 68-8. Intraoperative photograph of optic nerve of a child with glaucoma showing advanced optic neuropathy (ie, large central cupping, thinned peripheral neuroretinal rim, loss of optic nerve fiber layer color, and small papillary vessels).

- Confirming or excluding the diagnosis and etiology of glaucoma
- Determining other ocular anomalies
- Obtaining additional systemic medical information needed to plan for an examination under anesthesia.

If one can confidently exclude the diagnosis of glaucoma, or if an older child with glaucoma can be thoroughly examined while awake, examination under anesthesia may not be indicated.

INTRAOCULAR PRESSURE ELEVATION

IOP levels and measurement in children with glaucoma will be discussed next.

DIAGNOSTIC EXAMINATION

The ophthalmic evaluation of the child with suspected glaucoma should address the following objectives:

OFFICE EXAMINATION

History and Equipment

Taking history from parents and caretakers can be especially valuable in evaluating patients too young to provide any useful verbal information. Information should be gathered regarding pregnancy, labor and delivery, possible signs and symptoms of glaucoma, evidence of systemic abnormality, possible trauma, drug and medication exposure,

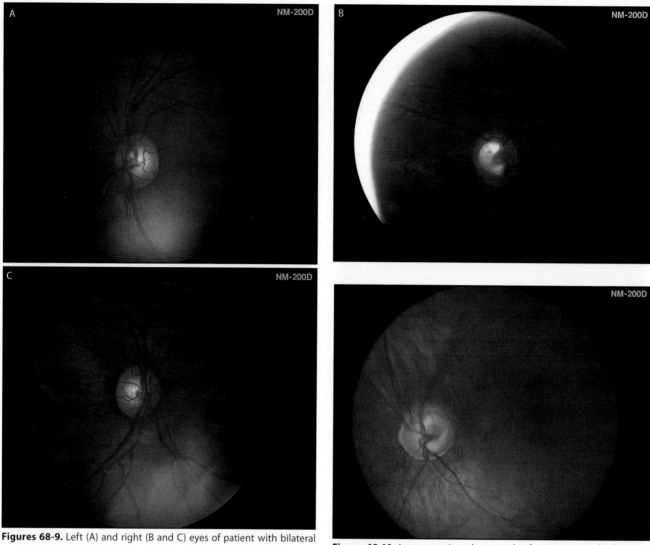

Figures 68-9. Left (A) and right (B and C) eyes of patient with bilateral asymmetric glaucoma showing initial asymmetry in optic neuropathy with the left eye affected to a greater degree (B) and subsequent reversal in cupping of left eye months after successful surgical treatment (C).

Figure 68-10. Intraoperative photograph of optic nerve of left eye of a child with well-controlled glaucoma for 2 years showing stable optic neuropathy, large central cup, and thinned and grey nerve fiber layer with steep walls of the cup.

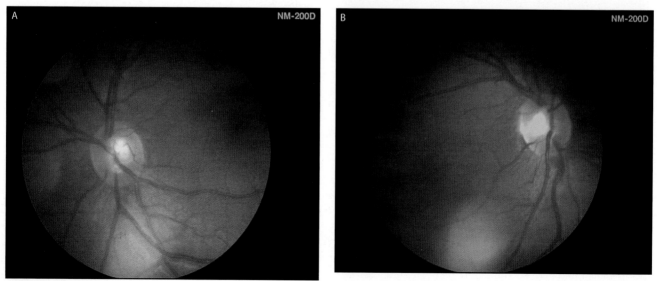

Figures 68-11. Left (A) and right (B) intraoperative optic nerve photographs of patient with asymmetric (worse right eye) optic neuropathy due to bilateral glaucoma.

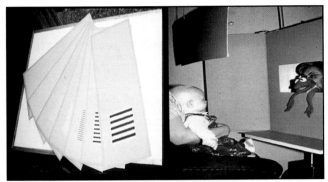

Figure 68-12. This illustrates the performance of the Teller Acuity Card procedure (on the right side of the figure) that provides a behavioral test of resolution vision in preverbal infants and children. The infant is "forced" to choose between increasing spatial frequency gratings versus an isoluminant grey target on each card (left side of figure).

TABLE 68-3. EXAMINATION UNDER GENERAL ANESTHESIA: SUGGESTED SEQUENCE
1. External examination (brief)
2. Tonometry (as early as possible after induction and before intubation)
3. Corneal diameter measurement
4. Anterior segment examination
5. Koeppe gonioscopy
6. Fundus examination (optic disc)
7. Optic disc photography

and pertinent family history. In addition to commonly used office equipment, the use of a portable slit-lamp, millimeter ruler, Tono-Pen (Medtronic Solan, Jacksonville, FL) and/or Perkins tonometer (Haag-Streit, Mason, OH), and Koeppe diagnostic gonioscopic lenses (Ocular Instruments, Bellevue, WA) may be valuable.

Assessment of Vision and Ocular Adnexa

Examination begins with an assessment of the general overall appearance and visual function. In infants, the ability to monocularly fix and follow well and the absence of nystagmus suggest good visual function. Visual acuity can be evaluated with Teller Acuity Cards (Precision Vision, La Salle, IL) in infancy, and eventually visual fields can be evaluated in children older than about 7 years, respectively (Figure 68-12). The penlight and direct ophthalmoscope are useful instruments for inspecting the adnexa and corneas. It may be useful to delay use of the portable slit-lamp until after tonometry has been attempted to maximize the opportunity for measuring IOP in an unanesthetized, undisturbed infant. During the external examination, one looks for abnormalities (eg, lid malformations) to suggest congenital syndromes that may include glaucoma (Table 68-3) and for signs of lacrimal system obstruction that may explain epiphora. The use of visual evoked potentials is becoming increasing useful in the evaluation of optic neuropathies including glaucoma.

Corneal Examination

The corneas are examined for abnormalities in shape, size, clarity, symmetry, curvature, and thickness. In the presence of corneal epithelial edema, the corneal surface lacks its normal luster and produces an irregular penlight reflection off its bedewed surface. Because corneal opacification obscures details of the underlying pupil and iris, the relative visibility of these intraocular structures helps to quantify the

degree of corneal haze or opacity and is well evaluated with the direct ophthalmoscope. In the worst cases, the cornea appears opaque white or pearly gray and completely hides any view of the pupil. In moderately severe cases, the cornea appears bluish and allows visualization of the pupil but few iris details. Corneal diameter can be estimated using a millimeter rule.[29] The examiner may notice a difference in the overall size of one cornea compared to the other, even when corneal diameter measurements seem similar between the fellow eyes. Because the area of a circle varies as the square of its radius, it seems reasonable that the observer's eye may more easily note differences in area than in diameter of a patient's 2 corneas (Figures 68-13 and 68-14).

Tonometry and Intraocular Pressure

The best IOP measurements are those obtained on a cooperative patient using only topical anesthesia, because IOP may be falsely elevated in a struggling patient or in a patient who is squeezing his or her lids and is often unpredictably altered by systemic sedatives and anesthetics (see the "Examination Under Anesthesia" section). Sometimes, tonometry can be achieved on a sleepy or hungry infant taking a bottle in the parents' arms (Figure 68-15). Among various instruments used to measure IOP in children, the Perkins applanation tonometer and the Tono-Pen (a hand-held Mackay-Marg-type tonometer [Reichert Technologies, Depew, NY]) rank highly in terms of accuracy and ease of use in these patients.[30,31] The Pulsair (Reichert Technologies), a hand-held noncontact tonometer, has also been successfully used to measure IOP in children.[30,31] The slit-lamp-mounted Goldmann applanation tonometer may be useful in older, cooperative children.

Studies of IOP in unanesthetized infants and children suggest that normal values lie below the mean pressures for normal adults. Pensiero and colleagues (using a Pulsair noncontact tonometer) reported a mean IOP of 9.59 ± 2.3 mm Hg in premature/newborn infants. They found that the mean IOP rose gradually with increasing age of the subjects, reaching 13.95 ± 2.49 mm Hg by age 7 to 8 years and remaining essentially constant at that level through the middle teenage

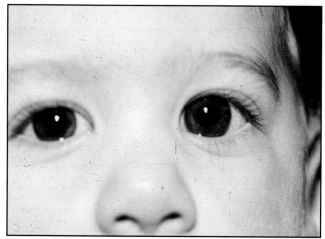

Figure 68-13. Patient with unilateral buphthalmos showing asymmetric involvement due to infantile glaucoma of the left eye. This patient has normal acuity for age in the affected left eye when corrected for the anisometropia due to the globe enlargement.

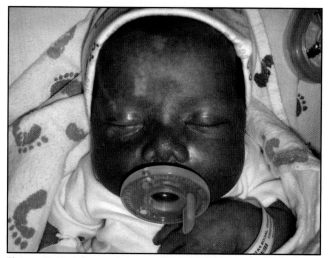

Figure 68-15. Infant with Sturge-Weber syndrome and bilateral glaucoma who, when pacified, is able to have office tonometry accomplished.

years. A mean IOP of 10.11 ± 2.2 mm Hg in normal premature infants using a Pulsair tonometer while Perkins applanation tonometry found the mean IOP of unanesthetized newborns to be 11.24 ± 2.4 mm Hg.[32] Others have reported mean IOP using the Perkins tonometer as low as 5.89 and as high as 18 mm Hg in infants and young children.[30,31,33] Infants with primary infantile glaucoma commonly present with unanesthetized IOPs between 30 and 40 mm Hg, although occasionally values above or below this range occur. Often, pressure measurements are confounded by a failure to cooperate, requiring measurement under anesthesia or sedation. The mean IOP in a group of struggling infants has been reported as 28.3 mm Hg by Perkins tonometry, more than twice the value (10.8 mm Hg) obtained in the same infants while quiet.[30,31,33] Falsely elevated IOP measurements may either falsely alarm or falsely reassure the examiner. For example, measuring high IOP in both eyes of an intermittently struggling infant with unilateral glaucoma may obscure the actual

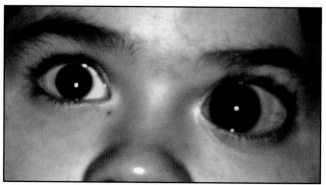

Figure 68-14. Patient with unilateral buphthalmos showing asymmetric involvement due to infantile glaucoma of the left eye. After multiple surgical procedures, the left eye has worse than 20/200 visual acuity due to glaucomatous optic neuropathy and amblyopia.

IOP asymmetry between the eyes. The examiner might erroneously attach less importance to the elevated IOP in the glaucomatous eye, secure in the belief that it matched the falsely elevated IOP in the normal eye (Table 68-4).

Anterior Segment Examination

Following tonometry (or attempts at it), use of the portable slit-lamp allows more detailed inspection of the cornea and the remainder of the anterior segment. An abnormally deep anterior chamber or abnormalities of the iris may be additional clues to glaucoma in some cases (eg, aniridia, Axenfeld-Rieger syndrome). Gonioscopy provides the most important anatomic information in the clinical examination regarding the mechanism of the glaucoma and may sometimes be performed using Koeppe contact lenses (Reichert Technologies) and a portable slit-lamp or loupes in the office. Angle evaluation is then usually repeated in greater detail under anesthesia.

Fundus Examination

Fundus examination centers on evaluation of the optic discs, although associated findings such as choroidal hemangioma (suggesting Sturge-Weber syndrome) can add useful information regarding the type of glaucoma present. If infant movements preclude direct ophthalmoscopic evaluation of the discs, indirect ophthalmoscopy using a 14 diopter (D) lens or a direct ophthalmoscope together with a 20 D condensing lens. As with gonioscopy, disc examination should be repeated under anesthesia, unless normal findings and pressures have obviated this next step. Photography of the optic nerve can be accomplished using such cameras as the Nidek handheld fundus camera (Gamagori, Japan).

Refraction and Perimetry

Determination of refractive errors using cycloplegic retinoscopy or automated refraction can be helpful, especially when they are asymmetric in the setting of unilateral or

TABLE 68-4. INTRAOCULAR PRESSURE AND SEDATIVES/ANESTHETICS

Sedative/ Anesthetic Agent	Route of Administration	Usual Effect on IOP
Chloral hydrate	Oral or rectal	↔
Methohexital (Brevital)	Rectal, IM, IV	± ↓
Midazolam	Same as above	± ↓
Ketamine	IM	± ↑
Halothane (and similar agents)	Inhalation	
Oxygen	Inhalation	↓-↓↓↓
Nitrous oxide/ oxygen	Inhalation	↓
Succinylcholine	IV	↑↑↑
Endotracheal intubation		↑↑↑

IM: intramuscular; IV: intravenous.

aphakic glaucoma; in this case, relative myopia of the affected eye or increasing myopia supports the diagnosis of glaucoma. Older children (beginning at 6 or 7 years of age) can also undergo subjective visual field examinations, allowing assessment of the extent of initial field loss as well as stability of the remaining visual field over time (as one attempts to control the glaucoma). Goldmann visual field testing is our choice for younger children because the tester may constantly encourage the patient and may briefly suspend testing when fixation wanders or attention wanes. Teenaged patients often perform well on standard automated perimetry programs, such as the Humphrey 24-2.

When one or more findings of the initial examination confirm or raise suspicions of childhood glaucoma, the administration of anesthesia is usually justified, both for a more complete examination as well as for probable surgical intervention.

EXAMINATION UNDER ANESTHESIA

General Anesthesia Versus Office Sedation

General anesthesia in the operating room has advantages over sedation or anesthesia administered elsewhere because it allows surgical intervention without further delay once the diagnosis of glaucoma is confirmed. An exception may be the use of chloral hydrate to facilitate office tonometry in the following patients:

- Patients felt unlikely to actually have glaucoma.
- Patients in whom the need for further surgical intervention seems unlikely or in whom decision making depends heavily upon obtaining IOP unaltered by inhaled anesthetics.

Chloral Hydrate Sedation

Oral chloral hydrate sedation has been used by clinicians (pediatricians, pediatric ophthalmologists, radiologists, and dentists) for many years and may be particularly useful to the ophthalmologist when IOP determination is pivotal to decision-making in the office setting. Chloral hydrate seems to minimally alter IOP recorded in children.[32] It has been stated that chloral hydrate is an effective short-term sedative that infrequently causes toxicity when administered orally at appropriate dosages with no serious systemic side effects with oral doses as high as 100 mg/kg for the first 10 kg, then 50 mg/kg for each additional kg body weight.[32] Recently, major medical centers have begun to formalize the setting under which conscious sedation may be performed (in compliance with JCAHO standards). Key suggested guidelines include the following:

- Preprocedure evaluation of the patient by a physician prior to administration of medication
- Informed consent to include risks of conscious sedation
- Minimum of 2 personnel available (the operator, or physician performing the examination, as well as the monitor, or assistant trained to monitor the patient)
- Patient monitoring (and documentation on flowsheet) to include continuous pulse oximetry as well as other vital signs and level of consciousness (recorded at least every 10 minutes)
- Minimum equipment available to include emergency airway equipment (eg, oxygen and suction), pulse oximeter, blood pressure monitor, and cardiac arrest cart

In many centers, this may be so burdensome as to preclude outpatient sedation in favor of only examination under anesthesia.

Sequence of Examination Under Anesthesia

A logical sequence for examination under anesthesia begins with brief external examination followed by IOP measurements (Figure 68-16). Tonometry should be performed during the earliest possible moments after induction and before endotracheal intubation (Figures 68-17 through 68-19). One may then proceed with corneal diameter measurements followed by slit-lamp examination of the anterior segment and Koeppe gonioscopy and fundoscopy (Ocular

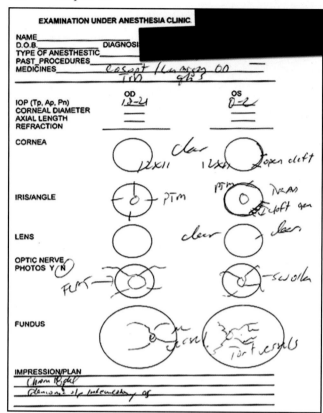

Figure 68-16. This is the exam under anesthesia documentation we use in the operating room from which continuous clinical data can be recorded for evaluation over time.

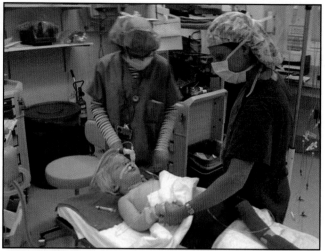

Figure 68-17. Figure showing complexity of examination of children under anesthesia. It is important to measure IOP during induction, prior to complete anesthesia.

Instruments). Pupil dilation is performed only if results of the aforementioned examination are reassuring enough to obviate surgery. In this case, optic disc photography is also helpful in following children with glaucoma. Great care should be taken during administration of anesthesia and examination under anesthesia to avoid drying or damage to the corneal epithelium, as this may increase the difficulty and risk of subsequent surgical intervention (especially goniotomy).

Tonometry Under Anesthesia and Sedation

An unfortunate consequence of the anesthesia required for adequate examination is that IOP measurements are variably altered by sedatives, narcotics, and inhaled anesthetic agents (see Table 68-4). There are no to minimal changes in IOP recorded after high-dose oral chloral hydrate (100 mg/kg for the first 10 kg, then 50 mg/kg for each additional kg body weight) was given to a group of 50 normal children under 6 years, as well as to a smaller group of children with glaucoma. The mean IOP under chloral hydrate for normal eyes was 5.6 mm Hg by Perkins tonometry and 14.7 mm Hg by digital pneumotonometry, while glaucomatous eyes

measured 19.5 and 28.5 mm Hg, respectively. Others have reported IOP in nonglaucomatous children under chloral hydrate ranging from 11 to 17 mm Hg by Mackay-Marg tonometry.[32,34] Ketamine has been variously reported to raise and to minimally affect the pressure in children.[34]

Although there are conflicting reports, inhaled anesthetics (eg, halothane and enflurane) are generally agreed to lower IOP measurements variably.[35-37] The normal IOP in an infant under halothane anesthesia is reported to be 9 to 10 mm Hg, with a pressure of 20 mm Hg or greater considered suspicious for glaucoma.[35-37] IOP elevation is consistently reported after administration of succinylcholine as well as with tracheal intubation.[38] Even administration of 100% oxygen alone slightly lowers IOP (as does breathing nitrous oxide-oxygen mixtures).[38]

Fortunately, although IOP measurements influenced by sedatives and anesthetics may vary greatly from true awake readings, high preanesthetic IOPs usually remain in an abnormal range, even under anesthesia. Asymmetric IOP measurements between fellow eyes more reliably indicate abnormality than do borderline IOP readings in both eyes taken under anesthesia. IOP measurements under anesthesia should never be taken as the sole proof of glaucoma; if they are elevated in the setting of an otherwise negative glaucoma evaluation, conservative management and close observation are warranted. In contrast, when corneal and optic nerve abnormalities suggest glaucomatous damage, low IOP readings may be cause for repeat examination prior to surgical intervention, but should not provide false reassurance (see Table 68-4).

Ophthalmologists may have ready access in the operating room to Shiotz tonometry but not to the Perkins applanation or Tono-Pen tonometers. While IOP measurement with Schiotz tonometry may be employed during examination under anesthesia, this technique has definite disadvantages. Because indentation tonometry is influenced by both scleral

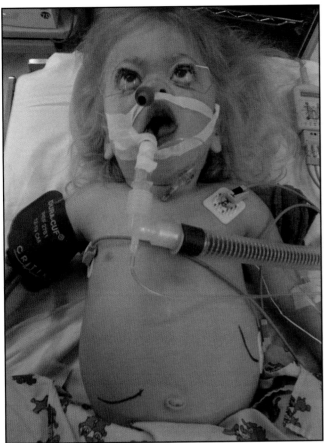

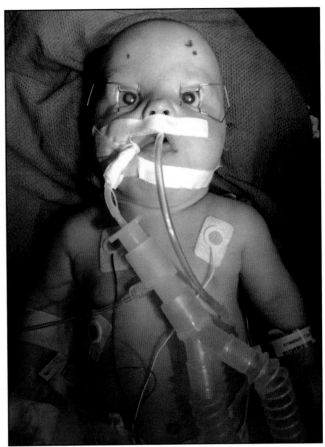

Figure 68-18. Child with mucopolysaccharidosis (Hurler syndrome) during examination under anesthesia for bilateral cloudy corneas. This patient did have trabeculodysgenesis and glaucoma in both eyes. The markings on the abdomen show evidence of hepatosplenomegaly.

Figure 68-19. Intraoperative photograph of a child with bilateral microphthalmia, cataracts, and glaucoma prior to examination under anesthesia and lensectomy/vitrectomy.

rigidity and corneal curvature and thickness, IOP recorded in infants using Schiotz tonometry may differ significantly from that recorded by applanation, depending upon the size and thickness of the cornea. For a given Schiotz pressure (1955 calibration), the corresponding applanation IOP may be from 5 mm Hg higher to 7 mm Hg lower.

Anterior Segment Examination

Corneal diameter measurements under anesthesia are made using a caliper ordinarily used for strabismus and other surgeries with similar precision. Anterior segment examination with a portable slit-lamp should be performed.

Gonioscopy Under Anesthesia

If the cornea is clear enough to permit it, gonioscopy should be performed using Koeppe gonioscopy lenses of proper size, together with a handheld binocular microscope and Barkan focal illuminator (Reichert Technologies), or a portable slit-lamp (Figures 68-20 through 68-22). Placing a Koeppe lens

onto each eye at the same time facilitates comparison of the angle features in the fellow eyes.

Gonioscopic findings in normal infants and young children differ significantly from those of adults. Of the visible angle structures, the uveal meshwork (extending forward from peripheral iris onto corneoscleral meshwork) differs most greatly between the 2 age groups. In normal infants younger than 1 year of age, the uveal meshwork is so delicate that the juncture of scleral spur and ciliary body band appears crisp and distinct. In later years, the uveal meshwork loses its early homogeneous, sheet-like appearance and becomes a more coarse, lacy, and open structure. In dark-eyed individuals, pigmentation of the uveal meshwork with increasing age increases visibility of this lacy structure.

The iris in infantile glaucoma often shows a more anterior insertion than that of the normal infant, with altered translucency of the angle face producing an indistinct ciliary body band, trabecular meshwork (TM), and scleral spur. The scalloped border of the iris pigment epithelium and the meshwork itself may be unusually prominent in infantile glaucoma, visible through the translucent peripheral iris

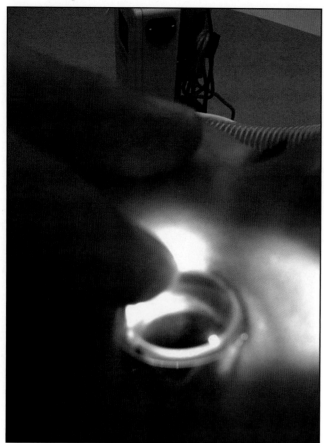

Figure 68-20. Intraoperative photography of use of Koeppe goniolens (Ocular Instruments) to examine the angle while under anesthesia (a high flat insertion of the iris in the angle can be seen).

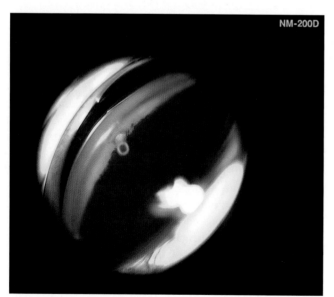

Figure 68-22. Intraoperative photography of use of Koeppe goniolens to examine the angle while under anesthesia showing a high flat insertion of the iris, clear trabeculodysgenesis, multiple persistence of fetal trabecular processes, and diffuse pigmentary disturbance.

stroma as if viewed through a "morning mist."[39,40] Juvenile open-angle glaucoma (JOAG) patients usually demonstrate a

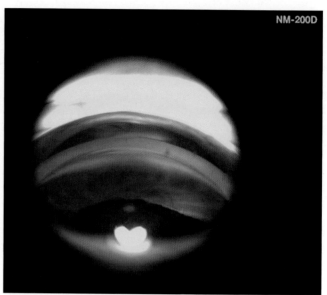

Figure 68-21. Intraoperative photography of use of Koeppe goniolens to examine the angle while under anesthesia showing a colobomatous pupillary border of the iris with ectropion uvea and a broad sweeping concave peripheral iris with a high insertion into the angle.

normal-appearing open angle, often with a prominent, lacy uveal meshwork.

Fundus Examination and Possible Surgery

After gonioscopy, direct ophthalmoscopy through a Koeppe lens (and undilated pupil) usually affords an excellent view of the optic nerves. At this point, if sufficient evidence suggests glaucoma, one may proceed directly to appropriate surgical intervention. Otherwise, if glaucoma is excluded or conservative management is indicated (as in the case of borderline pressures in the absence of suggestive corneal, angle, or optic nerve abnormalities), the pupils can be dilated (Figure 68-23). Pupil dilation facilitates photographic documentation of disc cupping, as well as cycloplegic refraction (although the latter can usually be performed with equal ease in the office setting, obviating prolonged anesthesia). Examination under anesthesia can often be accomplished entirely without endotracheal intubation in slightly older infants and children, until the need for surgical intervention has been confirmed in the operating room. If surgery is deferred, wake-up and recovery time for the patient may be minimized.

VISUAL FIELD TESTING IN CHILDREN

Standard Goldmann or automated perimetry can be performed on children with glaucoma, but like all clinical evaluations in the pediatric population, are age-dependent.[37] Most developmentally normal children are able to provide valid and reliable data on perimetry at about 10 years of age, albeit many need practice sessions. In a

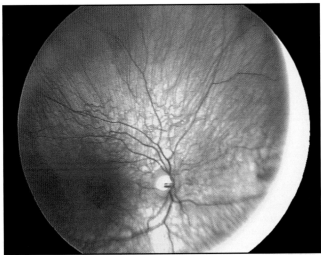

Figure 68-23. Intraoperative fundus photograph using a Retcam (Clarity Medical Systems, Inc, Pleasanton, CA) showing glaucomatous optic neuropathy and peripheral retinal pigment epithelial hypopigmentation.

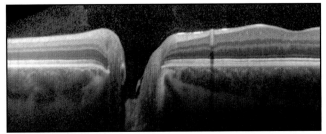

Figure 68-24. OCT of the normal optic nerve in a child with unilateral glaucoma.

group of 13 children between the ages of 4 and 14 years with congenital glaucoma and 10 age-matched healthy children, localized visual field defects (eg, paracentral scotoma, nasal step, and arcuate scotoma) were determined.[38] Specific visual field defects were found only in bilateral cases.[38] Paracentral scotoma was found in 1 of 12 eyes with bilateral congenital glaucoma.[38] Nasal steps were found in 6 of 12 eyes with bilateral congenital glaucoma.[38] Arcuate scotoma were found in 4 of 12 eyes with bilateral congenital glaucoma.[38] In another report, long-term functional results in 102 eyes of 59 patients with childhood glaucoma with specific reference to the pattern of optic nerve damage were studied.[39] Optic disc photography and quantitative perimetry were used to judge the degree of damage that had been sustained.[39] There was a predilection for initial visual field damage in the arcuate area followed by further arcuate and nasal field loss similar to the pattern of visual field loss seen in adult glaucoma. In children, as in adults, neural tissue appeared to be lost preferentially at the vertical disc poles.[39] The selective pattern of glaucomatous optic nerve damage seemed not to depend upon the age of the optic nerve structures.[39]

OPTICAL COHERENCE TOMOGRAPHY IN CHILDREN

This is an exciting clinical and research tool and will have a tremendous impact on the understanding, diagnosis, and treatment of glaucoma in infants and children. Other chapters in this volume discuss this technology in detail. We have been able to acquire reliable Stratus optical coherence tomography (OCT; Carl Zeiss Meditec, Dublin, CA) data from outpatients as young as 3 years of age. Now that handheld OCT technology is becoming available, the use

of this in the operating room will assist the clinician in diagnosis and management. Some early reports on OCT and children have been completed. In one report, 156 eyes of 79 patients were enrolled. Fifty-two eyes (33.3%) met criteria for glaucoma, and 104 (66.7%) were normal. There were 44 female (55.6%) and 35 male (44.3%) subjects whose ages ranged from 3 to 17 years old. The OCT-3 (Carl Zeiss Meditec, Dublin, CA) was used to obtain a fast macular thickness map as well as a fast retinal nerve fiber layer (NFL) map of each eye. There was a statistically significant difference in macular thickness and NFL thickness when normal eyes were compared against those with glaucoma in all quadrants studied (all $p \leq 0.001$). The authors concluded that OCT may prove valuable in the early diagnosis of glaucoma and that the difference between normal and glaucomatous eyes in children is similar to that reported in adults[41] (Figures 68-24 through 68-26).

PRIMARY CONGENITAL OPEN-ANGLE GLAUCOMA

Definition

Primary congenital open-angle glaucoma (trabeculodysgenesis), commonly referred to as congenital glaucoma or infantile glaucoma, is a specific inherited developmental defect of the TM and anterior chamber angle in which the angle appears to be open in the sense that the iris and corneoscleral TM are separated.[5,42] It is a significant cause of childhood blindness and is the most common type of glaucoma in infants. Characteristically, it manifests itself in the neonatal or infantile period with clouding and enlargement of the cornea, buphthalmos, epiphora, photophobia, and blepharospasm. Because of its relative rarity, it is often misdiagnosed and confused with inflammatory or infectious processes affecting the conjunctiva, cornea, and lids.[13,43] Approximately 25% of patients are diagnosed at birth, more than 60% are diagnosed by age 6 months, and more than 80% will have their onset within the first year of life.[13,43] Primary infantile glaucoma can occur in later childhood, then commonly termed *juvenile glaucoma*. This type is usually not associated with buphthalmos and corneal enlargement, although these can continue to occur until ages 6 to 8 years.[44]

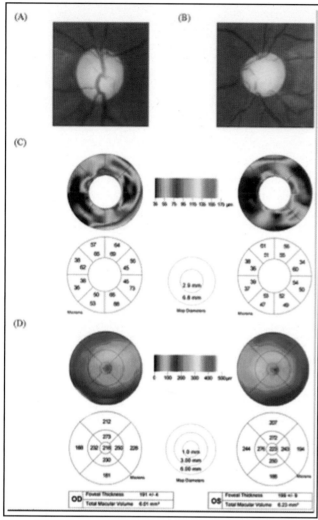

Figure 68-25. Report of OCT of the optic nerve (optic nerve head analysis) in a child with glaucoma.

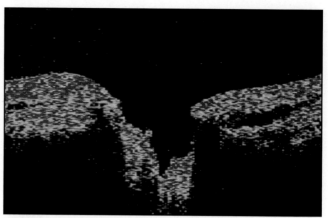

Figure 68-26. OCT of the abnormal optic nerve in the child in Figure 68-30 with unilateral glaucoma.

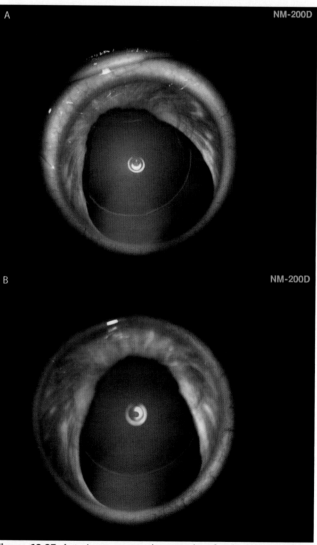

Figure 68-27. Anterior segment photographs of right (A) and left (B) eyes of a child with uveal coloboma, mild spherophakia, absence of lens zonules inferonasally, minimal lens subluxation, and secondary ocular hypertension without glaucomatous optic neuropathy.

Primary congenital glaucoma (PCG) can be distinguished from secondary infantile glaucoma by the absence of easily recognizable congenital abnormalities of the iris (such as aniridia), obvious obstructions of the TM (such as iridocorneal dysgenesis), and other metabolic inflammatory or congenital diseases of the eye (Figures 68-27 through 68-31).

Demographics

Primary infantile glaucoma occurs in approximately 0.01% of children (1 out of 10 000 births) and results in blindness in 2% to 15% of individuals (Table 68-5).[9,10] It is bilateral in 60% to 80% of patients and occurs more frequently in males (65%) than females (35%).[45-47] There is no racial or geographic predilection.

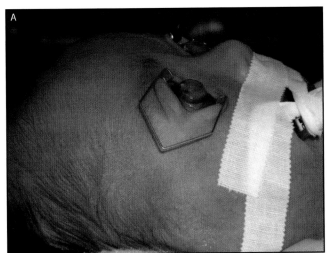
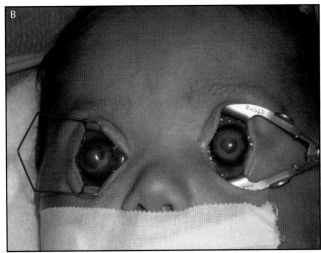

Figure 68-28. Figures of anterior segment photographs of lateral (A) and frontal views (B) of eyes of a newborn, full-term infant with severe, congenital anterior segment dysgenesis, glaucoma, buphthalmos, and corneal thinning with impending perforation. This child had to have emergency bilateral corneal transplantation, lensectomy, anterior vitrectomy, and tube implantation in both eyes.

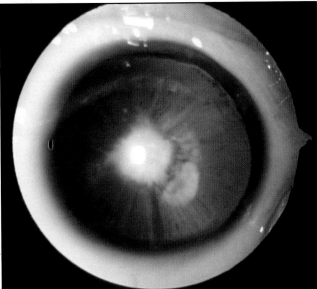

Figure 68-29. Anterior segment photograph of child with complicated aniridia, irido-corneo-trabeculodysgenesis, central cataract, lenticulocorneal adhesion, and glaucoma. This child had to have corneal transplantation, lensectomy, anterior vitrectomy, and tube implantation in both eyes.

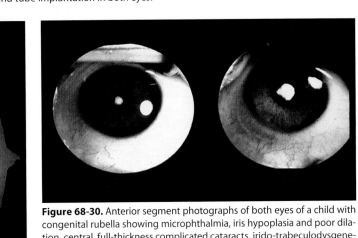

Figure 68-30. Anterior segment photographs of both eyes of a child with congenital rubella showing microphthalmia, iris hypoplasia and poor dilation, central, full-thickness complicated cataracts, irido-trabeculodysgenesis, and glaucoma. (Reprinted with permission from David B. Schaffer, MD.)

Figure 68-31. Anterior segment photograph of a child with familial ectopia lentis, irido-corneo-trabeculodysgenesis, iris hypoplasia, lens subluxation, and zonular dehiscence. This child had to have lensectomy and anterior vitrectomy, and then IOP was controlled on topical medications alone.

Inheritance

Most cases of PCG occur sporadically. However, an autosomal recessive form with variable expressivity has been described.[48,49] The fact that PCG occurs in parent and sibling with approximate equal frequency, has an unequal distribution by gender, and occurs in multiple siblings of healthy parents supports an autosomal recessive inheritance pattern that is polygenic, multifactorial, and has variable penetrance.[48-50]

Adult primary open-angle glaucoma (POAG) does not appear to be associated with primary infantile glaucoma.

TABLE 68-5. VISUAL LOSS IN PRIMARY CONGENITAL GLAUCOMA
Amblyopia
Anisometropia
Strabismic corneal scarring
Myopic astigmatism
Cataracts
Optic nerve damage

Steroid-induced elevations of IOP, a risk factor for adult POAG, occur no more frequently among parents of infants with primary infantile glaucoma than in the nonaffected general population.[51,52]

Hafez and colleagues[53] examined the correlation between human leukocyte antigen (HLA) and PCG. Family studies revealed an autosomal recessive gene predisposing to congenital glaucoma with strong linkage to the HLA-B8 antigen.[53]

Because of the known occurrence of primary congenital open-angle glaucoma in siblings and in offspring of parents with childhood glaucoma, it is important to counsel parents about the probability of future offspring having the disease and to examine and follow the younger and older siblings of patients who have this glaucoma. The chance of a second child having the disease is approximately 1% to 3%. If 2 children have the disease, the likelihood that subsequent children will be affected increases to as much as 25%. Frequent examinations of these infants are important, especially during the first 6 to 12 months of life. A single examination during the first month of life is inadequate.

Pathogenesis

The exact etiology of PCG still remains obscure. Originally, Barkan[54] and later Worst[55] proposed that an imperfect, thin glass-like membrane covered the anterior chamber angle and blocked aqueous outflow. To date, the presence of this membrane has not been established histopathologically. Most authorities now believe that the site of obstruction is the TM rather than an overlying membrane.[56]

A major obstacle to our understanding the etiology of primary infantile glaucoma is our lack of knowledge about the normal development of the anterior chamber angle. Allen, Burian, and Braley postulated that the anterior chamber angle normally forms by cleavage of mesoderm and that incomplete separation of the layers results in the formation of abnormal TM and, subsequently, infantile glaucoma.[57] Others[58,59] postulated that the anterior chamber angle was formed by mesodermal atrophy rather than cleavage and failure of this process resulted in retention of abnormal tissue in the TM that blocked aqueous

outflow or by posterior sliding of uveal tissues in relation to the cornea and sclera and a repositioning of the various layers within the uveal tract along the inner side of the sclera.[58,59] Anderson and colleagues[60] suggested that premature or excessive formation of collagenous beams within the TM prevents the normal posterior sliding of the ciliary body and peripheral iris, which results in an anterior insertion of the uvea into the TM with compression of the anterior trabecular spaces and blockage of aqueous outflow. This theory[60] is consistent with the theory of Maumenee,[61] who suggested that the abnormal insertion of the longitudinal ciliary muscle into the TM compresses the trabecular sheets when the muscle contracts. Shields[62] has noted a similar microscopic appearance of the anterior chamber angle in eyes of patients with Axenfeld-Rieger's syndrome, although the ultrastructural appearance in these cases suggests that the compactness of the TM may be due to failure of the intertrabecular spaces to develop, rather than to subsequent mechanical compression.

The concept of a fundamental defect in cellular development was supported by Smelser and Ozanics[62,63] who proposed that normally there is a gradual rearrangement of mesodermal cells to form the anterior chamber angle and that failure of this process results in structural changes of the uveal meshwork, which result in aqueous obstruction. The developmental process may be modulated by neural crest cells, which appear to be the precursors to many of the anterior chamber structures. Kupfer and Kaiser-Kupfer proposed that it is the faulty migration or differentiation of these cells that may result in the defects seen in the various types of congenital glaucoma.[63] The occasional association of PCG with other systemic anomalies may be explained in part by a common neural crest origin of the affected tissues.

It, therefore, appears that a true Barkan's membrane probably does not exist and that PCG results from a developmental arrest of anterior chamber tissue derived from neural crest cells. Structurally, this is manifested by the high insertion of ciliary body and iris into the posterior portion of the TM. The actual mechanism of aqueous outflow obstruction is uncertain and may result from compression of the trabecular beams, abnormal development of the TM or Schlemm's canal, or the persistence of some precursor material in the anterior chamber angle.

Clinical Manifestations

The clinical appearance of an infant with PCG is often striking. The child normally presents during the first months of life with a history of epiphora, blepharospasm, and photophobia (Figure 68-32). This is often accompanied by moderate tearing, and in older infants, by rubbing of the eyes. The photophobia appears to be related to corneal edema. The symptoms can be gradual in onset or occur suddenly as a result of rupturing of Descemet's membrane.

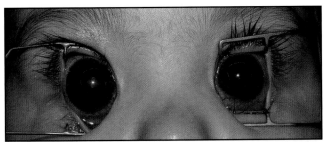

Figure 68-32. Anterior segment photograph of a child born with high IOP, irido-trabeculodysgenesis, iris hypoplasia, buphthalmos, and anterior cortical cataracts in both eyes. This child had bilateral 360-degree goniotomies followed by bilateral tube implantation, iridectomies then lensectomy, and anterior vitrectomy in both eyes. IOP is controlled now without topical medications.

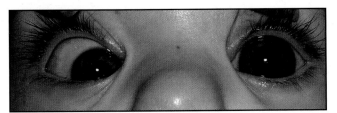

Figure 68-33. Anterior segment photograph of child with bilateral trabeculodysgenesis, asymmetric buphthalmos (OS worse than OD), and bilateral glaucoma well controlled after 360 degrees of trabeculotomy in both eyes.

TABLE 68-6. CLINICAL CHARACTERISTICS OF INFANTS AND CHILDREN WITH PRIMARY INFANTILE GLAUCOMA	
Clinical Characteristics of Infants	**%**
Problems noted by parents	
Tearing	55
Photophobia	41
Tearing and photophobia	32
Corneal haze	41
Corneal enlargement	32
Signs noted by initial physician	
Corneal haze	83
Corneal/global enlargement	58
Corneal clouding and/or enlargement	92
Bilateral involvement	58
Male/female	54/46

Reproduced with permission from *Pediatrics*, Vol 77, Pages 399-404, Copyright 1986 by the AAP.

Although common, these symptoms are frequently not present. In a study by Seidman and colleagues,[64] epiphora or photophobia were present in only half of the cases, and the combination was present in approximately one-third. Parents were as likely to notice signs of glaucoma (corneal clouding and enlargement) as they were to notice symptoms.

The classic signs (Table 68-6) of PCG include corneal enlargement, enlargement of the globe, corneal clouding, and cupping of the optic disc. In children with bilateral enlarged corneas, particularly in the absence of visible corneal edema, recognition may be delayed as parents believe their baby's big eyes enhance his or her appearance (Figure 68-33). When local areas of corneal opacification are present, associated curvilinear breaks of Descemet's membrane, Haab's striae, are almost always found. The anterior chamber of an affected eye can be strikingly deep compared to the usual shallow infantile anterior chamber.

The severity of presenting signs and symptoms varies from patient to patient presumably because of differences in the elevation of IOP. Infants born with grey edematous and enlarged corneas presumably have had high IOP even before birth, while those infants in whom signs are present with minimal symptoms may have had a gradual rise in IOP after birth. In some cases of bilateral glaucoma, the characteristic signs are much more evident in one eye than the other and, when the infant is initially examined, the diagnosis in the less affected eye may not be suspected.

Nystagmus is seldom noted in primary congenital open-angle glaucoma, although it is common in aniridia and in glaucoma secondary to surgery for congenital cataracts. When nystagmus does occur in congenital glaucoma, it is usually due to severe early loss of vision and is often infantile nystagmus syndrome.

The Diagnostic Examination

Some of the clinical findings in congenital glaucoma such as buphthalmos, enlarged corneal diameter, and corneal edema can be seen on gross inspection and do not require complicated examinations and techniques. The differential diagnosis of congenital glaucoma is listed in Table 68-7. Each of these conditions can be distinguished by means of a thorough ophthalmic evaluation, which includes tonometry, measurement of corneal diameter, gonioscopy, and funduscopic examination.

It is important to note that determining the presence or absence of PCG is not always easy. There are equivocal cases in which some of the features may be missing and some of the evidence may be weak. The correct diagnosis and further decision as to the proper form of treatment necessitate considering all the factors.

Differential Diagnosis

The diagnosis of PCG is very straightforward when the classic triad of symptoms (epiphora, blepharospasm, and photophobia) and signs (corneal enlargement, corneal haze, and buphthalmos) are present. Interpretation of the child's eye problem with respect to glaucoma is more difficult in the

TABLE 68-7. DIFFERENTIAL DIAGNOSIS OF SYMPTOMS AND SIGNS IN PRIMARY INFANTILE GLAUCOMA

I. Conditions sharing signs of epiphora and red eye

  A. Conjunctivitis

  B. Congenital nasolacrimal duct obstruction

  C. Corneal epithelial defect/abrasion

  D. Ocular inflammation (uveitis, trauma)

II. Conditions sharing signs of corneal edema or opacification

  A. Corneal dystrophy

    1. Congenital hereditary endothelial dystrophy

    2. Posterior polymorphous dystrophy

  B. Obstetrical birth trauma with Descemet's tears

  C. Storage disease

    1. Mucopolysaccharoidoses

    2. Cystinosis

  D. Congenital anomalies

    1. Sclerocornea

    2. Peter's anomaly

  E. Keratitis

    1. Maternal rubella keratitis

    2. Herpetic

    3. Phlectenular

  F. Idiopathic (diagnosis of exclusion only)

III. Conditions sharing signs of corneal enlargement

  A. Axial myopia

  B. Megalocornea

IV. Conditions sharing sign of optic nerve cupping (real or apparent)

  A. Physiologic optic nerve cupping

  B. Optic nerve coloboma

  C. Optic atrophy

  D. Optic nerve hypoplasia

  E. Optic nerve malformation

---

entertained to confirm a diagnosis. A red eye plus epiphora and blepharospasm suggests an ocular infection or inflammation. In the absence of positive findings, a therapeutic trial or careful observation may be indicated.

Buphthalmos and corneal enlargement may be due to a congenital anomaly. Megalocornea is a rare x-linked recessive condition of abnormal corneal enlargement, usually greater than 14 mm, with a deep anterior chamber, iridodonesis, normal IOP, absence of Haab's striae, and no optic nerve cupping.[65] Enlargement is practically always bilateral and symmetrical. Corneas may be thin but there is absence of photophobia, discomfort, edema, or clouding. Families have been reported in which some members have megalocornea and others have primary infantile glaucoma.[65] Careful follow-up is necessary to search for possible increased IOP changes indicative of primary infantile glaucoma.

Axial myopia can mimic a large buphthalmic eye and is commonly associated with corneal enlargement. Funduscopic examination, however, is quite characteristic with a tilted insertion of the optic nerve, myopic crescent, and retinal pigmentary and choroidal abnormalities.

Corneal edema or opacities can be caused by breaks in Descemet's membrane, corneal dystrophies, or with abnormalities in metabolism such as storage diseases of mucopolysaccharides, gangliosides, or sphingomyelin. Birth trauma may result in vertical breaks in Descemet's membrane with resultant corneal edema. Obstetrical corneal trauma is usually unilateral (left greater than right because of the higher incidence of left occipital anterior presentation) and is associated with signs of skin bruising as a result of the trauma. It is often stated that Descemet's membrane breaks from trauma are vertically oriented while those caused by increased IOP are horizontal. However, traumatic injuries can also be curvilinear and run diagonally across the cornea, but there is no corneal enlargement and IOPs are normal.

Corneal dystrophic changes that most closely mimic primary congenital open-angle glaucoma are severe infantile posterior polymorphous dystrophy (and congenital hereditary endothelial dystrophy). In severe infantile posterior polymorphous dystrophy, the patient often experiences a period of photophobia in the first year of life. A diffuse irregular thickening and opacification at the level of Descemet's membrane is found. The posterior surface of the cornea sometimes resembles alligator skin but the corneal diameters are normal. Some temporary elevation of IOP may occur, but the symptoms and disturbance of the corneas do not appear to be related to the IOP. It is an autosomal recessive condition.

Congenital hereditary endothelial dystrophy (CHED) is characterized by diffusely opacified and thickened corneal stroma. Abnormalities are seen clinically at the level of Descemet's membrane. Metabolic diseases that produce corneal opacification are usually associated with obvious

absence of these pathognomic signs and other entities such as those listed in Table 68-7.

In the absence of corneal haze or buphthalmos, abnormalities of the ocular surface or drainage system should be considered. Epiphora alone suggests nasolacrimal duct obstruction, and a lacrimal duct probing should be

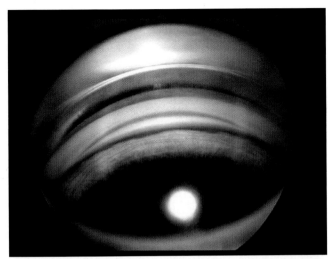

Figure 68-34. Illustration of goniotomy with an incision in the anterior TM and resultant gonioscopic view of channel in the peripheral angle observed after a successful goniotomy (ice cream scoop-like appearance).

TABLE 68-8. SURGICAL RESULTS IN CONGENITAL GLAUCOMA (AGE < 1 YEAR)				
	Date	Eyes	Success (%)	
			1st	2nd
Goniotomy				
Barkan[8]	1953	185	80	
Haas[13]	1955	253	77	
Bietti[67]	1966	321	82	
Shaffer[70]	1967	100	85	
Morin[76]	1980	171	56	76
Anderson[81]	1982	16	81	100
McPherson[95]	1983	24	33	83
Trabeculotomy				
Harms[90]	1969	30	93	
Gregerson[80]	1977	21	100	88
Anderson[97]	1982	25	76	100
McPherson[80]	1983	23	83	

systemic abnormalities. Such entities as oculo-cerebral-renal syndrome of Lowe, mucopolysaccharidosis, cystinoses, and corneal lipidosis can produce corneal clouding, mimicking the corneal edema of primary infantile glaucoma.[66] It is important to remember that, although PCG is the most common form of glaucoma in early life, it is not the only form, and that the signs associated with this entity, such as corneal enlargement, breaks in Descemet's membrane, and edematous cornea, are abnormalities that can also be associated with the other types of glaucomas.

Treatment

There are multiple treatment modalities available to aid in the control of IOP in PCG. The primary intervention is surgical and the initial procedure is usually a goniotomy or trabeculotomy (Figure 68-34). Pharmacologic agents, however, are often necessary to optimize pressure control.

MEDICAL TREATMENT

Indications

Even though PCG usually requires a surgical intervention, the role of pharmacological agents is significant. First, most patients are placed on some form of topical or oral medication to reduce IOP in preparation for surgery. In those patients who have significant corneal edema, preoperative management of the IOP has been advocated to clear the cornea, which increases surgical safety and reduces complications. This is especially important if goniotomy is to be attempted. Secondly, medical therapy is often used as a temporizing measure to control IOP between surgical procedures or to enhance control in those borderline situations where deferral of surgery is necessary. Lastly, in those patients with severe disease who have been unresponsive to surgical interventions, medications can be used to reduce IOP to the level that may preserve some visual function. Because surgery is performed in the vast majority of patients with primary infantile glaucoma, there are no long-term studies using medical treatment alone[9,67,68] (Table 68-8).

Carbonic Anhydrase Inhibitors

Acetazolamide (Diamox) is usually well tolerated by infants and children and it often effectively lowers IOP in these patients when it is administered orally as 10 to 15 mg/kg/day, divided every 6 to 8 hours.[69] Parents sometimes note diarrhea, diminished energy levels, and loss of appetite in their children on this therapy, thus requiring dosage adjustment or discontinuation. Metabolic acidosis has also been reported in infants, and it may be ameliorated with oral bicitra (1 milleequivalent/kg/day). In general, however, younger patients tolerate acetazolamide better than older ones: 77% of patients younger than 40 years are able to tolerate acetazolamide milliequivalents.[65,67,69]

Miotics

Historically, miotics have been of limited value in treating childhood glaucomas.[70] In cases of congenital glaucoma, the abnormal insertion of the ciliary muscle into the TM has been blamed for the poor response of IOP to miotics.[71] Nonetheless, miotics have been useful in achieving miosis just before and after goniotomy.[72,73] Whereas pilocarpine 2% every 6 to 8 hours has been used in treating congenital glaucoma, stronger miotics, such as phospholine iodide, have also been administered in infants, with less ocular irritation than that observed in adults.[71] Phospholine iodide therapy has sometimes been accompanied by diarrhea and requires extreme care in the concurrent use of succinylcholine for general anesthesia. Older children often experience severe visual blurring attributable to myopia induced by even dilute miotics. If they are effective in treating the glaucoma, miotics in these children may be better tolerated when the induced myopia is rendered stable, so that it can be compensated by spectacles. To this end, higher concentrations (eg, pilocarpine 2% to 4%) or longer-acting formulations (eg, pilocarpine Ocusert) may be useful.

Beta-Adrenergic Antagonists (Beta-Blockers)

Topical beta-blockers have been available for the treatment of glaucoma since the introduction of timolol in 1978.[38,74] Several studies have examined the role of timolol in treating uncontrolled childhood glaucomas, often after previous surgical intervention.[38,74] Reported success rate with timolol alone ranges from less than 10% to almost 50% in various studies with most stable on the 0.25% twice-daily concentration, and all subjects with adverse reactions (10%) were using 0.5% timolol.[38,71]

In multiple series of patients, most of whom were younger than 20 years of age, 72%[69,70] were controlled without further surgery for up to 2.5 years on regimens including timoptic 0.25% or 0.5% twice daily, with an overall IOP decline of 30.7%. Systemic side effects occurred in only 4% of the patients in this series. In earlier studies, the addition of timolol 0.25% or 0.5% to the regimen of young patients with severe uncontrolled glaucoma resulted in stabilization of glaucoma in about one-third of patients without further surgery for up to 2.5 years. Systemic adverse side effects were reported in none of 34 patients and in 5 of 28 patients (18%), respectively, in these studies.[69-71]

The most severe systemic adverse effects occurring in children on topical timolol therapy have included acute asthma attacks, bradycardia, and apneic spells (the latter in neonates). Plasma timolol levels measured in children on 0.25% timolol (ranging from 3.5 ng/mL in a 5-year-old to 34 ng/mL in a 3-week-old) vastly exceeded those in adults on 0.5% timolol (0.34 to 2.45 ng/mL). The use of punctal occlusion in adults further lowered mean 1-hour plasma timolol levels by 40% in the adult patients in this study (from 1.34 to 0.9 ng/mL). The high plasma timolol levels in children may be explained by a child's volume of distribution for the drug, which is much smaller than that of an adult. For example, whereas the ocular volume of a neonate is about 50% that of an adult (reaching full size by about age 2 years), the average 3.5-kg newborn infant has a body mass only one-twentieth that of a small adult male (70 kg), with a blood volume relatively even smaller.

When timolol is used in small children, treatment should always begin with 0.25% drops, excluding those children with a history of asthma or bradycardia. Topical beta-blockers should be used with extreme caution in neonates with particular attention paid to the possibility of apnea. It may be reasonable to observe children for adverse systemic effects for 1 to 2 hours in the office after an initial dose of beta-blocker has been given, before prescribing the beta-blocker for outpatient use. Punctal occlusion, when feasible, should be performed by parents or caretakers.[7]

Few data are available on the use of topical beta-blockers other than timolol in the treatment of childhood glaucoma. Based on experience in adults, betaxolol, as a relatively beta 1-selective agent, may be less prone to precipitating acute asthma attacks (which may present as coughing) than the nonselective beta-blockers. The remaining nonselective beta-blockers should be approached in a fashion similar to timolol regarding risks and probable efficacy. As in adults, beta-blockers used in children often have an additive effect to carbonic anhydrase inhibitors (acetazolamide) in treating children with glaucoma.

Adrenergic Agonists

Epinephrine compounds have been used in infants and children with glaucoma, but there are few published data to suggest optimal dosing schedules or the magnitude of the IOP decrement to be expected from these drugs.

Furthermore, these drugs are relegated to secondary importance because of their potential for systemic toxicity (eg, tachyarrhythmias, hypertension) and for their ocular side effects (eg, irritation, reactive hyperemia, epinephrine oxidation deposits), together with their limited effectiveness.[38,71] Topical dipivefrin (Propine), as an epinephrine pro-drug, should theoretically have fewer systemic side effects in children than epinephrine. Based on adult studies, little additional pressure-lowering effect would be expected with the use of Propine or epinephrine together with a nonselective beta-blocker.[37,43,62] No data are available regarding the use of the alpha-2 agonist apraclonidine (Iopidine) in children with glaucoma. This drug is useful in the setting of goniotomy to minimize intraoperative hyphema.

SURGICAL TREATMENT

Although surgical intervention provides the most definitive treatment for most forms of childhood glaucoma, there are significant challenges, especially in young children (Table 68-9). If the diagnosis of glaucoma has been secured in the office, medical therapy (especially oral acetazolamide) can be used preoperatively to clear the cornea maximally for gonioscopy, fundus examination, and surgery. Anesthesia itself poses significant risks, especially in neonates. The infant eye, with a smaller palpebral fissure, less rigid and

TABLE 68-9. INDICATIONS FOR SURGERY IN CHILDHOOD GLAUCOMAS

I. Angle surgery

  A. Goniotomy (may repeat one or more times)

    1. Primary congenital/infantile open-angle glaucoma

    2. Other primary glaucomas (generally poor success)

      a. Axenfeld-Rieger syndrome

      b. Lowe's syndrome

      c. Neurofibromatosis

      d. Sturge-Weber syndrome

      e. Other

    3. Selected secondary glaucomas

      a. Maternal rubella syndrome

      b. Open-angle glaucoma after congenital cataract surgery

      c. Uveitic glaucoma (especially with juvenile rheumatoid arthritis)

    4. Prophylaxis against acquired glaucoma in aniridia

    5. Early onset JOAG

  B. Trabeculotomy (may repeat one time)

    1. Same as for goniotomy, but preferred in the presence of corneal opacification.

    2. Performed by some surgeons after 2 goniotomies have failed.

    3. May be combined with trabeculectomy.

II. Peripheral iridectomy (secondary pupillary block glaucoma)

III. Filtration surgery

  A. Combined trabeculotomy/trabeculectomy

    1. When trabeculotomy cannot be completed (failure to cannulate Schlemm's canal)

    2. Failed previous angle surgery (2 goniotomies and/or trabeculotomies)

    3. Low likelihood of success with angle surgery alone (eg, chronic aphakic glaucoma)

  B. Trabeculectomy (almost always with intraoperative mitomycin C)

    1. Any glaucoma in an eye with reasonable visual potential and unscarred conjunctiva after angle surgery has failed

    2. Low likelihood of success with angle surgery (would usually favor III A)

  C. Combined cataract removal/trabeculectomy

    1. Not usually recommended (suggest cataract first, then glaucoma surgery)

    2. Consider for older child with intact posterior capsule

IV. Drainage implant (seton) surgery

  A. Failed trabeculectomy with intraoperative mitomycin C and reasonable visual potential

  B. High risk for complications with filtration surgery (eg, Sturge-Weber syndrome)

  C. High risk for failure with trabeculectomy from scarring (eg, after multiple conjunctival surgeries)

V. Cyclodestructive procedures

  A. Laser cycloablation (Nd:YAG or diode)

    1. Failed angle surgery (or angle surgery not possible) and minimal visual potential

    2. Failed trabeculectomy and/or seton with poor central vision

    3. Anatomy precluding trabeculectomy or seton (eg, disorganized anterior segment after trauma, sclerocornea)

    4. In patients who are gravely ill, or when follow-up and postoperative care cannot be assured, or prolonged intubation poses life-threatening risk

    5. High risk for complications with intraocular surgery (eg, Sturge-Weber)

  B. CCT

    1. Same as for cycloablation but in phakic patients with small or normal-sized eyes

    2. Repeat therapy in selected quadrants after previous CCT

often thinned sclera, and limbal tissue (especially in buphthalmic eyes), behaves differently from an adult eye during surgery. Postoperatively, difficulties may be encountered in protection of the operated eye from inadvertent injury, compliance with postoperative medications, and monitoring of the eye for possible surgical complications and response to surgery. Family members should be informed preoperatively of the long-term prognosis, multiple visits, and likely additional anesthetics that will be needed postoperatively, as well as the likelihood that further surgery may be needed to control glaucoma. Often, the first examination under anesthesia can be followed immediately by the first indicated surgical procedure, thereby avoiding time delay in controlling IOP and avoiding at least one additional anesthesia.

Goniotomy

With the aim of incising the uveal TM under direct visualization, goniotomy is the surgical procedure of choice in most cases of PCG. Trabeculotomy ab externo, covered later in this chapter, is an alternative procedure that is especially useful when corneal clouding prevents an optimal view of the angle structures by gonioscopy.

In 1893, the Italian ophthalmologist Carlo deVincentiis described a new operation that attempted to open Schlemm's canal by incising the angle tissues (without visualization of the angle).[72] Because of a high complication rate and poor results in adults with open-angle glaucoma, this operation was initially abandoned. With the advent of clinical gonioscopy, Barkan[72] modified the technique in 1938 as an operation for PCG, naming it *goniotomy* (Greek: gonio = angle + tomein = to cut).[75] With this effective operation for congenital glaucoma, the dismal prognosis for this disease dramatically improved. The technique for performing goniotomy has remained essentially unaltered for more than 50 years—a testament to its importance and widespread use as the initial procedure for PCG. Whereas the goal of goniotomy is to remove obstructing tissue and to open a route for aqueous humor to exit the anterior chamber into Schlemm's canal, the precise mechanism by which pressure reduction occurs remains obscure. Successful goniotomy does appear, however, to lower IOP as a result of improved facility of aqueous outflow.[76-79]

Goniotomy enjoys its greatest success in the therapy of PCG but it may also be used in other primary developmental glaucomas, although with a lower success rate. Examples of these other primary glaucomas include those associated with Sturge-Weber syndrome, neurofibromatosis, Lowe's syndrome, Axenfeld-Rieger syndrome, and aniridia, among others. In addition, several secondary glaucomas may respond favorably to goniotomy in some cases. These include aphakic glaucoma presenting early after congenital cataract surgery and glaucoma complicating chronic anterior uveitis. Goniotomy also deserves special consideration as a prophylactic procedure in congenital aniridia.[80-83]

If the diagnosis of glaucoma has been confirmed before anesthesia and if goniotomy is the preferred surgical procedure, oral acetazolamide therapy for at least several days preoperatively may help to maximize corneal clarity by lowering IOP. Topical antibiotics may also be used for 1 to 2 days preoperatively. Pilocarpine 1% or 2% should be placed onto the eye(s) to be operated just before surgery to aid in protecting the crystalline lens from injury during surgery. Miochol may be injected into the anterior chamber, if necessary, to promote further miosis.

Goniotomy is performed using a surgical goniolens and a goniotomy knife. There are several available goniolenses in addition to the round-domed Barkan goniolens (Reichert Technologies), including the Lister modification that includes irrigation, or the Swan-Jacobs lens (Reichert Technologies), which incorporates a handle and facilitates use of a microscope. Several types of goniotomy knives are also available. A nontapered Swan knife (or needle-knife; Katena Eye Instruments, Denville, NJ) enters the anterior chamber easily and cuts in either direction. Alternatively, a disposable 23- or 25-gauge needle attached to a syringe containing hyaluronic acid (Healon [Abbott Medical Optics, Abbott Park, IL]) may be used, allowing the anterior chamber to be deepened before incision and to be maintained upon instrument removal. Enthusiastic use of Healon may acutely increase corneal edema by increasing IOP, thereby degrading the surgeon's view of the angle structures (Table 68-10).

To perform goniotomy safely and effectively, the surgeon must ensure a degree of corneal clarity sufficient to allow an adequate view of the angle structures. If corneal epithelial (but not stromal) edema obscures an adequate angle view, the epithelium can be removed with the edge of a No. 15 Bard-Parker blade (Katena Eye Instruments) from a window of cornea nearest the surgeon (after sterile preparation of the eye and placement of a lid speculum has taken place). This cornea epithelia removal is best performed after applying topical proparacaine, followed by 70% isopropyl alcohol (on a swab) to the appropriate section of epithelium.[71,84] Often, corneal stromal edema persists even after epithelial removal; in this setting, trabeculotomy may be preferred.

The surgeon may use a binocular operating loupe or operating microscope to view the angle for goniotomy. The surgeon should be positioned opposite the portion of the angle to be operated (ie, to the temporal side of the patient for nasal goniotomy), with the patient's head slightly rotated away from the surgeon. Elschnig-O'Connor (Katena Eye Instruments) or Moody locking fixation forceps (Katena Eye Instruments) are usually placed on the superior and inferior rectus muscles when a nasal or temporal goniotomy is planned. If the lids seem tight, a small lateral single-snip canthotomy can be helpful. Apraclonidine 1% may be placed on the limbus overlying the angle to be operated, and then the operating goniolens is applied to the cornea. Healon may be helpful in preventing air bubble formation under the Barkan goniotomy lens, and the lens may be stabilized with a nontoothed fine forcep in the positioning holes of the lens.

The goniotomy knife or needle is placed through peripheral clear cornea 1 mm from the limbus, opposite the midpoint of the intended goniotomy, in a plane parallel to the iris. The knife or needle is guided over iris tissue (not pupil) to engage TM in its anterior third, just posterior to Schwalbe's line. A circumferential incision is then made

TABLE 68-10. GONIOTOMY: KEY POINTS IN SURGICAL TECHNIQUE	
Key Point	Comment
Select patients with favorable surgical prognosis	PCG, aphakic glaucoma early after cataract surgery, uveitic glaucoma
Confirm adequate corneal clarity	Use medical therapy preoperatively, perform gonioscopy under anesthesia just before surgery
Position patient and surgeon for optimal access to surgical site	Easiest first goniotomy is nasal, with surgeon seated on temporal side, patient's head turned slightly away from the surgeon
Stabilize globe adequately for surgery	Place locking forceps on insertions of appropriate rectus muscle pair (usually superior and inferior recti)
Improve angle view if suboptimal	Consider scraping portion of corneal epithelium (glycerin marginally helpful); reposition eye, microscope, goniolens (Healon under lens helpful)
Make entry into anterior chamber	25-gauge needle on Healon syringe easiest; enter parallel to iris plane opposite angle to be operated; use miochol first if pupil not miotic
Guide needle (or knife) safely to engage angle	Pass over iris (not pupil), engaging angle tissue just below Schwalbe's line, in anterior-most uveal tissue for incision meshwork
Make angle incision smoothly and of adequate extent (4 to 5 clock-hours)	Keep incision superficial, watch for cleft formation and posterior iris movement; have assistant rotate eye in same plane to gain access to additional angle
Remove needle (or knife) safely from eye	Keep instrument over iris tissue, move swiftly, inject Healon if needed to maintain anterior chamber
Refill chamber and close entry site	Balanced salt solution useful to deepen anterior chamber; single 10-0 Vicryl adequate to close

(right to left for a right-handed surgeon) for about 4 to 5 clock-hours, and the knife or needle is carefully and quickly withdrawn from the eye over iris tissue at all times. The incision should be superficial with no grating or scraping sensation noted. A deeper cleft with exposure of whiter tissue may be noted in the wake of the incision, with a widening of the angle and a posterior movement of peripheral iris in some cases. The assistant may help the surgeon to extend the angle accessible to goniotomy by rotating the eye clockwise and counterclockwise, respectively, at the surgeon's request. After knife withdrawal, blood often egresses from the angle incision, stopping when the chamber is refilled with balanced salt solution. A single suture of 9-0 or 10-0 Vicryl ([Ethicon, Inc, Somerville, NJ]; or 10-0 nylon in an older child, with the knot buried) secures the corneal wound if leakage occurs (Figure 68-35).

Postoperative treatment with a topical antibiotic-steroid (and miotic) is continued for 1 week. If bilateral goniotomies are needed, they may be performed during one anesthesia, provided that the first eye was uncomplicated and all instruments are sterilized, all drapes, gowns and gloves replaced, and the fellow eye reprepared and draped in sterile fashion

following the first procedure.[85] Key points in the surgical technique of goniotomy are summarized in Table 68-10. Common errors are listed in Table 68-11.

Mild to moderate hyphemas commonly occur after goniotomy but almost always clear rapidly without sequelae over several days. Other complications following goniotomy are rare and include iridodialysis, cyclodialysis, the appearance of small peripheral anterior synechiae (PAS) in the incised angle, damage to the crystalline lens, and retinal detachment in eyes with high myopia.[86] Cardiopulmonary arrests (nonfatal) occurred during anesthesia in 1.8% of cases in a series of 401 goniotomies.[86]

The results of goniotomy should be evaluated weekly in the immediate postoperative period and are often evident by 3 to 6 weeks. Gonioscopy after successful goniotomy often reveals a widened angle in the previous incision site, with improved visibility of the ciliary band and scleral spur. This appearance suggests that an opening has been created in the uveal meshwork with little injury to the underlying tissues. Scattered PAS in the bed of the goniotomy may partially, or significantly, obscure a view of the incised angle. Because 4 to 5 clock-hours of angle tissue are incised with a single

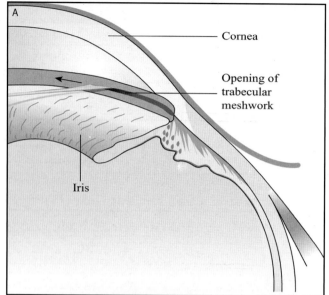

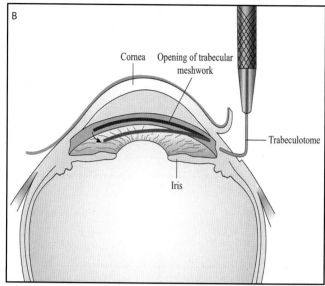

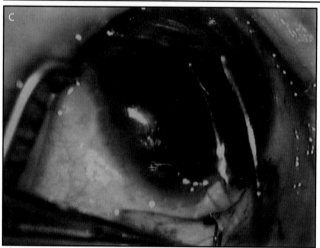

Figure 68-35. (A, B) Illustration of trabeculotomy with external to internal tract in the anterior chamber through the TM. (C) Actual anterior segment photograph of successful trabeculotome entering the anterior chamber.

goniotomy, repeat procedures in untreated portions of the angle may enhance IOP control in selected cases. Goniotomy may fail to control infantile glaucoma in some instances due to improper placement and depth of the angle incision, or the obliteration of the incision by PAS. Rarely, a third or even fourth goniotomy procedure may control glaucoma.

The success of goniotomy in controlling glaucoma varies with the etiology of the glaucoma. The best results—80% to more than 90% success after 1 to 2 procedures—are achieved in infants with PCG presenting between 3 months and 1 year of age.[76-79]

Procedures Related to Goniotomy

Scheie reported a modification of goniotomy termed goniopuncture, which involved passage of a goniotomy knife through the TM and sclera to the subconjunctival space following a standard goniotomy. However, scarring of the limbal incision limited the usefulness of goniopuncture.

The neodymium:YAG laser has been used to perform trabeculopuncture by directing laser energy gonioscopically at the TM in order to penetrate through to Schlemm's canal.[87,88] Success was reported with this procedure in 6 of 8 eyes with juvenile glaucoma over a 6-month follow-up period.[87,88] A technique requiring a large limbal incision, direct goniotomy has also been described, but it has been superceded by trabeculotomy.[89]

Trabeculodialysis, a modification of goniotomy in which the TM is scraped or retracted from the scleral sulcus after a standard goniotomy incision, has been effective in the treatment of children with glaucoma secondary to anterior uveitis (60% IOP control reported in a series of 23 such patients). Argon laser trabeculoplasty is not effective in the treatment of childhood glaucomas, nor is it possible to perform in young patients.

Trabeculotomy Ab Externo

Trabeculotomy ab externo, performed by cannulating Schlemm's canal from an external approach and then tearing through the TM into the anterior chamber, creates a direct communication between the anterior chamber and Schlemm's canal. Burian and Smith independently described trabeculotomy ab externo in 1960 as an alternative procedure to goniotomy.[90-93] The technique was later modified by Harms and Dannheim,[90] McPherson,[91] Aldave et al,[92] and Yang et al.[93] Success rates varying from 73% to 100% have been reported for this procedure in congenital glaucoma.[90-93] In a series of 71 patients (most with primary infantile glaucoma), Akimoto and colleagues[94]

TABLE 68-11 GONIOTOMY: COMMON ERRORS IN SURGICAL TECHNIQUE	
Common Error	**Consequence**
Poor patient selection	Surgical success unlikely; time and effort of goniotomy could be better spent
Angle view suboptimal	Increased likelihood of damage to cornea, iris, or crystalline lens; decreased chance of incision in angle tissue
Globe position not stable	Same as above
Pupil not miotic	Increases danger of crystalline lens damage
Entry wound too anterior	Angle tissue may be difficult to reach or incise; corneal endothelium may be injured
Entry wound too posterior	Needle (or knife) may engage iris upon entry; crystalline lens damage more likely; chamber may collapse as excessive lifting is needed to engage angle
Angle incision too anterior	Angle tissue may not be entered; surgery likely will be ineffective
Angle incision too posterior	Iridodialysis, cyclodialysis, and hyphema more likely to occur; angle tissue itself may not be incised
Anterior chamber collapse upon instrument withdrawal from eye	Needle (knife) more likely to injure cornea, iris, and crystalline lens; significant hyphema more likely to occur

recently reported total success probabilities of one or more trabeculotomies of 92.5% and 76.5%, at 5 and 10 years, respectively. Conjunctival scarring is the salient disadvantage of trabeculotomy. However, trabeculotomy's advantage is that it is little affected by an edematous or scarred cornea (see Figure 68-35).

In the surgical technique described by McPherson and McFarland[95] and McPherson and Berry,[96] a limbal-based conjunctival flap and a partial-thickness triangular or rectangular scleral flap are created as for standard trabeculectomy. Pilocarpine may be used preoperatively to induce miosis. After a paracentesis (and injection into the anterior chamber of a small amount of viscoelastic), a radial scratch incision is made across the sclero-limbal junction in the bed of the scleral flap. This scratch incision is gradually deepened under high magnification until Schlemm's canal is visualized just anterior to the circumferential fibers of the scleral spur (near the posterior aspect of the limbal gray zone). Often, a small amount of blood or aqueous humor will reflux through the cut ends of Schlemm's canal, and the internal wall of the canal will appear slightly pigmented. To confirm the identity of the canal, a 5-0 or 6-0 nylon suture may thread easily to both the left and the right sides of the radial incision. If resistance is met, the suture may need to be repositioned, the radial incision deepened, or a second parallel radial incision made beneath the same scleral flap to aid in locating Schlemm's canal. (The presence of the suture in Schlemm's canal may sometimes be confirmed by gonioscopy using a Zeiss 4-mirror lens [Ocular Instruments].) Once the canal has been located, the internal arm of a trabeculotome should be passed gently into the canal (to the

right side first for a right-handed surgeon) as far as possible without meeting resistance and using the parallel external arm as a guide (see Figure 68-35). The internal arm is then gently rotated into the anterior chamber, with care to avoid entry into peripheral cornea or beneath the iris plane. Rotation of the trabeculotome into the anterior chamber tears through the intervening TM (see Figure 68-35) and requires very little force. Rotation should be halted once about 75% to 80% of the internal arm of the trabeculotome is visible in the anterior chamber. The anterior chamber may shallow slightly and blood may egress from the torn TM as the trabeculotome is removed from the eye along its path of entry. In a similar fashion, the trabeculotome should be placed into the left side of the radial incision and the procedure repeated to the left. By leaving a portion of intact TM underlying the radial incision into Schlemm's canal, one hopes to prevent prolapse of the iris into the wound. The scleral flap is then sutured with 10-0 nylon, while the Tenon's capsule and conjunctival layers may be closed with a running suture of 8-0 or 10-0 Vicryl, as for standard trabeculectomy.[96] Postoperatively, patients are treated with topical antibiotics and steroids, together with low-dose pilocarpine for 1 to 2 weeks. While hyphema occurs commonly after trabeculotomy, rarer complications include inadvertent filtering blebs, choroidal detachment, iridotomy, damage to the lens, creation of a false passage into the anterior chamber or suprachoroidal space, and infection.

One proposed modification of trabeculotomy involves the use of a nylon or Prolene suture (Ethicon, Inc) to perform a 180- or 360-degree trabeculotomy at one surgery, using 1 or 2 external incisions into Schlemm's canal.[97,98] Although

TABLE 68-12. TRABECULOTOMY: KEY POINTS IN SURGICAL TECHNIQUE		
Key Point	**Comment**	**Related Complication**
Select patient well	Same as for goniotomy but may have opacified cornea	Surgical success unlikely, increased time to IOP control
	Spares superior conjunctiva for later filtration surgery	Superior scarring may predispose later filter to failure
Consider temporal approach	Facilitates finding and cannulating Schlemm's canal	Schlemm's canal may not be found if dissection not carried well into limbal gray zone
Dissect conjunctival and scleral flap very anteriorly		Chamber may shallow and hyphema occur, precluding canal cannulation to the opposite side
	Maintains anterior chamber access and facilitates second trabeculotome passage	Schlemm's canal may be transected and "missed" and anterior chamber entered if deep incision quickly made
	Transverse fibers of Schlemm's canal easier to see if exposed gradually without canal transection	Metal trabeculotome may make false passage and canal can be missed altogether
Make paracentesis and inject Healon	Facilitates confirmation of true Schlemm's canal rather than false corneal or scleral passage	Excess force allows trabeculotome to rotate in incorrect plane into cornea or iris/ciliary body tissue
Gradually deepen radial scratch incision	TM is delicate and easy to tear through	Failure to facilitate aqueous outflow will prolong uncontrolled IOP
Rotate trabeculotome gently into anterior chamber	Consider converting to trabeculectomy if Schlemm's canal not found after several attempts	

intriguing, the early results of 360-degree trabeculotomy are similar to those reported for more conventional trabeculotomy procedures and are not without its own special complications.[97,98] The effects of the trabeculotomy should be determined 3 to 4 weeks after surgery, usually under anesthesia. Although a trabeculotomy may be repeated in a different portion of the angle, it may be reasonable to combine the second procedure with a trabeculectomy if no beneficial effect was noted following the first trabeculotomy. Key points in the surgical technique are listed in Table 68-12.

Combined Trabeculotomy-Trabeculectomy

If Schlemm's canal has not been successfully annulated and/or previous similar trabeculotomy procedures have failed to control IOP, the trabeculotomy can be combined with a trabeculectomy by removal of a full-thickness block of limbal tissue in the bed of the scleral flap, followed by peripheral iridectomy as in standard trabeculectomy. If conversion to trabeculectomy seems likely, one may apply an antimetabolite such as mitomycin C to the sclera at the site of intended scleral flap formation prior to dissection of the scleral flap (as described for adult trabeculectomy).[99-102] If mitomycin C has been applied, use of a rectangular partial-thickness scleral flap with a rather secure closure and a subsequent separate running closure of both Tenon's and conjunctival layers with 10-0 Dexon (Ethicon, Inc) or Vicryl is preferred. Postoperative care should be as for pediatric trabeculectomy in this case.

Goniotomy Versus Trabeculotomy

Each of these procedures has staunch advocates who espouse the advantages of one technique over the other. Reported success has been similarly high with both procedures in favorable cases of glaucoma (eg, previously unoperated eyes with PCG with onset postnatally, but before 1 year of life).[103,104] If the cornea is clear, goniotomy has certain advantages over trabeculotomy: there is no conjunctival scarring and the operating time is shorter with goniotomy than with trabeculotomy. On the other hand, the microsurgeon experienced in adult glaucoma surgery may find trabeculotomy a more familiar procedure than goniotomy.

Peripheral Iridectomy

Several types of pupillary block glaucoma occur in children. After cataract surgery, pupillary block glaucoma may respond to peripheral iridectomy (with or without anterior vitrectomy or synechialysis). Glaucoma associated with advanced cicatricial retinopathy of prematurity may similarly improve with iridectomy alone or coupled with lens removal. In these cases, peripheral iridectomy should proceed essentially as described for adults.[105-107]

Filtering Surgery

Filtering surgery is usually employed when goniotomy and/or trabeculotomy either fails or, as is the case in many secondary glaucomas, is very unlikely to succeed. Many such surgical procedures have been attempted over the years to treat children with glaucoma, including iridencleisis, cyclodiathermy, thermal sclerostomy (Scheie procedure), and standard trabeculectomy.[38,108-110] Success rates were usually poor. For example, Cadera and colleagues[108] reported a 52% success at IOP control (defined as IOP < 22 mm Hg) with thermal sclerostomy and trabeculectomy in a series of 24 children (average age 4 years) followed for several years. Similarly poor success with thermal sclerostomy (54% overall; 37% per surgery)[29,91] and with trabeculectomy (50%), respectively, and complications in 20% of trabeculectomies, including vitreous loss, scleral collapse, ectasia, retinal detachment, and endophthalmitis; no patients in this series achieved better than 20/200 vision have been reported.[29,91,105]

Many factors contributed to poor outcome from trabeculectomy in children, including lower scleral rigidity, more rapid healing and exuberant scarring processes, and enlargement of glaucomatous eyes with thinning and distortion of intraocular anatomy. In addition to these physiologic considerations, there are difficulties in postoperative management in children as well as visual loss from amblyopia even if glaucoma has been controlled. The use of intraoperative beta irradiation to the surgical site has improved the success of trabeculectomy. In a large retrospective series of 66 eyes[111] (in patients younger than 18 years of age with congenital glaucoma), IOP was controlled (IOP < 21 mm Hg) in approximately 40% of eyes after standard trabeculectomy compared with > 65% after irradiation-augmented trabeculectomy. No complications were attributed to the use of this low-dose beta irradiation.[111]

Subconjunctival 5-fluorouracil (5-FU) has been administered postoperatively in children after trabeculectomy, resulting in successful filtration, but its administration usually requires multiple sequential anesthesias and is limited by corneal epithelial toxicity, as in adults.[112,113]

More recently, the intraoperative use of mitomycin C has greatly enhanced the success of trabeculectomy in controlling glaucoma in adults at high risk for surgical failure, presumably by limiting postoperative scarring by Tenon's capsule and scleral fibroblasts.[114,115] Early results of mitomycin C-augmented trabeculectomy in children are somewhat encouraging. Using 0.5 mg/mL mitomycin C for 5 minutes without major complications, in one report, IOP was controlled (IOP < 21 mm Hg) in 8 of 10 eyes in a series of 8 patients with a mean age of 4 years and an average 14-month follow-up.[116]

Because of a high incidence of hypotony, a probe tip (a modified Hoskins lens [Ocular Instruments]) for the diode laser (Iris Medical [Iridex, Mountain View, CA]) that allows postoperative laser suture lysis of scleral flap sutures, with the patient supine, has been developed.[110-112] Suture lysis is performed within 1 week after surgery to titrate IOP during the early healing phase after trabeculectomy. A delay in suture lysis allows patients to recover fully from anesthesia, allows time to evaluate the eye's early response to the filtration surgery, and still seems effective in enhancing filtration in these patients. (The use of absorbable [eg, 10-0 Vicryl] or releasable sutures in the trabeculectomy flap might also encourage the success of trabeculectomy in children.)

The response of very young children to mitomycin C-augmented trabeculectomy is extremely variable with some patients scarring rapidly despite antifibrotic therapy, whereas others develop hypotony with large avascular filtration blebs.

In addition to postoperative laser suture lysis, postoperative subconjunctival 5-FU may be used after trabeculectomy with mitomycin C to further retard healing and enhance filtration. We have used subconjunctival 5-FU (5 mg) delivered in the quadrant adjacent to the bleb periodically every 1 to 2 weeks for up to 2 months after trabeculectomy with mitomycin C in selected infants at high risk for failure. The use of mitomycin C seems to prolong the postoperative period during which laser suture lysis and 5-FU may be effective in enhancing filtration.

Hypotony, flat anterior chamber, choroidal detachment, and crystalline lens opacification are the most common complications noted after trabeculectomy with mitomycin C in recent series.[49] In addition, we have encountered retinal and preretinal hemorrhages, which are sometimes impressive, after mitomycin C-augmented trabeculectomy in children. Similar, "decompression" hemorrhages have been reported after standard trabeculectomy in young patients[50] and they usually resolve spontaneously without serious sequelae.[114,115,117,118] The use of intraoperative topical mitomycin C during filtering surgery may improve the overall success of this type of surgery in difficult cases of childhood glaucoma. Nevertheless, the application of even small amounts of this potent alkylating agent to a child's eye raises the theoretical concern of long-term carcinogenicity (seen in rodents after systemic mitomycin C application). Because mitomycin C has been administered mainly in the palliative therapy of cancers, no data exist regarding the risk of secondary malignancy in people after exposure to systemic mitomycin C. However, the total amount of mitomycin C applied topically to the sclera and Tenon's capsule before irrigation does not usually exceed 40 to 60 jxg in most instances; this represents, at most, 0.3% of the chemotherapeutic dose (for a single cycle of therapy) for a 70-kg adult.[114,115,117,118] Evidence from trabeculectomy specimens further suggests at least a 48-fold dilution of mitomycin C concentration as it enters ocular tissue.[119]

Despite the absence of prospective data, it seems reasonable to extrapolate from the oncologic literature that the ophthalmic administration of mitomycin C poses a small risk of systemic toxicity, both acute and delayed. The small risk may be justified by intraoperative mitomycin's potential for helping to preserve visual function in difficult glaucomas. Because we do not know the long-term ocular sequelae of topical mitomycin C application to the sclera and Tenon's capsule of young children with glaucoma, caution is advised in repeating mitomycin C filters in children with glaucoma. One must weigh the potential and the as yet unknown long-term risks of mitomycin C against those of other alternative procedures.

Drainage Implant (Seton) Surgery

Despite improvements in trabeculectomy in children, this procedure still fails to control IOP in a number of difficult cases. Remaining surgical options include cyclodestructive and drainage implant (seton) procedures. Whereas the Molteno valve implant (Molteno Glaucoma Drainage Devices, Dunedin, New Zealand) has been used in children for more than a decade, early experience is now also available for several other setons, including the Baerveldt (Abbott Medical Optics) and Ahmed valves (New World Medical, Rancho Cucamonga, CA; Figures 68-36 through 68-39). Reported success and complication rates vary widely.[120-124]

Using a 2-stage single-plate Molteno implant procedure, Molteno and colleagues reported a 95% success rate (IOP <20 mm Hg), with a low complication rate (10%), in patients with advanced childhood glaucomas.[55] Several studies have exclusively included younger children, with a lower reported success of IOP control. Lloyd and colleagues achieved a 56% success rate after placement of 1 or 2 single-plate Molteno implants in 16 children under 13 years old; most of these patients required concurrent antiglaucoma medications.[56] Hill and colleagues[125] reported a 62% success (5< IOP >22 mm Hg) after a 2-stage 1- or 2-plate Molteno implant procedure in 70 eyes (patients younger than 21 years old) followed for at least 6 months; nonetheless, 83% of patients needed further glaucoma or other surgery and complications were common. In another relatively large group of 49 children younger than 12 years of age, others report a 68% success rate at IOP control using a single-plate Molteno implant in one stage.[120] In all of the aforementioned series, Molteno implants were used with ligation or other reversible partial blockade of the connecting tube if single-stage implantation was used. Some

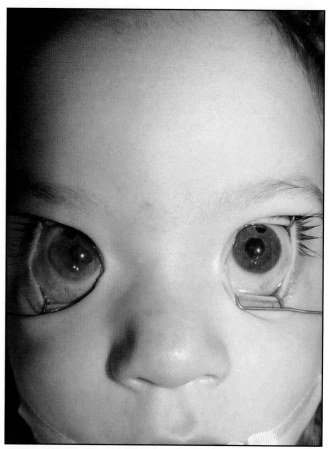

Figure 68-36. A child with bilateral trabeculodysgenesis, buphthalmos, and glaucoma, poorly controlled after 360 degrees of trabeculotomy in both eyes, who then had subsequent filtering procedures in both eyes with iridectomies. Both failed and were followed by bilateral tube placement. The child is now stable with the addition of topical medications.

surgeons placed the Molteno tube under a host partial-thickness trabeculectomy-type scleral flap, whereas more recently, many have favored using a full-thickness donor scleral graft.

Complications seen with Molteno implantation in children include not only those encountered after trabeculectomy, but also those specific to seton implantation. Most common among the latter in many series were contact between the tube and corneal endothelium (tube-cornea touch), erosion of the tube externally through the conjunctiva, migration of the tube, and cataract formation or progression. Interestingly, motility disturbances, reported in adults after seton surgery, have not yet been reported in children.[120]

In a report of Molteno and Baerveldt implants used to treat severe uncontrolled glaucoma in a series of 20 patients younger than 10 years, with a mean follow-up of 2 years, IOP control (IOP 21 mm Hg without further surgery) was achieved in 80%, although 75% of these controlled patients also required glaucoma medical treatment. In addition to complications found in other series, chronic inflammation was noted in 20% of cases. Similarly, high rates of success have been reported using the Baerveldt (86%)[63] and the Ahmed (85%) implants, respectively.[126]

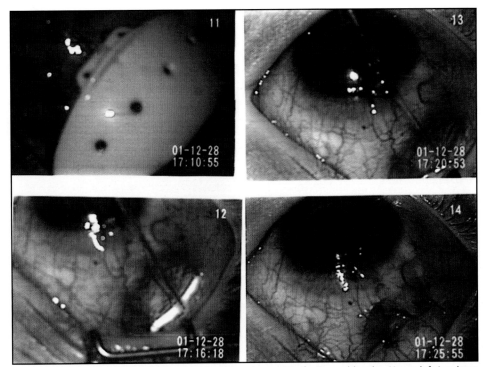

Figure 68-37. Intraoperative photomontage of the placement of a Baerveldt tube. Upper left is a large winged plate, upper right plate is placed 12 to 14 mm from the limbus and, the bottom left, secured with sutures through positioning holes and episclera. The bottom right tube is tied off with 6-0 Vicryl as posteriorly as possible on the tube prior to insertion in the anterior chamber to prevent hypotony.

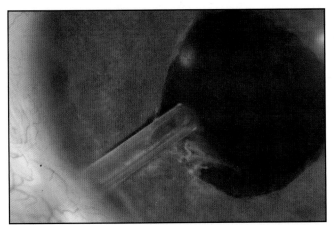

Figure 68-38. Anterior segment photograph of a Baerveldt tube in the anterior chamber. The length of this tube is about 2.0 to 2.5 mm too long and over the pupil causing optical distortion and shadowing on the retina.

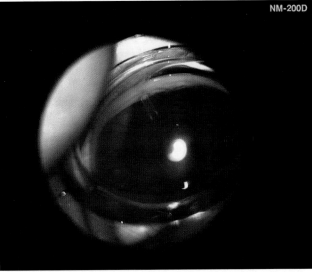

Figure 68-39. Gonioscopic photograph of a Baerveldt tube in the anterior chamber. Although the length of this tube is about 1.0 to 1.5 mm too long, it is well positioned away from the iris and cornea with an unobstructed opening.

Seton implantation can successfully control glaucoma in children, although many patients need postoperative glaucoma medications. Postoperative care of these patients is arduous, many complications occur, and long-term effects of drainage implants in the eyes of children are not yet known. Although many different seton designs and methods of implantation are available, published experience suggests that the Molteno, Baerveldt, and Ahmed implants can control IOP in children with difficult glaucomas (especially those with extensive scarring or in whom trabeculectomy has failed). The anticipated IOP decrement would be expected to increase with the surface area of the implant's reservoir. Hence, the single-plate Molteno (135 square mm), Ahmed (185 square mm), and smallest Baerveldt (200 square mm) implants should have intermediate IOP-lowering ability, whereas the double-plate Molteno and larger Baerveldt setons might be reserved best for cases with exceedingly high preoperative pressures. Ligation of the Molteno and Baerveldt tubes for one-stage implantation is recommended; the Ahmed valve may be used without ligation. In children with eyes scarred from previous surgeries, a fornix-based approach may be beneficial, securing the tube of the implant under a full-thickness donor scleral graft.

Combined Filtration and Cataract Surgery

Although surgery for cataract removal in the setting of severe or uncontrolled glaucoma is relatively frequent in adults, the analogous situation in children is fortunately very rare. Children who present with PCG usually have clear lenses, while those with congenital cataracts usually have normal IOP. Glaucoma most often arises in young children with cataracts a while after cataract surgery has been completed. Children do present with concurrent glaucoma and cataracts in the following unusual settings:

- With primary glaucoma and associated cataracts (ie, Lowe syndrome)

- With chronic uveitis and coexisting secondary glaucoma and cataract (ie, as seen in juvenile rheumatoid arthritis)

- In other unusual cases of secondary glaucoma and cataract (eg, post-traumatic or steroid-induced)

It is usually not recommended to combine cataract and glaucoma surgery in most children because of postoperative hypotony and ciliary body shutdown, secondary choroidal detachment, and subsequent bleb scarring and failure in these cases. In nonuveitic cases of cataract and glaucoma, it is generally recommended to do cataract surgery first with subsequent filtration, implant placement, or cyclodestructive procedures (the latter as a last resort). In the rare instance of an older child with cataract and a quiet eye, one might consider extracapsular cataract removal with preservation of the posterior capsule and concurrent filtration surgery (with a tightly sutured scleral flap). In patients with uveitic glaucoma and cataract in whom lensectomy and anterior or more extensive vitrectomy will be employed, a goniotomy (as the glaucoma procedure of choice) before cataract surgery may be the best sequence of procedures. Although goniotomy can be effective even in children with uveitis who are aphakic, postoperative hyphema may gain access to the vitreous cavity in aphakic but not phakic eyes. If angle surgery has failed, and filtration surgery is needed, removal of the cataract first, followed by glaucoma surgery as a second procedure (an adequate filtering bleb, arduous to achieve, may easily fail following cataract surgery), may be the best course of action (Figure 68-40).

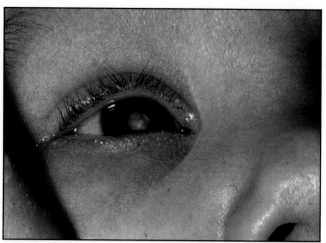

Figure 68-40. An infant with a unilateral congenital cataract prior to lensectomy and vitrectomy. These infants need to be followed for secondary glaucoma for a lifetime. This incidence of glaucoma in these patients has been reported to be as high as 30% over the course of their lives.

Cyclodestructive Procedures

The surgical procedures described in this chapter all share the goal of increasing facility of aqueous outflow from the eye, either through the angle structures or via a fistula or tube placed into the anterior chamber. In contrast, cyclodestructive procedures reduce the rate of aqueous production by injuring the ciliary processes; results are often unpredictable, and complications are frequent. Cyclodestruction nonetheless constitutes a valid means of attempting control of otherwise vision-threatening glaucoma in children, once medical and other surgical means have been exhausted or have proven inadequate to the task.[79,127]

Cyclocryotherapy ([CCT]; freezing the ciliary processes from an external approach) has been used as therapy for difficult childhood glaucomas for many years, and it is applied with a similar technique to that used in adults. Unfortunately, overall success (IOP control without severe visual loss or phthisis) has been fairly poor (30% in a large series of children with advanced congenital glaucoma).[79,127] In children, cryotherapy should be applied to a maximum of 180 degrees of the circumference of the eye at one session, using 6 or 7 freezes (60 s each at -80°C) with a 2.5-mm diameter cryoprobe centered about 2.5 mm from the limbus.[14] In retreatments, at least one quadrant of the ciliary body should be left untouched; no treatment is available if chronic postoperative hypotony or phthisis occurs.[14] Aside from the risks of hypotony or phthisis, uveitis, cataract formation, and attendant visual loss are the major problems with CCT.

Trans-scleral cyclophotocoagulation (CPC) with the neodymium:yttrium-aluminium-garnet (Nd:YAG) laser has recently reduced IOP in comparable fashion to CCT. With the continuous-wave Nd:YAG laser, successful IOP control ($3 < \text{IOP} < 19$ mm Hg) in 56% of adults with

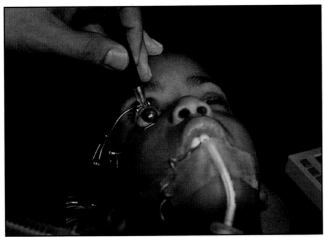

Figure 68-41. A child undergoing cyclodestruction with the contact diode laser.

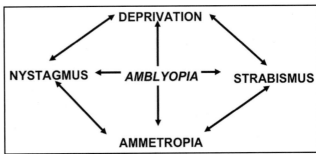

Figure 68-42. Dynamic processes involved in visual system development in infants and children that are associated with glaucoma and combine to determine the final visual outcome in most patients.

severe glaucoma after trans-scleral CPC[120,123]; phthisis or severe hypotony occurred in 10%. This procedure is performed using a spherical-tipped probe, placed with its anterior edge 0.5 to 1.5 mm from the limbus and perpendicular to the eye; 32 to 40 applications of 7 to 9 watts for 0.5 to 0.7 s are applied for 360 often sparing the 3- and 9-o'clock positions.

Early experience with Nd:YAG contact trans-scleral CPC in young children with advanced, uncontrolled glaucoma suggests effective IOP reduction in 50%, with a 70% retreatment rate. Significant advantages of Nd:YAG trans-scleral CPC over CCT in adults (and likely also in children) include fewer transient IOP rises, a less exuberant uveitic response, and less pain postoperatively. Similar complications have nonetheless been reported with both procedures.

The Iris Medical G-Probe can be used with the diode laser in performing trans-scleral CPC (Figure 68-41). This procedure seems comparable to the contact Nd:YAG technique for CPC in adults, with reported IOP reduction (>20% from baseline IOP) in 56% of subjects after 2 years. The technique in this series involved placement of 16 to 18 applications of 2 s each) to 3 quadrants with the Iris Medical G-probe, with variable power settings (mostly 1500 to 2000 mW). Using transillumination to guide diode trans-scleral CPC in 5 buphthalmic eyes, Lehmann and colleagues[110,117] reported at least a 25% IOP reduction in 4 of them after a minimum 6-month follow-up period.[69] Further experience with this therapy in children may prove it a worthy alternative to CCT and Nd:YAG CPC.

Long-Term Follow-Up of Children With Glaucoma

Even children whose glaucoma is well controlled after surgical therapy (with or without adjunctive medical therapy) deserve lifetime follow-up. Loss of IOP control may occur months or even decades after initial successful control

with surgery and may be asymptomatic in the older child/ young adult. In addition, young children with glaucoma often face vision-threatening difficulties, such as corneal scarring, anisometropia and resultant amblyopia, even after IOP control has been achieved (Figure 68-42). Children with glaucoma that is controlled without medications should be followed at least every 6 months, and young children, or those in whom IOP has been controlled for less than 2 years, should probably be evaluated at least every 3 or 4 months. During these office examinations, the correlates of adequate IOP control include the following:

- Stable visual function, refractive error, and optic nerve appearance

- Corneas that are free of edema and are stable in size

- Children who are free of epiphora, excessive photophobia, and blepharospasm

In contrast, even if the IOP is less than 20 mm Hg, deteriorating vision, progressive myopia, and optic nerve cupping, and/or increases in corneal size, edema, or ocular symptomatology suggest that control of glaucoma may be inadequate for the long-term.

Medical and surgical therapy for childhood glaucomas has challenged ophthalmologists for many years. Despite tremendous advances in medical, laser, and surgical technology over the past quarter century, we are still humbled by our inability to preserve sight in many children with glaucoma.

Prognosis

As a group, patients with PCG respond well to therapy with more than 80% achieving reasonable IOP control. The rate of success of control of IOP is related to the age of the patient at the initial diagnosis and surgery.[76,128-131] If glaucoma was present at birth, the cure rate is only 55%. If, however, it presents later during the third or fourth month, the long-term success rate increases to almost 100%. This favorable outlook continues for cases presenting within the first year of life. Lifetime surveillance is warranted even in children whose glaucoma is cured after surgery; at least 10% of them will demonstrate a later recurrence of

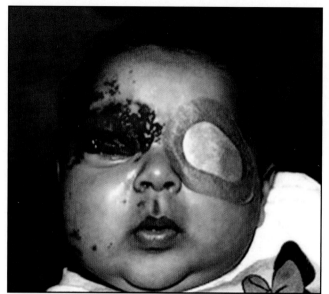

Figure 68-43. A child with severe hemangioma of the face. This is showing one of the most important treatments of visual system rehabilitation in infants and children—a patch over the preferred eye.

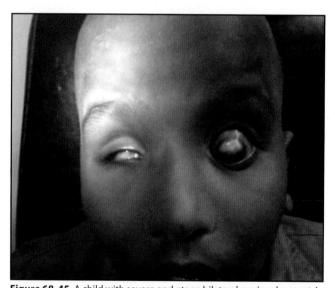

Figure 68-45. A child with severe end-stage bilateral eye involvement. In addition to the buphthalmos and cloudy corneas, this child had bilateral optic nerve hypoplasia, chorioretinal and iris coloboma, lenticulo-irido-trabeculo-corneo dysgenesis, micro cornea, cornea plana, and sclerocornea.

glaucoma.[76,128-131] The prognosis is poor for those who present after age 2 (Figures 68-43 through 68-45).

The cornea can clear remarkably in eyes in which IOPs have been normalized. The faster the IOP is controlled, the quicker the cornea will clear. Improved appearance, however, does not necessarily correlate with the return of normal vision. Optical irregularities because of breaks in Descemet's membrane or persistent stromal haze can have profound effects on visual development. The residual optical disturbance can often be appreciated on ophthalmoscopic and retinoscopic examination.

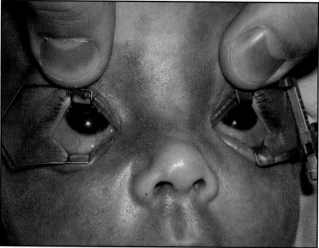

Figure 68-44. A child with Sturge-Weber hemangioma and bilateral glaucoma. In addition to the buphthalmos and cloudy corneas, one can see the conjunctival hyperemia due to a fine network of episcleral vessels that may interfere with all types of surgery on the eye.

Glaucomatous cupping of the optic nerve can decrease in size when IOP is reduced early in life. It is not uncommon to see a striking reduction in depth and diameter of the optic cup in the immediate postoperative period after IOP is reduced to normal. In some eyes, the optic nerve heads have returned to completely physiologic form. Atrophy, however, when present, has been irreversible. Myopia from enlargement of the globe usually is not reversible. One of the major causes of visual loss in unilateral glaucoma is the anisometropic amblyopia that results. This must be treated aggressively with frequent refractions and patching therapy to obtain the best visual outcome.[93,124,131-136]

ACKNOWLEDGMENTS

I acknowledge Drs. Sharon Freedman and Edward Buckley for their work on this chapter in earlier editions. Much of the text remains the same due to the diligence of these authors in updating their experience with this disease. Their previous work made the job of updating this chapter easy for me.

REFERENCES

1. Khandekar R, Al Awaidy S, Ganesh A, Bawikar S. An epidemiological and clinical study of ocular manifestations of congenital rubella syndrome in Omani children. *Arch Ophthalmol.* 2004;122: 541-545.
2. Haas J. Principles and problems of therapy in congenital glaucoma. *Invest Ophthalmol.* 1968;7:140-146.
3. Morin JD, Bryars JH. Causes of loss of vision in congenital glaucoma. *Arch Ophthalmol.* 1980;98:1575-1576.
4. Waring GO 3rd, Rodrigues MM, Laibson PR. Anterior chamber cleavage syndrome. A stepladder classification. *Surv Ophthalmol.* 1975;20:3-27.
5. Bordeianu CD. The pathogenic classification of glaucomas. *Oftalmologia.* 1992;36:331-342.

6. Chitsazian F, Tusi BK, Elahi E, et al. CYP1B1 mutation profile of Iranian primary congenital glaucoma patients and associated haplotypes. *J Mol Diagn.* 2007;9:382-393.

7. Goldberg I. Glaucoma—diagnostic hints. *Aust Fam Physician.* 1991;20:150-151, 154-162.

8. Beck AD. Diagnosis and management of pediatric glaucoma. *Ophthalmol Clin North Am.* 2001;14:501-512.

9. Consultation section. Cataract surgical problem. *J Cataract Refract Surg.* 2003;29:2261-2268.

10. Tabbara KF, Ross-Degnan D. Blindness in Saudi Arabia. *JAMA.* 1986;255:3378-3384.

11. Taylor RH, Ainsworth JR, Evans AR, Levin AV. The epidemiology of pediatric glaucoma: the Toronto experience. *J AAPOS.* 1999;3:308-315.

12. Kwitko ML. Congenital glaucoma. A clinical study. *Can J Ophthalmol.* 1967;2:91-102.

13. Wagner RS. Glaucoma in children. *Pediatr Clin North Am.* 1993;40:855-867.

14. Le Rebeller MJ, Lagoutte F. [Spontaneous resolution of a case of congenital glaucoma]. *Bull Soc Ophtalmol Fr.* 1975;75:555-559.

15. Nagao K. What's your diagnosis? Congenital glaucoma. *J Pediatr Ophthalmol Strabismus.* 2009;46:74, 82.

16. Worst JG. Congenital glaucoma. Remarks on the aspect of chamber angle, ontogenetic and pathogenetic background, and mode of action of goniotomy. *Invest Ophthalmol.* 1968;7:127-134.

17. Kupfer C, Ross K. The development of outflow facility in human eyes. *Invest Ophthalmol.* 1971;10:513-517.

18. Idrees F, Vaideanu D, Fraser SG, Sowden JC, Khaw PT. A review of anterior segment dysgeneses. *Surv Ophthalmol.* 2006;51:213-231.

19. Alward WL. Biomedicine. A new angle on ocular development. *Science.* 2003;299:1527-1528.

20. Townsend WM. Congenital corneal leukomas. 1. Central defect in Descemet's membrane. *Am J Ophthalmol.* 1974;77:80-86.

21. Quigley HA. Descemet's membrane ruptures. *Arch Ophthalmol.* 1982;100:844.

22. Sampaolesi R, Caruso R. Ocular echometry in the diagnosis of congenital glaucoma. *Arch Ophthalmol.* 1982;100:574-577.

23. Tarkkanen A, Uusitalo R, Mianowicz J. Ultrasonographic biometry in congenital glaucoma. *Acta Ophthalmol (Copenh).* 1983;61:618-623.

24. Gupta A, Kekunnaya R, Ramappa M, Vaddavalli PK. Safety profile of primary intraocular lens implantation in children below 2 years of age. *Br J Ophthalmol.* 2011;95:477-480.

25. Richardson KT, Shaffer RN. Optic-nerve cupping in congenital glaucoma. *Am J Ophthalmol.* 1966;62:507-509.

26. Busanyova B, Gerinec A. The problems of pediatric glaucoma. *Bratisl Lek Listy.* 2008;109:280.

27. Hetherington JN. Surgery for glaucoma in the young. *Trans Ophthalmol Soc N Z.* 1975;27:28-29.

28. Richardson KT. Optic cup symmetry in normal newborn infants. *Invest Ophthalmol.* 1968;7:137-140.

29. Wallace DK, Plager DA. Corneal diameter in childhood aphakic glaucoma. *J Pediatr Ophthalmol Strabismus.* 1996;33:230-234.

30. Lasseck J, Jehle T, Feltgen N, Lagreze WA. Comparison of intraocular tonometry using three different non-invasive tonometers in children. *Graefes Arch Clin Exp Ophthalmol.* 2008;246:1463-1466.

31. Martinez-de-la-Casa JM, Garcia-Feijoo J, Saenz-Frances F, et al. Comparison of rebound tonometer and Goldmann handheld applanation tonometer in congenital glaucoma. *J Glaucoma.* 2009;18:49-52.

32. Radtke ND, Cohan BE. Intraocular pressure measurement in the newborn. *Am J Ophthalmol.* 1974;78:501-504.

33. Bresson-Dumont H. [Intraocular pressure measurement in children]. *J Fr Ophtalmol.* 2009;32:176-181.

34. Wygnanski-Jaffe T, Barequet IS. Central corneal thickness in congenital glaucoma. *Cornea.* 2006;25:923-925.

35. Ausinsch B, Munson ES, Levy NS. Intraocular pressures in children with glaucoma during halothane anesthesia. *Ann Ophthalmol.* 1977;9:1391-1394.

36. Blumberg D, Congdon N, Jampel H, et al. The effects of sevoflurane and ketamine on intraocular pressure in children during examination under anesthesia. *Am J Ophthalmol.* 2007;143:494-499.

37. Cibis GW. Congenital glaucoma. *J Am Optom Assoc.* 1987;58:728-733.

38. Bussieres JF, Therrien R, Hamel P, Barret P, Prot-Labarthe S. Retrospective cohort study of 163 pediatric glaucoma patients. *Can J Ophthalmol.* 2009;44:323-327.

39. Reme C, d'Epinay SL. Periods of development of the normal human chamber angle. *Doc Ophthalmol.* 1981;51:241-268.

40. Fledelius HC, Christensen AC. Reappraisal of the human ocular growth curve in fetal life, infancy, and early childhood. *Br J Ophthalmol.* 1996;80:918-921.

41. Hess DB, Asrani SG, Bhide MG, Enyedi LB, Stinnett SS, Freedman SF. Macular and retinal nerve fiber layer analysis of normal and glaucomatous eyes in children using optical coherence tomography. *Am J Ophthalmol.* 2005;139:509-517.

42. Walton DS. Primary congenital open angle glaucoma: a study of the anterior segment abnormalities. *Trans Am Ophthalmol Soc.* 1979;77:746-768.

43. Spaeth GL. Congenital glaucoma. *Pediatrics.* 1991;88:1075-1076.

44. Sarfarazi M. Recent advances in molecular genetics of glaucomas. *Hum Mol Genet.* 1997;6:1667-1677.

45. Kotb AA, Hammouda EF, Tabbara KF. Childhood blindness at a school for the blind in Riyadh, Saudi Arabia. *Ophthalmic Epidemiol.* 2006;13:1-5.

46. Papadopoulos M, Cable N, Rahi J, Khaw PT. The British Infantile and Childhood Glaucoma (BIG) Eye Study. *Invest Ophthalmol Vis Sci.* 2007;48:4100-4106.

47. Qiao CY, Wang LH, Tang X, Wang T, Yang DY, Wang NL. Epidemiology of hospitalized pediatric glaucoma patients in Beijing Tongren Hospital. *Chin Med J (Engl).* 2009;122:1162-1166.

48. Weissschuh N, Schiefer U. Progress in the genetics of glaucoma. *Dev Ophthalmol.* 2003;37:83-93.

49. Vogt G, Horvath-Puho E, Czeizel AE. A population-based case-control study of isolated primary congenital glaucoma. *Am J Med Genet A.* 2006;140:1148-1155.

50. Gencik A. Epidemiology and genetics of primary congenital glaucoma in Slovakia. Description of a form of primary congenital glaucoma in gypsies with autosomal-recessive inheritance and complete penetrance. *Dev Ophthalmol.* 1989;16:76-115.

51. Jerndal T, Munkby M. Corticosteroid response in dominant congenital glaucoma. *Acta Ophthalmol (Copenh).* 1978;56:373-383.

52. Basdekidou C, Dureau P, Edelson C, De Laage De Meux P, Caputo G. Should unilateral congenital corneal opacities in Peters' anomaly be grafted? *Eur J Ophthalmol.* 2011;21:695-699.

53. Hafez M, Moustafa EE, Mokpel TH, Settein S, el-Serogy H. Evidence of HLA-linked susceptibility gene(s) in primary congenital glaucoma. *Dis Markers.* 1990;8:191-197.

54. Barkan O. Pathogenesis of congenital glaucoma: gonioscopic and anatomic observation of the angle of the anterior chamber in the normal eye and in congenital glaucoma. *Am J Ophthalmol.* 1955;40:1-11.

55. Worst JG. Pathogenesis and treatment of congenital glaucoma. *Ophthalmologica.* 1965;149:118-120.

56. Biglan AW. Glaucoma in children: are we making progress? *J AAPOS.* 2006;10:7-21.

57. Burian HM. Goniotomy and congenital glaucoma. *Am J Ophthalmol.* 1964;58:143-144.

58. Ozeki H, Shirai S, Majima A, Sano M, Ikeda K. Clinical evaluation of posterior embryotoxon in one institution. *Jpn J Ophthalmol.* 1997;41:422-425.

59. Langenberg T, Kahana A, Wszalek JA, Halloran MC. The eye organizes neural crest cell migration. *Dev Dyn.* 2008;237:1645-1652.

60. Anderson KL, Lewis RA, Bejjani BA, et al. A gene for primary congenital glaucoma is not linked to the locus on chromosome 1q for autosomal dominant juvenile-onset open angle glaucoma. *J Glaucoma.* 1996;5:416-421.

61. Maumenee AE. Further observations on the pathogenesis of congenital glaucoma. *Am J Ophthalmol.* 1963;55:1163-1176.

62. Shields MB. Axenfeld-Rieger syndrome: a theory of mechanism and distinctions from the iridocorneal endothelial syndrome. *Trans Am Ophthalmol Soc.* 1983;81:736-784.

63. Kupfer C, Kaiser-Kupfer MI. Observations on the development of the anterior chamber angle with reference to the pathogenesis of congenital glaucomas. *Am J Ophthalmol.* 1979;88:424-426.

64. Seidman DJ, Nelson LB, Calhoun JH, Spaeth GL, Harley RD. Signs and symptoms in the presentation of primary infantile glaucoma. *Pediatrics.* 1986;77:399-404.

65. Kraft SP, Judisch GF, Grayson DM. Megalocornea: a clinical and echographic study of an autosomal dominant pedigree. *J Pediatr Ophthalmol Strabismus.* 1984;21:190-193.

66. Rezende RA, Uchoa UB, Uchoa R, Rapuano CJ, Laibson PR, Cohen EJ. Congenital corneal opacities in a cornea referral practice. *Cornea.* 2004;23:565-570.

67. Chandler PA. Diagnosis and management of glaucoma. *Sight Sav Rev.* 1970;40:31-36.

68. Terraciano AJ, Sidoti PA. Management of refractory glaucoma in childhood. *Curr Opin Ophthalmol.* 2002;13:97-102.

69. Koraszewska-Matuszewska B. [Pharmacotherapy of congenital glaucoma in young children]. *Klin Oczna.* 1999;101:393-396.

70. Grigor'eva VN, Ustinova EI. [Our experience in the treatment of congenital glaucoma]. *Oftalmol Zh.* 1968;23:248-252.

71. Turach ME, Aktan G, Idil A. Medical and surgical aspects of congenital glaucoma. *Acta Ophthalmol Scand.* 1995;73:261-263.

72. Barkan O. Technic of goniotomy for congenital glaucoma. *Arch Ophthalmol.* 1949;41:65-82.

73. Kulkarni SV, Damji KF, Fournier AV, Pan I, Hodge WG. Endoscopic goniotomy: early clinical experience in congenital glaucoma. *J Glaucoma.* 2010;19:264-269.

74. Heimann K, Peschgens T, Merz U, Hoernchen H, Wenzl T. [Depression of respiration via toxic effects on the central nervous system following use of topical brimonidine in an infant with congenital glaucoma]. *Ophthalmologe.* 2007;104:505-507.

75. Scheie HG. Goniotomy in treatment of congenital glaucoma. *Arch Ophthalmol.* 1949;42:266-282.

76. Shaffer RN. Prognosis of goniotomy in primary infantile glaucoma (trabeculodysgenesis). *Trans Am Ophthalmol Soc.* 1982;80:321-325.

77. Murthy KR. Irrigating needle goniotomy. *Indian J Ophthalmol.* 1987;35:271-273.

78. Arnoult JB, Vila-Coro AA, Mazow ML. Goniotomy with sodium hyaluronate. *J Pediatr Ophthalmol Strabismus.* 1988;25:18-22.

79. Fu P, Yang L, Bo SY, Na X. A national survey on low vision and blindness of 0 - 6 years old children in China [in Chinese]. *Zhonghua Yi Xue Za Zhi.* 2004;84:1545-1548.

80. Alsheikheh A, Klink J, Klink T, Steffen H, Grehn F. Long-term results of surgery in childhood glaucoma. *Graefes Arch Clin Exp Ophthalmol.* 2007;245:195-203.

81. Blake EM. The surgical treatment of glaucoma complicating congenital aniridia. *Trans Am Ophthalmol Soc.* 1952;50:47-53.

82. Ch'ng S, Tan ST. Facial port-wine stains—clinical stratification and risks of neuro-ocular involvement. *J Plast Reconstr Aesthet Surg.* 2008;61:889-893.

83. Moreker M, Parikh R, Parikh SR, Thomas R. Aniridia associated with congenital aphakia and secondary glaucoma. *Indian J Ophthalmol.* 2009;57:313-314.

84. Tamcelik N, Ozkiris A. A comparison of viscogoniotomy with classical goniotomy in Turkish patients. *Jpn J Ophthalmol.* 2004;48:404-407.

85. Wheeler DT, Stager DR, Weakley DR Jr. Endophthalmitis following pediatric intraocular surgery for congenital cataracts and congenital glaucoma. *J Pediatr Ophthalmol Strabismus.* 1992;29:139-141.

86. Litinsky SM, Shaffer RN, Hetherington J, Hoskins HD. Operative complications of goniotomy. *Trans Sect Ophthalmol Am Acad Ophthalmol Otolaryngol.* 1977;83:78-79.

87. Yumita A, Shirato S, Yamamoto T, Kitazawa Y. Goniotomy with Q-switched Nd-YAG laser in juvenile developmental glaucoma: a preliminary report. *Jpn J Ophthalmol.* 1984;28:349-355.

88. Epstein DL, Melamed S, Puliafto CA, Steinert RF. Neodymium:YAG laser trabeculopuncture in open-angle glaucoma. *Ophthalmology.* 1985;92:931-937.

89. Bayraktar S, Koseoglu T. Endoscopic goniotomy with anterior chamber maintainer: surgical technique and one-year results. *Ophthalmic Surg Lasers.* 2001;32:496-502.

90. Harms H, Dannheim R. Trabeculotomy—results and problems. *Bibl Ophthalmol.* 1970;81:121-131.

91. McPherson SD Jr. Results of external trabeculotomy. *Am J Ophthalmol.* 1973;76:918-920.

92. Aldave AJ, Yellore VS, Vo RC, et al. Exclusion of positional candidate gene coding region mutations in the common posterior polymorphous corneal dystrophy 1 candidate gene interval. *Cornea.* 2009;28:801-807.

93. Yang M, Guo X, Liu X, et al. Investigation of CYP1B1 mutations in Chinese patients with primary congenital glaucoma. *Mol Vis.* 2009;15:432-437.

94. Akimoto M, Tanihara H, Negi A, Nagata M. Surgical results of trabeculotomy ab externo for developmental glaucoma. *Arch Ophthalmol.* 1994;112:1540-1544.

95. McPherson SD Jr, McFarland D. External trabeculotomy for developmental glaucoma. *Ophthalmology.* 1980;87:302-305.

96. McPherson SD Jr, Berry DP. Goniotomy vs external trabeculotomy for developmental glaucoma. *Am J Ophthalmol.* 1983;95:427-431.

97. Beck AD, Lynch MG. 360 degrees trabeculotomy for primary congenital glaucoma. *Arch Ophthalmol.* 1995;113:1200-1202.

98. Verner-Cole EA, Ortiz S, Bell NP, Feldman RM. Subretinal suture misdirection during 360 degrees suture trabeculotomy. *Am J Ophthalmol.* 2006;141:391-392.

99. Colev G, Calin A, Ciglinian R. Trabeculectomy and trabeculotomy in the treatment of infantile glaucoma [in Romanian]. *Rev Chir Oncol Radiol O R L Oftalmol Stomatol Ser Oftalmol.* 1977;21:139-141.

100. Luntz MH, Livingston DG. Trabeculotomy ab externo and trabeculectomy in congenital and adult-onset glaucoma. *Am J Ophthalmol.* 1977;83:174-179.

101. Luntz MH. Trabeculotomy-trabeculectomy for early-onset glaucoma. *Ophthalmology.* 2000;107:624-625.

102. Sidoti PA, Belmonte SJ, Liebmann JM, Ritch R. Trabeculectomy with mitomycin-C in the treatment of pediatric glaucomas. *Ophthalmology.* 2000;107:422-429.

103. Anderson DP, Khalil M, Lorenzetti DW, Saheb NE. Abnormal blood vessels on the optic disc. *Can J Ophthalmol.* 1983;18:108-114.

104. Luntz MH. The choice of surgical procedure in congenital, infantile, and juvenile glaucoma. *Todays OR Nurse.* 1991;13:25-26.

105. Scheie HG. Results of peripheral iridectomy with scleral cautery in congenital and juvenile glaucoma. *Trans Am Ophthalmol Soc.* 1962;60:116-139.

106. Mizuno K, Fukuyo T. AB interno iridectomy combined with pars plicata lensectomy. *Jpn J Ophthalmol.* 1984;28:416-420.

107. Medow N, Crouch E, Wilson R. Pediatric aphakic glaucoma. *J Pediatr Ophthalmol Strabismus.* 2004;41:5-9.

108. Cadera W, Pachtman MA, Cantor LB, Ellis FD, Helveston EM. Filtering surgery in childhood glaucoma. *Ophthalmic Surg.* 1984;15:319-322.

109. Bhola R, Keech RV, Olson RJ, Petersen DB. Long-term outcome of pediatric aphakic glaucoma. *J AAPOS.* 2006;10:243-248.

110. Tanimoto SA, Brandt JD. Options in pediatric glaucoma after angle surgery has failed. *Curr Opin Ophthalmol.* 2006;17:132-137.

111. Miller MH, Rice NS. Trabeculectomy combined with beta irradiation for congenital glaucoma. *Br J Ophthalmol.* 1991;75:584-590.

112. Zalish M, Leiba H, Oliver M. Subconjunctival injection of 5-fluorouracil following trabeculectomy for congenital and infantile glaucoma. *Ophthalmic Surg.* 1992;23:203-205.

113. Al-Mobarak F, Khan AO. Complications and 2-year valve survival following Ahmed valve implantation during the first 2 years of life. *Br J Ophthalmol.* 2009;93:795-798.

114. Snir M, Lusky M, Shalev B, Gaton D, Weinberger D. Mitomycin C and 5-fluorouracil antimetabolite therapy for pediatric glaucoma filtration surgery. *Ophthalmic Surg Lasers.* 2000;31:31-37.

115. Chakrabarti S, Komatireddy S, Mandal AK, Balasubramanian D. Gene symbol: CYP1B1. Disease: glaucoma, primary congenital. *Hum Genet.* 2003;113:556.

116. Meyer G, Schwenn O, Pfeiffer N, Grehn F. Trabeculotomy in congenital glaucoma. *Graefes Arch Clin Exp Ophthalmol.* 2000;238:207-213.

117. Agarwal HC, Sood NN, Sihota R, Sanga L, Honavar SG. Mitomycin-C in congenital glaucoma. *Ophthalmic Surg Lasers.* 1997;28:979-985.

118. al-Hazmi A, Zwaan J, Awad A, al-Mesfer S, Mullaney PB, Wheeler DT. Effectiveness and complications of mitomycin C use during pediatric glaucoma surgery. *Ophthalmology.* 1998;105:1915-1920.

119. Sarfarazi M, Akarsu AN, Hossain A, et al. Assignment of a locus (GLC3A) for primary congenital glaucoma (Buphthalmos) to 2p21 and evidence for genetic heterogeneity. *Genomics.* 1995;30:171-177.

120. Freedman J, Rubin B. Molteno implants as a treatment for refractory glaucoma in black patients. *Arch Ophthalmol.* 1991;109:1417-1420.

121. Cunliffe IA, Molteno AC. Long-term follow-up of Molteno drains used in the treatment of glaucoma presenting in childhood. *Eye (Lond).* 1998;12(pt 3a):379-385.

122. Brandt JD, Casuso LA, Budenz DL. Markedly increased central corneal thickness: an unrecognized finding in congenital aniridia. *Am J Ophthalmol.* 2004;137:348-350.

123. Al-Mobarak F, Khan AO. Two-year survival of Ahmed valve implantation in the first 2 years of life with and without intraoperative mitomycin-C. *Ophthalmology.* 2009;116:1862-1865.

124. Naked in front of the eyedoctor: life through the eyes of a glaucoma patient. *Bull Soc Belge Ophtalmol.* 2009:55-58; discussion 53.

125. Hill R, Ohanesian R, Voskanyan L, Malayan A. The Armenian Eye Care Project: surgical outcomes of complicated paediatric glaucoma. *Br J Ophthalmol.* 2003;87:673-676.

126. Mandal AK, Bhatia PG, Bhaskar A, Nutheti R. Long-term surgical and visual outcomes in Indian children with developmental glaucoma operated on within 6 months of birth. *Ophthalmology.* 2004;111:283-290.

127. Langseth FG. Transscleral cyclophotocoagulation. A laser treatment for glaucoma. *AORN J.* 1988;48:1122-1125, 1127.

128. Lister A. Congenital glaucoma [in Polish]. *Klin Oczna.* 1966;36:517-526.

129. Chew E, Morin JD. Glaucoma in children. *Pediatr Clin North Am.* 1983;30:1043-1060.

130. Cronemberger S, Lourenco LF, Silva LC, Calixto N, Pires MC. Prognosis of glaucoma in relation to blindness at a university hospital. *Arq Bras Oftalmol.* 2009;72:199-204.

131. Tourame B, Ben Younes N, Guigou S, Denis D. Congenital glaucoma: future of vision and pressure. Results of an 11-year study [in French]. *J Fr Ophtalmol.* 2009;32:335-340.

132. Kargi SH, Koc F, Biglan AW, Davis JS. Visual acuity in children with glaucoma. *Ophthalmology.* 2006;113:229-238.

133. Kirwan C, O'Keefe M. Paediatric aphakic glaucoma. *Acta Ophthalmol Scand.* 2006;84:734-739.

134. Robaei D, Huynh SC, Kifley A, Mitchell P. Correctable and noncorrectable visual impairment in a population-based sample of 12-year-old Australian children. *Am J Ophthalmol.* 2006;142:112-118.

135. O'Malley Schotthoefer E, Yanovitch TL, Freedman SF. Aqueous drainage device surgery in refractory pediatric glaucoma: II. Ocular motility consequences. *J AAPOS.* 2008;12:40-45.

136. Haddad MA, Sampaio MW, Oltrogge EW, Kara-Jose N, Betinjane AJ. Visual impairment secondary to congenital glaucoma in children: visual responses, optical correction and use of low vision AIDS. *Clinics (Sao Paulo).* 2009;64:725-730.

69

Unusual Pediatric Glaucomas

Vicki M. Chen, MD and David S. Walton, MD

In this section, primary childhood glaucoma associated with systemic or ocular abnormalities will be described. See Table 69-1 for a complete listing of these types of childhood glaucoma.

PRIMARY GLAUCOMAS ASSOCIATED WITH SYSTEMIC DISEASES

Primary infantile glaucoma is associated with an astounding number of diverse systemic conditions (Table 69-1). While glaucoma associated with nevus flammeus is relatively common, each of the other listed causes is quite uncommon. Some conditions are nonhereditary (eg, rubella syndrome and fetal alcohol syndrome), while others clearly are hereditary (eg, Lowe syndrome, hepatocerebral renal syndrome, and neurofibromatosis).

Congenital Rubella Syndrome

The well-known diverse ocular complications of the maternal rubella syndrome may occur in up to 50% of neonates born to mothers infected during the first trimester.[1,2] Ophthalmic findings include pigmentary retinopathy (25% to 40%), cataracts (14% to 30%), microphthalmia (10%), optic nerve atrophy (10%), keratitis or corneal haze (8%).[1,3-6] Infantile glaucoma is probably the least common of these secondary ocular anomalies, occurring in an estimated 5% to 10% of affected children.[3,6]

Congenital rubella infantile glaucoma is often detected in infancy secondary to corneal opacification and is usually bilateral (Figures 69-1A and B).[7] It must be differentiated from permanent rubella leucomas and transient corneal opacification seen in some infants. In addition to corneal haze and enlargement, these children often possess diaphanous hypoplastic irides, along with other aforementioned ocular findings (Figure 69-1C). Glaucoma may also present

later in life, particularly in microphthalmic patients; therefore continued vigilance is necessary.[6] Gonioscopy of children with rubella glaucoma reveals abnormalities similar to that seen in hereditary infantile glaucoma, with an anterior iris insertion, pigmentary changes, and increased opacification of the inner tissue of the filtration angle making visualization of the scleral spur and ciliary body very difficult.[3]

Treatment of this glaucoma by goniosurgery is often successful at all ages, providing an additional similarity to hereditary infantile glaucoma.

Nevus Flammeus of the Eyelids With Glaucoma

Nevus flammeus of the face is a well-known component of Sturge-Weber syndrome, Klippel-Trenaunay-Weber syndrome, and cutis marmorata telangiectasia congenita (see Chapter 49). In Sturge-Weber syndrome, glaucoma is associated with a facial nevus flammeus and a leptomeningeal vascular defect. Usually, a side of the face is affected (68% to 78%),[8,9] but bilateral involvement also occurs (Figure 69-2A). When the facial nevus is bilateral, glaucoma also is often bilateral. With intracranial involvement, seizures, hemiparesis, and hemianopsia may occur. Children without intracranial involvement, observed to have nevus flammeus not involving the upper eyelid, seem to be at no risk for glaucoma.[10,11] On examination, it is appropriate to remember the neural crest origin of components of the vascular system, meninges, pigmentation tissues, trabecular meshwork (TM), iris, as well as other tissues.

The glaucoma complicating these vascular diseases is usually of early onset and may often be congenital. In the absence of early intraocular pressure (IOP) measurements, enlargement of the cornea and globe indicates the presence of glaucoma during the first 2 to 3 years of life. Because of frequent unilateral involvement, the examiner should take

Kahook MY, Schuman JS, eds.
Chandler and Grant's Glaucoma, Fifth Edition (pp 661-679).
© 2013 SLACK Incorporated.

TABLE 69-1. THE CHILDHOOD GLAUCOMAS

I. Primary (developmental) glaucomas

  A. Primary congenital glaucoma (PCG)

    1. Newborn PCG

    2. Infantile PCG

    3. Late-recognized PCG

  B. Juvenile open-angle glaucoma (JOAG)

  C. Primary angle-closure glaucoma (PACG)

  D. Primary glaucomas associated with systemic diseases

    1. Sturge-Weber syndrome

    2. Neurofibromatosis (NF-1)

    3. Stickler syndrome

    4. Oculocerebrorenal syndrome (Lowe)

    5. Rieger syndrome

    6. SHORT syndrome

    7. Hepatocerebrorenal syndrome (Zellweger)

    8. Marfan syndrome

    9. Rubinstein-Taybi syndrome

    10. Infantile glaucoma with retardation and paralysis

    11. Oculodentodigital dysplasia

    12. Glaucoma with microcornea and absent sinuses

    13. Mucopolysaccharidosis

    14. Trisomy 13

    15. Caudal regression syndrome

    16. Trisomy 21 (Down syndrome)

    17. Cutis marmorata telangiectatica congenita

    18. Walker-Warburg syndrome

    19. Kniest syndrome (skeletal dysplasia)

    20. Michels syndrome

    21. Nonprogressive hemiatrophy

    22. PHACE syndrome

    23. Soto syndrome

    24. Linear scleroderma

    25. GAPO syndrome

    26. Roberts' pseudothalidomide syndrome

    27. Wolf-Hirschhorn (4p-) syndrome

    28. Robinow syndrome

    29. Nail-Patella syndrome

    30. Proteus syndrome

    31. Fetal hydantoin syndrome

    32. Cranio-cerebello-cardiac (3C) syndrome

    33. Brachmann-de Lange syndrome

    34. Rothmund-Thomson syndrome

    35. 9p deletion syndrome

    36. Phakomatosis pigmentovascularis (PPV)

    37. Nevoid basal cell carcinoma syndrome (Gorlin syndrome)

    38. Epidermal nevus syndrome (Solomon syndrome)

    39. Androgen insensitivity, pyloric stenosis

    40. Diabetes mellitus, polycystic kidneys, hepatic fibrosis, hypothyroidism

    41. Diamond-Blackfan syndrome

  E. Primary glaucomas with profound ocular anomalies

    1. Aniridia

      a. Congenital aniridic glaucoma

      b. Acquired aniridic glaucoma

    2. Congenital ocular melanosis

    3. Sclerocornea

    4. Congenital iris ectropion syndrome

    5. Peters anomaly syndrome

    6. Iridotrabecular dysgenesis (iris hypoplasia)

    7. Posterior polymorphous dystrophy

    8. Idiopathic or familial elevated venous pressure

    9. Congenital anterior (corneal) staphyloma

    10. Congenital microcoria

    11. Congenital hereditary endothelial dystrophy

    12. Axenfeld-Rieger anomaly

(continued)

TABLE 69-1. THE CHILDHOOD GLAUCOMAS (CONTINUED)

II. Secondary (acquired) glaucomas

  A. Traumatic glaucoma

    1. Acute glaucoma

      a. Hyphema

      b. Ghost cell glaucoma

    2. Glaucoma related to angle recession

    3. Arteriovenous fistula

  B. Glaucoma with intraocular neoplasms

    1. Retinoblastoma

    2. Juvenile xanthogranuloma (JXG)

    3. Leukemia

    4. Melanoma of ciliary body

    5. Melanocytoma

    6. Iris rhabdomyosarcoma

    7. Aggressive iris nevi

    8. Medulloepithelioma

    9. Mucogenic glaucoma with iris stromal cyst

  C. Glaucoma related to chronic uveitis

    1. Open-angle glaucoma

    2. Angle-blockage mechanisms

      a. Synechial angle closure

      b. Iris bombé with pupillary block

      c. TM endothelialization

  D. Lens-related glaucoma

    1. Subluxation-dislocation with pupillary block

      a. Marfan syndrome

      b. Homocystinuria

      c. Weill-Marchesani syndrome

      d. Axial-subluxation high myopia syndrome

      e. Ectopia lentis et pupillae

      f. Spherophakia

    2. Phacolytic glaucoma

  E. Glaucoma following lensectomy for congenital cataracts

    1. Pupillary-block glaucoma

    2. Infantile aphakic open angle glaucoma

  F. Glaucoma related to corticosteroids

  G. Glaucoma secondary to rubeosis

    1. Retinoblastoma

    2. Coats' disease

    3. Medulloepithelioma

    4. Familial exudative vitreoretinopathy

    5. Subacute/chronic retinal detachment

    6. Retinopathy of prematurity (ROP)

  H. Angle-closure glaucoma

    1. Retinopathy of prematurity

    2. Microphthalmos

    3. Nanophthalmos

    4. Retinoblastoma

    5. Persistent hyperplastic primary vitreous

    6. Congenital pupillary iris-lens membrane

    7. Topiramate therapy

    8. Central retinal vein occlusion

    9. Ciliary body cysts

  I. Malignant glaucoma

  J. Glaucoma associated with increased venous pressure

    1. Sturge-Weber syndrome

  K. Intraocular infection-related glaucoma

    1. Acute recurrent toxoplasmosis

    2. Acute herpetic iritis

    3. Maternal rubella infection

    4. Endogenous endophthalmitis

  L. Glaucoma secondary to unknown etiology

    1. Iridocorneal endothelial syndrome (ICE)

GAPO: growth retardation, alopecia, pseudoanodontia (failture of tooth eruption), and progressive optic atrophy; PHACE: posterior fossa brain malformations, hemangiomas of the face (large or complex), arterial anomalies, cardiac anomalies, and eye abnormalities; SHORT: short suture, hyperextensibility of joints or hernia (inguinal) or both, ocular depression, Rieger anomaly, teething decay. Reprinted with permission from Yeung H, Walton DS. Clinical classification of childhood glaucomas. *Arch Ophthalmol.* 2010;128(6):680-684.

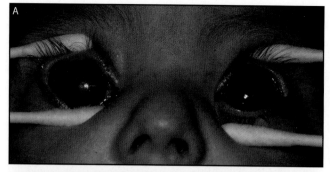

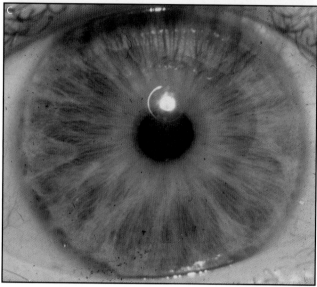

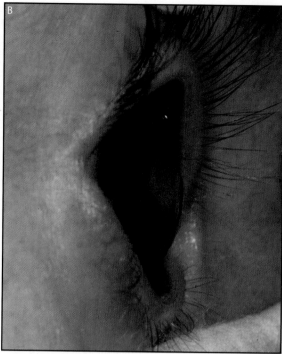

Figure 69-1. (A) Bilateral corneal haze, dense centrally. (B) Sagittal view demonstrating keratopathy involving peripheral cornea. (C) The iris stroma of a 9-year-old girl with rubella glaucoma was porous and associated with a granular transillumination.

advantage of the opportunity to compare IOP in affected and unaffected eyes, as symmetry is often marked.[12]

Children seen with this type of glaucoma usually have moderately advanced glaucoma associated with decreased visual acuity, anisometropia, and disc abnormalities. The bulbar conjunctiva usually shows fine tortuous vessels. The episclera will show a more uniform grid of permanent vessels, abnormal by their number and size. The cornea is usually enlarged, but breaks in Descemet's membrane (Haab's striae) are infrequent. The anterior chamber is usually deep. The iris of the involved eye possesses a more compact and often more pigmented than seen in the contralateral normal eye. With bilateral occurrence, the presence of bilateral iridal melanosis is less obvious than the heterochromia seen in unilateral cases. The lenses are clear. The fundi often appear diffusely red, suggesting the presence of an associated capillary hemangioma. Vascular anomalies can be demonstrated on fluorescein angiography. Ultrasonography for choroidal thickness will show thickening of the choroid in the presence of a typical choroidal hemangioma in this condition. Blood vessel abnormalities of retinal vessels are not seen. If the IOP is excessive, glaucomatous cupping and atrophy develop, as in other glaucomas.

In 32 patients having nevus flammeus of the upper lid with glaucoma in whom we have performed gonioscopy, all have had open angles and have had little in the angle to suggest a vascular abnormality. In general, when the glaucomatous eyes were compared with the contralateral normal eyes, except for peculiarities of Schlemm's canal, the principal recognizable abnormality was similar to that which we believe is characteristic of ordinary congenital open-angle glaucoma. The iris was commonly attached farther forward in glaucomatous eyes than in normal eyes, but never hiding the scleral spur, and the level of attachment of the iris was variable, causing the insertion of the iris to appear wavy as one scanned circumferentially.

When blood has refluxed into Schlemm's canal during gonioscopy in some eyes having glaucoma with hemangioma, we have had the impression that the distribution in Schlemm's canal has been abnormal and different from the ordinary congenital open-angle glaucoma (Figure 69-2B). In some eyes, no distinct line of blood, but only a diffuse reddish glow, was seen deep in the corneoscleral meshwork. In eyes in which the blood in Schlemm's canal could be seen in more distinct lines, Schlemm's canal appeared to wander at a varying distance anterior to the scleral spur or to be broken up into multiple channels.

Measurements of episcleral venous pressure vessels in hemangioma of the lid with glaucoma show 2 categories of patients. One type has inconspicuous vessels on the globe with normal pressure. The other type has elevated episcleral venous pressure and the vessels appear abnormally prominent. According to tonography, there is obstruction to aqueous outflow in both types.

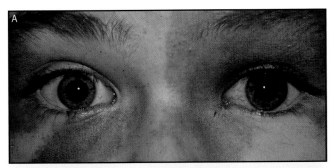

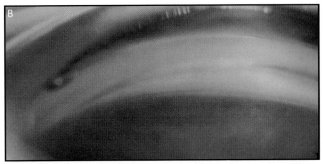

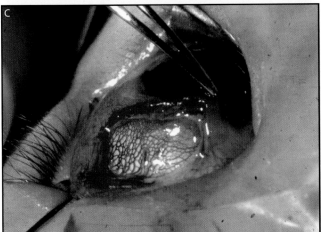

Figure 69-2. (A) Sturge-Weber syndrome. Heterochromia OS with tortuous conjunctival vessels and diffuse eyelid involvement. (B) Reflux of blood into Schlemm's canal, line is irregular, observe reddish hue of corneoscleral TM suggestive of abnormal vasculature. (C) Note diffuse anastomotic episcleral blood vessels seen at surgery.

A noteworthy peculiarity about the IOP in this condition is that, when the patient changes from sitting to recumbent position, the IOP undergoes a greater change than in other types of glaucoma or in normal eyes. When the patient lies down, the IOP in the eye affected by hemangioma may increase by several mm Hg. However, if the patient remains in the recumbent position, the IOP drops again in 15 to 30 minutes, approaching what it was in the sitting position. Presumably, the rise in IOP is due to a rapid distention of an intraocular hemangioma, probably in the choroid, after which the eye gradually returns to its steady-state IOP as a result of slow expulsion of an equal and compensatory volume of aqueous humor. When the eye is in a steady state, tonography indicates abnormal resistance to aqueous outflow to be responsible for the glaucoma.

Glaucoma treatment should first be medical therapy, especially in young children who might be expected to have fewer good results with filtration surgery. Beta-blockers, miotics, and carbonic anhydrase inhibitors (CAIs) are frequently helpful. If medical control proves inadequate, then surgery must be attempted. Goniotomies performed during childhood in 6 patients by us have been uncomplicated, but even multiple goniotomies have proven unsuccessful in controlling this type of glaucoma. Filtration surgery, in light of the poor results that can be expected with a goniotomy procedure, must be considered in the presence of uncontrolled glaucoma in these patients, and filtration surgery is sometimes successful. Trabeculectomy with use of intraoperative mitomycin C is the treatment of choice. Reasonably tight closure of the

scleral flap with or without releasable sutures is appropriate, given the risk for rapid operative or postoperative uveal effusions.[13] Consideration should be given to performing sclerotomy over the ciliary body at the time of surgery to allow immediate and postoperative choroidal drainage. The trabeculectomy surgeon will be impressed with the dense grid of episcleral vessels present at the flap and sclerostomy site (Figure 69-2C). These can be managed well with an underwater diathermy tip. Five patients under the age of 9 years with glaucoma associated with a nevus flammeus and who required trabeculectomy surgery with adjunctive use of mitomycin-C, successful control of the glaucoma was achieved without medication in each of these patients.[14]

Our experience with cycloablative procedures, usually cyclocryotherapy, in a few patients suggests that it can also be helpful and that it is not more problematic in this glaucoma than in other types of glaucoma.

Iridocorneal Goniodysgenesis With Glaucoma

Under iridocorneal goniodysgenesis, we include all congenital ocular abnormalities that tend to combine malformations of the cornea, iris, and filtration angle. The abnormality may be predominantly corneal (as in embryotoxon) or may involve both cornea and iris (Axenfeld's anomaly and Peters' anomaly). In Rieger's anomaly, the angle is involved, as well as the cornea and iris, and glaucoma is more likely. This eye condition can be associated with systemic abnormalities, including abnormalities of the teeth (hypodontia, microdontia, oligodontia), mid-face (hypertelorism, maxillary hypoplasia), pituitary (empty sella syndrome, isolated growth hormone deficiency, parasellar arachnoid cyst), cardiovascular system (atrial septal defect), genitalia (hypospadia, anal stenosis), and excessive periumbilical skin (Rieger's syndrome).[15]

Axenfeld-Rieger syndrome is frequently transmitted as a heterogeneous autosomal dominant disorder. Recent cytogenetic studies have found an array of genetic defects in families with Axenfeld-Rieger syndrome, including deletions of 4q25 (Rieger syndrome type 1 or RIEG1), 13q14 (Rieger syndrome type 2 or RIEG2), 6p25 (FOXC1), and possibly 16q24. The region coding for RIEG1, also known as PITX2, is a type of homeobox transcription gene with widespread multisystem involvement during embryologic development.[15-17] The loss of this gene may help to explain the diversity of anomalies associated with Axenfeld-Rieger syndrome.

Whether or not glaucoma develops in an eye with typical iridocorneal goniodysgenesis depends upon the degree of obstruction of outflow of aqueous humor, either by iridocorneal tissue overlying the TM or apparently in certain cases by abnormalities in the outflow channels themselves (Figure 69-3). The conspicuous processes seen bridging the filtration angle face do not seem to contribute to the obstruction to outflow of aqueous humor. As expected, goniotomy surgery, which strips these processes, frequently does not treat the complicating glaucoma successfully.

For discussion, we have divided cases of iridocorneal dysgenesis into 3 groups, representing different degrees of severity. In actuality, these conditions in the various categories probably are related in some instances. For example, we know that separating cases according to whether or not the pupil is involved is artificial because, in 2 families, we have seen pairs of individuals (mother and son, and a pair of sisters) with iridocorneal dysgenesis with glaucoma, but with the pupils normal in one and abnormal in the other member of each pair. The categories are for convenience in description.

EMBRYOTOXON WITHOUT ATTACHMENTS TO THE IRIS

Probably the mildest and most common abnormality one may consider under iridocorneal dysgenesis is simple embryotoxon, or marginal corneal dysplasia, occurring without other evident abnormality. Embryotoxon is an abnormal thickening of the peripheral rim of Descemet's membrane (Schwalbe's line). The thickening has a refractile glassy character. This thickening may be in the form of a uniform, circumferential, prominent ridge on the inner surface of the cornea, but more commonly, it varies in thickness and sometimes is abnormally prominent in only one sector. It often varies in thickness so much that it has a beaded appearance.

One can often see embryotoxon very well with the slit-lamp biomicroscope through clear cornea adjacent to the limbus, but only by gonioscopy can one be sure whether there are associated structural abnormalities in the angle. Embryotoxon without other abnormality and without glaucoma is noted in adults as an incidental finding on routine examination and also in infants and children when slit-lamp or gonioscopic examination is performed.

We have seen no eye in which we could relate embryotoxon to glaucoma, unless in addition to the embryotoxon

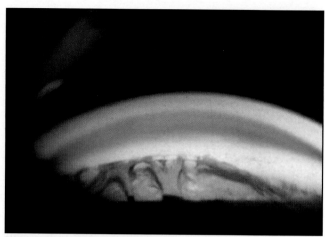

Figure 69-3. Iridocorneal goniodysgenesis: forward attachment of iris stromal processes to a central displaced and prominent Schwalbe's line (posterior embryotoxon) is common with this anomaly.

there were congenital attachments across the angle between iris and cornea, as we will describe next.

EMBRYOTOXON WITH CONGENITAL ATTACHMENTS BETWEEN PERIPHERAL IRIS AND CORNEA, BUT PUPIL NORMAL

In iridocorneal dysgenesis having these qualifications, the principal feature is congenital bridging of the angle between Schwalbe's line and peripheral iris by strands of tissue. The stroma of the iris may be normal, atrophic, or split, and the lens may or may not be cataractous, but the pupil is normal. The strands bridging the angle can usually be seen conclusively only by gonioscopy. These strands are variable in character. In some eyes, they consist of refractile avascular material like ropes of Descemet's membrane; in other eyes, they consist of avascular iris stroma, with or without pigmentation, and in still other eyes, of iris stroma together with iris blood vessels.

We have found congenital iridocorneal bridges of this sort with normal pupils in the following circumstances:

- In adult or children's nonglaucomatous eyes

- In eyes having what seemed to be adult open-angle glaucoma

- In eyes having congenital or childhood glaucoma

These anomalies are also seen in arteriohepatic dysplasia (Alagille syndrome). In this syndrome, posterior embryotoxon is a near constant abnormality and is frequently associated with multiple bridging angle processes and less frequent corectopia. This syndrome is an autosomal dominant condition with congenital cholestasis, facial defects, cardiovascular anomalies, and skeletal defects. The anterior segment anomalies are accompanied by other ocular defects, including pigmentary retinopathy, but glaucoma does not seem to complicate this syndrome.

EMBRYOTOXON WITH CONGENITAL ATTACHMENTS BETWEEN PERIPHERAL IRIS AND CORNEA, PLUS ABNORMALITIES OF THE PUPIL

This combination of congenital abnormalities consists of a combination of posterior embryotoxon (posterior marginal dysplasia of the cornea), with attachments across the angle from iris to cornea and TM, often with hypoplasia of the stroma of the iris, which may give the iris a dark appearance, plus a considerable variety of possible abnormalities of the pupil, including eccentric pupil (corectopia), pinpoint pupil, slit-like pupil, ectropion of the pigment layer of the iris at the pupil (ectropion uveae), and multiple holes in the iris, inaccurately called polycoria. (Eyes with polycoria may show progressive changes in the iris that may behave like essential atrophy of the iris.) If the angle face can be seen through the processes, it is usually not possible to define the TM, scleral spur, and ciliary body band. In their places, a uniform plane of white tissue is typically seen. These malformations occasionally are associated with microphthalmia or cataract.

This most conspicuous form of iridocorneal goniodysgenesis that involves the pupil and iris as well as the angle often has a hereditary basis, with similar conditions occurring in relatives as seen in Rieger's syndrome.[18]

Children with these associated defects of the pupil, iris, angle, and peripheral cornea are at significant risk (50%) for glaucoma, which may be present in infancy or be later acquired.[15] Those patients with progressive anterior segment changes characterized by degeneration of the iris and associated blockage of the angle by peripheral iris tissue are especially at risk. These degenerative changes with development of glaucoma or worsening of glaucoma usually occur in the first 5 years of life.

When the anterior segment defects possess a dense central corneal opacification, the presence of Peters anomaly should be considered. In this condition, which is often bilateral and may be hereditary, a dense central leukoma is present with the attachment of iris processes at the periphery of the opacity. A cataract may be present. The angle is usually open but abnormal with scattered bridges of tissue from the iris root to the TM. These patients also are at risk for glaucoma. We have frequently seen moderate IOP elevations in infancy in this condition slowly improve over the first 5 years of life.

Treatment of children with glaucoma complicating iridocorneal goniodysgenesis should be initiated with medical therapy. Such treatment is more often helpful with cases of glaucoma that develop later in childhood. Beta-blockers and CAIs have been helpful. When the glaucoma is present from infancy, medical therapy generally is inadequate for satisfactory IOP control but may be useful before glaucoma surgery to decrease the IOP or as an adjunct to therapy after glaucoma surgery.

Goniosurgery should always be considered in these forms of trabecular dysgenesis, especially in infancy. Better control may be achieved with continued medical therapy for a period of time, but in our experience, definitive glaucoma control with goniosurgery is rarely achieved. Best results with goniosurgery can be expected in those eyes with less severe defects, such as those with iris processes alone, unassociated with iris abnormalities. Failure of goniosurgery to help with one eye may be useful information in deciding against goniosurgery for a fellow eye.

Trabeculectomy with adjunctive use of mitomycin C has been helpful in these patients and now represents the surgical treatment of choice.

The Oculocerebrorenal (Lowe) Syndrome

Lowe syndrome is a rare x-linked recessive disease characterized by mental retardation, hypotonia, systemic acidosis, rickets, and ocular defects, including glaucoma. The condition is caused by mutation of the OCRL-1 gene located at Xq26.1.[19] The most constant defects are cataracts, which are characteristically bilateral, irregularly dense, thin, and are associated with extreme miosis (Figure 69-4). Glaucoma occurs less frequently than cataracts (47% to 64%). In a recent review of 7 patients with Lowe syndrome,[19] 5 patients (71%) were found to have glaucoma. Of those 10 eyes, 6 eyes presented with increased IOP prior to lensectomy. Gonioscopy revealed an open angle with normal grey TM without abnormal iris processes. The ciliary body bands were abnormally narrow and visibility of the scleral spur was variable and often limited.[19]

Treatment of glaucoma associated with Lowe syndrome is difficult. Goniotomy frequently fails to control IOP. It also has been associated with extensive postoperative bleeding. Medical therapy consisting of a beta-blocker and a CAI is appropriate as first-line treatment. There is an appropriate reluctance to recommend an oral CAI in the presence of a condition complicated already by systemic acidosis and rickets. Patients with Lowe syndrome will be on supplemental base therapy (eg, Bicitra/Polycitra-Baker Norton). The dose of this supplement usually can be increased to take into account the effect of the oral CAI to allow its use for this ocular indication. Consultation with the patient's pediatrician is recommended.

Neurofibromatosis

Neurofibromatosis type 1 (NF-1) is a multisystem disorder inherited by autosomal dominant transmission with its gene on chromosome 17 (17qll.2). NF-1 is one of the most

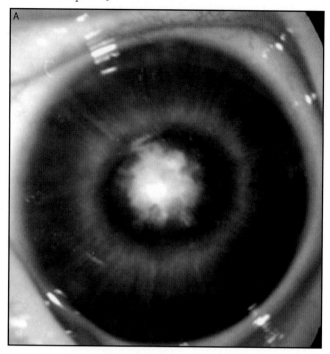

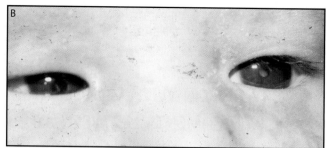

Figure 69-4. (A) Cataract irregularly dense. (B) Extreme miosis and bilateral cataracts in a child with Lowe syndrome.

common inherited disorders, and its systemic and ocular defects are well-known, including café-au-lait spots, optic nerve gliomas, and Lisch nodules (Figure 69-5A). Childhood glaucoma may be one of the least common ocular complications of this disease, but when present, it usually occurs as a congenital glaucoma.

An infant with NF-1 and glaucoma may show no nonocular stigmata of this disease. Even café-au-lait spots, abundant later in childhood, may not be apparent before 1 year of age. Proptosis from optic nerve gliomas may occur and present as a pseudo-ptosis. Glaucoma, however, almost always is associated with the development of a plexiform neuroma of the upper lid, producing a characteristic s-curve deformity (Figure 69-5B). The glaucoma may be bilateral, but this is unusual.

The globe of the involved eye is usually enlarged, as is the cornea. This enlargement may be striking and be associated with high myopia, even in the first months of life. The degree of enlargement often seems to be in excess of what would be expected secondary to the elevated IOP alone. On further examination, abnormal pale subconjunctival tissue may be present, suggesting a neurofibroma of the conjunctiva. The iris of the affected eye typically possesses a uniform stroma. Though no Lisch nodules would be expected in early life, they also seem not to occur in the irides of eyes affected with glaucoma compared to fellow nonglaucoma eyes. An ectropion uveae, however, is a characteristic pupillary rim abnormality seen in these eyes (Figure 69-5C). Although this abnormality is often considered to be congenital, it is characteristically quite subtle in infants and not recognized easily. During the first year of life, the width of the pigment layer will widen over the iris, making it easily recognizable, especially when the iris is blue.

Gonioscopy often reveals a striking deformity that has been seen in each of 6 eyes cared for by DSW. The iris leaf appears straight rather than convex and inserts anteriorly on the TM. Scleral spur and the ciliary body band are typically not present. The exposed TM band is usually narrow.

Treatment of infantile neurofibromatosis glaucoma should initially consist of a trial of medical therapy. The visual prognosis for these eyes may be poor if high myopia and glaucoma are present simultaneously. Short-term use of oral CAIs seems appropriate. Goniosurgery characteristically fails to affect the IOP favorably. Trabeculectomy with adjunct use of antimetabolites offers the best chance for successful surgery.

Stickler Syndrome, Rubinstein-Taybi Syndrome, and Marfan Syndrome

Patients with Stickler syndrome (hereditary progressive arthro-ophthalmopathy) and the Rubinstein-Taybi syndrome may present with glaucomatous disease that resembles primary infantile glaucoma.[20] Importantly, goniotomy is an effective treatment for glaucoma in these conditions. Stickler's syndrome also may be associated with a congenital infantile open-angle glaucoma, which is less responsive to goniotomy than when the glaucoma is congenital. Infantile glaucoma is rarely seen with Marfan syndrome.

Zellweger Spectrum Disorders

Infantile glaucoma is seen in the hepatocerebrorenal syndrome. This autosomal recessive disorder is characterized by striking hypotonia, inability to feed, characteristic faces, and early death. Elevated very-long chain fatty acids (VLFAs) are indicative of the peroxisomal agenesis found in this condition.[21] We have examined 4 patients with this disease. Glaucoma was present in one; gonioscopy revealed poor definition of the scleral spur and ciliary body band without abnormal processes. The posterior segment exam revealed typical equatorial black spots at the level of the retinal pigment epithelium, which are possibly pathognomonic for this condition. No glaucoma therapy was administered, but medical therapy may be appropriate under some circumstances.

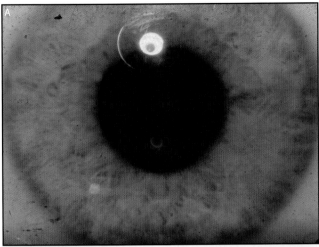

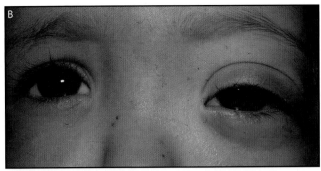

Figure 69-5. (A) Lisch nodules in a patient with neurofibromatosis type I. (B) S-curved deformity of the left upper eyelid due to plexiform neuroma with glaucoma and ocular enlargement OS. (C) Ectropion uvea, heterochromia, and secondary glaucoma OS.

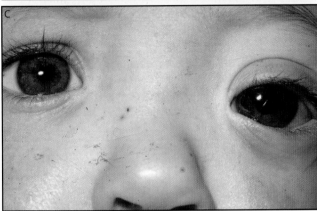

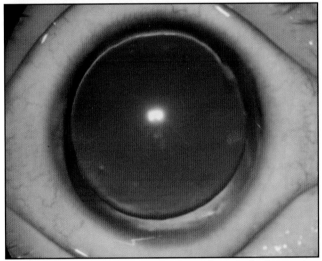

Figure 69-6. Aniridia. A young child with aniridia typically shows a clear cornea and lens and will rarely have glaucoma in infancy.

PRIMARY GLAUCOMA WITH PROFOUND OCULAR ANOMALIES

Childhood glaucoma is seen in the presence of other primary ocular disorders (Table 68-10).

Congenital Aniridia

Congenital aniridia is a hereditary disease of the eye with multiple congenital and acquired defects that become complicated by glaucoma in 6% to 75% of affected patients.[22] Aniridia may occur sporadically or be familial. Approximately one-third of aniridia cases arise sporadically and two-thirds are familial. The genetic defect has been isolated to the paried box gene (PAX6) found at 11p13. When a chromosomal deletion occurs involving the short arm of chromosome 11, aniridia occurs as the ocular component of a systemic syndrome (known as WAGR) consisting of retardation, genital anomalies, and an increased risk for Wilms tumor before age 8. Recent advancements in molecular genetics have revealed a strong association of the deletion of the WT1 (Wilms tumor) gene located near the PAX6 gene on the short arm of chromosome 11. Muto and colleagues[23] studied 102 aniridic patients and found concurrent defects in WT1 in 30%. Of those patients with deletion of WT1, 45% developed Wilms tumor, whereas patients without involvement of WT1 did not.[24] Aniridia has also occurred in association with cerebellar ataxia. Extreme hypoplasia of the iris resembling the ocular appearance of hereditary aniridia has also been seen in trisomy 13 and Meckel syndrome.

Aniridia is usually represented by an obvious iris defect, decreased visual acuity with nystagmus, peripheral corneal epitheliopathy (aniridic pannus), small corneas, cataracts, small discs, foveal hypoplasia, optic nerve hypoplasia, and frequent glaucoma (Figure 69-6). Near-complete absence of the iris on slit-lamp examination is characteristic; a narrow rim of the iris, however, is often detectable. On gonioscopy, the iris stump becomes more obvious, is often of variable width, and presents circumferentially in a plane perpendicular to the visual axis. A small percentage of patients will possess an intact iris, making the recognition of aniridia less certain; on examination, such irides are always abnormal (Figure 69-7). The affected iris stroma is characteristically smooth

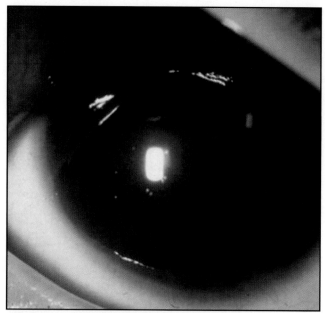

Figure 69-7. Peripheral opacification of the cornea is important evidence of aniridia. Atypically, some patients with aniridia have partial or complete irides; corectopia and defects in the stroma are present.

and homogeneously lacking normal crypts; furthermore, the collarette is usually absent or incomplete and located adjacent to the pupillary border. Mild corectopia is characteristic with symmetrical displacement in each eye. A partial ectropion uveae also is usually present, often located nasally or inferiorly.

The corneas in aniridia are small, often with horizontal diameters of 10.5 to 11.0 mm. The epithelial layer is constantly abnormal. In young patients, this defect is represented by an opacification of the peripheral cornea circumferentially, but usually more marked inferiorly. Fine subepithelial radial blood vessels are usually present in this opacity. This corneal opacity in aniridia is best located after applanation tonometry due to the bright fluorescein staining of the involved abnormal epithelium. The stromal and Descemet's membrane endothelial cell layers are normal. By 10 years of age, equatorial lens opacities are usually present, which progress often to be visually significant by the late teenage years. The ciliary processes and the zonules of the lens are well exposed to view by gonioscopy in aniridia. In eyes that have not been subjected to surgery, these structures as a rule appear normal.

GLAUCOMA IN ANIRIDIA

We believe that glaucoma occurs in 50% to 75% of patients with aniridia.[25] The presence or absence of glaucoma and its severity correlate well with the extent of gonioscopically visible obstruction of the filtration portion of the corneoscleral TM. The filtration area is covered by the stump of the iris approximately in proportion to the severity of the glaucoma. In some eyes, only the stromal portion of the iris stump is forward and adherent, covering the ciliary band, scleral spur,

and to a variable extent the TM, but in other eyes the whole thickness of the iris stump, including the pigment layer, is turned forward and is adherent to the angle wall. In those patients who do not have glaucoma, the TM is not so significantly covered by the stump of the iris and the structures of the angle wall appear more normal.

Gonioscopy of more than 75 patients with aniridia by the senior author has provided the following observations:

- In aniridia in eyes without glaucoma, the filtration portion of the TM has very little or no covering by iris tissue in most of its circumference. If some covering is present, it is usually in the superior aspect of the angle. The ciliary band usually does show variable covering by iris tissue, but in nonglaucomatous eyes the ciliary body band usually appears wider than in eyes that have glaucoma. The scleral spur often can be seen in most of the circumference.

- In aniridia in eyes with mild glaucoma, we have seen extensive blockage of less than half of the angle, as will be described in the next paragraph, but, more commonly, we have seen circumferential involvement of the angle. In this stage, one sees multiple, thin sawtooth extensions of iris stroma reaching across the scleral spur and attaching on and anterior to the filtration area of the TM. These extensions are often in the form of a sheet in some areas and perforated in other areas; they usually possess little pigment. In young children, these processes often have blood vessels that extend anteriorly in the sheet and can be seen to turn abruptly on the TM and run parallel to scleral spur and join other vessels from other similar extensions of iris stroma. These vessels do not characteristically branch and are less evident after early childhood. When these vessels are seen on the TM, mild glaucoma is usually present. In many areas, the peripheral iris stroma appears to be pulled up onto the ciliary body band; a mild concavity of the anterior iris leaf may be present and an inner separation of the iris stroma from the pigment epithelium may be seen.

- In aniridia in eyes with moderate to severe glaucoma, most of the filtration area of the TM is covered by forward attachment of the iris stroma tissue covering at least the posterior half of the TM in any meridian. Involvement superiorly again is most severe, usually with no recognizable TM in evidence. At this stage, the former anterior surface of the iris stroma now lies essentially parallel to the angle wall over much of its area. In meridians of most severe change, the former iris stromal stump is shifted completely onto the angle wall. At such sites, the iris pigment epithelium may be left behind and is seen draped across the ciliary processes, remaining on a plane perpendicular to the visual axis. The anterior border of the iris tissue on the TM is often fairly uniform and wavy as one views around the circumference of the angle; the iris appears to have come to rest. Vessels are not in evidence at this stage.

Our observations on glaucoma associated with aniridia suggest that the IOP usually tends to become elevated later in childhood than is usual in ordinary congenital open-angle glaucoma. What primarily suggests this is in glaucoma associated with aniridia, the corneas are not usually enlarged. Generally, it is thought to be a normal characteristic of an infant's eye in the first 2 years of life to be subject to stretching and enlargement, with attendant rupturing of Descemet's membrane, when the IOP is excessive. Because enlargement of the globe and ruptures of Descemet's membrane are seen in many types of glaucoma of early life, including secondary glaucomas, it is likely that the aniridic eye would behave in a similar fashion if significant glaucoma were present in early life, unless the aniridic eye possesses greater-than-usual resistance to such changes. These observations support our belief that, in most instances, glaucoma in aniridia develops later in childhood rather than during infancy. Among these patients, it has been rare for glaucoma to occur during the first year of life and unusual for glaucoma to develop in patients younger than 5 years of age. When it does occur, the angle abnormalities may be different than those seen in the more usual situation of glaucoma acquired in later childhood or in the teenage years. Most of our observations in aniridia are in patients during the first decade of life. Based on this selected population, it is our belief that the active stage of angle progression and development of glaucoma occurs during late childhood, rather than during the adult years.

TREATMENT OF ANIRIDIA

Treatment of glaucoma associated with aniridia is usually medical (Table 69-2). The glaucoma associated with aniridia, unlike congenital glaucoma, does commonly respond to treatment with pilocarpine and other miotic drops. Because there is no sphincter pupillae, it is assumed that in aniridia the miotic drops cause lowering of IOP by their effect on the ciliary muscle, inducing an improvement in facility of aqueous outflow through those portions of the TM that are unobstructed.

Goniotomy procedures are disappointing in eyes with frank glaucoma. In 15 glaucomatous eyes in our series, we found that with a goniotomy knife under direct observation, the covering iris stroma, and an anterior veil that often precedes it, can be nicely dissected off the TM, exposing the scleral spur and ciliary body band, producing a permanent change in the angle. However, none of the eyes, even with multiple operations, was cured by goniosurgery. In some cases, a temporary improved response to miotic therapy has been obtained.

Trabeculectomy with use of mitomycin C has been successful in 3 of 4 eyes treated in our series of aniridia patients. A standard procedure is done; iridectomy is usually unnecessary. Because the lens and cornea are unprotected by an

TABLE 69-2. MANAGEMENT OF GLAUCOMA IN ANIRIDIA	
Stage of Aniridia	**Treatment Considerations**
Normal IOP, stable exam, no evidence of progressive angle closure	Frequent observation
Normal IOP or early rise in IOP, progressive angle closure	Consider prophylactic goniotomy (refer to pediatric ophthalmologist); medical therapy for elevated IOP
Glaucoma with advanced angle closure	Medical treatment with aqueous suppressants and miotics; trabeculectomy with adjuvant antimetabolites (mitomycin C)

iris, careful postoperative observation is mandatory to prevent injury to these tissues that might occur from loss of the anterior chamber.

PROPHYLACTIC GONIOTOMY

Founded on our observations that suggest that the TM may be near normal in early childhood and then worsens when congenital synechiae become impervious to aqueous humor, or more commonly when iris stroma becomes drawn up on the TM, we have attempted early preventive surgery. We speculate that removal of attachments early may prevent changes in the filtration tissue that appear not to be corrected by removal of the synechial iris attachments and stroma at a later stage. Patients selected for this procedure have been young children who do not have glaucoma, but who on gonioscopy show extensive early bridging of synechial iris extensions across the scleral spur, and who usually have been observed to be undergoing a worsening of this angle abnormality.

This preventive or prophylactic goniosurgery has been performed with a goniotomy knife under direct observation. The anterior border of the tissue extending onto the TM is engaged with the tip of the knife, and then, with movements of the knife parallel to the visual axis as well as circumferential, the tissue is stripped off the angle wall, and a deep sulcus is created between the iris stump and the TM, leaving the latter appearing beautifully clean. Once a decision for surgery is made, 2 operations at separate hospitalizations are performed on a single eye to produce the desired change in more than half of the circumference of the angle.

The results of this procedure are encouraging. Fifty-five eyes in 33 patients have been operated upon in this way. This series includes a patient whose IOPs were beginning to rise. In each case, an exposure of the TM, except for isolated strands, has been produced (Figure 69-8). Postoperative

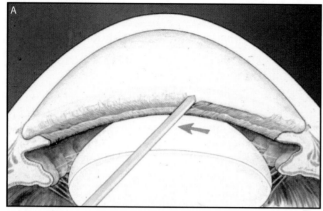

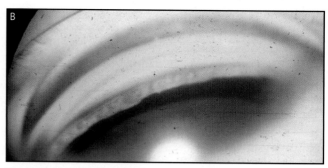

Figure 69-8. (A, B) After prophylactic goniosurgery for aniridic glaucoma, the separation of the iris stump from the angle seen on gonioscopy is permanent. (C) Angle defects in aniridia are progressive and should be monitored with gonioscopy.

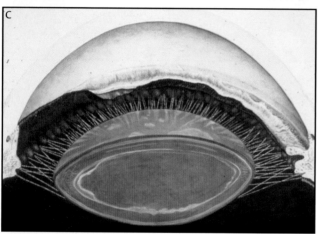

follow-up now ranges from less than 1 year to 26 years. IOPs above normal have developed in only 2 of these patients. One patient had glaucoma in one eye before prophylactic operation on the other eye. No postoperative complications have been encountered, except for the transient presence of blood in the anterior chamber in the immediate postoperative period.

When considering this procedure, it is important to explain clearly to the child's parents that it is a preventive rather than therapeutic step and, though results are encouraging, that its potential benefit still is unproved. Because of the small cornea in aniridia, with its peripheral zone of opacification, and because of the broad exposure of the clear lens in the anterior chamber in these children, we recommend that it be performed only by those surgeons who do goniotomy-type surgery regularly and who are familiar with the characteristics of angle changes in aniridia that are associated with glaucoma. Because of the shallowness of the anterior chamber in the first year of life, this surgery is best postponed until after this period. While considering whether a young child with aniridia is a candidate for this procedure, we usually perform gonioscopy at 6-month intervals under general anesthesia to evaluate what changes, if any, are occurring in the angle.

Weighing against the idea of early surgical intervention that is intended to be preventive is the knowledge that, when

the glaucoma is mild, medical treatment may suffice for reasonable control. We do not yet know enough to be able to predict far in advance which cases will ultimately fail medical treatment.

Glaucoma With Congenital Iris Ectropion Syndrome

A number of disorders that cause glaucoma in children are associated with iris abnormalities (Table 69-3). The occurrence of glaucoma with a congenital ectropion uveae without neurofibromatosis is an important but unusual cause of childhood glaucoma (Figure 69-9). The development of an iris ectropion is also seen in patients with the Axenfeld-Rieger syndrome, ICE syndromes, partial aniridia, as well as in neurofibromatosis (NF-1). Glaucoma associated with a congenital ectropion of the iris, iridogoniodysgenesis, represents a recognizable cause of childhood glaucoma apart from entities considered within the Axenfeld-Rieger spectrum of disorders. This glaucoma is nonhereditary, unilateral, and unassociated with any systemic defects. The condition is usually recognized by an investigation of the abnormal pupil. The associated glaucoma is most often present in early childhood and persists, but it may also be acquired. Each of 5 patients with this entity cared for by the author had glaucoma at a young age, but none were examined until after the second year of life.

On examination, corneal symmetry is typical without striking unilateral corneal enlargement as seen with other unilateral early onset glaucomas. Breaks in Descemet's membrane also are not usually present, suggesting further that IOP elevations in infancy are usually not great if present. The associated ptosis is mild. Striking abnormalities of the iris and filtration angle are present. The pupil is reactive but typically surrounded by an apparent ectropion uveae with the presence of dark iris pigment epithelium on the anterior surface of the iris. This defect is of variable width, may be partial, and, in my experience, has been stable. The unpigmented iris surface is smooth and without crypts or

TABLE 69-3. DEVELOPMENTAL DISORDERS WITH IRIS ABNORMALITIES AND GLAUCOMA	
Axenfeld-Rieger's syndrome	Bilateral, autosomal dominant, variable degree of angle, iris, and pupil involvement
Peters anomaly	Bilateral, some cases inherited, attachment of iris processes to dense central leukoma
Neurofibromatosis (NF-1)	Autosomal dominant, Lisch nodules, ectropion uveae
Aniridia	Autosomal dominant or sporadic with deletion of chromosome 11, residual iris stump (variable), angle closure (progressive in some cases)
Congenital ectropion uveae (iridogoniodysgenesis)	Not inherited, unilateral with corneal enlargement, no systemic manifestations, affected iris smooth without crypts
Familial (congenital) hypoplasia of the iris	Autosomal dominant, irides appear dark due to thin iris stroma, no polycoria or corectopia

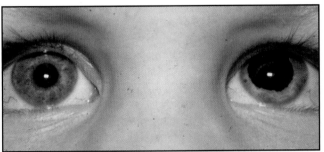

Figure 69-9. Glaucoma with congenital ectropion uveae. The unilateral abnormal iris stroma and pupillary ectropion are evident in this disorder. Gonioscopy revealed anterior insertion of the iris.

circumferential folds. It shares a similar color with the fellow eye but the character of the stromal architecture differs greatly from the normal opposite eye. On gonioscopy, the iris inserts anteriorly on the TM partially or completely circumferentially. The scleral spur and ciliary body band are not present. Some prominence of Schwalbe's line may be present. Pathological examination of iris and angle specimens from 2 of our patients has confirmed endothelialization of the angle and anterior iris surface.

Treatment of children with this type of primary glaucoma should be initiated with medical therapy. However, in our experience, this has not proven adequate. Goniosurgery has failed to provide improved control of the IOP following each of 6 operations performed by DSW. Filtration surgery, in contrast, has been rewarding for these patients and is, at present, the initial glaucoma surgery of choice.

Iridotrabecular Dysgenesis (Familial Hypoplasia of the Iris)

Iridotrabecular dysgenesis is a rare cause of childhood glaucoma inherited by autosomal dominant transmission. A family history of glaucoma involving numerous family members is important early evidence of this type of glaucoma.

On slit-lamp examination, the iris stroma appears porous and thinned, allowing the visualization of the darker posterior iris pigment epithelium. When brown, these irides appear rust-colored and when blue appear gray. Corectopia and iris hole formation do not occur. Gonioscopy is variable but always abnormal. Extra tissue obscuring the view of the scleral spur and ciliary body band may be present, or this tissue may seem to consist of fine processes directed from the iris root to the TM. The eye pressures are variable in this disease and may become progressively more elevated in childhood.

This entity must be distinguished gonioscopically from patients with an Axenfeld-Rieger anomaly and from patients with congenital glaucoma associated with iris defects. While the former entity may share autosomal dominant inheritance, gonioscopy will show the expected array of abnormal processes characteristic of the Axenfeld anomaly. Patients with congenital glaucoma with iris defects are usually sporadic in occurrence, and the irides appear abnormal by their very uniform character and absence of crypts and by the near constant enlargement of the pupils and minor ectropion of the pupillary frill. Anterior segment enlargement also is present with this glaucoma, which is severe early in life.

Treatment of children with glaucoma associated with congenital iris hypoplasia should be initiated with medical therapy. When surgery is necessary, goniotomy should be performed, followed by filtration surgery when necessary.

Four young children with this entity cared for by DSW have been controlled with topical beta-blockers in 2, while goniotomies with continued use of a beta-blocker have been satisfactory for a third patient. The fourth patient required filtration surgery after failed goniotomies at 8 years of age.

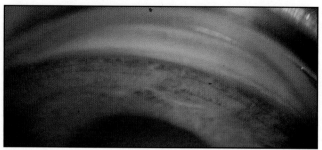

Figure 69-10. Juvenile glaucoma. On gonioscopy, the angle structures appear normal. The ciliary body band is easily distinguished from the TM.

JUVENILE OPEN-ANGLE GLAUCOMA

Adult open-angle glaucoma usually affects patients older than 50 years of age. Phenotypically, JOAG is the occurrence of open-angle glaucoma in children, often with the development of significant elevation of IOP by 10 years of age, although in some cases, IOP may not elevate until early adulthood. Clinically, this glaucoma is often associated with moderate amounts of myopia. Transmission of this disease is by autosomal dominant inheritance, and the gene locus has been linked to the TM inducible glucocorticoid response (TIGR) gene, also known as MYCO (formerly GLC1A gene) on the long arm of chromosome 1q21-q31.[23]

Candidate children who later develop glaucoma usually have normal IOP during the first 5 years of age then develop a slow progression of IOP before 10 years of age. Anterior segment enlargement is not seen. On examination by slit-lamp biomicroscopy and gonioscopy, no abnormality is found (Figure 69-10).

Children with JOAG must be differentiated from late-recognized cases of congenital glaucoma and from sporadic cases of other types of juvenile glaucoma. Late-recognized cases of congenital glaucoma are characterized by anterior segment enlargement, often associated with breaks in Descemet's membrane, suggesting the presence of glaucoma early in life. Other causes of juvenile glaucoma frequently demonstrate recognizable abnormalities on gonioscopy as well as frequent iris defects.

Treatment of JOAG is appropriately initiated with medical therapy. Miotics cause symptomatic blurring of vision and frequent headaches. A beta-blocker and a CAI will frequently, but temporarily, control the IOP in these patients. Goniotomy is the initial surgical glaucoma treatment of choice. If a second procedure does not produce adequate control, then trabeculectomy with adjunctive use of an antimetabolite in these young patients is indicated. Medical therapy followed by glaucoma surgery, if necessary, should be considered before the occurrence of disc damage and field loss, and when patients have been identified early and have developed uncontrolled IOP. See Chapter 50 for further information on this entity.

SECONDARY PEDIATRIC GLAUCOMA

The general ophthalmologist or pediatric ophthalmologist may infrequently see children with primary glaucoma, but can expect to see patients with a secondary glaucoma more frequently in the management of childhood ocular illness. Table 69-1 lists the diverse and multiple types of secondary pediatric glaucomas that collectively occur with significant frequency.

Traumatic Glaucoma

The principles that are understood in respect to adult traumatic glaucoma apply also to childhood (see Chapter 43). The most frequent cause of glaucoma after trauma in childhood is a recurrent hyphema. With such an occurrence, children must be cared for aggressively to control the IOP to prevent corneal staining, iris atrophy, permanent mydriasis, and optic nerve injury.

Initial glaucoma treatment should include a beta-blocker and CAI. Early anterior chamber washout should be performed when IOP control is not achieved by medical therapy. When anterior chamber paracentesis and washout are performed, the surgeon should remember that complete clearing of the anterior chamber is unnecessary to achieve at least temporary IOP control. Following the initial release of blood from the anterior chamber, an air injection aids the further evacuation of blood. Use of viscoelastics is not recommended. Consideration should be given to the use of tissue plasminogen activator (τ-PA). Entry of instruments into the eye to assist evacuation of a resistant blood clot is risky and rarely helpful.

Following successful initial care of patients with glaucoma complicating a hyphema, careful follow-up is indicated for potential recurrent glaucoma associated with further breakup of clots of blood and in the long-term related to permanent filtration angle defects.

Neoplastic Glaucoma

Glaucoma associated with a neoplasm in childhood is seen most frequently secondary to a retinoblastoma. Other causes are listed in Table 69-1 and include leukemia and juvenile xanthogranuloma of the iris.

Though retinoblastoma may occur with tumor cells in the anterior chamber, this is unusual. The occurrence of glaucoma is most frequently secondary to rubeosis and closure of the angle but also may occur secondary to pupillary block when the lens is pushed forward by the posterior segment mass (Figure 69-11). Treatment of glaucoma is usually directed to the neoplasm present. Medical therapy for the glaucoma is appropriate when necessary.

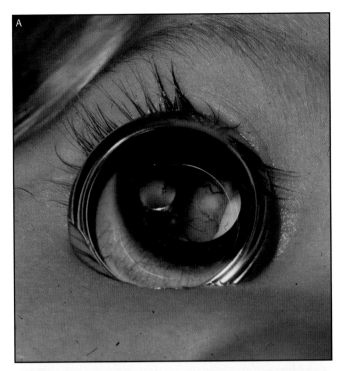

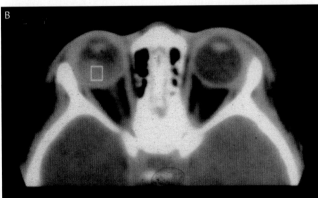

Figure 69-11. Glaucoma with retinoblastoma. (A) This young boy presented with signs of glaucoma and intraocular hemorrhage. (B) CT scan suggested a retinoblastoma (intraocular calcification), which was confirmed on pathological examination.

Uveitic Glaucoma

Glaucoma is a common complication of anterior uveitis in children (see Chapter 42). It may be acute and seen with acute uveitis complicating herpetic uveitis and recurrent posterior segment toxoplasmosis. The most common cause of secondary glaucoma is chronic uveitis associated with juvenile idiopathic arthritis (JIA).[26]

Children with chronic anterior uveitis require frequent re-examination, including tonometry. Increasing inflammation may cause relative hypotony, while control of the inflammation may reveal increasing obstruction of aqueous outflow by the occurrence of an elevated IOP. Prevention of glaucoma by way of control of the intraocular inflammation is an important goal of treatment. When topical steroids are tapered, special caution must be exercised to be sure that recurrent episodes of increased inflammation do not occur. Correspondingly, when treatment is increased, the increased risk for glaucoma must be recognized. Frequent follow-up examinations every 6 weeks throughout childhood are recommended.

When glaucoma occurs with chronic anterior uveitis, the inflammatory disease typically has been present for at least 1 or 2 years.[26] If evidence of pupillary block is present, the mechanism causing the glaucoma is obvious, and immediate iridectomy with or without goniosynechialysis is indicated as dictated by intraoperative gonioscopy. When pupillary block is not present, the mechanism of the glaucoma is less obvious, and the potential risk of steroids causing an elevated IOP needs to be considered. Long-term use of steroids before the development of glaucoma might be evidence against this etiology. However, it is often difficult to determine with certainty that steroids are not contributing to the glaucoma.

In most instances, the complicating glaucoma is an open angle-type associated with recognizable angle defects. When these abnormalities are found, the causal role of steroids seems less likely. In most cases, it will remain important to continue the steroid at an appropriate level for control of the inflammation. On gonioscopy, the angle in chronic anterior uveitis is typically found open, associated with unusual opacification of the TM and ciliary body band inferiorly. Scattered pigment dust may be seen along with a variable number of sawtoothed peripheral anterior synechiae (PAS) attaching the peripheral iris to the TM.

Treatment of the uveitic childhood glaucoma should be initiated with medical therapy consisting of a beta-blocker and a CAI when necessary. Strong miotics are contraindicated, but weak miotics (eg, pilocarpine HCl 0.5%) may be helpful if used infrequently (eg, bedtime daily).

Surgical treatment of childhood uveitic glaucoma is appropriately approached with caution. Goniotomy is the preferred initial procedure. For 31 eyes in 31 children treated with standard goniotomy, 71% achieved control of the IOP with a mean follow-up duration of 10.3 ± 6.4 years. Complete success, defined as IOP < 21 mm Hg without any medications, was achieved in 68% of patients.[26] Similar findings were reported by Freedman and colleagues[27] in a retrospective study of 16 eyes of 12 patients. The success rate was reported at 75%, with 75% of patients on 1.4 ± 1.1 medications.[28]

We do not favor initial seton implant surgery for glaucoma associated with uveitis because of the chronic intraocular inflammation associated with these devices. Filtration surgery with use of antimetabolites is an important surgery treatment for patients who are unresponsive to goniotomy.

Lens-Induced Glaucoma

The occurrence of glaucoma associated with the shape and position of the crystalline lens is an important cause of

TABLE 69-4. ACUTE LENS-INDUCED GLAUCOMAS OF CHILDHOOD (ANGLE CLOSURE)

Ectopia lentis	Pupillary block mechanism (particularly after pupillary dilation); perform iridectomy.
Marfan syndrome	
Homocystinuria	
Trauma	
Following cataract surgery	Children operated prior to age 2 years at increased risk. Pupillary block from residual lens tissue. History of pupillary block postoperatively.

glaucoma in children. The glaucoma may develop acutely or be chronic (Table 69-4).

Typically, with ectopia lentis complicating Marfan syndrome or homocystinuria, flow through the pupil is obstructed by entry of the lens partway through the pupil. Pupillary block occurs with collapse of the anterior chamber and further repositioning of the lens against the back of the cornea. Acute glaucoma occurs abruptly, which is painful and often associated with vomiting. Immediate care is necessary.

Glaucoma in these patients may be precipitated by a routine eye examination associated with pupillary dilation. Predisposed patients may best be examined during morning hours with instruction to avoid a face-down position until normal pupil size returns. A free lens in the eye gravitates, causing entry into the pupil in a face-down position.

Prevention of pupillary block in ectopia lentis can be successful by making these patients aware of the risks, using miotics selectively, and most importantly by creating a peripheral iridectomy. In the presence of a peripheral iridectomy, a patient will only be at risk for recurrence of pupillary block if the crystalline lens enters the anterior chamber. This event is much more frequent in patients with homocystinuria than in patients with Marfan syndrome.

Treatment of the acute pupillary block glaucoma complicating ectopia lentis is challenging. Pain medication should be administered. Medical therapy consisting of a beta-blocker, CAI, and osmotic agents is appropriate but has typically little IOP benefit. Effective treatment consists of relieving the pupillary block.

The anterior segment must be examined carefully. The anterior chamber will be flat and the pupil will be dilated. If the pupillary border is visible, an attempt may be made with a muscle hook to break the pupillary block by pushing the crystalline lens posteriorly at one edge of the pupil. In spite of the elevated IOP, a surprising amount of indentation of cornea against the lens can be achieved. It is only necessary to move the lens away from the cornea a small amount for this maneuver to be successful. The cornea can

be nicely protected by a soft contact lens. When the pupillary block is broken, aqueous will rush into the newly forming anterior chamber, forcing the lens posteriorly. The aqueous will then dissect peripherally and separate the iris away from the peripheral cornea and eventually from the angle. Gonioscopic observation of these events is important to ensure that the angle opens. Miotics and thymoxamine may accelerate this process.

Occasionally, the iris may wrap itself around the equator of the lens circumferentially. On examination, the eye with this arrangement may not appear very different. Careful inspection of the iris, however, will reveal a dilated pupil with no visible pigmentary frill, and examination of the anterior segment with a gonioscopy lens will reveal that the iris is wrapped around the equator of the lens. The lens in this position is in a fossa created by the iris and cannot be pushed posteriorly to break the pupillary block.

Large incisions into the eye in preparation for an anterior lensectomy would be expected to be complicated by prolapse of iris and other complications. To treat this problem, placement of a very beveled (long) paracentesis into the anterior chamber directed to the border of the iris against the lens is recommended. Follow this entry with a smooth rounded spatula placed between the lens and the iris directed posteriorly until the retrolenticular aqueous is reached. With slight rotation of the spatula away from the lens, the pupillary block will be released followed by a rush of aqueous into the anterior chamber, soon followed by movement of the lens posteriorly.

Aphakic Glaucoma

Young children who have surgery for congenital cataracts are at significant risk for glaucoma. The mechanism of this glaucoma is secondary to pupillary block or secondary to chronic changes in the TM leading to an impairment of aqueous outflow.

Children who develop glaucoma after cataract surgery usually are those who require cataract surgery before 2 years of age. When occurring secondary to pupillary block, the glaucoma usually occurs within 3 months after cataract surgery. If a surgical iridectomy remains patent after cataract surgery, this type of complicating glaucoma does not occur.

In recent years, with the use of vitreous cutting instruments, the technique of childhood cataract surgery has evolved such that removal of the lens can be accomplished more completely and with more confidence. In spite of these advances, young children remain at significant risk for glaucoma with an occurrence rate of approximately 20%.[29] Glaucoma is often not present until 1 to 2 years or more following the cataract surgery. On gonioscopy, abnormalities are consistently found in these patients with open angles. The abnormalities seen consist of an anterior insertion of the iris at the level of the posterior TM associated with fine PAS and a variable fine pigment deposition on the TM. The

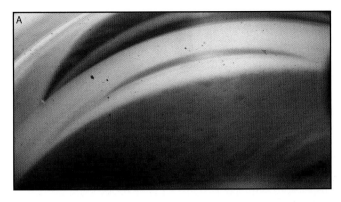

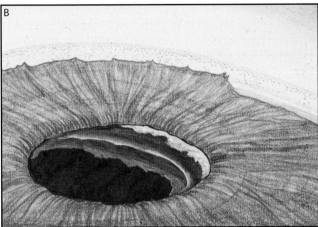

Figure 69-12. Aphakic glaucoma. On gonioscopy, abnormal synechial attachment of the iris anterior to the level of the posterior TM is seen and is typical of this glaucoma. (A) Residual lens tissue is also present. (B) Schematic of angle abnormality.

residual exposed TM often appears glazed with loss of the silk screen appearance of the normal TM (Figure 69-12).

Young patients who develop open-angle glaucoma following congenital cataract surgery more often have a history of secondary lens surgery for pupillary obstruction by residual lens tissue than those patients who do not develop this complication. Children who have congenital cataracts and who do not have lensectomy rarely develop glaucoma unless lens degeneration occurs. The mechanism of this glaucoma associated with a relatively open angle remains uncertain. Chronic inflammation following lens surgery may be a factor, but evidence of this inflammation on examination is not usually present. The release of lens proteins into the anterior chamber may be an additional provocative factor (see Chapter 47). The presence and effect of cytokines produced by residual lens epithelial cells deserves continued study in an attempt to further understand the mechanism of this glaucoma.

Treatment of aphakic open-angle glaucoma in young children is difficult. Medical therapy should be initiated with use of a beta-blocker and CAI. Miotics do not seem to be helpful. DSW has tried goniotomy surgery for 13 eyes and has considered 11 to be failures. Trabeculectomy with use of mitomycin C has been helpful for 10 of 15 eyes. With failure of goniotomy

and trabeculectomy surgery, Seton implant surgery is indicated. Cycloablation has a role in an attempt to save some eyes when other procedures and therapies have failed.

Secondary Angle-Closure Glaucoma in Children

Angle-closure glaucoma is an important cause of secondary glaucoma in childhood. A review of the childhood secondary glaucomas listed in Table 69-1 reveals multiple causes for this mechanism of glaucoma. These include neoplasm, uveitic glaucoma, lens-induced glaucoma, aphakic glaucoma, retinopathy of prematurity, and others.

GLAUCOMA ASSOCIATED WITH RETINOPATHY OF PREMATURITY

Retinopathy of prematurity (ROP) is of special importance because of the very frequent occurrence of glaucoma complicating cicatricial ROP and surgery for retinal detachment complicating ROP.

When ROP is complicated by glaucoma, it is usually angle-closure glaucoma. In our experience, the age of onset of this complication ranges from 4 months to 22 years. Most cases occur after 1 year of age. Typically, these eyes show advanced retinal abnormalities and possess variable amounts of equatorial perilenticular and retrolenticular membrane formation. The latter abnormality, if incomplete, is predictably more severe temporally and can be followed posteriorly to fuse with an organized mass of vitreous and retina. In some cases, it may be so severe as to involve the whole retrolenticular space uniformly. The severity usually is asymmetric. The corneas are often small and steep. Myopia is a constant finding and is more marked in the most severely affected eyes. The lenses are almost always clear and reveal the posterior abnormalities with brilliant clarity.

Of special importance to this discussion are the depths of the anterior chambers, which are almost always shallow in severely affected eyes. Careful inspection of the iris in these eyes may reveal noteworthy convexity of the iris leaf, greater than can be accounted for by the shape of the anterior lens surface, which is in fact relatively flat. When the TM and other angle structures can be seen, they usually appear normal in the absence of glaucoma.

The onset of the glaucoma may be acute with pain in the eye, nausea, and vomiting. We have known the glaucoma to be severe and to cause gray segmental atrophy of the stroma of the iris or even complete necrosis of the entire iris, an entity known as acute ischemia secondary to glaucoma. Children with this condition are often treated for an acute gastrointestinal disturbance because of the associated vomiting or for a lid infection due to misinterpretation of lid swelling. Other children have presented with less acute symptoms consisting of eye rubbing, photophobia, and tearing.

We feel that embarrassment of the flow of aqueous humor between the lens and iris from the posterior chamber to the anterior chamber must be a significant factor in causing the angle to close, because in some cases this glaucoma has been cured by iridectomy. Presumably, iridectomy works in these cases as it does in ordinary angle-closure glaucoma, by circumventing the obstruction at the pupil and preventing abnormal accumulation of aqueous behind the iris. Whether the onset of embarrassment in the pupillary passage that causes angle-closure glaucoma in association with ROP is due to growth of the crystalline lens or is due to change in retrolental membranes causing the lens to move farther forward, we do not know. In one instance, we know that the precipitating factor that caused the angle finally to close was the use of mydriatic-cycloplegic drops for refraction. When iridectomy is performed in these eyes, the preoperative convexity of the iris is lost, and the iris conforms more closely to the lens surface and even takes on a concave curvature in its mid-periphery. When synechiae have not yet formed, the angle will appear strikingly more open.

The importance of an underlying anatomical or structural basis for angle-closure glaucoma in ROP is indicated by the fact that in some patients in whom the ROP has been considerably more severe in one eye than in the other, the anterior chamber has become shallow and angle-closure glaucoma has developed only in the eye with the more severe abnormality.

Because of the frequent acute onset of glaucoma in ROP and the potential benefit of iridectomy in preventing its occurrence, we have attempted to identify those patients who are at most risk for glaucoma. Severe posterior segment involvement, perilenticular membrane formation, shallow anterior chamber, narrow peripheral angle, iris leaf convexity, and most importantly progression of these anatomical findings are critical signs to be followed. We feel that prophylactic iridectomy should be seriously considered when these signs indicate a present and increasing risk of acute angle-closure glaucoma.

In eyes in which acute glaucoma has not been treated early by iridectomy, the disease has taken various courses. In young children in whom the eye was essentially blind before the onset of glaucoma, pain has sometimes been controlled medically, with aspirin and acetazolamide, until the IOP has decreased and the globe has become atrophic and painless. Alternatively, the glaucoma may persist and be asymptomatic. If this occurs and enucleation is not necessary, there is sometimes later a remarkable spontaneous deepening of the anterior chamber, and the eye has become soft despite permanent synechial closure of the angle.

The mechanism of the spontaneous variation in the depth of the anterior chamber that sometimes occurs in ROP has not been apparent to us on clinical examination, but we suppose that the deepening might be explained by contraction of a retrolental membrane attached to the lens.

Rubeosis of the iris may be expected in a high percentage of eyes with chronic retinal detachment secondary to ROP. When such eyes become uncomfortable, treatment by enucleation must be considered.

Treatment of angle-closure glaucoma associated with ROP is preferentially by iridectomy, with the same reasoning as in ordinary angle-closure glaucoma, but additional medical treatment or other types of surgery, including goniosynechialysis and lensectomy, may be indicated. This operation to open the angle after synechial closure has been surprisingly helpful even for eyes whose angles have been closed for an undetermined number of months.

We have observed a remarkable phenomenon after surgical peripheral iridectomies in ROP that we have not observed in any other condition in which this procedure has been tried. Peripheral iridectomies in ROP eyes frequently have become closed as a result of gradual drawing of the coloboma into the angle where it has become obliterated in contact with the angle wall. In some patients, this necessitates reoperation. Because of this occurrence after initially successful peripheral iridectomy, we recommend that a large peripheral or a sector iridectomy be done, which may also facilitate posterior segment examination.

MICROPHTHALMOS

It is important to remember that the glaucoma mechanism that occurs complicating ROP can also be seen in any microphthalmic eye. We have seen angle closure in primary microphthalmos, microphthalmos associated with congenital diffuse choroiditis, and in microphthalmos associated with anterior displacement of the lens and high myopia, but we have most frequently observed this as a complication of ROP.

REFERENCES

1. Givens KT, Lee DA, Jones T, et al. Congenital rubella syndrome: Ophthalmic manifestations and associated systemic disorders. *Br J Ophthalmol*. 1993;77:358-363.
2. Khandekar R, Al Awaidy S, Ganesh A, Bawikar S. An epidemiological and clinical study of ocular manifestations of congenital rubella syndrome in Omani children. *Arch Ophthalmol*. 2004;122(4):541-545.
3. Sears ML. Congenital glaucoma in neonatal rubella. *Br J Ophthalmol*. 1967;51(11):744-748.
4. Romano A, Weinberg M, Bar-Izhak, R, et al. Rate and various aspects of eye infection resulting from congenital rubella. *JPOS*. 1978;16(1):26-30.
5. Wolff SM. The ocular manifestations of congenital rubella: a prospective study of 328 cases of congenital rubella. *J Ped Ophthalmol*. 1973;10(2):101-141.
6. Boger WP III. Late ocular complications in congenital rubella syndrome. *Ophthalmology*. 1980;87:1244-1252.
7. O'Neill JF. The ocular manifestations of congenital infection: a study of the early effect and long-term outcome of maternally transmitted rubella and toxoplasmosis. *Trans Am Ophthalmol Soc*. 1998;96:813-879.
8. Pascual-Castroviejo I, et al. Sturge-Weber syndrome: study of 40 patients. *Pediatr Neurol*. 1993;9(4):283-288.

9. Japtap S, Srinivas G, Harsha KJ, Radhakrishnan N, Radhakrishnan A. Sturge-Weber Syndrome: clinical spectrum, disease course, and outcome of 30 patients. *J Child Neurol.* 2012;25.

10. Piram M, Lorette G, Sirinelli D, Herbretau D, Giraudeau B, Maruani A. Sturge-Weber syndrome in patients with facial port-wine stain. *Pediatr Dermatol.* 2012;29(1):32-37.

11. Tallman B, Tan OT, Morelli JG, et al. Location of port wine stains and the likelihood of ophthalmic and/or cental nervous system complications. *Pediatrics.* 1991;87(3):323-327.

12. Phelps CD. The pathogenesis of glaucoma in Sturge-Weber syndrome. *Ophthalmology.* 1978;85:276-286.

13. Bellows AR, Chylack LT Jr, Epstein DL, et al. Choroidal effusion during glaucoma surgery in patients with prominent episcleral vessels. *Arch Ophthalmol.* 1979;97:493-497.

14. Patrianakos TD, Nagao K, Walton DS. Surgical management of glaucoma with the Sturge Weber syndrome. *Int Ophthalmol Clin.* 2008;48:63-78.

15. Idrees F, Vaideanu D, Fraser SG, et al. Major review: a review of anterior segment dysgeneses. *Surv Ophthalmol.* 2006;51(3):213-231.

16. Mortemousque B, Amati-Bonneau P, Couture F, et al. Axenfeld-Rieger anomaly: a novel mutation in the Forkhead Box C1 (FOXC1) gene in a 4-generation family. *Arch Ophthalmol.* 2004;122:1527-1533.

17. Phillips JD. Four novel mutations in the PITX2 gene in patients with Axenfeld-Rieger syndrome. *Ophthalmic Res.* 2002;34:324-326.

18. Sturngaru MH, Dinu I, Walter MA. Genotype-phenotype correlations in Axenfeld-Rieger malformation and glaucoma patients with FOXC1 and PITX2 mutations. *Invest Ophthal & Visual Science.* 2007;48(1):228-237.

19. Walton DS, Katsavounidou G, Lowe CU. Glaucoma with the oculo-cerebrorenal syndrome of Lowe. *J Glaucoma.* 2005;14(3):181-185.

20. Grant WM, Walton DS. Distinctive gonioscopic findings in glaucoma due to neurofibromatosis. *Arch Ophthalmol.* 1968;79:127-134.

21. Ziakas NG, Ramsay AS, Lynch SA, et al. Stickler's syndrome associated with congenital glaucoma. *Ophthalmic Genet.* 1998;19:55-58.

22. Folz SJ, Trobe JD. The peroxisome and the eye. *Surv Ophthalmol.* 1991;35:353-368.

23. Muto R, Yamamori S, Ohashi H, Osawa M. Prediction by FISH analysis of the occurrence of Wilms tumor in aniridia. *Am J Med Genet.* 2002;108(4):285-289.

24. Chen TC, Walton DS. Goniosurgery for prevention of aniridic glaucoma. *Arch Ophthalmol.* 1999;117:1144-1148.

25. Nelson LB, Spaeth GL, Nowinski TS, Margo CE, Jackson L. Aniridia. a review. *Surv Ophthalmol.* 1984;28(6):621-642.

26. Yeung HH, Walton DS. Goniotomy for juvenile open-angle glaucoma. *J Glaucoma.* 2010;19(1):2-4.

27. Freedman SF, Rodriguez-Rosa RE, Rojas MC, et al. Goniotomy for glaucoma secondary to chronic childhood uveitis. *Am J Ophthalmol.* 2002;133:617-621.

28. Ho CL, Walton DS. Goniosurgery for glaucoma secondary to chronic anterior uveitis: prognostic factors and surgical technique. *J Glaucoma.* 2004;13(6):445-449.

29. Beck AD, Freedman SF, Lynn MS, et al. Glaucoma-related adverse events in the Infant Aphakia Treatment Study: 1-year results. *Arch Ophthalmol.* 2012;130(3):300-305.

SPECIAL CONSIDERATIONS

70

The Role of the
Cornea in Managing Glaucoma

Leon W. Herndon Jr, MD

In routine clinical practice, intraocular pressure (IOP) represents one of several important parameters used not only in the diagnosis of glaucoma but also for following the progression of this disease and its response to treatment. Certainly, its value as a diagnostic tool hinges upon the reliability of measurements taken. The technique used most commonly for this purpose is Goldmann (Haag-Streit, Bern, Switzerland) applanation tonometry (GAT) (Figure 70-1). In first describing their applanation tonometer, Goldmann and Schmidt discussed the effect of central corneal thickness (CCT) on IOP as measured by the new device.[1] They felt that variations in corneal thickness occurred rarely in the absence of corneal disease and assumed a CCT of 520 μm but acknowledged that, at least theoretically, CCT might influence applanation readings. They started from the hypothesis that the cornea might be considered as a sheath covered by 2 membranes between which almost nonshifting water is located. It has since become apparent that CCT is more variable among clinically normal patients than Goldmann and Schmidt[1] ever realized. Studies by Von Bahr[2,3] showed that there were large variations in CCT within a normal population, and studies by Ehlers and colleagues[4-6] demonstrated that this variation in CCT had an effect on applanation-measured IOP. Many studies have since looked at the influence of CCT on IOP measurement with most agreeing that there is an increase in measured IOP with increasing CCT. However, CCT alone accounts for only a small proportion of the interindividual variation in measured IOP. In a manometric study,[6] Ehlers and colleagues cannulated 29 otherwise normal eyes undergoing cataract surgery and correlated corneal thickness with errors in GAT. They found that GAT most accurately reflected true intracameral IOP when CCT was 520 μm and that deviations from this value resulted in an over- or underestimation of IOP by as much as 7 mm Hg per 100 μm. Johnson and colleagues[7] reported a patient with a CCT of 900 μm with a manometric IOP of 11 mm Hg, but when measured by applanation, the IOP had ranged from 30 to 40 mm Hg while the patient was receiving maximum medical therapy! In a manometric study with the Perkins tonometer (Haag-Streit, Mason, OH), Whitacre and colleagues[8] demonstrated an underestimation of IOP by as much as 4.9 mm Hg in thin corneas, with thick corneas producing an overestimation by as much as 6.8 mm Hg. This corresponded to a calculated range of 0.18 to 0.49 mm Hg of change in IOP for a 10-μm change in CCT from the mean CCT.

The Goldmann tonometer measures the force required to applanate the eye to 3.06-mm diameter. The force required is a combination of opposition to IOP plus the force needed to bend the cornea (less a small attraction due to surface tension). Therefore, simply stated, the thicker the cornea, the higher the force needed to bend and the thinner the cornea, the lower the force needed to bend. Hence, deviation from normal CCT results in a potentially incorrect indication of IOP.

DISEASE IMPLICATIONS

A number of studies have looked at the distribution of CCT according to diagnosis in primary open-angle glaucoma (POAG), normal-tension glaucoma (NTG), and ocular hypertension (OHT). There was found to be a significant difference in the mean CCT of these 3 groups. In a study by Shah and colleagues,[9] normal eyes had a mean CCT of 554 μm. The POAG eyes had a mean CCT of 550 μm, the NTG eyes had a mean CCT of 514 μm, and the OHT eyes had a mean CCT of 580 μm. Similarly, Copt and colleagues[10] measured the CCT among patients classified as having POAG, NTG, and OHT. In addition to confirming that

Kahook MY, Schuman JS, eds.
Chandler and Grant's Glaucoma, Fifth Edition (pp 683-688).
© 2013 SLACK Incorporated.

patients with OHT had thicker corneas than their control and POAG counterparts, they likewise found that patients classified as having NTG had thinner corneas.

Central corneal thickness has been recognized as a significant risk factor for progression of ocular hypertensive patients to POAG in the Ocular Hypertension Treatment Study (OHTS).[11] This study was the first to prospectively demonstrate that a decreased CCT predicts the development of POAG. Participants with a CCT of 555 μm or less had a 3-fold greater risk of developing POAG compared with participants who had a CCT of more than 588 μm. This inverse relationship was found across the ranges of baseline IOP and baseline vertical cup-disc ratios. Medeiros and colleagues[12] studied 98 eyes of 98 patients with pre-perimetric glaucomatous optic neuropathy. The diagnosis of glaucomatous optic neuropathy (GON) was based on masked assessment of optic disc stereo photographs. All patients had normal standard automated perimetry visual fields at baseline. Thirty-four patients developed repeatable visual field abnormality during follow-up. A thinner central cornea predicted the development of visual field conversion in both univariate and multivariate models. Mean CCT was significantly lower in converters than in nonconverters. Medeiros and colleagues also found that a CCT value of 545 μm was the best dividing point to separate patients who developed visual field conversion from the patients who did not. At 4-year follow-up, the cumulative probability of developing visual field conversion was 46% in patients with CCT less than 545 μm compared to 11% in patients with CCT of 545 μm or more. Herndon and colleagues[13] retrospectively examined the initial visit of consecutive POAG patients over a 5-year period. They found that a lower CCT was a powerful clinical factor associated with a worsened Advanced Glaucoma Intervention Study (AGIS) score, worsened mean deviation of visual field, increased vertical and horizontal cup/disc ratios, and increased number of glaucoma medications.

RACIAL DIFFERENCES IN CENTRAL CORNEAL THICKNESS

Until recently, most pachymetry studies were performed on predominately White populations. Foster and colleagues,[14] however, studied more than 1000 Mongolian patients in rural China and found that this population had CCT measurements that were 30 to 40 μm lower than the average CCT in surveys found in White groups. Kunert and colleagues[15] measured the CCT of 615 Indian patients who presented for refractive surgery evaluation and found this group to have a mean CCT of approximately 520 μm. Several investigators have provided further evidence that Black subjects, as a group, tend to have thinner corneas than their White counterparts. LaRosa and colleagues[16] reported thinner CCT values among Black male veterans compared with their White counterparts. Nemesure and colleagues,[17]

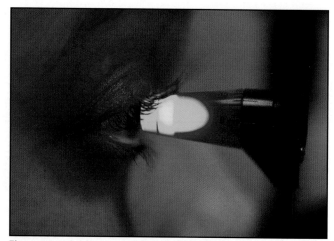

Figure 70-1. Goldmann applanation tonometry.

following a CCT survey of participants in the Barbados Eye Survey, reported that Black participants had thinner corneas (mean thickness 530 μm) than White participants (545 μm). Shimmyo and colleagues[18] performed a retrospective biometric review of patients at a large refractive surgery center, also finding that Black patients had thinner corneas than White patients seeking refractive surgery; they found no difference in CCT among White, Asian, and Hispanic patients in their population. This is in contrast to the findings of the population-based Los Angeles Latino Eye Study[19] that found CCTs among their Hispanic patients intermediate between values reported for Black and White populations. Herndon and colleagues[13] showed that Black persons with POAG had a significantly lower CCT (537 μm) compared to White persons (556 μm). These racial differences in CCT may in part explain the more advanced progression of glaucomatous disease at a relatively lower measured IOP among some groups.

CORNEAL REFRACTIVE SURGERY AND TONOMETRY

Laser-assisted in situ keratomileusis (LASIK) procedures are performed throughout the world among mostly young to middle-aged myopes. Myopia is a strong risk factor for the development of glaucoma,[20] and many of the patients undergoing LASIK today are destined genetically to develop glaucoma in the coming decades. Although we do not yet know how to correct a GAT measurement made on a LASIK-thinned cornea, it is clear that in many cases GAT will grossly under-estimate IOP. The problem will arise 10 or 15 years from now when patients neglect to inform their ophthalmologist that they had LASIK years ago, and a GAT measurement of 18 mm Hg is regarded as normal despite a 425-μm cornea.

One promising technology that may prove useful is the dynamic contour tonometer (DCT) (Pascal; Swiss Microtechnology AG, Port, Switzerland). This device consists of an electronic strain gauge embedded in a contoured

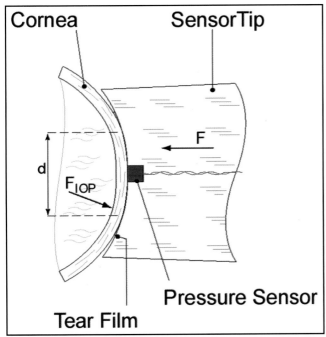

Figure 70-2. As opposed to forceful applanation, the contoured surface of the Pascal tonometer tip closely matches corneal shape. When this match is achieved, the law of Pascal states that tangential forces are theoretically neutralized.

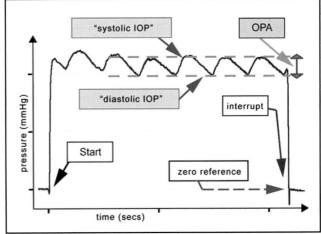

Figure 70-3. Ocular pulse amplitude is the difference in IOP between systole and diastole.

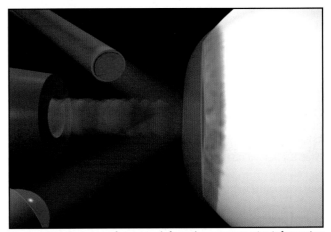

Figure 70-4. Emission of air jet to deform the cornea to give information on the ORA.

plastic tip. When in contact with the cornea, the tonometer tip creates a tight-fitting shell on the corneal surface without applanation of corneal tissue (Figure 70-2). The assumption is that the tonometer compensates for all forces exerted on the cornea, allowing the strain gauge to measure IOP largely independent of corneal properties. Studies have shown that the IOP measured by DCT is not altered after LASIK, unlike IOP measured by GAT.[21,22] Realini and colleagues[23] evaluated the diurnal IOP of 47 subjects with POAG and 38 normal control patients. They found no correlation between GAT and CCT and a weak inverse correlation between DCT and CCT in glaucoma eyes, which was different from the associations seen in normal controls. This finding might suggest that the collagen of the cornea is altered by glaucoma (or its treatment) altering the biomechanical properties of the cornea. DCT also provides a measurement called the ocular pulse amplitude (OPA), which may be a marker for overall ocular rigidity. OPA is the difference in IOP between systole and diastole (Figure 70-3). In studying the clinical utility of the OPA, Weizer and colleagues[24] found that an increased OPA was associated with a decreased severity of glaucoma. Kaufmann and colleagues[25] measured OPA in 223 healthy eyes and found that these readings were not affected by CCT or corneal curvature. The readings were, however, affected by IOP and axial length.

THE BIOMECHANICS FACTOR

Goldmann applanation tonometry measures IOP by flattening the cornea, which is not neutral in this measurement. Liu and Roberts[26] have shown that factors affecting corneal resistance include structural considerations, such as the amount of rigidity produced by the way the collagen beams in the tissue line up. The bendability of corneal tissue can also be affected by short-term factors, such as the presence of corneal edema. The ocular response analyzer (ORA; Reichert Technologies, Depew, NY) measures the corneal response to indentation by a rapid air pulse (Figure 70-4). The principles of the ORA are based on those of noncontact tonometry, in which the IOP is determined by the air pressure required to applanate the central cornea. The instrument makes 2 measurements of the corneal response to the pulse of air— the force required to flatten the cornea as the air pressure rises (force-in applanation, P1) and the force at which the cornea becomes flat again as the air pressure falls (force-out applanation, P2). The difference between the 2 pressures is termed *corneal hysteresis* (CH) (Figure 70-5). Corneal hysteresis is a direct measure of the cornea's biomechanical properties and may more completely describe the contribution of corneal resistance to IOP measurements than CCT alone.[27] The corneal resistance factor (CRF) is another measurement

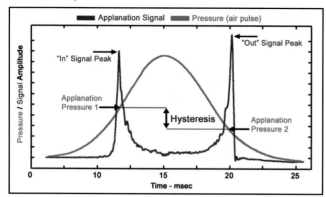

Figure 70-5. Profiles corresponding to an ORA measurement of IOP and corneal biomechanical properties.

of corneal biomechanical properties produced by the ORA and is derived from the formula P1 – *k*P2 where *k* is a constant. The CRF offers a measurement of corneal resistance and is a parameter that is relatively unaffected by changes in IOP. A feature of the ORA is that the maximum air pressure applied is not constant and is dependent on P1, a value determined by both the true IOP and the structural resistance of each individual eye. Kotecha and colleagues[28] recently assessed what effect this feature might have on CH values by measuring eyes before and after pharmacological reduction of IOP. The study found a weak but significant negative correlation between changes in CH and changes in IOP, such that higher values of CH were found at lower levels of IOP. Variations in maximum air pressure applied to the cornea may cause differing amounts of corneal indentation. Further work is needed to determine whether these variations alter the CH measurement.

The same study[28] also assessed the relationship between changes in P1 and P2 following the medical lowering of IOP and found that, for every unit change in P1, there was a corresponding proportional change in P2. This relationship was used to determine the constant *k* for the equation (P1 – *k*P2) to derive a parameter termed the corneal constant factor (CCF). Both the CCF and CRF are corneal parameters that are relatively unaffected by IOP, unlike CH. In this study,[28] CH, CCF, and CRF were positively associated with CCT, suggesting that thicker corneas exhibit greater viscoelastic properties. There was a negative association between both CCF and CRF and advancing age, possibly due to an age-related increase in cross-linking of collagen fibrils within the cornea leading to a stiffer structure. Congdon and colleagues[29] found that a lower CH was more associated with progression of visual field loss in their study than was a lower CCT.

Corneal hysteresis has been shown to be reduced in patients with keratoconus and Fuchs' endothelial dystrophy, conditions that cause a progressive decrease and increase in CCT, respectively. This finding may be an indication of the biomechanical similarities of such corneas in which alterations of stromal lamellar organization are known to

occur.[30,31] CH has also been shown to be markedly reduced in children with congenital glaucoma, especially in those with marked Haab's striae and larger corneal diameters.[32] Pepose and colleagues[33] have shown that following LASIK, CH and CRF show a marked reduction. This change in corneal biomechanical properties may be a result of the creation of the LASIK flap altering anterior stromal lamellar organization.

The effect of diabetes mellitus on the cornea may have clinical significance.[34] Stromal changes include structural alterations produced by collagen cross-linking.[35] In vitro studies show that collagen cross-linking causes increased stiffness of the cornea[36,37] that in turn may affect the measurement of IOP, causing overestimation of the true IOP.[38] Goldich and colleagues[39] compared the parameters of biomechanical response of the human cornea measured with the ORA in patients with diabetes mellitus and healthy control subjects. The results of their study showed that the CCT, CH, and CRF in diabetic eyes were significantly higher than in nondiabetic eyes. The results of the OHTS[40] suggest that there may be some protective effect of diabetes on the progression to POAG. Although this finding has been widely debated, the results of the Goldich study support it.

Researchers have investigated the possibility that a thick or thin cornea may tell us something about the back of the eye. It has been noted, for instance, that Black Americans have thinner corneas than White Americans and often have more advanced glaucoma,[16-18] so it is possible that a thinner cornea may indicate a thinner or more susceptible lamina cribrosa or optic nerve. Other research has found that ocular hypertensive patients with thinner corneas have thinner nerve fiber layers than ocular hypertensive patients with thicker corneas and healthy control subjects.[41] It is also possible that differences in corneal biomechanics may indicate more generalized structural differences between eyes. Wells and colleagues[42] investigated the relationship between acute IOP-induced optic nerve head deformation and CH and CCT in normal and glaucomatous eyes. They found that in glaucoma patients, CH but not CCT was associated with increased deformation of the optic nerve surface during transient elevations of IOP. This finding did not hold true in control patients, suggesting that glaucoma may modify the biomechanical properties of tissues supporting the optic nerve head. Quigley and colleagues[43] and Hernandez[44] have reported that there are alterations in the elastin of the optic nerve head in both human and experimental glaucoma and have suggested that differences in elastin function may have a part to play in susceptibility to glaucomatous injury. It remains unknown whether such elastin alterations relate to CCT differences. Two recent papers[45,46] suggest that there indeed may be an anatomical correlation between CCT and optic nerve susceptibility. Gunvant and colleagues[45] examined the relationship between CCT and optic disc topography, as determined by scanning laser ophthalmoscopy (SLO). They found that thinner corneas appear to be associated with larger and deeper optic disc cups in glaucoma patients. Kourkoutas and colleagues[46] investigated the relationship between CCT and optic disc topography, as determined by the Heidelberg Retina Tomograph (HRTII; Heidelberg Engineering, Heidelberg, Germany). They also found that there was a correlation between CCT and HRTII optic nerve head structural measurements in glaucoma patients. Finally, CCT shows a strong parent–child heritability.[47] Siblings and offspring of those with thin CCT are likely to have similarly thin CCT, and perhaps a more susceptible optic nerve head underlying the increased familial risk for glaucoma.

It has only recently become possible to measure the biomechanical properties of the cornea in vivo, and the importance of these properties rests primarily with its effects on IOP measurement. It is possible, however, that corneal biomechanics may give an indication of the structural integrity of the optic nerve head. Further work is required to determine precisely how we might be able to risk-stratify glaucoma patients based on their biomechanical properties.

CORRECTION ALGORITHMS

In the past few years, many practitioners have come to rely on several conversion tables that use an algorithm to adjust IOP measured with Goldmann based on CCT. What we've learned about corneal biomechanics indicates that this approach is not necessarily reliable. It may produce an accurate IOP for many patients but there is no way to know which patients those are. One 580-μm cornea may be altering the IOP reading very differently than another of the same thickness. Also, given the racial differences in CCT, one would likely need tables that take these differences into account. Confronted with the expanding evidence that CCT is an important ocular parameter that should be measured in clinical practice, clinicians understandably wonder what to do with the information.[13,40,41,45] A general recommendation supported by the data is that one can take far better care of patients simply by categorizing corneas as "thin, average, or thick," just as it is important to recognize that optic discs come in "small, medium, and large," allowing the clinician to interpret disc configurations accordingly.

IMPLICATIONS FOR CLINICAL PRACTICE

In clinical practice, the applanating pressure measured using an applanation tonometer is considered to be equal to the IOP. However, because further experimental studies show that this is not always true, a distinction can be made by denoting the measured applanating pressure as Goldmann's applanating pressure and as the true IOP. In the journal *Bulletin of Mathematical Biology*, Orssengo and Pye describe a theoretical mathematical model of the cornea for applanation tonometry where the cornea was modeled as a shell.[48] Theoretical equations for the deformation of a shell were used to derive the equation for predicting the true IOP. They considered the deformations of

the cornea due to both the intraocular and applanating pressures. The anterior cornea deforms radially inward due to the dominance of the applanating pressure, while away from the applanated area the cornea deforms radially outward due to the dominance of the IOP. The Goldmann tonometer simply measures the force needed to deform the cornea in a standardized manner. IOP is derived from the force measurement indirectly, based on a number of assumptions about corneal deformability. Corneal deformability in turn represents a summation of the cornea's curvature, elastic properties, surface tension, and the IOP. While CCT is a major component of corneal elasticity, it is likely not the only component. The mix of collagen types, corneal hydration, packing density of collagen fibrils, the extracellular matrix, and other factors undoubtedly vary among individuals; in some patients, these other factors may dwarf the effect of CCT on the accuracy of IOP estimation. A LASIK flap can be lifted easily a year or more after the procedure. Does this flap slide over its bed during applanation, altering corneal rigidity in ways we cannot imagine? There is evidence that the potent IOP-lowering effect of the prostaglandin analogs results not only from their impressive effects on outflow but also through an effect on the corneal extracellular matrix.[49,50]

FUTURE DIRECTIONS

We now grudgingly recognize that our ability to accurately measure IOP is far weaker than we've ever imagined—we have spent half a century believing that a flawed one-time measurement told us enough about our patients on which to base clinical decision making. A failure to question whether our measurement techniques were sufficiently accurate to guide patient care has led us to propose a variety of hypotheses to explain the outliers—patients who did not seem to fit the mold of a pressure-sensitive disease. As new technologies are developed to measure IOP with greater precision (and on a continuous basis), it seems likely that a much tighter dose-response relationship between glaucoma damage and IOP will be found. Incorporating corneal parameters into our thinking is but the beginning of this transformation.

REFERENCES

1. Goldmann H, Schmidt T. Uber applanationstonometrie. *Ophthalmologica.* 1957;134:221-242.
2. Von Bahr G. Measurements of the thickness of the cornea. *Acta Ophthalmol.* 1948;26:247-266.
3. Von Bahr G. Corneal thickness; its measurement and changes. *Am J Ophthalmol.* 1956;42:251-266.
4. Ehlers N, Hansen FK, Aasved H. Biometric correlations of corneal thickness. *Acta Ophthalmol (Copenh).* 1975;53:652-659.
5. Ehlers N, Hansen FK. Central corneal thickness in low-tension glaucoma. *Acta Ophthalmol (Copenh).* 1974;52:740-746.
6. Ehlers N, Bramsen T, Sperling S. Applanation tonometry and central corneal thickness. *Acta Ophthalmol (Copenh).* 1975;53:34-43.
7. Johnson M, Kass MA, Moses RA, et al. Increased corneal thickness simulating elevated IOP. *Arch Ophthalmol.* 1978;96:664-665.

8. Whitacre MM, Stein RA, Hassanein K. The effect of corneal thickness on applanation tonometry. *Am J Ophthalmol*. 1993;115:592-596.

9. Shah S, Chatterjee A, Mathai M, et al. Relationship between corneal thickness and measured IOP in a general ophthalmology clinic. *Ophthalmology*. 1999;106:2154-2160.

10. Copt RP, Thomas R, Mermoud A. Corneal thickness in ocular hypertension, primary open-angle glaucoma, and normal tension glaucoma. *Arch Ophthalmol*. 1999;117:14-16.

11. Gordon MO, Beiser JA, Brandt JD, et al. The Ocular Hypertension Treatment Study: baseline factors that predict the onset of primary open-angle glaucoma. *Arch Ophthalmol*. 2002;120:714-720.

12. Medeiros FA, Sample PA, Zangwill LM, et al. Corneal thickness as a risk factor for visual field loss in patients with preperimetric glaucomatous optic neuropathy. *Am J Ophthalmol*. 2003;136:805-813.

13. Herndon LW, Weizer JS, Stinnett SS. Central corneal thickness as a risk factor for advanced glaucoma damage. *Arch Ophthalmol*. 2004;122:17-21.

14. Foster PJ, Baasanhu J, Alsbirk PH, et al. Central corneal thickness and IOP in a Mongolian population. *Ophthalmology*. 1998;105: 969-973.

15. Kunert KS, Bhartiya P, Tandon R, et al. Central corneal thickness in Indian patients undergoing LASIK for myopia. *J Refract Surg*. 2003;19:378-379.

16. LaRosa FA, Gross RL, Orengo-Nania S. Central corneal thickness of Whites and African Americans in glaucomatous and nonglaucomatous populations. *Arch Ophthalmol*. 2001;119:23-27.

17. Nemesure B, Wu SY, Hennis A, et al. Corneal thickness and intraocular pressure in the Barbados eye studies. *Arch Ophthalmol*. 2003;121:240-244.

18. Shimmyo M, Ross AJ, Moy A, et al. IOP, Goldmann applanation tension, corneal thickness, and corneal curvature in Whites, Asians, Hispanics, and African Americans. *Am J Ophthalmol*. 2003;136:603-613.

19. Hahn S, Azen S, Ying-Lai M, et al. Central corneal thickness in Latinos. *Invest Ophthalmol Vis Sci*. 2003;44:1508-1512.

20. Mitchell P, Hourihan F, Sandbach J, et al. The relationship between glaucoma and myopia: the Blue Mountains Eye Study. *Ophthalmology*. 1999;106:2010-2015.

21. Kaufmann C, Bachmann LM, Thiel MA. IOP measurements using dynamic contour tonometry after laser in situ keratomileusis. *Invest Ophthalmol Vis Sci*. 2003;44:3790-3794.

22. Siganos DS, Papastergiou GI, Moedas C. Assessment of the Pascal dynamic contour tonometer in monitoring IOP in unoperated eyes and eyes after LASIK. *J Cataract Refract Surg*. 2004;30:746-751.

23. Realini T, Weinreb RN, Hobbs G. Correlation of IOP measured with Goldmann and dynamic contour tonometry in normal and glaucomatous eyes. *J Glaucoma*. 2009;18:119-123.

24. Weizer JS, Asrani S, Stinnett SS, et al. The clinical utility of dynamic contour tonometry and ocular pulse amplitude. *J Glaucoma*. 2007;16:700-703.

25. Kaufmann C, Bachmann LM, Robert YC, et al. Ocular pulse amplitude in healthy subjects as measured by dynamic contour tonometry. *Arch Ophthalmol*. 2006;124:1104-108.

26. Liu J, Roberts CJ. Influence of corneal biomechanical properties on IOP measurement: quantitative analysis. *J Cataract Refract Surg*. 2005;31:146-155.

27. Luce DA. Determining in vivo biomechanical properties of the cornea with an ocular response analyzer. *J Cataract Refract Surg*. 2005;31:156-162.

28. Kotecha A, Elsheikh A, Roberts CR, et al. Corneal thickness- and age-related biomechanical properties of the cornea measured with the ocular response analyzer. *Invest Ophthalmol Vis Sci*. 2006;47:5337-5347.

29. Congdon NG, Broman AT, Bandeen-Roche K, et al. Central corneal thickness and corneal hysteresis associated with glaucoma damage. *Am J Ophthalmol*. 2006;141:868-875.

30. Hayes S, Boote C, Tuft SJ, et al. A study of corneal thickness, shape and collagen organisation in keratoconus using videokeratography and X-ray scattering techniques. *Exp Eye Res*. 2007;84:423-434.

31. Meek KM, Leonard DW, Connon CJ, et al. Transparency, swelling and scarring in the corneal stroma. *Eye*. 2003;17:927-936.

32. Kirwan C, O'Keefe M, Lanigan B. Corneal hysteresis and IOP measurement in children using the Reichert ocular response analyzer. *Am J Ophthalmol*. 2006;142:990-992.

33. Pepose JS, Feigenbaum SK, Qazi MA, et al. Changes in corneal biomechanics and IOP following LASIK using static, dynamic, and noncontact tonometry. *Am J Ophthalmol*. 2007;143:39-47.

34. Sanchez-Thorin JC. The cornea in diabetes mellitus. *Int Ophthalmol Clin*. 1998;38:19-36.

35. Monnier VM, Sell DR, Abdul-Karim FW, et al. Collagen browning and cross-linking are increased in chronic experimental hyperglycemia: relevance to diabetes and aging. *Diabetes*. 1988;37: 867-872.

36. Wollensak G, Spoerl E, Seiler T. Stress-strain measurements of human and porcine corneas after riboflavin-ultraviolet-A-induced cross-linking. *J Cataract Refract Surg*. 2003;29:1780-1785.

37. Dupps WJ, Netto MV, Herekar S, et al. Surface wave elastometry of the cornea in porcine and human donor eyes. *J Refract Surg*. 2007;23:66-75.

38. Krueger RR, Ramos-Esteban JC. How might corneal elasticity help us understand diabetes and IOP? *J Refract Surg*. 2007;23:85-88.

39. Goldich Y, Barkana Y, Gerber Y, et al. Effect of diabetes mellitus on biomechanical parameters of the cornea. *J Cataract Refract Surg*. 2009;35:715-719.

40. Brandt JD, Beiser JA, Kass MA, et al. Central corneal thickness in the OHTS. *Ophthalmology*. 2001;108:1779-1788.

41. Henderson PA, Medeiros FA, Zangwill LM, et al. Relationship between central corneal thickness and retinal nerve fiber layer thickness in ocular hypertensive patients. *Ophthalmology*. 2005;112:251-256.

42. Wells A, Garway-Heath D, Poostchi A, et al. Corneal hysteresis but not central corneal thickness correlates with optic nerve surface deformation in glaucoma patients. *Invest Ophthalmol Vis Sci*. 2008;49:3262-3268.

43. Quigley HA, Brown A, Dorman-Pease ME. Alterations in elastin of the optic nerve head in human and experimental glaucoma. *Br J Ophthalmol*. 1991;75:552-557.

44. Hernandez MR. Ultrastructural immunocytochemical analysis of elastin in the human lamina cribrosa. Changes in elastic fibers in primary open-angle glaucoma. *Invest Ophthalmol Vis Sci*. 1992;33:2891-2903.

45. Gunvant P, Porsia L, Watkins RJ, et al. Relationships between central corneal thickness and optic disc topography in eyes with glaucoma. Suspicion of glaucoma, or ocular hypertension. *Clin Ophthalmol*. 2008;2:591-599.

46. Kourkoutas D, Georgopoulos G, Maragos A, et al. New nonlinear multivariable model shows the relationship between central corneal thickness and HRTII topographic parameters in glaucoma patients. *Clin Ophthalmol*. 2009;3:313-323.

47. Landers JA, Hewitt AW, Dimasi DP, et al. Heritability of central corneal thickness in nuclear families. *Invest Ophthalmol Vis Sci*. 2009;50:4087-4090.

48. Orssengo GJ, Pye DC. Determination of the true IOP and modulus of elasticity of the human cornea in vivo. *Bull Math Biol*. 1999;61:551-572.

49. Sen E, Nalcacioglu P, Yazici A, et al. Comparison of the effects of latanoprost and bimatoprost on central corneal thickness. *J Glaucoma*. 2008;17:398-402.

50. Hatanaka M, Vessani RM, Elias IR, et al. The effect of prostaglandin analogs and prostamide on central corneal thickness. *J Ocul Pharmacol Ther*. 2009;25:51-53.

71

Twenty-Four–Hour Intraocular Pressure Monitoring in Glaucoma

Brian J. Song, MD and Lama A. Al-Aswad, MD

Glaucoma is classically defined as an optic neuropathy leading to progressive visual field loss. Historically, glaucoma was often described as high pressure in the eye leading to blindness if left untreated.[1-3] Over the past few decades, it has been established that glaucoma is not simply a condition of elevated intraocular pressure (IOP). There are multiple risk factors (ie, age, race, family history) that are associated with glaucoma. Though elevated IOP is one of the major risk factors associated with the development of glaucoma, it is now known that glaucoma can occur at any IOP level. Over the past decade, fluctuations in IOP have been identified as a potentially greater risk factor for visual field loss than an elevated mean IOP itself.[4] While much recent research has focused on direct neuroprotection, IOP remains the only modifiable risk factor and effective target for therapy.[5-9] Consequently, the ability to accurately assess IOP is essential for diagnosis and determining the efficacy of treatment in patients with glaucoma.[10]

CIRCADIAN VARIATIONS IN INTRAOCULAR PRESSURE

Twenty-four-hour measurements of IOP have shown that IOP tends to fluctuate throughout the course of the day.[11-15] In addition, it is believed that patients with ocular hypertension and glaucomatous disease experience greater fluctuations in IOP than those with normal eyes.[16] Both short-term and long-term factors can affect the variability of the diurnal-IOP curve. Short-term factors such as eating and drinking can not only increase one's overall fluid volume, but the change in osmolarity that occurs (depending on what is consumed) can also cause IOP to rise.[17] In addition, changes in blood pressure and posture can also affect IOP.[17-19] As body position changes, there is a shift in body fluids that seems to alter ocular hemodynamics and perfusion pressure.[18] It is also known that maneuvers that cause an increase in intrathoracic pressure (ie, Valsalva) can also cause elevations in IOP.[20] Over the long term, IOP seems to be correlated with diurnal cortisol levels, as aqueous production is highest in the morning and trends downward throughout the day.[21] There is also limited evidence that IOP undergoes seasonal fluctuations as well.[22]

Previous studies have shown that IOP tends to be highest in the morning hours in both normal and glaucoma patients.[23] This peak appears to be followed by a steady decline throughout the day. IOP then peaks again during the nocturnal period, possibly because of the change in body position from upright to supine, despite the decreased production of aqueous humor during this time period.[19,24] Figure 71-1 depicts the 24-hour IOP curves in the sitting and supine positions in healthy, young individuals. Wilensky and colleagues[25] found that 50% of the time, the highest pressures were found between the hours of 5:00 PM and 8:00 AM. An increase in episcleral venous pressure in the supine sleeping position may be one explanation for this phenomenon.[26] As a result, decreasing episcleral venous pressure may be a worthwhile target in developing new therapies for these patients.[18] However, 2 studies[27,28] examining supine-IOPs found that nocturnal-IOPs were higher than diurnal-IOPs in healthy young individuals, implying that the nocturnal pressure spike cannot be completely explained by body positioning. Interestingly, these same studies also showed diurnal-IOP may actually be higher than the nocturnal-IOP in glaucoma patients. It should be noted that all such studies[29] that examine 24-hour diurnal fluctuations in IOP assume that awakening the patient from sleep to measure IOP does not otherwise alter the normal physiologic fluctuations in IOP.

Kahook MY, Schuman JS, eds.
Chandler and Grant's Glaucoma, Fifth Edition (pp 689-694).

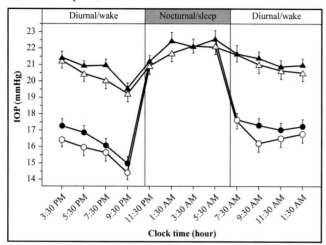

Figure 71-1. Profiles of 24-hour IOP variation in the 2 eyes of healthy, young subjects. Solid symbols represent IOP in the right eye and open symbols represent IOP in the left eye. Circles represent sitting IOP and triangles represent supine IOP. (This article was published in *Ophthalmology*, 112, Liu JH, Sit AJ, Weinreb RN, Variation of 24-hour IOP in healthy individuals: right eye versus left eye, 1670-1675, Copyright Elsevier 2005.)

CORNEAL BIOMECHANICS AND INTRAOCULAR PRESSURE

Central corneal thickness (CCT) is a well-established confounding factor that can impact the accuracy of applanation tonometry.[30] While thinner corneas tend to lead to an underestimation of true IOP, eyes with thicker corneas lead to an overestimation in IOP measurements. The Ocular Hypertension Treatment Study[10] (OHTS) highlighted the importance of CCT of corneal thickness by demonstrating an inverse relationship between CCT and the risk of developing glaucoma. Interestingly, it has been found that CCT also follows a diurnal pattern.[31] Like IOP, CCT is highest in the morning upon awakening and tends to decrease throughout the day. As a result, it is unclear what degree of measured diurnal IOP fluctuations are due to true variations in IOP versus variations in CCT. In addition to CCT, however, corneal biomechanics encompasses other properties, such as viscosity, elasticity, and hydration that can influence IOP measurement and evaluation.[32]

The concept of corneal hysteresis (CH), which can be likened to corneal stiffness, is gaining attention as a potentially more important biomechanical property that can affect IOP measurements during applanation tonometry.[33-36] CH is the difference between the force-in and force-out applanation pressures using a metered air pulse from a device called an ocular response analyzer (ORA; Reichert Technologies, Depew, NY).[37,38] While thicker corneas tend to be more rigid, there are exceptions as in Fuch's dystrophy where the cornea is thicker than normal but biomechanically floppy.[38,39] As a result, CH is likely to be a more useful measure of corneal resistance than CCT.[37] A

second property, corneal resistance factor (CRF), is defined as a linear function of the 2 peak pressures measured by the ORA and reflects corneal elasticity, whereas CH is more comparable to corneal viscosity.[38] As with CCT, there is a significant inverse relationship between IOP and CH.[40] Though it is still unclear whether people with thinner and/or less rigid corneas have a corresponding defect in structural integrity that predisposes them to glaucomatous damage, increasing evidence shows a correlation between decreased CCT and CH with glaucoma[41] with at least one report[42] in the literature demonstrating an association between CH and visual field progression.

IMPLICATIONS OF DIURNAL VARIATIONS IN INTRAOCULAR PRESSURE

In other organ systems, including the eye, the body is able to adapt and establish an equilibrium to some degree in the setting of chronic change. For example, chronic hypertension can promote atherosclerosis and other changes, such as left ventricular hypertrophy, but the majority of these patients tend to be asymptomatic for long periods of time. Over the course of many years, these alterations eventually lead to end-organ dysfunction, such as heart failure, renal failure, or retinopathy. In the setting of acute hypertensive crisis, however, patients are often symptomatic with complaints of blurry vision, headaches, and mental status changes, in part due to the body's inability to adapt to such an acute elevation in pressure.

In this sense, the concept of IOP and its role in glaucoma is analogous. Patients do not experience pain or other symptoms in the setting of chronic glaucoma, as a relative equilibrium is established in the setting of a higher IOP. Most patients are unaware of their peripheral vision loss as elevated IOP causes apoptosis of retinal ganglion cells over time, and many glaucoma patients retain good central vision even with moderate or advanced disease. It is usually during the acute glaucomas (ie, acute angle closure, and neovascular) that patients may actually complain of symptoms such as pain and photophobia, in part because the eye has not had time to adjust to the sudden and dramatic increase in IOP. Along this same line of thought, the body (and, in this case, the eye) does not appear to tolerate abrupt loading and unloading changes in pressure well. For these reasons, it is not surprising that fluctuations in IOP have been identified as a significant independent risk factor for glaucomatous vision loss compared to elevated mean IOP alone in some studies.[4,43-46]

Currently, the evidence is mixed in determining if fluctuations in IOP are truly an independent risk factor for visual field progression, although a growing number of studies seem to suggest this is the case. In a review by Singh and Shrivastava,[24] they point out that the severity of disease or the level of IOP may actually determine the magnitude of fluctuations as opposed to the fluctuations being the cause of worsening disease.[24] While it does appear that patients with glaucoma tend to experience larger fluctuations in IOP than healthy individuals, it is unclear whether larger variations in IOP are a cause or a consequence of glaucomatous disease.[16,24] Prospective studies are needed to resolve the question of whether diurnal variations in IOP are truly a causative factor for glaucomatous progression, but no such studies have been performed to date.

The challenges of measuring and managing IOP are 2-fold. The first is to detect the magnitude of diurnal variation that occurs in patients with glaucoma. While increasing the frequency of and staggering office visits at different times of the day can be helpful to detect such fluctuations, this strategy is ineffective in detecting the changes that occur when changing positions or during the nocturnal period. As a result, a single IOP measurement during a routine office visit may not accurately represent the actual state of a patient's diurnal IOP curve as a whole. However, in the absence of a method for continuous IOP measurement, true 24-hour IOP and its associated fluctuations cannot be measured.[24]

The second and perhaps more challenging aspect of managing IOP variations is to find ways to not only lower IOP but to decrease the enlarged fluctuations that occur in glaucoma patients to a more physiologic range. The ideal treatment modality would cause a uniform reduction in both diurnal and nocturnal IOP.[29] In general, antiglaucoma medications with a longer half-life, such as the prostaglandin analogs, seem to be more effective at restricting IOP fluctuations than shorter-acting agents, such as pilocarpine and alpha-adrenergics.[47-51] However, pharmacokinetic properties of a drug may not be the only factor that determines its ability to regulate fluctuations in IOP. Two recent studies[52,53] have found the carbonic anhydrase inhibitors to be more effective than the beta-blockers at decreasing nocturnal IOP. It should also be noted that there is a direct correlation between mean IOP and the range of diurnal fluctuations, with the largest fluctuations occurring in those with the highest mean IOP.[17,50] As a result, the most effective antiglaucoma medications at lowering IOP may also be the most effective at narrowing the degree of diurnal variations. The same effect is seen in patients who undergo laser trabeculoplasty; as the mean IOP is lowered due to the effect of the procedure, there is also a corresponding reduction in the diurnal range.[54] In a study comparing glaucoma patients on medical therapy with those who underwent trabeculectomy, it was found that those patients who underwent trabeculectomy had a smaller diurnal range than those who were being managed by medications alone (2.2 mm Hg versus 3.2 mm Hg, respectively).[55] However, the mean IOP of the surgical patients (10.5 mm Hg) was also lower than that of the medically managed patients (11.2 mm Hg), thus reinforcing the notion that mean IOP and diurnal range are directly related.[55,56]

METHODS FOR 24-HOUR INTRAOCULAR PRESSURE MONITORING

Goldmann applanation tonometry (GAT; Haag-Streit, Bern, Switzerland) is currently considered the gold standard for measuring IOP. The basis of GAT is the Imbert-Fick law that states that the pressure inside a sphere surrounded by an infinitely thin membrane can be measured by a counterpressure that just flattens the membrane.[57] By applying a force to an applanated area of the central cornea, IOP is then calculated by using this principle.[58] However, GAT is limited by the fact that it is a static measurement that records IOP at a single point in time while the patient is in a sitting position, which does not account for habitual changes in body position.

A more promising and dynamic method of measuring IOP may be Pascal Dynamic Contour Tonometry (DCT; Ziemer Ophthalmic Solutions, Port, Switzerland). This instrument is able to record 100 IOP measurements per second while measuring IOP fluctuations throughout the cardiac cycle, providing a dynamic measurement over a 5- to 8-second period. Unlike GAT, which flattens an area of the central cornea, the contact surface of the DCT is concave to better match the curved contour of the corneal surface. As a result, DCT reduces some of the potential confounding effects of corneal biomechanics on the IOP measurement. Subsequently, CCT affects IOP measurements in DCT to a much lesser degree than in GAT.[59-62]

Currently, continuous IOP monitoring requires the controlled setting of a sleep laboratory where patients' IOPs can be recorded at regular intervals throughout the day and night.[29] However, the ideal tool for measuring IOP would be a self-monitoring, telemetric device that allows a continuous recording in an ambulatory setting. It should be inexpensive, noninvasive, and convenient, and its accuracy would not be affected by corneal biomechanics. A recent review by Sit proposes 2 potential categories (temporary and permanent) for continuous IOP recording.[63] Temporary IOP recording devices would collect IOP data over a finite period of time (eg, 24 hours) using noninvasive methods. The first such device was proposed by Maurice[64] in 1951 in the form of an indentation tonometer that was mounted to a headband. A scleral applanator that could be used to make measurements by detecting changes on the scleral surface was reported by Cooper and colleagues in 1977.[65] However, there were problems with calibration and significant variability was seen depending on the degree of the individual's scleral rigidity.[63,65-68] It appears that the cornea undergoes changes in viscoelasticity and strain with changes in IOP.[63,69] As a result, another alternative that has been proposed is a pressure-sensing contact lens that undergoes changes that correspond with changes in IOP.[70-72]

The idea for a permanent implantable IOP monitor was first proposed by Collins in 1965.[73] One potential method to accomplish this would be the implantation of a permanent capacitive pressure monitor potentially as part of an intraocular lens during routine cataract surgery.[74-77] More recently, Walter and colleagues[76,77] have further developed this concept to allow the IOP monitor to transmit digital measurements to the external environment via radio frequency.[75] While this IOP sensor has shown promise in animal studies, it has yet to be evaluated in human trials. Another concept for permanent IOP recording proposed[78,79] in the 1980s is the use of a strain gauge on a scleral buckle that could measure changes in scleral circumference due to fluctuations in IOP, similar to the one proposed by Cooper originally. The main drawbacks of both proposed methods, however, are based on the invasive nature of both devices, as it would be difficult to justify surgery in a patient with glaucoma who did not have either a cataract or retinal detachment for the purpose of placing a permanent IOP recording device. While the potential for developing a continuous IOP monitor has been promising in in vivo experiments, there are still many challenges that will need to be overcome before this technology becomes clinically practical.

CONCLUSION

IOP continues to be the most important risk factor in the management and treatment of glaucoma patients today. It should be remembered that IOP is a dynamic phenomenon that must be considered in its entirety when selecting medications or making decisions about laser or surgical intervention. Until neuroprotective treatment modalities that are independent of IOP become available, measuring and managing IOP will remain the primary focus of treatment. With greater knowledge of the role of diurnal IOP variations and its associated factors (eg, corneal biomechanics), stabilization of these fluctuations may become a target of future treatment modalities. Clearly, the development of more comprehensive tools that are better able to measure the full spectrum of a patient's true IOP and any corresponding disease progression will be needed to answer these questions but, in the interim, the importance of mean IOP in the treatment and management of glaucoma should not be overlooked.

REFERENCES

1. Drance SM. Glaucoma-changing concepts. *Eye.* 1992;6:337-345.
2. Obstbaum SA, Cioffi GA, Krieglstein GK, et al. Gold standard medical therapy for glaucoma: defining the criteria identifying measures for an evidence-based analysis. *Clin Ther.* 2004;26(12):2102-2120.
3. Hitchings RA. Glaucoma: an area of darkness. *Eye.* 2009;23:1764-1774.
4. Asrani S, Zeimer R, Wilensky J, et al. Large diurnal fluctuations in intraocular pressure are an independent risk factor in patients with glaucoma. *J Glaucoma.* 2000;9(2):134-142.
5. The Collaborative Normal Tension Study Group. The effectiveness of intraocular pressure reduction in the treatment of normal tension glaucoma. *Am J Ophthalmol.* 1998;126(4):498-505.
6. AGIS Investigators. The relationship between control of intraocular pressure and visual field deterioration. *Am J Ophthalmol.* 2000;130(4):429-440.
7. Kass MA, Heuer DK, Higginbotham EJ, et al. The Ocular Hypertension Treatment Study: a randomized trial determines that topical ocular hypertensive medication delays or prevents the onset of primary open-angle glaucoma. *Arch Ophthalmol.* 2002;120(6):701-713.
8. Leske MC, Heijl A, Hussein M, et al. Factors for glaucoma progression and the effect of treatment: the early manifest glaucoma trial. *Arch Ophthalmol.* 2003;121(1):48-56.
9. Lichter PR, Musch DC, Gillespie BW, et al. Interim clinical outcomes in the Collaborative Initial Glaucoma Treatment Study comparing initial treatment randomized to medications or surgery. *Ophthalmology.* 2001;108(11):1943-1953.
10. Brandt JD, Beiser JA, Kass MA, Gordon MO. Central corneal thickness in the Ocular Hypertension Treatment Study (OHTS). *Ophthalmology.* 2001;108(10):1779-1788.
11. Liu JH, Kripke DF, Hoffman RE, et al. Nocturnal elevation of intraocular pressure in young adults. *Invest Ophthalmol Vis Sci.* 1998;39(13):2707-2712.
12. Liu JH, Kripke DF, Twa MD, et al. Twenty-four hour pattern of intraocular pressure in the aging population. *Invest Ophthalmol Vis Sci.* 1999;40(12):2912-2917.
13. Liu JH, Sit AJ, Weinreb RN. Variation of 24-hour intraocular pressure in healthy individuals: right eye versus left eye. *Ophthalmology.* 2005;112(10):1670-1675.
14. Weinreb RN, Liu JH. Nocturnal rhythms of intraocular pressure. *Arch Ophthalmol.* 2006;124(2):269-270.
15. Wilensky JT. Diurnal variations in intraocular pressure. *Trans Am Ophthalmol Soc.* 1991;89:757-790.
16. David R, Zangwill L, Briscoe D, et al. Diurnal intraocular pressure variations: an analysis of 690 diurnal curves. *Br J Ophthalmol.* 1992;76(5):280-283.
17. Wilensky JT. The role of diurnal pressure measurements in the management of open angle glaucoma. *Curr Opin Ophthalmol.* 2004;15(2):90-92.
18. Liu JH. Diurnal measurement of intraocular pressure. *J Glaucoma.* 2001;10(5 suppl 1):S39-S41.
19. Liu JHK, Zhang X, Kripke DF, Wienreb R. Twenty-four hour intraocular pressure pattern associated with early glaucomatous changes. *Invest Ophthal Vis Sci.* 2003;44(4):1586-1591.
20. Brody S, Erb C, Veit R, Rau H. Intraocular pressure changes: the influence of psychological stress and the Valsalva maneuver. *Biol Psychol.* 1999;51(1):43-57.
21. Weitzman ED, Henkind P, Leitman M, et al. Correlative 24-hour relationship between intraocular pressure and plasma cortisol in normal subjects and patients with glaucoma. *Br J Ophthalmol.* 1975;59(10):566-572.
22. Koga T, Tanihara H. Seasonal variation of intraocular pressure in normal and glaucomatous eyes. *Jpn J Clin Ophthalmol.* 2001;55(8):1519-1522.
23. Saccà SC, Rolando M, Marletta A, et al. Fluctuations of intraocular pressure during the day in open-angle glaucoma, normal-tension glaucoma and normal subjects. *Ophthalmologica.* 1998;212(2):115-119.
24. Singh K, Shrivastava A. Intraocular pressure fluctuations: how much do they matter? *Curr Opin Ophthalmol.* 2009;20(2):84-87.
25. Wilensky JT, Gieser DK, Mori MT, et al. Self-tonometry to manage patients with glaucoma and apparently controlled intraocular pressure. *Arch Ophthalmol.* 1987;105(8):1022-1025.
26. Friberg TR, Sanborn G, Weinreb RN. Intraocular and episcleral venous pressure during inverted posture. *Am J Ophthalmol.* 1987;103(4):523-526.
27. Orzalesi N, Rossetti L, Invernizzi T, et al. Effect of timolol, latanoprost, and dorzolamide on circadian IOP in glaucoma or ocular hypertension. *Invest Ophthalmol Vis Sci.* 2000;41(9):2566-2573.

28. Noël C, Kabo AM, Romanet JP, et al. Twenty-four-hour time course of intraocular pressure in healthy and glaucomatous Africans: relation to sleep patterns. *Ophthalmology.* 2001;108(1):139-144.

29. Bagga H, Liu JH, Weinreb RN. Intraocular pressure measurements throughout the 24 h. *Curr Opin Ophthalmol.* 2009;20(2): 79-83.

30. Doughty MJ, Zaman ML. Human corneal thickness and its impact on intraocular pressure measures: a review and metaanalysis approach. *Surv Ophthalmol.* 2000;44(5):367-408.

31. Kotecha A, Crabb DP, Spratt A, Garway-Heath DF. The relationship between diurnal variations in intraocular pressure measurements and central corneal thickness and corneal hysteresis. *Invest Ophthalmol Vis Sci.* 2009;50(9):4229-4236.

32. Liu J, Roberts CJ. Influence of corneal biomechanical properties on intraocular pressure measurement: quantitative analysis. *J Cataract Refract Surg.* 2005;31(1):146-155.

33. Sullivan-Mee M, Billingsley SC, Patel AD, et al. Ocular response analyzer in patients with and without glaucoma. *Optom Vis Sci.* 2008;85(6):463-470.

34. Molinari JF, Dancd DD. Corneal hysteresis: a useful tool in the diagnosis and management of primary open angle glaucoma. *Mil Med.* 2009;174(9):996-1000.

35. Abitbol O, Bouden J, Doan S, et al. Corneal hysteresis measure with the Ocular Response Analyzer in normal and glaucomatous eyes. *Acta Ophthalmol.* 2010;88(1):116-119.

36. Anand A, De Moraes CG, Teng CC, et al. Corneal hysteresis and visual field asymmetry in open angle glaucoma. *Invest Ophthalmol Vis Sci.* 2010;51(12):6514-6518.

37. Luce DA. Determining in vivo biomechanical properties of the cornea with an ocular response analyzer. *J Cataract Refract Surg.* 2005;31(1)156-162.

38. Pepose JS, Feigenbaum SK, Qazi MA, et al. Changes in corneal biomechanics and intraocular pressure following LASIK using static, dynamic, and noncontact tonometry. *Am J Ophthalmol.* 2007;143(1):39-47.

39. Broman AT, Congdon NG, Bandeen-Roche K, Quigley HA. Influence of corneal structure, corneal responsiveness, and other ocular parameters on tonometric measurement of intraocular pressure. *J Glaucoma.* 2007;16(7):581-588.

40. Kotecha A, Elsheikh A, Roberts CR, et al. Corneal thickness- and age-related biomechanical properties of the cornea measured with the ocular response analyzer. *Invest Ophthalmol Vis Sci.* 2006;47(12):5337-5347.

41. Abitbol O, Bouden J, Doan S, Hoang-Xuan T, Gatinel D. Corneal hysteresis measured with the ocular response analyzer in normal and glaucomatous eyes. *Acta Ophthalmol.* 2010;88(1):116-119.

42. Congdon NG, Broman AT, Bandeen-Roche K, et al. Central corneal thickness and corneal hysteresis associated with glaucoma damage. *Am J Ophthalmol.* 2006;141(5):868-875.

43. Bergea B, Bodin L, Svedbergh B. Impact of intraocular pressure regulation on visual fields in open-angle glaucoma. *Ophthalmology.* 1999;106(5):997-1004; discussion 1004-1005.

44. Nouri-Mahdavi K, Hoffman D, Coleman AL, et al. Predictive factors for glaucomatous visual field progression in the Advanced Glaucoma Intervention Study. *Ophthalmology.* 2004;111(9):1627-1635.

45. Caprioli J, Coleman AL. Intraocular pressure fluctuation: a risk factor for visual field progression at low intraocular pressures in the advanced glaucoma intervention study. *Ophthalmology.* 2008;115(7):1123-1129.

46. Lee PP, Walt JW, Rosenblatt LC, et al. Association between intraocular pressure variation and glaucoma progression: data from a United States chart review. *Am J Ophthalmol.* 2007;144(6): 901-907.

47. Larson LI, Mishema HK, Takamatsu M, et al. The effect of latanoprost on circadian intraocular pressure. *Surv Ophthalmol.* 2002;47(suppl 1):S90-S96.

48. Orzalesi N, Rossetti L, Bottoli A, et al. The effect of latanoprost, brimonidine and a fixed combination of timolol and dorzolamide on circadian intraocular pressure in patients with glaucoma or ocular hypertension. *Arch Ophthalmol.* 2003;121(4):453-457.

49. Parrish RK, Palmberg P, Sheu W, et al. A comparison of latanoprost, bimatoprost and travoprost in patients with elevated intraocular pressure: a 12-week randomized masked-evaluator multicenter study. *Am J Ophthalmol.* 2003;135(5):688-703.

50. Konstas AGP, Papapanos P, Ioannis T, et al. Twenty-four hour diurnal curve comparison of commercially available latanoprost 0.005% versus the timolol and dorzolamide fixed combination. *Ophthalmology.* 2003;110(7):1357-1360.

51. Konstas AG, Kozobolis VP, Tsironi S, et al. Comparison of the 24-hour intraocular pressure-lowering effect of latanoprost and dorzolamide/timolol fixed combination after 2 and 6 months of treatment. *Ophthalmology.* 2008;115(1):99-103.

52. Liu JHK, Medeiros FA, Slight RJ, Weinreb RN. Comparing diurnal and nocturnal effects of brinzolamide and timolol on intraocular pressure in patients receiving latanoprost monotherapy. *Ophthalmology.* 2009;116(3):449-454.

53. Tamer C, Oksuz H. Circadian intraocular pressure control with dorzolamide versus timolol maleate add-on treatments in primary open-angle glaucoma patients using latanoprost. *Ophthalmic Res.* 2007;39(1):24-31.

54. Agarwal HC, Sihota R, Das C, et al. Role of argon laser trabeculoplasty as primary and secondary therapy in open angle glaucoma in Indian patients. *Br J Ophthalmol.* 2002;86(7):733-736.

55. Medeiros FA, Pinheiro A, Moura FC, et al. Intraocular pressure fluctuations in medical versus surgically treated glaucomatous patients. *J Ocul Pharmacol Ther.* 2002;18(6):489-498.

56. Wilensky JT, Zeimer RC, Gieser DK, et al. The effects of glaucoma filtering surgery on the variability of diurnal intraocular pressure. *Trans Am Ophthalmol Soc.* 1994;92:377-381.

57. Markiewitz HH. The so-called Imbert-Fick law. *Arch Ophthalmol.* 1960;64(1):159.

58. Goldmann H, Schmidt T. On applanation tonography. *Ophthalmologica.* 1965;150(1):65-75.

59. Kaufmann C, Bachmann LM, Thiel MA. Intraocular pressure measurements using dynamic contour tonometry after laser in situ keratomileusis. *Invest Ophthalmol Vis Sci.* 2003;44(9):3790-3794.

60. Doyle A, Lachkar Y. Comparison of dynamic contour tonometry with goldmann applanation tonometry over a wide range of central corneal thickness. *J Glaucoma.* 2005;14(4):288-292.

61. Kotecha A, White ET, Shewry JM, et al. The relative effects of corneal thickness and age on Goldmann applanation tonometry and dynamic contour tonometry. *Br J Ophthalmol.* 2005;89(12): 1572-1575.

62. Boehm AG, Weber A, Pillunat LE, et al. Dynamic contour tonometry in comparison to intracameral IOP measurements. *Invest Ophthalmol Vis Sci.* 2008;49(6):2472-2477.

63. Sit AJ. Continuous monitoring of intraocular pressure. *J Glaucoma.* 2009;18(4):272-279.

64. Maurice DM. A recording tonometer. *Br J Ophthalmol.* 1958;42(6):321-335.

65. Cooper RL, Beale D. Radio telemetry of intraocular pressure in vitro. *Invest Ophthalmol Vis Sci.* 1977;16(2):168-171.

66. Cooper RL, Beale DG, Constable IJ. Passive radiotelemetry of intraocular pressure in vivo: calibration and validation of continual scleral guard-ring applanation transensors in the dog and rabbit. *Invest Ophthalmol Vis Sci.* 1979;18(9):930-938.

67. Cooper RL, Beale DG, Constable IJ, et al. Continual monitoring of intraocular pressure: effect of central venous pressure, respiration, and eye movements on continual recordings of intraocular pressure in the rabbit, dog, and man. *Br J Ophthalmol.* 1979;63(12):799-804.

68. Cooper RL, Grose GC, Wasser P, et al. Progress in continual eye pressure monitoring. *Aust J Ophthalmol.* 1983;11:143-148.

69. Elsheikh A, Wang D, Brown M, et al. Assessment of corneal biomechanical properties and their variation with age. *Curr Eye Res.* 2007;32(1):11-19.

70. Greene ME, Gilman BG. Intraocular pressure measurement with instrumented contact lenses. *Invest Ophthalmol.* 1974;13(4):299-302.

71. Leonardi M, Leuenberger P, Bertrand D, et al. First steps toward noninvasive intraocular pressure monitoring with a sensing contact lens. *Invest Ophthalmol Vis Sci.* 2004;45(9):3113-3117.

72. Pitchon EM, Leonardi M, Renaud P, et al. First in vivo human measure of the intraocular pressure fluctuation and ocular pulsation by a wireless soft contact lens sensor. *Invest Ophthalmol Vis Sci.* 2008;49:E-Abstract 687.

73. Collins CC. Miniature passive pressure transensor for implanting in the eye. *IEEE Trans Biomed Eng.* 1967;14(2):74-83.

74. Svedbergh B, Backlund Y, Hok B, et al. The IOP-IOL. A probe into the eye. *Acta Ophthalmol (Copenh).* 1992;70(2):266-268.

75. Schnakenberg U, Walter P, Bogel GV, et al. Initial investigations on systems for measuring intraocular pressure. *Sens Actuators A Phys.* 2000;85:287-291.

76. Walter P, Schnakenberg U, vom Bogel G, et al. Development of a completely encapsulated intraocular pressure sensor. *Ophthalmic Res.* 2000;32(6):278-284.

77. Walter P. Intraocular pressure sensor: where are we-where will we go? *Graefes Arch Clin Exp Ophthalmol.* 2002;240(5):335-336.

78. Wolbarsht ML, Wortman J, Schwartz B, et al. A scleral buckle pressure gauge for continuous monitoring of intraocular pressure. *Int Ophthalmol.* 1980;3(1):11-17.

79. Flower RW, Maumenee AE, Michelson EA. Long-term continuous monitoring of intraocular pressure in conscious primates. *Ophthalmic Res.* 1982;14(2):98-106.

72

The Role of Ocular Perfusion Pressure in the Pathogenesis of Glaucoma

Yvonne Ou, MD and Sanjay Asrani, MD

Although many risk factors, such as elevated intraocular pressure (IOP), have been implicated in the pathogenesis of open-angle glaucoma (OAG), the exact mechanisms remain unclear. There are 2 theories that have gained the most traction over time: the mechanical theory suggests that IOP directly damages the lamina cribrosa and retinal ganglion cell axons, whereas the vascular theory hypothesizes that insufficient ocular blood flow predisposes the optic nerve to damage, especially in the setting of increased IOP.[1,2] While these 2 theories are presented as distinct, they are not mutually exclusive, and in many clinical scenarios, both mechanisms may be at play.

In many glaucomatous conditions, including congenital glaucoma and secondary glaucomas such as angle-recession glaucoma, it is clear that increased IOP is a major factor in the development of glaucomatous optic neuropathy. According to the mechanical theory, increased IOP leads to biomechanical forces that stretch and collapse the laminar beams of the lamina cribrosa and result in posterior bowing.[3-5] The retinal ganglion cell axons are either damaged directly by increased IOP or indirectly by deformation of the laminar beams. It has also been shown that axoplasmic transport is impeded and that the retinal ganglion cells undergo apoptosis, although the exact mechanism of this relationship is still under investigation.[6-9]

However, elevated IOP cannot be the only risk factor involved in glaucomatous optic neuropathy because many patients diagnosed with glaucoma do not have elevated IOP. Systemic hypertension, atherosclerosis, vasospasm, and nocturnal hypotension have all been studied as potential risk factors.[2,10-13] However, the evidence is inconsistent and sometimes contradictory. In patients with normal-tension glaucoma (NTG), glaucomatous optic neuropathy occurs even when IOP is not in an elevated range. It has been hypothesized that patients with NTG have structural abnormalities that make them susceptible to nerve damage at normal IOP levels.[14,15] It has also been hypothesized that vascular risk factors, including migraine, significant blood loss requiring transfusion, Raynaud's phenomenon, and nocturnal hypotension, are risk factors involved in the development of glaucoma.

While the evidence regarding systemic blood pressure (BP) and glaucoma has been inconsistent, nocturnal hypotension and unstable ocular perfusion pressure (OPP) may be involved in the pathogenesis and progression of glaucomatous optic neuropathy. In several population-based studies,[10,16-18] lower diastolic BP and lower diastolic ocular perfusion pressure (DOPP) were identified as risk factors for glaucoma. In order to better understand the role of OPP in the pathogenesis of glaucoma, it is important to review the definition of OPP and the anatomy and physiology of ocular blood flow.

VASCULAR SUPPLY OF THE OPTIC NERVE

Perfusion pressure of a tissue is equal to the difference between arterial and venous pressure. In the eye, IOP is the surrogate for venous pressure and thus, BP and IOP are the main components of OPP. OPP is defined by the following different parameters:

- Systolic ocular perfusion pressure (SOPP = SBP – IOP) where SBP is the systolic BP
- Diastolic ocular perfusion pressure (DOPP = DBP – IOP) where DBP is diastolic BP

Kahook MY, Schuman JS, eds.
Chandler and Grant's Glaucoma, Fifth Edition (pp 695-698).
© 2013 SLACK Incorporated.

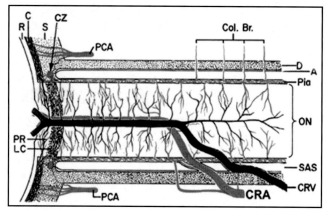

Figure 72-1. Blood supply of the anterior optic nerve. A, arachnoid; C, choroid; Col. Br., collateral branches supplying the optic nerve pial plexus; CRA, central retinal artery; CRV, central retinal vein; CZ, circle of Zinn and Haller; D, dura; LC, lamina cribrosa; ON, optic nerve; PCA, posterior ciliary artery; PR, prelaminar region; R, retina; S, sclera; SAS, subarachnoid space. (Reprinted by permission from Macmillan Publishers Ltd: *Eye.* Hayreh SS. Posterior ischaemic optic neuropathy: clinical features, pathogenesis, and management. 2004;18:1188-1206, copyright 2004.)

- Mean perfusion pressure (MPP = 2/3 of mean arterial pressure – IOP) where mean arterial pressure = DBP + 1/3 (SBP – DBP)

There are 3 major sources of blood supply to the optic nerve head (Figure 72-1):

1. Retinal (retinal arterioles including small branches of the central retinal artery)

2. Prelaminar (recurrent choroidal arteries)

3. Laminar (short posterior ciliary arteries)

While retinal circulation is characterized by low-flow and high-level of oxygen extraction, choroidal circulation is characterized by high-flow and low-level oxygen extraction. Additionally, retinal circulation is autoregulated and thus somewhat independent of perfusion pressure, whereas choroidal circulation is more dependent on perfusion pressure.[19]

Given the complexity of ocular blood flow, many mechanisms have been suggested to play a role in the poor perfusion of the optic nerve. These include alterations in the microvasculature and changes in retinal or choroidal blood flow that interfere with the delivery of nutrients or removal of waste products, failure in autoregulation, and release of toxic vasoactive substances that injure the optic nerve.[20] In particular, the failure in autoregulation has been suggested to result in ischemic damage and reperfusion injury to the optic nerve.[19]

A detailed discussion of the methods used to measure ocular blood flow is beyond the scope of this chapter, and one is directed to comprehensive reviews on this subject.[20,21] Methods include fluorescein angiography, laser and color Doppler imaging, and laser speckle phenomenon. There is evidence that there is reduced retinal blood flow and dye leakage from optic nerve capillaries, as well as abnormal retrobulbar flow velocities in glaucoma.[20]

EPIDEMIOLOGIC EVIDENCE

While large clinical trials have shown that lowering IOP slows progression of glaucomatous optic neuropathy, it is also clear that some glaucoma patients will continue to progress despite lowering of IOP. The Early Manifest Glaucoma Trial[22] (EMGT) demonstrated that lowering IOP resulted in decreasing the rate of progression in the treatment group (45%) as compared to the control group (62%). Subsequent analysis of data from the EMGT revealed that risk factors for disease progression included lower systolic perfusion pressure, lower systolic BP, and cardiovascular disease history.[23]

Vascular-related risk factors, including low OPP, have been associated with OAG in numerous large population-based studies throughout the world. In the Baltimore Eye Study,[10] systemic BP and IOP were significantly although modestly correlated. The authors hypothesized that earlier stages of hypertension might be protective against optic nerve damage because of increased perfusion but that later stages of hypertension would damage the optic nerve as peripheral resistance increased. Using age as a surrogate for the duration of hypertension, they showed that age modified the effect of systemic hypertension on the prevalence of primary open-angle glaucoma (POAG), with a stronger association as age increased. Perhaps most interestingly, lower diastolic perfusion pressure was strongly associated with a higher prevalence of POAG (Table 72-1).

Later studies supported this relationship between low OPP and prevalence of OAG. In the Rotterdam Study,[24] patients with an OPP lower than 50 mm Hg had a 4 times greater risk of developing OAG than those with a perfusion pressure of 80 mm Hg. This finding was supported in the Egna-Neumarkt Glaucoma Study,[17] which found that lower diastolic perfusion pressure was associated with hypertensive glaucoma.

More recently, 9-year follow-up data from the Barbados Eye Study[25] demonstrated that patients with low OPP at baseline had a significantly increased risk of developing OAG over time. The relative risks for the development of incident OAG ranged from 2.0 to 2.6 for systolic, diastolic, and mean OPP.

While the association between DOPP and OAG has been established, the relationship between SOPP and OAG is less definitive. In the Blue Mountains Eye Study,[26] there was a marginal association between elevated SOPP and prevalence of OAG. The Barbados Eye studies,[16,25] however, reported the opposite finding, with low SOPP increasing the relative risk of OAG at 4- and 9-year follow-up. The EMGT,[23] in which the authors controlled for IOP as well as IOP- and BP-lowering treatments, also revealed that lower SOPP was a significant risk factor for progression of glaucoma.

Study	Study Size (n)	Increased Prevalence of OAG
Baltimore Eye Study[10]	5308	2- to 6-fold
Egna-Neumarkt Study[17]	4297	3-fold[a,b]
Proyecto VER[18]	4774	4-fold
Barbados Eye Study[25]	4631	> 3-fold
Rotterdam Eye Study[24]	1329	< 4-fold[a]

TABLE 72-1. LOW DIASTOLIC OCULAR PERFUSION PRESSURE (< 55 MM HG) AND PREVALENCE OF OPEN-ANGLE GLAUCOMA

[a]High-tension glaucoma only.

[b]Low ocular perfusion pressure is defined as <68 mm Hg in this study.

Adapted from Werne A, Harris A, Moore D, BenZion I, Siesky B. The circadian variations in systemic blood pressure, ocular perfusion pressure, and ocular blood flow: risk factors for glaucoma? *Surv Ophthalmol.* 2008;53:559-567.

OAG: open-angle glaucoma.

VASCULAR DYSREGULATION AND OPEN-ANGLE GLAUCOMA

Given the definition of OPP, an abnormal OPP could be due to low blood pressure (SBP or DBP) or an elevated IOP. The relationship between BP and OAG is unclear as various studies have reported both positive and negative associations. It has been hypothesized that abnormal OPP due to vascular dysregulation is an underlying cause of glaucoma.[27] Vascular dysregulation may not only result in chronically low OPP, but also fluctuations and instability in OPP. Appropriate vascular autoregulation in healthy patients likely provides consistent ocular blood flow (OBF) over a wide range of perfusion pressures. On the other hand, in susceptible patients, any fluctuation in OPP (either due to systemic BP or IOP changes) results in abnormal OBF and possible compromise in optic nerve perfusion.[28] Gherghel and colleagues[29] demonstrated that OAG patients with progressive visual field damage and well-controlled IOP had lower OPP and low retrobulbar blood flow.

In normal-tension glaucoma (NTG), vascular factors are hypothesized to play a relatively more important role than mechanical factors in disease pathogenesis, although NTG patients may have increased susceptibility to structural damage at lower IOPs. In the Collaborative Normal Tension Glaucoma Study[30] (CNTGS), 20% of NTG patients had visual field progression despite 30% IOP lowering from baseline. NTG patients have lower systemic BPs and nocturnal hypotension compared to controls, although the nocturnal dip

TOPICAL MEDICATIONS AND OCULAR PERFUSION PRESSURE

Yvonne Ou, MD and Sanjay Asrani, MD

The treatment of glaucoma is currently focused on the lowering of IOP, even though elevated IOP is not the only risk factor in glaucomatous optic neuropathy. Ideally, a medication would both lower IOP and increase OPP. Conversely, a medication that insufficiently reduces IOP or decreases systemic BP would be suboptimal because of its detrimental effect on OPP

Our understanding of the effects of current topical medical therapy on parameters such as DOPP is growing. Quaranta and colleagues[1] demonstrated that latanoprost and dorzolamide decreased IOP and increased DOPP over a 24-hour period. Timolol and brimonidine both predictably had significant IOP-lowering effects, but brimonidine also caused a significant decrease in SBP and DBP, which resulted in a decrease in DOPP. This group[2] further investigated the effect of timolol-dorzolamide fixed combination and latanoprost on 24-hour IOP, SBP, DBP, and DOPP. They found that timolol-dorzolamide and latanoprost both significantly increased 24-hour DOPP with no difference in this effect between the 2 medications.[2] Although timolol-dorzolamide significantly reduced DBP, it counteracted this effect with a greater decrease in IOP, whereas latanoprost had minimal effect on DBP while reducing IOP. While these studies raise intriguing differences among topical medications in their effects on DOPP, patients with systemic hypertension and/or on BP-lowering medications were excluded. Larger studies with longer follow-up periods will be needed in order to more definitively tease out the effects of topical glaucoma medications on OPP and glaucoma progression.

REFERENCES

1. Quaranta L, Gandolfo F, Turano R, et al. Effects of topical hypotensive drugs on circadian IOP, blood pressure, and calculated diastolic ocular perfusion pressure in patients with glaucoma. *Invest Ophthalmol Vis Sci.* 2006;47:2917-2923.
2. Quaranta L, Miglior S, Floriani I, Pizzolante T, Konstas AG. Effects of the timolol-dorzolamide fixed combination and latanoprost on circadian diastolic ocular perfusion pressure in glaucoma. *Invest Ophthalmol Vis Sci.* 2008;49:4226-4231.

seems to be the more important factor.[31] Indeed, increased mean ocular perfusion pressure (MOPP) fluctuation was associated with nocturnal hypotension in a group of NTG patients.[19]

There have also been several studies examining the relationship between nocturnal dips in OPP on OAG progression, especially in NTG. Choi and colleagues[32] measured IOP, mean arterial pressure, and mean OPP (MOPP) in 113 NTG patients and found that 24-hour MOPP fluctuation was the greatest risk factor for glaucoma severity as determined by visual field parameters at initial presentation. The group went on further to show that 24-hour MOPP fluctuation was the most consistent risk factor for glaucomatous progression in a cohort of 101 NTG eyes.[33]

CONCLUSION

Mounting evidence is accumulating to suggest that vascular dysregulation and low OPP play important roles in glaucoma pathogenesis. Vascular dysregulation may involve low systemic BP, and thus low OPP. Impaired auto-regulation may result in the inability to adapt to increased IOP or decreased systemic BP. These mechanisms may be particularly important in NTG patients or in patients who have progressive glaucoma despite normalized IOP. As the field looks toward expanding current IOP-lowering thera-py as well as other treatment modalities, improving ocular perfusion dynamics may be a critical target.

REFERENCES

1. Yan DB, Coloma FM, Metheetrairut A, Trope GE, Heathcote JG, Ethier CR. Deformation of the lamina cribrosa by elevated intra-ocular pressure. *Br J Ophthalmol.* 1994;78:643-648.

2. Flammer J. The vascular concept of glaucoma. *Surv Ophthalmol.* 1994;38(suppl):S3-S6.

3. Bellezza AJ, Rintalan CJ, Thompson HW, Downs JC, Hart RT, Burgoyne CF. Deformation of the lamina cribrosa and ante-rior scleral canal wall in early experimental glaucoma. *Invest Ophthalmol Vis Sci.* 2003;44:623-637.

4. Burgoyne CF, Downs JC, Bellezza AJ, Suh JK, Hart RT. The optic nerve head as a biomechanical structure: a new paradigm for understanding the role of IOP-related stress and strain in the pathophysiology of glaucomatous optic nerve head damage. *Prog Retin Eye Res.* 2005;24:39-73.

5. Yang H, Downs JC, Sigal IA, Roberts MD, Thompson H, Burgoyne CF. Deformation of the normal monkey optic nerve head connec-tive tissue after acute IOP elevation within 3-D histomorphometric reconstructions. *Invest Ophthalmol Vis Sci.* 2009;50:5785-5799.

6. Quigley HA, Flower RW, Addicks EM, McLeod DS. The mecha-nism of optic nerve damage in experimental acute intraocular pressure elevation. *Invest Ophthalmol Vis Sci.* 1980;19:505-517.

7. Pease ME, McKinnon SJ, Quigley HA, Kerrigan-Baumrind LA, Zack DJ. Obstructed axonal transport of BDNF and its receptor TrkB in experimental glaucoma. *Invest Ophthalmol Vis Sci.* 2000;41:764-774.

8. Fagiolini M, Caleo M, Strettoi E, Maffei L. Axonal transport block-ade in the neonatal rat optic nerve induces limited retinal ganglion cell death. *J Neurosci.* 1997;17:7045-7052.

9. Vrabec JP, Levin LA. The neurobiology of cell death in glaucoma. *Eye (Lond).* 2007;21(suppl 1):S11-S14.

10. Tielsch JM, Katz J, Sommer A, Quigley HA, Javitt JC. Hypertension, perfusion pressure, and primary open-angle glaucoma. A population-based assessment. *Arch Ophthalmol.* 1995;113:216-221.

11. Deokule S, Weinreb RN. Relationships among systemic blood pressure, intraocular pressure, and open-angle glaucoma. *Can J Ophthalmol.* 2008;43:302-307.

12. Chung HS, Harris A, Evans DW, Kagemann L, Garzozi HJ, Martin B. Vascular aspects in the pathophysiology of glaucomatous optic neuropathy. *Surv Ophthalmol.* 1999;43(suppl 1):S43-S50.

13. Graham SL, Drance SM. Nocturnal hypotension: role in glaucoma progression. *Surv Ophthalmol.* 1999;43(suppl 1):S10-S16.

14. Park KH, Tomita G, Liou SY, Kitazawa Y. Correlation between peripapillary atrophy and optic nerve damage in normal-tension glaucoma. *Ophthalmology.* 1996;103:1899-1906.

15. Tomita G. The optic nerve head in normal-tension glaucoma. *Curr Opin Ophthalmol.* 2000;11:116-120.

16. Leske MC, Connell AM, Wu SY, Hyman LG, Schachat AP. Risk factors for open-angle glaucoma. The Barbados Eye Study. *Arch Ophthalmol.* 1995;113:918-924.

17. Bonomi L, Marchini G, Marraffa M, Bernardi P, Morbio R, Varotto A. Vascular risk factors for primary open angle glaucoma: the Egna-Neumarkt Study. *Ophthalmology.* 2000;107:1287-1293.

18. Quigley HA, West SK, Rodriguez J, Munoz B, Klein R, Snyder R. The prevalence of glaucoma in a population-based study of Hispanic subjects: Proyecto VER. *Arch Ophthalmol.* 2001;119:1819-1826.

19. Choi J, Jeong J, Cho HS, Kook MS. Effect of nocturnal blood pressure reduction on circadian fluctuation of mean ocular perfusion pressure: a risk factor for normal tension glaucoma. *Invest Ophthalmol Vis Sci.* 2006;47:831-836.

20. Flammer J, Orgul S, Costa VP, et al. The impact of ocular blood flow in glaucoma. *Prog Retin Eye Res.* 2002;21:359-393.

21. Grieshaber MC, Flammer J. Blood flow in glaucoma. *Curr Opin Ophthalmol.* 2005;16:79-83.

22. Heijl A, Leske MC, Bengtsson B, Hyman L, Hussein M. Reduction of intraocular pressure and glaucoma progression: results from the Early Manifest Glaucoma Trial. *Arch Ophthalmol.* 2002;120:1268-1279.

23. Leske MC, Heijl A, Hyman L, Bengtsson B, Dong L, Yang Z. Predictors of long-term progression in the early manifest glaucoma trial. *Ophthalmology.* 2007;114:1965-1972.

24. Hulsman CA, Vingerling JR, Hofman A, Witteman JC, de Jong PT. Blood pressure, arterial stiffness, and open-angle glaucoma: the Rotterdam Study. *Arch Ophthalmol.* 2007;125:805-812.

25. Leske MC, Wu SY, Hennis A, Honkanen R, Nemesure B. Risk fac-tors for incident open-angle glaucoma: the Barbados Eye studies. *Ophthalmology.* 2008;115:85-93.

26. Mitchell P, Lee AJ, Rochtchina E, Wang JJ. Open-angle glau-coma and systemic hypertension: the Blue Mountains Eye Study. *J Glaucoma.* 2004;13:319-326.

27. Grieshaber MC, Mozaffarieh M, Flammer J. What is the link between vascular dysregulation and glaucoma? *Surv Ophthalmol.* 2007;52(suppl 2):S144-S154.

28. Werne A, Harris A, Moore D, BenZion I, Siesky B. The circadian variations in systemic blood pressure, ocular perfusion pressure, and ocular blood flow: risk factors for glaucoma? *Surv Ophthalmol.* 2008;53:559-567.

29. Gherghel D, Orgul S, Gugleta K, Gekkieva M, Flammer J. Relationship between ocular perfusion pressure and retrobulbar blood flow in patients with glaucoma with progressive damage. *Am J Ophthalmol.* 2000;130:597-605.

30. The effectiveness of intraocular pressure reduction in the treat-ment of normal-tension glaucoma. Collaborative Normal-Tension Glaucoma Study Group. *Am J Ophthalmol.* 1998;126:498-505.

31. Meyer JH, Brandi-Dohrn J, Funk J. Twenty four hour blood pres-sure monitoring in normal tension glaucoma. *Br J Ophthalmol.* 1996;80:864-867.

32. Choi J, Kim KH, Jeong J, Cho HS, Lee CH, Kook MS. Circadian fluc-tuation of mean ocular perfusion pressure is a consistent risk factor for normal-tension glaucoma. *Invest Ophthalmol Vis Sci.* 2007;48:104-111.

33. Sung KR, Lee S, Park SB, et al. Twenty-four hour ocular perfusion pressure fluctuation and risk of normal-tension glaucoma progres-sion. *Invest Ophthalmol Vis Sci.* 2009;50:5266-5274.

Neuroprotection in Glaucoma

Yvonne Ou, MD and Stuart J. McKinnon, MD, PhD

Neuroprotection is a therapeutic modality that aims to slow or prevent neuronal death. In glaucoma, the target neuron is the retinal ganglion cell (RGC) and its axon. The ultimate goal of neuroprotection is to delay or prevent the loss of visual function. An advantage of the neuroprotective approach is that regardless of the mechanism of glaucomatous optic nerve damage and visual loss, this strategy targets the final common pathway of neuronal loss at the level of the RGC and its axonal projections. Some argue that, by definition, glaucoma neuroprotection is independent from intraocular pressure (IOP) lowering.[1] For the purposes of this discussion, we will follow this convention and define neuroprotection as therapy directed toward preserving RGC viability and function independent of IOP lowering.

PATHOGENESIS OF NEURONAL DEATH IN GLAUCOMA AND POSSIBLE THERAPEUTIC STRATEGIES

Although the exact mechanism of RGC death is unknown, several mechanisms have been proposed and studied. These include mechanical compression of RGC axons at the optic nerve head, decreased ocular perfusion pressure and ischemia, excitotoxicity, neurotrophic factor deprivation, oxidative stress, immune modulation, and exposures to molecules, such as nitric oxide, endothelin and, amyloid-β (Figure 73-1).[2] The actual mechanism is likely to be multifactorial.

In direct axonal injury, 2 paradigms are most commonly discussed. One hypothesis is that axonal degeneration begins at the distal ends of the injured axon and spreads in a retrograde fashion toward the cell body.[3] Alternatively, one or more focal injuries cause degeneration of the axon in both anterograde and retrograde directions, consistent with Wallerian degeneration. These mechanisms of axonal degeneration may not be

mutually exclusive, although the focal injury hypothesis likely plays a more important role in RGC axonal degeneration. It has been documented that axonal compression occurs as the axons pass through the lamina cribrosa of the optic nerve head, and it is hypothesized that this localized injury results in axonal transport disruption as well as glial activation, vascular ischemia, and hypoxia, all of which contribute to axonal degeneration.[4,5]

TARGETING APOPTOSIS

Despite the various proposed mechanisms of RGC death, the final common pathway likely involves apoptosis. This mode of programmed cell death has been seen in models of axotomy and optic nerve crush[6-8] and in models of experimental glaucoma.[9,10] It is thought that RGC death begins with damage at the lamina cribrosa and therefore the RGC axon, and then spreads to the dendrites and soma in the retina.[4,11] Morphologically, the dying RGCs demonstrate dendrite and soma shrinkage, chromatin condensation, intracellular and DNA fragmentation, and formation of apoptotic bodies.[12] Activation of a cascade of caspases, a class of cysteine proteases, culminates in apoptosis and cell death. Caspases are pro-proteins that become activated when the prodomain is cleaved off and these activated caspases subsequently digest cellular contents. Caspases are activated by 2 distinct pathways: an extrinsic and intrinsic pathway (Figure 73-2).[12] In extrinsic apoptosis, also called the death receptor pathway, members of the tumor necrosis factor (TNF) receptor superfamily are activated by the caspase cascade via proteolytic cleavage of procaspase 8. In intrinsic apoptosis, members of the Bcl2 gene family are recruited to the mitochondrial outer membrane, resulting in the release of cytochrome c, which complexes with a molecule called apoptosis inducing factor-1 and procaspase 9. This complex causes proteolytic cleavage of procaspase 9, which activates the caspase cascade. Although

Kahook MY, Schuman JS, eds.
Chandler and Grant's Glaucoma, Fifth Edition (pp 699-704).
© 2013 SLACK Incorporated.

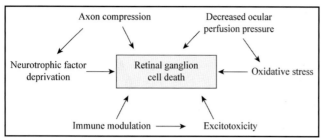

Figure 73-1. Possible mechanisms leading to RGC apoptosis in glaucoma. Proposed mechanisms of RGC death include axon compression at the optic nerve head and blockage of axonal transport, decreased ocular perfusion pressure, excitotoxicity, activation of astrocytes, macrophages, microglia, and exposure to molecules such as nitric oxide and amyloid-β. The role of cerebrospinal fluid pressure and its relationship to IOP is also under investigation. The actual mechanism is likely to include several different etiologies. (Reprinted with permission from Frankie-Lynn Silver, MD.)

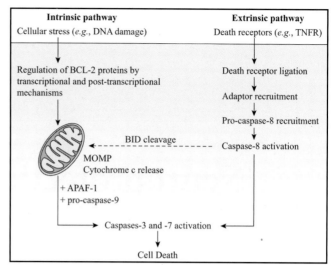

Figure 73-2. The intrinsic and extrinsic apoptosis pathways. The extrinsic pathway is engaged by ligation of death receptors (eg, members of the tumor necrosis factor receptor [TNFR] superfamily), which results in procaspase-8 activation. Executioner caspases-3 and -7 are then activated, resulting in cell death. In the intrinsic pathway, a repertoire of Bcl-2 proteins are activated, which results in mitochondrial outer membrane permeabilization (MOMP), cytochrome c release, and apoptosis inducing factor-1 (APAF-1)–dependent procaspase-9 activation. As with the extrinsic pathway, executioner caspases-3 and -7 are then activated. (Reprinted by permission from Macmillan Publishers Ltd: *Cell Death and Differentiation.* Chipuk JE, Green DR. Dissecting p53-dependent apoptosis. 2006;13:994-1002, copyright 2006.)

these 2 pathways operate through different mechanisms, they are not mutually exclusive and may share common elements.

Strategies to target RGC apoptosis via these pathways include application or local expression of neurotrophic factors, which will be discussed in more detail below. It has been shown that neurotrophic factors can inhibit apoptosis by activating intracellular signaling pathways, such as the extracellular signal-regulated kinase 1/2 (Erk1/2), the phosphatidylinositol-3 kinase (PI3K), and the janus kinase/signal transducer and activator of transcription 3 (JAK/STAT3) pathways. The former 2 pathways activate the cAMP-response-element binding protein (CREB), which promotes transcription of several prosurvival genes, including Bcl-2 and Bcl-XL. Brain-derived neurotrophic factor (BDNF) promotes RGC survival via the Erk1/2 pathway, whereas ciliary-derived neurotrophic factor (CNTF) promotes RGC survival via the JAK/STAT3 pathway. Intravitreal injection of BDNF delays RGC death after axotomy and may be associated with the suppression of caspase 3 activity.[13] Another strategy to target apoptosis is the use of caspase inhibitors. In rodent models of optic nerve axotomy and glaucoma, RGC apoptosis is reduced by intraocular administration of caspase inhibitors.[14-17]

TARGETING NEUROTROPHIC FACTORS

Neurotrophic factors promote neuronal survival and differentiation by activating survival signals and inhibiting apoptotic signaling cascades. It is hypothesized that blockage of axonal transport deprives RGCs from critical neurotrophic factors, resulting in RGC apoptosis. In the retina, the nerve growth factor family of neurotrophins includes BDNF, nerve growth factor (NGF), neurotrophin-3 (NT3), and neurotrophin-4/5 (NT4/5).[18] These neurotrophins bind to tyrosine receptor kinases (TRKs) or the p75NT receptor (p75NTR) to promote either cell survival or cell death, respectively (Figure 73-3). BDNF is a potent neurotrophic factor for RGCs, and its retrograde transport is inhibited when IOP was acutely elevated in rats.[19]

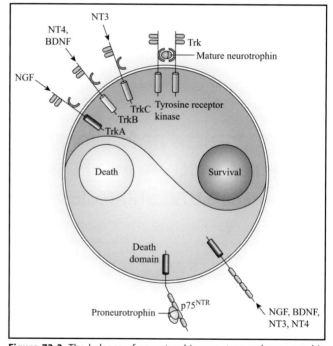

Figure 73-3. The balance of neurotrophin receptors and neurotrophin function. The actions of neurotrophins are mediated by 2 principal transmembrane-receptor signaling systems. Each neurotrophin receptor (TrkA, TrkB, TrkC, and p75NTR) is characterized by specific affinities for the neurotrophins (nerve growth factor [NGF], brain-derived neurotrophic factor [BDNF], neurotrophin 3 [NT3], and neurotrophin 4 [NT4]). Activation of the tyrosine receptor kinases (TRKs) promotes cell survival, whereas activation of the p75NT receptor (p75NTR) promotes cell death. (Reprinted by permission from Macmillan Publishers Ltd: *Nature Reviews Neuroscience.* Lu B, Pang PT, Woo NH. 2005;6:603-614, copyright 2005.)

Furthermore, the receptor for BDNF, TrkB, accumulated in the optic nerve head in the same model of experimental glaucoma.[20] However, it should be noted that there are endogenous sources of neurotrophins in the retina, and they may compensate in situations when retrograde axonal transport of brain-derived neurotrophins is blocked.[21-23] In a rat model of glaucoma, intravitreal injections of BDNF increased the number of surviving RGCs as compared to control eyes.[24] In a similar model, viral vectors overexpressing BDNF were intravitreally injected in glaucomatous rat eyes and reduced RGC loss.[25] Another study from the same group demonstrated that virally mediated overexpression of CNTF decreased RGC loss but not BDNF.[26]

TARGETING GLUTAMATE EXCITOTOXICITY

Glutamate is one of the major excitatory neurotransmitters in the brain and visual system. Excessive neurotransmission initiated by glutamate can be excitotoxic and result in cell death, first discovered in the retina.[27] There are 3 classes of ionotropic glutamate-gated ion channels: AMPA receptors, kainate receptors, and *N*-methyl-D-aspartate (NMDA) receptors,[28] the latter of which has been implicated in RGC loss. Under physiologic conditions, glutamate is released by presynaptic neurons, binds to postsynaptic receptors, and allows influx of cations and results in neurotransmission. However, overactivation of NMDA receptors due to excessive glutamate or receptor hyperactivity triggers Ca^{2+} influx into neurons and initiates cell death pathways.[28,29] Calcium influx results in mitochondrial membrane depolarization, release of cytochrome c into the cytosol, activation of caspases, and subsequent DNA fragmentation and apoptosis.

Despite the evidence that glutamate excitotoxicity results in RGC death, its role in glaucoma pathogenesis has been controversial. An early study[30] found increased levels of glutamate in the vitreous of glaucoma versus control patients, but later studies were unable to confirm this finding.[31-33] Certainly, it is also possible that injured or metabolically compromised RGCs may react to normal levels of glutamate abnormally.[28]

Memantine is a derivative of the antiviral amantadine and is an NMDA channel blocker, and preferentially blocks its activity if the ion channel is excessively open (ie, in high glutamate conditions). When there is an increased concentration of extracellular glutamate, more NMDA receptors are activated and open, and memantine is more effective at blocking them under these conditions. Memantine has been shown to prevent or reduce neuronal death in numerous animal models of central nervous system injury, including stroke, Alzheimer's disease, and traumatic brain injury. In experimental primate models of glaucoma, memantine-inhibited RGC death and neuronal shrinkage in the lateral geniculate nucleus.[34-37] However, primary endpoints were not reached in a human phase III clinical trial using memantine to treat primary open-angle glaucoma, and to date Food and Drug Administration (FDA) approval for use in glaucoma has not been granted.

TARGETING AMYLOID-β

Alzheimer's disease (AD) is the most common cause of dementia in the elderly,[38] characterized by progressive impairment in memory and cognitive function. As a neurodegenerative disease, major histologic features include neurofibrillary tangles and neuritic plaques. Amyloid precursor protein (APP) is a transmembrane protein expressed in the brain and RGCs and regulates neurite outgrowth, synaptogenesis, and cell survival. Cleavage of APP by β- and β-secretases produces amyloid-β, which plays a major role in AD pathogenesis.

Several studies[39-42] have raised the possibility that there may be a relationship between AD and glaucoma. It has been shown that there is a higher incidence of glaucoma in patients with AD when compared to age-matched control patients.[43] Structural studies[39,40] of optic nerves from AD patients have shown loss of RGCs. We have shown that caspase activation and altered metabolism of APP and amyloid-β contributes to RGC apoptosis in glaucoma.[14,44]

Currently, there are 2 classes of drugs approved to treat AD: acetylcholine esterase inhibitors (donepezil, rivastigmine, and galantamine) and an NMDA receptor antagonist (memantine). Other antiamyloid therapeutic strategies include decreasing amyloid-β production by inhibiting secretases or by interfering with amyloid-β aggregation using amyloid-β vaccination. In a rat glaucoma model, intravitreal injection of antibodies to amyloid-β or Congo red as well as β-secretase inhibitors decreased rates of RGC apoptosis.[44]

TARGETING NEUROINFLAMMATION

Recent evidence has focused attention on the possibility that inflammation plays a role in the pathogenesis of glaucoma. It has been demonstrated that activation of the classical complement cascade results in RGC death. In the classic complement cascade, C1q binds to an antigen and activates several proteases (C1r, C1s, C2-C4) that initiate opsonization and attract phagocytes that directly attack cell membranes via the membrane attack complex (MAC). During development, C1q localizes to developing synapses and regulates synapse elimination.[45] In AD, damaged neuronal processes show evidence of MAC activation, with concurrent increased expression of C1q.[46,47] C1q also binds to amyloid plaques in AD brains, reducing amyloid-β uptake and resulting in extracellular amyloid-β accumulation.[48] C1q upregulation can be detected in the retinas of murine, primate, and human glaucomatous eyes.[49] Recently, it was shown that complement activation in glaucoma resembles that seen in AD, raising the possibility that the normal developmental mechanism of complement-mediated synapse elimination becomes aberrantly reactivated in neurodegenerative diseases.[45] It is intriguing to hypothesize that C1q tags retinal synapses in glaucomatous eyes for elimination at early stages of disease and may drive dendritic atrophy and axon degeneration in glaucoma.

TARGETING TUMOR NECROSIS FACTOR SUPERFAMILY RECEPTOR PATHWAYS

Tumor necrosis factor alpha (TNF-α) is a nonglycosylated protein cytokine with a molecular weight of 17 kDa and a length of 157 amino acids. TNF-α is produced by mast cells, neutrophils, activated lymphocytes, endothelial cells, adipocytes, and smooth muscle cells, as well as by natural killer cells after their stimulation by lipopolysaccharides. Prior studies have shown that that TNF-α and its membrane-bound receptors may contribute to the pathophysiology of glaucoma, although the mechanism of action is poorly understood. TNF-α production was upregulated in cultured rat retinal glial cells exposed to elevated hydrostatic pressure and caused apoptosis in cocultured rat RGCs.[50] Immunohistochemical analysis has shown upregulation of TNF-α in the optic nerve head of human glaucoma patients, mainly in glia. Using a laser mouse glaucoma model,[51] Nakazawa and colleagues reported rapid upregulation of TNF-α, microglial activation, loss of optic nerve oligodendrocytes, and delayed loss of RGCs.[52] Intravitreal TNF-α injections produced similar effects. In this study, TNF receptor 2-knockout mice treated to induce elevated IOP showed minimal evidence of developing glaucoma compared to similarly treated wild-type mice.

TARGETING DECREASED OCULAR PERFUSION AND HYPOXIA

As discussed in Chapter 72, decreased ocular perfusion pressure may play a role in glaucomatous optic neuropathy. Insufficient autoregulation of optic nerve blood flow may lead to optic nerve ischemia and RGC loss. In several animal studies,[53,54] exogenous application of vasoactive peptide endothelin-1 resulting in decreased optic nerve blood flow can lead to RGC loss in the absence of elevated IOP.

Hypoxia of the retina has also been shown to result in RGC apoptosis.[55,56] The pathophysiology of neuronal hypoxic damage may involve several different mechanisms, including excitotoxic damage, calcium overload, and oxidative stress. Indeed, hypoxia-mediated mechanisms at work in the brain may play a role in glaucomatous optic neuropathy. Despite the fact that there is evidence of vascular abnormalities in glaucoma patients, including vasospasm, systemic hypotension, and abnormal blood flow characteristics,[57] there is scant direct evidence of retinal or optic nerve hypoxia in glaucomatous eyes. Recently, it was demonstrated that expression of hypoxia-induced factor 1a (HIF-1a) is upregulated in human glaucomatous retina and optic nerves compared to control patients.[58] HIF-1a is an oxygen-regulated transcription factor that serves as a master regulator of oxygen homeostasis.

The most well-studied pharmacologic agent class that may improve perfusion of the optic nerve are calcium channel blockers that cause vasodilation of the cerebral vasculature. This class of medication has been evaluated in the context of normal-tension glaucoma treatment. Prospective clinical studies[59-61] have shown that patients taking oral calcium channel blockers had fewer optic nerve and visual field changes as compared to control patients. However, concerns for systemic hypotension, especially nocturnal hypotension, have limited widespread use of this class of drugs.[62]

CONCLUSION

The field of neuroprotection in glaucoma is full of promise, but clinically proven strategies have remained elusive. While there has been accumulating laboratory evidence of the effectiveness of targeting RGC death as a treatment for glaucoma, data from randomized clinical trials are still lacking. However, the search for successful neuroprotective therapies that act independently of IOP lowering is critically important and continues to be an active area of research.

REFERENCES

1. Levin LA. Neuroprotection and regeneration in glaucoma. *Ophthalmol Clin North Am.* 2005;18(4):585-596, vii.
2. Kuehn MH, Fingert JH, Kwon YH. Retinal ganglion cell death in glaucoma: mechanisms and neuroprotective strategies. *Ophthalmol Clin North Am.* 2005;18(3):383-395, vi.
3. Cavanagh JB. The "dying back" process. A common denominator in many naturally occurring and toxic neuropathies. *Arch Pathol Lab Med.* 1979;103(13):659-664.
4. Quigley HA, Addicks EM, Green WR, Maumenee AE. Optic nerve damage in human glaucoma. II. The site of injury and susceptibility to damage. *Arch Ophthalmol.* 1981;99(4):635-649.
5. Quigley HA, Anderson DR. Distribution of axonal transport blockade by acute intraocular pressure elevation in the primate optic nerve head. *Invest Ophthalmol Vis Sci.* 1977;16(7):640-644.
6. Berkelaar M, Clarke DB, Wang YC, et al. Axotomy results in delayed death and apoptosis of retinal ganglion cells in adult rats. *J Neurosci.* 1994;14(7):4368-4374.
7. Garcia-Valenzuela E, Gorczyca W, Darzynkiewicz Z, Sharma SC. Apoptosis in adult retinal ganglion cells after axotomy. *J Neurobiol.* 1994;25(4):431-438.
8. Li Y, Schlamp CL, Nickells RW. Experimental induction of retinal ganglion cell death in adult mice. *Invest Ophthalmol Vis Sci.* 1999;40(5):1004-1008.
9. Quigley HA, Nickells RW, Kerrigan LA, et al. Retinal ganglion cell death in experimental glaucoma and after axotomy occurs by apoptosis. *Invest Ophthalmol Vis Sci.* 1995;36(5):774-786.
10. Garcia-Valenzuela E, Shareef S, Walsh J, Sharma SC. Programmed cell death of retinal ganglion cells during experimental glaucoma. *Exp Eye Res.* 1995;61(1):33-44.

11. Howell GR, Libby RT, Jakobs TC, et al. Axons of retinal ganglion cells are insulted in the optic nerve early in DBA/2J glaucoma. *J Cell Biol.* 2007;179(7):1523-1537.

12. Nickells RW, Semaan SJ, Schlamp CL. Involvement of the Bcl2 gene family in the signaling and control of retinal ganglion cell death. *Prog Brain Res.* 2008;173:423-435.

13. Klocker N, Kermer P, Weishaupt JH, et al. Brain-derived neurotrophic factor-mediated neuroprotection of adult rat retinal ganglion cells in vivo does not exclusively depend on phosphatidyl-inositol-3'-kinase/protein kinase B signaling. *J Neurosci.* 2000;20(18):6962-6967.

14. McKinnon SJ, Lehman DM, Kerrigan-Baumrind LA, et al. Caspase activation and amyloid precursor protein cleavage in rat ocular hypertension. *Invest Ophthalmol Vis Sci.* 2002;43(4):1077-1087.

15. Hanninen VA, Pantcheva MB, Freeman EE, et al. Activation of caspase 9 in a rat model of experimental glaucoma. *Curr Eye Res.* 2002;25(6):389-395.

16. Chaudhary P, Ahmed F, Quebada P, Sharma SC. Caspase inhibitors block the retinal ganglion cell death following optic nerve transection. *Brain Res Mol Brain Res.* 1999;67(1):36-45.

17. Kermer P, Ankerhold R, Klocker N, et al. Caspase-9: involvement in secondary death of axotomized rat retinal ganglion cells in vivo. *Brain Res Mol Brain Res.* 2000;85(1-2):144-150.

18. Johnson EC, Guo Y, Cepurna WO, Morrison JC. Neurotrophin roles in retinal ganglion cell survival: lessons from rat glaucoma models. *Exp Eye Res.* 2009;88(4):808-815.

19. Quigley HA, McKinnon SJ, Zack DJ, et al. Retrograde axonal transport of BDNF in retinal ganglion cells is blocked by acute IOP elevation in rats. *Invest Ophthalmol Vis Sci.* 2000;41(11):3460-3466.

20. Pease ME, McKinnon SJ, Quigley HA, et al. Obstructed axonal transport of BDNF and its receptor TrkB in experimental glaucoma. *Invest Ophthalmol Vis Sci.* 2000;41(3):764-774.

21. Vecino E, Garcia-Grespo D, Garcia M, et al. Rat retinal ganglion cells co-express brain derived neurotrophic factor (BDNF) and its receptor TrkB. *Vision Res.* 2002;42(2):151-157.

22. Spalding KL, Rush RA, Harvey AR. Target-derived and locally derived neurotrophins support retinal ganglion cell survival in the neonatal rat retina. *J Neurobiol.* 2004;60(3):319-327.

23. Seki M, Tanaka T, Sakai Y, et al. Muller cells as a source of brain-derived neurotrophic factor in the retina: noradrenaline upregulates brain-derived neurotrophic factor levels in cultured rat Muller cells. *Neurochem Res.* 2005;30(9):1163-1170.

24. Kalback W, Watson MD, Kokjohn TA, et al. APP transgenic mice Tg2576 accumulate Abeta peptides that are distinct from the chemically modified and insoluble peptides deposited in Alzheimer's disease senile plaques. *Biochemistry.* 2002;41(3):922-928.

25. Martin KR, Quigley HA, Zack DJ, et al. Gene therapy with brain-derived neurotrophic factor as a protection: retinal ganglion cells in a rat glaucoma model. *Invest Ophthalmol Vis Sci.* 2003;44(10): 4357-4365.

26. Pease ME, Zack DJ, Berlinicke C, et al. Effect of CNTF on retinal ganglion cell survival in experimental glaucoma. *Invest Ophthalmol Vis Sci.* 2009;50(5):2194-2200.

27. Lucas DR, Newhouse JP. The toxic effect of sodium L-glutamate on the inner layers of the retina. *AMA Arch Ophthalmol.* 1957;58(2):193-201.

28. Seki M, Lipton SA. Targeting excitotoxic/free radical signaling pathways for therapeutic intervention in glaucoma. *Prog Brain Res.* 2008;173:495-510.

29. Lipton SA, Rosenberg PA. Excitatory amino acids as a final common pathway for neurologic disorders. *N Engl J Med.* 1994;330(9):613-622.

30. Dreyer EB, Zurakowski D, Schumer RA, et al. Elevated glutamate levels in the vitreous body of humans and monkeys with glaucoma. *Arch Ophthalmol.* 1996;114(3):299-305.

31. Honkanen RA, Baruah S, Zimmerman MB, et al. Vitreous amino acid concentrations in patients with glaucoma undergoing vitrectomy. *Arch Ophthalmol.* 2003;121(2):183-188.

32. Levkovitch-Verbin H, Martin KR, Quigley HA, et al. Measurement of amino acid levels in the vitreous humor of rats after chronic intraocular pressure elevation or optic nerve transection. *J Glaucoma.* 2002;11(5):396-405.

33. Wamsley S, Gabelt BT, Dahl DB, et al. Vitreous glutamate concentration and axon loss in monkeys with experimental glaucoma. *Arch Ophthalmol.* 2005;123(1):64-70.

34. WoldeMussie E, Yoles E, Schwartz M, et al. Neuroprotective effect of memantine in different retinal injury models in rats. *J Glaucoma.* 2002;11(6):474-480.

35. Hare WA, WoldeMussie E, Lai RK, et al. Efficacy and safety of memantine treatment for reduction of changes associated with experimental glaucoma in monkey, I: functional measures. *Invest Ophthalmol Vis Sci.* 2004;45(8):2625-2639.

36. Hare WA, WoldeMussie E, Weinreb RN, et al. Efficacy and safety of memantine treatment for reduction of changes associated with experimental glaucoma in monkey, II: structural measures. *Invest Ophthalmol Vis Sci.* 2004;45(8):2640-2651.

37. Yucel YH, Gupta N, Zhang Q, et al. Memantine protects neurons from shrinkage in the lateral geniculate nucleus in experimental glaucoma. *Arch Ophthalmol.* 2006;124(2):217-225.

38. Reitz C, Brayne C, Mayeux R. Epidemiology of Alzheimer disease. *Nat Rev Neurol.* 2011;7(3):137-152.

39. Hinton DR, Sadun AA, Blanks JC, Miller CA. Optic-nerve degeneration in Alzheimer's disease. *N Engl J Med.* 1986;315(8):485-487.

40. Sadun AA, Bassi CJ. Optic nerve damage in Alzheimer's disease. *Ophthalmology.* 1990;97(1):9-17.

41. Bayer AU, Keller ON, Ferrari F, Maag KP. Association of glaucoma with neurodegenerative diseases with apoptotic cell death: Alzheimer's disease and Parkinson's disease. *Am J Ophthalmol.* 2002;133(1):135-137.

42. Tamura H, Kawakami H, Kanamoto T, et al. High frequency of open-angle glaucoma in Japanese patients with Alzheimer's disease. *J Neurol Sci.* 2006;246(1-2):79-83.

43. Bayer AU, Ferrari F, Erb C. High occurrence rate of glaucoma among patients with Alzheimer's disease. *Eur Neurol.* 2002;47(3):165-168.

44. Guo L, Salt TE, Luong V, et al. Targeting amyloid-beta in glaucoma treatment. *Proc Natl Acad Sci USA.* 2007;104(33):13444-13449.

45. Stevens B, Allen NJ, Vazquez LE, et al. The classical complement cascade mediates CNS synapse elimination. *Cell.* 2007;131(6):1164-1178.

46. Itagaki S, Akiyama H, Saito H, McGeer PL. Ultrastructural localization of complement membrane attack complex (MAC)-like immunoreactivity in brains of patients with Alzheimer's disease. *Brain Res.* 1994;645(1-2):78-84.

47. Emmerling MR, Watson MD, Raby CA, Spiegel K. The role of complement in Alzheimer's disease pathology. *Biochim Biophys Acta.* 2000;1502(1):158-171.

48. Webster SD, Yang AJ, Margol L, et al. Complement component C1q modulates the phagocytosis of Abeta by microglia. *Exp Neurol.* 2000;161(1):127-138.

49. Stasi K, Nagel D, Yang X, et al. Complement component 1Q (C1Q) upregulation in retina of murine, primate, and human glaucomatous eyes. *Invest Ophthalmol Vis Sci.* 2006;47(3):1024-1029.

50. Tezel G, Wax MB. Increased production of tumor necrosis factor-alpha by glial cells exposed to simulated ischemia or elevated hydrostatic pressure induces apoptosis in cocultured retinal ganglion cells. *J Neurosci.* 2000;20(23):8693-8700.

51. Tezel G, Li LY, Patil RV, Wax MB. TNF-alpha and TNF-alpha receptor-1 in the retina of normal and glaucomatous eyes. *Invest Ophthalmol Vis Sci.* 2001;42(8):1787-1794.

52. Nakazawa T, Nakazawa C, Matsubara A, et al. Tumor necrosis factor-alpha mediates oligodendrocyte death and delayed retinal ganglion cell loss in a mouse model of glaucoma. *J Neurosci.* 2006;26(49):12633-12641.

53. Orgul S, Cioffi GA, Bacon DR, Van Buskirk EM. An endothelin-1-induced model of chronic optic nerve ischemia in rhesus monkeys. *J Glaucoma.* 1996;5(2):135-138.

54. Chauhan BC, LeVatte TL, Jollimore CA, et al. Model of endothelin-1-induced chronic optic neuropathy in rat. *Invest Ophthalmol Vis Sci.* 2004;45(1):144-152.

55. Kitano S, Morgan J, Caprioli J. Hypoxic and excitotoxic damage to cultured rat retinal ganglion cells. *Exp Eye Res.* 1996;63(1):105-112.

56. Gross RL, Hensley SH, Gao F, Wu SM. Retinal ganglion cell dysfunction induced by hypoxia and glutamate: potential neuroprotective effects of beta-blockers. *Surv Ophthalmol.* 1999;43(suppl 1):S162-S170.

57. Flammer J, Orgul S, Costa VP, et al. The impact of ocular blood flow in glaucoma. *Prog Retin Eye Res.* 2002;21(4):359-393.

58. Tezel G, Wax MB. Hypoxia-inducible factor 1alpha in the glaucomatous retina and optic nerve head. *Arch Ophthalmol.* 2004;122(9):1348-1356.

59. Netland PA, Chaturvedi N, Dreyer EB. Calcium channel blockers in the management of low-tension and open-angle glaucoma. *Am J Ophthalmol.* 1993;115(5):608-613.

60. Sawada A, Kitazawa Y, Yamamoto T, et al. Prevention of visual field defect progression with brovincamine in eyes with normal-tension glaucoma. *Ophthalmology.* 1996;103(2):283-288.

61. Bose S, Piltz JR, Breton ME. Nimodipine, a centrally active calcium antagonist, exerts a beneficial effect on contrast sensitivity in patients with normal-tension glaucoma and in control subjects. *Ophthalmology.* 1995;102(8):1236-1241.

62. Hayreh SS, Zimmerman MB, Podhajsky P, Alward WL. Nocturnal arterial hypotension and its role in optic nerve head and ocular ischemic disorders. *Am J Ophthalmol.* 1994;117(5):603-624.

74

Adherence to
Glaucoma Medical Therapy

Lisa S. Gamell, MD and Gretta Fridman, MD

One of the great clinical challenges in the management of glaucoma is getting patients to adhere to a therapeutic regimen. C. Everett Koop, former United States Surgeon General, famously remarked, "Drugs don't work in patients who don't take them."[1] The magnitude of this problem has gained more attention in recent years, as evidenced by the increasing number of studies and publications designed to aid the physician in identifying and addressing the issue of poor adherence to glaucoma medical therapy.

Adherence to chronic therapy in glaucoma has been estimated to be at 70% or less.[2] It has been compared to other systemic conditions that are also asymptomatic to the patient and are associated with serious outcomes and for which monitoring is usually done at the doctor's office, such as arterial hypertension and hypercholesterolemia.[3-5] On the other hand, consistent reduction in intraocular pressure (IOP) has been reported to reduce a risk of glaucoma progression, decreasing the risk of optic nerve damage and visual field deterioration.[6-8]

In general, physicians have difficulty detecting whether or not patients are adherent with glaucoma medical therapy. Studies[5,9,10] have demonstrated that most physicians significantly overestimate their ability to identify patients who are not taking their medications, thereby limiting opportunities to assess and modify barriers to adherence. Many physicians underestimate the role of risk factors and their own influence on the patient's adherence. The risk factors for poor adherence have recently been classified into 4 categories: patient factors, provider factors, medication regimen, and situational factors.[11]

Patient factors include the patient's motivation and understanding of the health benefits of the treatment, remembering to administer drops, physical ability and dexterity for drop administration, and comorbidities—other systemic illnesses that may also require medication use. Many of the glaucoma patients are elderly with impaired visual acuity and other physical and cognitive ailments, limiting their ability to identify and instill drops correctly. In one study,[12] patients who had someone else administer the drops for them were more likely to find it difficult to remember taking their drops. Certain of these factors can be modified, such as clear labeling, large-print regimen handouts, and reminder phone calls. Other factors, such as a patient's level of education (which is associated with poor adherence) cannot be altered.

Provider factors include the patient's perception of the relationship with the physician, the ability to communicate and understand the medication regimen, as well as the satisfaction with the care received. Motivating patients to learn more about the disease and encouraging active participation in setting therapeutic goals can be achieved by the physician or office staff. Of note, not understanding the chronic nature of glaucoma medical treatment is a significant reason for patients discontinuing topical therapy.

Regimen factors include the cost of the medications, the complexity of the medication schedule, and side effects. Although cost is important in glaucoma therapy, it was not found to be a consistent factor significantly affecting adherence. One study[13] found the highest adherence to medication regimen when taking a prostaglandin analog, which also had one of the highest copayments. On average, the more complicated the dosing regimen, the higher the likelihood of adherence problems. In practice, balancing the cost of the medications may be difficult, while trying to simplify the regimen, such as using combination drops, and finding the medications that will minimize the side effects.

Situational factors consist of other life events interfering with the ability to administer medications. Major life changes, such as birth or death in the family, jobs with demanding schedules, travel, or being away from home are associated with poor adherence.[11] Most situational factors cannot be

Kahook MY, Schuman JS, eds.
Chandler and Grant's Glaucoma, Fifth Edition (pp 705-707).
© 2013 SLACK Incorporated.

directly modified by a physician, but rather influenced by increasing the patient's knowledge and understanding about the disease and the need for consistent treatment.

The Glaucoma Adherence and Persistency Study (GAPS) is the largest study to date looking at adherence to topical medication by the glaucoma patients.[2,9,13] GAPS used medication possession ratio (MPR) as the measure for adherence to therapy. MPR is the number of days of prescription supply dispensed divided by the number of days between the first and last prescription refill. An MPR of 1.0 indicates that the patient possessed all of the medication necessary for complete adherence. Any MPR less than 1.0 indicates less-than-complete adherence.

Data from 10,260 subjects[14] were analyzed. The mean MPR for the GAPS cohort was 0.64.[14] GAPS identified 8 of the following independent variables that lowered the MPR by up to 34%:

1. Hearing all of what you know about glaucoma from your doctor (compared with some or nothing)
2. Not believing that reduced vision is a risk of not taking medication as recommended
3. Having a problem paying for medications
4. Difficulty while traveling or being away from home
5. Not acknowledging stinging and burning
6. Being non-White
7. Receiving samples
8. Not receiving a phone call visit reminder

While a physician can attempt to address some of these barriers to adherence, others are inherent to the patient and cannot be modified. GAPS also identified different learning styles among patients to highlight the importance of a tailored, patient-centered approach.

The first step toward improved adherence is detection. Recognizing nonadherence can be a difficult task in the typically short encounter the physician has with the patient. Patients are reluctant to admit nonadherence as they do not want to be perceived as bad patients.[15] Using a 4-step adherence assessment interview as described by Hahn[15] can help a physician identify and address problems with adherence. The first step is to find out what the patient understands about his or her medication regimen by asking an open-ended question about taking medication. The second step is to explicitly acknowledge that taking medication is difficult and that forgetting or missing a dose is understandable. The third step is to ensure that the patient understands that treatment decisions depend on knowing the actual regimen adhered to by the patient. Thus, if the IOP is elevated at the time of the visit, it is important to convey to the patient that admission to the nonadherence might avoid the unnecessary escalation in therapy. The final step is to ask directly about adherence. It is important that this step would be the last in this sequence as direct questioning early on might lead to

---

WHAT DO WE ACTUALLY DO TO ENSURE ADHERENCE?

Lisa S. Gamell, MD

Talk to the patients. We ask open-ended questions when they come in for a visit, such as "So which medications are you using? And how often do you put them in?" These open-ended questions are more likely to elicit an honest response than asking "So are you using the timolol twice a day?" where you have already given the patient the right answer. We ask questions about the patient's daily schedule and lifestyle. This helps us tailor the drug regimen to the patient's schedule. We commonly write the eye drop instructions on a sheet, detailing the name of the drug, the cap color, which eye, and how many times a day the drug should be administered. If necessary, we write a schedule for the eye drops, specifying times as well. We ask patients to always bring all of their drops and their schedule with them to each visit.

What if the patient's pressure is high but the patient claims to be using the drops? We bring the patient back for an early-morning visit, when he or she should have recently used their drops. If the pressure is high, we administer the medication in the office. If the IOP comes down dramatically, he or she probably forgot to use the medication.

If we suspect a patient is nonadherent, we do have him or her return for more frequent visits, especially in the setting of more advanced disease. If they have a family member or close friend who can be involved and help them take greater interest in their ocular health, we often ask them to bring that person to one of the visits.

The best thing a physician can do to create an open dialogue about adherence is to not be judgmental. We will often ask patients if they are having trouble getting their medications in or are taking them on schedule. If they admit to an adherence problem, we ask what they think the issue is and what changes could be made to help make taking medication easier for them. Empowering the patient is an important step in building trust in the therapeutic relationship. Sometimes, their goal may be to not take medications at all, and the possibility of laser trabeculoplasty may be raised as a viable option. For others, the idea of a procedure, whether it be laser or incisional surgery, is enough to motivate adherence to medical therapy.

---

false assurance of adherence.[15] Once nonadherence is established, the specific barriers can be identified and addressed.

In order to improve a patient's adherence, his or her motivational factors have to be understood. If the perception of the need for treatment does not outweigh the concerns about the medication use, the patient is unlikely to be adherent. Therefore, education should be targeted toward increasing the patient's knowledge of the disease and its course. The manner in which this is done can play a dramatic role in altering adherence. All too often, physicians start out with a manufactured speech they give all of their patients. Although they may modify it to the patient's perceived education level, and even give an opportunity to ask questions at the end, this approach may not be very successful. Often, patients already have certain understandings and beliefs, which they may not know how to merge with the information provided. Instead, a better approach is to use *ask-tell-ask* dialogue. In this model, the physician first asks the patient about his or her current understanding and concerns about the disease and treatment. This gives the physician an opportunity to learn not only what the patient knows about the disease, but also any incorrect information the patient might believe. It also provides a framework for discussion, as the physician can add to the information the patient already possesses. After completing the *tell*, another *ask* is required to assess if the patient has understood and internalized the information, and give the patient the opportunity to clarify any concerns. It is important that open-ended questions are used to prompt the patient to verbalize comprehension.[15]

Being actively aware of the adherence barriers is the first step in battling nonadherence. Identifying patients at risk and the barriers at hand is the next logical step. Providers should design and implement strategies and interventions that work for their practice. Some strategies may include the following:

- Trying to address adherence problems early on

- Training office staff to educate patients about glaucoma and the importance of treatment

- Simplifying regimens, reviewing medications at each visit

- Assessing and reducing side effects

- Keeping a medication diary

- Using telephone reminders

- Large-print handouts that are easy for patients to understand

- Working with patients' insurance companies to minimize cost

- Being supportive and encouraging open communication[16]

Last, it is important to remember that patients can regress at any time, so adherence assessment is a long-term undertaking—just as is glaucoma medical therapy.

REFERENCES

1. Mansberger SL. Are you compliant with addressing glaucoma adherence? *Am J Ophthalmol.* 2010;149:1-3.

2. Friedman DS, Quigley HA, Gelb L, et al. Using pharmacy data to study adherence to glaucoma medications: methodology and findings of the Glaucoma Adherence and Persistence Study (GAPS). *Invest Ophthalmol Vis Sci.* 2007;48(11):5052-5057.

3. Rudd P, Ahmen S, Zachary V, et al. Improved compliance measures: applications in an ambulatory hypertensive drug trial. *Clin Pharmacol Ther.* 1990;48:676-685.

4. Gordon ME, Kass MA. Validity of standard compliance measures in glaucoma compared with an electronic eye drop monitor. In: Cramer JA, Spilker B, eds. *Patient Compliance in Medical Practice and Clinical Trials.* New York, NY: Raven Press; 1991:163-173.

5. Kass MA, Meltzer DW, Gordon M, et al. Compliance with topical pilocarpine treatment. *Am J Ophthalmol.* 1986;101:515-523.

6. Kass MA, Heuer DK, Higginbotham EJ, et al. The ocular hypertension treatment study: a randomized trial determines that topical ocular hypotensive medication delays or prevents the onset of primary open-angle glaucoma. *Arch Ophthalmol.* 2002;120:701-713.

7. Collaborative Normal-Tension Glaucoma Study Group. The effectiveness of intraocular pressure reduction in the treatment of normal-tension glaucoma. *Am J Ophthalmol.* 1998;126:498-505.

8. The AGIS Investigators. The Advance Glaucoma Intervention Study (AGIS): 7. The relationship between control of intraocular pressure and visual field deterioration. *Am J Ophthalmol.* 2000;130:429-440.

9. Gelb L, Friedman DS, Quigley HA, et al. Physician beliefs and behaviors related to glaucoma treatment adherence. The Glaucoma Adherence and Persistency Study. *J Glaucoma.* 2008;17:690-698.

10. Okeke CO, Quigley HA, Jampel HD, et al. Adherence with topical glaucoma medication monitored electronically the Travatan Dosing Aid study. *Ophthalmology.* 2009;116:191-199.

11. Tsai JC, McClure CA, Ramos SE, et al. Compliance barriers in glaucoma: a systematic classification. *J Glaucoma.* 2003;12:393-398.

12. Sleath B, Robin AL, Covert D, et al. Patient-reported behavior and problems in using glaucoma medications. *Ophthalmology.* 2006;113:431-436.

13. Nordstrom BL, Friedman DS, Mozaffari E, et al. Persistence and adherence with topical glaucoma therapy. *Am J Ophthalmol.* 2005;140:598-606.

14. Tsai JC. A comprehensive perspective on patient adherence to topical glaucoma therapy. *Ophthalmology.* 2009;116(11 suppl):s30-s36.

15. Hahn SR. Patient-centered communication to assess and enhance patient adherence to glaucoma medication. *Ophthalmology.* 2009;116(11 suppl):s37-s42.

16. Budenz DL. A clinician's guide to the assessment and management of nonadherence in glaucoma. *Ophthalmology.* 2009;116(11 suppl):s43-s47.

75

Epidemiology of Glaucoma

Michael B. Horsley, MD and M. Roy Wilson, MD, MS

In its broadest interpretation, epidemiology encompasses a vast field and includes the following issues related to disease:

- Occurrence and distribution
- Factors that influence that occurrence and distribution
- Health delivery and outcome measures

With respect to glaucoma, investigations related to epidemiology have been focused on determining occurrence and distribution and on investigating possible risk factors. The past decade has witnessed an explosion of knowledge in these areas. More recently, various outcome measures related to having glaucoma and to treating it have received increasing attention.

Knowledge derived from epidemiological studies contributes to a better understanding of the disease, assists in clinical decision-making, and allows a better appreciation of the individual and societal impact of having the disease. This chapter focuses on epidemiological aspects of primary open-angle glaucoma (POAG). Other types of glaucoma (eg, pigmentary, exfoliation, and primary angle-closure) have distinguishing epidemiological features and are discussed in other chapters of this edition.

OCCURRENCE AND DISTRIBUTION

It is estimated that at least 2.79 million Americans 40 years of age and older have POAG.[1] Due to a rapidly aging population, by 2020 this number is predicted to increase by 50%.[1] In addition, approximately 400,000 Americans are currently believed to be bilaterally blind from glaucoma.[1]

Glaucoma is second only to cataract in causing blindness in the world. Recent reports[2,3] have suggested the mean prevalence for POAG worldwide in 2010 to be 1.96%, or nearly 48 million people. It is also postulated that this total will increase to more than 58 million people in the next decade. More than 5.9 million people worldwide will be bilaterally blind from POAG in 2020.[1]

Estimates of the prevalence of POAG can be relied upon with confidence only if standardized sampling methodology is used, if the diagnosis is based upon evidence of optic nerve and/or visual field damage, and if appropriate evaluations, including gonioscopy, are performed on a large proportion of subjects. In recent years, well-designed population-based studies have been conducted to determine the prevalence of POAG in many areas of Europe, the United States, the Caribbean, Australia, and Asia. This increase in epidemiologically sound glaucoma prevalence data provides greater confidence in the global estimates of the numbers of people affected.

The overall prevalence of POAG worldwide is estimated to be approximately 2%.[1] During the past few decades, multiple population-based studies have attempted to define the prevalence of POAG in select populations. In the Baltimore Eye Survey[4] (1985-1988), the prevalence of POAG in the White population ranged from 0.92% for those older than 40 years of age and up to 2.16% for those older than 80 years of age. For Black Americans in that study, the range was from 1.23% to 11.26% in the same age categories. For the Beaver Dam Eye Study[5] (1988-1990) and in the Rotterdam Study[6] (1990-1993), the overall prevalence was 2.1%. The Barbados Eye Study[7] (1988-1992) showed an overall prevalence of POAG of 6.67% (7.0% in Black persons, 3.3% in multiracial persons, and 0.8% in White persons). More recent studies have yielded prevalence estimates of 2.1% in Segovia, Spain[8]; 1.62% to 1.7% in southern India (Andhra Pradesh Eye Disease Study)[9,10]; 0.5% in Mongolia[11]; 2.9% in Temba, South Africa[12]; 2.3% in Thailand[13]; 1.7% in Melbourne, Australia[14]; and 2.7% in Thessaloniki, Greece.[15] From the 2000 Census figures and a meta-analysis of recent population-based studies, the prevalence of POAG was estimated at 1.86% in the United States.[16] These aforementioned studies are particularly noteworthy for using highly standardized methodology and for defining glaucoma on the basis of optic nerve and/or visual field damage. Gonioscopy was performed as part of the evaluation in the Baltimore Eye Study,[4] the Andhra

Kahook MY, Schuman JS, eds.
Chandler and Grant's Glaucoma, Fifth Edition (pp 709-716).
© 2013 SLACK Incorporated.

Pradesh Eye Disease Study,[9,10] and in the studies performed in Thailand,[13] Mongolia,[11] and Temba.[12] An assessment of anterior chamber depth was made with a slit-lamp in the Beaver Dam Study[5] and with a penlight using the method of Van Herick in the Rotterdam Study,[6] but gonioscopy was not performed. The Segovia Study[8] performed anterior segment biomicroscopy to evaluate the angle structures. Without gonioscopy or an evaluation with anterior segment imaging, cases of chronic angle-closure glaucoma may be misclassified as open-angle glaucoma (OAG).

More recently, Quigley and Broman[1] summarized the prevalence of glaucoma worldwide. The prevalence of OAG in patients older than 40 years of age for the 8 regions in their study were as follows: Africa (4.2%), Japan (3.3%), Latin America (3.2%), Europe (2.0%), India (1.8%), China (1.4%), Middle East (1.3%), and Southeast Asia (1.2%).

It has long been established that the prevalence of glaucoma increases with age.[17-20] Prevalence estimates have generally been 3 to 8 times higher in the oldest age groups compared with people in their 40s. In addition, the Ocular Hypertensive Treatment Study[21] and the European Glaucoma Prevention Study[21] found that age had a relative risk of 1.22 to 1.32 per decade for the development of glaucoma in patients with ocular hypertension.[21]

A racial disparity in glaucoma prevalence also exists. The Baltimore Eye Survey[4] was performed in a racially mixed population, and it found the prevalence of POAG among Black persons to be 3 to 4 times higher than among White persons. Also, a higher prevalence has been reported among Black persons in St. Lucia[22] and Barbados,[7] West Indies, than among Black persons in Baltimore, Maryland.[4] Prevalence of 8.8% were found among Black individuals 30 years of age and older in St. Lucia and 7.0% among Black individuals 40 years of age and older in Barbados. Currently, we do not know whether the observed differences among Black individuals in the West Indies compared with Black individuals in Baltimore reflect an inherently higher rate of disease among the West Indians or are related to differences in design of the studies.

Data from Baltimore[4] and from the West Indies[7,22] suggest that there is likely a high prevalence among Black people of African descent. A number of clinic-based studies[21,23] and population-based general ophthalmology surveys[22,24] have certainly suggested a high prevalence among some African populations.[21-24] However, these results have not been uniformly consistent, and it is likely that there are wide variations in prevalence of POAG and other types of glaucoma among the various regions of Africa.[25]

Two recent studies have focused on the prevalence of POAG in the Hispanic population: Proyecto VER[26] and the Los Angeles Latino Eye Study (LALES).[27] Proyecto VER used 1990 census data from Arizona to estimate the overall POAG prevalence at 1.97% for Hispanics in that state. Of note, this study described a steeper slope of increase in prevalence with age as compared to previous reports in

other populations. In the LALES population-based study, Hispanics of primarily Mexican ancestry older than 40 years of age from 6 census tracts in Los Angeles, CA, were identified. The overall prevalence of POAG was 4.74%. In the Arizona study, all adults older than 40 years of age in the home of a self-described Hispanic were included. This population, therefore, may have included Hispanics of other nationalities as well as American Indians. As with the data on Black individuals in Baltimore[4] versus the West Indies,[7,22] there was a significant disparity in prevalence in these 2 studies. Whether this difference is due to study design or differences in prevalence in different Hispanic subpopulations is yet to be determined.

Previous population-based general ophthalmology surveys and clinic-based data from various regions of Asia indicated a high proportion of cases of glaucoma to be of the angle-closure variety.[28] However, a nationwide glaucoma survey[29] conducted in Japan found an OAG prevalence of 2.62% and only 0.34% for POAG. More recently, the Tajimi Study[30] (2000 to 2001) found an overall prevalence of POAG of 3.9% in this central Japanese city. Another interesting finding of this study[30] was that the large majority (92%) of subjects determined to have POAG had an IOP less than 21 mm Hg.

Although our knowledge of race-specific prevalence for POAG is less than complete, there is an even greater dearth of incidence data. Whereas prevalence reflects the number of cases in a given population at a given time, incidence reflects the number of new cases that develop in a given population within a given time frame. In a disease such as POAG, which is chronic and has a relatively low incidence, large cohorts and long follow-up periods are necessary to obtain a sufficient number of newly diagnosed cases to ensure valid estimates. Thus, only a few population-based studies to determine glaucoma incidence have been attempted. One such study[31] performed in Dalby, Sweden, found an incidence of between 0.19% and 0.24% per year. The Barbados Eye Study[32,33] recently reported its 9-year incidence report of OAG at 4.4% (0.49% per year). They also found the 9-year incidence of bilateral blindness in this population, based on the World Health Organization (WHO) criteria, to be 1.0% (0.11% per year); 14.3% of these cases were attributable to POAG. Finally, a follow-up of the Rotterdam Study found that the 5-year incidence of probable POAG was 1.2% (0.24% per year) and that of definite glaucoma was 0.6% (0.12% per year) in patients older than 55 years of age.[34]

Factors That Influence Occurrence and Distribution of Primary Open-Angle Glaucoma

It is well accepted that most diseases do not occur randomly throughout a population but that the frequency varies in different subgroups of people. It is important to

TABLE 75-1. RISK FACTORS FOR PRIMARY OPEN-ANGLE GLAUCOMA
Intraocular pressure
Age
Race/ethnicity (greater in Black and Hispanic populations)
Family history of primary open-angle glaucoma
Central corneal thickness
Possible risk factors: Cup/disc ratio Myopia Systemic hypertension Adult-onset diabetes mellitus

understand what causes this uneven distribution. In doing so, risk factors for the disease can be identified (Table 75-1).

Identifying risk factors is important because this information may lead to the development of strategies for disease screening and prevention and may be useful for identifying people for whom close medical supervision is indicated. Strictly defined, a factor can be considered a risk factor only if it truly predates disease occurrence. However, from a clinical perspective, it is often difficult to differentiate normal from very early disease. In fact, this determination is often dependent on how the disease is defined. Glaucoma is usually defined by the presence of characteristic visual field defects and sometimes, in the absence of visual field defects, by the appearance of optic nerve damage. How often this diagnosis is made in marginal cases is influenced by the sensitivity of available diagnostic tests. Thus, determining whether abnormalities in certain parameters (eg, optic nerve parameters, such as nerve fiber layer loss) are indicative of increased susceptibility to developing glaucoma or are signs of early disease may pose a dilemma. From a practical standpoint, the distinction is unimportant. Individuals manifesting such abnormalities must be closely monitored for signs of clinically significant disease development in either situation.

Current thinking regarding risk factors for glaucoma is influenced by data collected in 2 large recently completed clinical trials of treatment versus observation of subjects with ocular hypertension.[35,36] There is general agreement that IOP, age, race, central corneal thickness (CCT), and family history of glaucoma are risk factors for POAG. The relevance of optic nerve parameters, refractive status, and various systemic factors, such as diabetes, systemic hypertension, migraine, and arteriosclerotic and ischemic vascular diseases as factors that affect glaucoma risk, is less certain.

Elevated IOP is generally accepted as a risk factor for POAG. It is perhaps the most important of the risk factors

in that it is the only factor for which a causal mechanism has been ascribed and is the only factor currently amenable to modification. A causal role of IOP in glaucoma is supported by considering examples of experimentally induced high IOP in animals that result in typical glaucomatous cupping,[37,38] examples of acute angle closure and unilateral secondary glaucoma in which glaucomatous damage occurs in the eye with elevated IOP, and examples of normal but asymmetric IOPs that result in asymmetrical cupping and visual field loss with greater damage on the side with the higher IOP.[39,40] However, it must be recognized that a 1-to-1 relationship between elevated IOP and glaucoma does not exist. For example, glaucomatous damage may occur despite normal or even low IOP levels.

The efficacy of lowering IOP in preventing progressive glaucomatous damage was demonstrated in the Early Manifest Glaucoma Trial.[35] Two hundred fifty-five patients with POAG were randomized to laser trabeculoplasty plus topical betaxolol or no immediate treatment. Patients who were treated early had half the progression risk of the control patients, and the initial IOP reduction was the major factor influencing this improved outcome. Also, the results of the Collaborative Normal Tension Glaucoma Study[41] showed that IOP plays a major role in glaucomatous nerve progression, even in the subgroup of eyes with statistically normal IOPs. In a 13-year follow-up to the Ocular Hypertension Treatment Study,[36] those patients who had received ocular hypotensive medical treatment immediately after ocular hypertension was diagnosed had a 16% chance of developing POAG versus 22% for the group who received delayed treatment.

Population-based studies[3-7,14-16,20,27] have established that glaucoma prevalence increases with age. Although age-specific incidence rates of POAG in normal populations have not yet been determined, the Collaborative Glaucoma Study[20] found that visual field defects developed at a rate 7 times higher in people 60 years of age and older compared to people younger than 40 years. The exact causal mechanisms responsible for increased susceptibility of older people to POAG is not known. IOP tends to increase with age, but this is not likely to be a primary explanation. The magnitude of the IOP increase with age is not great, and this age-related rise has not been consistently demonstrated among all populations. For example, among Japanese, IOP apparently decreases with age whereas POAG increases with age.[29] There is a study that even found an inverse correlation between IOP and age when accounting for blood pressure change.[42] This suggests that there are other vascular or mechanical factors at play in addition to the well-established risk factor of increased IOP leading to glaucomatous nerve changes in older patients who develop POAG.

The race-specific incidence data in the Barbados Eye Study[7] suggest a large disparity in the development of POAG for Black individuals compared to White individuals. In addition to these results, the magnitude of the racial disparity in the prevalence data strongly suggests that Black persons develop glaucoma at a higher rate than White persons. Among the hypotheses offered to explain this increased susceptibility among the Black population are that Black individuals have higher IOPs,[43] thinner CCTs,[44] larger cup/disc ratios,[45,46] higher prevalence of diseases that may cause ischemia of the optic nerve head,[47] and medical undersurveillance compared to White individuals.[48,49] Data do not unequivocally support any of these hypotheses, and the exact biological, anatomical, or social factors that may be operational in placing the Black population at greater risk of developing glaucoma are not yet known.

It is well established that family members of subjects with POAG have an underlying susceptibility to the development of the disease. Exactly how much more at risk a family member is compared to the general population is not known with certainty. The Baltimore Eye Survey[4] solicited information on the history of glaucoma in relatives and reported age-adjusted associations with POAG subjects. Odds ratios for having a history of glaucoma were found to be 3.69 for siblings and 2.17 for parents.[50] However, these estimates are susceptible to recall bias because people with glaucoma are probably more likely to recall the disease or to attribute all vision disorders to glaucoma. Many ocular parameters, such as cup/disc ratio, IOP, and POAG, were shown to be influenced by genetics through the work of the Salisbury Eye Evaluation.[51] They found that family members of patients with POAG had a larger cup/disc ratio and higher IOPs and concluded that cup/disc ratio was highly heritable and IOP moderately heritable.

The genetic basis for juvenile glaucoma is more firmly established than for POAG. An autosomal dominant inheritance pattern has been documented in several large multigeneration families for juvenile glaucoma.[52,53] The genetic factors influencing POAG appear to be far more complex than those for juvenile glaucoma. The search for genetic markers associated with POAG has recently yielded some exciting developments as a number of both chromosomal and genetic associations have been established.[54] These associations are discussed in other chapters of this book.

The Ocular Hypertension Treatment Study[55] further clarified and added to our knowledge of risk factors of POAG. Central corneal thickness was found to be a powerful predictor for development of POAG.[55] In addition, this study showed that race (ie, Black American), older age, larger vertical or horizontal cup/disc ratio, and higher IOP were risk factors. CCT has been proven to be an independent risk factor for progression of ocular hypertension to POAG in multiple subsequent studies.[56-61] In addition, it has been described as a risk factor for the presence of glaucoma in the Barbados Eye Study,[61] the Rotterdam Study,[62] as well as the Los Angeles Latino Eye Study.[63] However, a thin CCT was not associated with glaucoma in 2 large population-based studies.[30,64] The use of CCT measurement as a screening parameter for POAG remains a subject of controversy. The explanation of why CCT is a risk factor for glaucoma is still not known. One theory is that when the CCT is thinner, the measured IOP is lower than the true higher IOP. But, the OHTS trial showed that there was a strong independent risk of CCT. Further studies are needed to understand if there is a biomechanical correlation of CCT and its effect on the optic nerve head's susceptibility to glaucomatous damage.

Data regarding the possible role of other factors in the development of POAG are conflicting. Associations between myopia and POAG have been observed,[65,66] but it is possible that these associations were influenced by selection bias because people who have refractive errors are more likely to seek eye care and have a higher probability of being diagnosed as having glaucoma.

Various optic nerve parameters such as large cup/disc ratio,[21,67,68] asymmetric cupping,[69,70] disc hemorrhages (DHs),[41,71-73] and loss of the nerve fiber layer[74] have been declared risk factors for development of glaucoma. With regard to the optic nerve, discs with large cup/disc ratios also tend to be larger with proportionally more neural rim tissue.[75] Thus, a determination of the cup/disc ratio must consider the size of the optic disc. Also, in some cases, a large cup/disc ratio as well as the other parameters listed above may represent signs of early glaucoma. In the Ocular Hypertension Treatment Study,[55] a larger horizontal and vertical cup/disc ratio was considered to be a risk factor for the presence of glaucoma.

Optic DHs are transient and thus are difficult to assess as a risk factor for glaucomatous damage. Even though DHs are an established risk factor for disease progression in glaucoma, not all patients experience advancement in glaucomatous damage after a DH.[76] A recent report[77] showed that the presence of a DH in patients with worse visual fields at baseline predicts further global deterioration of visual field by more than 5 decibel within 4 years. Although many clinicians may wish to advance treatment in patients with DHs, 70% of patients in the Blue Mountain Eye Study[78] who presented with DHs had no other signs of glaucoma. More studies are needed to understand the role of DHs in glaucomatous vision loss and how this should impact practice guidelines.

Positive associations between blood pressure and IOP[79] and between blood pressure and POAG[80] have been reported. Although the evidence for systemic hypertension being a risk factor for glaucoma is not strong, the hypothesis that microcirculatory effects on the optic disc may possibly lead to increased glaucoma susceptibility is biologically plausible. The Rotterdam Study[81] reported an association of systemic hypertension with high-tension glaucoma but not with normal-tension glaucoma. The Baltimore Eye Survey[82] reported modest, positive associations of systolic and diastolic blood pressure with POAG, but the 95% confidence intervals of the odds ratios for these associations included 1.00, the value of no association. However, lower perfusion pressure (blood pressure – IOP) was strongly associated with an increased prevalence of POAG. Although not yet clearly documented, these results suggest that POAG may be associated with an alteration in factors related to ocular blood flow.

The role of diabetes as a risk factor for POAG remains controversial. The Blue Mountain Eye Study[83] as well as others[84-87] have found diabetes and POAG to be correlated. But, the Baltimore Eye Survey[4] did not detect this association. As with myopia, self-selection into the health care system may also have influenced some of the associations found between diabetes and glaucoma. The possible role of arteriosclerotic and ischemic vascular diseases is also unclear. Migraine and peripheral vasospasm may be important in the development of some cases of glaucoma, particularly those with IOP in the normal or low range, although definitive evidence has been lacking up to this point. Further study is needed to clarify the role of all of these factors in the development of glaucoma.

Data are conflicting as to whether POAG is more frequently associated with men or women. Some studies show a higher prevalence in women,[17,86] others in men,[7,19] and some with no appreciable difference between genders.[4,5,14,22,26,27] The possible relevance of general exposures such as diet, stress, alcohol consumption, and cigarette smoking has been inadequately studied, and the scant data available are not convincing enough to warrant further consideration of any of these exposures at this time.[19,87] It is interesting to note that IOP among the Japanese has not been found to increase with age as in Western populations studied.[29] One hypothesis to explain this apparent discrepancy has been that IOP is related to body build and that Japanese typically do not develop obesity with age as do many Americans and Europeans. Such an anthromorphologic consideration does not explain why glaucoma prevalence increases with age among the Japanese. Nonetheless, it suggests that anthromorphology may be an area worthy of further study.

HEALTH DELIVERY AND OUTCOME MEASURES

IOP is believed to be an important causal factor in glaucomatous damage. It is the risk factor most amenable to modification, and the primary goal in treatment of glaucoma has traditionally been to lower the IOP. The efficacy of medications, laser treatments, and incisional surgeries in lowering IOP has been extensively documented. Most clinicians who take care of patients with glaucoma have had the unpleasant experience of witnessing the blinding sequelae of glaucoma left untreated. Understandably, clinicians have enthusiastically embraced the various modalities to lower IOP and undoubtedly, many patients will have been saved from blindness. Many studies, such as the Ocular Hypertension Treatment Study,[36] Collaborative Normal-Tension Glaucoma Study (CNTGS),[41] Early Manifest Glaucoma Trial (EMGT),[35] and Collaborative Initial Glaucoma Treatment Study (CIGTS),[88] have proven that by lowering IOP, glaucomatous damage can

be decreased. The CNTGS[41] showed that the rate of visual field (VF) loss was slowed in eyes with IOP reduction of 30% compared to eyes that did not have pressure reduction. In the EMGT, there was a rate of progression of 45% in the treated group versus 62% in the untreated group. The EMGT also showed that, through the use of argon laser trabeculoplasty plus betaxolol, IOP was reduced by 20% and the risk of worsening glaucoma was decreased by 50%. CIGTS[88] showed that, with an improved IOP control, VF loss was reduced in both the medical and surgical groups.

With the tightening of the health care budget, the government, health insurers, and health provider organizations have begun the process of critically assessing the value of services provided. In this arena of health service research, the goal of glaucoma treatment has focused on lowering IOP to potentiate the preservation of vision. A recent article[89] analyzed the cost-effectiveness of routine office-based identification of POAG as well as the subsequent medical treatment. It found that diagnosing POAG was highly cost-effective when factoring in quality-adjusted life years and the cost per year of sight gained for the patients.

Quality of life is an outcome measure that is gaining increasing notice in glaucoma studies. Glaucoma affects many areas of a patient's life, both psychologically and physically. It has recently been found to be an independent risk factor for depression and is more severe in patients with more advanced glaucomatous vision loss.[90] Also, a study[91] that analyzed determinants of serious falls among elderly glaucoma patients found that using topical medications was the greatest single factor. Many studies[92-94] have found that a patient's perceived visual disability was highly correlated with the level of binocular visual field loss. Among the questionnaires that have been developed to better assess the effect of glaucoma on quality of life is the GQL-15.[95] By focusing this questionnaire on daily activities that may be especially troublesome for patients with glaucoma, even patients with mild glaucoma showed a statistically significant difference in quality of life assessment as compared to controls. In addition, as with the results of the CIGTS study,[96] glare, peripheral vision, and dark adaptation affect quality of life scores in the early stages of glaucoma. From the results of these studies, there is a trend to include visual function and quality of life as a key outcome measure in the treatment of glaucoma. Although the more recently developed questionnaires tend to correlate with visual field loss, suggesting that the quality of life changes are correlated with disease progression, improvements are needed in both the methods of collecting and analyzing quality of life data to ensure that other variables that can affect quality of life have been accounted for.[97]

Two large recent studies have evaluated quality of life in patients with glaucoma (the Salisbury Eye Evaluation[98] and the Los Angeles Latino Eye Study[27]). One found that patients with bilateral glaucoma had significant difficulty on the Activities of Daily Vision Scale[98] and the other that those with central VF loss had lower scores on the National Eye

Institute Visual Function Questionnaire.[99] Undoubtedly, there are numerous other quality-of-life issues that have not yet been investigated, and the potential impact that glaucoma has on quality of life is likely greater than previously appreciated.

An argument has been raised that optimal initial treatment of glaucoma should be surgical rather than medical. Initial studies[100,101] comparing trabeculectomy versus topical treatment to lower IOP showed promising results for early surgical intervention; however, many newer topical treatment modalities have surfaced since these early studies. CIGTS[102] was designed to further investigate this question. At 8-year follow-up, a comparable decrease in vision was noted in both the initial surgical (21.3%) and initial medicine (25.5%) groups, concluding that due to the patient's strict IOP control, VF was minimized in both groups. Also, diabetics may benefit from early surgery, and those with severe VF loss initially may have improved outcomes from an earlier surgical course. Furthermore, although an increase in cataract and local eye symptoms was found in the surgical group, most quality-of-life measurements were similar in both groups. Many factors come into play when deciding the initial step in glaucoma treatment, such as cost of medications; life expectancy; ability to adhere to a treatment regimen and follow-up schedule; and level of current glaucomatous damage. In conclusion, as with many chronic diseases in medicine, a patient-focused approach is needed when deciding upon the most appropriate glaucoma treatment plan.

CONCLUSION

The past decade has witnessed an explosion of information related to epidemiological aspects of glaucoma. Cross-sectional population-based surveys and clinical trials have provided reliable age and race-specific prevalence data as well as risk factors. The focus for the next decade will likely shift. Factors that influence not only glaucoma development but also progression and other outcomes will be further investigated. The accumulation of such epidemiological data in combination with contributions from the basic sciences and clinical practice will bring us that much closer to the goal of designing intervention programs that can prevent, or at least control, the debilitating outcomes associated with glaucoma.

REFERENCES

1. Quigley HA, Broman AT. The number of people with glaucoma worldwide in 2010 and 2020. *Br J Ophthalmol.* 2006;90(3):262-267.
2. Goldberg I. How common is glaucoma worldwide? In: Weinreb R, Kitazawa Y, Krieglstein G, eds. *Glaucoma in the 21st Century.* London: Mosby; 2000:1-9.
3. Friedman DS, Wolfs RC, O'Colmain BJ, et al; Eye Diseases Prevalence Research Group. Prevalence of open-angle glaucoma among adults in the United States. *Arch Ophthalmol.* 2004;122(4):532-538.
4. Tielsch JM, Sommer A, Witt K, Katz J, Royall RM. Blindness and visual impairment in an American urban population: the Baltimore Eye Survey. *Arch Ophthalmol.* 1990;108:286.
5. Klein BE, Klein R, Sponsel WE, et al. Prevalence of glaucoma: the Beaver Dam Eye Study. *Ophthalmology.* 1992;99:1499.
6. Dielemans I, Vingerling JR, Wolfs RC, Hofman A, Grobbee DE, de Jong PT. The prevalence of primary open-angle glaucoma in a population-based study in the Netherlands. *Ophthalmology.* 1994;101:1851-1855.
7. Leske MC, Connell AMS, Schachat AP, et al. The Barbados Eye Study. Prevalence of open angle glaucoma. *Arch Ophthalmol.* 1994;112:821-829.
8. Anton A, Andrada MT, Mujica V, et al. Prevalence of primary open-angle glaucoma in a Spanish population. The Segovia Study. *J Glaucoma.* 2004;13:371-376.
9. Dandona L, Dandona R, Srinivas M. Open-angle glaucoma in an urban population in southern India. *Ophthalmology.* 2000;107:1702-1709.
10. Ramakrishnan R, Nirmalan RK, Krishnadas R, et al. Glaucoma in a rural population of southern India. *Ophthalmology.* 2003;10:1484-1490.
11. Foster PJ, Baasanhu J, Isbirk PH, et al. Glaucoma in Mongolia. A population based survey in Hovsgoll Province, Northern Mongolia. *Arch Ophthalmol.* 1996;114:1235-1241.
12. Rotchford AP, Kirwan JF, Muller MA, et al. Temba Glaucoma Study: a population-based cross-sectional survey in urban South Africa. *Ophthalmology.* 2003;110:376-382.
13. Bourne RR, Sukudom P, Foster PJ, et al. Prevalence of glaucoma in Thailand: a population based survey in Rom Klao District, Bangkok. *Br J Ophthalmol.* 2003;87(9):1069-1074.
14. Wensor MD, McCarty CA, Stanislavsky YL, et al. The prevalence of glaucoma in the Melbourne Visual Impairment Project. *Ophthalmology.* 1998;105:733-739.
15. Topouzis F, Wilson MR, Harris A, et al. Prevalence of open-angle glaucoma in Greece: the Thessaloniki Eye Study. *Am J Ophthalmol.* 2007;144(4):511-519.
16. Friedman DS, Wolfs RC, O'Colmain BJ, et al. Prevalence of open-angle glaucoma among adults in the United States. *Arch Ophthalmol.* 2004;122:532-538.
17. Bengtsson B. The prevalence of glaucoma. *Br J Ophthalmol.* 1981;65:46-49.
18. Hollows FC, Graham PA. Intraocular pressure, glaucoma, and glaucoma suspects in a defined population. *Br J Ophthalmol.* 1986;50:570-585.
19. Kahn HA, Milton RC. Revised Framingham Eye Study: prevalence of glaucoma and diabetic retinopathy. *Am J Epidemiol.* 1989;111:769.
20. Armaly MF, Krueger DE, Maunder L, et al. Biostatistical analysis of the collaborative glaucoma study. I. Summary report of the risk factors for glaucomatous visual-field defects. *Arch Ophthalmol.* 1980;98:2163-2171.
21. Coleman AL, Miglior S. Risk factors for glaucoma onset and progression. *Surv Ophthalmol.* 2008;53(suppl 1):S3-S10.
22. Mason RP, Kosoko O, Wilson MR, et al. National survey of the prevalence and risk factors of glaucoma in St. Lucia, West Indies. Part I: prevalence findings. *Ophthalmology.* 1989;65:1363-1368.
23. Kragha I. Prevalence of glaucoma in an eye hospital in Nigeria. *Am J Optom Physiol Opt.* 1987;64:617-620.
24. Neumann E, Zauberman H. Glaucoma survey in Liberia. *Am J Ophthalmol.* 1965;59:8-12.
25. Verrey JD, Foster A, Wormald R, et al. Chronic glaucoma in Northern Ghana. A retrospective study of 397 patients. *Eye.* 1990;4:115-120.
26. Quigley HA, West SK, Rodriguez J, Munoz B, Klein R, Snyder R. The prevalence of glaucoma in a population-based study of Hispanic subjects: Proyecto VER. *Arch Ophthalmol.* 2001;119:1819-1826.

27. Varma R, Ying-Lai M, Francis BA, et al; Los Angeles Latino Eye Study Group. Prevalence of open-angle glaucoma and ocular hypertension in Latinos: the Los Angeles Latino Eye Study. *Ophthalmology*. 2004;111(8):1439-1448.

28. Congdon N, Wang F, Tielsch JM. Issues in the epidemiology and population-based screening of primary angle-closure glaucoma. *Surv Ophthalmol*. 1992;36:411-423.

29. Shiose Y, Kitazawa Y, Tsukahara S, et al. Epidemiology of glaucoma in Japan: a nationwide glaucoma survey. *Jpn J Ophthalmol*. 1991;35:133-136.

30. Iwase A, Suzuki Y, Araie M, et al; Tajimi Study Group, Japan Glaucoma Society. The prevalence of primary open-angle glaucoma in Japanese: the Tajimi Study. *Ophthalmology*. 2004;111(9): 1641-1648.

31. Bengtsson E. Incidence of manifest glaucoma. *Br J Ophthalmol*. 1989;73:483.

32. Leske MC, Wu SY, Hennis A, Honkanen R, Nemesure B; BESs Study Group. Risk factors for incident open-angle glaucoma: the Barbados Eye Studies. *Ophthalmology*. 2008;115(1):85-93.

33. Hennis AJ, Wu SY, Nemesure B, Hyman L, Schachat AP, Leske MC; Barbados Eye Studies Group. Nine-year incidence of visual impairment in the Barbados Eye Studies. *Ophthalmology*. 2009;116(8): 1461-1468.

34. de Voogd S, Ikram MK, Wolfs RC, Jansonius NM, Hofman A, de Jong PT. Incidence of open-angle glaucoma in a general elderly population: the Rotterdam Study. *Ophthalmology*. 2005;112(9): 1487-1493.

35. Leske MC, Heijl A, Hussein M, Bengtsson B, Hyman L, Komaroff E; Early Manifest Glaucoma Trial Group. Factors for glaucoma progression and the effect of treatment: the early manifest glaucoma trial. *Arch Ophthalmol*. 2003;121(1):48-56.

36. Kass MA, Gordon MO, Gao F, et al. Is there a penalty for delaying treatment of ocular hypertension? The Ocular Hypertension Treatment Study. *Arch Ophthalmol*. 2010;128(3):276-287.

37. Quigley HA, Addicks EM. Chronic experimental glaucoma in primates: II. Effect of extended intraocular pressure elevation on optic nervehead and axonal transport. *Invest Ophthalmol Vis Sci*. 1980;19:137.

38. Gaasterland O, Tanashima T, Kuwabara T. Axoplasmic flow during chronic experimental glaucoma. I. Light and electron microscopic studies of the monkey optic nerve head during development of glaucomatous cupping. *Invest Ophthalmol Vis Sci*. 1978;17:838.

39. Cartwright MJ, Anderson DR. Correlation of asymmetric damage with asymmetric intraocular pressure in normal-tension glaucoma (low-tension glaucoma). *Arch Ophthalmol*. 1988;106:898.

40. Crichton A, Drance SM, Douglas GR, et al. Unequal intraocular pressure and its relation to asymmetric visual field defects in low-tension glaucoma. *Ophthalmology*. 1989;96:1312.

41. Collaborative Normal-Tension Glaucoma Study Group. Comparison of glaucomatous progression between untreated patients with normal-tension glaucoma and patients with therapeutically reduced intraocular pressures. *Am J Ophthalmol*. 1998;126(4):487-497.

42. Chang TC, Congdon NG, Wojciechowski R, et al. Determinants and heritability of intraocular pressure and cup/disc ratio in a defined older population. *Ophthalmology*. 2005;112(7):1186-1191.

43. Coulehan JL, Helzlsouer KJ, Rogers KD, et al. Racial differences in intraocular tension and glaucoma surgery. *Am J Epidemiol*. 1980;11:759.

44. Aghaian E, Choe JE, Stamper RL. Central corneal thickness of Caucasians, Chinese, Hispanics, Filipinos, African Americans, and Japanese in a glaucoma clinic. *Ophthalmology*. 2004;111(12): 2211-2219.

45. Beck RW, Messner DK, Musch DC, Martonyi CL, Lichter PR. Is there a racial difference in physiologic cup size? *Ophthalmology*. 1985;92:873.

46. Chi T, Ritch R, Stickler D, Pitman B, Tsai C, Hsieh FY. Racial differences in optic nervehead parameters. *Arch Ophthalmol*. 1989;107:836.

47. Steinmann W, Stone R, Nichols C, et al. A case-control study of the association of sickle cell trait and chronic open-angle glaucoma. *Am J Epidemiol*. 1983;118:288.

48. Javitt JC, McBean AM, Nicholson GA, Babish JD, Warren JL, Krakauer H. Undertreatment of glaucoma among black Americans. *N Engl J Med*. 1991;325:1418.

49. Kahn KL, Brooten D, Campbell R, et al. Health care for black and poor hospitalized Medicare patients. *JAMA*. 1994;271:1169.

50. Tielsch JM, Katz J, Sommer A, Quigley HA, Javitt JC. Family history and risk of primary open-angle glaucoma: the Baltimore Eye Survey. *Arch Ophthalmol*. 1994;112:69-73.

51. Chang TC, Congdon NG, Wojciechowski R, et al. Determinants and heritability of intraocular pressure and cup/disc ratio in a defined older population. *Ophthalmology*. 2005;112(7):1186-1191.

52. Johnson AT, Drack AV, Kwitek AE, Cannon RL, Stone EM, Alward WL. Clinical features and linkage analysis of a family with autosomal dominant juvenile glaucoma. *Ophthalmology*. 1993;100:524.

53. Richards JE, Lichter PR, Boehnke M, et al. Mapping of a gene for autosomal dominant juvenile-onset open-angle glaucoma to chromosome Iq. *Am J Hum Gen*. 1994;54:62.

54. Alllingham RR, Liu Y, Rhee DJ. The genetics of primary open-angle glaucoma: a review. *Exp Eye Res*. 2009;88(4):837-844.

55. Gordon MO, Beiser JA, Brandt JD, et al. The Ocular Hypertension Treatment Study: baseline factors that predict the onset of primary open-angle glaucoma. *Arch Ophthalmol*. 2002;120(6):714-720.

56. Leske MC, Wu SY, Hennis A, Honkanen R, Nemesure B; BESs Study Group. Risk factors of incident open-angle glaucoma: the Barbados Eye Studies. *Ophthalmology*. 2008;115(1):85-93.

57. Medeiros FA, Sample PA, Weinreb RN. Corneal thickness measurements and frequency doubling technology perimetry abnormalities in ocular hypertensive eyes. *Ophthalmology*. 2003;110:1903-1908.

58. Medeiros FA, Sample PA, Zangwill LM, et al. Corneal thickness as a risk factor for visual field loss in patients with preperimetric glaucomatous optic neuropathy. *Am J Ophthalmol*. 2003;136:805-813.

59. Medeiros FA, Sample PA, Weinreb RN. Corneal thickness measurements and visual function abnormalities in ocular hypertensive patients. *Am J Ophthalmol*. 2003;135:131-137.

60. Zeppieri M, Brusini P, Miglior S. Corneal thickness and functional damage in patients with ocular hypertension. *Eur J Ophthalmol*. 2005;15:196-201.

61. Nemesure B, Wu SY, Hennis A, et al. Corneal thickness and intraocular pressure in the Barbados Eye Studies. *Arch Ophthalmol*. 2003;121:240-244.

62. Wolfs RC, Klaver CC, Vingerling JR, et al. Distribution of central corneal thickness and its association with intraocular pressure: the Rotterdam Study. *Am J Ophthalmol*. 1997;123:767-772.

63. Francis BA, Varma R, Chopra V, Lai MY, Shtir C, Azen SP; Los Angeles Latino Eye Study Group. Intraocular pressure, central corneal thickness and prevalence of open-angle glaucoma: the Los Angeles Latino Eye Study. *Am J Ophthalmol*. 2008;146(5):741-746.

64. Vijaya L, George R, Paul PG, et al. Prevalence of open-angle glaucoma in a rural south Indian population. *Invest Ophthalmol Vis Sci*. 2005;46:4461-4467.

65. Perkins ES, Phelps CS. Open angle glaucoma, ocular hypertension, low tension glaucoma, and refraction. *Arch Ophthalmol*. 1982;100:1464.

66. Mitchell P, Hourihan F, Sandbach J, Wanj JJ. The relationship between glaucoma and myopia: the Blue Mountain Eye Study. *Ophthalmology*. 1999;106(10):2010-2015.

67. Armaly MF. Cup/disc ratio in early open-angle glaucoma. *Doc Ophthalmol*. 1969;26:526.

68. Hart WM Jr, Yablonski M, Kass MA, Becker B. Multivariate analysis of the risk of glaucomatous visual field loss. *Arch Ophthalmol.* 1979;97:1455.

69. Yablonski ME, Zimmerman TJ, Kass MA, et al. Prognostic significance of optic disc cupping in ocular hypertension patients. *Am J Ophthalmol.* 1980;89:585.

70. Ocular Hypertension Treatment Study Group and the European Glaucoma Prevention Study Group. The accuracy and clinical application of predictive models for primary open-angle glaucoma in ocular hypertensive individuals. *Ophthalmology.* 2008;115(11):2030-2036.

71. Krakau T. Disc hemorrhages and the etiology of glaucoma. *Acta Ophthalmol.* 1989;67:31-33.

72. Ishida K, Yamamoto T, Sugiyama K, Kitazawa Y. Disk hemorrhage is a significantly negative prognostic factor in normal tension glaucoma. *Am J Ophthalmol.* 2000;129:707-714.

73. Gordon J, Piltz-Seymour JR. The significance of optic disc hemorrhages in glaucoma. *J Glaucoma.* 1997;6:62-64.

74. Budenz DL, Anderson DR, Feuer WJ, et al; Ocular Hypertension Treatment Study Group. Detection and prognostic significance of optic disc hemorrhages during the Ocular Hypertension Treatment Study. *Ophthalmology.* 2006;113:2137-2143.

75. Quigley HA, Katz J, Derick RJ, Gilbert D, Sommer A. An evaluation of optic disc and nerve fiber layer examinations in monitoring progression of early glaucoma damage. *Ophthalmology.* 1992; 99:19-28.

76. Quigley HA, Brown ME, Morrison JD, Drance SM. The size and shape of the optic disc in normal human eyes. *Arch Ophthalmol.* 1990;108(1):51-57.

77. Prata TS, De Moraes CG, Teng CC, Tello C, Ritch R, Liebmann JM. Factors affecting rates of visual field progression in glaucoma patients with optic disc hemorrhage. *Ophthalmology.* 2010;117(1):24-29.

78. Healey PR, Mitchell P, Smith W, Wang JJ. Optic disc hemorrhages in a population with and without signs of glaucoma. *Ophthalmology.* 1998;105(2):216-223.

79. Klein BEK, Klein R. Intraocular pressure and cardiovascular risk variables. *Arch Ophthalmol.* 1981;99:837-839.

80. Leighton DA, Phillips CI. Systemic blood pressure in open-angle glaucoma, low tension glaucoma, and the normal eye. *Br J Ophthalmol.* 1972;56:447-453.

81. Dielemans I, Vingerling JR, Algra D, Hofman A, Grobbee DE, de Jong PT. Primary open-angle glaucoma, intraocular pressure, and systemic blood pressure in the general elderly population. The Rotterdam Study. *Ophthalmology.* 1995;102:54-60.

82. Tielsch JM, Katz J, Sommer A, Quigley HA, Javitt JC. Hypertension, perfusion pressure, and primary open-angle glaucoma: a population-based assessment. *Arch Ophthalmol.* 1995;11(13): 216-221.

83. Mitchell P, Smith W, Chey T, Healey PR. Open-angle glaucoma and diabetes: the Blue Mountains eye study, Australia. *Ophthalmology.* 1997;104(4):712-718.

84. Nielsen NV. The prevalence of glaucoma and ocular hypertension in type 1 and type 2 diabetes mellitus. *Acta Ophthalmol.* 1983;61:662-672.

85. Katz J, Sommer A. Risk factors for primary open angle glaucoma. *Am J Prev Med.* 1988;4:110-114.

86. Mitchell P, Smith W, Attebo K, Healey PR. Prevalence of open-angle glaucoma in Australia. The Blue Mountains Eye Study. *Ophthalmology.* 1996;103(10):1661-1669.

87. Wilson MR, Hertzmark E, Walker AM, Childs-Shaw K, Epstein DL. A case-control study of risk factors in open-angle glaucoma. *Arch Ophthalmol.* 1987;105:1066-1071.

88. Musch DC, Lichter PR, Guire KE, Standardi CL. The Collaborative Initial Glaucoma Treatment Study: study design, methods, and baseline characteristics of enrolled patients. *Ophthalmology.* 1999;106(4):653-662.

89. Rein DB, Wittenborn JS, Lee PP, et al. The cost-effectiveness of routine office-based identification and subsequent medical treatment of primary open-angle glaucoma in the United States. *Ophthalmology.* 2009;116(5):823-832.

90. Skalicky S, Goldberg I. Depression and quality of life in patients with glaucoma: a cross-sectional analysis using the Geriatric Depression Scale-15, assessment of function related to vision, and the Glaucoma Quality of Life-15. *J Glaucoma.* 2008;17(7):546-551.

91. Glynn RJ, Seddon JM, Krug JH Jr, Sahagian CR, Chiavelli ME, Campion EW. Falls in elderly patients with glaucoma. *Arch Ophthalmol.* 1991;109:205.

92. Nelson P, Aspinall P, Papasouliotis O, et al. Quality of life in glaucoma and its relationship with visual function. *J Glaucoma.* 2003;12:139-150.

93. Gutierrez P, Wilson MR, Johnson C, et al. Influence of glaucomatous visual field loss on health-related quality of life. *Arch Ophthalmol.* 1997;115:777-784.

94. Iester M, Zingirian M. Quality of life in patients with early, moderate and advanced glaucoma. *Eye.* 2002;16:44-49.

95. Goldberg I, Clement CI, Chiang TH, et al. Assessing quality of life in patients with glaucoma using the Glaucoma Quality of Life-15 (GQL-15) questionnaire. *J Glaucoma.* 2009;18(1):6-12.

96. Janz NK, Wren PA, Lichter PR, et al; The CIGTS Group. Quality of life in newly diagnosed glaucoma patients. *Ophthalmology.* 2001;108:887-898.

97. Spaeth G, Walt J, Keener J. Evaluation of quality of life for patients with glaucoma. *Am J Ophthalmol.* 2006;141(1 suppl):S3-S14.

98. Freeman EE, Muñoz B, West SK, Jampel HD, Friedman DS. Glaucoma and quality of life: the Salisbury Eye Evaluation. *Ophthalmology.* 2008;115(2):233-238.

99. McKean-Cowdin R, Wang Y, Wu J, Azen SP, Varma R; Los Angeles Latino Eye Study Group. Impact of visual field loss on health-related quality of life in glaucoma: the Los Angeles Latino Eye Study. *Ophthalmology.* 2008;115(6):941-948.

100. Jay JL, Allan D. The benefit of early trabeculectomy versus conventional management in primary open-angle glaucoma relative to severity of disease. *Eye.* 1989;3:528-535.

101. Midgal C, Hitchings R. Control of chronic simple glaucoma with primary medical, surgical, and laser treatment. *Trans Ophthalmol Soc UK.* 1986;105:653-656.

102. Musch DC, Gillespie BW, Lichter PR, Niziol LM, Janz NK; CIGTS Study Investigators. Visual field progression in the Collaborative Initial Glaucoma Treatment Study the impact of treatment and other baseline factors. *Ophthalmology.* 2009;116(2):200-207.

Financial Disclosures

Dr. Ron A. Adelman has no financial or proprietary interest in the materials presented herein.

Dr. Iqbal "Ike" K. Ahmed is a consultant for/receives consulting fees from Ade Therapeutics, Ace Vision Group, Alcon, Allergan, Aquesys, Carl Zeiss Meditec, Clarity Medical Systems, Ivantis, EndoOptiks, Eyelight, iScience, Glaukos, Ono Pharma, Pfizer, SOLX, Stroma, and Transcend Medical. He is a speaker for/receives honoraria from Alcon, Abbott Medical Optics, Allergan, Carl Zeiss Meditec, Clarity Medical Systems, iScience, and New World Medical. He receives research grants and support from Alcon, Allergan, Aquesys, Carl Zeiss Meditec, Ivantis, iScience, and Transcend Medical.

Dr. Lama A. Al-Aswad has no financial or proprietary interest in the materials presented herein.

Dr. R. Rand Allingham has no financial or proprietary interest in the materials presented herein.

Dr. Michael A. Alunni has not disclosed any relevant financial relationships.

Dr. Cristan M. Arena has no financial or proprietary interest in the materials presented herein.

Dr. Sanjay Asrani has no financial or proprietary interest in the materials presented herein.

Dr. Ramesh S. Ayyala has no financial or proprietary interest in the materials presented herein.

Dr. Priti Batta has no financial or proprietary interest in the materials presented herein.

Dr. Carla I. Bourne has no financial or proprietary interest in the materials presented herein.

Dr. Zvia Burgansky-Eliash has no financial or proprietary interest in the materials presented herein.

Dr. Pratap Challa has no financial or proprietary interest in the materials presented herein.

Dr. Vicki M. Chen has no financial or proprietary interest in the materials presented herein.

Dr. Garry P. Condon has not disclosed any relevant financial relationships.

Dr. Ian P. Conner has no financial or proprietary interest in the materials presented herein.

Dr. Daniel Cotlear has no financial or proprietary interest in the materials presented herein.

Dr. Marshall N. Cyrlin is a speaker for Alcon Laboratories and Merck & Co, Inc. He is also a consultant for Alcon Laboratories. He is an investigator for Refocus Group.

Dr. David K. Dueker has no financial or proprietary interest in the materials presented herein.

Dr. Jay S. Duker receives research support from Carl Zeiss Meditec and Optovue. He is a consultant for EMD/Serono, Neovista, Novartis Pharmaceuticals Corp, Optos, QLT Phototherapeutics Inc, and Thrombogenics. He is also a stockholder in EyeNetra, Hemera Biosciences, Ophthotech, and Paloma Pharmaceuticals.

Dr. David L. Epstein has financial interest through Duke University Patent Policies. He is a founder of Aerie Pharmaceuticals, Inc. He is on the Glaukos scientific advisory board and is a consultant to GrayBug, LLC.

Lindsey S. Folio has no financial or proprietary interest in the materials presented herein.

Dr. Gretta Fridman has no financial or proprietary interest in the materials presented herein.

Dr. Lisa S. Gamell has no financial or proprietary interest in the materials presented herein.

Dr. Morton F. Goldberg has no financial or proprietary interest in the materials presented herein.

Dr. Modi Goldenfeld has no financial or proprietary interest in the materials presented herein.

Dr. Leon W. Herndon Jr has no financial or proprietary interest in the materials presented herein.

Dr. Richard W. Hertle is associated with Austin Bioinnovation Institute of Akron and Oxford University Press.

Dr. Michael B. Horsley has no financial or proprietary interest in the materials presented herein.

Dr. Farhan A. Irshad has no financial or proprietary interest in the materials presented herein.

Dr. Annisa L. Jamil has no financial or proprietary interest in the materials presented herein.

Dr. Murray A. Johnstone has no financial or proprietary interest in the materials presented herein.

Dr. Deval Joshi has no financial or proprietary interest in the materials presented herein.

Dr. Malik Y. Kahook has received consulting and/or research support from Alcon, Allergan, Merck, Bausch & Lomb, Regeneron, Genentech, Actelion, AMO, Merck, Glaukos, Ivantis, and the State of Colorado. He has ownership and/or intellectual property interests with AMO, Oasis, Dose Medical, ClarVista Medical, ShapeOphthalmics, ShapeTech, and Innovative Laser Solutions.

Dr. Mahmoud A. Khaimi has no financial or proprietary interest in the materials presented herein.

Dr. David A. Lee has no financial or proprietary interest in the materials presented herein.

Dr. Cynthia Mattox has no financial or proprietary interest in the materials presented herein.

Dr. Stuart J. McKinnon has no financial or proprietary interest in the materials presented herein.

Dr. Shlomo Melamed has not disclosed any relevant financial relationships.

Dr. Kimberly V. Miller has no financial or proprietary interest in the materials presented herein.

Dr. Peter A. Netland has no financial or proprietary interest in the materials presented herein.

Dr. Yvonne Ou has no financial or proprietary interest in the materials presented herein.

Dr. Mina B. Pantcheva has no financial or proprietary interest in the materials presented herein.

Dr. Marcos Reyes is an occasional speaker for Allergan and Alcon.

Dr. Douglas J. Rhee is an ad hoc consultant for Alcon, Allergan, Aquesys, Ivantis, Merck, and Santen. He provides research for Alcon, Aquesys, and Merck.

Dr. Claudia U. Richter has no financial or proprietary interest in the materials presented herein.

Dr. Sarwat Salim is a lecturer for Alcon and Merck.

Dr. Steven R. Sarkisian Jr is a consultant for iScience; Sight Sciences, Inc; Alcon; Ivantis; and Optous. He receives research support from Glaukos, Transcend, Alcon, Aquesys, and Aeon Astron.

Dr. Timothy Saunders has no financial or proprietary interest in the materials presented herein.

Dr. Joel S. Schuman receives royalties for intellectual property owned by Massachusetts Institute of Technology and Massachusetts Eye and Ear Infirmary and licensed to Carl Zeiss Meditec, Inc. He receives grant/research support from the NIH.

Dr. Sumit P. Shah has no financial or proprietary interest in the materials presented herein.

Dr. M. Bruce Shields is a consultant for OPKO Health, Inc.

Dr. Bradford J. Shingleton is a lecturer and receives grant support from Alcon Laboratories, Inc and Allergan, Inc. He is a consultant for Bausch & Lomb Surgical, iScience, Ocular Therapeutix, and Transcend Medical.

Dr. Richard J. Simmons has no financial or proprietary interest in the materials presented herein.

Dr. Brian J. Song has no financial or proprietary interest in the materials presented herein.

Dr. Jeffrey R. SooHoo has no financial or proprietary interest in the materials presented herein.

Dr. Joshua D. Stein has no financial or proprietary interest in the materials presented herein.

Dr. David P. Tingey has no financial or proprietary interest in the materials presented herein.

Dr. Angela V. Turalba has no financial or proprietary interest in the materials presented herein.

Dr. George Ulrich provides paid consulting services for Heidelberg Engineering.

Dr. E. Michael Van Buskirk has no financial or proprietary interest in the materials presented herein.

Dr. David S. Walton has no financial or proprietary interest in the materials presented herein.

Dr. Martin Wand has no financial or proprietary interest in the materials presented herein.

Dr. Guy Aharon Weiss has no financial or proprietary interest in the materials presented herein.

Dr. Janey L. Wiggs has no financial or proprietary interest in the materials presented herein.

Dr. M. Roy Wilson has no financial or proprietary interest in the materials presented herein.

Dr. Jeremy B. Wingard has no financial or proprietary interest in the materials presented herein.

Dr. Gadi Wollstein has no financial or proprietary interest in the materials presented herein.

Index